ILLUSTRATED TEXTBOOK OF

PEDIATRIC EMERGENCY & CRITICAL CARE PROCEDURES

ILLUSTRATED TEXTBOOK OF

PEDIATRIC EMERGENCY & CRITICAL CARE PROCEDURES

EDITORS

Ronald A. Dieckmann, M.D., M.P.H.
Professor of Pediatrics and Medicine
University of California, San Francisco
Director
Pediatric Emergency Medicine
San Francisco General Hospital
San Francisco, California

Debra H. Fiser, M.D.
Professor and Chairman
Department of Pediatrics
Chief
Department of Pediatric Critical Care Medicine
University of Arkansas for Medical Sciences
Arkansas Children's Hospital
Little Rock, Arkansas

Steven M. Selbst, M.D.
Associate Professor of Pediatrics
University of Pennsylvania School of Medicine
Director
Emergency Department
Children's Hospital of Philadelphia
Philadelphia, Pennsylvania

with 891 illustrations

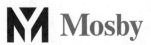 Mosby

St. Louis Baltimore Boston Carlsbad Chicago Naples New York Philadelphia Portland
London Madrid Mexico City Singapore Sydney Tokyo Toronto Wiesbaden

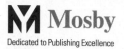

Vice President and Publisher: Anne S. Patterson
Senior Developmental Editor: Kathryn H. Falk
Administrative Assistant: Robin Sutter
Project Manager: Deborah Vogel
Project Specialist: Mary Cusick Drone
Manuscript Editors: Susan Thornton, Jodi Willard
Layout Artist: Gail Hudson
Designer: Pati Pye
Manufacturing Manager: Theresa Fuchs

FIRST EDITION

Copyright © 1997 by Mosby-Year Book, Inc.

Printed in the United States of America
Composition by Carlisle Communications, Ltd.
Lithography/color film by Top Graphics
Printing/binding by Courier Companies, Inc.

Mosby-Year Book, Inc.
11830 Westline Industrial Drive
St. Louis, Missouri 63146

Library of Congress Cataloging-in-Publication Data

Illustrated textbook of pediatric emergency & critical care procedures
/ editors, Ronald A. Dieckmann, Debra H. Fiser, Steven M. Selbst.
    p. cm.
  Includes bibliographical references and index.
    ISBN 0-8016-8102-2
    1. Pediatric emergencies.   2. Pediatric emergencies—Atlases.
  3. Pediatric intensive care.   4. Pediatric intensive care—Atlases.
  I. Dieckmann, Ronald A.   II. Fiser, Debra H.   III. Selbst, Steven M.
    [DNLM: 1. Emergencies—in infancy & childhood.   2. Emergency
Medicine—methods.   3. Critical Care—in infancy & childhood.
4. Critical Care—methods.   WS 205 I29 1996]
RJ370.I44 1996
618. 92'0025—dc21
DNLM/DLC
for Library of Congress   96-46924
                                   CIP

96 97 98 99 00 / 9 8 7 6 5 4 3 2 1

Part Editors

F. Keith Battan, M.D.
Associate Professor
Department of Pediatrics
University of Colorado School of Medicine
Associate Medical Director
Emergency Department
The Children's Hospital
Denver, Colorado
Part Editor—Nonvascular Access Techniques

Richard M. Cantor, M.D.
Associate Professor
Departments of Emergency Medicine and Pediatrics
SUNY Health Science Center at Syracuse
Medical Director
Central New York Poison Control Center
Syracuse, New York
Part Editor—General Considerations

George Foltin, M.D.
Assistant Professor of Clinical Pediatrics
New York University School of Medicine
Director
Department of Pediatric Emergency Medicine
Bellevue Hospital Center
New York, New York
Part Editor—Cardiopulmonary Resuscitation Techniques

Marianne Gausche, M.D.
Associate Professor of Medicine
UCLA School of Medicine
Director
Emergency Medical Services
Department of Emergency Medicine
Harbor-UCLA Medical Center
Torrance, California
Part Editor—Trauma Techniques

Jonathan Grisham, M.D.
Assistant Clinical Professor of Pediatrics
University of California, San Francisco
San Francisco, California
Attending Physician
Emergency Department
Children's Hospital Oakland
Oakland, California
Part Editor—Wound Care

Alfred D. Sacchetti, M.D.
Assistant Clinical Professor
Section of Emergency Medicine
Thomas Jefferson University
Philadelphia, Pennsylvania
Research Director
Department of Emergency Medicine
Our Lady of Lourdes Medical Center
Camden, New Jersey
Part Editor—Ophthalmology Techniques

Contributors

Evaline A. Alessandrini, M.D.
Assistant Professor
Department of Pediatrics
University of Pennsylvania School of Medicine
Division of Emergency Medicine
The Children's Hospital of Philadelphia
Philadelphia, Pennsylvania

Carolyn A. Altman, M.D.
Assistant Professor
Department of Pediatrics
Baylor College of Medicine
Houston, Texas

Bruce J. Andersen, M.D., Ph.D.
Chairman
Department of Neurosurgery
Brooklyn Hospital Center
New York University School of Medicine
Brooklyn, New York

Dean B. Andropoulos, M.D.
Assistant Clinical Professor
Departments of Anesthesia and Pediatrics
University of California
San Francisco, California
Staff Anesthesiologist and Associate Intensivist
Department of Anesthesiology and Critical Care
Children's Hospital Oakland
Oakland, California

M. Douglas Baker, M.D.
Associate Professor
Department of Pediatrics
University of Pennsylvania School of Medicine
Associate Director
Division of Emergency Medicine
Children's Hospital of Philadelphia
Philadelphia, Pennsylvania

Jill M. Baren, M.D.
Assistant Professor of Surgery (Emergency Medicine) and
Pediatrics
Yale University School of Medicine
Attending Physician
Pediatric and Adult Emergency Departments
Yale–New Haven Hospital
New Haven, Connecticut

F. Keith Battan, M.D.
Associate Professor
Department of Pediatrics
University of Colorado School of Medicine
Associate Medical Director
Emergency Department
The Children's Hospital
Denver, Colorado

Louis M. Bell, M.D.
Associate Professor
Department of Pediatrics
University of Pennsylvania School of Medicine
Associate Director
Division of Emergency Medicine
The Children's Hospital of Philadelphia
Philadelphia, Pennsylvania

Phillip L. Berry, M.D.
Professor
Department of Pediatrics
University of Arkansas for Medical Sciences
Director
Section of Pediatric Nephrology
Arkansas Children's Hospital
Little Rock, Arkansas

Frederick A. Boop, M.D.
Assistant Professor
Department of Neurosurgery and Anatomy
University of Arkansas for Medical Sciences
Little Rock, Arkansas
Chief
Division of Pediatric Neurosurgery
Arkansas Children's Hospital

Joan Bothner, M.D.
Assistant Professor
Department of Pediatrics
University of Colorado School of Medicine
Medical Director
Emergency Department
The Children's Hospital
Denver, Colorado

Charles M. Bower, M.D.
Assistant Professor
Department of Otolaryngology
University of Arkansas for Medical Sciences
Arkansas Children's Hospital
Little Rock, Arkansas

Russell U. Braun, M.D., M.P.H.
Assistant Clinical Professor of Medicine
University of California, San Francisco
San Francisco, California
Medical Director
Department of Emergency Medicine
Highland General Hospital
Oakland, California

Judith E. Brill, M.D.
Associate Professor of Pediatrics and Anesthesiology
Department of Pediatrics
UCLA School of Medicine
Chief
Division of Critical Care
Director
Pediatric ICU
UCLA Medical Center
Los Angeles, California

Raeford E. Brown, Jr., M.D.
Professor of Anesthesiology and Pediatrics
Executive Vice Chairman
Department of Anesthesiology
University of Arkansas for Medical Sciences
Little Rock, Arkansas

Greg S. Buchert, M.D.
Department of Emergency Medicine
Children's Hospital of Orange County
Orange, California

James M. Callahan, M.D.
Instructor in Pediatrics
Department of Pediatrics
University of Pennsylvania School of Medicine
Fellow
Emergency Department
The Children's Hospital of Philadelphia
Philadelphia, Pennsylvania

Richard M. Cantor, M.D.
Associate Professor
Departments of Emergency Medicine and Pediatrics
SUNY Health Science Center at Syracuse
Medical Director
Central New York Poison Control Center
Syracuse, New York

Gail N. Carruthers, M.D.
Assistant Clinical Professor
Department of Emergency Medicine
University of Southern California
Assistant Director
Department of Emergency Medicine
Long Beach Memorial Medical Center and Miller Children's Hospital
Long Beach, California

Rachel L. Chin, M.D.
Assistant Professor of Surgery
University of California, San Francisco
Attending Physician
Emergency Department
San Francisco General Hospital
San Francisco, California

Kathryn D. Clark, M.D.
Assistant Professor
Department of Pediatrics
University of Colorado School of Medicine
Attending Physician
Emergency Department
The Children's Hospital
Denver, Colorado

Kathleen Connors, M.D.
Assistant Professor
Department of Emergency Medicine
SUNY Health Science Center at Syracuse
Syracuse, New York

Arthur Cooper, M.D.
Associate Professor of Clinical Surgery
College of Physicians and Surgeons of Columbia University
Chief
Pediatric Surgical Critical Care
Harlem Hospital Center
New York, New York

Andrew J. Costarino, Jr., M.D.
Associate Professor of Anesthesia and Pediatrics
Department of Anesthesia and Critical Care Medicine
University of Pennsylvania School of Medicine
The Children's Hospital of Philadelphia
Philadelphia, Pennsylvania

Kevin Coulter, M.D.
Associate Professor of Pediatrics
University of California, San Francisco
Medical Director
Children's Health Center
San Francisco General Hospital
San Francisco, California

J. Thomas Cross, M.D., M.P.H.
Assistant Professor
Department of Pediatrics and Internal Medicine
Infectious Disease Division
School of Medicine in Shreveport
Louisiana State University Medical Center
Shreveport, Louisiana

Bonnie C. Desselle, M.D.
Assistant Professor
Division of Critical Care Medicine
Louisiana State University School of Medicine
New Orleans, Louisiana
Department of Pediatrics
University of Tennessee
LeBonheur Children's Medical Center
Memphis, Tennessee

Rhonda Dick, M.D.
Associate Professor
Department of Pediatrics
Chief
Section of Emergency Medicine
University of Arkansas for Medical Sciences
Arkansas Children's Hospital
Little Rock, Arkansas

Ronald A. Dieckmann, M.D., M.P.H.
Professor of Pediatrics and Medicine
University of California, San Francisco
Director
Pediatric Emergency Medicine
San Francisco General Hospital
San Francisco, California

John P. Dormans, M.D.
Associate Professor of Orthopaedic Surgery
University of Pennsylvania School of Medicine
Chief
Division of Orthopaedic Surgery
The Children's Hospital of Philadelphia
Philadelphia, Pennsylvania

Dennis Robert Durbin, M.D.
Assistant Professor
Department of Pediatrics and Epidemiology
University of Pennsylvania School of Medicine
Attending Physician
Emergency Department
The Children's Hospital of Philadelphia
Philadelphia, Pennsylvania

Christopher C. Erickson, M.D.
Associate Professor
Department of Pediatric Cardiology
University of Arkansas for Medical Sciences
Arkansas Children's Hospital
Little Rock, Arkansas

Joel A. Fein, M.D.
Assistant Professor
Department of Pediatrics
University of Pennsylvania School of Medicine
Attending Physician
Emergency Department
The Children's Hospital of Philadelphia
Philadelphia, Pennsylvania

Edward Gerard Fernandez, M.D.
Instructor
Critical Care Medicine
Department of Pediatrics
University of Minnesota
Minneapolis, Minnesota

Debra H. Fiser, M.D.
Professor and Chairman
Department of Pediatrics
Chief
Department of Pediatric Critical Care Medicine
University of Arkansas for Medical Sciences
Arkansas Children's Hospital
Little Rock, Arkansas

George Foltin, M.D.
Assistant Professor of Clinical Pediatrics
New York University School of Medicine
Director
Department of Pediatric Emergency Medicine
Bellevue Hospital Center
New York, New York

Thomas M. Foy, M.D.
Pediatric Gastroenterology
Cardinal Glennon Children's Hospital
St. Louis, Missouri

Timothy C. Frewen, M.D.
Department of Pediatrics
Children's Hospital of Western Ontario
London, Ontario
Canada

Norbert Froese, M.D.
Assistant Professor
Department of Anesthesia
University of British Columbia
Assistant Professor
British Columbia's Children's Hospital
Vancouver, British Columbia
Canada

Bradley P. Fuhrman, M.D.
Professor of Pediatrics
Chief
Pediatric Critical Care
Children's Hospital of Buffalo
Buffalo, New York

Gayle Garvin, R.N.
Surgical Clinical Nurse Specialist
Children's Hospital Oakland
Oakland, California

Marianne Gausche, M.D.
Associate Professor of Medicine
UCLA School of Medicine
Director
Emergency Medical Services
Department of Emergency Medicine
Harbor-UCLA Medical Center
Torrance, California

Alan Gelb, M.D.
Professor of Medicine
University of California, San Francisco
Chief
Department of Emergency Services
San Francisco General Hospital
San Francisco, California

Marc Gorelick, M.D.
Assistant Professor
Department of Pediatrics and Epidemiology
University of Pennsylvania School of Medicine
Attending Physician
Emergency Department
The Children's Hospital of Philadelphia
Philadelphia, Pennsylvania

Thomas P. Green, M.D.
Professor and Division Head
Children's Memorial Hospital
Northwestern University Medical School
Chicago, Illinois

Jonathan Grisham, M.D.
Assistant Clinical Professor of Pediatrics
University of California, San Francisco
San Francisco, California
Attending Physician
Emergency Department
Children's Hospital Oakland
Oakland, California

Emily B. Hak, Pharm.D., B.C.N.S.P.
Associate Professor
Department of Clinical Pharmacy
The University of Tennessee, Memphis
Memphis, Tennessee

Russell Howard Harris, M.D.
Assistant Professor
Department of Surgery
Thomas Jefferson University Hospital
Philadelphia, Pennsylvania
Chief
Emergency Department
Our Lady of Lourdes Medical Center
Camden, New Jersey

William H. Hawk, M.D.
Attending Physician
Emergency Department
Children's Hospital Oakland
Oakland, California

Philip L. Henneman, M.D.
Associate Professor
Department of Medicine
UCLA School of Medicine
Vice Chairman
Department of Emergency Medicine
Harbor-UCLA Medical Center
Torrance, California

Lynn J. Hernan, M.D.
Assistant Professor of Pediatrics and Anesthesia
Department of Pediatrics
State University of New York at Buffalo
Division of Pediatric Critical Care
Children's Hospital of Buffalo
Buffalo, New York

Mark Joseph Heulitt, M.D.
Associate Professor
Department of Pediatrics
Division of Critical Care Medicine and Neonatology
University of Arkansas for Medical Sciences
Arkansas Children's Hospital
Little Rock, Arkansas

Steven L. Hickerson, M.D.
Infectious Disease Division
Trinity-Mother Francis Health System
Tyler, Texas

Dee Hodge III, M.D.
Assistant Clinical Professor of Pediatrics
University of California, San Francisco
Director
Emergency Department
Children's Hospital Oakland
Oakland, California

James Hopkins, M.D.
Attending Physician
Emergency Department
Children's Hospital Oakland
Oakland, California

Stanley H. Inkelis, M.D.
Associate Professor of Pediatrics
UCLA School of Medicine
Director
Pediatric Emergency Medicine
Department of Emergency Medicine
Harbor-UCLA Medical Center
Torrance, California

S. Marshal Isaacs, M.D.
Assistant Professor of Surgery
University of California, San Francisco
Attending Physician
Emergency Department
San Francisco General Hospital
Medical Director
Department of Public Health
Paramedic Division
San Francisco Fire Department
San Francisco, California

Richard F. Jacobs, M.D.
Horace C. Cabe Professor of Pediatrics
Chief
Pediatric Infectious Diseases
Department of Pediatrics
University of Arkansas for Medical Sciences
Arkansas Children's Hospital
Little Rock, Arkansas

Ramon W. Johnson, M.D.
Attending Physician
Department of Emergency Medicine
Long Beach Memorial Medical Center
Long Beach, California

Beth Carol Kaplan, M.D.
Assistant Professor of Surgery
University of California, San Francisco
Attending Physician
Emergency Department
San Francisco General Hospital
San Francisco, California

Karl H. Karlson, Jr, M.D.
Associate Professor
Department of Pediatric Pulmonology
Eastern Virginia Medical School
Children's Hospital of King's Daughters
Norfolk, Virginia

Susan B. Kirelik, M.D.
Attending Physician
Pediatric Emergency Medicine
Carepoint, PC
Columbia Aurora Medical Center
Columbia Rose Medical Center
Denver, Colorado

William J. Koenig, M.D.
Assistant Clinical Professor
Department of Emergency Medicine
University of Southern California
Medical Editor
Journal of Emergency Medical Services (JEMS)
Medical Director
Emergency Department
Memorial Hospital Medical Center
Long Beach, California

Nanette C. Kunkel, M.D.
Assistant Professor of Pediatrics
Department of Pediatrics
University of Utah
Attending Physician
Emergency Department
Primary Children's Hospital
Salt Lake City, Utah

Jane M. Lavelle, M.D.
Assistant Professor
Department of Pediatrics
University of Pennsylvania School of Medicine
Attending Physician
Division of Emergency Medicine
Children's Hospital of Philadelphia
Philadelphia, Pennsylvania

Carol A. Ledwith, M.D.
Attending Physician
Emergency Department
The Children's Hospital
Denver, Colorado

Daniel L. Levin, M.D.
Professor of Clinical Pediatrics
University of Texas Southwestern Medical Center at Dallas
Pediatric Intensive Care Unit and Pediatric Trauma Intensive Care Unit
Children's Medical Center of Dallas
Dallas, Texas

Roger J. Lewis, M.D., Ph.D.
Assistant Professor of Medicine
UCLA School of Medicine
Director of Research
Department of Emergency Medicine
Harbor-UCLA Medical Center
Torrance, California

Stephen Ludwig, M.D.
Professor
Department of Pediatrics
University of Pennsylvania School of Medicine
Associate Chairman for Medical Education
Children's Hospital of Philadelphia
Philadelphia, Pennsylvania

Robert Luten, M.D.
Professor of Surgery
University of Florida, Jacksonville
Director
Pediatric Emergency Medicine
University Hospital of Jacksonville
Jacksonville, Florida

Thomas Malinowski, R.C.P.
Department of Pediatrics
School of Medicine
Loma Linda University Medical Center
Loma Linda, California

Jacalyn S. Maller, M.D.
Clinical Assistant Professor
Department of Pediatrics
University of Pennsylvania School of Medicine
Attending Physician
Emergency Department
Children's Hospital of Philadelphia
Philadelphia, Pennsylvania

George B. Mallory, Jr., M.D.
Associate Professor
Department of Pediatrics
Medical Director
Pediatric Lung Transplant Program
Washington University School of Medicine
St. Louis Children's Hospital
St. Louis, Missouri

Mariann Manno, M.D.
Attending Physician
Department of Emergency Medicine
University of Massachusetts Medical Center
Worcester, Massachusetts

James D. Marshall, M.D.
Assistant Professor of Pediatrics, Critical Care and Clinical
Pharmacology
Department of Pediatrics
University of Missouri, Kansas City
The Children's Mercy Hospital
Kansas City, Missouri

Constance McAneney, M.D.
Assistant Professor of Clinical Pediatrics
University of Cincinnati College of Medicine
Attending Physician
Department of Emergency Medicine
Children's Hospital Medical Center
Cincinnati, Ohio

M. Michele Moss, M.D.
Associate Professor and Vice-Chairman
Department of Pediatrics
Divisions of Critical Care and Cardiology
University of Arkansas for Medical Sciences
Medical Director
Pediatric Intensive Care Unit and Pediatric Transport Service
Arkansas Children's Hospital
Little Rock, Arkansas

Deborah Mulligan-Smith, M.D.
Associate Clinical Professor
Community Health and Family Medicine
University of Florida College of Medicine
Medical Director
Emergency Medical Services for Children
North Broward Hospital District
Broward General Medical Center
Ft. Lauderdale, Florida

Pamela Joy Okada, M.D.
Fellow, Pediatric Emergency Medicine
Department of Pediatrics
Division of Pediatric Emergency Medicine
The University of Texas Southwestern Medical Center at
Dallas
Dallas, Texas

Kristin Outwater, M.D.
Pediatric Intensive Care Unit
St. Luke's Hospital
Saginaw, Michigan

Michele C. Papo, M.D., M.P.H.
Assistant Professor of Pediatrics and Anesthesiology
State University of New York
Associate Director
Pediatric Intensive Care Unit
Division of Pediatric Critical Care
Children's Hospital of Buffalo
Buffalo, New York

Ronald M. Perkin, M.D.
Professor and Associate Chairman
Department of Pediatrics
Loma Linda University School of Medicine
Director
Pediatric Critical Care, Inpatient Respiratory Services and
Sleep Disorders Center
Loma Linda University Children's Hospital
Loma Linda, California

Michelle Perro, M.D.
Assistant Clinical Professor of Pediatrics
University of California, San Francisco
Attending Physician
Emergency Department
Children's Hospital Oakland
Oakland, California

Curtis B. Pickert, M.D.
Assistant Professor
Departments of Pediatrics and Anesthesiology
University of Kansas School of Medicine, Wichita
Medical Director
Pediatric ICU
Wesley Medical Center
Wichita, Kansas

David Plummer, M.D.
Associate Professor
Department of Emergency Medicine
University of Minnesota
Attending Physician
Emergency Department
Hennepin County Medical Center
Minneapolis, Minnesota

Tom B. Rice, M.D.
Chief
Pulmonary/Critical Care Division
Department of Pediatrics
Medical College of Wisconsin
Milwaukee, Wisconsin

Mary Workman Rutherford, M.D.
Associate Director
Emergency Department
Children's Hospital Oakland
Oakland, California

Alfred D. Sacchetti, M.D.
Assistant Clinical Professor
Section of Emergency Medicine
Thomas Jefferson University
Philadelphia, Pennsylvania
Research Director
Department of Emergency Medicine
Our Lady of Lourdes Medical Center
Camden, New Jersey

Mary R. Salassi-Scotter, R.N., M.N.Sc.
Instructor
College of Nursing
University of Arkansas for Medical Sciences
Director
Department of Nursing Education
Arkansas Children's Hospital
Little Rock, Arkansas

Morton Elliot Salomon, M.D.
Associate Professor of Pediatrics
Albert Einstein College of Medicine
Director
Department of Emergency Services and Pediatric Emergency
Services
North Central Bronx Hospital
Montefiore Medical Center
Bronx, New York

John P. Santamaria, M.D.
Associate Clinical Professor of Pediatrics
University of South Florida School of Medicine
Director
Wound and Hyperbaric Center
St. Joseph's Hospital
Attending Physician
Pediatric Emergency Service
Tampa Children's Hospital at St. Joseph's
Tampa, Florida

Thomas A. Scaletta, M.D.
Associate Director
Adult Emergency Services
Department of Emergency Medicine
Cook County Hospital
Chicago, Illinois

Stephen M. Schexnayder, M.D.
Assistant Professor
Departments of Pediatrics and Internal Medicine
Division of Pediatric Critical Care Medicine
University of Arkansas for Medical Sciences
Arkansas Children's Hospital
Little Rock, Arkansas

Gordon E. Schutze, M.D.
Associate Professor
Departments of Pediatrics and Pathology
University of Arkansas for Medical Sciences
Arkansas Children's Hospital
Little Rock, Arkansas

Joanna J. Seibert, M.D.
Director
Pediatric Radiology
University of Arkansas for Medical Sciences
Little Rock, Arkansas

Steven M. Selbst, M.D.
Associate Professor of Pediatrics
University of Pennsylvania School of Medicine
Director
Emergency Department
Children's Hospital of Philadelphia
Philadelphia, Pennsylvania

Kathy N. Shaw, M.D., M.S.
Associate Professor
Department of Pediatrics
University of Pennsylvania School of Medicine
Acting Division Chief
Division of Emergency Medicine
Children's Hospital of Philadelphia
Philadelphia, Pennsylvania

Steven W. Shirm, M.D.
Associate Professor
Department of Pediatrics
University of Arkansas for Medical Sciences
Arkansas Children's Hospital
Little Rock, Arkansas

Narenda C. Singh, B.Sc., M.B., B.S.
Director
Pediatric Critical Care
Department of Pediatrics
Children's Hospital of Western Ontario
London, Ontario
Canada

Karl A. Sporer, M.D.
Assistant Professor of Surgery
University of California, San Francisco
Attending Physician
Emergency Department
San Francisco General Hospital
San Francisco, California

Curt M. Steinhart, M.D.
Professor of Pediatrics, Surgery, and Anesthesiology
Chief
Section of Pediatric Critical Care Medicine
Co-Director
Pediatric Intensive Care Unit
Department of Pediatrics
Medical College of Georgia
Augusta, Georgia

Gregory L. Stidham, M.D.
Associate Professor
Department of Pediatrics
University of Tennessee
Director
Department of Critical Care
LeBonheur Children's Medical Center
Memphis, Tennessee

Paul C. Stillwell, M.D.
Director
Pediatric Pulmonology
Department of Pediatrics
Cleveland Clinic Foundation
Cleveland, Ohio

Kimo C. Stine, M.D.
Assistant Professor
Section of Pediatric Hematology-Oncology
Department of Pediatrics
University of Arkansas for Medical Sciences
Arkansas Children's Hospital
Little Rock, Arkansas

Stephanie A. Storgion, M.D.
Associate Professor of Pediatrics
Division of Critical Care Medicine
The University of Tennessee, Memphis
LeBonheur Children's Medical Center
Memphis, Tennessee

Eustacia Su, M.D.
Assistant Professor of Emergency Medicine and Pediatrics
University of Oregon
Attending Physician
Emergency Department
Oregon Health Sciences
Portland, Oregon

Michael F. Sweeney, M.D.
Assistant Professor of Anesthesiology
Director
Pediatric Critical Care
ECMO Program
Department of Anesthesiology and Pediatrics
University of Minnesota Hospital and Clinic
Minneapolis, Minnesota

Robert L. Sweeney, D.O.
Chairman
Department of Emergency Medicine
Jersey Shore Medical Center
Neptune, New Jersey
Spring Lake, New Jersey

Ann Thompson, M.D.
Professor of Pediatrics
Department of Pediatric Critical Care Medicine
Children's Hospital of Pittsburgh
Pittsburgh, Pennsylvania

Luis O. Toro-Figueroa, M.D.
Associate Professor
Department of Pediatrics, Critical Care Pediatrics
UT Southwestern Medical Center
Medical Director
Department of Respiratory Care
Children's Medical Center of Dallas
Dallas, Texas

Adalberto Torres, Jr., M.D.
Assistant Professor
Department of Pediatric Critical Care
University of Arkansas for Medical Sciences
Arkansas Children's Hospital
Little Rock, Arkansas

Edward J. Truemper, M.D.
Assistant Professor
Department of Pediatrics
Medical College of Georgia
Augusta, Georgia

Nicholas Tsarouhas, M.D.
Assistant Professor of Clinical Pediatrics and Surgery
University of Medicine and Dentistry of New Jersey/
Robert Wood Johnson Medical School
Division Head
Division of Pediatric Emergency Medicine
Department of Emergency Medicine
Cooper Hospital University Medical Center
Camden, New Jersey

Michael Tunik, M.D.
Assistant Professor of Clinical Pediatrics
New York University School of Medicine
Associate Director
Department of Pediatric Emergency Medicine
Bellevue Hospital Center
New York, New York

Mark W. Uhl, M.D.
Pediatric Intensivist
Department of Pediatrics
Carolinas Medical Center
Charlotte, North Carolina

Daved van Stralen, M.D.
Medical Director
Pediatric Critical Care Transport
Loma Linda University Children's Hospital
Medical Director
Program in Emergency Medical Care
Department of Cardiopulmonary Sciences
School of Allied Health Professions
Loma Linda University
Loma Linda, California

Stephanie A. Walton, M.D.
Attending Physician
Department of Emergency Medicine
Children's Hospital of Los Angeles
Los Angeles, California

Patricia A. Webster, M.D.
Assistant Professor
Pediatric Critical Care
Director of Pediatric Transport Service
Department of Pediatrics
School of Medicine in Shreveport
Louisiana State University Medical Center
Shreveport, Louisiana

John Robert Williams, M.D.
Instructor/Fellow
Department of Pediatric Emergency Medicine
The Children's Hospital
University of Colorado School of Medicine
Denver, Colorado

Robert H. Winokur, M.D.
Clinical Instructor
Department of Emergency Medicine
UCLA School of Medicine
Attending Physician
Emergency Department
Long Beach Memorial Medical Center and Miller Children's
Hospital
Long Beach, California

George Anthony Woodward, M.D.
Assistant Professor
Department of Pediatrics
Medical Director
Section of Transport Medicine
Attending Physician
Emergency Department
University of Pennsylvania School of Medicine
Children's Hospital of Philadelphia
Philadelphia, Pennsylvania

Timothy S. Yeh, M.D.
Clinical Professor of Pediatrics
University of California, San Francisco
San Francisco, California
Chief
Division of Critical Care Medicine
Children's Hospital Oakland
Oakland, California

Douglas Yoshida, M.D.
Assistant Professor of Surgery
University of California, San Francisco
Attending Physician
Emergency Department
San Francisco General Hospital
San Francisco, California

Kimberly R. Zimmerman, M.D.
Director of Pediatric Emergency Medicine
Los Angeles County-University of Southern California
Medical Center
Los Angeles, California

To Patty, Lauren, Marlowe, and Hayley, who provided the love and laughter to make it all happen.

RD

To Marty, Wesley, and Kathryn, whose patience, love, faithful support, and encouragement made this project a success.

DF

To my wife, Andrea, and my children, Lonn and Eric, for their love, encouragement, and understanding. To my parents for their support and devotion.

SMS

Foreword

M. Joycelyn Elders, M.D.

U.S. Public Health Service
Professor of Pediatrics and Endocrinology
University of Arkansas School of Medicine and Arkansas Children's Hospital
Little Rock, Arkansas

Pediatric emergency medicine and pediatric critical care medicine are relatively new specialties in pediatrics and are bringing much needed attention to the care of sick and injured children. While I was Surgeon General, I was most concerned with a pattern of neglect toward the unique needs and special requirements of children's health services. We have often followed critical care procedures, methodologies, and medicine dosage schedules that have been developed for adults and scaled down for children, without critical scientific evaluations in pediatric patients. Most physicians have not been well trained in the care of pediatric emergencies and critical care procedures, and there are few textbooks devoted to these topics. Not all children have the opportunity to receive care in a pediatric intensive care unit or from a physician specially trained in emergency medicine. Therefore it is very important that there be a textbook or "bible" readily available in every emergency department, intensive care unit, and physician's office where patients with pediatric emergencies receive care.

This illustrated textbook by Dieckmann, Fiser, and Selbst will be an excellent reference for the emergency physician and pediatric intensivist and for the training of house officers and fellows. It is also an important textbook for the library of pediatricians in practice who must care for pediatric emergencies before transport to an intensive care unit and for many others caring for children. This is a badly needed text and I believe the authors have done an excellent job discussing not only how emergencies are diagnosed, but also how they are managed. The authors have taught us not only how to approach a critically ill or injured child and how to evaluate consciousness and manage pain and sedation appropriately, but also how to perform these emergency and critical care procedures: establish airways, deliver ventilation, and appropriately and properly deal with vascular and nonvascular access techniques and hemodynamic monitoring. More than 875 photographs and drawings are used to illustrate procedures, techniques, and appropriate monitoring. Special techniques relevant to each system have been covered. Important emergencies for each system, as well as a step-by-step method on how to deal with these emergencies, are addressed. This textbook is unique in that it provides a single, comprehensive, well-illustrated, and ready reference source for pediatric emergency medicine and critical care procedures.

The *Illustrated Textbook of Pediatric Emergency and Critical Care Procedures* will mean as much to pediatricians, emergency physicians, family physicians, and intensivists as Stanbury's *Inherited Basis of Metabolic Disease* means to physicians in endocrinology and metabolism. This is a highly desirable textbook, and I think that it will be found in almost all emergency departments, intensive care units, and physicians' offices that care for children. Not many textbooks are essential in this age of computers and ready library access, but this book will be one we will want within our reach.

Foreword

Roger Barkin, M.D., M.P.H.

Professor of Surgery
University of Colorado Health Sciences Center
Denver, Colorado

Pediatric emergency medicine and pediatric critical care medicine have evolved rapidly, reflecting the escalating knowledge, experience, and technology that focus on the care of children. The uniqueness of these specialties rests in the urgency of intervention and the breadth of acute medical and traumatic conditions encountered. Building on the knowledge base of our colleagues' caring for adults has facilitated the expansion of our clinical expertise in children's services. The growing body of knowledge that has created the foundations of these fields has now been delineated in numerous textbooks about pediatric emergency medicine and pediatric critical care medicine.

The emergency department and the critical care unit face unpredictable challenges, and unique diagnostic and analytical skills are required of the practitioner to approach the patient in a professional, speedy, and deliberate manner. Procedures must supplement the cognitive process to ensure timely interventions. Concomitantly, the clinician must be sensitive to the emotional needs, concerns, and anxieties of the child and family as they find themselves, usually unexpectedly, in an unfamiliar setting.

Within this stressful environment, the clinician faces a world of highly technical diagnostic, therapeutic, and monitoring options and the necessity to perform a vast array of procedures.

No textbook to date has ventured into this relatively uncodified arena of pediatric practice. In the *Illustrated Textbook of Pediatric Emergency and Critical Care Proce-* *dures,* Drs. Dieckmann, Fiser, and Selbst have brought together a uniquely talented group of subspecialist clinicians to establish order and clarity in the procedural requirements of the emergency department and critical care unit. The result is a groundbreaking, substantive, and expansive book that does a superb job of providing the practitioner with clear and specific guidelines for pediatric emergency and critical care procedures.

The *Illustrated Textbook of Pediatric Emergency and Critical Care Procedures* is uniformly formatted to facilitate access during high stress moments. The information is presented in a highly graphic fashion, using over 875 illustrations of children requiring emergency and critical care procedures. Although individual biases do exist, reflecting different experiences and education, the techniques depicted are accompanied by appropriate documentation to allow the reader to pursue areas of controversy.

The *Illustrated Textbook of Pediatric Emergency and Critical Care Procedures* is important in providing a common basis for discussion and rigorous evaluation, ultimately creating a better consistency of approach. This textbook will provide all practitioners with a single procedural reference on which to base the clinical practices of pediatric emergency medicine and pediatric critical care medicine and to assist in those difficult situations in which assessment must be combined with technical skills to minimize morbidity and maximize patient outcomes.

Foreword

J. Michael Dean, M.D.

Professor of Pediatrics
University of Utah School of Medicine
Salt Lake City, Utah

It has been nearly two decades since I decided to enter the field of pediatric critical care medicine, and these two decades have witnessed an exciting transformation of critical care and pediatric emergency medicine. From the days of the mid-1970s, when there were only a half dozen or so pediatric intensive care units in the United States, and when emergency departments were staffed by general pediatricians and largely unsupervised residents, we can now look at a landscape of subspecialty boarded pediatric emergency physicians and pediatric critical care physicians, a myriad of textbooks, and a large body of knowledge.

In tandem with the explosion of these two specialties into pediatrics, a plethora of textbooks appeared, many of which are now in their second, third, or fourth editions. These textbooks can be loosely classified into two types. The first type of textbook, the so-called "definitive" textbook, generally exceeds 2000 pages, is comprehensive in its treatment of pathophysiology of critical and emergency illness, and looks ponderously respectable on the bookshelf of critical care and emergency department physicians. Unfortunately these books tend not to make their way to the bedside, since in the busy clinical environment clinicians often do not have time to devote to reading the scholarly, beautifully referenced chapters that reside in such books. The second group of books may be loosely called "handbooks"; they attempt to concisely convey to the bedside clinician the bare necessities with which to proceed in the emergency or critical care environment. These books are ever-present in emergency departments and intensive care units and provide a valuable resource for the harried house officer at 2:00 AM, who is trying to decide what set of orders to write for a patient with a critical illness or injury.

Finally, there are a variety of sources for information about procedures that we carry out in the critical care and emergency department areas, but these sources of information tend to be highly topical. Thus one would not expect to find a single textbook that would explain how to perform a rectal examination and how to place a pulmonary artery catheter. Furthermore, these types of books tend to be rather precisely focused on procedures and contain little information about the underlying diseases and situations in which such procedures might be used.

The *Illustrated Textbook of Pediatric Emergency and Critical Care Procedures* fills a void in a remarkable way. This textbook is expressly about procedures, but it combines the discussion of procedures with a context that is scholarly and well written. Thus the reader does not simply look up a procedure to perform but has the opportunity to see the context in which such a procedure should be performed. There is a great deal that is scholarly about this textbook, with its vast numbers of illustrations and tables; it also contains large numbers of references so that the interested reader can pursue more in-depth reading about various subjects. More important, the editors have made an effort to think of virtually any procedure that might be carried out in the context of pediatric emergency and critical care. Thus in this single textbook, one finds details as mundane as how to take vital signs, how to approach the distressed child, and details of physical restraint, as well as issues that are as technical as how to set up an ECMO circuit, how to place an arterial or pulmonary arterial catheter, or how to perform jugular bulb catheterization. Not to leave out any particular issues, there are clear instructions about where to anesthetize the perineum for a delivering mother in the emergency department, details about the performance of a tracheostomy, and a wealth of information about a high number of procedures of all types.

As I read the *Illustrated Textbook of Pediatric Emergency and Critical Care Procedures,* I was struck with the scope of the material. I tried to think of any emergency or critical care procedure that I could not find in this book, and I was unable to come up with one. The textbook also includes details that normally do not make it into textbooks for physicians and a wealth of useful information that will be of great assistance in running or operating a pediatric intensive care or emergency department. For example, one finds details about antiseptic solutions, various types of hospital policies such as universal precautions and how to take temperatures, as well as the weaknesses of various temperature-taking technologies.

In short, this is a textbook that, despite its large size, will find its way to the bedside and will be used by physicians, nurses, respiratory therapists, and all other health-care professionals who participate in the care of children in the emergency department or intensive care unit. This is an eminently useful book, but more important, it is eminently usable. The *Illustrated Textbook of Pediatric Emergency and Critical Care Procedures* addresses important issues and will be a wonderful resource for clinicians taking care of children in emergency departments and intensive care units.

Preface

Pediatric emergency medicine and pediatric critical care medicine are relative newcomers to the family of medical subspecialties, both formally anointed as unique practice areas in the 1990s. Both subspecialties have enjoyed quite a flourish of popularity. The spotlight on children's emergency and critical care services comes from many directions: enhanced hospital interest in pediatric emergency and critical care services, new federal and state grants for research and program support, appearance of a critical mass of original literature, and heightened public awareness and expectations of physicians' and hospitals' capabilities to treat acutely ill and injured children. These developments have occurred in concert with dramatic improvements in medical science and technology. Indeed, the diagnostic and treatment possibilities for acutely ill and injured children in emergency departments and critical care units now include a vast array of new procedures, techniques, and devices—many utterly unheard of only a few years ago.

Until the publication of this textbook, physicians performing emergency and critical care procedures on children had to extrapolate from adult emergency medicine references, ambulatory pediatric references, and anecdotes. No previous book has addressed emergency and critical care procedures with an exclusive focus on children. Moreover, no other reference to date has merged the procedural domains of pediatric emergency medicine and pediatric critical care medicine. Yet the union of emergency and critical care procedures in the *Illustrated Textbook of Pediatric Emergency and Critical Care Procedures* is a natural one, given the overlapping and complementary nature of the subspecialty practices and the shared practical responsibilities in immediate care of the acutely ill and injured child.

The *Illustrated Textbook of Pediatric Emergency and Critical Care Procedures* has a broad vision: to provide a single, comprehensive, and graphic reference that offers to the harried practitioner all relevant pediatric information at once. Hence this volume is written for all health-care personnel who perform, teach, and evaluate children's emergency and critical care—including the pediatric emergency physician, pediatric critical care specialist, pediatrician, emergency physician, family physician, surgeon, anesthesiologist, general critical care specialist, nurse, and prehospital provider. The *Illustrated Textbook of Pediatric Emergency and Critical Care Procedures,* although not by any means the last word in this rapidly evolving practice environment, establishes a solid foundation for prudent current procedural practice, ongoing re-evaluation, and revision.

Throughout the text, the editors have attempted to enforce clarity and simplicity. The procedures are accompanied by over 875 original illustrations to provide essential information in a visual format. There are references to indicate available literature support; the scientific underpinnings, however, are shaky—a key factor in the conception and production of this book. Nonetheless, the chapters offer the most detailed representations of the current empiric foundations of pediatric emergency and critical care available from the current literature. To accomplish such a mammoth task the editors have drawn on the expertise of over 125 recognized authorities in pediatric emergency and pediatric critical care medicine across the United States. The finely crafted contributions from these subspecialist leaders provide the heart and lifeblood to the *Illustrated Textbook of Pediatric Emergency and Critical Care Procedures.*

The book has 152 chapters, divided into twenty-eight parts, reflecting the natural divisions of knowledge and techniques. Parts I and II deal with epidemiology, the developmentally appropriate approach to the distressed child, and general procedural considerations. Part III addresses sedation and pain management. Parts IV through IX depict procedures essential to the ABCs of emergency care: airway, breathing, and circulation. Parts X through XVII present procedures pertinent to organ-specific medical and surgical conditions. Parts XVIII and XIX present key diagnostic procedures; and Part XX reviews toxicologic techniques. Parts XXI through XXV focus on trauma care. Part XXVI presents dental procedures; and Part XXVII, blood component therapy. Last, Part XXVIII describes a detailed medicolegal approach to examination and evidence collection for child victims of sexual or physical abuse.

The *Illustrated Textbook of Pediatric Emergency and Critical Care Procedures* is organized and written for usability and ease of access. It is designed for use on the physician's desktop or in the clinical area, within the fingertips of the busy practitioner. Although it may function as a library reference, its real place is near the bedside of the patient. When combined with finesse and compassion from the practitioner, the book will have its greatest use in the management of the youngest, most challenging, and most vulnerable members of our patient population.

Ronald A. Dieckmann, M.D., M.P.H.
San Francisco

Debra H. Fiser, M.D.
Little Rock

Steven M. Selbst, M.D.
Philadelphia

Acknowledgments

The *Illustrated Textbook of Pediatric Emergency and Critical Care Procedures* owes its existence to a long list of valued friends, colleagues, and mentors. First, we extend our thanks to Laurel Craven from Mosby, a long time ally of pediatric emergency medicine and the original Developmental Editor for the book. Her vision and support of the project were instrumental in its conception and early development. We thank Kathy Falk, Senior Developmental Editor, Kimberley Cox, Robin Sutter, Mary Drone, and other staff members at Mosby for translating thousands of pages of hieroglyphics into a beautiful textbook. We also thank our contributors—all academic specialists in pediatric emergency medicine and pediatric critical care medicine—who taught us the true breadth of art and science for pediatric procedures. Their state-of-the-art chapters give the book its substance and creativity. And last, we extend our thanks to special individuals in San Francisco, Little Rock, and Philadelphia.

In San Francisco, Joan Hu deserves special recognition and gratitude. As a clever and committed assistant, she commandeered an ocean of correspondence and manuscripts over four years, somehow with endless good humor and aplomb. And thanks to Moses Grossman, esteemed Chief of Pediatrics at San Francisco General Hospital for over 40 years, who edited with Delmer Pascoe in 1973 the first book about pediatric emergency medicine, *Quick Reference to Pediatric Emergencies*. He can rightfully be viewed as a "grandfather" of the specialty and has been a dear friend, teacher, and patron for many years. Last, to Alan Gelb, Chief of Emergency Services at San Francisco General Hospital, who has given freely his wisdom, support, and friendship.

RD

In Little Rock, the critical care medicine faculty, including Michele Moss, Mark Heulitt, Al Torres, and Steve Schexnayder, deserve particular recognition, not only for their significant individual contributions to this work, but also for their tolerance of the inevitable internal distractions that the project created for many months. Thanks also to Elizabeth Holley for her skillful administrative assistance in organizing the last stages of this project. A final thanks goes to Robert H. Fiser, Chairman of Pediatrics for the University of Arkansas for Medical Sciences from 1975-1994 for his unfailing inspiration and encouragement.

DF

In Philadelphia, Patricia Parkinson and Sharon Saunders are recognized for their tremendous efforts to prepare the manuscripts of numerous authors and facilitate smooth communication with our publishers. We have sincere appreciation for their upbeat spirit, diligence, meticulous attention to detail, and constant encouragement. Thanks to our mentors and friends, Elias Schwartz, M.D., Stephen Ludwig, M.D., and Edward Charney, M.D. (in memoriam), for their support and guidance. We also thank the very talented nursing staff of the emergency department and intensive care unit staff and the pediatric housestaff at the Children's Hospital of Philadelphia. They inspired us by the high-quality, humane, and compassionate care that they gave to their patients.

SMS

Contents

Part XXI Trauma Techniques

Part XXII Orthopedic Techniques

PART 1

APPROACH TO THE ACUTELY ILL OR INJURED CHILD

1   Epidemiology of Pediatric Emergency Care

Ronald A. Dieckmann

Children experience a wide array of acute illnesses and injuries, many of them unique to the vulnerable anatomy, immature immunology and physiology, and normal exploratory behavior of youth. Fortunately, most pediatric emergencies are minor and can be readily managed with simple first aid measures at home or in school or by a primary medical provider in a community office, clinic, or hospital pediatric ambulatory practice. Sometimes pediatric illness or injury is of high acuity or life-threatening, and the more sophisticated medical capabilities of the emergency department (ED) are needed for immediate treatment.

The overall epidemiology of pediatric emergencies, however, is not known, because of the ambiguities in the definition of "emergency," because of the community-to-community variabilities in ED use, and because at the present time our illness and injury information systems cannot monitor and track the aggregate numbers and types of pediatric emergencies, patient demographics, complaint categories, emergency procedures, and outcomes. There is simply no uniform, comprehensive reporting system or categorization methodology for pediatric emergencies and emergency procedures that describes precisely pediatric emergency care in all of the myriad care settings in a community, region, or state. Nonetheless, many pieces of the epidemiologic picture of pediatric emergencies are available to establish a reasonable background.

EMERGENCY DEPARTMENT USE PATTERNS AND PATIENT DEMOGRAPHICS

Although population-based data describing the incidence and epidemiology of pediatric emergencies are scant, a site-specific national survey completed in 1994 does provide the most accurate picture to date of children cared for in hospital EDs. The National Center for Health Statistics reported the first National Hospital Ambulatory Medical Care survey (NHAMCS) from a 12-month sampling of approximately 89.8 million ED visits to nonfederal, short-stay, or general hospitals.[8] The study separates visits to hospital EDs from visits to hospital ambulatory care departments and hence focuses specifically on unscheduled ED care. Overall, 41.7% of ED patients were under 24 years of age, and 25.1% were under 15 years of age. The NHAMCS data show that care of children is a major part of ED business.

The American College of Emergency Physicians reports that countrywide about one third of approximately 80 million ED patients per year are children. The majority are seen in about 5000 general EDs, and the rest in about 60 pediatric EDs in children's hospitals.[1] A Massachusetts analysis of children in two hospitals, one a general ED and the other the pediatric ED at Boston Children's Hospital, indicated that 23% of general ED patients were below age 18 years and had a mean age of 7.93 years, compared to a mean age of 6 years

in the pediatric ED. Far fewer children over 6 months and under 3 years were seen in the general ED compared to the pediatric ED. On the other hand, patients older than 6 years were more common in the general ED.[12] Therefore type of ED appears to influence ED use and users' demographic characteristics.

The NHAMCS indicates that the younger the children, the more likely it is that they are male. Among ED patients under 15 years, males outnumber females 42.7 to 37, measured in visits per 100 children per year in the general population; whereas females outnumber males 46.6 vs. 39.8 per 100 children in the 15- to 24-year category. Population-adjusted use rates of the ED by race reveal that Blacks come to the ED significantly more frequently than Whites in both pediatric age categories, 54.5 vs. 37.5 per 100 children in the under 15 years group, and 56.4 vs. 42.2 in the 15- to 24-year group.

The NHAMCS data pertain only to ED pediatric patients, who may be significantly different in their demographic characteristics from children with emergency conditions cared for in private offices or clinics. Several physician surveys have found an important role for pediatricians in out-of-hospital management of many moderate-to-severe childhood emergencies, including meningitis, severe asthma, severe dehydration, seizures, altered mental status, anaphylaxis, and cardiopulmonary arrest.[5,16] Illnesses seem to predominate in office and clinic pediatric emergency experiences, whereas injuries are the most common childhood complaints in EDs. Other data suggest that children with many minor acute conditions easily treatable in the office or clinic are often managed in the ED. In the NHAMCS, persons 15 to 24 years, when compared to five other age groups, had the highest rates of nonurgent ED visits (i.e., 26.3 per 100 visits), and persons under 15 years had the second highest rate (i.e., 24.2), compared to a 19.8 average for all age groups. Because of the high proportion of office and clinic "off-hours," easier access to the ED and patient and provider convenience may explain this important and costly level of overuse.[2]

PREHOSPITAL AND IN-HOSPITAL EPIDEMIOLOGY

In the prehospital setting, about 10% of ambulance runs are for infants, children, and adolescents.[7,18] This rate is variable, however, depending on the geographic location of the Emergency Medical Services (EMS) system. Trauma represents a disproportionately high proportion of pediatric prehospital complaints, comprising approximately 50% to 65% of transported cases.[6,9] One study of rural pediatric EMS found 64% trauma cases.[17] The most frequent injury mechanisms are motor vehicle crashes, falls, and burns. Among prehospital illness complaints, the most common are seizures, respiratory problems, and toxic exposures. The epidemiology of prehospital pediatrics is age dependent, with illness complaints more common among younger children and injury more common with increasing age. One study showed that medically handicapped children under 21 years of age were transported by ambulance 2.5 times as frequently as nonhandicapped patients.[20]

The in-hospital setting provides a high acuity picture of the epidemiology of pediatric emergencies. Overall, less than 10% of pediatric ED visits result in hospitalization.[4] Only 5% of injured children appear to require hospitalization.[19] However, these data vary widely in different communities, depending on transfer rates, primary physician ED use patterns, and the overall socioeconomic status of the population.[5] A comparison of pediatric illness admission patterns in three New York cities revealed that, in general, Boston children were admitted twice as frequently as Rochester children and five times as frequently for certain conditions such as otitis media, respiratory infections, croup, and toxic ingestions.[13]

Another factor in ED pediatric hospitalization rates may be the type of hospital (i.e., whether it is in a general or a pediatric hospital). One review found a 3.8% pediatric admission rate from the general ED versus an 11% rate for a pediatric ED. Although such experience may vary widely in different geographic locations, these data suggest that EDs in children's hospitals see sicker children than general EDs. In the same study, the most common admission diagnoses from the general ED were seizures, respiratory distress, and abdominal pain; from the pediatric ED, the most likely specific diagnoses were abdominal pain, poisoning, seizures, and asthma.[12]

INJURIES

Injuries are the most common reason for pediatric presentations to the ED, and unintentional injuries are the leading cause of death in children over 1 year of age.[14] In the NHAMCS, persons 15 to 24 years had a higher injury-related visit rate at 18.9 visits per 100 persons than individuals in all other five age categories (average rate = 12.6). Of a 1-year cohort of children presenting to a pediatric ED in an Hawaiian children's hospital, 33% had injury complaints (i.e., trauma, burns, water-related events, or child abuse).[9] There may be significant differences between general EDs and pediatric EDs with respect to frequency of injury complaints in children; one analysis indicates that 41% of children in a general ED had injury complaints, compared to only 22% in a pediatric ED.

Death and hospital discharge data indicate that serious pediatric injuries most frequently involve motor vehicles, with the child being either an occupant or a pedestrian, except in infancy, when homicide is most prominent. Occupant injuries are the most important problems among teens and young adults, whereas pedestrian and bicycle deaths associated with motor vehicles are most common in younger age categories. Burns, drownings, and violent deaths from homicide and suicide are also extremely important severe mechanisms in childhood injury mortality.[4]

One large study of pediatric injuries cared for in Massachusetts EDs showed that sprains, lacerations, and contusions were the most common problems.[6] Another revealed that sprains, lacerations, fractures, and mild head injuries accounted for 90% of pediatric trauma in a general ED. Lacerations on the head and face accounted for 60% of all lacerations; and the phalanx was the most common fracture site, followed by radius/ulna.[12]

ILLNESSES

Site-specific epidemiology for pediatric illness emergencies is poorly documented. Wheezing-related illness conditions were the most common noninjury complaints in the Hawaiian children's hospital 1-year cohort, representing 14% of all presentations.[9] In the comparative Massachusetts study, illness complaints varied significantly with ED type. In both the general and pediatric ED, however, fever and respiratory distress were the most frequent complaints. Upper respiratory infection (URI) and sore throat were more common in general ED pediatric patients than in pediatric ED patients, whereas fever, respiratory distress, abdominal pain, and gastroenteritis were more common in the pediatric ED. The causes of fever in the general ED were, in decreasing frequency, otitis media, viral syndromes, URIs, and pneumonia.[12]

Respiratory illness is the leading reason for hospitalization of children. Asthma, pneumonia, and bronchiolitis together represent about one third of pediatric hospitalizations.[10] Central nervous system problems, primarily seizures, and gastroenteritis are also important reasons for hospitalization. Deaths from illness during the neonatal period are most frequently due to congenital anomalies or birth-related conditions. Most postneonatal noninjury mortality in childhood is secondary to Sudden Infant Death syndrome (SIDS). The overwhelming majority of unexpected pediatric (under 18 years of age) out-of-hospital cardiopulmonary arrests occur in children under 2 years of age, and most of those are from SIDS.[3] Overall, pediatric death from illness is more common than from injury (27,652 vs. 21,133 cases in 1988); but after age 12 months, injury is much more likely (19,840 vs. 6354 cases in 1988).[11]

PROCEDURES

No study to date has documented the exact types and frequency of pediatric emergency procedures. In the 1994 NHAMCS, the most common overall ED procedures were intravenous infusions, wound care, orthopedic care; eye, ear, nose, and throat care; bladder catheterization; and nasogastric tube/gastric lavage. Two pediatric reports have emphasized the importance of ED pediatric procedural skills involving care of musculoskeletal injuries, immobilization, laceration repair, administration of effective sedation and analgesia, and accurate diagnosis of infectious diseases.[12,15]

In 1992, the National Subboard of Pediatric Emergency Medicine, the regulatory authority for specialists in pediatric emergency medicine and a joint subboard of the American Board of Pediatrics and the American Board of Emergency Medicine, empirically derived a comprehensive list of important procedures in pediatric emergency medicine. This procedures list, outlined in Box 1-1, was intended to outline the expected knowledge base for physician applicants for subboard certification. It represents the subboard's consensus

BOX 1-1   PROCEDURES FOR THE PEDIATRIC EMERGENCY PHYSICIAN, NATIONAL SUBBOARD OF PEDIATRIC EMERGENCY MEDICINE

I. Resuscitation procedures

Orotracheal intubation
Nasotracheal intubation
Cricothyrotomy
Replacement of tracheostomy tube
Oxygen delivery
Bag-valve-mask ventilation
Pulse oximetry
Capnometry
Spirometry

II. Cardiovascular

Peripheral vein catheter
Intraosseous needle insertion
Internal and external jugular vein catherization
Femoral and subclavian vein catheterization
Saphenous vein cutdown
Umbilical vein catheterization
Catheterization of the radial artery
Central artery catheterization
Umbilical artery catheterization
Countershock/defibrillation

III. Trauma

Tube thoracostomy
Thoracotomy
Peritoneal lavage
Pericardiocentesis
Thoracentesis
Physical restraints
Burns
Anesthetics
  Local
  Regional
Incision and drainage of abscesses
Incision and drainage of paronychia
Incision and drainage of pilonidal cysts
Evacuation of subungual hematomas

IV. Foreign body removal

Nose
Ear
Rectum
Vagina
Soft tissue
Eye
Pharynx

V. Orthopedics

Dislocations
Fracture immobilization
Reduction of fractures with vascular compromise

VI. Nonvascular access

Endotracheal administration of drugs
Administration of drugs by inhalation
Intramuscular administration
Intranasal administration
Rectal administration
Sublingual administration
Subcutaneous/intradermal administration
Topical/transdermal administration

VII. Diagnostic and therapeutic procedures

Abdominal

Anoscopy
Gastric intubation
Gastrostomy tube replacement
Paracentesis
Reduction of rectal prolapse
Inguinal hernia reduction

Dentistry

Reimplantation of a tooth
Splinting of a tooth
Temporomandibular jaw dislocation

Ear

Cerumen removal
Incision and drainage of auricular hematomas
Tympanocentesis

Genitourinary

Paraphimosis reduction
Suprapubic aspiration
Suprapubic cystotomy
Urethral catheterization

Musculoskeletal

Arthrocentesis

Neurologic

Lumbar puncture
Subdural tap
Ventriculoperitoneal shunt tap

Nose

Cauterization for epistaxis
Incision and drainage of septal hematomas
Packing for epistaxis

Obstetric

Culdocentesis
Vaginal delivery
Incision and drainage of bartholin abscesses

Continued.

BOX 1-1 PROCEDURES FOR THE PEDIATRIC EMERGENCY PHYSICIAN, NATIONAL SUBBOARD OF PEDIATRIC EMERGENCY MEDICINE—cont'd

Opthalmologic

Application of an eye patch
Conjunctival irrigation
Contact lens removal
Eversion of eyelids
Fluorescein instillation
Slit-lamp examination
Tonometry (Schiotz)

Toxicology

Gut decontamination

Ultrasonography

---

opinion of the desired scope of pediatric emergency procedures. The emergency procedures list, along with a similar list of pediatric critical care procedures developed by the National Subboard of Pediatric Critical Care and shown in Box 2-2, in Chapter 2, represents an inclusive index of all commonly performed procedures in pediatric emergency and pediatric critical care medicine. Competency in performing the listed procedures is viewed by both subboards as fundamental for subspecialist credentialing. Likewise, other specialty boards consider many pediatric emergency and critical care procedures to be essential skills for their own practitioners.

REFERENCES

1. American College of Emergency Physicians: The role of the emergency physician in the care of children, *Ann Emerg Med* 19:435-436, 1990.
2. Committee on Pediatric Emergency Medicial Services, Division of Health Care Services, Institute of Medicine: *Emergency medical services for children,* Washington DC, 1993, National Academy Press, p 57.
3. Dieckmann RA, Vardis R: High-dose epinephrine in pediatric out-of-hospital cardiopulmonary arrest, *Pediatrics* 95(6):901-913, 1995.
4. Fifield GC, Magnuson C, Carr WP, et al: Pediatric emergency care in a metropolitan area, *J Emerg Med* 267:495-507, 1984.
5. Fuchs S, Jaffe DM, Christoffel KK: Pediatric emergencies in office practice: prevalence and office preparedness, *Pediatrics* (83):931-939, 1989.
6. Gallagher SS, Finison K, Guyer B, et al: The incidence of injuries among 87,000 Massachusetts children and adolescents: results of the 1980-1981 statewide childhood injury prevention surveillance system, *Am J Public Health* 74:1340-1347, 1984.
7. Kallsen GW: Epidemiology of prehospital pediatric emergencies. In Dieckmann RA, editor: *Pediatric emergency care systems: planning and management,* Baltimore, 1992, Williams & Wilkins, pp 153-158.
8. McCaig LF: National Hospital Ambulatory Medical Care Survey: 1992 Emergency Department summary: vital and health statistics of the Centers for Disease Control and Prevention/National Center for Health Statistics, March 2, 1994, p 245.
9. Meador SA: Age-related utilization of advanced life support services, *Prehospital Disaster Med* 6(1):9-14, 1991.
10. National Center for Health Statistics: Detailed diagnoses and procedures, national hospital discharge survey, 1990: vital and health statistics, series 13, No. 113, DHHS Pub No. (PHS) 92-1774, Hyattsville Md, June, 1992, US Dept of Health and Human Services.
11. National Center for Health Statistics: Mortality files, Hyattsville Md, November, 1992, US Dept of Health and Human Services, Centers for Disease Control and Prevention.
12. Nelson DS, Walsh K, Fleisher G: Spectrum and frequency of pediatric illness presenting to a general community hospital emergency department, *Pediatrics* 90 (1):5-10, 1992.
13. Perrin JM, Homer CJ, Berwick DM, et al: Variations in rates of hospitalization of children in three urban communities, *N Engl J Med* 320:1183-1197, 1989.
14. Rivara FP, Baker SP: Epidemiology of pediatric trauma. In Dieckmann RA, editor: *Pediatric emergency care systems: planning and management,* Baltimore, 1992, Williams & Wilkins, pp 80-90.
15. Sacchetti A, Carraccio C, Warden T, et al: Community hospital management of pediatric emergencies: implications foe pediatric emergency services, *Am J Emerg Med* 15:19-27, 1986.
16. Schweich PJ, DeAngelis C, Duggan AK: Preparedness of practicing pediatricians to manage emergencies, *Pediatrics* (88):223-229, 1991.
17. Seidel JS, Henderson DP, Ward P, et al: Pediatric prehospital care in urban and rural areas, *Pediatrics* 88:681-690, 1991.
18. Tsai A, Kallsen G: Epidemiology of pediatric prehospital care, *Ann Emerg Med* 16:284-292, 1987.
19. Yamamoto LG, Wiebe RA, Matthews WJ: A one-year prospective ED cohort of pediatric trauma, *Ped Emerg Care* 7:267-274, 1991.
20. Yamamoto LG, Wiebe RA, Wallace JM, Sia CC. The Hawaii EMS-C project data. I. Reducing pediatric emergency morbidity and mortality; II. Statewide pediatric emergency registry to monitor morbidity and mortality, *Pediatr Emerg Care* 8(2):70-78, 1992.

2 Epidemiology of Pediatric Critical Care

Judith E. Brill

Pediatric intensive care units (PICUs) were developed in the early 1970s in response to growing needs for postoperative intensive care for children, advances in pediatric trauma care, and improvements in postresuscitative pediatric respiratory care. Effective, organized intensive care for both neonates and adults had evolved earlier, and highly favorable results of such efforts highlighted the need for similar units for older infants and children.[8]

Use patterns for PICUs indicate that approximately 200 per 100,000 children in the general population require critical care each year and that the current demand for PICU beds is significant.[7] There is approximately one bed for every 20,000 children in the United States, which is a higher level of overall PICU bed/population ratio than in most westernized countries. For example, in Australia there is one bed for every 60,000 children.[9] Such differences may be due to governmental centralization of intensive care services in Australia and elsewhere, in contrast to largely disorganized regionalization processes for pediatric critical care in the United States, which have evolved piecemeal and rarely by statute.[11]

Who are the patients occupying these costly, technologically advanced tertiary beds? What are their illness and injury conditions? And what have been the benefits of providing intensive care to infants and children? The first two epidemiologic questions can be answered in part by data from large, organized PICU systems. The question of efficacy is far more difficult to answer, because only a few centers in the past decade have followed surviving patients to assess long-term morbidity and mortality outcomes.[5,6]

PICU USE

The PICU patient differs from her adult counterpart in that he or she does *not* suffer from self-imposed or degenerative diseases. More often than not, the child is "an innocent victim of some malady afflicting a developing physiologic system."[7] In 1986 more than 22,000 children 19 years and younger died of injuries in the United States; injuries cause more deaths than all diseases combined. These deaths were largely the result of motor vehicle crashes, homicides, suicides, drownings, and fires and burns. More than 30,000 children suffer permanent disabilities from injuries each year.[4] The financial, emotional, and social effects of injuries on the individual, families, and society as a whole are enormous. The cost of injuries to children exceeds $7.5 billion each year; but since this figure does not take into account future productivity losses for fatalities, it is probably much higher.[4] As the level of violence in our society increases, injuries and admissions to PICUs will increase accordingly. Other injuries, such as those caused by farm equipment in rural areas, also result in many PICU admissions; these injuries are probably more amenable to injury prevention efforts than are the many penetrating injuries caused by the escalation of violence involving firearms in our communities. The overall incidence of critical illness in the community and the cost of such events in dollars are not as well documented as the incidence and cost of injury, but they appear to be significant countrywide and rising in many areas.

The makeup of the patients in an individual PICU varies, depending on whether or not the PICU is in a hospital that receives specialized patient groups (e.g., trauma, burn, spinal cord injury, or bone-marrow transplantation patients or children requiring advanced surgical procedures, such as cardiac surgery or organ transplantation). The PICU population may also be affected by the availability of other special services at the hospital such as extracorporeal membrane oxygenation (ECMO). ECMO is used in neonates with meconium aspiration syndrome, congenital diaphragmatic hernia, or group B streptococcal pneumonia, but is now increasingly used for older children with respiratory failure resulting from infection or aspiration or following open heart surgery. The hospital's geographic location and the pattern of use in the region (i.e., transport from referring institutions or via the emergency department [ED]) also significantly influence the mix of patients in the PICU.

EPIDEMIOLOGY

Despite some differences between institutions, it appears that respiratory problems continue to account for a significant number of the patients in the PICU (30%), according to the Ross Planning Associates survey of 1985 that collected data from 106 hospitals that had four or more PICU beds (self-defined).[11] Postoperative patients accounted for 36% of admissions to PICUs. According to the survey, 48% of patients required ventilatory assistance, 97% received cardiac or respiratory monitoring, and 35% invasive hemodynamic monitoring. The acuity of patients admitted to PICUs has increased recently, and patients with lower acuity and in need of fewer interventions and nursing hours are, in many institutions, being triaged to monitored beds in observation units or "step-down" units. Certain diagnoses that were seen frequently in PICUs only one decade ago (e.g., Reye syndrome, epiglottitis, or salicylate intoxication) are rarely seen today. Conversely, new diagnoses have emerged such as human immunodeficiency virus.

The major admission categories in the PICU include the injuries described above, as well as immersion injuries, ingestions, and burns. Box 2-1 lists the most frequent diagnoses among children in the University of California, Los Angeles Medical Center PICU, from 1990-1993. Illnesses include respiratory insufficiency resulting from upper airway obstruction, asthma, bronchiolitis, and pneumonia. Children with cardiac anomalies are frequent patients in PICUs, either following corrective or palliative surgical

---

BOX 2-1 FREQUENT ADMISSION DIAGNOSES TO PEDIATRIC INTENSIVE CARE UNITS

Trauma

Motor vehicle crashes (auto vs. pedestrian, passenger)
Burns
Homicides (penetrating injuries, shaken-baby syndrome,
    other abuse)
Suicides
Drownings

Ingestions

Respiratory insufficiency

Upper airway obstruction
Bronchiolitis
Status asthmaticus
Chronic lung disease, including bronchopulmonary
    dysplasia
Pneumonia
Adult respiratory distress syndrome

Cardiac disease

Congenital heart disease
Cardiomyopathy
Postcorrective or palliative heart surgery
Dysrhythmias

CNS

Hydrocephalus
Seizures, including idiopathic epilepsy and febrile seizures
Head trauma
Catastrophic CNS events (stroke, hemorrhage, increased
    intracranial pressure)
Post neurosurgical procedures (VP shunt, dorsal rhizotomy,
    hemispherectomy)

Neuromuscular failure (e.g., Guillain Barré syndrome,
    Werdnig Hoffman disease)

Hepatic failure

Acute fulminant hepatic failure
Variceal bleeding
Hepatic encephalopathy
Orthotopic liver transplantation

Renal failure

Acute renal failure (e.g., hemolytic uremic syndrome,
    acute tubular necrosis)
Chronic renal failure
Renal transplantation

Sepsis

Miscellaneous diagnoses

Sudden infant death syndrome
Infant botulism
Hypovolemic shock
Second-degree gastroenteritis
Psychomotor retardation with acute disease (e.g., cerebral
    palsy with aspiration pneumonia)
Chronically ventilated patient
HIV
Congenital anomalies
Childhood malignancies
Bone-marrow transplantation
ECMO

Compiled on the basis of admission diagnoses to UCLA Pediatric Intensive Care Unit, 1990-1993.
CNS, Central nervous system; *VP,* ventriculoperitoneal; *HIV,* human immunodeficiency virus; *ECMO,* extracorporeal membrane oxygenation.

procedures or because they need treatment for other superimposed medical problems (e.g., pneumonia).

Patients with cardiomyopathies now constitute a growing group of PICU patients as they await an available heart for transplantation. Patients with central nervous system (CNS) disease in the PICU include those with meningitis/encephalitis, hydrocephalus, seizures, head trauma, or other catastrophic CNS events such as stroke or hemorrhage from arteriovenous malformations or aneurysms. Advances in epilepsy surgery now allow patients with intractable seizures to benefit from hemispherectomy or lobectomy and require many PICU days. Children with hepatic or renal failure may enter the PICU many times and require PICU care following orthotopic liver transplantation or renal transplantation. The septic child, the immunocompromised patient, the child undergoing induction chemotherapy for malignancy, the transplant patient, or the previously healthy host with meningococcemia are other important PICU candidates.

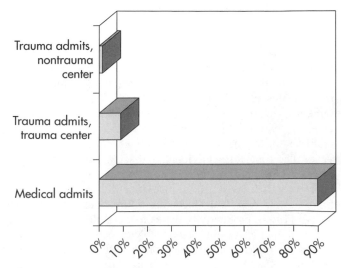

FIG. 2-1 1992 PICU admissions, northern and central California.

A number of other "miscellaneous" diagnoses provide variety in the population of children cared for in PICU, including infant botulism, hemolytic uremic syndrome, child abuse and neglect, sudden infant death syndrome, acute fulminant hepatic failure, unusual poisonings, malignancies, and congenital anomalies of varying severity.

In some PICUs a majority of beds will be used by surgical patients because of advanced surgical techniques offered in that institution. However, as noted in Fig. 2-1, the overwhelming majority of pediatric patients requiring intensive care have medical diagnoses. In a 1-year consecutive sampling by the Pediatric Intensive Care Network of Northern and Central California, trauma represented only 10% of PICU cases. Nine percent of the patients were in pediatric trauma centers, and 1% in pediatric critical care centers there were not identified as pediatric trauma centers.

CRITICAL CARE PROCEDURES

Infants and children requiring intensive care are constantly subjected to painful and invasive procedures, including intravenous cannulation, suprapubic bladder aspiration, urinary bladder catheterization, venipuncture, arterial line or central line placement, bone marrow aspiration, chest tube insertion, lumbar puncture, paracentesis, thoracentesis, laryngoscopy and endotracheal intubation, bronchoscopy, placement of intracranial pressure monitor, pericardiocentesis, suctioning, suturing, and dressing changes.[1,2,10] Newer techniques for the PICU include sedation and analgesia, advanced monitoring, improved ventilation, and sepsis management. Box 2-2 outlines a comprehensive list of pediatric critical care procedures, derived by the National Subboard of Pediatric Critical Care. This list, like the emergency procedures list in Box 1-1, represents the recommended knowledge base for specialists in the field, but also serves as a compendium of all pediatric critical care procedures.

> **BOX 2-2   PROCEDURES LIST: PEDIATRIC CRITICAL CARE MEDICINE**
>
> | | |
> |---|---|
> | Percutaneous arterial puncture | Initiation and/or management of peritoneal dialysis |
> | Percutaneous arterial cannulation | Initiation and/or management of hemodialysis |
> | Arterial cutdown | Management of patient with liver failure |
> | Peripheral venous cutdown | |
> | Central venous cannulation | Management of disseminated intravascular coagulation |
> | Bedside pulmonary artery catheterization | Initiation and management: of total parenteral nutrition |
> | Endotracheal intubation | |
> | Replacement of tracheostomy tubes | Defibrillation cardioversion |
> | | Management of a patient with a cardiac pacemaker |
> | Fiberoptic bronchoscopy | |
> | Initiation and maintenance of ventilation on a respirator | Pericardiocentesis |
> | | Management of burn patient |
> | Initiation and maintenance of PEEP 10 cm H_2O | Thoracentesis |
> | | Chest tube placement |
> | High-frequency ventilation | Paracentesis |
> | Management of patient with epiglottitis | Cardiopulmonary resuscitation |
> | Management of patient with intracranial pressure monitor | Management of septic shock |
> | Brain death/organ donor patient | |

REFERENCES

1. Bauchner H, May A, Coates E: Use of analgesic agents for invasive medical procedures in pediatric and neonatal intensive care units, *J Pediatr* 121:647, 1992.
2. Brill JE: Control of pain, *Crit Care Clin* 8:203, 1992.
3. Carpenter CCJ: Oral rehydration: is it as good as parenteral therapy? *N Engl J Med* 306:1103, 1982.
4. Division of Injury Control, Center for Environmental Health and Injury Control, Centers for Disease Control: Childhood injuries in the United States, *Am J Dis Child* 144:627, 1990.
5. Downes J: The future of pediatric critical care medicine, *Crit Care Med* 21:S307, 1993.
6. Downes J: The historical evolution, current status, and prospective development of pediatric critical care, *Crit Care Clin* 8:1, 1992.
7. Fuhrman B, Zimmerman J: The pediatric critical care patient. In Fuhrman B, Zimmerman J, editors: *Pediatric critical care,* St. Louis, 1992, Mosby.
8. Rogers M: Introduction: the development of pediatric intensive care. In Rogers M, editor: *Textbook of pediatric intensive care,* Baltimore, 1987, Williams & Wilkins.
9. Shann F: Pediatric intensive care around the world: Australia, *Crit Care Med* 21:S405, 1993.
10. Southall DP, Cronin BC, Harmann H, et al: Invasive procedures in children receiving intensive care, *Br Med J* 306:1512, 1993.
11. Yeh T: Regionalization of pediatric critical care, *Crit Care Clin* 8:23, 1992.

3 Approach to the Distressed Child

John P. Santamaria

GENERAL CONSIDERATIONS

The optimal approach to the ill or injured child is determined by patient age, acuity of illness or injury, and developmental stage. It is imperative to establish rapport with parent(s) or caretaker(s). Attention to parental concerns greatly affects overall perceived quality of care to the child and enhances the quality of the medical encounter for the child, caretaker, and physician. Dealing with family members who may seem unreasonable or overprotective is a part of caring for children. Only on rare occasions does critical illness or injury preclude physician efforts to create a friendly and understanding milieu, because of requirements for rapid therapeutic interventions. Almost always the few extra minutes and added mental effort by the physician to prepare himself or herself, the child, and the caretaker for a diagnostic or therapeutic procedure is well rewarded.

Essential qualities in a skilled physician-child and physician-caretaker encounter include:

- **Respect.** The child's self-esteem depends partly on his perception of how others treat him and his parents. Address the child by his or her name, rather than boy or girl. It is helpful to ask a child what he likes to be called.
- **Gentleness.** A child quickly perceives and appreciates a physician's *understanding, calm,* and *gentle* manner. In a stressful situation, children and their parents may seem unpleasant, uncooperative, and hostile. The physician should anticipate such behavior in distressed circumstances; they should not impair physician poise, professionalism, and objectivity.
- **Self-confidence.** A self-assured physician instills trust and security and rapidly establishes a better-controlled therapeutic environment.
- **Sympathy.** Sympathy is conveyed by word or touch and alleviates the child's or parents' feelings of fear, pain, or worry. Tell them that it is alright to cry.
- **Kindness.** Giving a child a syringe to use as a squirt gun or letting him or her play with a stethoscope, for example, establishes trust.
- **Honesty.** Even little children know the difference. Do not say, "this won't hurt," if it will. If a child is told to expect brief pain with local injection of an anesthetic, and experience confirms the physician's forewarning, he is more likely to remain calm after explanations of pain or no pain in subsequent procedures. Some truths can be terrifying; honesty must be tempered with tenderness.
- **Optimism.** Suggestions of well-being, hope, and recovery can be quite soothing. Some practitioners are able to use suggestion successfully as a sole modality for analgesia. These qualities are universally appreciated and will enhance effective data collection and examination, compliance with requests, and mutual satisfaction.

ANATOMIC, PHYSIOLOGIC, AND DEVELOPMENTAL CONSIDERATIONS

The ill and injured child has important anatomic and developmental differences from those of an adult. Elements to distinguish include:

Growth and Development

An appreciation for major developmental milestones will help the examiner know how to interact best with the patient and evaluate appropriateness of behavior. Major milestones are noted in Fig. 3-1, the test form for the DENVER II, which is the revised version of the Denver Developmental Screening Test.

The greatest rate of physical growth occurs in the first year of life. Birth weight doubles by 6 months and triples by 1 year. Weight of older children can be approximated using the following formula:

$$\text{Weight in kilograms} = (2 \times \text{age in years}) + 8$$

The younger the child, the greater the body surface area/body weight ratio. Therefore, insensible heat losses are exaggerated in cold exposure, submersion injury, or during exposure for examination or procedures. The young child's immature thermoregulatory system requires close monitoring and support of core temperature to detect serious heat or fluid losses from the skin and to avert untoward iatrogenic hemodynamic effects.

The child's large head relative to body size contributes to the relatively high incidence of head injury. Although the cranium is thicker in early childhood, the brain is more loosely attached to the periosteum, predisposing to shaken-baby syndrome. Also, heat and fluid losses from the uncovered head can be rapid. A skull cap fashioned from simple stockinette can help avoid such problems (Fig. 3-2).

Airway

The glottis is anterior and superior in the small child compared to the adult. The trachea is short, with the most narrow part distal to the vocal cords at the level of the cricoid cartilage. Therefore ensure proper head positioning during intubation, select an endotracheal tube size to allow for a small air leak, and carefully auscultate breath sounds after the cords are passed to avoid mainstem bronchus intubation.

Cardiovascular System

The young child's highly responsive vasculature preserves blood pressure through early stages of shock primarily through tachycardia and peripheral vasoconstriction. Carefully observe for evidence of poor organ perfusion to recognize reversible compensated shock early. Tachycardia, cool skin, and delayed capillary refill are key early signs of

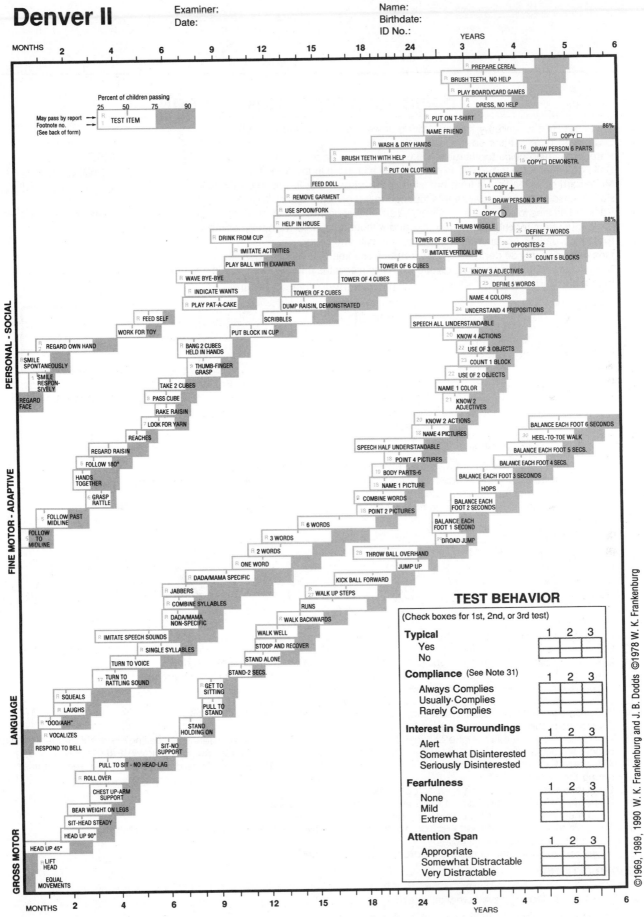

FIG. 3-1   A, Denver developmental screening test.

(From Hoeckelman RA, et al: *Primary pediatric care,* ed 3, St. Louis, 1996, Mosby. Courtesy William K. Frankenburg, M.D.)

Continued.

DIRECTIONS FOR ADMINISTRATION

1. Try to get child to smile by smiling, talking or waving. Do not touch him/her.
2. Child must stare at hand several seconds.
3. Parent may help guide toothbrush and put toothpaste on brush.
4. Child does not have to be able to tie shoes or button/zip in the back.
5. Move yarn slowly in an arc from one side to the other, about 8" above child's face.
6. Pass if child grasps rattle when it is touched to the backs or tips of fingers.
7. Pass if child tries to see where yarn went. Yarn should be dropped quickly from sight from tester's hand without arm movement.
8. Child must transfer cube from hand to hand without help of body, mouth, or table.
9. Pass if child picks up raisin with any part of thumb and finger.
10. Line can vary only 30 degrees or less from tester's line. $\checkmark$
11. Make a fist with thumb pointing upward and wiggle only the thumb. Pass if child imitates and does not move any fingers other than the thumb.

12. Pass any enclosed form. Fail continuous round motions.	13. Which line is longer? (Not bigger.) Turn paper upside down and repeat. (Pass 3 of 3 or 5 of 6)	14. Pass any lines crossing near midpoint.	15. Have child copy first. If failed, demonstrate.

When giving items 12, 14, and 15, do not name the forms. Do not demonstrate 12 and 14.

16. When scoring, each pair (2 arms, 2 legs, etc.) counts as one part.
17. Place one cube in cup and shake gently near child's ear, but out of sight. Repeat for other ear.
18. Point to picture and have child name it. (No credit is given for sounds only.)
    If less than 4 pictures are named correctly, have child point to picture as each is named by tester.

 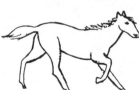 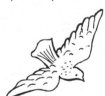 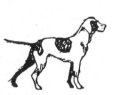 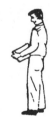

19. Using doll, tell child: Show me the nose, eyes, ears, mouth, hands, feet, tummy, hair. Pass 6 of 8.
20. Using pictures, ask child: Which one flies?... says meow?... talks?... barks?... gallops? Pass 2 of 5, 4 of 5.
21. Ask child: What do you do when you are cold?... tired?... hungry? Pass 2 of 3, 3 of 3.
22. Ask child: What do you do with a cup? What is a chair used for? What is a pencil used for? Action words must be included in answers.
23. Pass if child correctly places <u>and</u> says how many blocks are on paper. (1, 5).
24. Tell child: Put block **on** table; **under** table; **in front of** me, **behind** me. Pass 4 of 4. (Do not help child by pointing, moving head or eyes.)
25. Ask child: What is a ball?... lake?... desk?... house?... banana?... curtain?... fence?... ceiling? Pass if defined in terms of use, shape, what it is made of, or general category (such as banana is fruit, not just yellow). Pass 5 of 8, 7 of 8.
26. Ask child: If a horse is big, a mouse is __? If fire is hot, ice is __? If the sun shines during the day, the moon shines during the __? Pass 2 of 3.
27. Child may use wall or rail only, not person. May not crawl.
28. Child must throw ball overhand 3 feet to within arm's reach of tester.
29. Child must perform standing broad jump over width of test sheet (8 1/2 inches).
30. Tell child to walk forward, ∞ heel within 1 inch of toe. Tester may demonstrate. Child must walk 4 consecutive steps.
31. In the second year, half of normal children are non-compliant.

OBSERVATIONS:

FIG. 3-1, cont'd. **B,** Denver developmental screening test.

(From Hoeckelman RA, et al: *Primary pediatric care,* ed 3, St. Louis, 1996, Mosby.)

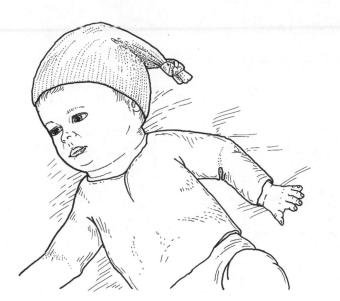

FIG. 3-2   Heat loss reduction by use of stockinette skull cap.

hypovolemia. Blood pressure, while specific, is quite insensitive to volume loss and may be normal in the face of serious volume deficits (see Chapter 4).

Musculoskeletal System

Compliant chest and relatively unprotected abdominal walls contribute to high risk of intrathoracic and intraabdominal

injuries. Rib fractures and external signs of injury are often absent, even when significant trauma has occurred. Likewise, splenic, renal, and hepatic injuries must be suspected even in the absence of abdominal bruises.

Developmental Differences

See Chapter 6.

CONSENT

Obtaining consent for life-saving emergency procedures is unnecessary. If, in the opinion of the treating physician, need for medical intervention is imminent, do not delay provision of appropriate care. Less clear-cut clinical situations demand other considerations.

The American College of Emergency Physicians has developed a policy statement on evaluation and treatment of minors to clarify decision pathways so that appropriate care is rendered without delay. This document serves as a practical guideline and assists health-care facilities in developing a consent policy as required by the Joint Commission on Accreditation of Healthcare Organizations. Figs. 3-3 through 3-5 depict the appropriate initial approach to obtaining consent, the approach under conflict, and the approach in different settings of time criticality.

The medical care in question may not constitute a true emergency (category I in algorithms), but it still may be deemed to be in the best interest of the minor child by the treating physician. A child may qualify for consenting to his

FIG. 3-3   Consent: initial approach.

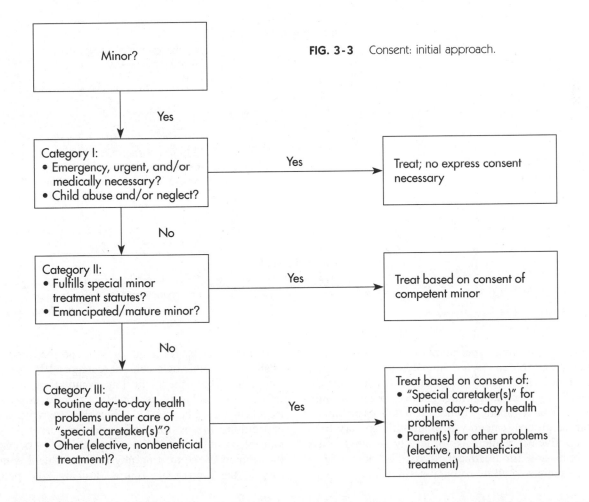

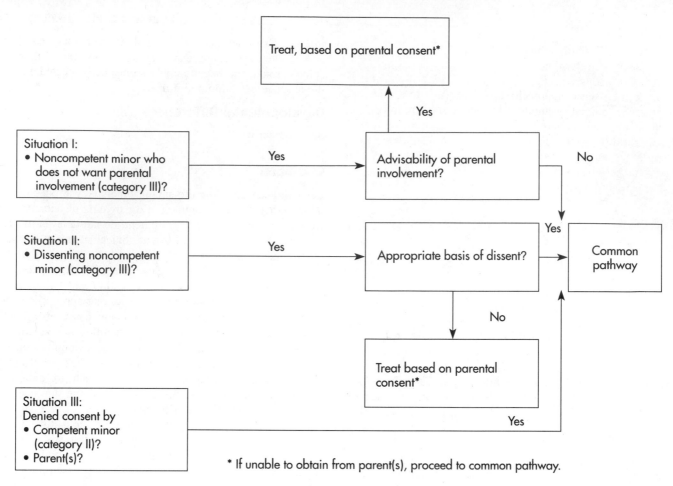

FIG. 3-4 Consent: conflict situations.

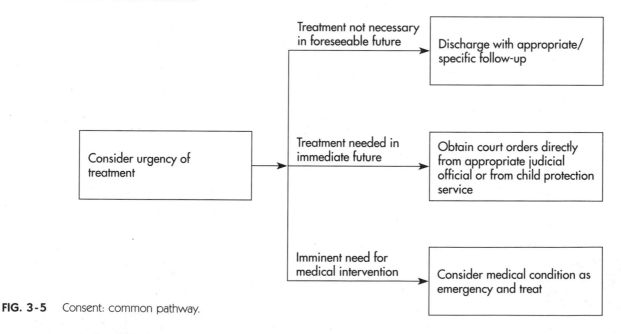

FIG. 3-5 Consent: common pathway.

own treatment by meeting "special minor treatment statutes" (e.g., sexually transmitted disease, human immunodeficiency virus, drug-related treatments), consideration as an "emancipated minor" (e.g., self-supporting, married, pregnant, military recruit), or as a "mature minor." Guidelines for inclusion into these groups (category II in algorithms) vary from state to state. Even if a minor is not legally required to ask parental permission for treatment, it is often advisable to persuade the patient to allow parental notification.

If imminent danger is not present and the minor does not qualify to give his own consent (category III), determine the time-criticality of the medical intervention. In cases in which only a brief delay is acceptable, obtain a court order for treatment (see Chapter 152). Establish in writing the most expeditious means to obtain such an order in advance; valuable time is wasted if no preplanning has occurred. If in the opinion of the treating physician treatment is not necessary in the foreseeable future, discharge the patient with appropriate follow-up. Instructions should always stress the importance of returning for further care if the clinical condition worsens.

A common-sense approach should prevail. It is not the intent of the judicial system to delay necessary care to minors if parental consent cannot be obtained. Courts have routinely upheld the physician's judgment of what constitutes emergency intervention. Clear documentation in the medical record of the physician's decision process and of attempts to obtain parental consent is imperative important.

HISTORY

Box 3-1 outlines a basic approach to the collection of historical data. Sometimes, when critical injury or illness is present, history taking may follow or occur concurrently with treatment. However, when distress is not severe in a child requiring a diagnostic or therapeutic procedure, a slow, friendly, and methodic approach is desirable. Assume a comfortable, relaxed position for the interview. Introduce yourself by name with a handshake. This is a direct and expeditious way to create a nonthreatening environment. Age-appropriate play may help the younger child. Humor can be tricky. When successful, it may relieve tension, but as any comedian can attest, a joking statement can be unappreciated or misconstrued. Physicians, with few exceptions, are not comedians. Children know the difference.

A good way to convey respect and concern is to apologize for time spent waiting, even if the waiting time was short. "I'm sorry to keep you waiting." Convey your desire to help simply by asking, "What can I do to help you?" This is perhaps the most important single question for overall patient and family satisfaction.

Invite the historian to relate the circumstances leading to the medical visit without interruption. Whenever possible, the historian initially should be the child. Clarify confusing points by reiterating the important aspects of the history in chronologic order. Next, collect a problem-oriented review of symptoms and past medical history (FADISM)[2] (Box 3-1).

Attempt to make the parent and child feel comfortable with the decision to seek medical care. It is counterproductive to infer that a visit is unnecessary while it is in progress. In fact, many of the visits that physicians declare are unnecessary visits are only so judged after the benefit of trained history collection, physical examination, and adjunctive testing. It is unreasonable to expect the same judgment from a parent with an apparently ill or injured child.

Allow the informant to answer one question fully before asking the next. Failure in this regard implies impatience or disrespect. Do not be accusatory.

PHYSICAL EXAMINATION

Respect the child's modesty but *do not compromise the examination* (Box 3-2). "The child should be completely undressed, but not necessarily all at once."[1] Try to leave diaper (self-defense) and underwear in place except for examination of these parts. Save examination of the head and neck, especially the ears and mouth, for last. These are usually the most anxiety-provoking in young children. Give generous doses of praise after a patient has undergone an anxiety-provoking part of the physical examination or procedure. Even if the child cries and struggles, praise and reward his efforts. Praise and reward are appropriate at all ages and should be tailored to the developmental stage of the child.

Perform physical examination of the child under age 2 in a parent's arms whenever possible. Although the neonate may not even know the difference, the parent will feel more in control and involved if maintaining close contact with the child. As the child differentiates self from others and parents from strangers, he becomes frightened if taken away from the parent, even for a brief time. Especially in the first year of life when object permanence is incompletely developed, keep times away from parents, even for procedures, minimal.

Knowledge of developmental stages is key to successful evaluation (Fig. 3-1). Keep the bed rails up when a child can roll over. Use a cage crib or constant adult supervision when a child is capable of climbing. By approximately 9 months of age the child has acquired a pincer grasp; if small objects are left within reach, the differential diagnosis can be expanded in many presentations to include aspiration or ingestion of small objects.

The preschooler has usually accumulated negative experi-

BOX 3-1   **INITIAL CONTACT: HISTORY**

Introduce yourself and assume a comfortable position.
Call patient by name and establish friendly, nonthreatening contact (e.g., handshake, age-appropriate play).
Open-ended opener (e.g., I'm sorry to keep you waiting. What can I do to help you?)
Restate your understanding of what you have been told.
Ask questions to expand and clarify the History of Present Illness and Review of Systems.
Past medical history F-A-D-I-S-M₁
    Family history
    Allergies
    Diet (infant) / last meal
    Immunizations
    Social history
    Medications
    Medical illnesses / surgery / hospitalizations

BOX 3-2   **PRIORITIES IN THE PHYSICAL EXAMINATION OF AN ILL OR INJURED CHILD**

- Cervical spine precautions—
    A, Airway
    B, Breathing
    C, Circulation
- Apparent disability
- Complete exposure
- Vital signs, including weight (or length)
- Initial assessment: stable vs. unstable
- Mental status, hydration, disfigurement, active bleeding
- Secondary survey toe-to-head (save most noxious parts for last)

ences and resists physical examination and conveys his thoughts verbally. It is the incomplete understanding and persistence of "magical" thinking that makes it so difficult to reason with children at this age.[2] Attempt to cajole and win their cooperation, but realize that these efforts may be in vain. At this point, complete the examination in a sympathetic yet firm manner. Provide discussions and explanations of procedures just before they are performed to minimize frightening fantasies.[5]

The school-age child has better understanding of the medical visit and requires more detailed explanations of procedures than younger children. Although command of language is quite good at this age, it is important to speak clearly and use appropriate vocabulary. Make the child an active participant in the examination and ask him or her to make decisions when appropriate; the choice of being examined in the sitting or standing position may be appropriate for an 8-year-old.

Teenagers generally prize their privacy, especially when being examined. Sensitivity to this need can take many forms. Palpate the abdomen under a bed sheet. Draw curtains in the room before beginning the examination. The more self-conscious teenager is also less likely to ask questions than the younger school-age child, yet will have many of the same concerns. Providing a play-by-play of physical examination findings, especially if normal, will allay fears that may not be expressed. Box 3-2 summarizes the key points of an examination.

CREATING AN APPROPRIATE ENVIRONMENT

Creating the appropriate environment to perform a diagnostic or therapeutic procedure on an ill or injured child reduces the need for chemical and physical restraint; enhances success of the procedure; and improves the quality of the experience for child, caretaker, and medical personnel. Issues related to the appropriate physical environment, equipment, and staffing must be considered.

Sights and sounds of a bustling medical facility further stress the ill child and his family. A physical environment that provides privacy and treatment for children, away from adult patients, is desirable. Proper equipment is necessary to the optimal performance of any medical procedure. For the pediatric patient, appropriate-sized equipment must be available and organized in a way that is familiar to medical personnel should an emergency arise. Ideally pediatric procedures are performed by physicians and nurses having specific interest, training, and experience with children. The use of light and color, as well as familiar graphics and symbols, is helpful in shifting patient focus away from illness. However, smiling faces, playful behavior, and demeanors conveying competency, warmth, efficiency, and caring are less often emphasized, although immeasurably more important than decorative walls.[4]

Even in busy medical centers, the presentation of a critically ill or injured child may not be a daily event. It is best for the team to rehearse in advance their approach to these patients. Preparation for critical cases, in which coordination of personnel is key to optimal care, includes "mock runs" or other didactic sessions to emphasize: (1) what his or her role will be in advance; (2) where appropriate equipment, supplies, medications are and how they work; (3) leadership hierarchy; (4) consultation or activation procedure for other key team members (e.g., trauma surgeon); (5) general order of interventions to anticipate sequential procedures; and (6) physical placement of team members around child.

REFERENCES

1. Barness LA: History and physical examination. In Kaye R, Oski FA, Barness LA, editors: *Core textbook of pediatrics,* Philadelphia, 1988, JB Lippincott.
2. Fraiberg SH: *The magic years,* New York, 1959, Charles Scribner's Sons.
3. Grossman M, Dieckmann R: *Pediatric emergency medicine: a clinician's reference,* Philadelphia, 1991, JB Lippincott.
4. Santamaria JP: Design considerations in pediatric emergency care. In Riggs L, editor; *Emergency department design,* Dallas, 1993, American College of Emergency Physicians.
5. Seidel JS, Henderson DP: Approach to the pediatric patient in the emergency department. In Barkin RM, editor: *Pediatric emergency medicine, concepts and clinical practice,* St. Louis, 1992, Mosby.

4 Vital Signs

Deborah Mulligan-Smith

Respiratory rate, pulse, blood pressure, and temperature are referred to as the four vital signs. Historically these objective measurements have been the major physiologic parameters available to the clinician for evaluation of cardiopulmonary status. Although this past era has brought dramatic technologic advances in cardiopulmonary assessment and monitoring, vital signs still play an important role. However, obtaining and interpreting vital signs accurately in children, especially in a busy Emergency Department (ED), can be problematic. Obtaining children's vital signs requires appropriate equipment and the knowledge of normal ranges for age.

RESPIRATION

As the result of a maturation process of respiratory control initiated in utero, normal ventilation is effortless. Infants and children have anatomic variants from adults that make them more vulnerable to respiratory dysfunction. Breathing is controlled through the respiratory centers in the pons and medulla. These centers are influenced from a variety of sources, including peripheral and cortical chemoreceptors, mechanoreceptors throughout the respiratory tree, juxtapulmonary (type J receptors) capillary receptors, lung irritant receptors, reticular activating system, and voluntary centers in the cerebral cortex. Input from these sources modifies respiratory effort and patterns of respiration.[2,8]

Active inspiration involves the contraction of respiratory muscles, thereby increasing intrathoracic volume. Diaphragmatic movement accounts for the majority of change in the intrathoracic volume. Unlike the diaphragm of the older child or adult, which assumes a dome-shaped cylinder when these muscles are stretched to maximum length, the infant's diaphragm takes on a flatter configuration, which is less effective in moving large lung volumes. The normal tidal volume of children is 5 to 7 ml/kg compared to 7 ml/kg (500 ml) in adults. In addition, the smaller, thin, elastic chest walls of infants are more compliant. Expiration results through the contraction of both the internal intercostal muscles and the abdominal wall muscles. This dynamic process pulls the rib cage downward and inward, increases intraabdominal pressure, and pushes the diaphragm upward.[2,5,8,15]

Immaturity of the infant's central nervous system and less functional respiratory reserve make him or her especially susceptible to ventilatory malfunction.[4] Also, the infant's medullary center is more sensitive to metabolic abnormalities. Hence, respiratory depression can result from myriad causes, from hypoxemia to anemia or hypothermia. Tachypnea may be a response to hypoxemia or a clinical manifestation of shock. (Refer to Table 4-1 for normal respiratory rates for age.) On the other hand, periodic breathing, in which the regular rhythm of breathing is interrupted by brief, cyclic episodes of apnea, is normal in the sleeping newborn.

Table 4-1 Age-Appropriate Normal Respiratory Rates

Age	Normal respiratory rates/min
Birth	30-60
Infant (1-6 months)	30-40
Infant (6-12 months)	20-30
1-6 years	20-25
Over 6 years	16-20

Therefore both the rate and pattern of respiration have age-related differences.[2,4,5]

Indications and Contraindications

Document rate and effort of respirations at the time of initial evaluation. This is not a static measurement. With the ill child, obtain comparative measures. Respiratory emergencies require evaluation and stabilization. Respiratory illness is the most common underlying pediatric medical emergency leading to cardiopulmonary arrest. The only relative contraindication to assessment of the respiratory rate and pattern is airway obstruction for which an immediate artificial airway is imperative.[5-7,15]

Equipment

Equipment includes a timing mechanism and stethoscope. Sophisticated cardiorespiratory monitors are also useful but are not necessary for taking basic vital signs. Efficiency of respiration can be measured more precisely with pulse oximeters, capnometry, and peak expiratory flow meters (clinically useful in children older than 5 years), as discussed in Chapter 23.[2,5,9,12]

Technique

The respiratory rate is the number of inspirations in 1 full minute. Establishing an accurate respiratory rate depends on the patient's developmental age. If the child is older than 6 months but younger than 2 years of age, assess him or her at a comfortable distance. These youngsters feel most secure in the parent's lap. Ask the parent to expose the child's chest and abdomen for purposes of observation.

The respiratory assessment includes observation, palpation of chest/abdominal excursions, and/or auscultation. Establish the rate, rhythm, and/or depth of respirations. Note skin and lip color, nasal flaring, grunting, head bobbing, stridor, wheezing, retractions, quality of voice, shape of the chest (e.g., barrel), subcutaneous emphysema, posture (e.g., hunched over, tripod), level of activity, and mental status[2-5,8,15] (Fig. 4-1).

Specific descriptions provide objective information for precise communication about illness acuity and serial evaluations of response to therapy. For example, indicate if stridor occurs at rest, if wheezing is inspiratory and expiratory,

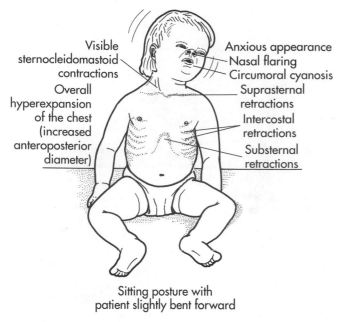

Visible sternocleidomastoid contractions

Overall hyperexpansion of the chest (increased anteroposterior diameter)

Anxious appearance
Nasal flaring
Circumoral cyanosis
Suprasternal retractions
Intercostal retractions
Substernal retractions

Sitting posture with patient slightly bent forward

Fig. 4-1 Possible physical findings observed in a child with respiratory distress.

Table 4-2 Diagnostic Possibilities Associated with Change in Respirations

↑ Respirations	↓ Respirations
Acute salicylate intoxication	Anemia
Cerebral infarction	Fatigue
Congenital heart disease	Drugs and toxins
Crying	Hypoglycemia
Diabetes	Hypothermia
Drugs and toxins	Intracranial pathology
Encephalitis	Irritability
Exercise	Metabolic alkalosis
Fear	Neuromuscular disorders
Hyperthermia	
Hypoxia	
Inborn errors of metabolism	
Metabolic acidosis	
Pain	
Pneumothorax	
Psychogenic	
Pregnancy	
Shock	
Stress	
Urinary bladder distention	

where retractions are present (supraclavicular, intercostal, substernal), and mental status (e.g., alert, sleepy, confused, unresponsive).[13,16]

Remarks

The normal respiratory rate decreases with age (see Table 4-1). Regardless of the etiology, respiratory dysfunction produces notable aberrations in the rate and pattern of breathing. A respiratory rate greater than 60 breaths/min in any age child is abnormal.[3,15] The respiratory demand for oxygen consumption and carbon dioxide elimination is higher in children because of their increased metabolic rate. Look for signs of respiratory failure (e.g., circumoral cyanosis, anxious appearance, and suprasternal retractions). If respiratory failure is present, separate the child from the parent or caretaker to facilitate aggressive interventions to restore stability. Table 4-2 summarizes common causes of abnormal respiratory rates.[4,5,7,13,16]

Apnea, or cessation of breathing, occurs in premature infants and young newborns as a response to a variety of factors. Some but not all are pathologic. Apnea of prematurity may occur in 50% of premature infants. Irregular breathing in the otherwise well infant may be a "healthy sign." Significant apnea is usually associated with evidence of hypoxia (bradycardia, change in color, or muscle tone).[2,6]

The infant chest wall is highly compliant, which allows it to be sucked in (retractions) while the abdomen is simultaneously expanding. This breathing pattern, described as "see-saw" or "rocking respirations," makes the newborn more vulnerable to muscle fatigue, leading to respiratory failure. Therefore repeat evaluation of the ill-appearing infant is mandatory. The infant who initially presents with a respiratory rate of 80 respirations/min that falls to 60/min may appear to have improved, but to the contrary is on a perilous downward trend.[4,7,13,15]

Head bobbing, nasal flaring, grunting, retractions, altered

respiratory rate, wheezing, and/or stridor suggest respiratory dysfunction. Nasal flaring is commonly noted in the infant in respiratory distress and is specific for hypoxia.[3]

An expiratory grunt is produced by early closure of the glottis at the end of expiration, thus raising functional residual capacity. Grunting is a phenomenon observed with lung diseases that cause accumulation of interstitital/alveolar fluid.[2,8]

Careful observation of the child's respiratory effort can help discern restrictive from obstructive or upper from lower airway problems. The pediatric patient's airway is small. Airway resistance is inversely proportional to the fourth power of the radius.

$$\text{Resistance} = 1/\text{radius}^4$$

A decrease in radius by one half causes a sixteenfold increase in resistance; a 1-mm rim of edema in a 5-mm cross-section area results in a 75% loss of airway. The upper airway may easily become obstructed by body fluids, foreign bodies, or active constriction. The physical findings suggesting upper airway obstruction include prolonged inspiration; inspiratory stridor (a crowing sound); and suprasternal, supraclavicular, and subcostal retractions. In lower airway obstruction the expiration phase is prolonged, and retractions and expiratory wheezing are present.[*]

PULSE

Cardiac output is heart rate times stroke volume. It is the volume of blood ejected by the heart per minute. Increase in heart rate is the single most important mechanism for increasing cardiac output in the infant/child. As blood is

---

[*]References 2, 5, 7, 12, 14, and 15.

forced into the aorta during systole, it moves forward in the vessels and sets up a pressure wave that travels down the arteries. This pressure wave creates a palpable pulse as it expands the arterial walls. It travels 10 times faster than the blood itself. In the young child the pulse is felt in the radial artery at about 0.1 seconds after the peak of systolic ejection into the aorta. Thorough pulse evaluation can provide information about cardiac rate, rhythm, and possible disease states.[2,8]

Indications and Contraindications

Assess and document the presence, character, and rate of pulse. There are no contraindications.

Equipment

Only a watch/clock with a second hand or digital readout is usually required. A stethoscope is needed for the auscultation method. Electrocardiograms provide precise documentation of heart rate, rhythm, and electrical conduction. If continuous monitoring is necessary, use a cardiorespiratory monitor or pulse oximeter.[1,2,4,9,12]

Technique

The pulse rate varies with age, body temperature, and level of anxiety. Create a comfortable, safe environment for the patient who is older than 6 months but younger than 3 years of age by asking the calm parent to hold the child in his or her lap, whenever possible. Approach the child from a safe distance and at the patient's eye level. Unless the child is seriously distressed, leave the toddler's clothing on rather than risk a negative interaction.

Assess pulse using palpation or auscultation. The pulse palpation method provides information regarding heart rate and character of the pulse.[2,9,12]

Use the radial pulse to assess these parameters in the older child and adult. Infants have a large head on a short neck and chubby wrists, thereby making the brachial or femoral arteries easier sites of assessment. To feel the brachial pulse, place the pads of the index and middle fingers on the medial aspect of the biceps muscle, in the antecubital fossa, and slightly flex the elbow. Compress the artery until a maximum pulsation is detected. (Do not use the thumb as it is possible to sense one's own thumb pulse for the patient's.)[9,12]

Palpate the cardiac apex to determine heart rate. It does not accurately measure pulse. The absence of precordial activity does not directly correlate with absent cardiac activity.[2,8,9,12]

An alternative to palpation is the auscultation method of evaluation. Simply auscultate over the cardiac precordium with a stethoscope.

Observe the pulsations of the anterior fontanel to obtain heart rate in undistressed infants.[2,9]

Measure the pulse rate over a 1-minute interval and document as the number of beats per minute. If circumstances preclude a full 1-minute assessment time, document the pulse rate over a 15-second interval and multiply by 4. Start the count at 0 seconds or the pulse will be inaccurate by an additional 4 beats/min. The heart rate of newborn infants is subject to wide variation. The rate may increase to 170 with irritability or dramatically decrease to 90 with peaceful sleep. As with respiratory rate, the heart rate fluctuates less

Table 4-3   Age-Appropriate Range of Normal Pulse Rates

Age	Resting pulse rate (per minute)
Newborn	120-160
Infant (less than 1 year)	80-140
2 year	80-130
3-6 year	80-120
7 years to adolescence	70-110

and decreases as the child grows older. Table 4-3 contains the normal range of pulse rates by age.[2,5,9,12,16]

The character of the pulse describes its rhythm and amplitude. Standard practice for evaluation of pulse amplitude is to grade it from 0 to 3, with zero being an absent pulse; 1, a diminished pulse; 2, a normal pulse; and 3, a bounding pulse.[8]

Remarks

Bradycardia almost always means hypoxia and advanced respiratory failure. Act instantly to improve oxygenation and ventilation. Tachycardia may indicate hypoxia, but it may also denote volume loss, fear, anxiety, or fever. Although it is sensitive to hypoxia, it is nonspecific. Reduction in heart rate with therapy may be an important measure of improvement.[4,7,15]

Diminished pulses (*pulsus parvus*) may suggest diminished cardiac output. Causes may include decreased stroke volume (shock, heart failure) or mechanical obstruction to left ventricular output (aortic stenosis, pericardial tamponade, cardiomyopathy). With *bounding pulses* there is a perceptible rapid rise, brief peak, and rapid fall. Bounding pulses may result from hyperkinetic states such as anxiety, fever, and anemia or abnormally rapid runoff of blood as in patent ductus arteriosus or arteriovenous communication. To diagnose *pulsus alternans* the rhythm must be regular. This beat-to-beat variability in the amplitude of the pulse is evidence of left-sided cardiac decompensation.[2,8,9,12]

Pulsus paradoxus is the cyclic diminution of systolic pressure with inspiration. Increased pulsus paradoxus occurs when mechanical forces on the pericardium (e.g., hemopericardium) restrict blood return and reduce cardiac output transiently during inspiration. It is occasionally noted in severe cases of status asthmaticus, with marked increases in intrathoracic pressure. Sphygmomanometry is usually necessary. Pump the sphygmomanometer cuff to occlude the peripheral pulse. As the cuff pressure falls, note the pressure at which the first Korotkoff sound is heard. This should be heard only during expiration. Continue to decrease the cuff pressure until the first sound is detected during both inspiration and expiration. Pulsus paradoxus is present if the absolute difference between this pressure and the first is greater than or equal to 10.

Is the rhythm of the pulse regular, irregular, sporadically irregular, or regularly irregular? This information may provide clues to various cardiac arrhythmias. The *bigeminal pulse* is actually an irregular rhythm. The normal beat alternates with a premature contraction. The stroke volume of the premature contraction is diminished, and the pulse pressure alternates in volume.[2,8,11,15]

ARTERIAL BLOOD PRESSURE MEASUREMENTS

The homeostatic relationship between cardiac output and peripheral vascular resistance is measurable as arterial blood pressure. The pressure in the large arteries rises to a peak value, the systolic pressure, and falls to a minimum value, the diastolic pressure. Effective perfusion pressure is the mean intraluminal pressure of the arterial system minus the mean pressure of the venous system. Flow through the cardiovascular system is equal to effective perfusion pressure/resistance. Peripheral vascular resistance varies. *Therefore a normal blood pressure cannot be relied on to assess adequate perfusion.* This is especially true in pediatrics.[2,5,6,12,15]

Children have tremendous cardiovascular compensatory mechanisms. Despite large volume losses, normal blood pressure can be maintained through vasoconstriction, tachycardia and increased cardiac contractility, which collectively support a transient state of "compensated shock." With a normal blood pressure and relatively mild elevations in pulse and respirations, the patient may appear stable. As hypovolemia evolves into "decompensated" shock, the child "precipitously" may deteriorate into cardiac arrest. Therefore blood pressure is helpful but quite insensitive as a measure of cardiovascular performance.[5-7,15]

The pulse pressure is the difference between the systolic and diastolic pressures. The mean pressure is the average pressure throughout the cardiac cycle. A quick estimate can be made by adding the diastolic pressure to one third of the pulse pressure.[5,15]

Indications and Contraindications

Measure and document arterial blood pressure in all ill patients and as indicated in all patients 2 years of age and older. Use timed repeated determinations in the seriously distressed child. Continuous blood pressure monitoring is necessary for the unstable patient (see Chapter 26). Relative contraindications include the presence of an arteriovenous shunt, intravenous line in the designated extremity, circumferential burns, lymphedema, or any site where there is the potential for circulatory compromise.[1,5,7,10,14]

Equipment

See detailed discussion in Chapter 36.

Remarks

Volume status can be assessed by use of *orthostatic vital signs*. Relative contraindications include the patient in shock who requires immediate medical management or patient findings that prohibit physical maneuvers (e.g., suspected spinal cord injury, pelvic fractures).[5-7,15] Record the blood pressure and pulse after the patient has been in the supine position for 2 to 3 minutes. Next ask the patient to stand. (The sitting position may be used with the legs dependent, although this is less accurate than the supine-to-standing measurement.) Record the blood pressure and pulse after the patient has been standing for 1 minute. Prepare to lay the patient down should she develop syncope.[2,9,12]

The test is positive if the patient is symptomatic; the heart rate increases by 20 beats/min (30 beats/min in adults); bradycardia ensues, or blood pressure decreases by 20 mm Hg (25 mm Hg for the adult patient). Orthostatic hypotension reflects a multitude of potential disorders, including hypovolemia, blood loss, pregnancy, drugs (e.g., phenothiazines, antihypertensives, nitrates, diuretics), nervous system disorders, and metabolic abnormalities. A thorough history and physical examination aid the clinician in making the diagnosis and formulating an appropriate treatment plan.[2,5-7,12,15]

REFERENCES

1. Aoki B: *Principles in the stabilization and transport of critically ill children,* Oakland, Calif, 1984, Children's Hospital Oakland.
2. Behrman R, editor: *Nelson textbook of pediatrics,* Philadelphia, 1992, Saunders.
3. Carlo W, Martin MB, Bruce NB, et al: Alae nasi activation decreases nasal resistance in preterm infants, *Pediatrics* 72:338-343, 1983.
4. Carroll J: Disordered control of breathing in infants and children, *Pediatr Rev* 2:51-65, 1993.
5. Chameides L, editor: *Pediatric advanced life support,* 1994, AHA.
6. Eichelberger M: *Pediatric trauma.* St. Louis, 1993, Mosby.
7. Fleisher G, Ludwig S, editors: *Pediatric emergency medicine,* Baltimore, 1995, Williams & Wilkins.
8. Guyton A: *Textbook of medical physiology,* ed 8, Philadelphia, 1991, Saunders.
9. Lohr JA: *Pediatric outpatient procedures,* Philadelphia, 1991, JB Lippincott.
10. Ornato J: Hemodynamic monitoring during CPR, *Ann Emerg Med* 22: 289-294, 1993.
11. Park M, Menard S: Accuracy of blood pressure measurement by the dinamap monitor in infants and children, *Pediatrics* 79:907-913, 1987.
12. Roberts J, Hedges J: *Clinical procedures in emergency medicine,* ed 2, Philadelphia, 1991, Saunders.
13. Rudoph A: *Rudolph's pediatrics,* ed 19, Norwalk, Conn, 1991, Appleton & Lange.
14. Saipe C: Respiratory emergencies in children, *Pediatr Ann* 19:637-646, 1990.
15. Silverman BK, editor: *Advanced pediatric life support: the pediatric emergency medicine course,* 1993, ACEP/AAP.
16. Uhari M, Nuutinen M, Turtinin J, et al: Pulse sounds and measurement of diastolic blood pressure in children, *Lancet* 338:159-161, 1991.

5 Temperature Taking

Kevin Coulter

The accurate measurement of body temperature is a key element in the evaluation of ill and injured children. Abnormal temperature may be a manifestation of an infectious, inflammatory, or malignant disease; an alteration in body metabolism; or a dysfunction of thermoregulation. Obtaining body temperature has long been a routine part of initial vital sign assessment in both the Emergency Department (ED) and the Pediatric Intensive Care Unit (PICU). Ongoing monitoring of body temperature provides an important measure of response to therapy (e.g., rewarming for hypothermia) and ensures an appropriate thermal environment for ongoing treatment, especially in infants who are particularly vulnerable to rapid heat loss.

The body temperature can be measured by a variety of different instruments and techniques with different degrees of sensitivity and specificity. These span the spectrum from the time-honored but inaccurate method of tactile estimation of forehead temperature to the most accurate technique of inserting indwelling catheters into the viscera or vascular tree of critically ill or injured patients.

This chapter discusses the most common temperature-taking techniques for infants and children in the ED or PICU: glass thermometry, electronic digital thermometry, infrared emission detection tympanic thermometry, and rectal probes. Chapter 93 discusses temperature control and monitoring in the neonate.

Indications

Unless the individual requires immediate resuscitation, measure a temperature as part of the initial assessment of any infant or child. In the ED, important triage decisions derive from an abnormal temperature (either hyperthermia or hypothermia), particularly in younger children and infants in whom there is special concern for bacteremia. The preferred method of temperature taking depends on the age of the child; the nature of the presenting illness or injury; and acceptance of the procedure by the child, parent, and medical staff.

The axilla is the preferred site for taking initial temperatures in the premature neonate. This site is safe and easily accessible. Axillary temperatures are a reliable reflection of core body temperature in newborn nurseries where the ambient temperatures are carefully controlled. When properly performed, axillary temperatures correlate reasonably well with rectal temperatures—the present gold standard.[6] Skin probes are usually satisfactory after a baseline temperature determination. In normal-weight neonates, the rectum is also an acceptable site for initial temperature taking (see Chapter 93).

Obtain *oral* temperatures in the cooperative child older than 3 years. The lateral sublingual pockets are easily accessible for thermometer placement. Because of proximity to the sublingual branch of the lingual artery, oral temperatures may detect rapid changes in body temperature more quickly than axillary or rectal temperatures.

Rectal temperatures are the widely regarded gold standard for temperature measurement. In many offices and hospitals, the rectum is the preferred site for all infants and toddlers under 3 years of age. It is the most reliable site for patients presenting in shock or coma, with altered level of consciousness, or with oral injury or disease.

Infrared emission detection tympanic membrane thermometry (TMT) represents a recent advance in the technology of temperature taking. This technique has gained a high level of popularity in EDs because of its speed, cleanliness, lack of contact with mucous membranes, noninvasiveness, patient and nurse acceptance, and minimal risk of disease transmission. However, the TMT literature suggests a variable degree of sensitivity and specificity.*

TMT appears to be reasonably accurate in older infants and children but not as accurate as in adults.[14] Cerumen, otitis media, or tympanostomy tubes do not affect tympanic temperatures.[11] The disadvantage of TMT is the apparent discrepancy between TMT and rectal-based techniques in identifying children with fever, especially in children under 3 months.[2,12] There is a reported range of sensitivity of TMT (i.e., the probability that TMT will detect a real fever) relative to rectal thermometry of 0% to 97%; specificity (i.e., the probability that a real fever is present if TMT is high) is better between 74% and 100%.[1] TMT is low relative to rectal temperature, although studies using rectal temperature as the gold standard are controversial, because TMT temperatures change earlier than rectal temperatures when there are real changes in core temperature. The principle advantages of TMT compared to the other sites are that it is faster, safer, and simpler.

Rectal probes are useful in the ED or PICU for ongoing monitoring of temperatures in unstable children. The most common indications are: (1) hypothermic children with rectal temperatures $<35°$ C who require continuous temperature monitoring during rewarming, and (2) critically ill or injured infants and young children, who are especially vulnerable to dangerous heat loss because of large body surface area. Rectal probes are also useful in children who are difficult to move because of severe injuries or burns. At least one study has demonstrated the accuracy of TMT as an alternative to an indwelling rectal probe in tracking pulmonary arterial temperatures in children in the PICU.[10]

Contraindications

The only absolute contraindication to temperature taking is cardiopulmonary arrest or instability, in which immediate therapeutic interventions take precedence. However, under

---

*References 1-4, 7-9, 14, and 15.

such conditions, temperature taking is still imperative after initial resuscitation.

There are contraindications to specific temperature taking techniques, as outlined in the following paragraphs.

Axillary temperatures are actually skin temperature recordings. Although they are usually reliable in neonates, the skin may be an inaccurate site when there is ambient temperature variability or bundling.[5] It also may be insensitive for detecting fever in older infants and children, and it is totally insensitive for detecting core temperature in hypothermic conditions because of peripheral vasoconstriction. Axillary temperatures are time consuming, sometimes taking up to 10 minutes before recording peak temperature. *Therefore the axilla is not an appropriate site for measuring temperature in the seriously ill or injured child.*[11]

Oral temperatures cannot be reliably obtained in most children younger than 3 years because of their inability to cooperate. Also, temperature recordings from the mouth may be altered by tachypnea or by the consumption of hot or cold fluids.[13] *Do not use oral temperatures in children suffering from shock, altered mental status, or oral trauma.*

Avoid rectal temperatures in the premature neonate because of the risk of rectal perforation. Other contraindications to rectal temperatures include neutropenia, rectal trauma and/or bleeding, hemorrhoids, and suspicion of sexual abuse.

Currently the only relative contraindication to TMT is age. As noted earlier, there is not sufficient experience with young infants under 3 months old, where it may be insensitive to fever. Patients with prior ear surgery (with the exception of tympanostomy tubes) or widespread tympanic scarring may have alterations of tympanic blood flow that alter temperature recordings.[11]

The contraindications to rectal probes are the same as for rectal thermometry: premature neonate, neutropenia, rectal trauma and/or bleeding, hemorrhoids, and suspicion of sexual abuse.

Complications

Inadequate cleaning of reusable glass thermometers after mucosal contact may result in the spread of infection.

A glass thermometer may break in the rectal canal of a vigorously struggling child. The small amount of mercury present does not pose any danger, but broken glass may injure the rectum.

Perforation of the rectum in neonates has been reported without breakage of the thermometer.

Equipment

Glass thermometers are manufactured according to strict specifications and are precisely calibrated. After 1 year's use they may become inaccurate because of distortion of the glass.

Electronic digital thermometers consist of a metal probe covered with a disposable sheath. The probe is connected to a microprocessor unit that detects changes in the temperature of the probe. These changes are translated into an electronic digital readout. Peak temperature is usually reached within 40 seconds. Digital thermometers are placed in the same anatomic locations described for glass thermometers.

TMT measures infrared emissions from the tympanic membrane. There is a known gradient of temperature in the auditory canal, with maximum temperature at the TM, and then a gradual temperature decrease laterally to outside air. Hence, aiming the instrument at auditory canal skin rather than at the TM may cause a spuriously low recording. Three TMT recordings in the same ear, taking the highest measurement, decrease error rates.

The TMT infrared beam is transmitted to a microprocessor unit. There the heated energy is measured and converted through specified conversion factors into core, rectal, or oral equivalent temperatures. Digital temperature readouts are given in 3 seconds. The ear probes are mounted on lightweight handles that resemble otoscopes.

Rectal probes are elongated, flexible, sheathed devices with electronic recording capability. They are inserted approximately 3 cm into the rectum and are directly attached to a monitor to provide a continuous digital display of rectal temperature.

Techniques

When taking axillary temperatures, first pat the axilla dry. Place the end of the glass or digital thermometer in the upper part of the axilla facing anteriorly. Then bring the arm down over the thermometer and completely cover it. Leave mercury thermometers in place at least 5 minutes, although peak readings may require 10 minutes.

Place oral glass or digital thermometers far under the tongue in the lateral sublingual pocket after ensuring that the mercury has been shaken down. Leave glass thermometers in place for 3 to 5 minutes.

To take a rectal temperature, first place the child in a prone position on the parent's lap or the examination table. Gently spread the buttocks and insert the lubricated thermometer into the rectum in a slightly anterior direction. Do not insert the thermometer more than 1.5 cm in infants or 2.5 cm in older children. Keep the child comfortably restrained.

For TMT, place a plastic cover over the probe and insert in the auditory meatus until a seal is obtained, as shown in Fig.

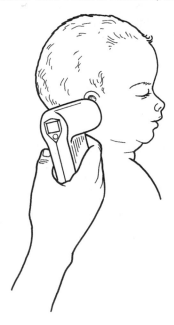

Fig. 5-1   Placement of tympanic membrane thermometer probe in ear of child.

5-1. For right-handed operators, the right ear may be easier than the left and visa versa.[3] For infants younger than 6 months of age, take the temperature in the supine position; older children can sit upright or in their parent's lap. Apply traction to the pinna during insertion of the probe, pulling posteriorly in infants under 1 year of age and posteriorly and superiorly in older children. Point the probe toward the contralateral temple. Press the scan button and read the temperature off the digital display screen.

To place a rectal probe, simply lubricate the device and then gently insert about 3 cm into the rectal vault. Connect the probe to the display monitor.

Remarks

Regardless of the technique, accurate temperature taking requires proper equipment, appropriate operator technique, and cooperation of the patient. TMT offers a quicker and less frightening alternative to traditional techniques for the anxious child, but the method still needs to be validated.

REFERENCES

1. Brennan DF, Falk JL, Rothrock SG, et al: Reliability of infrared tympanic thermometry in the detection of rectal fever in children, *Ann Emerg Med* 25:21-30, 1995.
2. Chamberlain JM, Grandner J, Rubinoff JL, et al: Comparison of a tympanic thermometer to rectal and oral thermometers in the pediatric emergency department, *Clin Pediatr* 30(suppl):24-29, 1991.
3. Chamberlain JM, Terndrup TE, Alexander DT, et al: Determination of normal ear temperature using an infrared emission detection thermometer, *Ann Emerg Med* 25:15-20, 1995.
4. Freed GL, Fraley JK: Lack of agreement of tympanic membrane temperature assessments with conventional methods in a private practice setting, *Pediatrics* 89:384-386, 1992.
5. Grover G, Berkowitz CD, Lewis RJ, et al.: The effects of bundling on infant temperature, *Pediatrics* 94:669-673, 1994.
6. Kresch MJ: Axillary temperature as a screening test for fever in children, *J Pediatr* 104:596-599, 1984.
7. Mayfield SR, Bhatia J, Nakamura KT, et al: Temperature measurement in term and preterm neonates, *J Pediatr* 104:271-275, 1984.
8. Muma BK, Treloar DJ, Wurmlinger K, et al: Comparison of rectal, axillary, and tympanic membrane temperatures in infants and young children, *Ann Emerg Med* 20:41-44, 1991.
9. Pontious S, Kennedy AH, Shelley S, et al: Accuracy and reliability of temperature measurement by instrument and site, *J Pediatr Nurs* 9:114-123, 1994.
10. Romano MJ, Fortenberry JD, Autrey E, et al: Infrared thermometry in the pediatric intensive care unit, *Crit Care Med* 21:1181-1185, 1993.
11. Schuman AJ: Tympanic thermometry: temperatures without tears, *Contemp Pediatr* 8:54-73, 1991.
12. Stewart JV, Webster D: Re-evaluation of the tympanic thermometer in the emergency department, *Ann Emerg Med* 21:158-161, 1992.
13. Tandberg D, Sklar D: Effect of tachypnea on the estimation of body temperature by an oral thermometer, *N Engl J Med* 308:945-946, 1983.
14. Terndrup TE: An appraisal of temperature assessment by infrared emission detection tympanic thermometry, *Ann Emerg Med* 21:1483-1492, 1992.
15. Yetman RJ, Coody DK, West MS, et al: Comparison of temperature measurements by an aural infrared thermometer with measurements by traditional rectal and axillary techniques, *J Pediatr* 122:769-773, 1993.

PART II

GENERAL CONSIDERATIONS

6 Preparation for a Procedure

Richard M. Cantor

The Emergency Department (ED) and in-hospital setting expose children with even minor illnesses or injuries to many stressful experiences involving themselves and their families.[5] A sensitive, caring approach by all health-care providers reduces stress for patients and families, as well as for caregivers. An approach aimed at enhancing a child's and family's coping skills not only ameliorates anxiety, but also facilitates care delivery and successful performance of diagnostic and therapeutic procedures.

Indications

The approaches outlined within this chapter are applicable to any and all clinical scenarios in pediatric emergency and critical care.

Contraindications/Complications

There are no contraindications or complications.

Equipment

Environmental Characteristics. There are many common problems in the emergency and critical care environments of the hospital that contribute to psychologically bad outcomes, including[4]:

1. Inflicting painful stimuli, without warning.
2. De-emphasizing holding, cuddling, and other reassuring social behaviors.
3. Providing uncomfortably bright and constant lighting.
4. Using physical restraints in a common and "routine" manner without regard to individual needs and assessment.
5. A lack of consistency among the child's caretakers.
6. Using conversations among large numbers of people without involving the child or family.
7. Denying access to the child by his or her parents and the consequent development of an adversarial relationship between the parent and the caregiver regarding health information specific to the child.
8. Depersonalizing treatment in general.
9. Failing to use appropriate conscious sedation and analgesia (see Part III).

Factors that promote a more receptive ED or pediatric intensive care unit (PICU) experience include:

1. Constantly reinforcing the concept that caring, concern, and gentleness remain basic tenets from which all care flows.
2. Considering the ill or injured child as an ill or injured family member.
3. Addressing the child and family members by name; personalized introduction by the caregiver.
4. An organized approach in providing care and procedures with consideration of patient needs and priorities.
5. Familiarization on the part of the caregiver with various methods of patient stress relief/release, including pharmacologic and nonpharmacologic options.
6. Acknowledging the child as an individual during necessary bedside conversations and including of the child in these conversations in an age-appropriate manner.

Techniques

Preparation of Children and Adolescents for Procedures. The caregiver must approach each child in the ED or PICU as an individual with age-specific developmental characteristics that may impact the clinical encounter.[1-3] Table 6-1 summarizes key characteristics of the major age groups and several useful strategies.

INFANTS (0 TO 1 YEAR). In some ways, infants represent the population easiest to examine, but in other ways they are the most difficult. Lack of language development in this population prohibits any chance of discussion of the procedure at hand. The major fears of infants relate to separation from parents and exposure to strangers. Stranger anxiety is a developmental milestone that occurs most often in children over the age 6 to 9 months. Procedure preparation within this age group entails providing consistent caretakers and a concerted attempt to decrease parental anxiety, which transmits easily to the infant. Minimal separation from the parents is key.

TODDLERS (1 TO 3 YEARS). The major concerns of this age child relate to separation from parents and loss of control of environment. Toddlers are apt to understand more than they may or can express. They have a developed sense of self and remain quite egocentric. The toddler's experience with physicians mostly relates to the memory of negative stimuli (i.e., immunizations ["shots"] during well-child care visits).

Prepare the toddler for a procedure in a time frame that is proximal to the event itself, since preparation too far in advance only heightens anxiety. Keep explanations very simple and choose words carefully (Table 6-2). If possible, let the toddler play with equipment, and use objects of play to demonstrate the procedure. Providing familiar objects (e.g., personal dolls, blankets) fosters a more secure environment. Keep the parents in the room. Recognize that any intrusive procedure may provoke an intense reaction that, in most cases, relates more to an expression of fear of injury than the perception of pain.

PRESCHOOLERS (3 TO 5 YEARS). Major fears of this developmental period include bodily injury, mutilation, and a loss of control. This age group is extremely sensitive to the unknown, the dark, and being left alone. It is impossible at this age to differentiate a "good" hurt (beneficial treatment) from a "bad" hurt (illness or injury). Since these children are apt to interpret any communication quite literally, they are often unable to abstract and interpret what might happen to

Table 6-1 Age-Specific Developmental Guidelines to Facilitate Procedures

Age group	Characteristic	Provider strategy
Infancy	Parental attachment	Involve parent in procedure, keep in sight
	Stranger anxiety	Make advances nonthreatening
	Sensorimotor learning	Use soothing measures during procedure
	Muscle control	Restrain adequately
	Past memories	Keep frightening objects away
	Gesture imitation	Model desired behavior
Toddler	Egocentric	Relate the procedure to sight and smell
	Behavioral negativity	Expect resistance, ignore tantrums
	Limited language skills	Use few, simple commands; use toys
	Poor time concept	Keep preparation time short; tell child when done
	Need for independence	Allow whatever choices possible
Preschool	Egocentric	Demonstrate equipment
	Better language skills	Encourage child to verbalize fears
	Poor time conception	Keep preparation time brief
	Illness viewed as punishment	Be clear as to why the procedure is being done
	Fears of bodily harm	Point out on drawing or doll location of event
	Need for initiative	Give choices when possible
School age	Interest in knowledge	Explain reason for procedure, equipment
	Better time concepts	Fully prepare for procedure
	Increased self-control	Suggest coping mechanisms (deep breathing)
	Need for industry	Allow responsibility for simple tasks
Adolescent	Narcissism	Provide privacy and describe outcome
	Concerned with present	Discuss immediate benefits of procedure
	Striving for independence	Allow decision making
		Accept regressive behavior as coping means

Table 6-2 Selecting Nonthreatening Words or Phrases to Communicate About Procedures

Instead of this	Say this
Shot, bee sting, stick	Medicine under the skin
Test	See how (body part) is working
Incision	Special opening
Edema	Puffiness
Stretcher	Rolling bed
Stool	Child's usual term
Dye	Special medicine
Pain	Hurt, "owie," "boo-boo"
Deaden	Numb, make sleepy
Cut, fix	Make better
Take (as in temperature)	See how warm you are
Put to sleep anesthesia	Special sleep
Catheter	Tube
Monitor	TV screen
Electrodes	Stickers, ticklers

their bodies as a result of the procedure. Therefore unreasonable fears are commonplace among preschoolers.

Keep explanations simple and concrete for these children with a careful choice of vocabulary. Avoid words like "cut," "take out," and "a little stick," without a full explanation of their intended meanings. When discussing anesthesia with the parents of these children, avoid the phrase "put to sleep." Using pictures or demonstrating actual equipment may augment verbal explanations, which may be insufficient. Emphasize to the child that he or she has not done anything wrong and is not being punished and that the procedure in question is necessary to help the child be "healthier." Be concrete with these children and explain what they will see, hear, feel, smell, or taste. Carefully avoid linking evaluations of the child with comments about his or her behavior during the procedure (e.g., he is not "a good boy" for holding still, but rather, "that was good holding still").

SCHOOL-AGE CHILDREN (5 TO 10 YEARS). School-age children are extremely sensitive to the expectations of important people in their lives and react quite negatively to any failure on their part to live up to these expectations. In an attempt to please, these children may appear to understand the situation with which they are presented, when in reality they do not comprehend what is about to happen. The school-age child is often reluctant to ask questions or admit not knowing something that adults expect him to know. Within this age group, the meaning of death may already have a concrete basis.

In preparation for the procedure, ask the child to explain what he or she understands. Using body diagrams, pictures, and models facilitates the explanation. In selected situations, give the child a choice of whether or not he or she wants a parent present during the procedure. Emphasize that it is "normal" to be uncomfortable or frightened of things never experienced before. Reassure the child that he or she did nothing wrong and that the procedure(s) at hand are unrelated to his or her actions.

ADOLESCENTS (10 TO 19 YEARS). The adolescent is often concerned with a loss of control, alteration in body image, and separation from his peer group. This age group has a tendency toward hyperresponsiveness to pain. Therefore reactions are often disproportionate to the event, and even minor illnesses or injuries may be magnified. A persistence of some magical thinking (perception of guilt related to their illness or problem) may contribute to a negative interaction as well. Adolescents demand some degree of involvement in the decision making because they often project the future and see long-term consequences related to the procedure. The adolescent reacts not only to what he or she is told but also to the manner by which it is presented. Therefore, make every attempt to explore tactfully what adolescents know and what they do not know, since they are easily concerned with any perception of ignorance on their part. Allow the adolescent to foster the perception of control within the procedural environment. It may be possible, and in some cases preferable, to separate the adolescent from his parent as a means of affirming his need to exert independence and individuality.

PARENTAL INVOLVEMENT. Involve the parents in all facets of care delivered to their children within the ED or ICU. Separation of the child and parent during an emergency visit coincides with a heightened degree of anxiety in child and parent and may prove counterproductive. Provide a full explanation of the necessity of the procedure to the parents, and pay strict attention to the degree of parental comprehension and intelligence. Use diagrams to demonstrate the actual equipment for the benefit of the parents.

In many teaching hospitals, residents carry out procedures with or without supervision by attending physicians. In these circumstances, the most senior person must maintain a level of control and authority both for the benefit of the resident and the parents to enhance the confidence level surrounding the procedure. Many studies have shown that parents are in no way appeased by brief explanations and rapid separation from their child during a procedure. Outline clear-cut guidelines for parental behavior and positioning during the procedure before the event, with warning that variances may necessitate removal from the situation. Most important, stress that what is being done is for the child's benefit and in no way impacts or diminishes the concern or sensitivity of the parent involved. When explaining the procedure to a child's parents, maintain a calm and caring interchange since the child often observes this directly. A parent's comfort level is directly proportional to how well the environment allows maintenance of his or her accustomed parental role in the care of the child.

REFERENCES

1. Anderson CJ: Integration of the Brazelton Neonatal Behavioral Assessment Scale into routine neonatal nursing care, *Issues Comp Pediatr Nurs* 9:341-345, 1986.
2. Belmont HS: Hospitalization and its effects upon the total child, *Clin Pediatr* 47:2-10, 1970.
3. Hammer SJ: The child in the Emergency Department. In Grossman M, Dieckmann RA, editors: *Pediatric emergency medicine: a clinician's reference,* Philadelphia, 1991, JB Lippincott.
4. Kissoon N: The critically ill child in the pediatric emergency department, *Ann Emerg Med* 18:59-62, 1989.
5. Nelson DS, Walsh K: Spectrum and frequency of pediatric illness presenting to a community hospital emergency department, *Pediatrics* 90:5-10, 1992.

7 Immunization

Richard M. Cantor

The Emergency Department (ED) provider, as well as the pediatric intensive care unit provider, now increasingly administer vaccines to unimmunized or possibly under immunized children. Although the decline of infectious diseases over the past 50 years resulted from the use of widespread immunization, unfortunately with success have come both parental complacency and unwarranted fears. In some urban areas up to 50% of children under 2 years of age are underimmunized, a factor that significantly contributed to measles epidemics reported from 1989 to 1991.[3] The reemergence of both measles and pertussis as public health issues has resulted in revisions of current recommendations for administration of a second dose of measles vaccine during childhood. In addition to parental complacency, other factors have contributed to the underimmunization problem. Unfounded fears related to side effects of vaccines, especially diphtheria-tetanus-pertussis (DTP), have also adversely impacted immunization rates and vaccine production. Media reports that the DTP vaccine causes sudden infant death syndrome and that the pertussis vaccine itself causes permanent neurologic damage have discouraged routine immunization. However, current data indicate that the benefits far outweigh the risks of standard immunization. Both the National Childhood Vaccine Injury Act (NCVIA) of 1986 and the Vaccine Compensation Amendments of 1987 provide fair compensation for children inadvertently injured and greater protection from liability for vaccine manufacturers and providers. The practitioner must fully inform families of the risk and benefits of the vaccine itself and record and report any form of postvaccine complication.

Indications

Timing of Immunobiologic Administration. Table 7-1 presents current recommendations for the age of administration of selected vaccines.[2]

Contraindications

Familiarity with conditions or circumstances that are true contraindications or precautions to vaccinations is imperative. ED personnel miss many opportunities for immunization because of improper interpretation of contraindications. National standards for pediatric immunization practices outline true contraindications and precautions to vaccinations (Table 7-3). True contraindications include a history of anaphylactic reaction to the vaccine or a vaccine constituent or the presence of a moderate or severe illness with or without temperature elevation. Ordinarily, do not give immune-compromised patients live vaccines. Also, a history of encephalopathy within 7 days of administration of DTP or diphtheria-tetanus-acellular pertussis (DTaP) precludes further doses of either vaccine. Give human immunodeficiency virus patients or patients with known immunodeficiency inactivated polio vaccine (IPV) rather than oral polio vaccine

(OPV). Do not give women known to be pregnant measles-mumps-rubella (MMR) vaccine due to the theoretic risk to the fetus. The most important conditions often inappropriately interpreted as contraindications to vaccination are the presence of diarrhea and minor upper respiratory illnesses, which are not true contraindications to OPV.

The most common dilemma is timing and use of the available form of tetanus vaccines. Currently three forms of tetanus vaccine are available: tetanus toxoid, tetanus immune globulin (TIG-human), and tetanus antitoxin (usually horse serum). Use tetanus toxoid for routine primary immunization, which provides protective antitoxin levels for 10 years or more. For a child undergoing complicated wound management and in situations in which existing patient immunity is in question, consider TIG. For persons who have received two previous doses of tetanus toxoid, a booster dose of the toxoid can be given. When tetanus toxoid and TIG are to be given concurrently, use a separate syringe and a different site for each. Table 130-1 in Part XXIV summarizes current recommendations for tetanus prophylaxis and wound management.

Techniques

Definitions. The following products, appropriately termed immunobiologics, are presently available for active or passive immunization or therapy:

1. *Vaccine* (Table 7-4): A suspension of live (usually attenuated) or inactivated microorganisms administered to induce immunity and prevent infectious disease or its sequelae. Vaccines may contain highly defined antigens (*Haemophilus influenzae* b) or complex incompletely defined antigens (e.g., *Bordetella pertussis*).

2. *Toxoid* (see Table 7-4): A modified bacterial toxin that has been made nontoxic but retains the ability to stimulate the formation of antibodies (e.g., tetanus toxoid).

3. *Immune globulin (IG)* (Table 7-5): Sterile solution containing antibodies from human blood obtained by fractionation of large pools of blood plasma. IG is primarily indicated for routine maintenance of immunity in certain immunodeficient persons and passive immunization against measles and hepatitis A. IG does not contribute to the transmission of hepatitis B virus, HIV, or other infectious diseases.

4. *Intravenous immune globulin (IGIV):* A product derived from blood plasma from a donor pool similar to the IG pool, but prepared for intravenous use. Use IGIV for replacement therapy in primary antibody deficiency disorders, Kawasaki disease therapy, immune thrombocytopenic purpura, and hypogammaglobulinemia and some cases of HIV.

5. *Specific immune globulin:* Specific preparations obtained from donor pools preselected for a high antibody content against a specific antigen (e.g., hepatitis B

Table 7–1   Recommended Schedule for Routine Active Vaccination of Infants and Children[a]

Vaccine	At birth (before hospital discharge)	1–2 months	2 months[b]	4 months	6 months	6–18 months	12–15 months	15 months	4–6 years (before school entry)
Diphtheria-tetanus-pertussis[c]			DTP	DTP	DTP			DTaP/DTP[d]	DTaP/DTP
Polio, live oral			OPV	OPV	OPV[e]				OPV
Measles-mumps-rubella							MMR		MMR[f]
Haemophilus influenzae type b conjugate									
HbOC/PRP-T[c,g]			Hib	Hib	Hib		Hib[h]		
PRP-OMP[g]			Hib	Hib			Hib[h]		
Hepatitis B[i]									
Option 1	HepB	HepB[j]				HepB[j]			
Option 2		HepB[j]		HepB[j]		HepB[j]			

Data from General recommendations on immunization, *MMWR* 43:1-33 1994.

[a]See Table 7-2 for the recommended immunization schedule for infants and children up to their seventh birthday who do not begin the vaccination series at the recommended times or who are >1 month behind in the immunization schedule.

[b]Can be administered as early as 6 weeks of age.

[c]Two DTP and Hib combination vaccines are available (DTP/HbOC [TETRAMUNE]; and PRP-T [ActHIB, OmniHIB] which can be reconstituted with DTP vaccine produced by Connaught).

[d]This dose of DTP can be administered as early as 12 months of age, provided that the interval since the previous dose of DTP is at least 6 months. *Diphtheria and tetanus toxoids and acellular pertussis vaccine (DTaP) is currently recommended only for use as the fourth and/or fifth doses of the DTP series among children age 15 months through 6 years (before the seventh birthday).* Some experts prefer to administer these vaccines at 18 months of age.

[e]The American Academy of Pediatrics (AAP) recommends this dose of vaccine at 6 to 18 months of age.

[f]The AAP recommends that two doses of MMR should be administered by 12 years of age, with the second dose being administered preferentially at entry to middle school or junior high school.

[g]HbOC: HibTITER (Lederle Praxis); PRP-T: ActHIB, OmniHIB (Pasteur Merieux); PRP-OMP: PedvaxHIB (Merck, Sharp, and Dohme). A DTP/Hib combination vaccine can be used in place of HbOC/PRP-T.

[h]After the primary infant Hib conjugate vaccine series is completed, any of the licensed Hib conjugate vaccines may be used as a booster dose at 12 to 15 months of age.

[i]For use among infants born to HBsAg-negative mothers. The first dose should be administered during the newborn period, preferably before hospital discharge, but no later than age 2 months. Premature infants of HBsAG-negative mothers should receive the first dose of the hepatitis B vaccine series at the time of hospital discharge or when the other routine childhood vaccines are initiated. (All infants born to HBsAg-positive mothers should receive immunoprophylaxis for hepatitis B as soon as possible after birth.)

[j]Hepatitis B vaccine can be administered simultaneously at the same visit with DTP (or DTaP), OPV, Hib, and/or MMR.

immune globulin, varicella-zoster immune globulin, rabies immune globulin, tetanus immune globulin).

6. *Antitoxin* (see Table 7-5): A solution of antibodies derived from the serum of animals immunized with specific antigens (e.g., diphtheria antitoxin and botulinum antitoxin).

Administration of Vaccines

GENERAL INSTRUCTIONS. Persons administering vaccine must minimize risks for spreading disease. Use a separate needle and syringe for each injection. Do not mix different vaccines in the same syringe unless specifically licensed for such use. To avoid unnecessary local or systemic effects and to guarantee optimal efficacy, do not deviate from the recommended routes of administration for each immunobiologic[1] (Figs. 7-1 to 7-4).

Administer *subcutaneous* injections into the thigh of infants and the deltoid area of older infants and adults (also see Chapter 45). The preferred sites for intramuscular injections are the anterolateral aspects of the upper thigh and deltoid of the upper arm (also see Chapter 46). The use of the buttock is contraindicated in the routine active vaccination of infants, children, or adults because of the potential risk of injury to

the sciatic nerve. Intradermal injection sites are generally on the volar surface of the forearm, with the exception of the human diploid cell rabies vaccine (HDCV) for which reactions are less demonstrable when administered in the deltoid area. Insert the needle with the full bevel intradermally until the injected solution raises a small bleb (see Chapter 45).

SKIN TESTING

Recent Centers for Disease Control and Prevention (CDC) data confirm that reported cases of tuberculosis (TB) are on the rise in the United States. Although children of all ages are susceptible, infants and postpubertal adolescents are at highest risk. Case rates for all ages are highest in urban and nonwhite populations. The highest rates of infection are currently among minority groups (i.e., first-generation immigrants from high-risk countries, Hispanics, Blacks, Asians, American Indians, and Alaskan Natives), the homeless, and institutionalized persons. Additional risk factors for progression to active TB disease among infected persons include recent close contact with an infectious case; recent skin test conversion; immunodeficiency, particularly that associated with HIV infection; Hodgkin's disease; lymphoma; diabetes

Text continued on p. 35.

Table 7–2 Recommended Accelerated Immunization Schedule for Infants and Children 7 Years of Age Who Start the Series Late* or Who Are 1 Month Behind in the Immunization Schedule† (i.e., Children for Whom Compliance With Scheduled Return Visits Cannot be Assured)

Timing	Vaccine(s)	Comments
First visit (≥4 mos of age)	DTP‡, OPV, Hib,§,‡ Hepatitis B, MMR (should be given as soon as child is age 12-15 months)	All vaccines should be administered simultaneously at the appropriate visit
Second visit (1 month after first visit)	DTP§, HIB,§,‡ Hepatitis B	
Third visit (1 month after second visit)	DTP§, OPV, Hib§,‡	
Fourth visit (6 weeks after third visit)	OPV	
Fifth visit (≥6 months after third visit)	DTaP§ or DTP, Hib,§,‡ Hepatitis B	
Additional visits (Age 4–6 years) (Age 14–16 years)	DTaP‡ or DTP, OPV, MMR Td	Administer preferably at or before school entry Repeat every 10 years through-out life

From *MMWR* 43:11, 1994. *DTP*, Diphtheria-tetanus-pertussis; *DTaP*, diphtheria-tetanus-acellular pertussis; *Hib, Haemophilus influenzae* type b conjugate; *MMR*, measles-mumps-rubella; *OPV*, poliovirus vaccine, live oral, trivalent; *Td*, tetanus and diphtheria toxoids (for use among persons ≥7 years of age).
*If initiated in the first year of life, administer DTP doses 1, 2, and 3 and OPV doses 1, 2, and 3 according to this schedule; administer MMR when the child reaches 12-15 months of age.
†See individual ACIP recommendations for detailed information on specific vaccines.
‡Two DTP and Hib combination vaccines are available (DTP/HbOC [TETRAMUNE]; and PRP-T [ActHIB, OmniHib] which can be reconstituted with DTP vaccine produced by Connaught). DTaP preparations are currently recommended only for use as the fourth and/or fifth doses of the DTP series among children 15 months through 6 years of age (before the seventh birthday). DTP and DTaP should not be used on or after the seventh birthday.
§The recommended schedule varies by vaccine manufacturer. For information specific to the vaccine being used, consult the package insert and ACIP recommendations. Children beginning the Hib vaccine series at age 2-6 months should receive a primary series of three doses of HbOC [HibTITER] (Ledere-Praxis), PRP-T [ActHIB, OmniHIB] (Pasteur Merieux; SmithKline Beecham; Connaught), or a licensed DTP-Hib combination vaccine; or two doses of PRP-OMP [PedvaxHIB] (Merck, Sharp, and Dohme). An additional booster dose of any licensed Hib conjugate vaccine should be administered at 12-15 months of age and at least 2 months after the previous dose. Children beginning the Hib vaccine series at 7-11 months of age should receive a primary series of two doses of an HbOC, PRP-T, or PRP-OMP-containing vaccine. An additional booster dose of any licensed Hib conjugate vaccine should be administered at 12-18 months of age and at least 2 months after the previous dose. Children beginning the Hib vaccine series at ages 12-14 months should receive a primary series of one dose of an HbOC, PRP-T, or PRP-OMP-containing vaccine. An additional booster dose of any licensed Hib conjugate vaccine should be administered 2 months after the previous dose. Children beginning the Hib vaccine series at ages 15-59 months should receive one dose of any licensed Hib vaccine. Hib vaccine should not be administered after the fifth birthday except for special circumstances as noted in the specific ACIP recommendations for the use of Hib vaccine.

Table 7–3 Contraindications and Precautions to Vaccinations

True contraindications and precautions	Not contraindications (vaccines may be administered)
General for all vaccines (DTP/DTaP, OPV, IPV, MMR, Hib, hepatitis B)	
Contraindications	*Not contraindications*
Anaphylactic reaction to a vaccine contraindicates further doses of that vaccine	Mild to moderate local reaction (soreness, redness, swelling) following a dose of an injectable antigen
Anaphylactic reaction to a vaccine constituent contraindicates the use of vaccines containing that substance	Mild acute illness with or without low-grade fever
Moderate or severe illness with or without a fever	Current antimicrobial therapy
	Convalescent phase of illnesses
	Prematurity (same dosage and indications as for normal, full-term infants)
	Recent exposure to an infectious disease
	History of penicillin or other nonspecific allergies or family history of such allergies

DTP, Diptheria-tetanus-pertussis; *DTaP*, diphtheria-tetanus-acellular pertussis; *OPV*, oral polio vaccine; *IPV*, inactivated polio vaccine; *MMR*, measles-mumps-rubella; *Hib, Haemophilus influenzae* type B.
This information is based on the recommendations of the Advisory Committee on Immunization Practices (ACIP) and those of the Committee on Infectious Diseases (Red Book Committee) of the American Academy of Pediatrics (AAP). Sometimes these recommendations vary from those contained in the manufacturer's package inserts. For more detailed information, providers should consult the published recommendations of the ACIP, AAP, and the manufacturer's package inserts.

Table 7–3   Contraindications and Precautions to Vaccinations*—cont'd

True contraindications and precautions	Not contraindications (vaccines may be administered)
DTP/DTaP	
Contraindications	*Not contraindications*
Encephalopathy within 7 days of administration of previous dose of DTP	Temperature of <40.5° C (105° F) following a previous dose of DTP
	Family history of convulsions
Precautions	Family history of sudden infant death syndrome
Fever of ≥40.5° C (105° F) within 48 hours after vaccination with a prior dose of DTP	Family history of an adverse event following DTP administration
Collapse or shocklike state (hypotonic-hyporesponsive episode) within 48 hours of receiving a prior dose of DTP	
Seizures within 3 days of receiving a prior dose of DTP	
Persistent, inconsolable crying lasting ≥3 hours within 48 hours of receiving a prior dose of DTP	
OPV	
Contraindications	*Not contraindications*
Infection with HIV or a household contact with HIV	Breast-feeding
Known altered immunodeficiency (hematologic and solid tumors; congenital immunodeficiency; and long-term immuno-suppressive therapy)	Current antimicrobial therapy
Immunodeficient household contact	Diarrhea
Precaution	
Pregnancy	
IPV	
Contraindication	
Anaphylactic reactions to neomyin or streptomycin	
Precaution	
Pregnancy	
MMR	
Contraindications	*Not contraindications*
Anaphylactic reactions to egg ingestion and to neomycin	Tuberculosis or positive PPD skin test
Pregnancy	Simultaneous TB skin testing
Known altered immunodeficiency (hematologic and solid tumors; congenital immunodeficiency; and long-term immunosuppressive therapy)	Breast-feeding
	Pregnancy of mother of recipient
	Immunodeficient family member or household contact
Precaution	Infection with HIV
Recent immune globulin administration	Nonanaphylactic reactions to eggs or neomycin
Hib	
Contraindication	*Not a contraindication*
None identified	History of Hib disease
Hepatitis B	
Contraindication	*Not a contraindication*
Anaphylactic reaction to common baker's yeast	Pregnancy

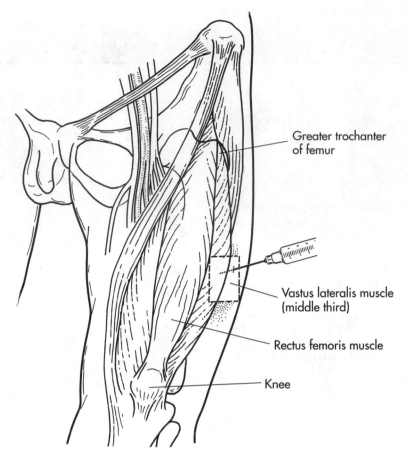

Fig. 7-1 Intramuscular injection sites in children: vastus lateralis.

Greater trochanter of femur

Vastus lateralis muscle (middle third)

Rectus femoris muscle

Knee

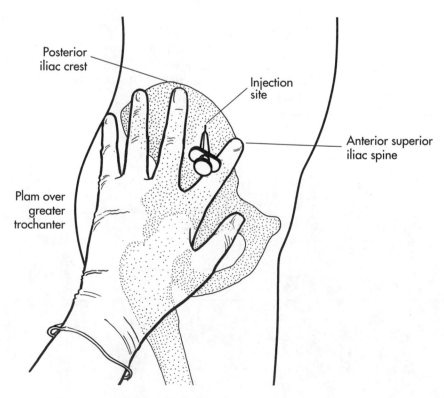

Fig. 7-2 Intramuscular injection sites in children: ventrogluteal.

Posterior iliac crest

Injection site

Anterior superior iliac spine

Plam over greater trochanter

Table 7-4   Licensed Vaccines and Toxoids Available in the United States, by Type and Recommended Route of Administration

Vaccine	Type	Route
Adenovirus[a]	Live virus	Oral
Anthrax[b]	Inactivated bacteria	Subcutaneous
Bacillus of Calmette and Guérin (BCG)	Live bacteria	Intradermal/percutaneous
Cholera	Inactivated bacteria	Subcutaneous or intradermal[c]
Diphtheria-tetanus-pertussis (DTP)	Toxoids and inactivated whole bacteria	Intramuscular
DTP-*Haemophilus influenzae* type b conjugate (DTP-Hib)	Toxoids, inactivated whole bacteria, and bacterial polysaccharide conjugated to protein	Intramuscular
Diphtheria-tetanus-acellular pertussis (DTaP)	Toxoids and inactivated bacterial components	Intramuscular
Hepatitis B	Inactive viral antigen	Intramuscular
Haemophilus influenzae type b conjugate (Hib)[d]	Bacterial polysaccharide conjugated to protein	Intramuscular
Influenza	Inactivated virus or viral components	Intramuscular
Japanese encephalitis	Inactivated virus	Subcutaneous
Measles	Live virus	Subcutaneous
Measles-mumps-rubella (MMR)	Live virus	Subcutaneous
Meningococcal	Bacterial polysaccharides of serotypes A/C/Y/W-135	Subcutaneous
Mumps	Live virus	Subcutaneous
Pertussis[b]	Inactivated whole bacteria	Intramuscular
Plague	Inactivated bacteria	Intramuscular
Pneumococcal	Bacterial polysaccharides of 23 pneumococcal types	Intramuscular or subcutaneous
Poliovirus vaccine, inactivated (IPV)	Inactivated viruses of all three serotypes	Subcutaneous
Poliovirus vaccine, oral (OPV)	Live viruses of all three serotypes	Oral
Rabies	Inactivated virus	Intramuscular or intradermal[e]
Rubella	Live virus	Subcutaneous
Tetanus	Inactivated toxin (toxoid)	Intramuscular[f]
Tetanus-diphtheria (Td or DT)[g]	Inactivated toxins (toxoids)	Intramuscular[f]
Typhoid (parenteral)	Inactivated bacteria	Subcutaneous[h]
(Ty21a oral)	Live bacteria	Oral
Varicella[i]	Live virus	Subcutaneous
Yellow fever	Live virus	Subcutaneous

Data from General recommendations on immunization, *MMWR* 43:1-33, 1994.

[a]Available only to the U.S. Armed Forces.

[b]Distributed by the Division of Biologic Products, Michigan Department of Public Health.

[c]The intradermal dose is lower than the subcutaneous dose.

[d]The recommended schedule for infants depends on the vaccine manufacturer; consult the package insert and ACIP recommendations for specific products.

[e]The intradermal dose of rabies vaccine, human diploid cell (HDCV), is lower than the intramuscular dose and is used only for preexposure vaccination. **Rabies** vaccine, adsorbed (RVA) should not be used intradermally.

[f]Preparations with adjuvants should be administered intramuscularly.

[g]Td=tetanus and diphtheria toxoids for use among persons ≥7 years of age. Td contains the same amount of tetanus toxoid as DTP or DT, but contains a smaller dose of diphtheria toxoid. DT=tetanus and diphtheria toxoids for use among children <7 years of age.

[h]Booster doses may be administered intradermally unless vaccine that is acetone-killed and dried is used.

[i]A live, attenuated varicella vaccine is currently under consideration for licensure. This vaccine may be available for use through a special study protocol to any physician requesting it for certain pediatric patients with acute lymphocytic leukemia. Additional information about eligibility criteria and vaccine administration is available from the Varivax Coordinating Center; telephone: (215) 283-0897.

mellitus; chronic renal failure; malnutrition; and immunosuppression related to accompanying viral infection or induced by drugs (e.g., steroid therapy).

Indications

Current recommendations from the American Academy of Pediatrics Committee on Infectious Disease for tuberculin testing include the following high-risk groups:

1. Black, Hispanic, Asian, American Indian, and Alaskan native children
2. Children living in neighborhoods where the case rate is higher than the national average
3. Children from, or whose parents have immigrated from, high-risk areas of Asia, Africa, the Middle East, Latin America, or the Caribbean
4. Children in households with cases of TB

Schedules for TB skin testing coincide with routine annual physical examinations (i.e., at 12 to 15 months, before school entry (4 to 6 years), and at adolescence (14 to 16 years).

Contraindications

Use the 1-tuberculin unit (TU) strength only for patients suspected of having intense tuberculin hypersensitivity. Do not use the 250-TU preparation in any circumstances for the initial skin test. Annual testing of low-risk children is unnecessary.

Table 7-5   Immune Globulins and Antitoxins Available in the United States by Type of Antibody and Indication for Use

Immunobiologic	Type	Indication(s)
Botulinum antitoxin	Specific equine antibodies	Treatment of botulism
Cytomegalovirus immune globulin, intravenous (CMV-IGIV)	Specific human antibodies	Prophylaxis for bone marrow and kidney transplant recipients
Diphtheria antitoxin	Specific equine antibodies	Treatment of respiratory diphtheria
Immune globulin (IG)*	Pooled human antibodies	Hepatitis A preexposure and postexposure prophylaxis; measles postexposure prophylaxis
Immune globulin, intravenous (IGIV)	Pooled human antibodies	Replacement therapy for antibody deficiency disorders; immune thrombocytopenic purpura (ITP); hypogammaglobulinemia in chronic lymphocytic leukemia; Kawasaki disease
Hepatitis B immune globulin (HBIG)	Specific human antibodies	Hepatitis B postexposure prophylaxis
Rabies immune globulin (HRIG)†	Specific human antibodies	Rabies postexposure management of persons not previously immunized with rabies vaccine
Tetanus immune globulin (TIG)	Specific human antibodies	Tetanus treatment; postexposure prophylaxis of persons not adequately immunized with tetanus toxoid
Vaccinia immune globulin (VIG)	Specific human antibodies	Treatment of eczema vaccinatum, vaccinia necrosum, and ocular vaccinia
Varicella zoster immune globulin (VZIG)	Specific human antibodies	Postexposure prophylaxis of susceptible immunocompromised persons, certain susceptible pregnant women, and perinatally exposed newborn infants

Data from General recommendations on immunizations, *MMWR* 43:1-33, 1994.
*Immune globulin preparations and antitoxins are administered intramuscularly unless otherwise indicated.
†HRIG is administered around the wounds in addition to being injected intramuscularly.

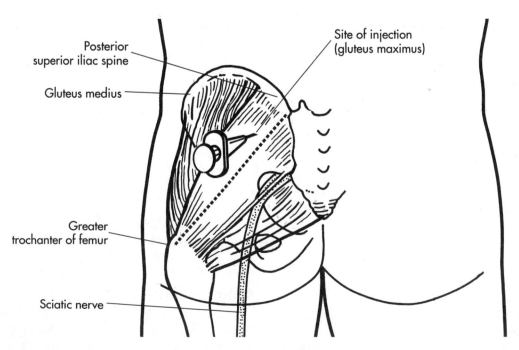

Fig. 7-3   Intramuscular injection sites in children: dorsogluteal.

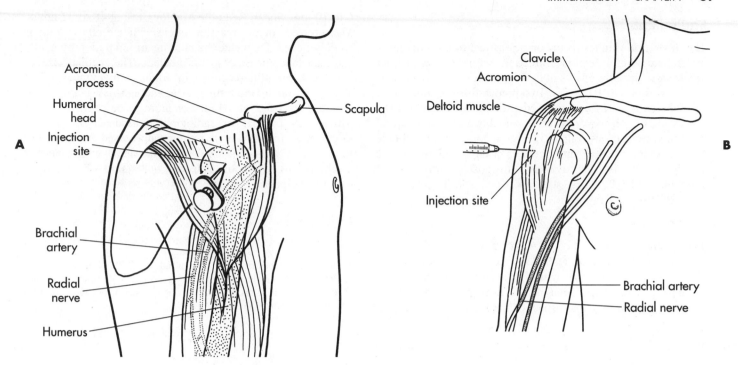

Fig. 7-4   Intramuscular injection sites in children: deltoid.

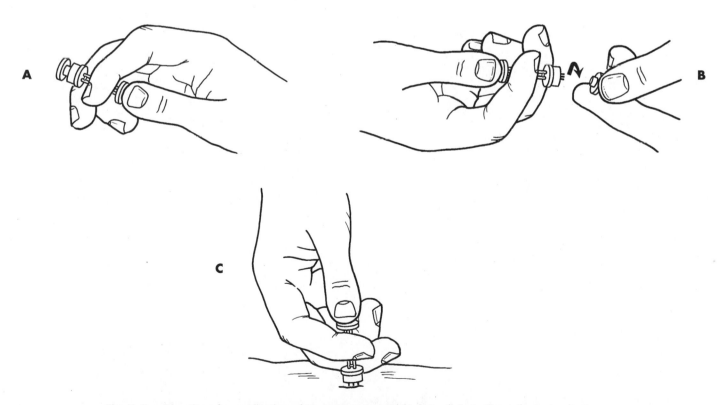

Fig. 7-5   Directions for application of Mono-Vacc test (old tuberculin). **A,** Grasp the test unit as you would a syringe, with your thumb on top and the stem between your first two fingers. **B,** While twisting the cap, carefully pull it away from the points. **C,** With skin taut, press the loaded points firmly into the cleansed site.

Equipment

The tuberculin skin test is the only practical tool for diagnosing tuberculous infection. Infection with *Mycobacterium tuberculosis* usually results in development of skin hypersensitivity within 2 to 10 weeks. Two preparations of tuberculin, old tuberculin (OT) and purified protein derivative (PPD), are available. However, OT is available only in multiple puncture preparations (Fig. 7-5). The standard dose of PPD is 5 TU (formerly called "intermediate strength") in 0.1 ml of solution. PPD is also available in unstandardized dose strengths of 1 TU ("first strength") and 250 TU ("second strength") per 0.1 ml.

Techniques

The Mantoux (intracutaneous) test of 5 TU-PPD (0.1 ml) is the standard tuberculin test. Aspirate the solution into a disposable plastic syringe with a No. 26-gauge, short-bevel needle no more than 1 hour before use. Inject the solution intradermally on the volar aspect of the forearm to produce a 6 to 10-mm wheal. Read the Mantoux test at 48 to 72 hours. Measurement of the reaction is easier if the elbow joint is slightly flexed. Delineate the margins of induration by gentle palpation and measure in millimeters. The median size of positive tuberculin reactions in adults with clinical TB is about 15 mm of induration. Among high-risk populations, consider reactions of 10 mm or more to be positive. If the patient has clinical or radiographic evidence of TB, is seropositive for HIV or is immunosuppressed from another cause, or is a known contact of an adult with acid-fast bacilli–positive sputum, consider a reaction of 5 mm or larger to be positive.

REFERENCES

1. Bergeson PS, Singer SA, Kaplan AM: Intramuscular injections in children, *Pediatrics* 70:944-948, 1982.
2. General recommendations on immunization, *MMWR* 43:1-33, 1994.
3. Hutchins SS: Measles outbreak among unvaccinated preschoolage children: opportunities missed by health care providers to administer measles vaccine, *Pediatrics* 83:369-374, 1989.

8 Fever Management

Richard M. Cantor

Fever is a manifestation of disease in the child and accounts for nearly 30% to 40% of after-hour Emergency Department (ED) visits. Reassure anxious parents that fever itself may be acceptable.[2,3] One can treat fever symptomatically quite effectively (Table 8-1). Fever may represent a reliable sign or symptom of disease and may be the first or sole finding of a disease process.[4] It is also easily detectable, verifiable, and quantifiable.

TEMPERATURE REGULATION IN THE PEDIATRIC PATIENT

The child regulates core temperature within a relatively narrow range, despite wide fluctuations in environmental temperature. The predominant regulatory center of body temperature lies within the preoptic region of the anterior hypothalamus.[1] There are multiple regions within this center, including a temperature-sensing region (the thermostat); a temperature-setting region (the set point); a detector region; and two effector regions (a heat gain and a heat loss area).

The thermostat measures body temperature by directly sensing the temperature of arterial blood perfusing the brain. The skin, spinal cord, and other parts of the brain also provide distal input. The set point represents an arrangement of neurons that determines the desired temperature of the body at any given instant. Serving as a reference point for the thermoregulatory mechanism, it possesses the ability to activate or deactivate heat-gain or heat-loss centers, depending on the specific circumstance.

The major mechanism for the production of heat is skeletal muscle metabolism. The sympathetic nervous system, with norepinephrine as the mediator, governs what is commonly referred to as nonshivering thermogenesis. If situations arise wherein this mechanism is inadequate to generate sufficient extra heat, shivering occurs. Recruitment of the masseter muscles is responsible for the familiar chattering of teeth that often accompanies a chill.

Mechanisms for heat loss are both evaporative and non-evaporative. Nonevaporative sources of heat loss between a child and the environment include radiation, conduction, and convection, which occur when the child is exposed to cool environments with or without highly conducted air movement. Varying the perfusion of the skin through vasodilation of the distal extremities primarily controls nonevaporative heat loss. Evaporative heat loss takes place through insensible perspiration, constant evaporation of water through the skin and respiratory interfaces, and sweating. Exposure to very hot or very humid environments essentially makes sweating the only mechanism for dissipating body heat.

Indications/Contraindications

Chapter 5 describes temperature ranges and complications in children and the techniques for temperature taking.

Technique

Correction of the Febrile State. There are advantages and disadvantages to symptomatic treatment of fever.[5] (Box 8-1 lists normal indications.) Arguments against treatment include:
1. Most instances of fever are brief and self-limited.
2. Fever can impair the growth or survival of invading microorganisms.
3. Fever may enhance the immunologic response.
4. Fever may itself enforce rest.
5. The treatment of fever may mask important clinical information.

Arguments favoring the symptomatic treatment of fever include:
1. There are undesirable metabolic effects of fever.
2. Fever may have deleterious cardiopulmonary effects.
3. Fever may have deleterious central nervous system effects.
4. Fever can precipitate seizures.
5. Fever may impair the immunologic response.
6. Fever depresses gastric motility.
7. Treatment of fever may make it easier to evaluate the patient.

Table 8-1 Drugs for the Treatment of Fever

Drug	Dose/route	Frequency	Comments
Acetaminophen	10-15 mg/kg PO, PR	Every 4 hours	Available as infant drops, suspensions, tabs, or suppositories
Ibuprofen	10 mg/kg PO	Every 6-8 hours	Only available as suspension or tabs
Aspirin	10 mg/kg PO, PR	Every 4 hours	Available as tabs or suppositories. Avoid in influenza or varicella

BOX 8-1 **INDICATIONS FOR SYMPTOMATIC TREATMENT OF FEVER**

Temperature > 104° F

Age between 6 months and 3 years

Age < 6 years with past history of seizures

Cardiopulmonary impairment

Renal or metabolic impairment

Fluid-electrolyte problems

Acute neurologic disease

Sepsis/shock

Impaired thermoregulation

Environmental heat illness

Sickle cell disease

REFERENCES

1. Cranston WI: Central mechanisms of fever, *Fed Proc* 38:49-55, 1979.
2. Ipp M: Physicians' attitudes toward the diagnosis and management of fever in children three months to two years of age, *Clin Pediatr* 32:66-70, 1993.
3. May A: Fever phobia: the pediatricians' contribution, *Pediatrics* 90:851-854, 1992.
4. Shmitt BD: Fever in childhood, *Pediatrics* 74:934-938, 1984.
5. Stein RC: Pathophysiologic basis for symptomatic treatment of fever, *Pediatrics* 59:92-97, 1977.

9 Universal Precautions

Richard M. Cantor

Use Universal Precautions (UPs) for all patient contacts that expose the health-care provider to blood, certain other body fluids (amniotic fluid, pericardial fluid, pleural fluid, synovial fluid, cerebrospinal fluid, semen, and vaginal secretions), or any other body fluid visibly contaminated with blood. Generally, UPs do not apply to feces, nasal secretions, sputum, sweat, tears, urine, and vomitus unless blood contaminates these secretions. UPs assume that *all* patients are carriers of infectious, contagious disease, since there is no reliable, immediate means to identify infected patients. Table 9-1 lists appropriate techniques for UPs.[1]

REFERENCE

1. Centers for Disease Control and Prevention: Centers for Disease Control recommendations for prevention of HIV transmission in health-care settings, *MMWR* 36:3S-18S, 1987.

Table 9-1 Summary of Universal Precautions

Type of precaution	Body substances considered high risk	Comments

Full precautions	Blood
	Semen
	Vaginal secretions
	Cerebrospinal fluid
	Synovial fluid
	Pleural fluid
	Peritoneal fluid
	Pericardial fluid
	Amniotic fluid
	Fluids not included unless they contain:
	  Visible blood
	  Feces
	  Nasal secretions
	  Sputum
	  Sweat
	  Tears
	  Urine and emesis
		UPs do not apply to breast milk or saliva, except in special situations:
		  Frequent exposure to breast milk
		  Dental procedures in which saliva may be contaminated with blood

Hand-washing	Immediately and thoroughly wash hands and skin surfaces that are contaminated with high-risk body fluids	Hand-washing is the single most important strategy for preventing infection transmission

Gloves	Must be worn when touching high-risk body fluids
	Use during phlebotomy depends on risk of exposure to blood and prevalence of blood-borne pathogens
	General guidelines include:
	  If operator has breaks in the skin
	  If operator is receiving training in phlebotomy
	  If hand contamination with blood is likely (uncooperative patient)
	  Fingersticks and/or heelsticks in infants and children
		Washing or disinfecting gloves for reuse is not recommended
		Disinfectants can deteriorate the glove
		Use gloves for digital examination of mucous membranes and endotracheal suctioning

Gowns or plastic aprons	Wear when it is likely that high-risk body substances will soil the clothing; change between patient contacts	

CDC, Centers of Disease Control and Prevention; *HIV*, human immunodeficiency virus; *HBV*, hepatitis B virus.

Continued.

Table 9-1   Summary of Universal Precautions—cont'd

Type of precaution	Body substances considered high risk	Comments
Masks and/or eye protection	Wear when likely that the eyes and/or nose and mouth will be splashed with body substances or when personnel are working directly over large, open skin lesions	Benefits of masks in preventing transmission of airborne infection is questionable UP system does not address masks, except for protection from splashes, since HIV and HBV are not airborne
Needle/syringe units and other sharp instruments	Do not remove, recap, or break used needles from disposable syringes; dispose all sharp instruments in a rigid, puncture-resistant container, preferably located near the site of use	Needle punctures are a leading cause of nosocomial transmission of bloodborne pathogens Gloves cannot prevent penetrating injuries caused by needles or other sharp instruments If recapping is necessary, use a one-handed scoop technique
Trash and linen	Bag securely in leakproof containers and dispose of or clean according to institutional policy	There is no evidence of casual or environmental transmission of HIV

10 Sterile Technique

Rachel L. Chin

Approximately ten million patients with traumatic wounds are treated annually in Emergency Departments (EDs) in the United States.[4,9] Wound infection occurs in about 6.5% of these patients.[8,9] When wound infection occurs, it has significant deleterious effects on healing, tissue strength, and cosmesis.[3] Proper sterile technique is crucial to achieve good wound closure, decrease transmittable diseases (for both child and physician), and prevent wound contamination. In addition, proper technique minimizes risk of iatrogenic infection of superficial and deep structures during procedures performed through intact skin.

Sterile technique includes: (1) use of appropriate body substance protective gear to decrease bilateral transmission of pathogens, (2) preparation of the skin, and (3) preparation and exploration of the wound.

Indications

Sterile technique is required for wound care ranging from minor abrasions to complicated lacerations. Sterile technique is also imperative for any invasive procedure that breaks the skin barrier.

Contraindications

There are no contraindications.

Complications

Complications are few and involve sensitivity of the skin to the cleaning solutions.

Equipment

- Sterile basin
- 35-ml syringe
- Pressurized irrigation device
- Sterile normal saline
- Antiseptic agents (Table 10-1)
- Sterile gloves
- Face mask and/or eye protection
- Sterile gown
- Sterile 4" × 4" gauze
- Sterile drape

Techniques

Protective Gear. To prevent iatrogenic infection of the patient and to protect the physician from potentially hazardous body substances, wear protective gear and use Universal Precautions (see Chapter 9). The type of protective gear depends on the procedure to be performed. The most invasive procedures require the most protective gear, whereas the simple bedside procedures require a minimal amount.

At the very least, sterile gloves should be worn for all procedures, except placement of peripheral intravenous catheters, for which nonsterile gloves and local sterile technique alone are sufficient. Procedures that involve large central

Table 10-1 Antiseptic Agents

Agent	Antibacterial efficacy	Tissue toxicity
Alcohol (70%)	10	10
Betadine surgical scrub*	9	8
pHisoHex*	8	8
Hydrogen peroxide	3	5
Quaternary ammonia	6	3
Hexachlorophene solution†	8	2
Betadine prep solution†	9	1
Shur-Clens (plurionic F-68)	1	0.5
Sterile water	0	0.5
Sterile saline	0	0

*A detergent preparation.
†An aqueous solution.

blood vessels or have the potential for splashing body substances require a mask. Common procedures requiring masks include central lines for the internal jugular and subclavian veins for the purposes of intravenous access or monitoring of central venous or pulmonary artery pressures. Femoral and external jugular intravenous lines may be placed without masks. Incision and drainage of abscesses require a mask because of the potential splashing of infected abscess material. Masks protect not only the mouth and nose, but must also shield the eyes. As an alternative to the eye shields, use glasses fitted with protective covers for the sides.

To ensure sterile procedure, most procedures that require a mask also require a sterile gown. (Exceptions include incision and drainage and amniocentesis in which the primary function of the mask is to protect the physician.) As with any surgical technique, the front of the gown above the waist is considered part of the sterile field; all other parts of the gown are nonsterile.

Finally, the hair must be covered for procedures that have the highest risk and degree of morbidity from iatrogenic infection, including placement of hyperalimentation lines and pulmonary artery (Swan-Ganz) catheters, in which infection can have dire consequences. Similarly, catheterization of the umbilical artery and epidural space must be performed with the highest level of protective gear. Hair coverings must cover all hair from the forehead to the back of the head and are not part of the sterile field.

Skin Preparation. Use any of several antiseptic agents for skin disinfection. Table 10-1 lists the antibacterial efficacy and tissue toxicity of several antiseptic agents commonly used in the hospital.[10]

Povidone-iodine and chlorhexidine are commonly used agents for application to intact skin because they are fast acting and have a broad spectrum of antimicrobial activity and a long shelf life.[4] Most preparations used to disinfect the skin are toxic to the defense system of the wound and may increase the incidence of wound infection.[7] *Therefore do not use skin preparation solutions directly into wounds.* Skin disinfection is distinct from debridement, irrigation, and preparation of the open wound and requires different solutions. The main purpose of skin preparation is to cleanse the periphery of the wound to decrease bacterial contamination of the wound without further damaging the traumatized tissues.

Povidone-iodine is generally available in a 10% solution, which is 1% free iodine. Apply the povidone-iodine preparation solution with a sterile pledget, then paint the surrounding intact skin in a circular motion. Paint the solution on the skin from the edges of the wound outward around the wound, and avoid contaminating the wound itself because the solution is toxic to subcutaneous tissues.

Begin examination of the injured site by assessing for sensory, motor, and vascular complications. If there are no associated major underlying injuries requiring use of the operating room, treat the wound in the ED.

Next, assess the wound for foreign bodies and devitalized tissue. Most wounds do not require removal of hair. Some areas of the body such as the scalp may require removal of some hair to keep it out of the wound. Clipping the hair or matting it down with some water-soluble lubricating gel is usually sufficient. Shaving is controversial. In preoperative wounds shaving increases the likelihood of wound infection.[1] Presently, there are no good data about infection rates with shaving in traumatic wounds. Never shave the eyebrows; they are slow to grow back and serve as valuable landmarks during suturing. Do not allow the small cut hairs to fall into the wound, where they may act as a nidus for infection and poor wound closure.

Wound Preparation and Exploration

ANESTHESIA/HEMOSTASIS. Often adequate anesthesia in combination with conscious sedation and/or narcotic analgesia is necessary for thorough cleansing, irrigation, foreign body removal, and debridement in large and complicated wounds. After an appropriate neurovascular examination, anesthetize the involved tissue. Sometimes a regional nerve block is needed instead of local infiltration (see Chapter 16). When bleeding is profuse and wound inspection is inadequate, apply a tourniquet, if possible, to ensure maximal exposure. Tourniquets are especially useful for hand wounds, but inflation time should be minimized (see Chapter 122) to avoid ischemic injury.

DÉBRIDEMENT. Débridement is a process of removing devitalized tissue or gross contaminants from the wound. The presence of any devitalized tissue in the wound will delay healing and significantly increase the risk of infection. Meticulously excise devitalized skin edges. Débridement may result in a larger tissue defect; if there is concern about viability of large areas of skin or muscle, prepare the wound for delayed primary closure.

WOUND CLEANSING. Forcefully irrigating a wound is one of the most important methods to decrease bacterial counts.[2,5,8] Wounds that are contaminated or appear 6 or more hours after injury are usually contaminated with bacteria greater than 10^5 organisms per gram of tissue.[6] On the highly vascularized areas of the face, scalp, and genitalia, the window for closure is longer. The number of bacteria rather than the bacteria type is the critical determinant of wound infection. Wounds often become infected after closure when levels are greater than 10^5 bacteria per gram of tissue.[6] Conversely, larger bacterial counts in wounds of well-vascularized areas may not develop infection.

Sterile saline is the best irrigating solution. There is no known advantage to more expensive solutions. The volume of irrigating solution must be enough to lower the concentration of bacteria. Clean wounds require little or no irrigation, whereas bite injuries and other contaminated wounds may require up to a liter of irrigation.

The most effective form of wound cleansing is high-pressure irrigation. Irrigating with pressures greater than 7 lb/in^2 (psi) significantly decreases the number of bacteria and the incidence of infection.[2,5,8] Although several commercial devices are available, a 19-gauge needle attached to a 35-ml syringe yields a force of 7 to 8 psi. Hold the device 1 to 2 inches from the wound and copiously irrigate without injecting directly into the wound.

When irrigating is complete, cover the sterile field with a sterile drape and close the wound. Part XXIV discusses wound closure techniques.

REFERENCES

1. Alexander JW, Fischer JE, Boyajian M, et al: The influence of hair-removal methods on wound infections, *Arch Surg* 118:347-352, 1983.
2. Brown LL, Shelton HT, Bornside GH, et al: Evaluation of wound irrigation by pulsatile jet and conventional methods, *Ann Surg* 187:170-173, 1978.
3. Bucknall TE: The effect of local infection upon wound healing: an experimental study, *Br J Surg* 67:851-855, 1980.
4. Edlich RF, Rodeheaver GT, Morgan RF, et al: Principles of emergency wound management, *Ann Emerg Med* 17:1284-1302, 1988.
5. Gross R, Cutright DE, Bhasker SN: Effectiveness of pulsating water jet lavage in treatment of contaminated crushed wounds, *Am J Surg* 124:373-377, 1972.
6. Mulliken JB, Management of wounds. In May HL, editor: *Emergency medicine*, 1984, John Wiley & Sons, pp 283-298.
7. Rodeheaver G, Bellamy W, Kody M, et al: Bactericidal activity and toxicity of iodine-containing solutions in wounds, *Arch Surg* 117:181-186, 1982.
8. Rodeheaver GT, Pettry D, Thacker JG, et al: Wound cleansing by high-pressure irrigation, *Surg Gynecol Obstet* 141:357-362, 1975.
9. Simon B: Principles of wound management. In Rosen P, Barki RM, Braen RG, editors: *Emergency medicine: concepts and clinical practice*, ed 3, St. Louis, 1992, Mosby, pp 303-318.
10. Zukin DD, Grisham J: Wound care. In Grossman M, Dieckmann RA, editors: *Pediatric emergency medicine*, Philadelphia, 1991, JB Lippincott, pp 321-330.

PART III

CONSCIOUS SEDATION AND PAIN MANAGEMENT

11 Physical Restraint

Steven M. Selbst

It is necessary to restrain many young children for painful procedures. In general, this may heighten, not reduce, fear or anxiety in the child, if not properly done. However, appropriate immobilization of the child may help the physician perform the procedure, reduce pain by enabling the successful performance with fewer attempts,[13] and hence improve the quality of the experience for child, parent, and physician.

Proper physical restraint ensures the child's safety, protects her or him from self-injury, and facilitates more rapid completion of the procedure.[14] Appropriate sedation and analgesia for painful procedures should be given along with restraint, and the parent's help enlisted if possible. After restraining the patient, verbal reassurance and relaxation techniques should also be used. Multiple strategies to prepare the child and parent for a painful procedure will minimize distress.

Physical restraint is also important to manage some violent patients. This must be done carefully to protect the patient and staff. Adhere to state laws and regulations of the Joint Commission on the Accreditation of Healthcare Organizations (JCAHO) whenever such restraint is applied.

Indications

Restrain a child who needs a procedure that requires immobilization of part or all of the body. Do not attempt a painful procedure on a child who is moving and improperly restrained. Ensure full immobilization so that the child does not get the idea that more vigorous movement will gain him or her freedom. Restrain a child in an appropriate position to reveal a desired anatomic area (e.g., intervertebral space for lumbar puncture). Likewise, consider restraint of a child to suture a laceration; remove a foreign body from skin, nose, or ears; aspirate an abscess; treat a paronychia; evaluate a subungual hematoma; or perform an otherwise painful or frightening procedure. Use developmental status and intensity of the procedure to determine the type of restraint. It is most often the infant, toddler, or preschooler who needs physical restraint. A school-age child can often cooperate without restraint.

Even in the absence of a painful procedure, restrain a large adolescent who demonstrates violent behavior that could result in injury to himself or herself or others. Restraint is also indicated to preempt violent behavior when calm discussion fails to alleviate the patient's anxiety or diffuse the situation.[2] Chemical sedation may be indicated before the use of physical restraint.

Contraindications

There are no absolute contraindications to proper restraint of a child. Do not use brute force or other means of restraint as a substitute for appropriate relaxation techniques, careful and honest explanation, an empathic approach to the child, or indicated sedatives, analgesics, and anesthetics. Use great caution when restraining a child who has abnormal vital signs, airway, or breathing problems. Do not restrain an angry patient just for convenience or punishment, since this may cause physical harm and result in litigation.[8]

Complications

Complications from proper restraint of a child are rare and usually insignificant. Significant complications are almost always due to the underlying condition. However, airway obstruction may result from restraint of a child for lumbar puncture. If the child is held tightly with the torso flexed to expose the spine and intervertebral processes, apnea and respiratory arrest can result.[16] Young infants and those with respiratory distress, hypotension, limited chest expansion, and airway anomalies are at greatest risk.[5] Consider use of a pulse oximeter during the lumbar puncture or for patients receiving conscious sedation or with potential breathing problems, and carefully observe the patient to minimize this risk.

Use of a papoose board, bed sheets, or adult hands to restrain a child may result in bruising, edema of some of the child's body parts, and transient vascular compromise of an extremity. To avoid these complications, do not hold the child too tightly or for excessively long periods, and use two pairs of hands when necessary.

The child (and personnel) can get excessively warm during restraint for a procedure. Ensure proper ventilation and assess the child's comfort during the restraint process. If a caregiver is an assistant, prepare the caregiver and provide a chair to avoid vasovagal syncope.

A violent patient or staff member who assists with a violent patient may suffer injury during the restraint procedure. This can be minimized by having an appropriate number of sufficiently trained personnel. The physician of record is liable for injuries that a patient incurs from restraint by the staff.[1] However, the Emergency Department staff also risks litigation for failing to intervene with an active or potentially violent patient.[8] Proper monitoring and humane care must follow physical restraint to avoid complications. Temporarily release one of the four restraint points every 15 minutes to prevent circulatory obstruction. Also, consider an organic etiology for the patient's violent behavior, since failure to do so may result in further complications. Finally, restraint during the second and third trimester of pregnancy may result in further discomfort such as increased urinary frequency, pruritus, and aortocaval obstruction by the gravid uterus.[7] Supine restraint carries a small risk of aspiration.[6]

Equipment

Use commercially available papoose boards to restrain non-violent children if possible. These come in small size for ages 2 to 6 years, large size for children ages 6 to 12 years, and extra-large size for teenagers and adults. Alternatively, use immobilization devices designed for stabilization of injured children. Use hospital bed sheets and 2- or 3-inch wide adhesive tape for other immobilization techniques.

One can purchase papoose boards with additional apparatus such as head and arm immobilizers that attach to or slide under the papoose board for special needs. Place a foam pad or sheet on the papoose board for additional comfort.

Leather restraints are the safest for violent patients. Do not use bed sheets, intravenous tubing, and other improvised devices, since these may result in injury to the patient or inadequate immobilization. Do not use locking restraints, since the need for keys is dangerous in the event of a fire or deteriorating medical condition.[6]

Techniques

Try to establish rapport with the child and family first. Explain the need for restraint to the caregivers and to the child if old enough to understand (usually over 1 year of age). Children understand more than they say. Avoid casual teasing, condescension, and exclusion of the child.[11,14] While restraining, warn the child honestly about the procedure but allow for the possibility that it may not hurt as much as she thinks.[11]

Let caregivers ask questions and offer alternative approaches. However, do not offer the child choices that do not exist. Allow caregivers who can remain calm to be nearby and to reassure the child. Do not ask caregivers to participate in the actual restraint of the patient.[12]

Allow time for sedatives or analgesics to be effective before applying restraints or performing the procedure.[14] However, do not allow a long delay between explaining the procedure, applying restraints, and performing the task. Anticipation is often the worst part of the procedure.[11]

Restraint by Hospital Personnel. Have a single assistant grasp the young child and immobilize her. If unsuccessful, get additional help rather than struggle with a large or strong child. In some situations, have one assistant hold the head while the other immobilizes the arms and legs. Hold the child firmly so that movement is not possible, but not so forcefully that injury results.

For lumbar puncture, place the child in the lateral recumbent position, have an assistant tuck one arm under the child's legs at the popliteal fossa, and tuck the other arm under the child's upper back, just below the neck. Ask the assistant to pull the child toward her to make the patient's intervertebral spaces more prominent (Fig. 11-1). "Curl" the child's trunk as much as possible without interfering with ventilation. Monitor the patient with pulse oximeter and frequent reassessment by the assistant after the patient is draped for the procedure. Alternatively, perform lumbar puncture with the child sitting, with maximum flexion of the spine. Have an assistant hold the infant's hands between her flexed legs with one hand, while flexing the infant's head with the other hand (Fig. 11-2).

To restrain the patient for other procedures, have the

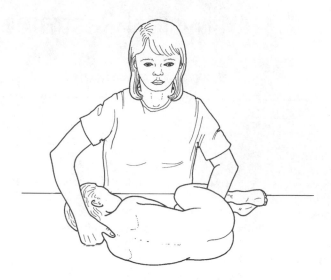

FIG. 11-1   Child properly restrained for lumbar puncture (curled position).

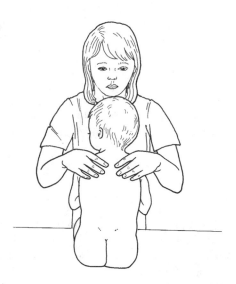

FIG. 11-2   Child properly restrained for lumbar puncture (sitting position).

assistant hold the involved body part firmly but without inflicting excessive pain. Fig. 11-3 shows examples of specific restraint positions. Ask the assistant to lean over the child if possible to prevent movement of other body parts not directly involved in the procedure (such as legs or arms).

Mummy Wraps. Use hospital bed sheets to immobilize the child. Fold a bed sheet on itself so the width extends from the child's axillae to her heel. Then stand the child on the stretcher and place a bed sheet behind her back, under the axilla, and in front of her arms. Tuck the bed sheet behind one arm and around the child's back. Then wrap the sheet around the back, across the front of the child while she stands (Fig. 11-4). With the child now wrapped in the sheet, lay her supine on the stretcher. Place strong tape over the child and sheet and attach tape to stretcher rails to immobilize her. One extremity can be left out of the mummy wrap, if desired, for a procedure.[9]

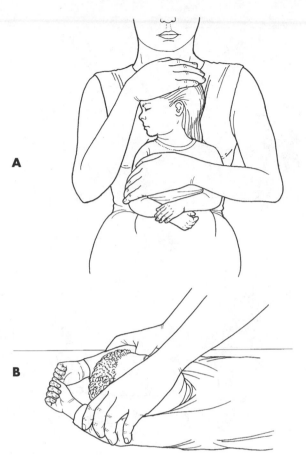

FIG. 11-3   Restraint of child for **A,** ear examination; and **B,** ear or throat examination.

Papoose. Place the papoose board in the center of the stretcher and place the child supine on the board. Restrain one or both arms with adjustable straps made of Velcro. The board has three sets of flaps to immobilize the upper arms, the abdomen and trunk, and the legs (Fig. 11-5, *A*).

Close the middle or abdominal flaps tightly, but allow for comfort (Fig. 11-5, *B*). Next, close the lower flaps snugly over the legs (Fig. 11-5, *C*). Finally, close the upper flaps over the shoulders and arms (Fig. 11-5, *D*).

Adjust the papoose board for selective exposure or restraint of body parts. Apply the padded Velcro head strap to limit head movement if desired (Fig. 11-5, *E*), or expose the legs, keeping the upper two flaps secured to perform a procedure on the lower extremities (Fig. 11-5, *F*). If needed, keep the lower two flaps secured while extending one or both arms through openings in chest flaps (i.e., for suturing, injections, vascular access) (Fig. 11-5, *G* [1]). Attach the child's arm(s) by Velcro straps to an immobilizing board that is perpendicular to the papoose board (Fig. 11-5, G [2]).

To expose the back, place the child prone on the papoose board, with the head and lower leg straps secured (Fig. 11-5, *H*). Apply a head immobilizer to the papoose board when the head strap is insufficient to achieve complete immobilization of the head (Fig. 11-5, *I*).

One may substitute a pediatric immobilizer designed to stabilize trauma patients for the papoose board (Fig. 11-6).

The Violent Patient. Approach the violent patient carefully. Attempt to diffuse a potentially explosive situation with calm discussion. However, do not continue to engage in lengthy conversation with a disoriented patient. Avoid provocation by arguments, sarcasm, or ridicule. After deciding to

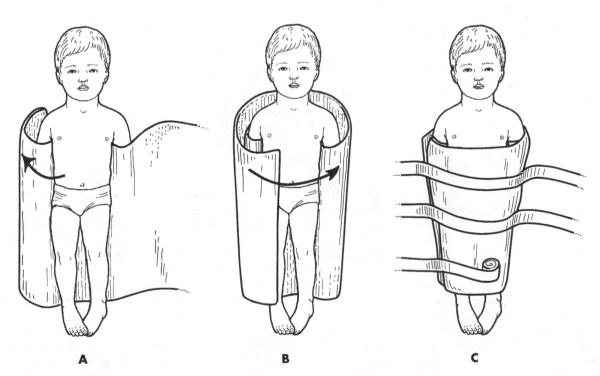

FIG. 11-4, A to C   Mummy wrap of a child with a bed sheet.

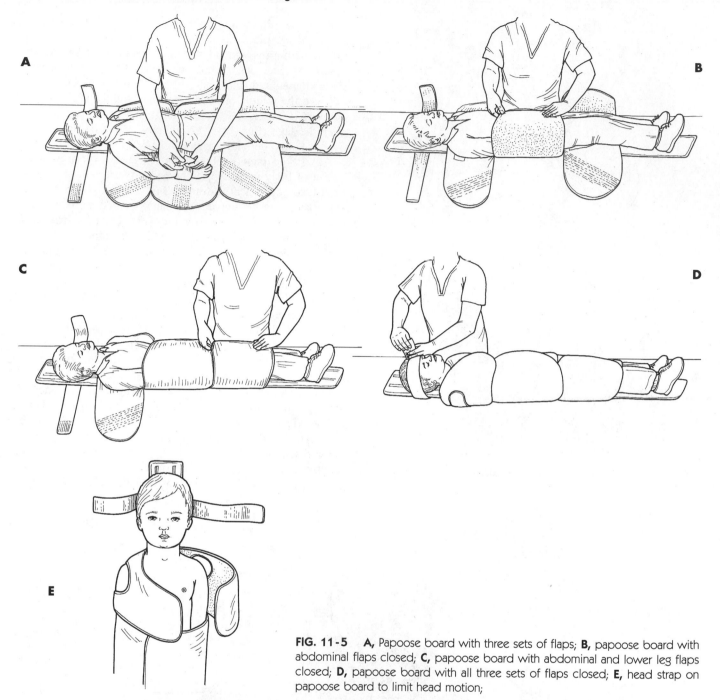

FIG. 11-5 **A,** Papoose board with three sets of flaps; **B,** papoose board with abdominal flaps closed; **C,** papoose board with abdominal and lower leg flaps closed; **D,** papoose board with all three sets of flaps closed; **E,** head strap on papoose board to limit head motion;

use leather restraints, contact security guards or other person-nel who have expertise in managing difficult patients. Do not allow them to immediately rush into the patient's room, but allow the patient to see the additional staff. This may convince the patient that staff will not tolerate her behavior and that there are enough staff to prevent her from losing control and harming herself.[2] This show of force may be enough to gain her cooperation. Remove jewelry, ties, and weapons before entering the room so the patient cannot use these to her advantage.[8]

Use five people to restrain the adolescent safely in the supine position.[10] Have one person seize each limb and the team leader hold the head to prevent biting.[15] If the adoles-cent is obviously pregnant, elevate the right hip with the patient on her side to avoid aortocaval obstruction.[7] Have one staff member always visible to reassure the patient that this process is for her own good. Explain the reason for the restraint. If the patient is a female, always have one female staff member present. If the patient is swinging a chair or other dangerous object, subdue her with a mattress from the stretcher or by throwing a blanket over her.[2,8] Do not approach a patient with a gun; call the police instead.

Do not leave the restrained patient alone. Every 15 minutes take and document vital signs and assess and document the adolescent's mobility, circulation, posture, and needs for micturition and defecation or change in position.[15] The 1995 JCAHO standard on restraints requires each hos-pital to develop and follow a policy on their use. Past

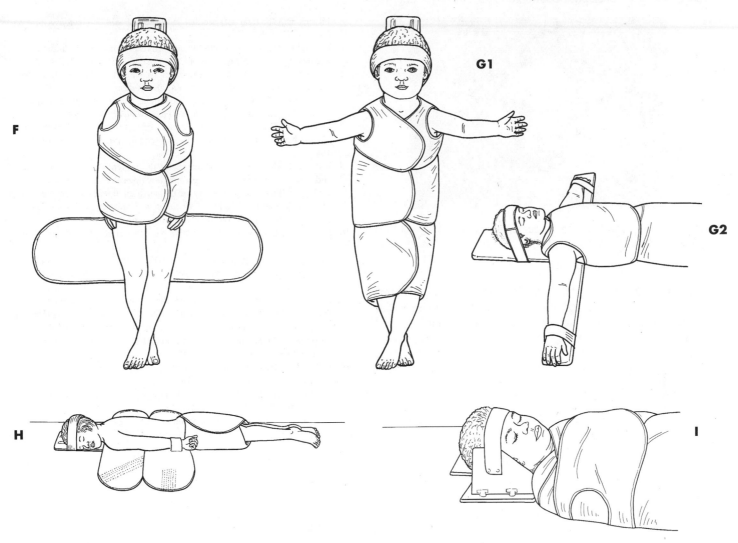

FIG. 11-5, cont'd   **F,** legs exposed for procedure—upper body immobilized in papoose; **G1,** and **G2,** child restrained with arms extended for procedure; **H,** prone position, back exposed, head and legs restrained; and **I,** head immobilizer attaches to papoose for maximal immobilization.

regulations of JCAHO required that an order by a physician (verbal or written) be obtained within 1 hour of the restraint procedure. Write a progress note about the actions taken and document carefully how the procedure was undertaken. The restraint order should be valid for no more than 12 hours and should not be a PRN order.

To remove a patient from restraints, gather adequate personnel, and free only one limb at a time. Debrief the patient while freeing her, and observe her behavior to be certain she has regained control.

Remarks

Even in a busy Emergency Department, do not treat children harshly or abruptly. Balance the desire to finish the procedure promptly with the need to reassure the child and make the experience tolerable.[12] Choose words of explanation carefully while restraining a child; always be sympathetic and empathic. An age-appropriate, empathic explanation, rather than cold impersonal instructions about an impending painful procedure, will help reduce pain behavior.[4] If possible, allow a child to read about a procedure, or permit brief role playing just before restraint. This reduces pulse rates and other physiologic responses to pain.[3]

Restraint alone provides no analgesia or anesthesia. Use medications, relaxation techniques, and other means to relieve procedural pain (see Chapters 12 to 14).

It may be necessary to physically restrain a violent adolescent to prevent injury to the patient or others. Always demonstrate concern for the patient and try not to appear punitive during the procedure. Following the restraint, continue to deliver humane, careful medical care, acting in the patient's best interest.[15]

Do not apply leather or other restrictive chest straps, since they can interfere with ventilation.[10] Do not use arm-leg or leg-leg two-point restraints because they permit the patient to fall from the stretcher.[6] Supine restraint with the head elevated is preferable to patients and more readily permits medical treatment. Prone restraint is more controlling. Use

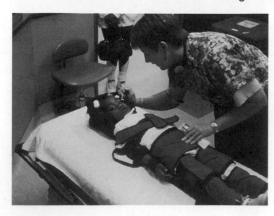

FIG. 11-6   Restraint with a pediatric immobilizer designed for a patient with suspected injury.

this approach only for the most agitated and violent patients or those at risk for regurgitation.[6] Apply a Philadelphia collar to the patient's neck to keep her from biting or head banging.[8]

REFERENCES

1. Blumenreich P, Lippmann S, Bacani-Oropilla T: Violent patients—are you prepared to deal with them? *Postgrad Med* 90:201-206, 1991.
2. Dubin WR: Evaluation and managing the violent patient, *Ann Emerg Med* 10:481-484, 1981.
3. Fassler D: The fear of needles in children, *Am J Orthopsychiatry* 55:371-377, 1985.
4. Fernald C, Corry J: Empathic vs. directive preparation of children for needles, *Child Health Care* 10:44-47, 1981.
5. Klein JO, Feigin RD, McCracken GH Jr: Report of the task force on diagnosis and management of meningitis, *Pediatrics* 78S:966, 1986.
6. Lavoie FW: Consent, involuntary treatment, and the use of force in an urban emergency department, *Ann Emerg Med* 21:25-32, 1992.
7. Raskin VD, Dresner N, Miller W: Risks of restraints versus psychotropic medication for pregnant patients (letter), *Am J Psych* 148:1760, 1991.
8. Rice MM, Moore GP: Management of the violent patient: therapeutic and legal considerations, *Emerg Clin North Am* 9:13-30, 1991.
9. Ruddy R: Illustrated techniques of pediatric emergency procedures. In Fleisher G, Ludwig S, editors: *Textbook of pediatric emergency medicine,* Baltimore, 1993, Williams & Wilkins, pp 1566-1569.
10. Scaletta T: Management of combative patients (letter), *Am J Emerg Med* 12:257, 1994.
11. Selbst SM: Sedation and analgesia. In Fleisher G, Ludwig S, editors: *Textbook of pediatric emergency medicine,* Baltimore, 1993, Williams & Wilkins, pp 55-64.
12. Selbst SM: Pain management in the emergency department. In Schechter NL, Berde CB, Yaster M, editors: *Pain in infants, children, and adolescents,* Baltimore, 1993, Williams & Wilkins, pp 505-518.
13. Selbst SM: Managing pain in the pediatric emergency department, *Pediatr Emerg Care* 5:56-63, 1989.
14. Selbst SM, Henretig FM: The treatment of pain in the emergency department, *Pediatr Clin North Am* 36:965-978, 1989.
15. Tardiff K: Management of the violent patient in an emergency situation, *Psych Clinc North Am* 11:539-549, 1988.
16. Weisman LE, Merenstein GD, Steenbarger JR: Effect of lumbar puncture position on the sick neonate, *Am J Dis Child* 137:1077-1079, 1983.

12   Pharmacologic Agents

James M. Callahan

Pain is "an unpleasant sensory and emotional experience associated with actual or potential tissue damage, or described in terms of such damage."[58] Different people experience varying amounts of discomfort from similar stimuli, depending on their past experience and emotional state.[114] "No one feels another's pain and physicians have to believe the patient's words or reactions to know if he is having pain ... pain, like a disease, is not an abstraction with an existence outside a person; a person must feel the pain and the complaint is the balance between cause, sensation and reaction."[100]

From early infancy acute pain serves as a warning that, if heeded, can lead to the prevention of serious injury or alert an individual of the need to seek medical attention. Parents often seek care for their children in the Emergency Department (ED) in an attempt to relieve pain caused by a variety of conditions. Most patients in pediatric intensive care units (PICUs) have painful conditions or undergo painful procedures. Intensity of pain varies from the relatively mild (e.g., acute otitis media) to the severe pain associated with a major fracture or a vasoocclusive crisis in a child with sickle cell disease. A patient's pain can help guide the emergency physician or intensive care physician to the correct nature and location of a patient's problem.[90] Once it has served these functions, pain is no longer useful, and its safe and effective relief should be a high priority in the emergency care of children.

Diagnostic and therapeutic procedures may also be painful. Anxiety often accompanies pain, as a result of trauma, illness, or a procedure, in children who unexpectedly find themselves in a foreign environment being cared for by strangers. Even procedures that are painless may be frightening to small children, who lack the cognitive ability to understand the necessity of holding very still in a loud, cold, confined space such as a magnetic resonance imaging (MRI) or computed tomographic (CT) scanner. Relief of anxiety and fear is also a humane goal in caring for acutely ill or injured children. Effective anxiolysis and sedation permit accomplishment of procedures in a more accurate, safe, and rapid manner.

Young children may not be able to verbalize their feelings or communicate that they are experiencing pain. Parents are the best predictors of the distress their children will experience during procedures. Using their knowledge may help to reduce pain-related stress.[87] The age and developmental stage of the child impact the pain experience greatly. Younger children often exaggerate the size and power of needles in drawings of physicians and hospitals.[41] Older children may be better able to understand why they have pain or why a procedure is necessary. They may also better understand the significance of their injury or illness and report that similar problems produce more unpleasant feelings.[14] Hence, health-care providers must quickly recognize pain and anxiety in children and adequately address them.

Pain management in pediatric patients has only recently begun to attract national attention. Children, both hospitalized and in EDs, often receive inadequate or no analgesia. Beyer, DeGood, Ashley, et al.[18]; Eland and Anderson[39]; and Schechter, Allen, and Hanson[86] showed that they often have little or no postoperative analgesia and are much less likely than adults to receive it for similar diagnoses. Undertreatment is especially common in infants and younger children.[86] Anand and colleagues[6-8] have shown that neonates were often not given effective anesthesia and analgesia for cardiac surgery and that effective analgesia both lessened the stress response in these patients and decreased complications. Children in PICUs often are not given adequate analgesia or sedation before procedures.[99]

Children in ED settings have not fared much better. Selbst and Clark[91] showed that children with sickle cell crises, lower extremity fractures, and second- and third-degree burns were much less likely to receive analgesics than adults. Again children less than 2 years old were even less likely than older children to receive analgesics. Schechter[83] has pointed out that physicians routinely prescribe analgesics for otitis in adults whereas this practice is not common in children. A recent retrospective study of multiple trauma victims showed that only 53% of children with long bone fractures received analgesics in the ED.[44]

The reasons for this underuse of appropriate analgesia in children are many; but few, if any, are well founded.[69,84,85,89,90] Children, especially infants, are not able to communicate that they are in pain to the professionals caring for them. Crying is a nonspecific response to many stimuli. To justify inappropriate withholding of humane analgesia or sedation, it has been argued in the past that children, especially infants, may not feel or remember pain.

Fear of side effects and addiction have limited the use of narcotic analgesics. Narcotic-induced respiratory depression and cardiovascular effects are dose-related. Careful titration of doses usually prevents these complications. The reversibility of narcotic-associated respiratory depression with naloxone makes it very attractive for administration in an ED.[70,90] Porter and Jick[72] reported only four cases of addiction in over 11,000 patients who received narcotics for acute pain. Fear of addiction must not impede appropriate treatment of acute pain in children.

ED and PICU staffs may not address pain adequately as the patient may have other needs that are more urgent or other more acutely ill patients may divert the attention of physicians and nurses away from the pain of a less critically ill child.[90] Pediatricians, emergency medicine, and critical care physicians may be reluctant to administer analgesics because of lack of knowledge of these agents. Rana[73] has noted the lack of attention to pain management in major pediatric textbooks. Medical schools and residency training programs often lack formal education in pain management for students and house officers.[69,85] Physicians who deal with children in acute-care settings must recognize the pain these children are experiencing and their duty as caring professionals to alleviate it.

Sedation techniques for pediatric patients are also underused. Until recently, EDs rarely employed sedation for procedures in children, and physical restraint was the standard.[88] Hawk has indicated that there is "no single drug or combination of drugs . . . used routinely in pediatric emergency departments to sedate children."[53] For painless procedures, Cook, Bass, Nomizu, et al.[34] found that chloral hydrate; a mixture of meperidine, promethazine, and chlorpromazine (DPT); and pentobarbital were the most commonly used sedatives.

Most pediatric emergency medicine physicians are not satisfied with their current sedation regimen.[53] New drugs and new routes of administration have greatly expanded sedation and analgesia options for physicians who care for children in emergency settings. Physicians must use feasible, safe, and efficacious methods for sedating children with appropriate ED and PICU operational and procedural protocols (including monitoring requirements), staff education, and pediatric resuscitation equipment and drug availability for optimal application.

An important goal of sedation and analgesia in children is to make sure the agent fits the clinical situation. Painless procedures do not require the use of an analgesic for sedation. Analgesia is typically produced by narcotics at lower doses, whereas doses required for sedation approach those that lead to respiratory depression. These agents are less than ideal choices for sedation for painless procedures.[114,120] Conversely, although pure sedatives like the benzodiazepines may decrease the crying and agitation associated with painful procedures, there is no evidence that they inhibit the sensation of pain. Therefore, do not use sedatives alone for patients undergoing painful procedures or for children with painful conditions.

Indications

Analgesia. Pain is one of the most common reasons for children to enter the Emergency Department.[90,91] Diagnosis of the underlying cause is important, but do not neglect symptomatic pain relief unless it is contraindicated. Traumatic conditions including fractures, lacerations, contusions, and sprains and strains are all painful. Physicians have traditionally underused analgesics in children with these conditions.[44,91] These children deserve analgesia, as well as appropriate wound or fracture care. Treat mild pain with peripherally acting, pure analgesics such as acetaminophen, aspirin, or nonsteroidal antiinflammatory drugs (NSAIDs). Treat more severe pain with oral or parenteral narcotics or possibly a parenteral NSAID, ketorolac (Tables 12-1 and 12-2). Local or topical anesthetics may be the only immediate analgesia needed for small laceration repair. However, prescribe peripherally acting, pure analgesics for even small wounds at discharge.

Children with a wide variety of painful syndromes, including chest pain, abdominal pain, or chronic pain syndromes, enter the ED episodically. If it is the patient's first visit to the ED, if the character of the pain has changed, or if there are new associated findings, seek an underlying cause. If the cause is known, or even if no organic cause is apparent, analgesics are indicated for treatment. Modify treatment choices depending on the severity, location, and cause of the pain. Reassurance that a serious medical condition is not present and that deterioration will not occur may be helpful if these statements are appropriate. Finding a cause, if possible, may go a long way to relieve pain or at least make it tolerable in many patients. Specific treatment besides analgesics may be indicated, depending on the cause (e.g., NSAIDs for costochondritis or antibiotics for sinusitis causing headache).

Patients with sickle cell disease often enter the ED in vasoocclusive crisis. These children deserve quick and aggressive pain management. If pain is mild, use oral opioids and acetaminophen or NSAIDs. For moderate-to-severe pain or if oral medicines at home have not controlled the pain, parenteral (i.e., intravenous) opioids are the drugs of choice.

Table 12-1 Commonly Used Oral Analgesics

Agent	Dose/route	Remarks
Aspirin	10–15 mg/kg PO q4h	No liquid formulation Associated with Reye's syndrome in patients with varicella and influenza Least expensive Gastrointestinal (GI) irritation and inactivation of platelets
Acetaminophen	10–15 mg/kg PO or PR q4h	More expensive than aspirin Wide safety margin Multiple formulations, can lead to dosing errors by parents
Ibuprofen	10 mg/kg PO q6h	More expensive than aspirin or acetaminophen Gastric irritation and inactivation of platelets can occur Must be used with caution in patients with preexisting renal disease or hypovolemia
Codeine	0.5 to 1 mg/kg PO q4h	Given in combination with acetaminophen Opioid with opioid side effects Bitter taste
Hydrocodone	0.1–0.2 mg/kg PO q3–6h	More expensive, but better tasting than codeine Also given with acetaminophen

Table 12-2   Parenteral Analgesics

Agent	Dose/route	Remarks
Ketorolac	1 mg/kg (max 60 mg) load and then 0.5 mg/kg (max 30 mg) q6h IV	Only parenteral NSAID GI upset and platelet inactivation Renal effects possible Expensive
Morphine	0.08-0.15 mg/kg IV q3h (max 10 mg)	Reduced dose in infants (0.025 to 0.03 mg/kg up to 6 months of age) Dosing interval may need to be increased in infants as well Respiratory depression reversed with naloxone
Meperidine	0.5-1 mg/kg IV (max 100 mg)	Repeated doses can lead to tremors, dysphoria, seizures Less Oddi sphincter spasm than morphine
Nalbuphine	0.1 mg/kg IV q3–4h	Less Oddi sphincter spasm than morphine
Fentanyl	1–2 μg/kg IV q1–2hr	Microgram dosing can lead to dosing errors and complications Very short duration of action Large doses and rapid administration associated with ventilatory compromise secondary to chest wall rigidity and/or glottic closure

Morphine sulfate 0.1 to 0.15 mg/kg and meperidine 1 to 2 mg/kg IV are the most common choices. Meperidine may not be as good as morphine, because its intermediate metabolite, normeperidiene, is a cerebral irritant that occasionally produces mood abnormalities, dysphoria, and, rarely, seizures. Appropriate hydration is also indicated in the treatment of these children.[28] Ketorolac may be helpful in these cases when given in addition to opioids.

Many minor painful medical conditions can lead to ED visits. Otitis media, pharyngitis, and sinusitis all can be extremely painful. Local anesthetics may provide some relief in patients with otitis. Prescribe peripherally acting pure analgesics for these diagnoses. Adequate pain relief may require oral opioids in some children.

Burns are another cause of pain among children in EDs and intensive care units. Sunburn, scald burns from hot water or food, and flame burns all can be very painful. Treat small, first-degree and partial thickness burns with oral acetaminophen and NSAIDs. There is some evidence that NSAIDs not only are useful for analgesia in patients with burns but may also preserve vascular patency in the burned tissues and promote healing.[40] Traditionally physicians have used aspirin to treat sunburn.[92] At times, these patients may need oral opioids.

Children with larger burns, burns that are in sensitive areas, burns that require extensive débridement, and deeper partial-thickness and full-thickness burns need intravenous opioids after stabilization of their cardiorespiratory status. Again, NSAIDs may be useful in addition to opioids. Children with burns of this magnitude often require hospital admission and frequent dressing changes and debridement. Appropriate analgesia in the ED is imperative for these children because it may lessen the anxiety they experience during these frequent therapeutic procedures.

Traditionally one of the most neglected types of pain experienced by children in EDs and intensive care units has been procedure-related pain. Only a papoose and some form of "This will only hurt a little" or "Only for a minute" have preceded suturing, lumbar punctures, incision and drainage procedures, and many other diagnostic and therapeutic procedures. Physicians must acknowledge procedure-related pain in dealing with children in acute-care settings and then treat it or, if possible, prevent it in a humane and effective way. Premedication with analgesics and/or sedatives is effective and safe in pediatric oncology patients who undergo repeated procedures.[82,94] As long as the patient's cardiorespiratory status is stable and staff can adequately observe him or her, administer appropriate and adequate analgesia and sedation to a child who is undergoing procedures in the ED or intensive care unit.

Local infiltration with a small amount of anesthetic may be helpful for intravenous (IV) line insertion and lumbar punctures. Topical anesthetic creams probably have limited use in emergency departments because they must be left in place for a prolonged period to achieve their effect, but they may have expanded application in the PICU. In addition to local or topical anesthesia for laceration repair, sedatives or analgesics administered orally, nasally, or parenterally may be useful. Aid more involved and painful procedures (e.g., reduction of fractures and dislocations, extensive laceration repair, or burn débridement) by the use of intravenous opioids. Pain management for procedures both prevents or relieves suffering and allows safe and efficient completion of the procedure.[120]

Sedation. Indications for the use of sedative medications in the pediatric ED and PICUs are similar to those for analgesics. Children who have painful conditions or are undergoing painful procedures often may be very anxious and tense. As an adjunct to analgesics, especially when children are having painful procedures, sedative medications can be very useful. In addition to producing anxiolysis, many of these agents have amnestic properties and provide muscular relaxation that is useful when reducing fractures or dislocations.

Painless procedures such as CT scans often require that children remain still for long periods. Especially in young children, they may produce anxiety and some discomfort. Pure sedatives like the benzodiazepines, barbiturates, or even chloral hydrate may be useful when the procedure is not painful. Simple sedation allows for safe and efficient completion of the procedure.

Monitoring Guidelines. Parenteral analgesics (other than ketorolac) and sedatives all can lead to central nervous system and cardiorespiratory depression. There are multiple reports of complications related to these agents in children.[34,66,67,118] Fear of respiratory depression and associated complications is not unwarranted among physicians who treat children. However, they should not limit the appropriate use of analgesics and sedatives. Following published guidelines for monitoring may prevent respiratory depression or, at the very least, ensure early recognition so that appropriate intervention can prevent complications (Box 12-1).[5]

Key concepts for safely sedating children or giving parenteral analgesics are to use appropriate doses, be sure one assistant whose only responsibility is to monitor the child's cardiorespiratory status and vital signs is available, and have appropriate emergency equipment immediately available in case problems occur. Pulse oximetry gives much earlier and more reliable assessment of oxygen saturation than visual detection of cyanosis.[29,32,35] The use of pulse oximetry is mandatory during conscious sedation according to the guidelines of the American Academy of Pediatrics.[5] Use special care with pulse oximetry during MRI scanning, as pulse oximetry probes used during MRI have reportedly produced burns.[93] Use only oximeters approved for use during MR scanning; be sure to place the probe as far as possible from the magnetic coil, and uncoil the oximeter wire to prevent such burns.[5,93]

Use written, prospectively developed discharge criteria to decide when it is safe to send a patient home from the ED after he or she has received analgesics or sedation (see Box 12-1). Recommended criteria include that the patient's cardiovascular and airway function, including protective reflexes, is intact and stable and that the patient is arousable, is able to talk and sit without assistance (if age-appropriate), and is able to maintain hydration.[5] Younger patients who do not sit or talk must return to their presedation level of responsiveness before discharge. Following these criteria will ensure safe discharge of patients.

Contraindications

Absolute contraindications to the use of analgesics and sedatives are few. Many fears regarding the use of these agents are not well founded. History of an allergic reaction or adverse side effect related to the use of a specific analgesic or sedative is a contraindication to that specific agent. Unresponsiveness or profound shock are usually absolute contraindications.

Certain classes of patients may be more prone to adverse reactions (Box 12-2). These groups require special attention when administering narcotic analgesics or sedatives. Infants, especially those <6 months of age, seem to be more prone to the respiratory depression associated with many of these agents; prevent this reaction with dose reduction.[19,112,114,117] In addition, the use of narcotics and sedatives makes sedation an unreliable marker of impending respiratory depression.[114] Monitor patients with underlying respiratory disease more carefully when using agents that lead to respiratory depression. Use agents with sedative properties (opioids, benzodiazepines, and barbiturates) cautiously in patients with possible central nervous system (CNS) injury as they may cloud the assessment of the neurologic status of these patients.

Stabilize the cardiopulmonary status of patients with multiple trauma before administering these agents. In patients suspected of having surgical conditions of the abdomen,

---

BOX 12-1 **MONITORING REQUIREMENTS IN CHILDREN AFTER CONSCIOUS SEDATION**

Health-care personnel

Training for personnel in at least pediatric basic life support; advanced life support skills are preferable, as are skills in obtaining vascular access.

Support person whose only role is to monitor vital signs and airway patency.

Monitoring

Obtain and record vital signs.

Continuous monitoring of oxygen saturation (pulse oximetry) and heart rate.

Intermittent recording of respiratory rate and blood pressure by support personnel.

Equipment

Functioning suction apparatus.

Oxygen source capable of providing 90% FiO_2 and positive pressure ventilation (e.g., bag-valve-mask device with high-flow oxygen source).

Discharge criteria

Patient can talk and sit up without assistance (preferably able to ambulate).

Cardiovascular function and airway patency are adequate and stable.

Hydration status is adequate.

Adapted from AAP Committee on Drugs: *Pediatrics* 89:1110–1115, 1992.

opioid analgesics may mask progression of abdominal symptoms. However, some relief of pain and anxiety may improve
the physical examination. In these patients use drugs cautiously and discuss pain and sedation with surgical consultants. The following sections discuss specific contraindications for agents.

Complications

The sections on specific agents discuss complications in
depth; this section highlights major issues. The most common and potentially most serious complication associated
with narcotic analgesics and sedative agents is respiratory
depression. Most sedative and analgesic agents decrease the
response to carbon dioxide and decrease minute ventilation
by decreasing respiratory rate and tidal volume.[19,26,36,51,117]
Certain classes of patients, especially infants, are more prone
to respiratory depressant effects. Adhere to recommended
doses, give these medications slowly, and closely monitor the
cardiorespiratory status of these patients to minimize side
effects. Reduce doses for patients with CNS or cardiopulmonary problems, and for those on other medications that may
be additive or synergistic (e.g., phenobarbital).

Opioid analgesics, benzodiazepines, and barbiturates can
lead to vasodilation and/or cardiac depression resulting in
hypotension.[36,117] Again, giving the medicines slowly, altering dosages when necessary, and using them with caution in
trauma patients and others who may be hypovolemic prevent
problems with these drugs. Closely monitor vital signs and
cardiorespiratory status.

Any medicines given intravenously can cause infiltration.
Diazepam and lorazepam, two of the sedative agents, often
cause phlebitis and pain on injection because of their carrier
compound.[9,115] Midazolam produces less pain on injection.[75,115] Aspirin and the NSAIDs can all inhibit platelet
function and lead to bleeding problems. Use these medicines
carefully in patients with cranial injuries, fresh open wounds,
or recent surgery. Opioid analgesics and sedatives can produce CNS depression, which may be prolonged in some
patients. At times, loss of protective airway reflexes can
occur, and aspiration can complicate therapy.

Technique

Analgesia. Physicians have used the concept of an "analgesic ladder" in the treatment of pain in cancer patients.[16,114]
This concept is applicable to the management of pain in other
pediatric patients as well. Use analgesic medicines in a way
that matches the potency of the agent with the severity of
pain. If pain persists or increases after use of a nonopioid
medicine for seemingly mild pain, add increasingly stronger
medicines to achieve good pain control. The analgesic ladder
model classifies pain as mild, moderate, or severe. Choose
agents according to this classification.

NONNARCOTIC ANALGESICS

Acetaminophen. For mild pain acetaminophen is the
drug of choice. It is the most commonly prescribed oral
analgesic and has a wide therapeutic ratio.[16,91,92,114] It is as
effective as aspirin for pain control.[83,92] It is well tolerated
with few side effects. It does not inhibit platelet activity or
precipitate bronchospasm in aspirin-sensitive patients. It
lacks the antiinflammatory effects of aspirin or the NSAIDs.

Acetaminophen is a peripherally acting, pure analgesic
that inhibits the generation of afferent pain signals.[114] The
usual dose is 10 to 15 mg/kg orally or rectally every 4 hours.
Acetaminophen and the NSAIDs have a ceiling effect so
increasing doses beyond the standard administration fails to
provide further pain relief.[16] If standard doses are not
effective, use more potent analgesics. Acetaminophen can be
combined with oral or parenteral opioids for the treatment of
moderate or severe pain, as these agents appear to be
synergistic in combination.[15,81]

Acetaminophen is an excellent choice for pain caused by
mild trauma and many medical conditions (e.g., otitis media). Multiple preparations are available and can sometimes
lead to confusion among parents regarding appropriate dosing.[83] Overdosage and toxicity may result if parents are
administering it at the same time they are administering
over-the-counter cold preparations that also contain acetaminophen. Caution parents about this and be sure to ask what
other medicines the child is taking. Acetaminophen, even at
recommended doses, if given around the clock for several
days has been reported to cause toxicity. Rectal suppositories
are available. Use them whole as the drug is unevenly
distributed in them. Toxicity is more often seen in patients
with a history of alcohol abuse as a result of induction of the
cytochrome p450 system, which can lead to the production of
toxic metabolites.

Aspirin. Aspirin is a peripherally acting analgesic with
antiinflammatory properties. It has the longest history of use
among the oral analgesics. It seems to decrease pain through
both antiinflammatory action and inhibition of a
prostaglandin-mediated peripheral pain pathway.[4,81] Give
aspirin in a dose of 10 to 15 mg/kg orally or rectally every 4
hours. Absorption is variable with rectal administration.[83]
There is no liquid form, but chewable tablets are available
for younger children.

Because of its antiinflammatory properties, aspirin is an
excellent choice for mild pain associated with mild orthopedic injuries such as sprains and strains. It is also a good
choice for myalgia, arthralgia, headache, and sunburn.[92]
Aspirin has more side effects than acetaminophen and therefore has fallen into some degree of disuse in recent years. If
one considers these side effects, one can safely use aspirin
for effective pain relief at a cost less than that of acetaminophen or the NSAIDs.

The most common side effect of aspirin use is gastric
irritation. Taking aspirin with milk or food may decrease the

epigastric distress experienced by these patients.[83] Some patients tolerate enteric-coated aspirin better.[92] Aspirin has been shown to precipitate bronchospasm in some children with asthma[92,113]; use it with caution in these patients. Aspirin also decreases levels of factor VII and irreversibly inactivates platelets.[16,83] Avoid its use in patients for whom bleeding may be a problem. Aspirin's link to Reye's syndrome in patients with influenza and varicella has also limited its indications and overall popularity.

Nonsteroidal Antiinflammatory Drugs. The nonsteroidal antiinflammatory drugs (NSAIDs) are the most commonly prescribed class of medications in the United States today.[63] There are a large number of agents in five different classes based on their chemical structure. Like that of aspirin, the first of the NSAIDs, their mechanism of analgesic action involves the inhibition of the production of prostaglandins and related compounds and the prevention of inflammation.[23] The U.S. Food and Drug Administration (FDA) has approved only naproxen, ibuprofen, choline-magnesium salicylate, and tolmetin for use in children. Choline-magnesium salicylate, ibuprofen, and naproxen are available in palatable liquid preparations.

The dose of ibuprofen is 10 mg/kg every 6 to 8 hours orally.[16,23,81] Give tolmetin in a dose of 5 to 7 mg/kg orally every 6 to 8 hours.[16] Naproxen's dose is also 5 to 7 mg/kg, but give it every 8 to 12 hours.[16] Give choline-magnesium salicylate in a dose of 10 mg/kg orally every 6 to 8 hours.[16,114] The oral NSAIDs seem to be better tolerated than aspirin with less gastric upset. Their effect on platelets is reversible. Choline-magnesium salicylate seems to be especially well tolerated and causes little change in bleeding time.[114] They remain more expensive than aspirin or acetaminophen, and liquid ibuprofen still requires a prescription in many states. They are especially useful for dysmenorrhea, headaches, musculoskeletal problems, and pain associated with inflammation of mild to moderate severity.[89]

The NSAIDs have rarely produced more severe side effects. A few reports cite renal effects, including nephrosis, papillary necrosis, and tubulointerstitial nephritis, which on occasion has led to end-stage renal disease.[63,76] Previous renal disease and volume depletion may predispose patients to these problems. Their inhibition of prostaglandin synthesis adversely effects renal and intrarenal blood flow. Chronic use in pediatric patients with rheumatologic disease has produced hepatic dysfunction and an increase in hepatic enzymes.[23] Long-term use of NSAIDs has also caused ulcers of the stomach, duodenum, and small intestine.[3]

Ketorolac is an NSAID available for parenteral administration. It seems to be especially effective for moderate-to-severe musculoskeletal and visceral pain, including biliary and renal colic.[81] It is also effective for headaches, including migraines, and sickle cell crisis (vasoocclusive crisis). It may have an opioid-sparing effect in some patients. Currently its only approved use is intramuscular administration in patients older than 12 years of age with an initial dose of 30 to 60 mg followed by 15 to 30 mg every 6 hours. Intravenous use has produced good results without an increase in side effects.[25,60,71] It does not cause the cardiorespiratory depression seen with opioid analgesics. Consider using ketorolac with a loading dose of 1 mg/kg IV to a maximum of 60 mg

followed by 0.5 mg/kg IV (maximum 30 mg) every 6 hours. It does seem to inhibit platelet aggregation and may cause gastrointestinal, renal, and hepatic effects similar to those produced by the oral NSAIDs. As with oral NSAIDs, there are reports of allergic reactions; use both ketorolac and oral NSAIDs with great caution in patients with asthma, as they may induce bronchospasm.

NARCOTIC ANALGESICS. When nonnarcotic analgesics are not effective in controlling pain, add narcotic analgesics. For obviously severe pain, proceeding directly to the use of intravenous opioid medications is appropriate if the patient's respiratory and hemodynamic status will tolerate it. Narcotic analgesics bind to opioid receptors in the brain and spinal cord as well as at peripheral sites.[59,81] They cause a decrease in the sensation of pain, making it more tolerable and less distressing. There does not appear to be a ceiling effect. Increasing dosages leads to increasing analgesia, but the higher the dose the more likely the patient is to experience side effects, including sedation; nausea and vomiting; smooth muscle spasm, including urinary retention; and respiratory depression.[9,79,81] Sedation usually precedes respiratory depression. This relationship is not an exact one; carefully monitor the cardiorespiratory status of patients receiving opioids. At equivalent analgesic dosages, all narcotic agents produce similar amounts of respiratory depression and other side effects.[117]

Codeine. Codeine is an opioid that retains most of its effectiveness when given orally.[89,117] It is useful for the treatment of mild to moderate pain (e.g., that associated with severe otitis media or dental abscess) and as an antitussive agent.[81,83,89,117] It is available in liquid form alone or in combination with acetaminophen. Prescribing it in combination with acetaminophen is usually cheaper and allows the synergistic effect of these two agents to decrease the amount of narcotic needed for adequate pain relief.[117] Decreasing the amount of narcotic decreases side effects, especially sedation. Give codeine at a dose of 0.5 to 1 mg/kg with acetaminophen 10 mg/kg orally every 3 to 4 hours.

Hydrocodone. Hydrocodone is an oral analgesic that is more potent than codeine and also available in a liquid preparation combined with acetaminophen.[89] It is more palatable (less bitter) than acetaminophen and codeine preparations and produces less nausea and vomiting. The usual dose is 0.1 to 0.2 mg/kg orally every 3 to 6 hours. The liquid preparation has 2.5 mg hydrocodone/5 ml and 120 mg acetaminophen/5 ml. Administration of 0.2 mg/kg hydrocodone produces an approximate dose of 10 mg/kg acetaminophen.

Morphine. Morphine is the standard opioid analgesic and is the basis of comparison for other analgesics.[91,117] It is the drug of choice for severe pain, including severe procedural pain, in the pediatric emergency department and acute care settings.[81,89,92] Morphine provides both analgesia and some sedation. If more sedation or anxiolysis is desirable (e.g., during procedures), combine it with a benzodiazepine, although this combination significantly increases the risk of respiratory depression.[81,118] The intravenous route is preferable as it is less painful and the onset and duration of action are more rapid and predictable than those produced by intramuscular administration. The effect is also more easily titratable when it is used intravenously. The subcutaneous route is less painful than intramuscular injection, but the absorption of the drug is very unpredictable.[92]

The major side effect of morphine and all opioids, especially when given parenterally, is respiratory depression. In addition, they can cause sedation, venous dilation and pooling, nausea and vomiting, miosis, pruritus, smooth muscle spasm, and urinary retention.[81,89,92,117,120] The respiratory depression associated with these agents is exaggerated in young infants,[19,112,117] and prolongation of their half-life and elimination is the rule.[19,117] Use them very cautiously with reduced doses in infants and also in patients with multiple trauma, head, or abdominal injuries. Volume depletion makes the occurrence of hemodynamic side effects more common.

The usual dose of morphine is 0.08 to 0.15 mg/kg given intravenously over 4 to 5 minutes. The effect on pain is usually immediate, with peak effect in approximately 20 minutes.[92] Usual dosing interval is 3 to 4 hours. Dosing recommendations are only guidelines, and it is best to titrate the administered dose to the desired effect, watching closely for side effects. The maximum recommended dose is 10 mg. Patients who have chronic, painful syndromes (e.g., sickle cell disease) or who need to be admitted (e.g., burn patients) may benefit from a continuous infusion of morphine or other opioid or its administration by patient-controlled analgesia (PCA) pumps.[30,114] Use a starting dose of 0.01 to 0.04 mg/kg/h when giving morphine as a continuous infusion.

Meperidine. Meperidine is a synthetic narcotic with a slightly shorter half-life than that of morphine. It reaches its peak effect more quickly than morphine when given by the intramuscular route.[89,92,117] Its advantages when compared with morphine are few. It may cause less Oddi's sphincter spasm, and therefore some practitioners prefer it for the treatment of biliary colic.[117] Other side effects are very similar when given in equianalgesic doses to morphine. Normeperidine is one of the principal active metabolites of meperidine produced by the liver. When it accumulates, it can cause tremors, dysphoria, and seizures. To prevent these side effects, do not use meperidine by continuous infusion or repeated parenteral doses.[117,120] The usual dose is 0.5 to 1 mg/kg IV every 3 to 4 hours. Maximum dose is 125 mg.[89] Meperidine is also part of the lytic cocktail, DPT, in a one-time dose up to 2 mg/kg (see the discussion of sedation technique). Ordinarily morphine is the preferred agent. Meperidine should be reserved for patients who do not tolerate morphine.

Fentanyl. Fentanyl is a synthetic opioid agonist that is very lipophilic, is quickly removed from the plasma, and rapidly crosses the blood-brain barrier.[79,81,89,117] Because of these properties it has several very attractive characteristics for the acute care setting. It has a rapid onset of action (90 to 120 seconds)[79] and reaches a peak effect quickly. With a half-life of about 20 minutes it has a short, predictable duration of action of about 30 to 40 minutes.[21,79,81,89,117] It causes very little change in the hemodynamic status of most patients and is very useful in critically ill patients.[117] It is about 100 times more potent than morphine, so administer it cautiously. The recommended dose is only 1 to 2 µg/kg by slow IV infusion (over 5 minutes) every 1 to 2 hours.* Fentanyl may be given as a continuous infusion in the intensive care unit. Use 1 µg/kg/h as a starting dose and carefully titrate up as needed.

Like all narcotic analgesics, fentanyl can lead to respiratory depression, nausea and vomiting, bradycardia, and pruritus.[21,79] Because of its extreme potency and microgram dosing, its use is prone to medication errors and inadvertent rapid infusion by the flushing of residual drug left in intravenous lines. Use extreme care with this drug.

Infants less than 3 months of age may be more sensitive to the respiratory depressant effect of fentanyl, but those more than 3 months do not seem to be more sensitive than older children or adults.[54] There seems to be a smaller volume of distribution in infants than in older children or adults but increased elimination and possibly an increased concentration of protein-bound drug. This leads to lower plasma fentanyl concentrations in infants after its one-time administration. In one study infants tolerated larger doses of fentanyl than older children or adults in an operative setting.[95]

The respiratory depressant effects of fentanyl seem to be potentiated when it is administered in conjunction with a benzodiazepine such as midazolam.[13,118] An additional, disturbing side effect is the sudden occurrence of chest wall rigidity associated with the rapid infusion of fentanyl, especially in large doses.[33,79] Inability to ventilate patients, related to glottic closure, may result, either alone or in addition to chest wall rigidity.[11] Fentanyl only causes these effects when administered in the high doses required for anesthetic induction, but, when they occur, they often require naloxone and neuromuscular blockade with succinylcholine or pancuronium for effective treatment.[21,27] Fentanyl infusions in the intensive care unit setting have caused transient movement disorders and other neurologic abnormalities in children when they have been discontinued.[17,61] Addiction can result from long-term infusion.

Despite these concerns, fentanyl seems to be a safe, effective option for opioid analgesia in acute-care settings for children if proper safeguards are used. Its rapid onset and relatively short duration of action make it an excellent choice for treating procedure-related pain (e.g., laceration repair, orthopedic reductions, burn débridement). Its relative lack of hemodynamic effects makes it especially attractive. Fentanyl is safe to use in the general emergency department and among children with facial trauma requiring laceration repair.[21,27]

In Billmire, Neale, and Gregory's report[21] of fentanyl use for pediatric facial trauma, patients received 2 to 3 µg/kg of body weight over 3 to 5 minutes. Older children often required a lesser dose. Children less than 36 months of age often did not appear adequately sedated at the end of the infusion but became so after a few minutes without additional medicine. In 2000 children only three cases of apnea that required a narcotic antagonist and respiratory support occurred. Facial pruritus often led to facial scratching. It was often necessary to provide minimal restraint to prevent contamination of the field.[21]

Chudnofsky, Wright, Dronew, et al.[27] reported the safety

---

*References 21, 79, 81, 89, 114, and 117.

of fentanyl in the general ED. Again, the prevalence of serious side effects was very low (approximately 1%); most occurred in intoxicated patients or those receiving other sedative agents.

A novel and attractive delivery device for fentanyl will soon come to market. The lollipoplike device for the oral, transmucosal delivery of fentanyl citrate is a proven method for delivery of preanesthetic medication in children[45,46] and in the ED.[64] In the intensive care unit, postoperative emesis and preoperative side effects, including some hypoxemia, often occur. Lind, Marcus, Mears, et al. reported a significant incidence of nausea, pruritus, dizziness, and dry mouth in the emergency department without significant changes in vital signs or oxygen saturation.[64] There were few children in this study group, however. In all groups this device achieved effective sedation and analgesia. This route of fentanyl delivery deserves further evaluation in the pediatric emergency department setting.

Nalbuphine. Nalbuphine hydrochloride is a narcotic antagonist analgesic with mixed agonist and antagonist properties. It is structurally similar to oxymorphone and naloxone.[77] It may cause less Oddi's sphincter spasm than morphine in patients with pancreatitis and biliary tract disease. It also has a ceiling effect for its respiratory depression properties.[77] This means that when using higher doses for patients with severe pain, there may be less respiratory depression than with morphine.

The usual initial dose of nalbuphine is 0.1 mg/kg given IV every 3 to 4 hours with a maximum dose of 10 mg.[1] Although a member of the partial agonist class of drugs, nalbuphine does have respiratory depressant effects and can cause CNS depression, flushing, urticaria, nausea and vomiting, and hypotension. Give this drug cautiously and in lower dosages in patients with hepatic disease.

Nalaxone. Naloxone is a narcotic antagonist that can reverse the respiratory and CNS depressant effects of morphine and the other opioids. For patients with presumed opioid overdose, use a 1- to 2-mg/dose regardless of age (outside the neonatal period) to reverse respiratory depression. Repeat the dose to a total dosage of 10 mg, as needed. Give it intravenously, intramuscularly, or endotracheally in emergencies. In patients receiving opioids for therapeutic purposes, large doses (1 to 2 mg) may precipitate the sudden onset of severe pain and hypertension, flushing, and diaphoresis.

In these patients it is better to support their respirations as needed with assisted ventilation and give naloxone in increments of 0.01 to 0.1 mg/kg. Titrate the dose until the desired effect (e.g., improved respiratory rate, level of consciousness) results. The duration of action of naloxone is often shorter than that of the opioid analgesics, and repeated doses may be necessary.

Sedation. Sedative agents, either alone or in combination with analgesics, are also very useful. Sedation is a continuum from wakefulness to deep obtundation (i.e., general anesthesia). There are no universally accepted definitions for the various points along this continuum. In general, *conscious sedation* is a minimally depressed level of consciousness during which a patient maintains airway protective mechanisms and ability to respond to physical stimuli and follow commands.[5,81] *Deep sedation* refers to a more depressed level of consciousness from which a patient is not easily arousable and in which the risk of the loss of airway protective reflexes is substantial. With *general anesthesia* a patient is completely unconscious and loses all airway protective reflexes. Most often we seek a level of conscious sedation among children requiring sedation in the ED or the PICU.

However, patients can easily and rapidly move from a level of conscious sedation to deep obtundation, depending on drug dosages and amount and intensity of external stimuli.[24] Close monitoring according to the guidelines of the American Academy of Pediatrics is appropriate in all sedated children (see Box 12-1). An ideal sedative, besides being effective, would be easy to administer, be quick and predictable in its onset and duration of action, have no side effects, and lead to rapid recovery for rapid patient discharge. Unfortunately no such agent or agents exist. Tailor the choice of agent to the needs of the individual child and procedure. The care given in the administration of the agent and the quality of observation the patient receives are more important in determining outcome than the choice of agent.[24]

CHLORAL HYDRATE. Chloral hydrate is a pure sedative hypnotic used for pediatric sedation for over 100 years.[22] Hepatic alcohol dehydrogenase converts this drug to trichloroethanol, its active metabolite. Avoid chloral hydrate in patients with liver or kidney failure. The drug has CNS, respiratory, and cardiovascular depressant effects.[101,120] In usual doses it is very safe, but overdoses can have fatal results. The acute toxicity of this medicine worsens with concurrent use of benzodiazepines, barbiturates, or ethanol. Most deaths have resulted from resistant cardiac dysrhythmias with very large overdoses.[101] Recent reports have shown that respiratory failure may be of particular concern in patients with CNS abnormality and obstructive sleep apnea.[20,47]

Give chloral hydrate orally or rectally. It is a gastric irritant and has a disagreeable taste; do not prescribe it in patients with gastritis. Children often do not receive the fully prescribed dose or may quickly vomit a major portion of it. Rectal administration may alleviate some of these problems. Onset of sedation occurs 30 to 60 minutes after administration. Recovery time may be as long as an hour but, because of the long half-lives of trichloroethanol and trichloracetic acid, residual motor impairment and decreased activity level may last up to 1 day.[81] It is often necessary to give additional doses to achieve adequate sedation. Neonates metabolize chloral hydrate differently from older children and adults. Its prolonged half-life and the accumulation of its active metabolites result in prolonged sedation. Repeated doses have led to a direct hyperbilirubinemia.[101] Chloral hydrate's long onset of action makes it less desirable as a sedative agent in the emergency department. Also, it has no analgesic properties.

Although chloral hydrate facilitates completion of procedures among pediatric patients in emergency departments[22] and in ophthalmologic examinations,[43] its main role seems to be in sedation for painless diagnostic procedures such as CT and MRI scans. Initial doses of 60 to 120 mg/kg orally or rectally safely produced sedation in 80% to 96% percent of

Table 12-3   Oral Sedatives

Agent	Dose	Remarks
Chloral hydrate	60-120 mg/kg PO or PR (max 1-2 g); may repeat half of the initial dose 30 min later (to a total max of 150 mg/kg or 1-2 g)	Long onset of action and prolonged drowsiness and motor impairment are common Use with caution in neonates Overdoses can lead to arrhythmias
Midazolam	0.5 mg/kg PO	Mix with sweet flavors Onset of action in 20 to 30 minutes Has amnestic properties Reverse with flumazenil

patients in a number of series* (Table 12-3). When it is ineffective, repeat a dose of up to one half the original dose to a total maximum dose of 150 mg/kg. The recommended maximum dose of chloral hydrate is 1 to 2 g. The most frequently reported side effect in these series was vomiting. Paradoxic hyperactivity and airway problems (less than 5% in all series) were rare. Sedation failures were more common in children with neurologic disorders[80] and in those over 48 months of age.[49]

Recent reports have raised concerns about the carcinogenesis of chloral hydrate in animal experiments.[37,96] Steinberg[101] has pointed out that the dose-response relationship in rodents is nonlinear, and that only in animals exposed to high doses given over a long enough period to induce cellular necrosis have malignancies developed. In addition, epidemiologic studies of humans exposed to trichloroethylene (metabolized to chloral hydrate in humans) have not shown an increase in cancer or mortality rates. Steinberg[101] and the Committees on Drugs and Environmental Health, American Academy of Pediatrics[31] have both concluded that chloral hydrate is a safe drug for short-term sedation at the recommended dosages. Limiting its use for long-term sedation and in neonates may be prudent until results of further studies are available.

BENZODIAZEPINES. The benzodiazepines are centrally acting compounds that interact with the γ-aminobutyric acid (GABA) receptor complex. They enhance the action of GABA and inhibit its reuptake, leading to its accumulation.[75,81] Because of this property and other actions, they lead to sedation, hypnosis, anxiolysis, and centrally mediated skeletal muscle relaxation.[75,81,120] They produce anterograde amnesia, a desirable effect in pediatric sedation. They may also produce respiratory depression, depending on the dose given and the speed of administration. They have become the "sedatives of choice for most ED activities and are equally popular in the ICU setting."[81] With proper safeguards and monitoring, they are excellent choices for sedating pediatric patients.

The benzodiazepines have no analgesic properties; do not mistake a quiet, sedated state for a lack of pain. Given alone, the benzodiazepines are excellent sedatives for nonpainful procedures (e.g., CT scans or MRI). For painful procedures, use them in conjunction with analgesics and/or local anes-

thetics. The combination of benzodiazepines and opioid analgesics leads to a marked increase in respiratory depression and requires close monitoring. A competitive antagonist, flumazenil, that can reverse the side effects of the benzodiazepines is now available (discussed later).

Diazepam. Traditionally diazepam has been the most widely used of the benzodiazepines for procedural sedation.[81,115] Administer it orally, rectally, or intravenously. Intramuscular use results in erratic absorption.[81] The intravenous dose is 0.1 to 0.2 mg/kg by slow IV push. Slow administration decreases the occurrence of respiratory side effects and venous irritation (Table 12-4). Rectally, the dose is 0.5 mg/kg. The oral dose is 0.12 to 0.5 mg/kg. Diazepam has a long half-life of approximately 30 hours.

The main side effects associated with diazepam are respiratory depression and venous irritation and thrombophlebitis.[74,120] Diazepam leads to decreased minute ventilation, increased resting $Paco_2$, and decreased ventilatory response to increasing $Paco_2$.[26,36,51] In addition, it has produced decreases in systolic blood pressure. The venous irritation and sequelae associated with diazepam relate to the propylene glycol in its solvent. Administer by slow IV push into large vessels with adequate blood flow to minimize this irritation and later side effects.

Diazepam has a slow onset of action that can make it difficult to titrate to a desired effect.[115] Its long half-life and the accumulation of active metabolites when it must be given in repeated doses can cause prolonged recovery.[115] It is appropriate for use for longer procedures such as MRI scans.[81]

Lorazepam. Lorazepam is very similar to diazepam, except that it has a longer half-life and slightly slower onset of action. It produces reliable sedation for a longer period. It is appropriate for extended sedation, such as with intubated patients requiring prolonged transport, diagnostic procedures, or prolonged mechanical ventilation.[81] The usual IV or oral dose is 0.02 to 0.08 mg/kg, with a maximum single dose of about 5 mg. For chronic sedation, a repeat dose every 4 to 6 hours may be given.

Lorazepam has the same respiratory depressant effects as diazepam. Its injectable form also contains propylene glycol and can cause vascular irritation and complications. If IV access is a problem, give it intramuscularly; absorption is reliable after intramuscular administration. When using it intramuscularly, give 0.05 mg/kg up to a maximum of 4 mg.

Midazolam. Midazolam is a newer benzodiazepine that

---

*References 48, 49, 56, 68, 80, and 106.

Table 12-4 Parenteral Sedatives

Agent	Route	Remarks
Diazepam	0.1 to 0.2 mg/kg IV	Additive respiratory depression with opioids
		Vascular irritant
		Flumazenil effective for reversal
Lorazepam	0.02 to 0.08 mg/kg IV or IM	Additive respiratory depression with opioids
		Long half-life
		Vascular irritant
		Can be given IM
		Flumazenil effective for reversal
Midazolam	0.02 to 0.2 mg/kg IV	Additive respiratory depression with opioids
		Given in small increments and slowly titrated to desired effect
		Little vascular irritation
		Given PO or nasally
		Short half-life
		Flumazenil effective for reversal
Pentobarbital	4 to 6 mg/kg IV	Can cause respiratory depression not responsive to flumazenil or naloxone
"DPT"	Up to: 2 mg/kg meperidine	Often causes prolonged sedation
	1 mg/kg promethazine	Often ineffective
	1 mg/kg chlorpromazine	Given IM, difficult to titrate to effect
		Serious side effects reported by some authors

is, in many ways, more appropriate for use as a sedative for short procedures. Midazolam is water-soluble at acidic pH, and its injectable form is buffered to a pH of 3.5. This means that propylene glycol and other irritant compounds are unnecessary to keep it in solution. It is compatible with many IV solutions and other medicines and does not cause the venous irritation that diazepam and lorazepam cause.[75] At physiologic pH, midazolam becomes highly lipid-soluble and has a rapid onset of action (about 5 minutes when given IV) and very short half-life (1 to 4 hours), leading to rapid recovery.[75]

Midazolam is two to four times more potent than diazepam.[74,75,81,108,115] It provides deeper sedation and more amnesia than diazepam, especially with painful experiences. It has faster onset of action and more rapid recovery.[12,75,108,115] It causes little or no vascular irritation when given intravenously and produces fewer vascular complications.[12,74,115] It does cause respiratory depression and may have a more narrow therapeutic window than diazepam in this regard.

White, Vasconez, Mathes, et al.[115] reported a steeper dose-response curve for midazolam than for diazepam. Other investigators[42] have reported similar degrees of respiratory depression for equivalent doses of these medicines. Midazolam decreases minute ventilation and ventilatory response to hypercapnea and hypoxia, as do other benzodiazepines.[2,42,75] Combining midazolam with fentanyl or other opioids enhances its respiratory depressant effects and may cause severe complications including death.[118] Respiratory depression relates not only to the dose given but also to its speed of administration: the faster the administration, the more likely apnea will result.[75]

Midazolam is reportedly safe to use in general EDs, in the

Table 12-5 Alternative Routes of Administration for Midazolam

Route	Dose
Intravenous	0.02 to 0.2 mg/kg
Oral	0.5 mg/kg
Intranasal	0.3 to 0.4 mg/kg

PICUs, and in a variety of pediatric procedures.* As with all respiratory depressants, use vigilant monitoring for side effects including pulse oximetry and appoint one individual whose only responsibility is to monitor the patient.

The intravenous dose of midazolam is 0.02 to 0.2 mg/kg.[81,82,94,107] Start off with a very small dose given slowly (Table 12-5). Repeat this dose slowly until the desired level of sedation up to a maximum dose 0.1 to 0.2 mg/kg is achieved. In adolescents and adults the initial dose may be up to 2 mg; the total dose should not exceed 5 mg. For prolonged sedation in the PICU, give a loading dose of 0.05 to 0.2 mg/kg, followed with an infusion of 1 to 2 μg/kg/min. If it is given in conjunction with opioid analgesics, the respiratory depressant effects of the two drugs may be synergistic and lead to an increased rate of complications.[118]

Midazolam may be used orally as a premedicant before anesthesia[65] and before ED procedures in children.[55] In a study of its effect on anxiolysis before laceration repair, 0.2 mg/kg of midazolam given orally produced effective anxiolysis without serious side effects in children less than 6

---

*References 38, 55, 78, 82, 94, 107, and 119.

Table 12-6   *Reversal Agents*

Agent	Dose	Remarks
Naloxone	Child 1 to 2-mg/dose Adolescent/adult 2-mg/dose For reversal of respiratory depression associated with analgesic overdosing, may give 0.01 to 0.1 mg/kg as needed and titrate to desired effect	Repeat dose as necessary up to 10 mg Effective for all opioids Often shorter duration of action than opioid; repeat dosing may be necessary
Flumazenil	0.01 to 0.02 mg/kg Adult 0.2 mg Repeat q1min until desired effect achieved up to a maximum of 1 mg	Effective for all benzodiazepines Not to be used as part of "coma protocol" Do not give in patients who have seizures or increased (ICP) or possible mixed ingestion

years of age.[55] Absorption of midazolam is rapid after oral administration, but only 40% to 50% is available because of extensive first-pass biotransformation in the liver.[75] Peak plasma concentrations occur about 1 hour after administration. This would suggest a possible need for larger doses in some children.

In a randomized, double-blind, placebo-controlled trial of midazolam given orally as an anesthesia premedicant, no difference in the degree of sedation or anxiolysis was observed among children given 0.5 mg/kg, 0.75 mg/kg, or 1 mg/kg of midazolam orally.[65] There were no serious side effects noted in any of the groups; the researchers observed minor side effects, including loss of balance and head control, blurred vision, and dysphoric reactions, only at the higher two doses and not with 0.5 mg/kg of midazolam orally. This suggests that 0.5 mg/kg may be the optimal dose of oral midazolam in children. Mask its bitter taste with sweet carrier vehicles such as liquid acetaminophen, apple juice, or chocolate-cherry syrup.[65]

Administration of midazolam by the intranasal route allows rapid absorption of the drug while bypassing the portal circulation.[116] An intranasal dose of 0.2 to 0.3 mg/kg produced effective anxiolysis and sedation as a preanesthetic agent.[116] No significant side effects occurred. It is also a good amnestic at this dose via this route.[2] Plasma concentrations of midazolam given intranasally peak in about 10 minutes and are about 57% of the peak concentration when given intravenously.[111] Use midazolam at doses of 0.2 to 0.5 mg/kg intranasally before suturing pediatric patients in the emergency department.[105,119] When given at 0.4 mg/kg, it is very effective and free of significant adverse effects. However, intranasal administration reportedly causes burning, irritation, and lacrimation, especially when given in large volumes to older children.[64a] Using a lidocaine nasal spray before midazolam administration[64a] or mixing the nasal dose with a drop of vanilla flavoring[88] has reportedly decreased the unpleasantness of administration.

Flumazenil. Flumazenil competitively blocks the effects of benzodiazepines on GABA-mediated inhibitory pathways in the central nervous system.[110] It can reverse the sedative effects of this class of medications and, to a lesser extent, the respiratory effects (Table 12-6). Its safety record includes many years of use in humans. Adverse effects may occur when it is given to patients with mixed medication overdoses (especially involving tricyclic antidepressants), to patients addicted to benzodiazepines, or to patients treated with benzodiazepines for increased intracranial pressure or status epilepticus. It is an excellent agent for the reversal of procedure-related benzodiazepine oversedation.

Flumazenil effectively reverses the effects of diazepam, lorazepam, and midazolam. In patients without the predisposing factors mentioned, it has a large therapeutic index.[62,110] When given intravenously, it has a rapid onset of action and an elimination half-life of 0.7 to 1.3 hours. Its duration of action is about 2 hours.[62,110] It reverses the sedation associated with benzodiazepines and increases tidal volume and minute ventilation but not the slope of the CO_2 response curve.[52] The duration of action of the benzodiazepines may be longer than that of flumazenil and may require repeated doses. After flumazenil administration, continue close observation of the patient until all of the effects of the benzodiazepines have dissipated.

The usual intravenous dose of flumazenil in adult patients is 0.2 mg. Repeat every minute as needed up to a total dose of 1 mg. Most patients respond to 0.6 to 1 mg. In the event of resedation, repeat every 20 minutes. Do not give patients more than 3 mg in any single hour and titrate the dose slowly. Intravenous injection produces intravascular irritation and inflammation.[78] No one has conducted clinical trials of flumazenil in pediatric patients, but intravenous doses of 0.01 to 0.02 mg/kg have produced good results.

PHENOTHIAZINES. For many years, physicians have used phenothiazines in combination with opioids for pain relief and sedation. They were formerly thought to potentiate the analgesic effect of narcotics. In most cases this is probably not true, and, with some agents, there may actually be an antianalgesic effect. Many practitioners still use phenothiazines in combination with meperidine as part of a "lytic cocktail" for analgesia and sedation before pediatric procedures.

Hydroxyzine, when given orally or intramuscularly, increases the amount of analgesia obtained from an opioid analgesic.[57] The combination of morphine and hydroxyzine also increases the incidence of drowsiness compared with that produced by morphine alone. A drawback of using this combination is the limitation to oral or intramuscular administration. Intramuscular injection is painful and most young children do not readily accept it. The dose of hydroxyzine is 0.5 mg/kg orally (may be given every 6 hours) or 0.5 to 1 mg/kg intramuscularly every 4 to 6 hours. The maximum single dosage is 100 mg.

The lytic cocktail is a combination of the drugs meperidine, promethazine, and chlorpromazine, traditionally known as DPT for the trade names of these drugs (Demerol, Phenergan, and Thorazine). Sometimes the abbreviation MPC, is used.[102,104] Although some recommend against the use of this combination of drugs, it remains a popular choice for sedation both for ED procedures and for painless diagnostic procedures, according to two recent surveys.[34,53] Administer the combination with a maximum dosage of 2 mg/kg of meperidine and 1 mg/kg of both promethazine and chlorpromazine.

Concerns regarding the use of this combination are many. Promethazine has a marked antianalgesic effect when given with opioids.[79] In addition, serious side effects, including orthostatic hypotension, ventilatory depression, and prolonged sedation, have occurred since the first use of DPT as a premedication for cardiac catheterization in the 1950s.[97,98] All three drugs are known to lower the seizure threshold, and unremitting seizures have led to death after their use.[98] In Smith, Rowe, and Vlad's original work,[97] in 3 of 670 patients severe respiratory depression developed and one fatality occurred. Also, 1 patient had cardiorespiratory arrest immediately after the administration of the cocktail, but resuscitation was successful.[97]

In a more recent study in patients receiving DPT, 4 of 95 patients, including 1 receiving only 0.07 ml/kg (1.75 mg/kg

of meperidine), experienced severe respiratory depression. Two thirds of the individuals in this series remained sedated for more than 7 hours. However, other authors[102,103] have pointed out the relatively low incidence of serious side effects (0% to 0.6%) when using this combination in a pediatric ED. However, average time to ED discharge was about 5 hours after administration of these drugs, and total ED time was about 9 hours.[103] Sedation was inadequate for 29% of patients. Omitting chlorpromazine further decreases the efficacy of this technique.[104]

All in all, the disadvantages of this combination of drugs seem to make other techniques for sedation that are safer, more easily titratable to effect, and deliverable by a nonintramuscular route more attractive.

REMARKS

Pain and anxiety have always accompanied pediatric patients in EDs and acute-care settings. Only relatively recently have medical professionals acknowledged and addressed these sensations. Health care professionals who care for children must recognize pain and anxiety in their patients and treat them in a safe and effective way. Forcibly restraining a child without the benefit of appropriate sedation and analgesia is not appropriate with the pharmacologic techniques available today.

Professionals who deal with children in these settings must be open-minded and willing to incorporate new safe and effective techniques into their practice. Collaboration with and instruction from colleagues in dentistry, oncology, and anesthesia will promote the development of safe, effective,

Table 12-7 Usual Agents for Management of Pain and Sedation in Pediatric Patients

Procedure or situation*	Analgesia	Sedation
Burn care (major)	Morphine PO, IV	Lorazepam PO, IV, midazolam IN, PO, IV
Burn care (minor)	NSAID PO; codeine PO; morphine PO, IV	Midazolam IN, PO, IV
Central line placement	Local anesthetic; morphine PO, IV	Midazolam IN, PO, IV
Chest tube placement/removal	Local anesthetic; morphine PO, IV	Midazolam IN, PO, IV
I & D	Local anesthetic; morphine PO, IV	Midazolam IN, PO, IV
Laceration repair	Local anesthetic; morphine PO, IV; fentanyl IV	Midazolam IN, PO, IV
Digital nail removal	Local anesthetic (digital block), morphine PO, IV	Midazolam IN, PO, IV
IV placement	EMLA; local anesthetic	
Lumbar puncture	EMLA; local anesthetic	Midazolam IN, PO, IV
Sexual abuse examination		Midazolam IN, PO, IV; ketamine IV
Arthrocentesis	Local anesthetic; morphine PO, IV, fentanyl IV	Midazolam IN, PO, IV
Fracture/dislocation reduction	Local anesthetic; morphine IV; fentanyl IV	Midazolam IV
MRI/CT scans		Pentobarbital IV; chloral hydrate PO, PR; midazolam po, in, iv
Sickle cell crisis pain	NSAID PO, IV; codeine and acetaminophen PO; morphine PO, IV	
Otitis media	Local anesthetic; acetaminophen or NSAID PO; codeine PO	

*Specific agent and route of administration should be guided by your familiarity with the agent and the clinical response of the patient. PO, IN, or PR administration is usually better accepted by patients than IV administration. IV administration allows more precise titration to effect. Equianalgesic doses have similar degrees of complications, regardless of route of administration.

I & D, Incision and drainage; *NSAID,* nonsteroidal antiinflammatory drug; *IV,* intravenous; *IN,* intranasal; *EMLA,* eutectic mixture of local anesthetics; *MRI,* magnetic resonance imaging; *CT,* computed tomography.

and "patient-friendly" alternatives for analgesia and sedation in the pediatric patient. New routes of administration, as well as new agents need investigation.

There is no truly ideal sedative or analgesic agent for use in these settings. It is probably less important to know all of the agents than to know well and be very comfortable with one or two agents appropriate to each of the routine clinical situations. Choose the correct agent for the particular clinical situation. Use an analgesic if a procedure or condition is painful. Some sedatives are more appropriate for painless procedures. Even minor medical conditions and injuries (e.g., otitis media, minor lacerations) are painful; do not forget symptomatic analgesia while completing or prescribing definitive treatment.

The concept of the analgesic ladder aids in matching the potency of the prescribed analgesic with the severity of pain. If the first medicine used is not effective, add a second, possibly synergistic agent. In patients with moderate-to-severe pain, quickly get pain under control. Intravenous medicines are less painful and can be better titrated than medicines given intramuscularly.

No one has yet discovered the ideal sedative that will be easy to administer in a painless way; has a quick and predictable onset of action, a predictable duration of action, and a rapid recovery period; is always effective; and has no side effects. Use agents that approach this ideal as closely as possible. Painless routes of administration are preferable. Flavorings may make oral preparations more palatable. Dilution, flavorings, or pretreatment with lidocaine may make nasal administration better tolerated. The benzodiazepine reversal agent flumazenil has made these compounds even safer to use for procedural sedation.

Certain groups are at an increased risk of side effects from potent analgesics and sedatives. Infants, children with respiratory disease or neurologic dysfunction, and children who have suffered head injuries or who are multiple trauma victims all run a higher risk of respiratory or cardiovascular compromise when using these agents. This does not absolutely preclude the use of appropriate analgesics and sedatives in these children (Table 12-7). However, vigilant monitoring of cardiorespiratory and neurologic status is even more important in these patients. Closely monitor all patients according to published guidelines.[5]

"Few things a doctor does are more important than relieving pain. . . . Pain is soul destroying. . . . The quality of mercy is essential to the practice of medicine; here of all places, it should not be strained."[10] Children feel pain. They are anxious and frightened. As competent professionals and caring, humane people we must recognize this and treat them appropriately.

REFERENCES

1. Acute Pain Management Guideline Panel: Acute pain in infants, children and adolescents: operative and medical procedures, quick reference guide for clinicians, AHCPR Pub No 92-0020, Rockville, Md, Agency for Health Care Policy and Research, Public Health Service, US Department of Health and Human Services.
2. Alexander CM, Gross JB: Sedative doses of midazolam depress hypoxic ventilatory responses in humans, *Anesth Analg* 67:377-382, 1988.
3. Allison MC, Howatson AG, Torrance CJ et al: Gastrointestinal damage associated with the use of nonsteroidal antiinflammatory drugs, *N Engl J Med* 327:749-754, 1992.
4. Amadio P, Jr: Peripherally acting analgesics, *Am J Med* 77:17-26, 1984.
5. American Academy of Pediatrics Committee on Drugs: Guidelines for monitoring and management of pediatric patients during and after sedation for diagnostic and therapeutic procedures, *Pediatrics* 89:1110-1115, 1992.
6. Anand KJS, Aynsley-Green A: Metabolic and endocrine effects of surgical ligation of patent ductus asteriosus in the human preterm neonate: are there implications for further improvement of postoperative outcome? *Mod Probl Pediatr* 23:143-157, 1985.
7. Anand KJS, Hickey PR: Halothane-morphine compared with high dose sufentanil for anesthesia and postoperative analgesia in neonatal cardiac surgery, *N Engl J Med* 326:1-9, 1992.
8. Anand KJS, Sippell WG, Aynsley-Green A: Randomized trial of fentanyl anesthesia in preterm babies undergoing surgery: effects on the stress response, *Lancet* 1:62-66, 1987.
9. Anderson CTM, Zeltzer LK, Fancerik D: Procedural pain. In Schechter NL, Berde CB, Yaster M, editors: *Pain in infants, children and adolescents,* Baltimore, 1993, Williams & Wilkins.
10. Angell M: The quality of mercy, *N Engl J Med* 306:98-99, 1982.
11. Arandia HY, Patil VU: Glottic closure following large doses of fentanyl, *Anesthesiology* 66:574-575, 1987.
12. Aun C, Flynn PJ, Richards J et al: A comparison of midazolam and diazepam for intravenous sedation in dentistry, *Anaesthesiology* 39:589-593, 1984.
13. Bailey PL, Race NL, Ashburn MA, et al.: Frequent hypoxemia and apnea after sedation with midazolam and fentanyl, *Anesthesiology* 73:826-830, 1990.
14. Beales JG, Keen JH, Holt PJL: The child's perception of the disease and the experience of pain in juvenile chronic arthritis, *J Rheumatol* 10:61-65, 1983.
15. Beaver WT: Combination analgesics, *Am J Med* 77:38-53, 1984.
16. Berde C, Albin A, Glazer J, et al: Report of the subcommittee on disease-related pain in childhood cancer, *Pediatrics* 86:818-825, 1990.
17. Bergman I, Steves M, Burchart G, et al: Reversible neurologic abnormalities associated with prolonged intravenous midazolam and fentanyl administration, *J Pediatr* 119:644-649, 1991.
18. Beyer JL, DeGood DE, Ashley LC, et al: Patterns of postoperative analgesia use with adults and children following cardiac surgery, *Pain* 17:71-81, 1983.
19. Bhat R, Abu-Harb M, Chari G, et al. Morphine metabolism in acutely ill preterm newborn infants, *J Pediatr* 120:795-799, 1992.
20. Biban P, Baraldi E, Pettenazzo A et al: Adverse effect of chloral hydrate in two young children with obstructive sleep apnea, *Pediatrics* 92:461-462, 1993.
21. Billmire DA, Neale HW, Gregory RO: Use of IV fentanyl in the outpatient treatment of pediatric facial trauma, *J Trauma* 25:1079-1080, 1985.
22. Binder LS, Leake LA: Chloral hydrate for emergency pediatric procedural sedation: a new look at an old drug, *Am J Emerg Med* 9:530-534, 1991.
23. Brewer EJ, Jr, Arroyo I: Use of nonsteroidal anti-inflammatory drugs in children, *Pediatr Ann* 15:575-581, 1986.
24. Broennle AM, Cohen DE: Pediatric anesthesia and sedation, *Curr Opin Pediatr* 5:310-314, 1993.
25. Camu F, Overberge LV, Bullingham R et al. Hemodynamic effects of two intravenous doses of ketorolac tromethamine compared with morphine, *Pharmacotherapy* 10:122S-126S, 1990.
26. Catchlove RFH, Kafer ER: The effects of diazepam on the ventilatory response to carbon dioxide and a steady-state gas exchange, *Anesthesiology* 34:9-13, 1971.
27. Chudnofsky CR, Wright SW, Dronew SC, et al: The safety of fentanyl use in the emergency department, *Ann Emerg Med* 18:635-639, 1989.
28. Cohen AR: Hematologic emergencies. In Fleisher GR, Ludwig S, editors: *Textbook of pediatric emergency medicine,* ed 3, Baltimore, 1993, Williams & Wilkins.
29. Cohen DE, Downes JJ, Rapaely RC: What difference does pulse oximetry make? *Anesthesiology* 68:181-183, 1988.
30. Cole TB, Sprinkle RH, Smith SJ, et al: Intravenous narcotic therapy for children with severe sickle cell pain crisis, *Am J Dis Child* 140:1255-1259, 1986.
31. Committees on Drugs and Environmental Health: Use of chloral hydrate for sedation in children, *Pediatrics* 92:471-473, 1993.

32. Comroe JH Jr, Bothello S: The unreliability of cyanosis in the recognition of arterial anoxemia, *Am J Med Sci* 214:1-6, 1947.

33. Comstock MK, Seaman FL, Carter JG, et al: Rigidity and hypercarbia on fentanyl-oxygen induction, *Anesthesiology* 51:528, 1979 (abstract).

34. Cook BA, Bass JW, Nomizu S, et al. Sedation of children for technical procedures: current standard of practice, *Clin Pediatr* 31:137-142, 1992.

35. Cote CJ, Goldstein EA, Cote MA, et al: A single-blind study of pulse oximetry in children, *Anesthesiology* 68:184-188, 1988.

36. Dalen JE, Evans GL, Banas JS, Jr et al: The hemodynamic and respiratory effects of diazepam (Valium), *Anesthesiology* 30:259-263, 1969.

37. Daniel FB, DeAngelo AB, Stokes JA, et al: Hepatocarcinogenicity of chloral hydrate, 2-chloroaceteldehyde, dichloroacetic acid in the male B6C3F1 mouse, *Fundam Appl Toxicol* 19:159-168, 1992.

38. Diament MJ, Stanley P: The use of midazolam for sedation of infants and children, *Am J Roentgenol* 150:377-378, 1988.

39. Eland JM, Anderson JE: The experience of pain in children. In Jacox A, editor: *Pain: a sourcebook for nurses and other health professionals,* Boston, 1977, Little, Brown.

40. Ehrlich HP: Anti-inflammatory drugs in the vascular response to burn injury, *J Trauma* 24:311-318, 1984.

41. Fassler B, Wallace N: Children's fear of needles, *Clinical Pediatrics* 21:59-60, 1982.

42. Forster A, Gardoz JP, Suter PM et al: Respiratory depression by midazolam and diazepam, *Anesthesiology* 53:494-497, 1980.

43. Fox BES, O'Brien CO, Kangas KJ et al: Use of high dose chloral hydrate for ophthalmologic exams in children: a retrospective review of 302 cases, *J Pediatr Ophthalmol Strabismus* 27:242-244, 1990.

44. Friedland LR, Kulick RM: Emergency department analgesic use in pediatric trauma victims with fractures, *Ann Emerg Med* 23:203-207, 1994.

45. Friesen RH, Lockhart CH: Oral transmucosal fentanyl citrate for preanesthetic medication of pediatric day surgery patients with and without droperidol as a prophylactic anti-emetic, *Anesthesiology* 76:46-51, 1992.

46. Goldstein-Dresner MC, Davis PJ, Kretchman E, et al: Double-blind comparison of oral transmucosal fentanyl citrate with oral meperidine, diazepam, and atropine as preanesthetic medication in children with congenital heart disease, *Anesthesiology* 74:28-33, 1991.

47. Greenberg SB, Faerber EN: Respiratory insufficiency following chloral hydrate sedation in two children with Leigh disease (subacute necrotizing encephalomyelopathy), *Pediatr Radiol* 20:287-288, 1990.

48. Greenberg SB, Faerber EN, Aspirall CL: High dose chloral hydrate sedation for children undergoing CT, *J Comput Assist Tomogr* 15:467-469, 1991.

49. Greenberg SB, Faerber EN, Aspinall CL, et al: High dose chloral hydrate sedation for children undergoing MR imaging: safety and efficacy in relation to age, *Am J Roentgenol* 161:6319-6341, 1993.

50. Greenblatt DJ, Ehrenberg BL, Gunderman J, et al: Pharmacokinetic and encephalographic study of intravenous diazepam, midazolam and placebo, *Clin Pharmacol Ther* 45:356-365, 1989.

51. Gross JB, Smith L, Smith TC: Time course of ventilatory response to carbon dioxide after intravenous diazepam, *Anesthesiology* 57:18-21, 1982.

52. Gross JB, Weller RS, Conrad P: Flumazenil antagonism of midazolam-induced ventilatory depression, *Anesthesiology* 75:179-185, 1991.

53. Hawk W, Crockett RK, Ochsenschlager DW, et al: Conscious sedation of the pediatric patient for suturing: a survey, *Pediatr Emerg Care* 6:84-88, 1990.

54. Hertzka RE, Gauntlett IS, Fisher DM et al: Fentanyl-induced respiratory depression: effects of age, *Anesthesiology* 70:213-218, 1989.

55. Hennes HM, Wagner V, Bonadio WA, et al: The effect of oral midazolam on anxiety of preschool children during laceration repair, *Ann Emerg Med* 19:1006-1009, 1990.

56. Hubbard AM, Markowitz RI, Kimmel B, et al: Sedation for pediatric patients undergoing CT and MRI, *J Comput Assist Tomogr* 16:3-6, 1992.

57. Hupert C, Yacoub M, Turgeon LR: Effect of hydroxyzine or morphine analgesia for the treatment of postoperative pain, *Anesth Analg* 59:6190-6196, 1980.

58. International Association for the Study of Pain, Subcommittee on Taxonomy: Pain terms: a list with definitions and notes on usage, *Pain* 6:249, 1979.

59. Inturrisi CE: Role of opioid analgesics, *Am J Med* 77:27-37, 1984.

60. Kenny GNC, McArdle C, Aitken HH: Parenteral ketorolac: opiate sparing effect and lack of cardiorespiratory depression in the perioperative patient, *Pharmacotherapy* 10:127S-131S, 1990.

61. Lane JC, Tennison MB, Lawless ST, et al: Movement disorder after withdrawal of fentanyl infusion, *J Pediatr* 119:649-651, 1991.

62. Lauren PM, Schwilden H, Stoeckel H, et al: The effects of a benzodiazepine antagonist Ro 15-1788 in the presence of stable concentrations of midazolam, *Anesthesiology* 63:61-64, 1985.

63. Laxer RM, Silverman ED, Balfe JW, et al: Naproxen-associated renal failure in a child with arthritis and inflammatory bowel disease, *Pediatrics* 80:904-908, 1987.

64. Lind GH, Marcus MA, Mears SL, et al: Oral transmucosal fentanyl citrate for analgesia and sedation in the emergency department, *Ann Emerg Med* 20:1117-1120, 1991.

64a. Lugo RA, Fishbein M, Nahata MC, et al: Complications of intranasal midazolam, *Pediatrics* 92:638, 1993.

65. McMillan CO, Spahr-Schopfer IA, Sikichn N, et al: Premedication of children with oral midazolam, *Can J Anesth* 39:545-550, 1992.

66. Mitchell AA, Louik C, Lacouture P, et al: Risks to children from computed tomographic scan premedication, *JAMA* 247:2385-2388, 1982.

67. Nahata MC, Clotz MA, Krogg EA: Adverse effects of meperidine, promethazine, and chlorpromazine for sedation in pediatric patients, *Clin Pediatr* 24:558-560, 1985.

68. Neuman GG, Kushins LG, Ferrante S: Sedation for children undergoing magnetic resonance imaging and computed tomography, *Anesth Analg* 74:931-932, 1992 (letter).

69. Paris PM: No pain, no pain, *Am J Emerg Med* 7:660-662, 1989.

70. Paris PM: Pain management in the child, *Emerg Med Clin North Am* 5:699-707, 1987.

71. Pierce RJ, Fragen RJ, Pemberton DM: Intravenous ketorolac tromethamine versus morphine sulfate in the treatment of immediate postoperative pain, *Pharmacotherapy* 10:111S-115S, 1990.

72. Porter J, Jick H: Addiction rare in patients treated with narcotics, *N Engl J Med* 302:123, 1980 (letter).

73. Rana SR: Pain: a subject ignored, *Pediatrics* 79:309, 1987 (letter).

74. Reves JG: *Plastic Reconstr Surg* 81:711-712, 1988.

75. Reves JG, Fragen RJ, Vinik HR, et al: Midazolam: pharmacology and uses, *Anesthesiology* 63:310-324, 1985.

76. Robinson J, Malleson P, Lirenman D, et al: Nephrotic syndrome associated with nonsteroidal anti-inflammatory drug use in two children, *Pediatrics* 85:844-847, 1990.

77. Romagnoli A, Keats AS: Ceiling effect for respiratory depression by nalbuphine, *Clin Pharmacol Ther* 27:478-485, 1980.

78. Romazicon product information.

79. Ros SP: Outpatient pediatric analgesia: a tale of two regimens, *Pediatr Emerg Care* 3:228-230, 1987.

80. Rumm PD, Jakao RT, Fox DJ, et al: Efficacy of sedation of children with chloral hydrate, *South Med J* 83:1040-1042, 1990.

81. Sacchetti A, Schafermeyer R, Gerardi M, et al: Pediatric analgesia and sedation, *Ann Emerg Med* 23:237-250, 1994.

82. Sandler ES, Weyman C, Conner K, et al: Midazolam versus fentanyl as premedication for painful procedures in children with cancer, *Pediatrics* 89:631-634, 1992.

83. Schechter NL: Pain: acknowledging it, assessing it, treating it, *Contemp Pediatr* 4:15-46, 1987.

84. Schechter NL: Pain and pain control in children, *Curr Probl Pediatr* 15:6-67, 1985.

85. Schechter NL: The undertreatment of pain in children: an overview, *Pediatr Clin North Am* 36:781-794, 1989.

86. Schechter NL, Allen DA, Hanson K: Status of pediatric pain control: a comparison of hospital analgesic usage in children and adults, *Pediatrics* 77:11-15, 1986.

87. Schechter NL, Bernstein BA, Beck A, et al: Individual differences in children's response to pain: role of temperament and parental characteristics, *Pediatrics* 87:171-177, 1991.

88. Schuman AJ: A protocol for pediatric sedation, *Contemp Pediatr* 11:74-89, 1994.

89. Selbst SM: Managing pain in the pediatric emergency department, *Pediatr Emerg Care* 5:56-63, 1989.

90. Selbst SM: Pain management in the emergency department. In Schechter NL, Berde CB, Yaster M, editors: *Pain in infants, children and adolescents,* Baltimore, 1993, Williams & Wilkins.

91. Selbst SM, Clark M: Analgesic use in the emergency department, *Ann Emerg Med* 19:1010-1013, 1990.

92. Selbst SM, Henretig FM: The treatment of pain in the emergency department, *Pediatr Clin North Am* 36:965-978, 1989.

93. Shellock FG, Slimp GL: Severe burn of the finger caused by using a pulse oximeter during MR imaging, *Am J Roentgenol* 153:1105, 1989.

94. Sievers TD, Yee J, Foley ME, et al: Midazolam for conscious sedation during pediatric oncology procedures: safety and recovery parameters, *Pediatrics* 88:1172-1179, 1991.

95. Singleton MA, Rosen JI, Fisher DM: Plasma concentrations of fentanyl in infants, children and adults, *Can J Anaesth* 34:152-155, 1987.

96. Smith MT: Chloral hydrate warning, *Science* 250:359, 1990.

97. Smith C, Rowe RD, Vlad P: Sedation of children for cardiac catheterization with ataractic mixture, *Can J Anaesth* 5:35-43, 1985.

98. Snodgrass WR, Dodge WF: Lytic "DPT" cocktail: time for rational and safe alternatives, *Pediatr Clin North Am* 36:1285-1289, 1989.

99. Southall DP, Cronin BC, Hartmann H: Invasive procedures in children receiving intensive care, *Br Med J* 306:1512-1513, 1993.

100. Spiro HM: Visceral viewpoints: pain and perfectionism—the physician and the "pain patient," *N Engl J Med* 294:829-830, 1974.

101. Steinberg AD: Should chloral hydrate be banned? *Pediatrics* 92:442-446, 1993.

102. Terndrup TE, Carton RM, Madden CM: Intramuscular meperidine, promethazine, and chlorpromazine: analysis of use and complications in 487 pediatric emergency department patients, *Ann Emerg Med* 18:528-533, 1989.

103. Terndrup TE, Dire DJ, Madden CM, et al: A prospective analysis of intramuscular meperidine, promethazine and chlorpromazine in pediatric emergency department patients, *Ann Emerg Med* 20:31-35, 1991.

104. Terndrup TE, Dire DJ, Madden CM, et al: Comparison of intramuscular meperidine and promethazine with and without chlorpromazine: a randomized, prospective, double-blind trial, *Ann Emerg Med* 22:206-211, 1993.

105. Theroux MC, West DW, Corddry DH, et al: Efficacy of intranasal midazolam in facilitating suturing of lacerations in preschool children in the emergency department, *Pediatrics* 91:624-627, 1993.

106. Thompson JR, Schneider S, Ashwal S, et al: The choice of sedation for computed tomography in children: a prospective evaluation, *Radiology* 143:475-479, 1982.

107. Tolia V, Brennan S, Aravind MK, et al: Pharmacokinetic and pharmacodynamic study of midazolam in children during esophagastroduodenoscopy, *J Pediatr* 119:467-471, 1991.

108. Tolia V, Fleming SL, Kauffman RE: Randomized, double-blind trial of midazolam and diazepam for endoscopic sedation in children, *Dev Pharmacol Ther* 14:141-147, 1990.

109. Twersky RS, Hartung J, McClain J, et al: Intranasal midazolam: its effect on memory in pediatric patients, *Anesthesiology* 75A:919, 1991 (abstract).

110. Voetey Sr, Bosse GM, Bayer MJ, et al: Flumazenil: a new benzodiazepine antagonist, *Ann Emerg Med* 20:181-188, 1991.

111. Walbergh EJ, Wills RJ, Eckhert J: Plasma concentrations of midazolam in children following intranasal administration, *Anesthesiology* 74:233-235, 1991.

112. Way WL, Costley EC, Way EL: Respiratory sensitivity of the newborn infant to meperidine and morphine, *Clin Pharmacol Ther* 6:454-461, 1965.

113. Weinberger M: Analgesic sensitivity in children with asthma, *Pediatrics* 62:910-915, 1978.

114. Weisman SJ, Schechter NL: The management of pain in children, *Pediatr Rev* 12:237-243, 1991.

115. White PF, Vasconez LO, Mathes SA, et al: Comparison of midazolam and diazepam for sedation during plastic surgery, *Plastic Reconstr Surg* 81:703-710, 1988.

116. Wilton NCT, Leigh J, Roscu DR, et al: Preanesthetic sedation of preschool children using intranasal midazolam, *Anesthesiology* 69:972-975, 1988.

117. Yaster M, Deshpande JK: Management of pediatric pain with opioid analgesics, *J Pediatr* 113:421-429, 1988.

118. Yaster M, Nichols DG, Deshprude JK: Midazolam-fentanyl intravenous sedation in children: case report of respiratory arrest, *Pediatrics* 86:463-466, 1990.

119. Yealy DM, Ellis JH, Hobbs GD, et al: Intranasal midazolam as a sedative for children during laceration repair, *Am J Emerg Med* 10:584-587, 1992.

120. Zeltzer LK, Jay SM, Fisher DM: The management of pain associated with pediatric procedures, *Pediatr Clin North Am* 36:941-964, 1989.

13 Sedation and Pain Relief: Other Agents

Norbert Froese and Andrew J. Costarino, Jr.

KETAMINE

Ketamine, an intravenous anesthetic derived from the hallucinogen phencyclidine, can be administered in subanesthetic doses to produce conscious sedation, analgesia, and amnesia.

Children sedated with ketamine seem to be disconnected from their surrounding environment. This state, termed *dissociative anesthesia,* results from functional and electrophysiologic separation of the cortex from the limbic systems[10] and is believed to be a result of ketamine's interaction with central nervous system N-methyl-D-aspartate (NMDA) receptors.[27] Even when deeply sedated, children may appear to be awake with open eyes and may vocalize or display random movements.

The onset of sedation after intravenous administration of ketamine is rapid, occurring within minutes. After a single intravenous dose, its effect is intermediate in duration, lasting approximately 15 minutes, and is related to the redistribution of ketamine from the central nervous system to more peripheral sites. With repeated administration or continuous infusion, the effect of ketamine depends on its elimination half-life and is considerably prolonged. Clearance of ketamine occurs via hepatic metabolism, and in children the elimination half-life is between 1½ and 2 hours.[9]

The onset of sedation with ketamine is slower after intramuscular administration, occurring in 5 to 10 minutes, and the duration of action is lengthened. First-pass metabolism, which describes hepatic clearance of enterally absorbed ketamine before it reaches the systemic circulation, and incomplete absorption account for an increased dose requirement for ketamine administered by mouth. Sedation after oral administration occurs in 15 to 45 minutes and dissipates within 2 hours.[25]

Indications

Ketamine provides intense analgesia at subanesthetic doses; therefore, use it to provide sedation for painful procedures.

When ketamine is used in doses resulting in conscious sedation, respiratory rate, tidal volume, and minute ventilation are minimally affected. Pharyngeal and laryngeal function, as well as other airway protective reflexes such as coughing and swallowing, are relatively unimpaired with ketamine sedation,[10] and therefore the risk of airway compromise in spontaneously breathing patients is lower with ketamine than other sedative agents.

Ketamine indirectly stimulates the sympathetic nervous system, resulting in increases in heart rate, blood pressure, and cardiac output. This provides for an increased margin of safety when ketamine is administered to patients with decreased intravascular volume or impaired myocardial function. Pulmonary vascular resistance in children is not affected by ketamine sedation, and ketamine may be safely administered to patients with cyanotic heart disease.[16]

Contraindications

Do not use ketamine in circumstances where the personnel and equipment required for cardiorespiratory monitoring; advanced airway management, including tracheal intubation; and circulatory resuscitation are not immediately available. Ketamine is a potent sedative and ketamine-induced sedation may progress to loss of consciousness and general anesthesia. In this circumstance, airway protective reflexes are lost and ventilatory response to carbon dioxide is depressed,[14] leaving the patient at risk for hypoventilation, respiratory obstruction, and aspiration of gastric contents.[19]

Ketamine sedation may be contraindicated in patients with increased intracranial pressure. Although intracranial pressure has been shown to rise after administration of ketamine secondary to cerebral vasodilation and increases in cerebral blood flow,[10,24] other workers have failed to demonstrate a direct effect of ketamine on the cerebral vasculature and indict ketamine-induced hypoventilation and hypercarbia as the causes of the increased intracranial pressure.[20] More recent understanding of the role of NMDA receptor stimulation in secondary central nervous system injury leads to speculation about a possible neuroprotective role for ketamine via NMDA receptor blockade.

Complications

Emergence from ketamine-induced sedation can be associated with psychic disturbances, manifested as dysphoric dreams and hallucinations. This problem is less common in children than in adults and is rare in children less than 10 years old.[10] Nonetheless, prolonged emotional disturbances related to ketamine administration have been reported in patients as young as 3 years.[18] These phenomena can be reduced or eliminated with the concomitant administration of a benzodiazepine.[21,26] When used for this purpose, midazolam is preferred to diazepam.

Administration of ketamine stimulates salivary secretions, causing potential airway obstruction and tracheal aspiration of secretions. Excess salivation can effectively be prevented by prior administration of an antisialagogue such as atropine or glycopyrrolate.

Ketamine's increase in cardiac output and blood pressure occurs indirectly, via stimulation of the sympathetic nervous system, and cannot be relied on in hemodynamically unstable patients. In these patients, ketamine can cause circulatory deterioration, through either a direct cardiac depressant effect or sedation-induced reduction of endogenous catecholamine release. Therefore administer ketamine by titration of small doses with careful hemodynamic monitoring.

The random movements that occur with ketamine sedation decrease the usefulness of this drug as a sedative for imaging procedures.

Equipment

Minimum monitoring equipment for ketamine sedation consists of a pulse oximeter and noninvasive blood pressure measurement. In addition, keep electrocardiographic (ECG) monitoring, airway management, and vascular access equipment immediately available.[1]

Techniques

Intravenous administration of ketamine allows for precise titration of dose to effect. A total dose of 0.25 to 1 mg/kg provides analgesia and sedation for short procedures. Preventing excessive or inadequate sedation with ketamine is more difficult in intramuscular administration because of variable absorption and lack of titratability. A wide variety of intramuscular doses has been advocated, depending on desired goals. In Green et al., a study of 109 pediatric patients in an emergency department setting, consistent deep sedation was achieved with 4 mg/kg with only 4% of patients exhibiting a withdrawal response.[11]

Oral administration of ketamine has even less predicable results. Gutstein, Johnson, Heard, et al. studied oral ketamine administration in doses of 3 and 6 mg/kg as a sedative before induction of anesthesia in healthy children aged 1 to 7 years.[13] They found that a dose of 3 mg/kg did not reliably produce adequate sedation, yet 13 of 100 children given 6 mg/kg were described as "barely arousable" and deeply sedated. When administered in doses of 10 mg/kg, oral ketamine produces deep sedation,[25] requiring additional personnel and monitoring for safe administration.

Administer atropine 0.01 mg/kg or glycopyrrolate 0.005 mg/kg (maximum 0.25 mg) concomitantly with ketamine to decrease salivation. Consider giving a relatively low dose of midazolam, 0.05 mg/kg intravenously (IV), before ketamine administration to help prevent dysphoric effects.

NITROUS OXIDE

Nitrous oxide is a colorless gas that, when inhaled in appropriate concentrations with oxygen, can provide safe, effective analgesia and sedation. Its effects are proportional to its partial pressure in the cerebral circulation. It is poorly soluble in body fluids, causing small changes in nitrous oxide blood content to result in large changes in nitrous oxide partial pressure. This allows for rapid onset, as well as rapid termination, of its effects. Safe administration requires specialized equipment and patient cooperation.

Indications

Nitrous oxide is particularly useful for providing pain relief and sedation during short procedures that do not entail significant residual discomfort. Its effective use has been described in the pediatric population for simple laceration repair[6] and a variety of other minor surgical procedures.[12] Because of its administration by inhalation, oversedation is a lesser risk with nitrous oxide than with conventionally administered sedatives. Central nervous system nitrous oxide concentrations cannot exceed the partial pressure of the agent in the administered gas, and accumulation of nitrous oxide cannot occur. When it is used in concentrations of 50% or less, there is little risk of inducing anesthesia or loss of airway reflexes.[23]

Contraindications

Nitrous oxide concentrations of at least 30% are required to provide effective analgesia and concentrations of 50% may be necessary.[6] Therefore effective use of nitrous oxide prevents simultaneous administration of high concentrations of inspired oxygen to patients with respiratory disease. This problem is exacerbated at high altitude, where the decreased barometric pressure necessitates that an even greater fraction of the inspired gas be nitrous oxide to achieve equivalent analgesic and sedative effects.[17]

Do not administer nitrous oxide to patients with illness or injury conditions associated with closed nitrogen-containing spaces such as pneumothorax, bowel obstruction, decompression sickness, or blocked eustachian tubes. Similarly, do not use it for procedures requiring balloon-tipped vascular catheters such as pulmonary artery catheters. The rapid diffusion of nitrous oxide into a closed cavity, combined with the inability of nitrogen to leave the space quickly, causes an increase in volume of an expandable space such as a pneumothorax or an increase in pressure of a confined space, such as the middle ear.

Complications

Diffusion hypoxia, hypoxia due to the dilution of alveolar oxygen by nitrous oxide that leaves the blood stream immediately after discontinuation of nitrous oxide analgesia, is a classic complication of its use. However, diffusion hypoxia is unlikely when concentrations of nitrous oxide of 50% or less are used.[22]

Nausea and vomiting are uncommon complications of nitrous oxide sedation. Gamis, Knapp, and Glenski found an incidence of 1 in 34 cases in a prospective study of 30% nitrous oxide sedation in children.[6]

Nitrous oxide has little effect on respiration, heart rate, blood pressure, or cardiac output, provided additional sedative medications are not concomitantly used.

Equipment

The safe administration of nitrous oxide requires specialized equipment. Use a demand-type regulator, which requires inspiratory effort to begin gas flow, in conjunction with a face mask with older children and adults. Because younger children have difficulty opening the demand valve, use a valveless breathing circuit. Griffin, Campbell, and Jones[12] described the use of nasal masks to deliver continuous-flow nitrous oxide/oxygen to approximately 3000 children. These authors stressed the additional safety of leaving the mouth uncovered.

Nitrous oxide and oxygen can be derived from separate sources and combined in a mixer before patient delivery or can be delivered from a single cylinder of premixed 50:50 nitrous oxide/oxygen. Sources of pure gases can be either wall outlets or cylinders. When a mixer is used, safeguards to prevent inadvertent crossover of gases, such as standardized coloring of connecting hoses and tanks, the Diameter Index Safety system for wall outlets, and the Pin Index Safety system for cylinders, are mandatory.[3a] The mixer must be designed to prevent the administration of less than 20% oxygen and be equipped with a mechanism to shut off the nitrous oxide supply automatically in the event of loss of oxygen pressure. If premixed cylinders are used, prevent exposure of the cylinders to temperatures of less than −5.5° C, as the nitrous oxide and oxygen will separate in these conditions and may incompletely remix upon rewarming. In all cases, use a properly functioning and accurately calibrated oxygen analyzer placed in line with the administered gas as a safeguard against the delivery of a hypoxic gas mixture.

Concern about the safety of prolonged exposure of healthcare personnel to low concentrations of nitrous oxide has led to the recommendation that nitrous oxide delivery systems be equipped with gas scavenging devices.[3,4] This equipment reduces ambient concentrations of nitrous oxide in an Emergency Department (ED) to near-zero levels.[3]

The use of a pulse oximeter is desirable, but not required, with 50% nitrous oxide in oxygen for a healthy patient. Keep available advanced monitoring and resuscitative equipment.[1]

Techniques

Administer nitrous oxide for 3 to 5 minutes before beginning the procedure.

Self-administration of nitrous oxide via a face mask is the preferred method of delivery in older children and adults.[23] Oversedation is unlikely to occur with this technique, since loss of consciousness will cause the mask to fall off the face. In cases in which the patient's hands are unavailable to hold the mask, provide a mouthpiece and instruct the patient to breathe through the mouth only.[23] Younger patients are unable to self-administer nitrous oxide, and nasal masks have been used successfully in this population.[12]

PROPOFOL

Propofol is an alkylphenol intravenous anesthetic lacking analgesic properties that produces sedation when administered in subanesthetic doses. It is insoluble in water and is prepared as an emulsion in an aqueous solution of soy bean oil, glycerol, and egg phosphatide.

Indications

Propofol is well suited for providing sedation for imaging studies or other procedures not associated with significant pain.[5] It is rapidly cleared from the circulation. Its short duration of action of 5 to 10 minutes requires administration by continuous infusion, which allows for precise control of the level of sedation by adjustment of the infusion rate.

Contraindications

Propofol is a potent sedative associated with significant respiratory depression. Loss of consciousness, airway obstruction, and apnea can occur, as well as marked cardiovascular depression. Therefore, as for ketamine, do not use propofol in settings where the equipment and personnel required for providing deep sedation are unavailable.

Complications

Because of its lack of analgesic properties, propofol cannot be used effectively as a single agent for sedation for painful procedures. Pain at the site of injection is a frequent complication of propofol administration. Minimize this complication by using a large antecubital vein, as opposed to a hand

vein[15]; slowing the speed of injection[7]; or coadministering intravenous lidocaine either immediately before propofol or mixed in with it.

Equipment

Use an infusion pump to administer propofol accurately. Infusion pumps compatible with magnetic resonance imaging sites are available, although additional intravenous extension tubing may be required to maintain a minimal distance from the magnet. The use of variable-flow devices in the magnetic resonance imaging suite has been described.[2]

All equipment necessary for managing an unconscious patient, as described for ketamine, must be available when propofol sedation is undertaken.

Techniques

Use an initial bolus dose of 2 mg/kg to induce sedation, and an infusion of 100 µg/kg/min to prevent movement.[3,8] Give lidocaine, 1 mg/kg (IV), before the bolus injection of propofol to decrease the associated discomfort.

PENTOBARBITAL

Pentobarbital, a barbiturate with an intermediate duration of action, provides reliable dose-related sedation without analgesic effects. It can be administered via an intravenous, intramuscular, or oral route. Pentobarbital-induced sedation dissipates in 15 to 20 minutes after single-dose intravenous injection. As in ketamine, the duration of action is related to redistribution of the drug from the central nervous system to peripheral tissues. The elimination half-time of pentobarbital is 15 to 20 hours, with drug clearance taking place via hepatic metabolism.

Indications

Pentobarbital is commonly used to sedate children for imaging studies. When given in sedating doses to normal children, pentobarbital has minimal effect on cardiac function, with decreases in heart rate and blood pressure not exceeding those seen with natural sleep.

Contraindications

Pentobarbital can induce anesthesia, so keep appropriate equipment and personnel available during its use.

Pentobarbital, like all barbiturates, enhances porphyrin production and is therefore contraindicated in acute intermittent porphyria and porphyria variegata.[8]

Complications

Pentobarbital has no analgesic effect and in fact can increase pain perception, and thus is not useful as a sedative for painful procedures. Depression of inhibitory central nervous system centers, in addition to hyperalgesia, may produce a paradoxical increase in agitation and excitement during attempted sedation with pentobarbital.

The effect of pentobarbital on respiratory function is dose-related. In sedative doses, respiratory depression is minimal, similar to natural sleep. However, severe decrease in respiratory drive is seen with increasing doses with elimination of respiratory drive at doses three times the sleep dose.[8] Airway protective reflexes are eliminated with larger doses of pentobarbital. Rarely, pentobarbital causes cardiovascular depression and hypotension. Hence, exercise great caution when using this agent in hypovolemic patients or those with possible cardiovascular instability.

Equipment

Monitoring with pulse oximetry is mandatory during pentobarbital-induced sedation. Sometimes time-cycled noninvasive blood pressure monitoring is necessary. As with all conscious sedation, keep advanced monitoring and resuscitative equipment available.

Techniques

Intravenous administration of pentobarbital is advantageous because rapid onset of effect and complete absorption allow for careful titration of the dose to the desired effect, decreasing the risk of oversedation. Sedation occurs with doses of 2 to 4 mg/kg administered in aliquots of 1 mg/kg. Alternatively, give 2 to 4 mg/kg intramuscularly or 4 to 6 mg/kg orally. Oral and intramuscular administration have a slower and less predictable onset and effect.

REFERENCES

1. American Board of Pediatrics Committee on Drugs: Guidelines for monitoring and management of pediatric patients during and after sedation for diagnostic and therapeutic procedures, *Pediatrics* 89:1110-1115, 1992.
2. Bloomfield EL, Masaryk TJ, Caplin A, et al: Intravenous sedation for MR imaging of the brain and spine in children: pentobarbital versus propofol, *Radiology* 186:93-97, 1993.
3. Dula DJ, Skiendzielewski JJ, Snover SW: The scavenger device for nitrous oxide administration, *Ann Emerg Med* 12:759-762, 1983.
3a. Dorsch JA, Dorsch SE: *Understanding anesthesia equipment*, ed 2, Baltimore, 1984, Williams & Wilkins.
4. Dula DJ, Skiendzielewski JJ, Toyka M: Nitrous oxide levels in the emergency department, *Ann Emerg Med* 10:575-578, 1981.
5. Frankville DD, Spear RM, Dyck JB: The dose of propofol required to prevent children from moving during magnetic resonance imaging, *Anesthesiology* 79:953-958, 1993.
6. Gamis AS, Knapp JF, Glenski JA: Nitrous oxide analgesia in a pediatric emergency department, *Ann Emerg Med* 18:177-181, 1989.
7. Gillies GW, Lees NW: The effect of speed of injection on induction with propofol, *Anesthesiology* 67:386-388, 1989.
8. Goodman L, Gilman A: *The pharmacological basis of therapeutics,* ed 8, New York, 1991, Pergamon Press.
9. Grant IS, Nimmo WS, McNicol LR, et al: Ketamine disposition in children and adults, *Br J Anaesth* 55:1107-1111, 1983.
10. Green SM, Johnson NE: Ketamine sedation for pediatric procedures. Part 2. Review and implications, *Ann Emerg Med* 19:1033-1046, 1990.
11. Green SM, Nakamura R, Johnson NE: Ketamine sedation for pediatric procedures. Part I. A prospective series, *Ann Emerg Med* 19:1024-1032, 1990.
12. Griffin GC, Campbell VD, Jones R: Nitrous oxide-oxygen sedation for minor surgery: experience in a pediatric setting, *JAMA* 245:2411-2413, 1981.
13. Gutstein HB, Johnson KL, Heard MB, et al: Oral ketamine premedication in children, *Anesthesiology* 76:28-33, 1992.
14. Hamza J, Ecoffey E, Gross JB: Ventilatory response to CO_2 following intravenous ketamine in children, *Anesthesiology* 70:422-425, 1989.
15. Hannallah RS, Baker SB, Casey W, et al: Propofol: effective dose and induction characteristics in unpremedicated children, *Anesthesiology* 74:217-219, 1991.
16. Hickey PR, Hansen DD, Cramolini GM, et al: Pulmonary and systemic hemodynamic responses to ketamine in infants with normal and elevated pulmonary vascular resistance, *Anesthesiology* 62:287-293, 1985.
17. James MFM, Manson EDM, Dennett JE: Nitrous oxide analgesia at higher elevations, *Anaesthesiology* 337:285-288, 1982.
18. Meyers EF, Charles P: Prolonged adverse reactions to ketamine in children, *Anesthesiology* 49:39-40, 1978.
19. Penrose BH: Aspiration pneumonitis following ketamine induction for a general anesthetic, *Anesth Analg* 51:41-43, 1972.
20. Reich DL, Silvay G: Ketamine: an update on the first twenty-five years of clinical experience, *Can J Anaesth* 36:186-197, 1989.
21. Rita L, Seleny FL: Ketamine hydrochloride for pediatric premedication. II. Prevention of postanesthetic excitement, *Anesth Analg* 53:380-382, 1974.
22. Stewart R, Gorayeb M, Peleton G: Arterial blood gases before, during, and after nitrous oxide:oxygen administration, *Ann Emerg Med* 15:1177-1180, 1986.
23. Stewart RD: Nitrous oxide sedation/analgesia in emergency medicine, *Ann Emerg Med* 14:139-148, 1985.
24. Takeshita H, Okuda Y, Sari A: The effects of ketamine on cerebral circulation and metabolism in man, *Anesthesiology* 36:69-75, 1972.
25. Tobias JD, Phipps S, Smith B, et al: Oral ketamine premedication to alleviate the distress of invasive procedures in pediatric oncology patients, *Pediatrics* 90:537-541, 1992.
26. White PF, Way WL, Trevor AJ: Ketamine: its pharmacology and therapeutic uses, *Anesthesiology* 56:260-263, 1982.
27. Yamamura T, Harada K, Okamura A, et al: Is the site of action of ketamine the N-methyl-D-aspartate receptor? *Anesthesiology* 72:704-710, 1990.

14 · Nonpharmacologic Aids in Pain Management

James M. Callahan

A number of nonpharmacologic techniques are available to alleviate pain and anxiety in children. These range from simple, unsophisticated methods, such as verbal preparation, to more sophisticated interventions, such as hypnosis or transcutaneous electrical nerve stimulation (TENS). Many of these techniques may aid in gaining the trust and cooperation of the child and, ideally, provide a more satisfying outcome for the child, the family, and the health-care professionals involved.

Indications

Use nonpharmacologic means of reducing pain and anxiety whenever a child has perceived pain or requires a potentially painful procedure. Use these techniques with supplemental analgesics and anesthetics whenever possible.

Contraindications

There are no contraindications to nonpharmacologic aids for pain reduction. However, many have not been well studied in children, or in the setting of the Emergency Department (ED) and pediatric intensive care unit (PICU).

Complications

Other than potential minor complications of restraint such as edema, bruising, and transient vascular compromise, non-pharmacologic aids pose no problems. Consider additional sedation and analgesics to ensure that the child suffers the least possible pain.

Equipment

Obtain papoose boards of various sizes for some patients who need restraint. Consider transcutaneous electrical nerve stimulation (TENS) units. Use tape recorders, age-appropriate cassette tapes, and earphones to provide music during procedures. Paintings/murals on walls or ceilings may also distract patients. Finally, use your imagination to reduce pain and fear further in children who undergo procedures.

Techniques

Preparation. It is important that children know what to expect. Take time to talk to them and not at or around them. Establish rapport, then explain, in language they can understand, what is about to happen.[5] Be honest. Anticipated or expected stress is more easily dealt with and less anxiety-provoking than unexpected stress.[12] Give both procedural information (step-by-step description of what is going to happen) and sensory information ("this will feel cold"). Do the preparation shortly before the procedure so that a long time does not elapse in which anxiety can grow while patients wait. Prepare frightening instruments (needles, scalpels, and the like) out of sight of children.

Parental Involvement. Establish rapport with the parents of a child in the ED and enlist their support. Ross and Ross[8] reported that, among a survey of 9- to 12-year-olds, the factor that helped most in dealing with pain experiences was the presence of the patient's parent. Most parents want to be present when children undergo procedures in the ED,[2] and, with proper preparation and guidance regarding what to do, they can be a stabilizing force for the child.[1,2,5]

Make sure the parents know what to expect so they can help the child through the procedure. Give them a specific role to play (e.g., talking to the patient or rubbing his or her head). At the same time, do not expect parents to immobilize the child or take the place of adequate medical or ancillary personnel to provide proper observation of the child during sedation.

Restraint. Proper preparation, use of parental support, and appropriate analgesia and sedation may make restraint unnecessary. However, the use of physical restraints (e.g., papoose boards) may at times be appropriate. Restraints should ensure a child's safety, protect the child from self-injury, and allow the procedure to be accomplished as quickly as possible with the best possible technique and outcome.[5] Administer sedative or analgesic medications before applying restraints. Often children fall asleep once restrained, and the procedure begins if sedation and analgesia are adequate. Do not allow restraints to limit observation of the patient's respiratory and cardiovascular status. For further details, see Chapter 11.

Relaxation Techniques. Children have vivid imaginations that can often lead them into a fantasy world by storytelling or the use of guided imagery.[5] The distraction provided by such interventions may benefit the patient by decreasing anxiety and improving analgesia. The telling of a story or the singing of a song, especially if the story can involve the child with one of his or her favorite fictional characters, can often quiet a frightened child. The ensuing relaxation may be just enough, when added to pharmacologic techniques, to gain the child's cooperation or even induce a peaceful, sedated period. For truly painful procedures, do not use relaxation techniques alone, but only as an adjunct to appropriate analgesia and/or local anesthesia.

A recently reported easy and interesting technique decreases pain behaviors associated with immunizations in 4- to 7-year-olds. While they received injections, children were taught to blow out air repetitively "as if they were blowing bubbles."[4] Children who used this technique exhibited significantly fewer pain behaviors. This technique might

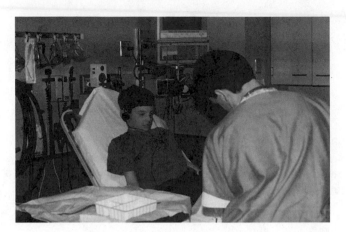

FIG. 14-1   Older child listening to music during a procedure.

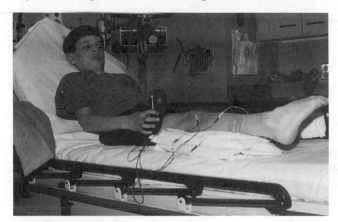

FIG. 14-2   TENS unit.

lead to similar results when applied to multiple minor procedures such as venipuncture and intravenous cannulation. It is easily taught and inexpensive and has no side effects.

Hypnosis is another relaxation technique recommended for use in pediatric patients experiencing pain or undergoing painful procedures. It is reportedly useful in patients with vasoocclusive crisis from sickle cell disease[11] and children and adolescents with cancer.[13] Although never studied, it could be very useful in pediatric patients in EDs.[5,9] Patients envision or "feel" a very pleasant sight or feeling or think of pain as a color painted over with a more pleasing color.[5,7] Suggest to the patient that, by some thought or action, he or she can actually decrease the pain being felt. In children with cancer-related pain, hypnosis is superior to other relaxation techniques.[13] Sometimes children require several sessions before they can master the imagery required to make this technique effective. This may limit its usefulness in some patients in an acute-care setting.

Music. Music has reduced the pain and anxiety associated with laceration repair in adult ED patients.[6] It decreased pain scores but did not significantly decrease anxiety scores. Almost all patients reported that the music was very beneficial, and all said they would use it again. Music is also effective when used as an adjunct when children are receiving immunizations.[3] Use headsets for older children (>10 years) to listen to music (Fig. 14-1). Younger children do not prefer earphones. Use a cassette tape without headset instead.

Transcutaneous Electrical Nerve Stimulation. Transcutaneous electrical nerve stimulation (TENS) units, which patients wear like portable radios and regulate themselves, produce electric currents that stimulate nerves and produce paresthesias.[5] Fig. 14-2 shows a TENS unit on a patient's arm. The units cause endorphin release and naloxone blocks their effects. There are no studies of the use of TENS in ED settings or in children. A randomized study in adults showed TENS to be effective as an adjunct to conventional therapy in patients with multiple rib fractures.[10] It may be useful in pediatric patients with fractures as well. Other uses merit investigation.

Remarks

Reassurance, restraint, and other nonpharmacologic techniques are quite helpful in achieving pain control in children. If medical staff are empathic and take the time needed to apply the techniques, significant pain can be prevented.

REFERENCES

1. Bauchner H: Procedures, pain, and parents, *Pediatrics* 87:563-565, 1991.
2. Bauchner H, Vinci R. Waring C: Pediatric procedures: do parents want to watch? *Pediatrics* 84:907-909, 1989.
3. Fowler-Kerry S, Lander JR: Management of injection pain in children, *Pain* 30:169-175, 1987.
4. French GM, Painter EC, Cowy DL: Blowing away shot pain: a technique for pain management during immunization, *Pediatrics* 93:384-388, 1994.
5. Henretig FM, Selbst SM: The treatment of pain in the emergency department, *Pediatr Clin North Am* 36:965-978, 1989.
6. Menegazzi JJ, Paris PM, Kersteen CH, et al: A randomized, controlled trial of the use of music during laceration repair, *Ann Emerg Med* 20:348-350, 1991.
7. Olness K: Hypnosis in pediatric practice, *Curr Probl Pediatr* 12:1-47, 1981.
8. Ross DM, Ross SA: The importance of type of question, psychological climate and subject set in interviewing children without pain, *Pain* 19:71-79, 1984.
9. Selbst SM: Managing pain in the pediatric emergency department, *Pediatr Emerg Care* 5:56-63, 1989.
10. Sloan JP, Muwanga CL, Waters EA, et al: Multiple rib fractures: transcutaneous nerve stimulation versus conventional analgesia, *J Trauma* 26:1120-1122, 1986.
11. Zeltzer L, Dash J, Holland JP: Hypnotically induced pain control in sickle cell anemia, *Pediatrics* 64:533-536, 1979.
12. Zeltzer LK, Jay SM, Fisher DM: The management of pain associated with pediatric procedures. *Pediatr Clin North Am* 36:941-964, 1989.
13. Zeltzer L, LeBaron S: Hypnosis and nonhypnotic techniques for reduction of pain and anxiety during painful procedures in children and adolescents with cancer, *J Pediatr* 101:1032-1035, 1982.

15 Local Anesthetics

Steven M. Selbst

Local anesthetics are extremely useful in the Emergency Department (ED) and pediatric intensive care unit (PICU). They have particular importance for reducing pain during procedures, especially wound care. Physicians caring for children should not assume that young children will not feel the pain of the procedure or that use of force and physical restraint is all that is required. Although some agents require a painful injection to induce local anesthesia, there are methods to alleviate the discomfort, and children should receive these agents as often as adults. Some agents can be applied topically on both intact skin and on wounds in limited situations.

AGENTS GIVEN BY SUBCUTANEOUS INJECTIONS

Lidocaine

Lidocaine is a local amide anesthetic that is metabolized in the liver and excreted by the kidney. Lidocaine interferes with nerve conduction. It binds at certain receptor sites in the nerve and slows or blocks the influx of sodium.[2,52] It gets into the interior of the cell and prevents depolarization by reducing membrane permeability to sodium.

Lidocaine is available in three concentrations: 0.5% solution (0.5 mg/ml lidocaine), 1% solution (10 mg/ml lidocaine), and 2% solution (20 mg/ml lidocaine). The higher concentration prolongs the duration of effect, but it does not increase anesthesia. It may increase the likelihood of motor blockade and systemic toxic effects.[60] Thus, since one can block pain sensation and not affect motor function by using dilute concentrations of local anesthetics, there is no advantage to using the 2% solution. The 0.5% solution may be useful for large wounds that require a large quantity of lidocaine, and in neonates.[60]

Lidocaine mixed with epinephrine causes vasoconstriction, which delays absorption and thus decreases lidocaine toxicity. It also increases the duration of effect.[55,60] However, it may lead to poor wound healing and possible infection because the vasoconstriction can cause hypoxia of tissues, which retards killing of *Staphylococcus aureus* by leukocytes.[51] The epinephrine may also lead to increased pain on injection[58] and ischemia to areas of end-arteriolar supply.

A level of lidocaine above 6 µg/ml is toxic.[49] However, lidocaine is less protein-bound in young children and therefore more likely to be toxic at a given dose per kilogram.[55] In early infancy, microsomal enzymes in the liver are deficient. Because of this, lidocaine may have prolonged duration of action, and toxicity can result after repeated doses without careful assessment of need. Infants may also be at greater risk for development of central nervous system (CNS) toxicity as a result of immaturity of the nervous system.[35]

Indications. Lidocaine is a safe anesthetic. It produces an effect quickly (5 to 10 minutes) and lasts long enough to allow most procedures to be completed (90 to 200 minutes).[60] Use lidocaine for local anesthesia for painful procedures such as wound repair, lumbar puncture, arterial puncture, intravenous catheterization, removal of foreign body from skin, and drainage of abscesses. Administration of lidocaine does not decrease the success rate of performing lumbar punctures in neonates.[42] Also consider the use of lidocaine for regional nerve blocks to make complicated wound repairs and for regional anesthesia for fracture reduction when given intravenously as a "mini Bier block"[21,39,52] (see Chapter 16).

Epinephrine is indicated with lidocaine in highly vascularized areas, such as the scalp, to help control profuse bleeding.

Contraindications. Do not use lidocaine if the patient has known allergy to the drug; switch to an ester. The need for this is quite rare. Do not use lidocaine combined with epinephrine in end organs such as the digits of the hands or feet, the penis, or the pinna of the ear.[2,60]

Complications. Allergic reaction to lidocaine is possible but rare. Reactions occur when it is accidentally injected intravenously, excessive total dosage is given, or poor excretion occurs. Serious toxicity from overdose is characterized by confusion, convulsions, and coma. Respiratory depression and vasomotor collapse leading to hypotension and bradycardia with cardiac arrest can occur. However, cardiac toxicity is extremely rare when lidocaine is used in small doses needed for wound repair.[47,60]

When lidocaine is combined with epinephrine, additional toxic effects such as tachycardia and syncope can occur with intravenous injection. Also, epinephrine rarely causes delay in wound healing and increased wound infections.[51]

When lidocaine is administered by jet injector, hematomas and bleeding at the injection site may occur. However, significant tissue damage is unlikely.[47]

Table 15-1 shows the toxic effects of lidocaine at varying concentrations in the blood.

Equipment. For local infiltration, use a 20-gauge needle and 5- or 10-ml disposable syringe to draw up the solution. Then for infiltration into the skin use a small needle (25-,

Table 15-1 Toxicity of Lidocaine by Blood Level

Concentration T (µg/ml)	
4 µg	Numbness of tongue, tinnitus, lightheadedness
6 µg	Visual disturbances
8 µg	Muscle twitching
10 µg	Seizures
15 µg	Coma
20 µg	Apnea

27-, or 30-gauge), preferably a longer needle (1⅝ to 2 inches) to produce "fanning" of the anesthetic. This causes less pain on injection and requires fewer needle punctures to infiltrate.[47,52,56] For deeper penetration, consider using a larger needle (22-gauge) for easier aspiration of blood.[2] If possible, use a syringe with a thumb ring for better control during infiltration and easier aspiration.[52] Use appropriate cleansing solution.

A jet injector (Syrijet) is also useful. This provides almost painless infiltration of 0.05 to 0.2 ml lidocaine to a depth of about 1.5 cm. Consider using this device to provide anesthesia for laceration repair, lumbar puncture, and abscess drainage.[10,46]

Technique. Prepare the patient for a painful procedure with carefully chosen words. It is important to be honest but is helpful to suggest that the child may not feel discomfort. A calm, reassuring approach may reduce the pain experience.[22] If possible, allow the parents to stay to hold or stay near the child without actually witnessing the procedure. Always prepare the lidocaine solution away from the patient. Hypnosis and other distraction techniques, such as providing music through earphones, may also help reduce pain[6,34] (see Chapter 14). Inquire about previous anesthesia and possible allergy to lidocaine before its use.

For local infiltration, cleanse the area well with alcohol or providone-iodine and drip a few drops of lidocaine solution into the wound a few minutes before infiltration.[52] Then, using a long, small needle, slowly infiltrate lidocaine at a rate of about 30 to 45 seconds per milliliter.[52] When injecting deep into tissue, use a larger needle to aspirate blood and prevent accidental injection into a vessel.[2] First rub the skin around the site of injection as this may reduce pain (according to the gate theory).[13] Pull the skin taut as you inject and remember, the deeper you inject, the less pain the patient is likely to feel.[5] Inject a small amount of lidocaine, since a large bolus causes distention of the tissue and is likely to cause more pain.[52] It may hurt less to infiltrate through the wound margins than through intact surrounding skin, and there is no evidence that this leads to more wound infections.[52] For a larger field, pull the needle out to the tip and inject again at a 90-degree angle to minimize the number of punctures. Puncture anesthetized tissue for further infiltration, but do not puncture the skin more than three times with the same needle.[52] Aspirate for blood with the syringe while injecting. Wait 5 to 10 minutes after infiltration before starting the procedure.[47]

Consider warming lidocaine before injection as this may alter the pain of infiltration.[13a] Consider mixing the solution with sodium bicarbonate with 10 parts lidocaine to 1 part sodium bicarbonate (8.4%, 1 mEq/ml) to raise the pH of the solution from about 6.2 to 7.0 or 7.4. This more alkaline solution has been shown to cause less burning on infiltration in adult subjects.[8,14] However, data in children are not available. Buffered lidocaine stays effective for up to 1 week after preparation and is therefore convenient to use.[9] Buffering does not alter the anesthetic efficacy or duration of effect of lidocaine.[14] Box 15-1 summarizes techniques to reduce pain of lidocaine administration.

When using the jet injector, clean the target surface and put the injector lightly but firmly at the skin site. Squeeze the trigger while holding the injector steadily (Fig. 15-1). Repeat

---

> **BOX 15-1   TECHNIQUES TO REDUCE PAIN OF SUBCUTANEOUS LIDOCAINE ADMINISTRATION**
>
> Prepare the medication away from the child.
> Buffer lidocaine with sodium bicarbonate (10:1).
> Rub skin around site of infiltration.
> Infiltrate through devitalized wound margin.
> Give further lidocaine through anesthetized skin.
> Use a small needle.
> Inject small amounts of lidocaine slowly.
> Wait for anesthesia effect before proceeding.

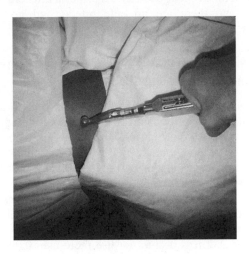

FIG. 15-1   Jet injector at skin site for local lidocaine infiltration for lumbar puncture.

if a wider area of anesthesia is needed. There is some pain associated with the jet injector, but it is brief.[10]

Give lidocaine for local anesthesia at a maximum dose of 3 to 5 mg/kg or 7 mg/kg if epinephrine is added. The 1% solution is adequate. Use a maximum dose of 5 mg/kg for infants and newborns, and use the 0.5% solution because complete analgesia and motor blockade can occur, even with dilute concentrations of local anesthetics.[60]

Remarks. Lidocaine is a highly useful agent for many procedures in the ED and ICU. Similar agents, such as 0.25% bupivacaine, have a longer duration of action and may help reduce pain for 6 hours after a wound is repaired.[50] Use this drug if the procedure is expected to be prolonged or significant postprocedure pain is anticipated. Use 0.5% to 1% procaine (an ester) if the patient is allergic to amide anesthetics (lidocaine, prilocaine, bupivacaine).[41,60]

OTHER INJECTABLE AGENTS

Diphenhydramine, 0.5% and 1%, has been found to produce local anesthesia when injected intradermally in adult volunteers for wound management.[20,25] Prepare diphenhydramine for injection by diluting a 50-mg/ml ampule with saline solution to make a 10- to 50-ml solution.[52] Although it is just as effective as lidocaine 1% for achieving local dermal anesthesia, the injection itself may be more painful with diphenhydramine.[20,25] Use of 0.5% diphenhydramine reduces this pain somewhat but may result in decreased anesthetic effect when used for facial lacerations.[20] The safety of diphenhydramine remains to be established, especially in areas with poor collateral perfusion. Skin necrosis has been reported.[25]

Injection of physiologic saline solution from a multidose vial subcutaneously may also provide a local anesthetic response for intravenous catheterization.[17,59] One report indicates that 0.9% benzyl alcohol additive (the bacteriostatic compound in multidose vials of physiologic saline solution) has anesthetic properties, whereas saline solution alone does not.[59] Thus, consider injecting 1 ml of subcutaneous saline solution with benzyl alcohol into the skin just before placement of an intravenous catheter. Anesthesia lasts only about 2 minutes, and there are no side effects and no pain on injection.

TOPICAL ANESTHETICS
Tetracaine/Adrenaline/Cocaine

Tetracaine/adrenaline/cocaine (TAC) is an effective topical anesthetic for wound repair. It is a clear solution of 0.5% of tetracaine, 1:2000 epinephrine, and 11.8% cocaine. Mix 60 ml of 2% tetracaine with 120 ml of 1:1000 epinephrine and 28.32 g of cocaine in the hospital pharmacy.[43,46,52] Dilute this combination with normal saline solution to make a volume of 240 ml and divide it into 3-ml aliquots.[11] Some physicians recommend adding cocaine in half that concentration (5.9%).[11] The maximum safe dose of TAC has not been established, but it is best to not use more than 0.09 ml/kg.[26] Because cocaine is the most toxic agent in TAC, some have used the solution without cocaine, but they have found it to be less effective.[44] Others recently attempted to determine whether cocaine alone would be as good as the TAC combination, while avoiding the potential toxicity of tetracaine. However, TAC was significantly better than cocaine alone for repair of small lacerations.[19]

Indications. Use TAC for simple wound repair instead of or in combination with local infiltration with lidocaine. Use TAC before cleaning the wound and suturing. TAC will not cause swelling or distortion of wound edges, which may occur with injection of local anesthetics. It is most effective when used on facial and scalp lacerations and less effective on truncal or extremity lacerations. Hagenberth, Altieri, Hawk, et al.[26] found that among patients with facial or scalp wounds, 81% of those treated with TAC had adequate anesthesia, compared with 87% for lidocaine-treated wounds. TAC was less effective on extremity or trunk wounds: only 43% of TAC-treated wounds achieved adequate anesthesia, compared with 89% of lidocaine-treated wounds. Increased vascularity of the face and scalp may make TAC more successful with these wounds. However, Anderson, Colecchi, Baronoski, et al.[3] found no difference between TAC and lidocaine in anesthesia effect (89% vs. 79%), and the location of the wound was irrelevant.[3] They found TAC superior to lidocaine for improving patient compliance with the suturing process. Others have noted that children who do not achieve adequate anesthesia with TAC can have a supplemental lidocaine injection. This infiltration is then less painful than if TAC were not used at all.[47,48] TAC is most helpful for young children, who may be fearful of a needle used for injected local anesthetic.

Contraindications. Since TAC is vasoconstrictive, do not use it on parts of the body where epinephrine is contraindicated, such as organs supplied by end arterioles (the penis, nose, pinna of the ear, digits, or skin flap).[46,48] Do not use it near the eye because the solution can cause corneal abrasions if it drips into the globe.[18]

Do not use TAC if the patient is allergic to any of its components. Since tetracaine and cocaine are "ester" local anesthetics, do not use TAC if the patient is allergic to para-aminobenzoic acid (PABA-)–containing suntan lotion.[60]

Most important, do not use TAC near mucous membranes because it is rapidly absorbed and can cause serious complications of cocaine toxicity, including death.[16] Be careful with TAC on large burns or abrasions because significant cocaine absorption can occur.

Complications. TAC is absorbed through open skin of wounds, and children may have measurable amounts of cocaine in blood or urine for 48 to 72 hours after use.[23,54] However, in one study there were no demonstrable clinical signs of cocaine toxicity in 51 children when TAC was used appropriately.[22]

If ingested, TAC causes disorientation, seizures, and death resulting from cocaine toxicity.[16-18] One child died after TAC was absorbed through nasal mucosal membranes during wound repair.[16]

One animal study showed increased wound infections with TAC,[7] but this was not found in a more recent study[40] or in human patients.[3,26,52]

Equipment. Use cotton swabs, gauze pads, or cotton balls for direct application of TAC to the wound. Alternatively, use a 3-ml syringe to directly drip TAC onto a wound. Keep additional gauze nearby to prevent it from dripping away from the wound.

Use disposable gloves when applying TAC as there may be some vasoconstriction to the provider's intact skin. However, TAC does not penetrate unbroken skin well.[46,60]

Technique. Apply TAC directly to the wound that needs repair by dripping a few drops onto the laceration.[32,36] Alternatively, "paint" TAC onto the laceration with a cotton swab[47] (Fig. 15-2). Then place about half of the 3-ml aliquot of TAC on a cotton ball or gauze pad and hold it firmly over the wound for 15 or 20 minutes.[40] Gauze may absorb too much TAC; thus cotton balls are preferable.[29] Note blanching of the skin near the wound, which indicates that vasoconstriction has occurred; then anesthesia near the wound margins should be satisfactory.[60]

Use TAC safely in a dose of 1 ml/1-cm wound but no more than 6 ml for a 6-cm wound.[36,52] A maximum dose is 0.09 ml/kg.[26] Box 15-2 reviews the use of TAC for laceration repair.

Remarks. TAC is a safe, highly effective anesthetic when used appropriately. It often allows laceration repair to be completed without the child's experiencing pain or fear. Even when complete anesthesia is not achieved, TAC is useful because subsequent injection of lidocaine is less painful. Use of TAC with conscious sedation may provide an especially effective combination for wound repair in young, agitated children with minor injuries.

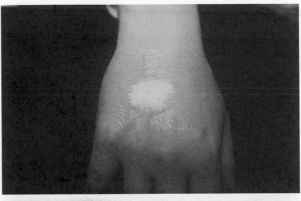

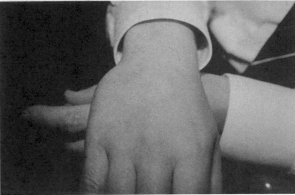

A

B

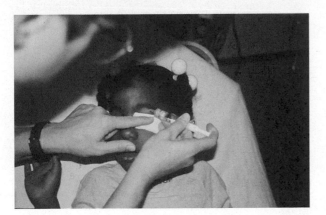

FIG. 15-2   "Painting" TAC onto a facial wound. *TAC,* Tetracaine/adrenaline/cocaine.

FIG. 15-3   **A** and **B,** Applying EMLA cream for IV placement. *EMLA,* Eutectic mixture of local anesthetics; *IV,* intravenous.

ANESTHETIC PATCHES AND CREAMS

Consider topical local anesthesia applied to intact skin before needle procedures. Unfortunately, available agents are not rapidly absorbed, and thus they are less useful in the ED setting because of the prolonged wait for anesthesia. Still, they are quite useful for scheduled procedures in the PICU.

Eutectic mixture of local anesthetics (EMLA) cream is a 1:1 oil/water emulsion of prilocaine 2% to 5% and lidocaine 2.5%. It must be applied at least 60 minutes before the procedure because lidocaine does not penetrate intact skin well.[16,46,60] In the animal model, EMLA does not affect wound healing,[39] but it has not been well studied for wound repair in children.

Indications. Use EMLA cream for scheduled lumbar punctures, intravenous catheter placement, drainage of paronychiae or perirectal abscess, bone marrow aspiration, arthrocentesis, arterial sticks, immunization, and accessing of subcutaneous drug reservoirs.[6,27,28,31,57] Although EMLA cream may reduce pain of needle puncture as well as lidocaine, children may still be uncooperative when they eventually see the needle to be used for the procedure.[60]

Contraindications. Do not use EMLA cream in emergencies when one must perform a procedure quickly. Never use it on broken skin or open wounds. Do not use EMLA on infants less than 1 month or those less than 12 months who are receiving treatment with methemoglobin-inducing agents.

Complications. Apply EMLA with an occlusive dressing (plastic wrap or Tegaderm) taped to the skin; there may be erythema of the skin surrounding the tape.[27,52,60] Pain may

occur when the taped dressing is removed. There are reports of increases in blood methemoglobin in young infants treated with this cream.[24] However, clinically significant problems are unlikely in infants older than 3 months who receive only a small amount of EMLA.[37]

Equipment. No special equipment other than the medication and occlusive dressing are necessary.

Technique. Apply half of a 5-g tube of the EMLA cream to the site of injection and cover it with occlusive dressing (Fig. 15-3, *A* and *B*). Write the time of application on the dressing. Keep this on the patient for 60 minutes before attempting the procedure. In preparation for venipuncture, ready multiple sites in case the first attempt is unsuccessful.[60] Larger application times up to 120 minutes may be better for deep procedures. Do not apply EMLA cream for more than 4 hours. Do not apply it to an area greater than 100 cm^2 for infants up to 10 kg, 600 cm^2 for children 10 to 20 kg, or 2000 cm^2 for patients who weigh more than 20 kg.

Remarks. EMLA cream may be helpful for some elective procedures, particularly in children who require frequent procedures. The cream may work best for procedures in which the child is unlikely to view the procedure needle and become agitated (e.g., lumbar puncture, bone marrow aspiration).[28,30,60] It may be difficult to keep the patch on the skin of a young, frightened child who perspires; this method may require additional nursing supervision.[48]

OTHER TOPICAL ANESTHETICS

Consider the use of LET instead of TAC for wound repair. LET is a solution of lidocaine (4%), epinephrine (0.05% to

Table 15-2 Characteristics of Local Anesthetics

	Concentration	Maximum safe dose	Onset	Duration/minutes	Use
Esters					
Procaine	0.5%–2.0%	7(9*) mg/kg	Slow	30–60	Infiltration/dental
Tetracaine	0.5%	0.75 mg/kg (2–3 Drops)	Slow	180–600	Topical for eyes
Amides					
Lidocaine	0.5%–2.0%	3–5 (7*) mg/kg	Rapid	60–120	Infiltration/skin
Bupivicaine	0.625%–0.25%	2 (3*) mg/kg	Slow	180–280	Infiltration/skin
Prilocaine	0.5%–1.5%	5 (7*) mg/kg	Slow	60–120	Topical/skin
Diphenhydramine	0.5%–1%	Unknown	Rapid		Infiltration/skin
Saline solution	0.9% Benzyl alcohol additive	—	Rapid	2	Infiltration/skin
TAC	2% Tetracaine 5.9% Cocaine 1:2000 Epinephrine	0.09 ml/kg	Rapid	45–60	Topical/skin
LET	4% Lidocaine 1% Epinephrine 0.5% Tetracaine	3 ml	Rapid	45–60	Topical/skin
EMLA cream	2.5% Prilocaine Lidocaine 2.5%	4-hour exposure limited application area/kg/weight	Very slow	60–120	Topical/skin

*With epinephrine. *TAC,* tetracaine/adrenal/cocaine; *EMLA,* eutectic mixture of local anesthetics. *LET,* lidocaine, epinephrine, tetracaine.

0.1%), and tetracaine (0.5%) that has been shown in two studies to provide an anesthetic effect equal to that of TAC.[20a,44a] It has been used successfully and safely for repair of uncomplicated scalp and facial lacerations in children.[20a,44a] LET can be made in gel form with hydroxyethyl cellulose. Apply the gel directly to the wound for 15 to 20 minutes before repair, or paint a 3-ml solution onto the wound with a cotton-tipped swab and place the remainder onto gauze and hold in place on the wound with tape. There is minimal absorption of the lidocaine, and the cost of LET is much less (perhaps ten times less) than that of TAC. The use of LET avoids the potential toxic effects of cocaine in TAC.

Consider application of lidocaine gel to the urethral meatus to reduce the pain of catheterization. Directly instill the jelly into the urethra with a cotton-tipped applicator moistened with benzocaine gel. For adolescent males, instill 5 to 10 ml of 2% lidocaine jelly, 3 to 5 ml for females.[52] Recommended doses for younger children are not known. Also, use the 2% jelly for skin wounds with embedded dirt or tattooing to reduce the pain of scrubbing.[52] Furthermore, one can mix lidocaine 2% jelly with a vasoconstrictor such as phenylephrine (Neo-Synephrine) spray. Use this on nasal mucosa for analgesia and vasoconstriction before insertion of a nasogastric (NG) tube.[60]

Adrenaline-cocaine gel is also available for topical use. One study showed that the gel provides excellent anesthetic efficacy for minor dermal lacerations in children.[12] The average dose used in that study was 0.35 ml of gel (containing 40 mg cocaine). There may be less risk of adverse reaction with this gel than with TAC, which may drip onto mucous membranes. No adverse reactions occurred in 35 children who received the gel.[12]

One can also use viscous lidocaine intraorally as it is marketed as a 2% compound and a 4% solution. Consider viscous lidocaine for management of painful oral lesions such as gingivostomatitis, pharyngitis, or dental pain. However, do not use this medication in infants with minor oral irritation or teething. Infants and young children cannot expectorate well, and lidocaine toxicity may develop. When lidocaine is applied to mucous membranes, blood levels of lidocaine approach that of the intravenous (IV) route,[1] and seizures have been reported to result from use of 2% viscous lidocaine in children.[35] Also, young children may have impaired swallowing after using oral lidocaine, and aspiration of food is possible. Tell older patients who use this medication to swish for no more than 1 or 2 minutes and expectorate.[4] Recommended dose for adults is 300 mg (15 ml of a 2% solution) used no more than every 3 hours for 2 or 3 days. Safe doses for children are not well established. Direct application to a sore oral lesion with a cotton swab reduces the dose and decreases toxicity.[4]

Benzocaine gel and liquid are available for topical application to oral lesions, gums sore from teething, and toothaches.[52] It is also useful before removal of anal and genital warts and in relief of the pruritus of poison ivy. It is water-soluble and poorly absorbed when applied topically.[60] However, when it is used often, significant absorption is possible, and systemic toxicity such as methemoglobinemia may result.[41] Because it is absorbed slowly, it can provide prolonged analgesia.[60]

Use a solution of benzocaine mixed with antipyrine and glycerin (Auralgan) to anesthetize the ear canal. This is helpful for severe otitis media, removal of a foreign body, or reduction of pain from a moving insect in the ear canal. Place the child supine with the head turned to the side. Drip 3 to 4 drops of the solution into the canal and hold the child for a few minutes. Covering the canal with cotton is optional and probably not necessary.

Use lidocaine aerosol spray (xylocaine 10% or 10-ml spray) for vocal cord anesthesia before intubation.[52] Use a solution of tetracaine (0.5% concentration) for surface anesthesia of the cornea.[52] Apply 2 to 3 drops directly to the eye when necessary for examination or removal of a foreign body. This produces little irritation to the eye. Repeat, if needed, as the solution quickly washes out, but do not discharge the patient with a prescription.

Also, consider using a topical spray of ethyl chloride before skin incision. For instance, it may be desirable to use this agent for incision of an abscess or paronychiae. Do not use it near electrocautery as ethyl chloride is flammable.[41] One can substitute a spray of 75% dichlorotetrafluoroethane and 25% ethylchloride (Fluroethyl), which is not flammable. These agents provide only very brief superficial anesthesia. To apply, invert the bottle/can 5 to 10 cm from the target area and direct a spray consistently until the area turns white. The spray is quite volatile and cools the skin to the point of freezing.

Generally do not use cocaine solution as a topical anesthetic. Because it is vasoconstrictive, some recommend it for relief of pain from nasal trauma and for use before passage of an NG tube, a nasotracheal tube, or an endoscope, but safe dosing guidelines for young children are not available. Some recommend 3 mg/kg of body weight.[53] One can apply a vasoconstrictor to the nasal mucosa before the cocaine to reduce absorption and toxicity.[45] However, systemic toxicity has occurred with 20 to 30 mg in adults.[48] The cocaine is rapidly absorbed through mucous membranes, and there are reports of seizures in a 2-month-old who received topical cocaine intranasally.[45] This infant received 0.6 to 0.7 mg/kg of cocaine.

Remarks. Several topical anesthetics are available for use on intact skin and open wounds and in reduction of the pain and fear associated with injectable anesthetics. Use these agents whenever possible before painful procedures (Table 15-2).

REFERENCES

1. Adriani J, Zepernick R: Clinical effectiveness of drugs used for topical anesthesia, *JAMA* 188:711-716, 1964.
2. Altman RS, Smith-Coggins R, Ampel LL: Local anesthetics, *Ann Emerg Med* 14:1209-1217, 1985.
3. Anderson AB, Colecchi C, Baronoski R, et al: Local anesthesia in pediatric patients: topical TAC versus lidocaine, *Ann Emerg Med* 19:519-522, 1990.
4. Anonymous: Viscous lidocaine, *Physicians desk reference*, ed 46, Montvale, NJ, 1992, Medical Economics Data.
5. Arndt KA, Burton C, Noe JM: Minimizing the pain of local anesthesia, *Plast Reconstr Surg* 76:676-679, 1983.
6. Arts SE, Abu-Saad HH, Champion GD, et al: Age-related response to lidocaine-prilocaine (EMLA) emulsion and effect of music distraction on the pain of intravenous cannulation, *Pediatrics* 93:797-801, 1994.
7. Barker W, Rodeheaver GT, Edgerton MT, et al: Damage to tissue defenses by a topical anesthetic agent, *Ann Emerg Med* 11:307-310, 1982.
8. Bartfield JM, Ford DT, Homer PJ: Buffered versus plain lidocaine for digital nerve blocks, *Ann Emerg Med* 22:216-219, 1993.
9. Bartfield JM, Homer RJ, Ford DT, et al: Buffered lidocaine as a local anesthetic: an investigation of shelf life, *Ann Emerg Med* 21:16-19, 1992.
10. Bennett CR, Mandell RD, Manheim LM: Studies on tissue penetration characteristics produced by jet injection, *J Am Dent Assoc* 83:625-629, 1971.
11. Bonadio WA, Wagner V: Half-strength TAC topical anesthetic, *Clin Pediatr* 27:495-498, 1988.
12. Bonadio WA, Wagner VR: Adrenaline-cocaine gel topical anesthetic for dermal laceration repair in children, *Ann Emerg Med* 21:1435-1438, 1992.
13. Bourke DZ: Counter-irritation reduces pain during cutaneous needle insertion, *Anesth Analg* 64:379, 1985 (letter).
13a. Brogan GX, Giarrusso E, Hollander JE, et al: Comparison of plain, harmed, and buffered notocaine for anesthesia of traumatic wounds, *Ann Emerg Med* 26:121-125, 1995.
14. Christoph RA, Buchanan L, Begalla K, et al: Pain reduction in local anesthetic administration through pH buffering, *Ann Emerg Med* 17:117-120, 1988.
15. Clark S, Radford M: Topical anesthesia for venipuncture, *Arch Dis Child* 61:1132-1134, 1987.
16. Dailey RH: Fatality secondary to misuse of TAC solution, *Ann Emerg Med* 17:159-160, 1988.
17. Daya MR, Barton BT, Schleiss MR, et al: Recurrent seizures following mucosal application of TAC, *Ann Emerg Med* 17:646-648, 1988.
18. Dronene SC: Complications of TAC, *Ann Emerg Med* 12:333, 1983 (letter).
19. Ernst AA, Crabbe LH, Winsemius KD, et al: Comparison of tetracaine, adrenaline and cocaine with cocaine alone for topical anesthesia, *Ann Emerg Med* 19:51-54, 1990.
20. Ernst AA, Marvez-Valls E, Mall G, et al: 1% lidocaine versus 0.5% diphenhydramine for local anesthesia in minor laceration repair, *Ann Emerg Med* 23:1328-1332, 1994.
20a. Ernst AA, Marvez E, Nick, TG, et al: Lidocaine, adrenaline, tetracaine gel vs. tetracaine adrenaline cocaine gel for topical anesthesia in linear scalp and facial lacerations in children ages 5 to 17 years, *Pediatrics* 95:255-258, 1995.
21. Farrell RG, Swanson LS, Walter JK: Safe and effective IV regional anesthesia for use in the emergency department, *Ann Emerg Med* 14:239-240, 1985.
22. Fernald C, Corry J: Empathic vs. directive preparation of children for needles, *Child Health Care* 10:44-47, 1981.
23. Fitzmaurice LS, Wasserman GS, Knapp JF, et al: TAC use and absorption of cocaine in a pediatric emergency department, *Ann Emerg Med* 19:515-518, 1990.
24. Frayling IM, Addison GM, Chattergee K et al: Methaemoglobinaemia in children treated with prilocaine-lignocaine cream, *Br Med J* 301:153-154, 1990.
25. Green SM, Rothrock SG, Gorchynski J: Validation of diphenhydramine as a dermal local anesthetic, *Ann Emerg Med* 23:1284-1289, 1994.
26. Hagenberth MA, Altieri MF, Hawk WH, et al: Comparison of topical tetracaine, adrenaline, and cocaine anesthesia with lidocaine infiltration for repair of lacerations in children, *Ann Emerg Med* 19:63-67, 1990.
27. Hallen B, Uppfeldt A: Does lidocaine-prilocaine cream permit pain-free insertion of IV catheters in children? *Anesthesiology* 57:340-342, 1982.
28. Halperin DL, Koren G, Attios D, et al: Topical skin anesthesia for venous, subcutaneous drug reservoir and lumbar punctures in children, *Pediatrics* 84:281-284, 1989.
29. Hanke BK: Advances in wound management in the emergency department, *Resid Staff Physician* 39:23-27, 1993.
30. Kapelushnik J, Koren G, Solh H, et al: Evaluating the efficacy of EMLA in alleviating pain associated with lumbar puncture: comparison of open and double-blinded protocols in children, *Pain* 42:32-34, 1990.
31. Lubens HM, Ausdenmoore RW, Shafer AD, et al: Anesthetic patch for painful procedures such as minor operations, *Am J Dis Child* 128:192-194, 1974.
32. Lyman JL, McCabe JB: Improving the effectiveness of TAC application, *Ann Emerg Med* 13:742, 1984 (letter).

33. Martin JR, Doezema D, Tandberg D, et al: The effect of local anesthetics on bacterial proliferation: TAC versus lidocaine, *Ann Emerg Med* 19:987-990, 1990.

34. Menegazzi JJ, Paris PM, Kersteen CH, et al: A randomized, controlled trial of the use of music during laceration repair, *Ann Emerg Med* 20:348-350, 1991.

35. Moferson HC, Caracccio TR, Miller H, et al: Lidocaine toxicity from topical mucosal application, *Clin Pediatr* 22:190-192, 1983.

36. Nichols FC, Macha P, Farnell MB: TAC topical anesthesia and minor skin lacerations, *Resid Staff Physician* 33:59-66, 1987.

37. Nilsson A, Engberg G, Hennenberg S, et al: Inverse relationship between age-dependent erythrocyte activity of methaemoglobin reductase and prilocaine-induced methaemoglobinaemia during infancy, *Br J Anaesth* 64:72-76, 1990.

38. Nykanen D, Kissoon N, Rieder M, et al: Comparison of a topical mixture of lidocaine and prilocaine (EMLA) versus 1% lidocaine infiltration on a wound healing, *Pediatr Emerg Care* 7:15-17, 1991.

39. Olney BW, Lugg PC, Turner PL, et al: Outpatient treatment of upper extremity injuries in childhood using intravenous regional anesthesia, *J Pediatr Orthop* 8:576-579, 1988.

40. Ordog GJ, Ordog C: The efficacy of TAC with various wound application durations, *Acad Emerg Med* 1:360-363, 1994.

41. Orlinsky M, Dean E: Local and topical anesthesia and nerve blocks of the thorax and extremities. In Roberts JR, Hedges JR, editors: *Clinical procedures in emergency medicine,* Philadelphia, 1991, WB Saunders.

42. Pinheiro JMP, Furdon S, Ochoa LF: Role of local anesthesia during lumbar puncture in neonates, *Pediatrics* 91:379-382, 1993.

43. Pryor GJ, Kilpatrick WR, Opp DR: Local anesthesia in minor lacerations: topical TAC vs. lidocaine infiltration, *Ann Emerg Med* 9:568-571, 1980.

44. Schaffer DJ: Clinical comparison of TAC anesthetic solutions with and without cocaine, *Ann Emerg Med* 14:1077-1080, 1985.

44a. Schilling CG, Bank DE, Borchert BA, et al: Tetracaine, epinephrine (adrenaline) and cocaine (TAC) vs. lidocaine, epinephrine, and tetracaine (LET) for anesthesia of lacerations in children, *Ann Emerg Med* 25:203-208,1995.

45. Schubert CJ, Wason S: Cocaine toxicity in an infant following intranasal instillation of a four percent cocaine solution, *Pediatr Emerg Care* 8:82-83, 1992.

46. Selbst SM: Managing pain in the pediatric emergency department, *Pediatr Emerg Care* 5:56-63, 1989.

47. Selbst SM: Pain management in the emergency department. In Schechter NL, Berde CB, Yaster M, editors: *Pain in infants, children, and adolescents,* Baltimore, 1993, Williams & Wilkins.

48. Selbst SM, Henretig FM: The treatment of pain in the emergency department, *Pediatr Clin North Am* 36:965-978, 1989.

49. Seldan R, Sasahara AA: Central nervous system toxicity induced by lidocaine, *JAMA* 202:908, 1967.

50. Spivey WH, McNamara RM, MacKenzie RS, et al: A clinical comparison of lidocaine and bupivacaine, *Ann Emerg Med* 16:752-757, 1987.

51. Stevenson TR, Rodehearer GT, Golden et al: Damage to tissue defenses by vasoconstrictors, *J Am Coll Emerg Physicians* 4:532-535, 1975.

52. Stewart RD: Local anesthesia. In Paris PM, Steward RD, editors: *Pain management in emergency medicine,* Norwalk, Conn, 1988, Appleton & Lange.

53. Stoelting RK, Miller RD: *Basics of anesthesia,* New York, 1984, Churchill Livingstone.

54. Terndrup TE, Walls HC, Mariani PJ, et al: Plasma cocaine and tetracaine levels following application of topical anesthesia in children, *Ann Emerg Med* 21:162-166, 1992.

55. Thompson AE, Frader JE: Pain management in children. In Paris PM, Stewart RD, editors: *Pain management in emergency medicine,* Norwalk, Conn, 1988, Appleton & Lange.

56. Tyler I: The relative pain inflicted by techniques used for insertion of needles, *Anesth Analg* 63:373-374, 1984 (letter).

57. Uheri M: A eutectic mixture of lidocaine and prilocaine for alleviating vaccination pain in infants, *Pediatrics* 92:720-721, 1993.

58. Weimer DR: Epinephrine pain with local anesthesia, *Plast Reconstr Surg* 73:997, 1984 (letter).

59. Wightman MA, Vaughan RW: Comparison of compounds used for intradermal anesthesia, *Anesthesiology* 45:687-689, 1976.

60. Yaster M, Tobin JR, Fisher QA, et al: Local anesthetics in the management of acute pain in children, *J Pediatr* 124:165-176, 1994.

16 Regional Anesthesia

Stephanie A. Walton and Dee Hodge III

Regional anesthesia is anesthesia to sensory nerves serving a particular anatomic region. It provides sensory block of a region without altering the normal anatomic features of the area to be repaired. Because less anesthetic agent is necessary for larger wounds, the regional technique is more advantageous than local infiltration. Once familiar with the body's sensory zones, the physician caring for children can readily employ these techniques in the Emergency Department (ED), pediatric intensive care unit (PICU), or office setting.

LOCAL ANESTHETIC AGENTS

There are two main classes of local anesthetic agents: the esters and amides. They stabilize neuronal membranes by inhibiting the ionic fluxes required for initiation and conduction of nerve impulses. The amide agents include the most commonly used anesthetics, lidocaine and bupivacaine; other amide agents are etidocaine and mepivacaine. If a child has exhibited an allergic reaction to an amide, then use an ester agent. The common ester agents include procaine and tetracaine.[6]

Epinephrine added to an agent increases its duration of action. Use only in areas with good perfusion. Avoid epinephrine-containing agents on areas in and around the fingers, toes, penis, ears, and nose.[16]

Buffered agents, particularly lidocaine, are less painful on injection than nonbuffered agents. To buffer lidocaine, add 1 ml sodium bicarbonate (44 mEq/50 ml) to 9 ml lidocaine for a total of 10 ml. It is possible to buffer the agent without compromising the efficacy.[2-4,10]

When using these agents, have pediatric resuscitation equipment and drugs on hand and have experience in their use.[1] Allow adequate time for the anesthetic to take effect. The area of anesthesia spreads from proximal to a distal sensory distribution. See Table 16-1 for discussion of the most commonly used agents.

Indications

Regional anesthesia produces profound analgesia with minimal physiologic or anatomic alteration. These techniques are especially useful in large or extensive lacerations that require the infiltration of large amounts of anesthetic agent for wound repair. These techniques are also useful in cosmetic repairs where local infiltration would cause distortion of tissues or loss of anatomic landmarks. Finally digital blocks are useful for wound débridement and nail bed repair. The discussions of specific blocks review specific indications.

Contraindications

There are few contraindications to regional anesthesia in children. They include infection at the site of puncture, history of bleeding disorder or coagulopathy, allergy to anesthetic agent, and degenerative axonal disease.[6,18] Patient uncooperativeness is a relative contraindication but is usually manageable with conscious sedation (Chapter 12).

Complications

Complications either are mechanical in nature or result from drug toxicity. Among the blocks commonly used in the ED, mechanical complications are rare. They are the result of incorrect needle placement and include hematomas, vascular compression ("compartment" syndrome), direct injury to nerve bundles, and pain from intraneural injection.

Adverse reactions to the anesthetic agents and toxicity are more common but also rare.[13,14,19] Adverse reactions of all the local anesthetic agents are similar (Table 16-2). These manifestations may sometimes be the result of inadvertent intravascular injection; to prevent intravascular injection, aspirate with the syringe. If there is blood return on aspira-

Table 16–1 Commonly Used Anesthetic Solutions

Agent	Maximum Dose (with Epinephrine)	Duration (minutes)	Comments
Lidocaine 1%, 1.5%, 2%	4–5 mg/kg (7 mg/kg)	60–120	Intermediate potency, rapid onset, metabolized by liver, excreted by kidneys, pH 6.5
Mepivacaine (Carbocaine) 1%, 1.5%, 2%	5 mg/kg) (6 mg/kg)	30–60	Intermediate potency, may buffer with bicarbonate, block longer than lidocaine, metabolized by liver, excreted by kidneys
Bupivacaine (Marcaine)	1.5 mg/kg (3 mg/kg)	3–4 times lido-	High potency, long duration, slower onset of action; caution in children under 12
Procaine, 1% (Novocaine)*		caine	Low potency, short duration of action
Tetracaine (Pontocaine)*			High potency, long duration, safety in children not established

*Esters.

Table 16–2 Adverse Reactions of Local Anesthetics

System/manifestation	Reaction
Central nervous system	Excitation to depression
	Nervousness
	Dizziness
	Tremors
	Drowsiness
	Unconsciousness and coma
Cardiovascular	Myocardial depression
	Hypotension
	Bradycardia to arrest
Allergic	Urticaria and edema
	Anaphylaxis

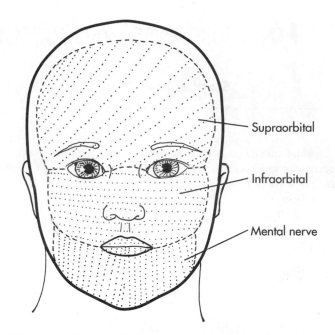

FIG. 16-1 Sensory distribution of the nerves of the face.

tion, reposition the needle and ensure that there is no blood return in the syringe. The absence of blood in the syringe does not guarantee that the needle is not intravascularly positioned.

Equipment

In general, a minimal amount of equipment is necessary to perform the regional blocks described in this chapter. A 5- to 10-ml syringe, a 25- to 27-gauge needle, and an anesthetic agent are the only supplies required for most blocks. Sections on specific techniques discuss the additional equipment needed for specific blocks.

SELECTED BLOCKS OF THE HEAD AND FACE

Refer to Table 16-3 for information on indications, equipment, and anesthetics.

Mental Nerve Block

The mental nerve emerges from the foramen of the mandible as a branch of the inferior alveolar nerve directly below the second lower premolar and supplies the skin and mucosal membrane of the lower lip (Figs. 16-1 and 16-2).

Technique. There are two approaches, the intraoral and extraoral routes. The intraoral approach produces less discomfort.

INTRAORAL. Pretreat the mucosa in the sulcus of the lower lip with a topical anesthetic such as cetacaine. Spray a small amount of cetacaine or apply a cetacaine-soaked swab for 2 to 3 minutes. Retract the lower lip and with a needle and syringe enter the sulcus at the gingival buccal mucosa, anterior and inferior to the second premolar (see Fig. 16-2, *A*). Inject 1 to 2 ml of anesthetic solution in and around the site after careful aspiration. Vigorously shake the lower lip as the needle enters the mucosa. This seems to help mask some of the discomfort of injection.

EXTRAORAL. Prepare the skin overlying the foramen. With the needle and syringe enter the skin directly over the foramen. Inject 1 to 2 ml of anesthetic solution into and around the site after careful aspiration (see Fig. 16-2, *A*).

Infraorbital Nerve Block

The infraorbital nerve exits from the infraorbital foramen and supplies the teeth and upper lip, as well as an area around the nose and the lower eyelid (see Fig. 16-1).

Table 16–3 Selected Blocks of the Head

Block	Indication	Equipment/anesthetic
Mental	Lacerations of the lower lip	25 to 27 gauge 1 to 1.5-2 in needle 5 ml syringe Viscous/spray lidocaine, 1 % or 2 % lidocaine with epinephrine

Infraorbital	Lacerations of the upper lip, lateral/in-ferior nose, and lower eyelid	25 to 27 gauge 1 to 1.5-2 in needle,
		    5 ml syringe,
		Viscous or spray lidocaine
		    1% or 2% lidocaine with epinephrine

Supraorbital	Lacerations of the forehead and ante-rior scalp	25 to 27 gauge 1 to 1.5-2 in needle, 1% or 2% lidocaine with epinephrine
Auricular	Lacerations of the auricle, débride-ment, hematoma evacuations	25 to 27 gauge 2.5-3 in needle, 1% lidocaine without epinephrine

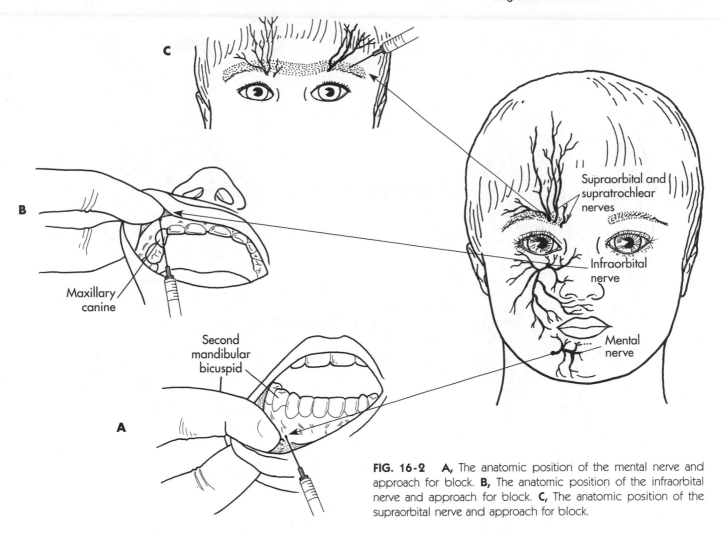

FIG. 16-2   A, The anatomic position of the mental nerve and approach for block. **B,** The anatomic position of the infraorbital nerve and approach for block. **C,** The anatomic position of the supraorbital nerve and approach for block.

Technique. There are two approaches for this block. The extraoral route produces less discomfort.

INTRAORAL. Apply a topical anesthetic such as cetacaine to the superior gingival sulcus just above the canine tooth (see Fig. 16-2, *B*). Spray a small amount of cetacaine or apply a cetacaine-soaked swab for 2 to 3 minutes. Palpate the infraorbital foramen beneath the orbital ridge. Evert the lip and vigorously shake it as the needle enters. With the needle, enter the superior gingival sulcus just medial to the canine tooth. Advance the needle toward the foramen using the free index finger to palpate the foramen as a marker. Inject 1 ml of anesthetic with an additional 0.5 to 1 ml to the right and left of the foramina.

EXTRAORAL. Prepare the overlying skin with alcohol. With the needle and syringe, enter the skin directly over the foramina. Inject 1 ml of anesthetic solution directly over the region and an additional 0.5 to 1 ml to the right and left.

Supraorbital and Supratrochlear Nerve Block

The supraorbital and supratrochlear nerves exit from the supraorbital foramina. They provide sensation to the anterior scalp and forehead (see Fig. 16-1).

Technique. Palpate the supraorbital foramina, then pull the brow up and away. Prepare the area. Inject 1 ml of

anesthetic over the foramen and an additional 0.5 to 1 ml lateral to the foramen. The supratrochlear nerve exits 0.5 to 1 cm medial to the supraorbital foramen. Without removing the needle, inject another 1 ml of anesthetic medial to the foramen. Using gentle pressure, press a finger against the lid. This reduces the chance of anesthetic's tracking down into the lid tissues (see Fig. 16-2, *C*).

An alternate method is to deposit anesthetic in a horizontal line extending across both supraorbital ridges. This technique is useful when the laceration crosses the midline.

Auricular Block

The auricle receives its sensory supply from the greater auricular nerve and the auriculotemporal nerve (Fig. 16-3, *A*).

Technique. Prepare the area in and around the ear. Begin just below the lobule in the sulcus behind the ear; with needle and syringe, enter the skin and deposit 3 to 5 ml of anesthetic in a track. Without removing the needle, redirect and lay a track anterior to the lobule and tragus (Fig. 16-3, *B*). Next remove the needle and enter the skin just superior to the helix. Lay a track of 3 to 5 ml just behind the helix. Redirect the needle and lay a track anterior to the tragus.[17] Complete anesthesia should occur in about 10 minutes.

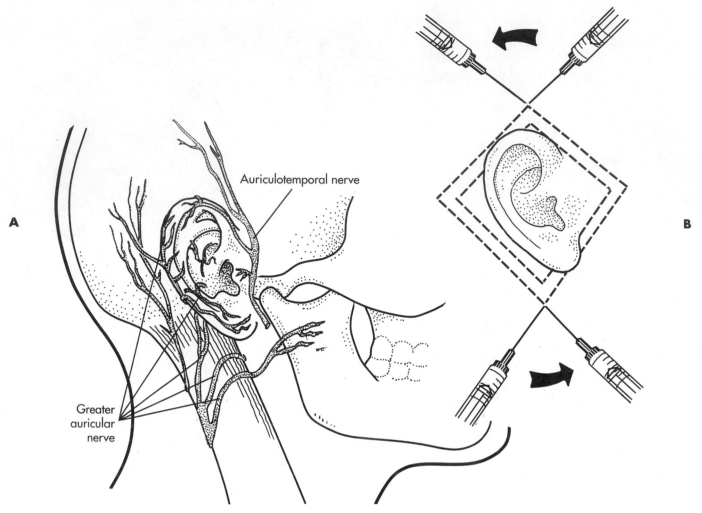

FIG. 16-3   **A,** Sensory nerve supply to the auricle. **B,** Approach for the auricular block.

SELECTED BLOCKS OF THE UPPER EXTREMITY

Use the median, ulnar, and radial blocks alone or in combination to provide effective anesthesia of the hand. Refer to Table 16-4 for discussion of indications, equipment, and anesthetic agents.

Median Nerve Block

The location of the median nerve is at the proximal flexor crease of the wrist between the tendons of the palmaris longus and the flexor carpi radialis. If the palmaris longus tendon is absent, the nerve lies just radial to the tendons of the flexor sublimis. Identify the tendons by opposing the thumb and the fifth digit while slightly flexing the wrist (Fig. 16-4). The median nerve supplies sensation to the palmar aspect of the first three and one half fingers, the dorsal half of those fingers, and the skin over the lateral part of the palm (Fig. 16-5, *A* and *B*).

   Technique. Place the extremity in the supine position. In young children immobilize the extremity with an armboard and place a small roll of gauze underneath the wrist to hold it in flexion. Next locate the site of injection. With needle, and syringe advance anesthetic down through the flexor retinaculum about 0.5 to 1 cm. If this produces paresthesias,

withdraw the needle slightly and, after careful aspiration, inject about 2 ml of anesthetic; then inject another 2 ml subcutaneously. If there are no paresthesias, inject 5 ml in and about the area. Anesthesia may not be complete for 20 minutes.

Ulnar Nerve Block

The ulnar nerve passes behind the medial epicondyle of the humerus. At the wrist its course becomes superficial and lies between the tendons of the flexor carpi ulnaris and the flexor digitorum superficialis. About 5 cm proximal to the wrist, the ulnar nerve divides into the dorsal and palmar branches. The radial artery lies lateral to the palmar branch. The larger dorsal branch supplies the dorsum of the little finger, the ulnar half of the fourth digit, and the ulnar aspect of the dorsum of the hand. The smaller palmar branch supplies the palmar aspect of the little finger, the palmar aspect of the ulnar half of the fourth finger, and the ulnar aspect of the palm (see Fig. 16-5, *A* and *B*). Blocking the ulnar nerve at the elbow provides complete ulnar anesthesia. Because of its division near the wrist, a wrist block may not provide complete anesthesia to both branches; however, it does usually provide anesthesia to the palmar branch.

Table 16–4   Selected Blocks of the Upper Extremity

Block	Indication	Equipment/Anesthetic
Median	Laceration and wound repair of the palmar aspect of the first three digits and the radial half of the palm	Armboard Roll gauze 25 to 27 gauge 1 to 1.5-in needle 10 ml syringe 2% lidocaine or bupivacaine
Ulnar	Laceration and wounds to the dorsal and palmar aspects of hand, fifth and ulnar side of the fourth finger	25 to 27 gauge 1 to 1.5-in needle 10 ml syringe 2% lidocaine or bupivacaine
Radial	Laceration and wounds on the dorsum of the thumb, second and third fingers, and radial aspect of the dorsum of the hand	25 to 27 gauge 1 to 1.5-in needle 10 ml syringe 1% or 2% lidocaine without epinephrine
Digital	Lacerations involving single fingers, nail bed repair, reduction of interphalangeal joint dislocations, or fractures of the phalanx	25 to 27 gauge 2.5-in needle, 10 ml syringe 1% lidocaine without epinephrine

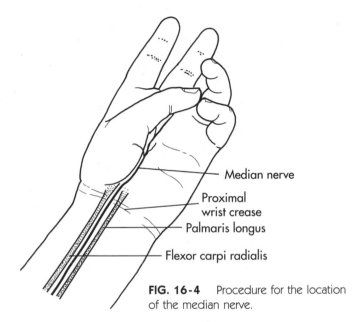

- Median nerve
- Proximal wrist crease
- Palmaris longus
- Flexor carpi radialis

FIG. 16-4   Procedure for the location of the median nerve.

Technique

ELBOW. Locate and palpate the ulnar nerve between the medial epicondyle and the olecranon. Inject 2 to 3 ml around, but not into, the nerve (Fig. 16-6, *A*). If this produces paresthesias, withdraw the needle slightly before injection.

WRIST. Locate the tendon of the flexor carpi ulnaris by asking the patient to ulnar deviate the wrist against resistance. Locate the pisiform bone on the ulnar flexor surface of the wrist. Palpate the tendon of the flexor carpi ulnaris at its attachment to the pisiform. Insert the needle into the skin just radial to and under the tendon at the proximal wrist crease. Insert to a depth of 1 to 2 cm. Aspirate to reduce the risk of an intravascular injection and then inject 3 to 5 ml of lidocaine. Withdraw the needle to just below the skin and infiltrate 5 ml of lidocaine from the flexi carpi ulnaris to the ulnar styloid (see Fig. 16-6, *B*). It may take up to 15 minutes for anesthesia to take effect.[12]

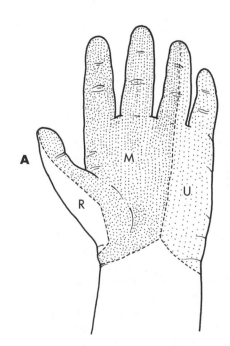

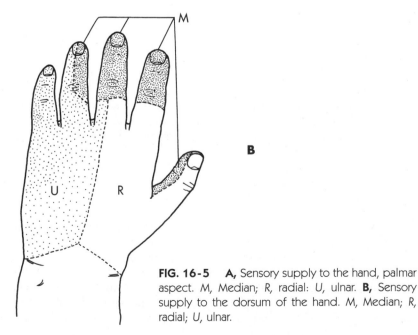

FIG. 16-5   **A,** Sensory supply to the hand, palmar aspect. *M,* Median; *R,* radial: *U,* ulnar. **B,** Sensory supply to the dorsum of the hand. *M,* Median; *R,* radial; *U,* ulnar.

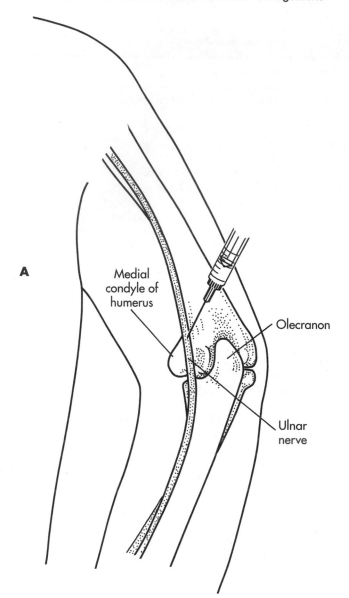

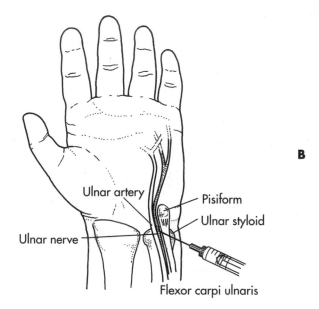

FIG. 16-6 **A,** Ulnar nerve block at the elbow. **B,** Ulnar nerve block at the wrist.

Radial Nerve Block

The radial nerve branches out at the level of the wrist to supply sensory innervation to the dorsal-radial aspect of the hand (see Fig. 16-5, *A* and *B*). It runs with the radial artery in the forearm.

Technique. Inject 10 ml subcutaneously in a track along the radial side of the wrist at the proximal skin crease just lateral to the radial artery and extending dorsilateral to the middle of the dorsum of the wrist (Fig. 16-7, *A* and *B*). This technique should block all sensory branches of the radial nerve. Time to anesthesia may be as long as 15 minutes.

Digital Blocks

There are two palmar and two dorsal nerves that lie on either side of the phalanges and supply sensation to the distal finger and fingertip. They derive from the common digital nerves, a branch of the ulnar and median nerves (Fig. 16-8).

Technique. Take care not to inject more than 2 to 4 ml of anesthetic solution into a digit. Never use epinephrine-containing agents. The ring technique causes local swelling

of the finger and therefore a temporary reduction in blood flow to the digit.

RING BLOCK. With the palm down, enter the dorsum of the proximal phalanx with the needle. Near the base, deposit a small wheal of anesthetic. Reposition and direct the needle down perpendicularly to the bone just past the base of the phalanx. Inject 0.5 to 1 ml on the palmar-lateral aspect of the finger. Withdraw the needle slightly and inject another 0.5 to 1 ml on the dorsal-lateral aspect of the finger. Repeat the procedure on the other side.

THE WEB SPACE BLOCK. The web space block has the advantage of producing less swelling. Therefore, there is little risk of compromise of the blood supply. It is also less painful than the ring block. With a needle, syringe, and anesthetic, enter the palmar aspect of the web space on both sides of the digit to a depth of about 0.5 cm and inject with about 1 ml of lidocaine (see Fig. 16-8). When using this block on the second and fifth digits, in addition to infiltration of the web space, do a half ring block on the ulnar side of the fifth digit and the radial side of the second digit. To block the

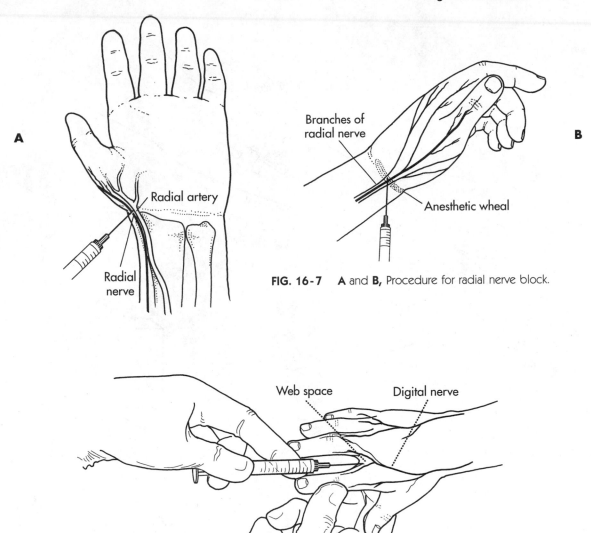

A

Radial artery

Radial nerve

Branches of radial nerve

Anesthetic wheal

B

FIG. 16-7   **A** and **B,** Procedure for radial nerve block.

Web space   Digital nerve

FIG. 16-8   Nerve supply to the digits and technique for web space block.

thumb, infiltrate the dorsum and sides in a half ring manner. Anesthesia will extend from the base of the finger to the tip over 15 minutes.

BIER BLOCK. The Bier block, which August Bier first described in 1908, is a technique that uses intravenous lidocaine and provides effective anesthesia of the upper extremity. It is indicated for closed reductions of upper extremity fractures, dislocations, and more extensive wound repairs. Its use has been successful in children as young as 2 years of age. The procedure is contraindicated in patients with peripheral vascular disease or with known allergies to lidocaine. This section describes the minidose Bier block, which uses a lower dose of lidocaine. Analgesia lasts from 30 to 90 minutes. Equipment needed includes two pneumatic

tourniquets, 0.5% lidocaine, rubber compression bandage (Esmarch), cottonette, syringes, angiocath, and tape.

Technique. Place the patient on a cardiorespiratory monitor and have resuscitation equipment readily available. First discuss the procedure with the child in an attempt to allay fears. Obtain intravenous access in an unaffected extremity. Consider sedation with a benzodiazepine. Place the child supine and wrap the upper arm (area for tourniquet placement) with cottonette. Place two inflatable tourniquets or blood pressure cuffs over the cottonette. Start an intravenous line in the affected limb distal to the distal tourniquet for lidocaine infusion (Fig. 16-9, *A*). The dorsum of the hand is the preferred site. Now exsanguinate the limb to rid the arm of excess blood standing in veins. Accomplish limb exsan-

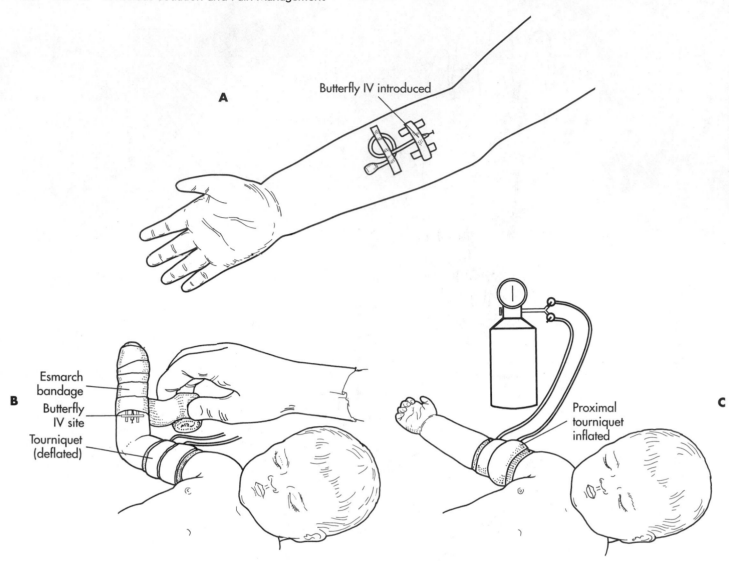

A, Butterfly IV introduced

B, Esmarch bandage / Butterfly IV site / Tourniquet (deflated)

C, Proximal tourniquet inflated

FIG. 16-9   Bier block: **A,** IV inserted into vein (preferred site is a dorsal vein in the hand). **B,** Elastic wrap applied and two blood pressure (BP) cuffs in place. **C,** Proximal cuff inflated.

guination by either of two techniques. In the first, elevate the limb for at least 30 seconds. This technique is less painful in the fractured arm. In the second, elevate the arm and wrap with bandage (Esmarch), starting from the hand and working up past the wrist and forearm to the elbow, taking care not to dislodge the intravenous (IV) line (Fig. 16-9, *B*). Both techniques produce effective anesthesia.

Next, rapidly inflate the proximal tourniquet to 100 mm Hg above systolic blood pressure. Rapid inflation minimizes blood flow and occludes the arterial system before the venous system, preventing engorgement of the arm with blood. Now inject 1.5 ml/kg of 0.5% lidocaine into the IV of the affected limb. Anesthesia should be complete in 5 minutes; if not, give additional lidocaine to a maximum of 3 ml/kg of body weight. Now begin the procedure. After injection of lidocaine, keep the tourniquet inflated for a minimum of 15 minutes for diffusion into surrounding tissues. This technique prevents large amounts of lidocaine from entering the systemic circulation, potentially producing toxicity.[7,11] Pain may develop under the proximal tourniquet; if it is unbearable, inflate the distal tourniquet as it lies over

an area of anesthesia and then deflate the proximal site. Deflate the tourniquet after the procedure is complete. Immediate return of perfusion to the extremity should occur. Return of sensation should follow. Observe the child for at least 1 hour after the procedure for signs of toxicity or complications of sedation. Complications include cardiac irregularity (usually from early release of lidocaine into circulation), thrombophlebitis, allergic reactions, tinnitus, and seizures or myoclonic twitching (usually the result of excessive systemic absorption of lidocaine).

SELECTED BLOCKS OF THE LOWER EXTREMITIES

Use the following blocks in combination to provide effective anesthesia to the foot. Refer to Table 16-5 for discussion of indications and equipment.

Nerve Block of the Toes

Technique. The nerve block of the toe is similar to the half ring block of the finger, described earlier. Insert the needle at a point on the dorsum of the toe in the midline

Table 16–5   Selected Blocks of the Lower Extremity

Block	Indication	Equipment/Anesthetic
Sole	Foreign body removal; wound débridement, laceration, and wound repair	25 gauge 1.5 to 2-in needle 10 ml syringe 2% lidocaine or bupivacaine
Dorsum	Wound débridement and laceration repair	25 gauge 1.5 to 2-in needle 10 ml syringe 1% lidocaine or bupivacaine
Digital	Nailbed repair, débridement and foreign body removal, reduction of interphalangeal joint dislocations or fractures of the phalanx	25 gauge 1.5-in needle 10 ml syringe 1% or 2% lidocaine without epinephrine

proximal to the point of injury. Raise a wheal of anesthetic in the midline. Now direct the needle medially and inject 1 to 2 ml along the side of the toe. Withdraw and redirect the needle laterally and inject another 1 to 2 ml along this side of the toe. Anesthesia should be complete in 10 minutes.

Anesthesia to the great toe requires an additional injection on the plantar surface because of its unique nerve supply. Proceed with the half ring block as described. Next, on the plantar surface, complete the ring block by inserting the needle near the base of the toe in the midline. Next, direct the needle medially and inject 0.5 to 1 ml of anesthetic. Now withdraw, redirect laterally, and inject another 0.5 to 1 ml of solution to complete the ring. Anesthesia should take place in 10 minutes.

Nerve Block to the Sole

The sole of the foot is a commonly injured area that tends to be difficult to anesthetize. Regional nerve blocks are much less painful than local infiltration. The nerve supply to the sole of the foot derives from two main nerves, the sural and the posterior tibial nerve. With both nerves blocked, complete anesthesia of the sole is possible.

The sural nerve supplies the posterior lateral aspect of the ankle and the heel, as well as the lateral aspect of the foot and the fifth toe. The posterior tibial nerve divides into the medial and lateral plantar branches, which supply sensation to the sole of the foot (Fig. 16-10, *A*).

Technique. The location of the posterior tibial nerve is between the Achilles tendon and the medial malleolus. Place the patient in the prone position. Locate the base of the medial malleolus and the Achilles tendon. Palpate the posterior tibial artery. Insert a 2-inch needle perpendicularly to the skin and lateral to the Achilles tendon at the upper border of the medial malleolus. Direct the needle lateral and posterior to the artery (Fig. 16-10, *B*). Advance the needle until it touches the tibia. If paresthesias result, withdraw slightly and inject up to 5 ml of anesthetic. If paresthesias do not result, inject 5 to 10 ml of anesthetic while slowly withdrawing the needle. Anesthesia is complete in 15 to 25 minutes.[15]

The sural nerve runs with the short saphenous vein behind the lateral malleolus. Place the patient prone and find the outer border of the lateral malleolus and the Achilles tendon. Insert the needle just lateral to the Achilles tendon at a level 1 cm above the lateral malleolus. Direct the needle superiorly to the lateral malleolus (Fig. 16-10, *C*). Infiltrate about 5 ml

of anesthetic in a fanlike manner between the Achilles tendon and the lateral malleolus. Anesthesia is complete in 10 to 15 minutes.

Nerve Block to the Dorsum of the Foot

The nerve supply to the dorsum of the foot includes the saphenous nerve, the superficial peroneal nerve, and the anterior tibial or deep peroneal nerve (see Fig. 16-10, *A*).

The saphenous nerve is a branch of the femoral nerve and courses parallel to the saphenous vein. It supplies the anteriomedial aspect of the ankle. The superficial peroneal nerve is a branch of the common peroneal nerve and supplies almost the entire dorsum of the foot. The anterior tibial nerve or the deep peroneal nerve is a branch of the popliteal nerve and courses between the tendons of the tibialis anterior and the extensor hallicus longus. It supplies sensation to a small area between the first two toes.

Technique. For the saphenous nerve block, position the patient supine with a roll under the calf. This relaxes the foot in a plantar-flexed position. Palpate the medial malleolus and locate the tendon of the extensor hallicus longus. At a point just 1 cm above the base of the medial malleolus and just medial to the tendon of the extensor hallicus longus, insert the needle perpendicularly until it reaches the tibia (Fig. 16-10, *D*). Withdraw the needle slightly and inject 2 ml of anesthetic. Now withdraw the needle to the subcutaneous tissue and inject another 2 ml toward the medial malleolus. Allow 5 to 10 minutes for anesthesia.

To block the superficial peroneal nerve, draw an imaginary line from the anterior border of the tibia to the lateral malleolus. Use 5 to 10 ml of anesthetic and lay down a track of anesthetic subcutaneously on that line between the two. Allow 5 to 10 minutes for anesthesia.

To block the anterior tibial nerve, locate the point midway between the lateral and the medial malleolus on the dorsum of the foot. Insert the needle until it reaches the tibia, and then withdraw slightly and inject 3 to 4 ml of anesthetic (Fig. 16-10, *D*). Anesthesia occurs in 5 to 10 minutes.

PENILE BLOCK

Penile blocks provide anesthesia to the penis for repair of lacerations. The sensory innervation of the penis arises primarily from the right and left dorsal nerves of the penis. These are terminal branches of the pudendal nerve. At the

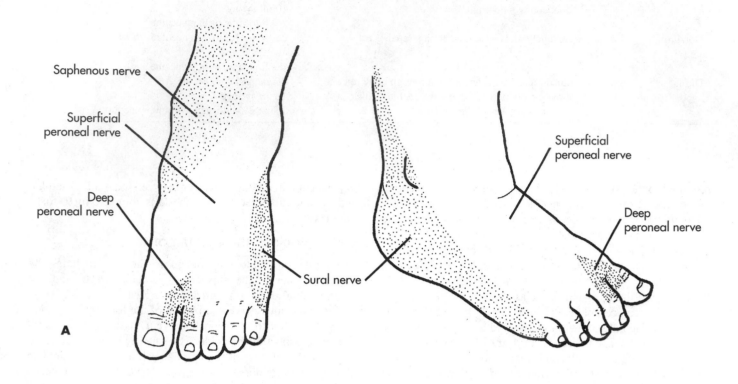

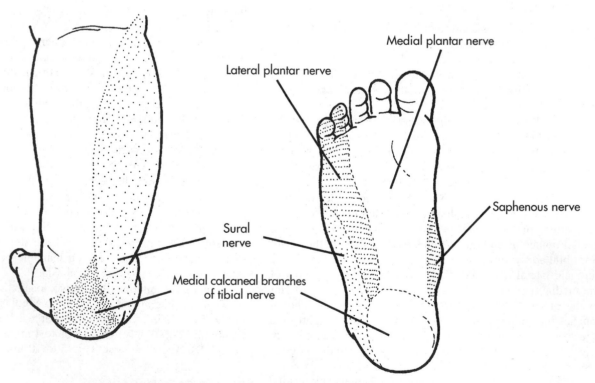

FIG. 16-10 **A,** The sensory distribution of the nerves of the foot.

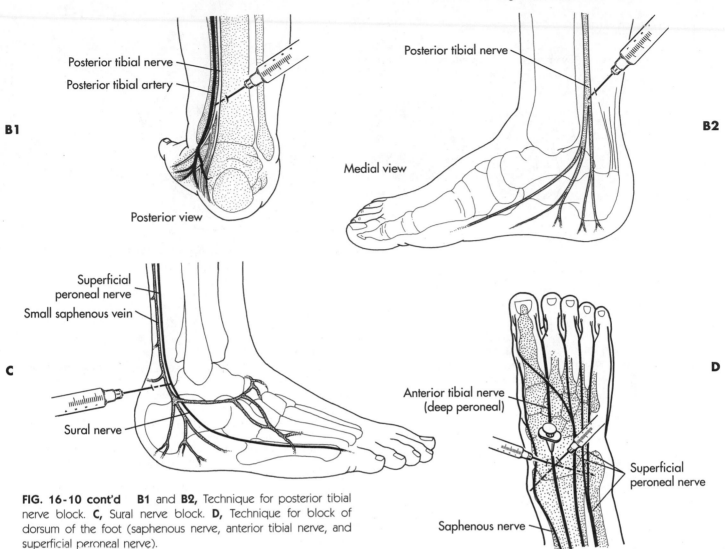

B1 and **B2**, Technique for posterior tibial nerve block. **Posterior view**, **Posterior tibial nerve**, **Posterior tibial artery**. **Medial view**, **Posterior tibial nerve**.

C, **Superficial peroneal nerve**, **Small saphenous vein**, **Sural nerve**.

D, **Anterior tibial nerve (deep peroneal)**, **Superficial peroneal nerve**, **Saphenous nerve**.

FIG. 16-10 cont'd   B1 and **B2,** Technique for posterior tibial nerve block. **C,** Sural nerve block. **D,** Technique for block of dorsum of the foot (saphenous nerve, anterior tibial nerve, and superficial peroneal nerve).

root of the penis, the dorsal nerves, arteries, and vein course 3 to 5 mm under the skin surface between Buck's fascia and the corpora cavernosa. The two nerves occupy positions at 10 and 2 o'clock (Fig. 16-11). In addition, the base of the penis receives sensory supply from the ilioinguinal nerve and the genitofemoral nerve. Achieve penile block either by a subcutaneous ring of local anesthetic or by specific block of the dorsal nerves. The ring technique is easier but requires more anesthetic.

Technique. Prepare the base of the penis and an area around the penis. Never use epinephrine-containing agents.

RING BLOCK. Envision a triangle encircling the penis with the apex located at the median raphe of the scrotum and the base located at the superior base of the penis. Use a 25 to 26 gauge needle 1 to 3 inches long, depending on the size of the patient. Begin at the superior base of the penis and lay a linear track of anesthetic deposited both intradermally and subcutaneously parallel to the base. Solution must be deposited at the base of the penis between the corpora cavernosa and the deep penile fascia. Remove the needle and lay a track

along the side of the penis from the superior wheal at the base of the penis to the triangle apex, the inferior site on the median raphe of the scrotum (Fig. 16-11). Next remove the needle and repeat for the other side of the triangle.[5,6] Anesthesia will extend from the base of the penis to the tip over 15 minutes.

DIRECT NERVE BLOCK. Identify by palpating the symphysis pubis and the corpora cavernosa at the penile root. Gently pull down on the penis. Insert the needle at either the 10 o'clock or the 2 o'clock site, 0.5 to 1 cm distal to the point where the penile root passes under the pubic arch (Fig. 16-12, *A*). Enter the skin and the fascia with the needle at an acute angle, directed slightly posteromedially (Fig. 16-12, *B*). Advance the needle until a give is felt when Buck's fascia is crossed. The tip of the needle should be freely mobile. If it is not, it is most likely embedded in the corpora cavernosum and should be withdrawn slightly. After aspiration, inject 0.1 ml/kg of anesthetic agent. Repeat the procedure at the second puncture site.[5,8,9] Allow 10 to 15 minutes for anesthesia to occur.

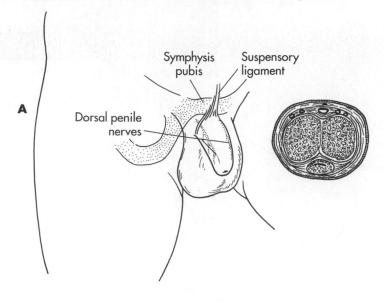

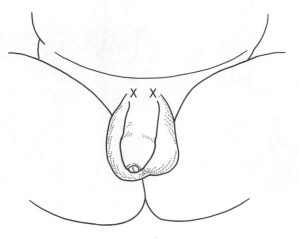

FIG. 16-11 **A,** Location of the dorsal penile nerves. **B** Subcutaneous wheal of anesthesia deposited in triangular fashion at base of penis.

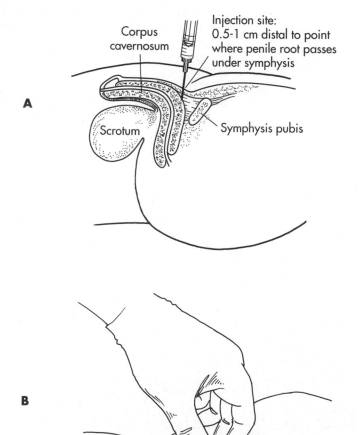

FIG. 16-12 **A** and **B,** Injection sites and technique for dorsal penile nerve block.

REFERENCES

1. American Academy of Pediatrics Committee on Drugs, *Pediatrics* 89:1110-1115, 1992.
2. Bancroft JW, Benenati JF, Becker GJ, et al: Neutralized lidocaine: use in pain reduction in local anesthesia, *J Vasc Interv Radiol* 3:107-109, 1992.
3. Bartfield JM, Ford DT, Honer PJ: Buffered versus plain lidocaine for digital nerve blocks, *Ann Emerg Med* 22:216-219, 1993.
4. Bartfield JM, Gennis P, Barbera J, et al: Buffered versus plain lidocaine as a local anesthetic for simple laceration repair, *Ann Emerg Med* 19:1387-1389, 1990.
5. Broadman LM, Hannallah RS, Belman B, et al: Post-circumcision analgesia—a prospective evaluation of subcutaneous ring block of the penis, *Anesthesiology* 67:399-402, 1987.
6. Dalens B: Regional anesthesia in children, *Anesth Analg* 68:654-672, 1989.
7. Farrell RG, Swanson SL, Walter JR: Safe and effective IV regional anesthesia for use in the emergency department, *Ann Emerg Med* 14:239-240, 1985.
8. Fontaine P, Toffler WL: Dorsal penile nerve block for newborn circumcision, *Am Fam Pract* 43:1327-1333, 1991.
9. Lau JTK: Penile block for pain relief after circumcision in children, *Am J Surg* 147:797-799, 1984.
10. Morris R, McKay W, Mushlin P: Comparison of pain associated with intradermal and subcutaneous infiltration with various local anesthetic solutions, *Anesth Analg* 66:1180-1182, 1987.
11. Onley BW, Lugg PC, Turner PL, et al: Outpatient treatment of upper extremity injuries in children using intravenous regional anaesthesia, *J Pediatr Orthop* 8:576-579, 1988.
12. Paris PM, Stewart RD: *Pain management in emergency medicine,* East Norwalk, Conn, 1988, Appleton & Lange.
13. Riez S, Nath S: Cardiotoxicity of local anaesthetic agents, *Br J Anaesth* 58:736-746, 1986.
14. Scott DB: Toxic effects of local anaesthetic agents on the central nervous system, *Br J Anaesth* 58:732-735, 1986.
15. Simon RR, Brenner BE: *Emergency procedure and techniques,* ed 2, Baltimore, 1987, Williams & Wilkins.
16. Todd K, Berk WA, Huang R: Effect of body locale and addition of epinephrine on the duration of action of a local anesthetic agent, *Ann Emerg Med* 21:723-726, 1992.
17. Trott A: *Wounds and laceration: emergency care and closure,* St. Louis, 1991, Mosby.
18. Yaster M, Tobin JR, Fisher QA, et al: Local anesthetics in the management of acute pain in children, *J Pediatr* 124:165-176, 1994.
19. Yaster M, Maxwell LG: Pediatric regional anesthesia, *Anesthesiology* 70:324-338, 1989.

AIRWAY TECHNIQUES

17 Upper Airway Obstruction

Timothy S. Yeh and Dean B. Andropoulos

Management of the patient with severe, acute upper airway obstruction requires an understanding of the mechanism of obstruction, as well as the differential diagnosis. The symptoms of obstruction of the proximal airway are the result of an acute change in airway resistance. Poiseuille's law relates the resistance produced by the *laminar* flow of gas in the airway inversely to the radius (r) raised to the fourth power. This is expressed as

$$\text{Resistance} = \frac{8lh}{\pi r^4} \qquad 1$$

where h = viscosity of gas, l = length of tube, and r = radius of tube.

With turbulent flow the radius is raised to the fifth power. Therefore absolute or relatively significant decreases in airway diameter can produce clinically important increases in airway resistance (as in an infant with a 5-mm airway in whom 1 mm of edema develops).[11]

Obstruction of the upper airway may manifest as changes in respiratory rate and character (retractions, grunting, nasal flaring), as well as associated findings of cardiac failure and pulmonary edema.[9,13] In addition obstruction in the extrathoracic (above the clavicles) and intrathoracic proximal airways produces the two cardinal symptoms of inspiratory stridor and expiratory wheezing, respectively.

Acute upper airway obstruction for the most part is due to acquired conditions (Box 17-1). However, in the newborn and infant, congenital abnormalities may be important and may become acutely symptomatic (Box 17-1). A careful history and physical examination can usually differentiate among three of the most common acquired causes of obstruction: epiglottitis, laryngotracheobronchitis, and bacterial tracheitis (Table 17-1).

PROCEDURES FOR MANAGING SEVERE, ACUTE UPPER AIRWAY OBSTRUCTION
Medical Therapy

The most basic principle of therapy is to *avoid upsetting* the child and thereby precipitating acute, complete airway obstruction. Allow patients who are in severe respiratory distress to assume a *position* of comfort (Fig. 17-1) and allow a parent to remain close at hand to *calm* or to hold the child. *Avoid needlesticks* and other upsetting procedures until the airway is secure. Provide *oxygen* for all patients in respiratory distress, but avoid causing upset by forcing it on the child. Often the child's parent can offer the mask or hold it gently on the child's face. It is important to observe the child closely with *cardiorespiratory monitoring* and *pulse oximetry;* however, do not delay definitive treatment of the specific abnormality causing severe, acute upper airway obstruction.

It is clear that appropriate *antibiotic therapy* and *drainage of abscesses* may be necessary for the treatment of certain

---

BOX 17–1 DIFFERENTIAL DIAGNOSIS OF COMMON CAUSES OF ACUTE UPPER AIRWAY OBSTRUCTION IN INFANTS AND CHILDREN

Congenital

Choanal atresia
Hypoplastic facial anomalies
Vocal cord paralysis
Aberrant vascular structures (rings and slings)
Laryngeal and tracheal webs and stenosis
Laryngotracheal malacia

Acquired

Infection

Epiglottitis
Laryngotracheobronchitis (croup)
Peritonsillar abscess
Retropharyngeal abscess
Diphtheria
Tonsillar and adenoidal hypertrophy
Bacterial tracheitis
Laryngeal papillomatosis

Trauma

Subglottic stenosis (secondary to prior airway manipulation)
Foreign body aspiration
Inhalation injuries (thermal and chemical)
External trauma (massive facial trauma, crush injuries to the larynx)

Miscellaneous

Extrinsic intrathoracic or cervical masses (tumor or lymphadenopathy)
Angioedema
Central nervous system depression with laxity of oropharyngeal soft tissue structures

---

infectious causes of acute upper airway obstruction. Although frequently used, *cool mist therapy* is not of proven benefit.[5]

The use of inhaled *racemic epinephrine* (0.05 ml/kg diluted to 3 ml with saline solution, nebulized q1-4h [prn]; maximum dose 0.5 ml) may be of benefit for patients with laryngotracheobronchitis.[5,8]

Corticosteroid therapy for laryngotracheobronchitis remains controversial.[12] Some practitioners have used doses of 0.1 to 0.2 mg/kg of dexamethasone (for four doses). However, a recent study recommended a single dose of 0.6 mg/kg of dexamethasone (orally [po], intramuscularly [IM], or intravenously [IV]).[17]

Table 17–1 History and Physical Examination

	Epiglottitis	Laryngotracheo-bronchitis	Bacterial tracheitis
Age	2-7 yr	3 mo-3 yr	All ages
Onset	Sudden	Gradual	Gradual
Fever	High	Low	High
Appearance	Toxic	Nontoxic	Toxic
Posture	Upright, leaning, forward, drooling	No preference	Upright
Cry	Muffled	Bark, stridor	Bark, stridor
Sore throat	Yes	No	Minimal

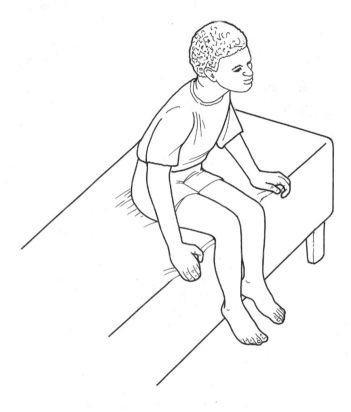

FIG. 17-1 Child in the "tripod" position or "position of comfort" frequently assumed by children with severe, acute upper airway obstruction.

Another adjunct for patients with severely narrowed airways is the use of a *helium-oxygen* mixture. Helium-oxygen has a lower viscosity than nitrogen-oxygen, producing more laminar, less turbulent flow through narrowed airways and thus reducing the work of breathing for the patient. It may be a useful adjunct before the onset of frank respiratory failure. However, some patients may be at increased risk for hypoxemia.[2,15]

Use a mask or head hood to deliver the helium-oxygen mixture since it is necessary to maintain a helium concentration greater than 60% to achieve clinical benefit. The helium-oxygen mixture is available preblended (80%:20%, 70%:30%, 60%:40%), and respiratory therapists can blend in additional oxygen at the bedside as needed. Follow pulse

oximetry continuously when using the 80%:20% mixture since the effective FIO_2 delivered is only approximately 20%.

In many cases of severe, acute upper airway obstruction, medical management alone is insufficient. In these instances it is necessary to perform one of the following interventions.

Adjunctive Methods

Oropharyngeal and Nasopharyngeal Airways.[3] Oropharyngeal and nasopharyngeal artificial airways are indicated for use in tonsillar and adenoidal hypertrophy as well as central nervous system depression with laxity of oropharyngeal soft tissue structures (see also Chapter 20). They are contraindicated in massive facial trauma and suspected abnormalities of the airway at or below the level of the glottis. Oropharyngeal artificial airways are not well tolerated in the conscious patient. In addition, oropharyngeal and nasopharyngeal artificial airways are seldom appropriate for long-term management of the obstructed upper airway. Instead, provide definitive therapy with a more secure airway such as an endotracheal or tracheostomy tube.

Continuous Positive Airway Pressure. There are few indications for the use of external continuous positive airway pressure (CPAP) devices in severe, acute upper airway obstruction. The primary effect of CPAP is to increase functional residual capacity (FRC), and it is therefore more likely to be of benefit in patients with lower airway and alveolar disease.[18] However CPAP and positive-pressure ventilation delivered by a bag-valve-mask device may be useful for first-line therapy to establish a patent airway in patients with acute epiglottitis who experience sudden obstruction before definitive airway establishment.[10]

Bag-Mask Ventilation. Bag-mask ventilation is essential for the delivery of high FIo_2 and positive pressure in preparation for definitive airway management for upper airway obstruction (see also Chapter 24). Bag-mask ventilation is contraindicated when a patient has *partial* airway obstruction with adequate air exchange and oxygenation (e.g., epiglottitis, foreign body, or laryngotracheobronchitis). Application of bag-mask ventilation in this situation may agitate the patient and increase the severity of obstruction. Use "blow-by" oxygen instead. Always institute bag-mask ventilation while preparing for definitive airway management.

Definitive Airway Management

Endotracheal Intubation.[1,7] Proceed to endotracheal intubation for the definitive management of severe, acute upper airway obstruction unresponsive to more conservative measures (see also Chapter 21). There are no absolute contraindications to endotracheal intubation for severe, acute upper airway obstruction. A relative contraindication exists for massive facial trauma since laryngoscopy may be difficult. Immediate surgical airway access may be necessary.

Rendering a patient unconscious and/or paralyzed for laryngoscopy and identifying the glottic opening may be difficult (e.g., in most cases of obstruction at or above the level of the vocal cords such as epiglottitis, massive facial trauma, retropharyngeal abscess, or atypical anatomy). Assure that the most skilled, experienced person performs the intubation, preferably an anesthesiologist. When possible, perform such intubations in the controlled setting of the operating room (OR), using a technique that maintains spontaneous ventilation (usually slow inhalation induction of anesthesia with halothane). In addition, have a surgeon present who is skilled in techniques of surgical airway management (i.e., rigid bronchoscopy, cricothyroidotomy, and tracheostomy). If the patient's condition precludes waiting to assemble OR staff and equipment, then the most skilled and experienced person available must proceed, using clinical judgment about use of sedation and paralysis. Prepare for emergency cricothyroidotomy should tracheal intubation attempts fail.

Specialized endotracheal intubation techniques (fiber-optic bronchoscopy, retrograde wire techniques, specialized laryngoscope blades) all require time to assemble equipment and highly skilled personnel and are often not useful for management of the acutely obstructed upper airway.

Cricothyroidotomy. Use cricothyroidotomy for definitive airway management of severe, acute upper airway obstruction when attempts at endotracheal intubation are unsuccessful or impossible (see also Chapter 22). Cricothyroidotomy is relatively contraindicated in severe neck trauma. If airway obstruction is due to a tracheal foreign body, cricothyroidotomy is unlikely to improve the condition.

Cricothyroidotomy is rarely necessary in the pediatric population and is fraught with technical difficulty because of small anatomic structures, especially in infants and young children. It is almost always possible to intubate the trachea by using direct laryngoscopy. Needle cricothyroidotomy may be effective in temporarily oxygenating the patient until it is possible to secure a surgical airway.[6] However adequate ventilation is difficult to achieve except by using special jet ventilation devices.[14,16] There are few reports of successful application of this technique in young children in the emergency situation. Therefore the techniques of surgical or percutaneous cricothyroidotomy are preferable to allow placement of a larger tube (3-mm inner diameter or larger) to accomplish both oxygenation and ventilation by using standard breathing circuits.[4]

REFERENCES

1. Berry FA: Acute airway obstruction, with special emphasis on epiglottitis and croup. In Berry FA, editor, *Anesthetic management of difficult and routine pediatric patients,* ed 2, New York, 1990, Churchill Livingstone, pp 243-266.

2. Butt WW, Koren G, England S, et al: Hypoxia associated with helium-oxygen therapy in neonates, *J Pediatr* 106:474, 1985.

3. Chameides L, Hazinski MF, editors: Pediatric airway management. In *Textbook of pediatric advanced life support,* Dallas, 1994, American Heart Association.

4. Chameides L, Hazinski MF, editors: Pediatric airway management. In *Textbook of pediatric advanced life support,* Dallas, 1994, American Heart Association.

5. Corkey CWB, Barker GA, Edmonds DF, et al: Radiographic tracheal diameter measurements in acute infectious croup: an objective scoring system, *Crit Care Med* 9:587, 1981.

6. Coté CJ, Eavey RD, Todres ID, et al: Cricothyroid membrane puncture: oxygenation and ventilation in a dog model using an intravenous catheter, *Crit Care Med* 16:615-619, 1988.

7. Coté CJ, Todres ID: The pediatric airway. In Coté CJ, Ryan JF, Todres ID, et al, editors: *A practice of anesthesia for infants and children,* ed 2, Philadelphia, 1993, WB Saunders.

8. Fogel JM, Berg IJ, Gerber MA, et al: Racemic epinephrine in treatment of croup: nebulization alone versus nebulization with intermittent positive pressure breathing, *J Pediatr* 101:1028, 1982.

9. Galvis AG, Stool SE, Bluestone DC: Pulmonary edema following relief of acute upper airway obstruction, *Ann Otolaryngol* 89:124, 1980.

10. Glicklich M, Cohen RD, Jona JZ: Steroids and bag and mask ventilation in the treatment of acute epiglottitis, *J Pediatr Surg* 14:247, 1979.

11. Jardine DS, Crone RK: Specific diseases of the respiratory system: upper airway. In Fuhrman BP, Zimmerman JJ, editors: *Pediatric critical care,* St. Louis, 1992, Mosby, p 425.

12. Kairys SW, Olmstead EM, O'Connor GT: Steroid treatment of laryngotracheitis: a meta-analysis of the evidence from randomized trials, *Pediatrics* 83:683, 1989.

13. Kanter RK, Watchko JF: Pulmonary edema associated with upper airway obstruction, *Am J Dis Child* 138:356, 1984.

14. Ravussin P, Bayer-Berger M, Monnier P, et al: Percutaneous transtracheal ventilation for laser endoscopic procedures in infants and small children with laryngeal obstruction: report of two cases, *Can J Anaesth* 34:83-86, 1987.

15. Skrinkas GJ, Hyland RH, Hutcheon MA: Using helium-oxygen mixtures in the management of acute airway obstruction, *Can Med Assoc J* 128:555, 1983.

16. Steward DJ: Percutaneous transtracheal ventilation for laser endoscopic procedures in infants and small children, *Can J Anaesth* 34:429-430, 1987.

17. Super DM, Cartelli NA, Brooks LJ, et al: A prospective randomized double-blind study to evaluate the effect of dexamethasone in acute laryngotracheitis, *J Pediatr* 115:323-329, 1989.

18. Venkataraman ST, Orr RA: Mechanical ventilation and respiratory care. In Fuhrman BP, Zimmerman JJ, editors: *Pediatric critical care,* St. Louis, 1992, Mosby, p 528.

18 Manual Maneuvers for Opening the Airway

Steven W. Shirm

The initial goal in the management of a critically ill patient is to secure a patent airway. Blood, vomitus, or secretions may potentially obstruct the airway; however, a functional suction apparatus usually handles this problem. In addition the tongue itself may cause partial or complete airway obstruction in the semiconscious or unconscious patient. When normal muscular control of the lower jaw and tongue is lost, the tongue can be posteriorly displaced against the posterior pharynx and compromise the airway (Fig. 18-1, *A*).

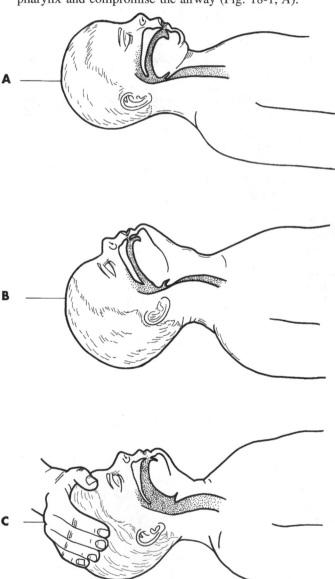

Indications and Contraindications

When the child has sustained head or neck trauma, assure that the airway is patent, but avoid hyperextension of the neck to prevent spinal cord injury. Because the infant's large head predisposes to hyperflexion of the cervical spine, use a towel roll under the shoulder in this age group to protect neutral spine positioning (see Fig. 24-4). Do not use the cervical spine-lift and head-tilt maneuvers as they are hazardous in the presence of cervical spine injury and provide less effective ventilation than the chin-lift or triple-airway maneuvers (Fig. 18-1, *B*).[1,2]

Techniques

The chin-lift is the most effective maneuver for opening an obstructed airway.[2] After suctioning thoroughly, place one hand on the infant's forehead to maintain a neutral or sniffing position (Fig. 18-1, *C*). Extend the child's head slightly if necessary. Place the fingers of the other hand under the bony portion of the chin and lift the mandible upward.[1] Use the thumb to manipulate the lower lip and assist with mask placement if spontaneous respirations are absent and bag-valve-mask-assisted ventilations are necessary (Fig. 18-2, *A*).

To perform the triple-airway maneuver, place two or three fingers of each hand at the angle of the mandible and manipulate the mandible caudad, anteriorly, and then cephalad, so that the mandible and lower teeth are anterior to the

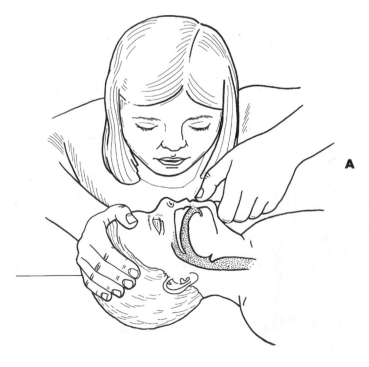

FIG. 18-1 **A,** Airway obstruction caused by hypotonia. **B,** Cervical hyperextension can obstruct an infant's airway and may be hazardous if cervical spine trauma is present. **C,** Sniffing position maximally opens the airway.

FIG. 18-2 **A,** Chin-lift maneuver.

upper jaw and teeth (Fig. 18-2, *B*). Tilt the head slightly if this maneuver alone does not adequately open the airway.[1]

Remarks

The triple-airway maneuver without head tilt is the safest maneuver for opening the airway when neck injury is suspected.[1]

REFERENCES

1. Chameides L, editor: Basic life support. In *Textbook of pediatric advanced life support,* Dallas, 1994, American Heart Association, pp 11-19.
2. Guildner CW: Resuscitation—opening the airway: a comparative study of techniques for opening the airway obstructed by the tongue, *J Am Call Emerg Phys* 5:588-590, 1976.

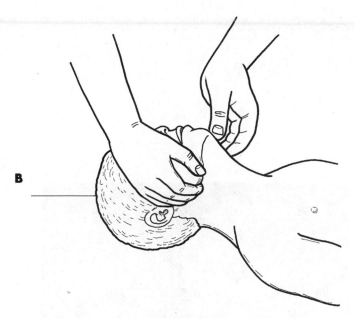

FIG. 18-2, cont'd   B, Triple-airway maneuver.

19 Emergency Maneuvers for Airway Obstruction by Foreign Body

Steven W. Shirm

Suspect aspiration of a foreign body when there is sudden onset of respiratory distress, which may include coughing, gagging, wheezing, or stridor. Aphonia, anxiety, and cyanosis may also be present.

Indications and Contraindications

Initiate maneuvers to clear the airway after witnessed aspiration or in the unconscious apneic patient whose airway remains obstructed despite the chin-lift or jaw-thrust maneuver. If the victim is able to speak and has an effective cough, attempts to dislodge the object by back blows or abdominal thrusts may cause a partial obstruction to become a complete airway obstruction. Consider maneuvers for removal of foreign bodies when the patient's cough is no longer effective (loss of sound) or respiratory distress increases.[3]

If the infant or child can speak, can cry, or has an effective cough, leave him or her in a position of comfort and give only supplemental oxygen as tolerated. Remove the foreign body in a controlled environment such as the operating room. If the patient loses cough effectiveness, experiences increased respiratory difficulty with stridor, or loses consciousness, initiate maneuvers to relieve an obstructed airway.[3]

When the victim is a child, use the Heimlich maneuver (a series of subdiaphragmatic abdominal thrusts). Increasing intrathoracic pressure expels the foreign body from the airway. For infants younger than 1 year of age, use back blows and chest thrusts to prevent possible intraabdominal injury caused by the Heimlich maneuver.[3]

Equipment

Most of these techniques do not require any supplies or equipment; however, it may be necessary in the most difficult cases to use a laryngoscope and Magill forceps (Fig. 19-1) for foreign body removal.

Technique

Position infants less than 1 year old so that they straddle the rescuer's forearm with the head and face dependent (Fig. 19-2). The rescuer should firmly support the infant's jaw and rest his or her own forearm on the thigh for support. Deliver up to five back blows between the infant's scapulae with the heel of the hand. Turn the child over, keeping the head in a dependent position (Fig. 19-3). Apply up to five chest thrusts by two fingers placed midsternum, one finger breadth below the intermammary line. After each series of five back blows and five chest thrusts, remove any visible object from the oropharynx. Repeat this sequence until it is possible to remove the object or the infant becomes unconscious.[3]

If the child is more than 1 year of age and conscious, perform the Heimlich maneuver. Stand behind the victim and

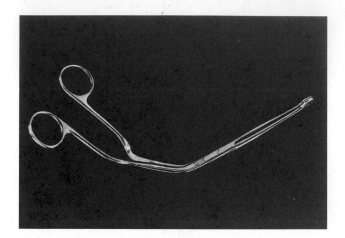

FIG. 19-1 Magill forceps.

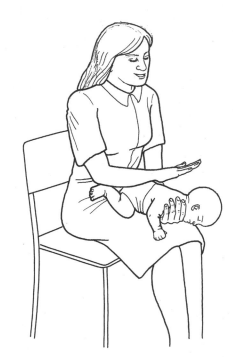

FIG. 19-2 Infant position for back blows.

place a fist midway between the navel and xiphoid process with the thumb firmly against the abdomen (Fig. 19-4). With the other hand, grasp the fist and with a quick, upward thrust, press the fist into the child's abdomen. Continue five distinct thrusts until the foreign body dislodges or the victim loses consciousness.[3]

If the child is unconscious, place him or her on the back.

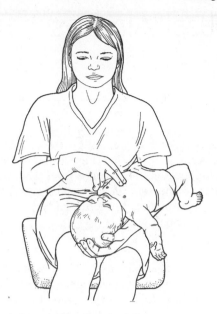

FIG. 19-3   Infant position for chest thrusts.

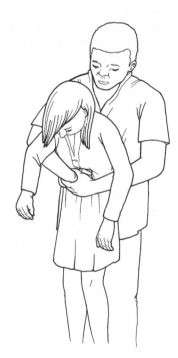

FIG. 19-4   Heimlich maneuver for conscious child, sitting or standing.

Stand at the feet if a child is on a bed, or kneel at the feet of a child who is on the floor. Straddle a larger child. With the heel of one hand on the child's abdomen midline above the navel and below the xiphoid process, place the other hand on the first hand. Perform a series of five distinct upward thrusts (Fig. 19-5).[3]

In the unconscious victim, after each series of chest thrusts or subdiaphragmatic thrusts, remove any visible foreign body by opening the victim's mouth and grasping the tongue and lower jaw between the forefinger and thumb and lifting anteriorly. Open the airway by manual maneuvers. If spontaneous respirations are absent, attempt to ventilate the patient. If unable to ventilate the patient, repeat the series of

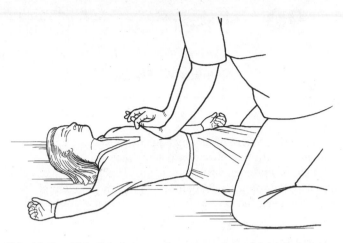

FIG. 19-5   Heimlich maneuver for unconscious child, lying supine.

back blows and chest thrusts or abdominal thrusts and again attempt to ventilate the patient.[3]

When an unconscious victim arrives at the hospital, attempt to ventilate the patient by using suction and simple maneuvers to open the airway. If unable to ventilate the patient, perform a series of back blows and chest thrusts or abdominal thrusts. If still unable to ventilate the patient, attempt visualization of the foreign body by direct laryngoscopy and removal with Magill forceps.

Place toddlers on a flat surface. Children older than 2 years may require elevation of the head on a towel in order to achieve the sniffing position. A straight laryngoscope blade provides better visualization of the glottis in infants and toddlers; a curved laryngoscope blade is preferable in older children and adults. Grasp the laryngoscope handle in the left hand, and insert the blade into the right side of the mouth to the base of the tongue. In order to visualize the glottic opening, use the tip of the straight blade to lift the epiglottis directly or insert the tip of the curved blade into the vallecula to displace the tongue anteriorly. Sweeping the blade and the handle to midline provides optimal visualization of the airway and creates a channel on the right side of the oral cavity through which to use Magill forceps to grasp and remove a visualized foreign body or through which to insert an endotracheal tube.[2]

If unable to visualize or remove the foreign body, use orotracheal intubation to dislodge a tracheal foreign body into a main stem bronchus, thus converting a complete airway obstruction to a partial obstruction.[1] If attempts at ventilation are still unsuccessful, consider needle cricothyrotomy or immediate bronchoscopy. Surgical cricothyrotomy and tracheotomy are options for skilled physicians (see also Chapter 22).[2]

REFERENCES

1. Brownstein D: Foreign bodies of the gastrointestinal tract and airway. In Barkin RM, editor: *Pediatric emergency medicine,* St. Louis, 1992, Mosby.
2. Chameides L, Hazinski MF, editors: Airway and ventilation. In *Textbook of pediatric advanced life support,* Dallas, 1994, American Heart Association.
3. Chameides L, Hazinski MF, editors: Pediatric basic life support. In *Textbook of pediatric advanced life support,* Dallas, 1994, American Heart Association.

20 Insertion of Oral and Nasal Airways

Steven W. Shirm

After establishment of airway patency by suction and manual maneuvers, the unconscious patient may require an airway adjunct to maintain airway patency. Use an oropharyngeal airway or nasopharyngeal airway to prevent the tongue from falling against the posterior pharyngeal wall and obstructing the airway.

Indications and Contraindications

Use an oropharyngeal airway only in an unconscious patient.[1] Oropharyngeal airways can induce emesis in a patient with an intact gag reflex. In addition to maintaining airway patency by supporting the tongue, an oral airway can prevent approximation of the teeth. This allows for oral suctioning and prevents occlusion of an oral endotracheal tube or oral gastric tube by the teeth.

Nasopharyngeal airways are less likely than oropharyngeal airways to induce gagging in responsive patients. Take care not to cause epistaxis during placement. Avoid nasopharyngeal airways in patients with suspected basilar skull fractures or bleeding disorders.

Complications

An improperly placed oropharyngeal airway can actually displace the tongue posteriorly and cause airway obstruction. An airway that is too long can induce emesis or laryngospasm.[3]

In children with prominent adenoidal tissue, epistaxis can complicate airway management. Mucus, blood, or vomitus can easily obstruct small-diameter nasopharyngeal airways.

Equipment

Oropharyngeal airways are made of plastic and consist of a proximal flange, a bite block, and a curved body that is hollow or channeled to provide an air passage or suction conduit (Fig. 20-1). Determine the proper size of oral airway by placing the flange at the level of the incisors with the tip of the airway reaching the angle of the mandible.[1] For approximate sizes, see Table 20-1.

Nasopharyngeal tubes are made of soft rubber and are available in sizes 12 to 36 (Fr) (Fig. 20-2). To determine the proper length, measure the distance from the tip of the nose to the tragus of the ear.[1] If a nasopharyngeal tube is not available, it is permissible to shorten an endotracheal tube to the appropriate length.[3]

Technique

Place the oropharyngeal airway by holding the tongue to the floor of the mouth with a tongue depressor and advancing the airway into position (Fig. 20-3).[1-3] Tape the oral airway in proper position to prevent expulsion by the tongue. The alternate method of inverting the airway (using the curved portion as a tongue depressor, advancing the airway, and rotating the airway 180 degrees when in position) is no longer recommended in children.[2] Placed in this way, the airway may damage the teeth and can lacerate the vascular mucosa and soft palate and cause hemorrhage, further compromising the airway.

Insert the nasopharyngeal airway in the nostril after lubrication and advance it along the floor of the nasopharynx until the flared end rests at the nasal orifice (Fig. 20-4). Be certain that the airway is not so large as to blanch the nasal ala because necrosis may result.[1]

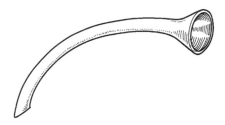

FIG. 20-2 Nasopharyngeal airway.

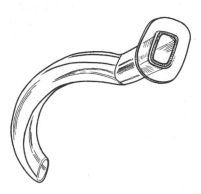

FIG. 20-1 Oropharyngeal airway.

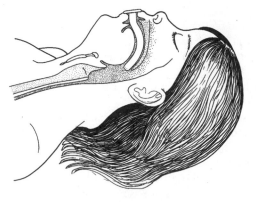

FIG. 20-3 Oropharyngeal airway in position.

Table 20-1   Selection of Appropriate Oropharyngeal Airway Size

Age	Weight (kg)	Airway choice		
Premature	1-2.5	Infant	00	35 mm
Neonate	3-5	Infant/small	0	35 mm
6 months	6-9	Small	1	40 mm
1-2 yr	10-13	Small	2	60 mm
4-6 yr	15-20	Medium	3	80 mm
8-10 yr	25-32	Medium/large	4/5	90 mm
12 yr	35-45	Large	5	100 mm
Adult	50-90	Large	6	100 mm

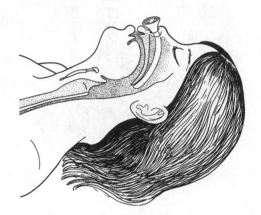

FIG. 20-4   Nasopharyngeal airway in position.

Remarks

Observe any patient with an oropharyngeal or nasopharyngeal airway closely with pulse oximetry and cardiac monitoring. These temporary airways do not replace intubation as definitive airway management, and many children who tolerate oral and nasal airways without resistance require endotracheal intubation.

REFERENCES

1. Chameides L, Hazinski MF, editors: Airway and ventilation. In *Textbook of pediatric advanced life support,* Dallas, 1994, American Heart Association.
2. Committee on Trauma: Airway management and ventilation. In *Advanced trauma life support course,* Chicago, 1989, American College of Surgeons, pp 33-41.
3. Coté CJ, Todres ID: The pediatric airway. In Coté CJ, Ryan JF, Todres ID, et al, editors: *A practice of anesthesia for infants and children,* Philadelphia, 1993, WB Saunders, pp 55-80.

21 Pediatric Emergency Airway Management

Ann Thompson

Emergency intubation often becomes necessary under adverse circumstances, without specific preparation, in settings where equipment and experienced personnel are very limited, for patients with physiologic instability. Successful placement without complications requires attention to the process of laryngoscopy and intubation, awareness of the physiologic effects and risks of the procedure, and development of an approach that minimizes undesirable effects.

Indications (Box 21-1)

Because respiratory failure may result from dysfunction at any point along the ventilatory pathway, make the decision to intubate after a full assessment of that child's central nervous system, airway structures, and functional integrity of the chest wall. The appropriate intervention depends on the pathophysiologic characteristics of the underlying problem and the degree of physiologic derangement. *Lower airway and pulmonary parenchymal disorders,* resulting in either hypoxemia or hypercarbia, are perhaps the most common reasons for intubation. *Upper airway obstruction,* inadequately responsive to treatment, or conditions in which respiratory failure is predictable by knowledge of a disease process (e.g., airway burns), are other indications; in these conditions, poor gas exchange may not appear until quite late. Although the need for intubation and respiratory support during resuscitation is obvious, patients with lesser degrees of *hemodynamic instability* or *anticipated instability* may also benefit from respiratory support to prevent cardiopulmonary collapse, to reduce the work of breathing, and to allow redistribution of precious cardiac output from respiratory muscles to other systems. *Neuromuscular weakness,* resulting from abnormalities of the neuromuscular junction, peripheral, or spinal motor nerves; primary muscle disorders; or structural abnormalities of the bony thorax, may also precipitate respiratory insufficiency. Often the result of arterial blood gas analysis in these patients reveals no abnormality, but measures of respiratory reserve indicate that patients have profoundly impaired ability to clear secretions or prevent massive atelectasis. *Central nervous system dysfunction* may result in hypoventilation, with hypercarbia and secondary hypoxemia and carbon dioxide retention, or loss of protective airway reflexes. Intubation is indicated to assure adequate ventilation and to prevent aspiration. Other indications include intubation to provide *therapeutic hyperventilation* and to improve *management of pulmonary secretions.*

Complications

Predictable consequences or risks attend laryngoscopy and intubation (Box 21-2).* Critically ill and injured children may not readily tolerate these iatrogenic problems.

Anticipate the difficult airway. Recognizing features that

*References 2, 7, 11, 12, 16, 17, 22, 26, and 44.

> **BOX 21-1   INDICATIONS FOR INTUBATION**
>
> 1. PaO_2 <60 mm Hg with $FIO_2 \geq 0.6$ (in absence of cyanotic congenital heart disease)
> 2. $PaCO_2$ >50 (acute and unresponsive to other intervention)
> 3. Upper airway obstruction, actual or imminent
> 4. Neuromuscular weakness (maximum inspiratory pressure less negative than -20 cm H_2O; vital capacity < 12-15 ml/kg)
> 5. Absent protective airway reflexes (cough, gag)
> 6. Hemodynamic instability (cardiopulmonary resuscitation [CPR], shock)
> 7. Therapeutic hyperventilation (intracranial hypertension, pulmonary hypertension, metabolic acidosis)
> 8. Pulmonary toilet
> 9. Emergency drug administration

> **BOX 21-2   COMPLICATIONS OF LARYNGOSCOPY AND INTUBATION**
>
> 1. Tachyarrhythmias and bradyarrhythmias
> 2. Impedance to systemic and jugular venous return
> 3. Hypertension or hypotension
> 4. Hypoxia
> 5. Hypercarbia
> 6. Increased intracranial, intragastric, and intraocular pressures
> 7. Injury to airway structures (from lips or nose to alveoli)
> 8. Regurgitation or vomiting with possible aspiration
> 9. Inadvertent placement of the tube into the esophagus, soft tissues, or cranial vault
> 10. Cervical spinal cord injury
> 11. Generation of significant pain and anxiety

signal a difficult airway helps prevent untoward events. Micrognathia, glossoptosis, facial clefts, midface hypoplasia, maxillary protrusion, facial asymmetry, a small mouth, limited temporomandibular movement, or a short or inflexible neck may interfere with effective manual ventilation and visualization of the larynx. Traumatic injury with midface instability, upper airway bleeding, edema, mass, or foreign body also complicates the procedure.

Children with severe hypoxemia or hypovolemia, increased intracranial pressure, myocardial dysfunction, full stomach, or serious preexistent underlying disorders present additional challenges. Many children who experience life-threatening illness have chronic problems that predispose them to physiologic instability. Approach these children with a plan specific to their underlying condition.

Equipment

Because the need for emergency airway support may not allow time for extensive preparation, it is essential that equipment adequate for a wide variety of circumstances be available and organized in advance (Box 21-3).

Many types of masks for manual ventilation are available. Correct use requires familiarity with the design of each (see Chapter 24). Suction equipment must be immediately accessible and functional. Oxygen is the one absolutely essential drug. In all but the most extreme emergencies, insert an intravenous catheter for drug infusion. A bag for manual ventilation, a well-fitting mask (sitting on the bridge of the nose and bony prominence of the chin), a laryngoscope with a *working* light, an assortment of blades, endotracheal tubes of the estimated correct size as well as others 0.5 to 1 mm larger and smaller in internal diameter, and a means of securing the tube once it is correctly positioned must be ready. The choice of laryngoscope blade depends largely on operator preference. In general, straight blades provide good exposure in young children; for adolescent patients many find the MacIntosh 3 preferable.

No formula guarantees selection of the correct endotracheal tube size. Table 21-1 provides one set of guidelines. In general, after infancy, the following formula works well:

$$\text{Tube size (mm ID)} = [\text{Age (yr)}/4] + 4$$

Select a tube that, under usual conditions, allows a leak between 15 and 30 cm H_2O pressure. In children who are very small or large for age, the formula may be more accurate when height age is substituted for chronological age. For a gross approximation of correct endotracheal tube size, select a tube of a diameter similar to the width of the child's fifth *fingernail* (not finger).[23] For children with very poor lung compliance or high airway resistance, a larger than expected tube may be necessary to achieve effective ventilation without a prohibitively large leak around the tube. Uncuffed tubes are usually preferable in children up to the age of about 8 years, because the cricoid ring, rather than the vocal cords, represents the narrowest point of the trachea and the inflated cuff may cause ischemia to the cricoid area. Since the narrowed cricoid area already simulates the function of the cuff, the inflated cuff usually provides no additional benefit. However, in children who require high ventilatory pressures, cuffs may be helpful.

Monitoring

Meticulous patient monitoring is essential during intubation. In addition to being attentive to signs of changing perfusion, color, neurologic status, and impending regurgitation, monitor heart rate and rhythm, systemic blood pressure, and arterial oxygen saturation. After intubation, demonstration of expired CO_2 may be extremely helpful, either by capnometry or by use of a disposable end-tidal CO_2 detector[2,3,25] (see Chapter 28). Also obtain early blood gas analysis and a chest radiograph to confirm tube placement.

Pharmacologic Agents

Although tracheal intubation is possible without the use of drugs, one can minimize much of the pain and anxiety and many of the noxious physical and physiologic consequences of the procedure by *judicious* use of anesthetic, analgesic, sedative, and neuromuscular blocking agents.* *In inexperienced hands, use of these agents may be lethal.* However, use of these agents by knowledgeable operators enhances patient safety and comfort. It is essential to match drug selection to the individual patient's needs and condition; never use adjunctive drugs for tracheal intubation during cardiopulmonary resuscitation.

Anticholinergic drugs decrease oral secretions and prevent bradycardia during laryngoscopy, especially in infants. Most patients benefit from the use of *sedative agents*. Commonly used drugs include intravenous anesthetics, anxiolytics, and narcotic analgesics. The choice in a particular child depends on the child's level of anxiety, hemodynamic and neurologic status, and underlying condition. *Neuromuscular blocking agents* cause reversible paralysis, facilitating visualization of the airway and atraumatic insertion of the endotracheal tube. However, do *not* use these agents if any uncertainty exists about the operator's ability to control ventilation by bag and mask, particularly in patients with upper airway obstruction. Table 21-2 lists common representative drugs in these categories along with benefits and disadvantages.

Technique

Endotracheal Intubation

EMERGENCY ORAL INTUBATION. On encountering the apneic patient, begin efforts to support ventilation. First, posi-

---

*References 2, 8, 15, 17, 18, 21, 28, 33, and 44.

Table 21-1   Guidelines for Endotracheal Tube and Laryngoscope Size*

Age	Internal diameter (ID)	Orotracheal length (cm) (at teeth)	Nasotracheal length (cm) (at nares)
Endotracheal tube size			
Premature	2.0-3.0	6-8	7-9
Newborn	3.0-3.5	9-10	10-11
3-9 Mo	3.5-4.0	11-12	11-13
9-18 Mo	4.0-4.5	12-13	14-15
1.5-3 Yr	4.5-5.0	12-14	16-17
4-5 Yr	5.0-5.5	14-16	18-19
6-7 Yr	5.5-6.0	16-18	19-20
8-10 Yr	6.0-6.5†	17-19	21-23
11-14 Yr	6.5-7.0†	18-20	22-24
14-16 Yr	7.0-7.5†	20-22	24-25

Laryngoscope blade size	
Premature infant	Miller 0
Newborn-2 Yr	Miller 1
2-6 Yr	Miller 2, Wis-Hippel 1.5
6-12 Yr	Miller 2, MacIntosh 2
12-Adult	Miller 2-3, MacIntosh 3

*Ideal tube size for an individual child varies according to specific anatomic features, as well as the child's size and weight. For children far from average size for age, tube size is likely to correspond best to the child's "height age." In most children, an air leak around the tube at 15 to 30 cm H_2O pressure is desirable.

†Cuffed tube.

tion the patient and open and clear the airway, manually if necessary, to remove large solid obstructions; then suction thoroughly with a Yankauer device or large-bore suction catheter. If the child is still breathing spontaneously but is in need of intubation and ventilatory support, consider use of pharmacologic support (see Table 21-2). Give drugs only after adequate monitoring and all necessary equipment are ready.

While medications take effect, maintain manual ventilation or support spontaneous ventilation with supplemental oxygen. Place the child supine, the head in the "sniffing" position, with the neck slightly flexed at the shoulders and the head slightly extended at the occipitoatlantoid junction (Fig. 21-1, A to D). The large occipitofrontal diameter of infants naturally results in good position in most cases. In older children a thin pillow under the occiput is usually sufficient to achieve good head positioning. Extreme neck extension is rarely necessary, is potentially traumatic, and may actually result in airway occlusion in young children. Have an assistant prepare specific intubation equipment as manual ventilation continues.

Although in most patients correct head position makes manual ventilation easy, it may be necessary to employ the "jaw thrust" or "triple-airway maneuver" (see Chapter 18) to prevent occlusion of the upper airway by the soft tissues of the mouth and pharynx. Place the mask on the bridge of the nose and bony prominence of the chin to prevent pressure on the eyes, soft tissues of the nose, branches of the trigeminal and facial nerves, or submandibular tissue. After preparing equipment and oxygenating the patient as well as possible, proceed with laryngoscopy and intubation.

In the flaccid patient in good position, the mouth naturally falls open. Achieve additional exposure by placing one's little finger on the chin and opening the mouth, or by using thumb and index fingers in scissors fashion between the teeth. Place the laryngoscope into the right corner of the child's mouth and sweep the blade toward the center and deep into the pharynx, moving the tongue leftward and out of the way. After advancing the laryngoscope to the base of the tongue, place the tip of the laryngoscope blade into the vallecula or onto the epiglottis itself and visualize the larynx by lifting the mandible with pressure on the laryngoscope handle directed toward the ceiling at a 45- to 60-degree angle to the child's chest. To prevent lip, tooth, or alveolar ridge injury, do not use the laryngoscope as a crowbar. Visualization of the larynx requires lifting along the line of the laryngoscope handle, not pivoting on a fulcrum (Fig. 21-1, C). If visualization of the vocal cords is difficult, an assistant may help by providing gentle cricoid pressure.

After visualizing the cords, advance the endotracheal tube from the right corner of the mouth, not along the laryngoscope blade, into the pharynx and through the vocal cords, aligning the appropriate marking with them. This marking is usually a bold or double line, 2 to 5 cm from the tip, depending on the size of the tube and varying from product to product. Resist the tendency to advance the tube a few more centimeters; this practice serves only to increase the frequency of main stem intubation with associated hypoxia and barotrauma.

Once the tube is in place, assure correct position by observing moisture condensation in the tube, good chest

Table 21-2   Drugs Facilitating Intubation

Type of drug	Drug	Dose	Duration	Comments*
Anticholinergic	Atropine	0.01-0.02 mg/kg IV	5-10 min	
	Glycopyrrolate	0.005-0.01 mg/kg	10-15 min	
Intravenous anesthetic	Thiopental	4-6 mg/kg IV	5-10 min	Anesthesia; apnea; potent myocardial depression, ↓venous tone: ↓CMRO$_2$; CBP; ↓ICP; ↓IOP
	Ketamine	1-2 mg/kg IV (IM)	10-15 min	Anesthesia; ↑HR; ↑Systemic BP; ↑ICP; ↑IOP; bronchodilation; hallucinations; usually maintain spontaneous respiration and protective airway reflexes; possible laryngospasm
Sedatives and narcotics	Diazepam	0.1-0.3 mg/kg IV	1-4 hr	Amnesia; sedation; minimal hemodynamic or respiratory depression: moderate ↓CMRO$_2$
	Midazolam	0.1-0.3 mg/kg IV, IN	1-2 hr	Amnesia; sedation or euphoria; hemodynamic stability; occasional respiratory depression; moderate ↓CMRO$_2$
	Fentanyl	5-10 μg/kg IV	0.5-1.5 hr	Analgesia; dose-related respiratory depression; cardiovascular stability; possible bradycardia or chest wall rigidity
	Morphine	0.1-0.3 mg/kg IV, IM	2-4 hr	Analgesia; respiratory depression; histamine release may cause ↓systemic arterial and venous tone and ↓BP
Neuromuscular blocking agents	Pancuronium	0.1-0.2 mg/kg IV	45-60 min	↑HR; possible mild ↑BP; prolonged effect in kidney failure
	Vecuronium	0.1-0.3 mg/kg IV	35-75 min	Minimal cardiovascular effect; prolonged effect in liver failure
	Atracuronium	0.5 mg/kg IV	20-30 min	Mild histamine release may cause ↓BP
	Succinylcholine	1-2 mg/kg IV	5-10 min	Bradycardia; massive K$^+$ release in neuromuscular disease, trauma, burns; masseter spasm, or frank malignant hyperthermia; myoglobinuria; possible ↑ICP, ↑IOP, ↑IGP

*$CMRO_2$, Cerebral metabolic rate for oxygen; *CBF*, cerebral blood flow; *ICP*, intracranial pressure; *IOP*, intraocular pressure; *HR*, heart rate; *BP*, blood pressure.

excursion, symmetric breath sounds, pink color, and good oxygen saturation. The most reliable means to ensure proper tube placement, after clear visualization of its passing between the vocal cords, is colorimetric or digital measurement of expired carbon dioxide though the tube* (see Chapter 28). CO$_2$ production may not occur during full cardiopulmonary arrest (i.e., false-negative end-tidal carbon dioxide result), so use several contributing bits of evidence.

When using a cuffed tube, inflate the cuff with the *minimum occlusive volume* (i.e., the minimal amount of air required to occlude a leak around the endotracheal tube at 25- to 40-cm H$_2$O airway pressure).[14] Additional volume serves only to increase pressure within the cuff and on the tracheal mucosa, risking ischemia of the mucosa and cartilage. Alternatively inflate the cuff to *minimal leak pressure,* the pressure at which a minimal audible leak occurs with positive pressure inflation to 20 to 25 cm H$_2$O. The theoretical risk of damage to the tracheal mucosa may be lower with the minimal leak technique; however, using minimal occlusion volume may decrease the risk of aspiration and may be necessary for adequate ventilation of children with very noncompliant lungs. After securing the tube (discussed later), document the tip position between the thoracic inlet and carina by chest radiograph.

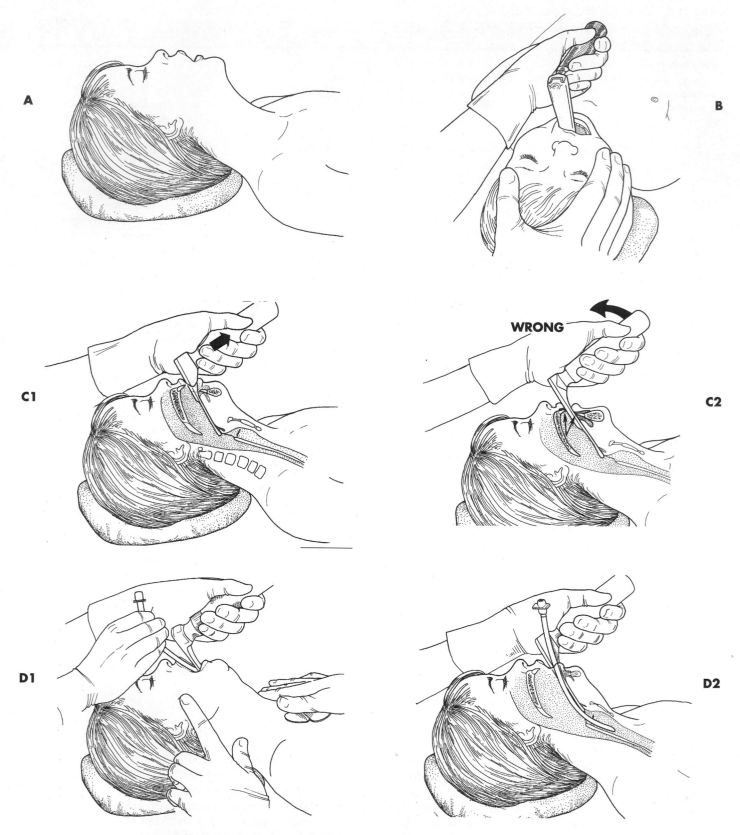

FIG. 21-1   **A,** In a flaccid child placed in the "sniffing" position, the mouth falls open.
B, Place the laryngoscope into the right corner of the mouth and advance into the pharynx,
sweeping the tongue leftward, until the tip of the blade is on the epiglottis or in the vallecula.
C, Lifting at a 45- to 60-degree angle along the handle of the layrngoscope, preventing
rotation onto the alveolar ridge or upper teeth, visualize the glottis. **D,** Advance the endotracheal
tube from the right corner of the mouth into the larynx.

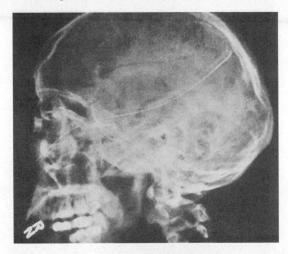

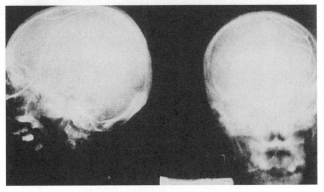

FIG. 21-2   Intracranial placement of endotracheal tube and nasogastric tube associated with basilar skull fracture. **A,** Endotracheal tube; **B,** nasogastric tube.

NASOTRACHEAL INTUBATION. Nasotracheal intubation may be desirable in awake patients, patients with oral abnormalities, those who require prolonged intubation, those troubled by profuse oral secretions or active gagging, or those who threaten an effective airway by excessive tongue movement or biting the tube. Box 21-4 summarizes contraindications (see also Fig. 21-2). In general, it is safest to perform nasotracheal intubation after stabilization with oral intubation and arrival of the patient in a controlled environment.

Position the awake patient (see previous discussion). Spray a topical vasoconstricting agent, such as phenylephrine 0.25% or oxymetazoline 0.05%, into the nasopharynx to minimize bleeding from local trauma. Advance a well-lubricated tube, usually of the same size as used orally, directly posteriorly along the floor of the nasal cavity (not cephalad) into the nasopharynx (Fig. 21-3). With the oral tube in the left corner of the mouth, proceed with laryngoscopy as described. Advance the nasal tube until its tip lies directly above the cords, anterior to the oral tube. Using Magill forceps, maneuver the tip into good position to enter the larynx; have the assistant remove the oral tube, and then advance the nasal tube into the larynx. On occasion there is difficulty advancing the tube, often because its curve directs the tip against the anterior tracheal wall; eliminate such difficulty by rotating the tube slightly or flexing the neck.

Blind nasal intubation is difficult in children. Although it is sometimes successful in cooperative, stable patients, it frequently takes longer, requires multiple attempts, and produces more complications than oral or nasal intubation under direct vision, even in adult patients.[37] The high, anterior position of the larynx in young children poses anatomic problems. Few major centers rely on it in critically ill children, but some experienced operators find this procedure a useful option in selected cooperative older children.

RAPID SEQUENCE INTUBATION. A child with a full stomach is at high risk for vomiting and aspirating gastric contents during intubation, particularly if protective airway reflexes

are impaired.[13] Patients who have eaten 4 to 6 hours before intubation are likely to have substantial gastric contents. Others at risk include those with bowel obstruction, either mechanical or functional; pharyngeal or upper gastrointestinal bleeding; tense abdominal distention resulting from any cause; or trauma or onset of illness within a few hours of eating. For most patients requiring intubation for other than elective intraoperative care, delaying intubation until the stomach empties is not feasible. In these patients minimize the danger of aspiration by the following steps (Box 21-5).

If the child is conscious and has effective protective airway reflexes, evacuation of gastric contents through a nasogastric or orogastric tube decreases the volume of retained material. This method lessens the risk of aspiration, but one can never assume that it has completely emptied the stomach. In a child with impaired airway reflexes, an attempt to pass a gastric tube may itself induce vomiting and is not indicated.

If the child appears to have a normal airway and an uncomplicated intubation is likely, perform rapid sequence intubation to minimize the risk of aspiration as well as the time between loss of protective reflexes and correct positioning of the endotracheal tube. Have the child spontaneously breathe 100% oxygen for 3 to 5 minutes, or, if old enough to cooperate, take four to five deep breaths. After "preoxygenation," give an anesthetic or sedative/analgesic combination by rapid intravenous infusion while an assistant applies

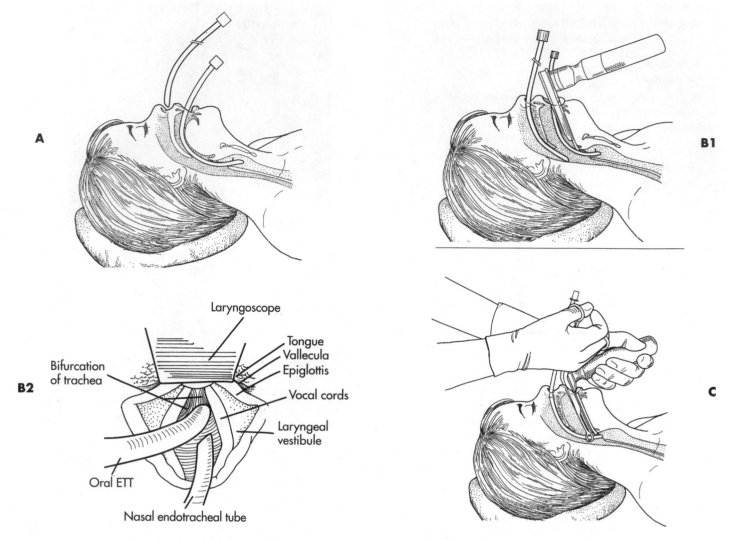

A

B1

B2

Laryngoscope

Tongue
Vallecula
Epiglottis

Bifurcation
of trachea

Vocal cords

Laryngeal
vestibule

Oral ETT

C

Nasal endotracheal tube

FIG. 21-3 **A,** Advance the nasotracheal tube into the right nare and directly posteriorly, along the floor of the nasal cavity. **B,** With manual ventilation continuing through to oral ETT, laryngoscopy provides visualization of the larynx. **C,** Using Magill forceps, advance the nasotracheal tube into position to replace the oral endotracheal tube, and then advance into the larynx as an assistant removes the oral tube. *ETT,* Endotracheal tube.

cricoid pressure (Fig. 21-4). As the child loses consciousness, administer a muscle relaxant as well. Have the child continue to breathe 100% oxygen until she or he becomes apneic, but *do not* ventilate manually, to prevent gastric distention. Once the patient is flaccid, proceed with laryngoscopy and oral intubation with a stylet in the endotracheal tube (ETT). After ascertaining correct tube position, inflate the cuff, if present; direct the assistant to release cricoid pressure; and begin manual ventilation. If difficulty accomplishing intubation occurs, if tube placement is uncertain, or if the child demonstrates progressive hypoxemia, begin manual ventilation between attempts with continuing cricoid pressure.

The "classic" combination of drugs for rapid sequence intubation is sodium thiopental (4 to 6 mg/kg) and succinylcholine (1 to 4 mg/kg) preceded by a defasciculating dose of a nondepolarizing relaxant such as pancuronium or vecuronium (about one tenth of the intubating dose). Ketamine or a mixture of a benzodiazepine and analgesic provides an alternative in hemodynamically unstable patients. The depolarizing relaxant succinylcholine acts quickly but has many

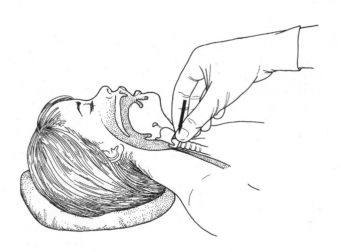

FIG. 21-4 Firm cricoid pressure occludes the esophagus, prevents regurgitation, and improves visualization of the larynx.

undesirable side effects (see Table 21-2). Nondepolarizing relaxants, given in two to three times the usual dose, produce good intubating conditions nearly as quickly, without many of these effects, but last much longer. The longer duration of action may pose problems when ventilation fails, and ventilation of the apneic child must occur by bag-valve-mask until spontaneous breathing resumes.

One must weigh the risk of aspiration against other aspects of the child's condition. In those with a predictably difficult airway, profuse upper airway bleeding, or upper airway obstruction, the risk of being unable to visualize the airway after drug administration precludes using this approach. In children suspected of severe intracranial hypertension, the rising Paco$_2$ associated with the onset of apnea may precipitate herniation.

FLEXIBLE FIBER-OPTIC BRONCHOSCOPY. Fiber-optic bronchoscopy provides an effective, safe, and atraumatic way of securing a difficult airway, especially in children with cervical spine instability, limited jaw mobility, or oropharyngeal abnormalities.[10,19,41] In most cases the nasal approach is preferable, both because it is more comfortable and because there is less risk of breaking the instrument. After administration of a topical vasoconstricting agent and local anesthetic, pass the endotracheal tube into the nasopharynx. Then thread the bronchoscope through the tube and advance it through the vocal cords. Next advance the endotracheal tube over the bronchoscope into good position and remove the bronchoscope. However unless equipment and skilled personnel are routinely available, the inherent delay makes this approach exceptional rather than routine. Also the child must be old enough to require a size 5 mm internal diameter tube or larger, since the bronchoscope does not fit into a smaller tube.

SPECIAL CIRCUMSTANCES

Increased Intracranial Pressure. In the child with central nervous system dysfunction, laryngoscopy and intubation are likely to precipitate or exacerbate intracranial hypertension.[5,12,36] Pain and anxiety increase cerebral blood flow; coughing or straining impedes jugular venous drainage; autonomic stimulation increases systemic pressure and, frequently, intracranial pressure (ICP) and may further add to the risk of hemorrhage in a child with a vascular malformation, coagulopathy, or bleeding into a tumor. Hypoxemia and hypercarbia that develop during the process of intubation also increase cerebral blood flow.

Given the life-threatening risks of systemic and intracranial hypertension in these patients, minimize stimulation and struggle (Box 21-6). In general this requires ensuring excellent oxygenation and ventilation, and intubating under protection of deep sedation or anesthesia with help from neuromuscular blockade. Perform a baseline neurologic assessment before drug administration and continue subsequent observations when drugs have worn off. Often subsequent diagnostic imaging (e.g., computed tomographic [CT] brain scan) requires a prolonged period of sedation and paralysis; if not, use short-acting drugs.

In those with suspected intracranial hypertension, initiate manual hyperventilation at once to lower ICP as much as possible before laryngoscopy. In the hemodynamically stable, normovolemic patient, thiopental 4 to 6 mg/kg results in fairly deep anesthesia and a rapid decline in cerebral metabolic rate for oxygen (CMRO$_2$), cerebral blood flow (CBF), and ICP. In other patients benzodiazepines in combination with narcotic analgesics cause less hemodynamic compromise but have less effect on CMRO$_2$. Lidocaine in doses below the seizure-producing threshold (1 to 1.5 mg/kg IV) also decreases CMRO$_2$, blocks the cerebral hypertensive response, and decreases cough.[32,34,39,43] Nondepolarizing relaxants are preferable, but succinylcholine is acceptable if one prevents fasciculation. In most cases oral intubation, at least initially, is preferable because it is possible to accomplish it rapidly without delays that result in prolonged stimulation, interruption of oxygen administration, or hypoventilation. Nasal intubation is contraindicated in patients with evidence of basilar skull fracture.[20]

Cervical Spine Instability. Spinal cord injury may result from either bony compression or fracture or disruption of cervical ligaments; in young children severe injury may occur without radiologic evidence of injury, simply as a result of severe ligamentous stretch after acceleration/deceleration events.[29] In addition congenital anatomic abnormalities, penetrating wounds, or mass lesions may compromise spinal column integrity. In such patients the usual neck flexion and head extension associated with laryngoscopy present the risk of additional damage.[45]

The best approach to intubation in these patients is controversial and uncertain. Although Advanced Trauma Life Support (ATLS) guidelines suggest blind nasotracheal intubation in spontaneously breathing patients,[1] the difficulty of

BOX 21-6 INTUBATION IN PATIENTS WITH INCREASED INTRACRANIAL PRESSURE

Goal

Minimize factors that exacerbate increased intracranial pressure (ICP).
Prevent pain and anxiety.
Prevent coughing, straining.
Limit automatic stimulation and alterations in systemic blood pressure.
Prevent hypercarbia and hypoxia.

Procedure

Oxygenate with 100% oxygen.
Initiate manual hyperventilation.
Consider likelihood of difficult airway and need to avoid relaxant.

Patients with associated cardiovascular compromise or hypovolemia

Administer diazepam or midasolam (0.2-0.3 mg/kg), fentanyl (5-10 mg/kg), and lidocaine (1-1.5 mg/kg).
Administer neuromuscular relaxant, e.g., vecuronium (0.1 mg/kg).
Perform orotracheal intubation.

Patients with no associated cardiovascular compromise

Administer osmotic or loop diuretic.
Administer thiopental (4-6 mg/kg) and lidocaine (1-1.5 mg/kg).
Administer neuromuscular relaxant.
Continue manual hyperventilation to full drug effect.
Perform orotracheal intubation.

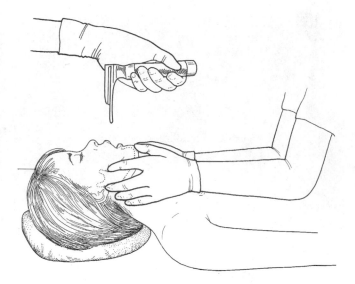

FIG. 21-5 To stabilize the cervical spine in suspected neck injury, an assistant immobilizes the head and neck in a neutral position.

struction from poor pharyngeal muscle tone may result from a variety of drugs or from central nervous system depression. Where the disorder is likely to be transient, a nasopharyngeal airway may provide adequate relief (see Chapter 20). However in many situations where edema, inflammation, trauma, or a mass lesion is likely to cause progressive obstruction, intubation is essential.

During preparation allow the child to assume whatever position is most comfortable. Provide supplemental oxygen and approach the child calmly and gently until she or he can accept a mask. Initially support spontaneous breathing with continuous positive airway pressure and then by gradually assisting breaths. Even in cases of severe obstruction, manual ventilation usually provides effective temporary support, at least for oxygenation, as long as one coordinates efforts with the child's. Do nothing that compromises the child's ability to breathe, until certain that airway control is possible.[6] In particular, neuromuscular blocking agents are dangerous. Do not use them until after controlling the airway. However, *careful* titration of sedative agents may make it easier to assist the child's breathing and to establish an artificial airway. Once adequate ventilatory support is possible, lower the child to a supine position and intubate orally. In most cases use a tube 0.5 to 1 mm smaller in internal diameter than predicted by the child's age. When the child's condition and available personnel permit, it is often best to accomplish intubation in the operating room under general anesthesia.

Facial and Laryngotracheal Injury. Face and neck injuries are enormously variable and present special challenges to airway control. In some cases breathing is not impaired, and there is no urgent need to intervene beyond providing supplemental oxygen. In others the approach depends on the extent of airway compromise, presence of bleeding into the airway, stability of facial structures, and likely progression of swelling and airway distortion.

First, clear the mouth of blood and debris. If bony structures of the face allow effective bag and mask ventilation and bleeding is controllable, perform orotracheal intubation as described with full-stomach precautions. If, however,

accomplishing this in children, and the violent and potentially injurious struggle it is likely to elicit in them, make it a less than desirable approach.[42]

In general direct efforts to maintaining a neutral position and minimizing voluntary movement through heavy sedation and/or paralysis. Have an assistant immobilize the child's head and neck in a neutral position (Fig. 21-5) with one hand over each ear. Because succinylcholine administration in patients with spinal cord injury may produce severe hyperkalemia, arrhythmias, and asystole (reported to occur any time from 48 hours to 6 to 9 months after injury), a nondepolarizing relaxant is safest. After drug administration orotracheal intubation proceeds as described, achieving airway exposure by lifting the mandible vigorously, rather than by manipulating the neck. If the available time, expertise, and equipment permit, flexible fiberoptic laryngoscopy may facilitate intubation with minimal movement.[27] On occasion associated facial or airway trauma prohibits orotracheal intubation and makes cricothyrotomy or primary tracheostomy essential.[40,46] However the high incidence of complications of tracheostomy in children without an endotracheal tube in place limits these choices to times when orotracheal intubation and cricothyrotomy are unsafe or unsuccessful.

Upper Airway Obstruction. Transient upper airway ob-

mask pressure on the face exacerbates obstruction, awake intubation is necessary, as in the case of other causes of upper airway obstruction. If profuse bleeding obscures the airway, oral injuries prevent successful laryngoscopy, or the child's struggle threatens to exacerbate intracranial hypertension or cervical cord injury, secure a surgical airway (see Chapter 22). Avoid nasogastric and nasotracheal tubes if basilar skull fracture is possible.

A history of anterior neck trauma and/or hoarseness, stridor, subcutaneous emphysema, or other evidence of air leak raises the possibility of *laryngotracheal injury.* Administration of aerosolized epinephrine may temporarily decrease airway edema to provide time to evaluate the airway and plan specific intervention directed to preventing sudden, complete obstruction. In most cases, awake oral intubation, with judicious sedation and topical anesthesia, under direct laryngoscopy or, ideally, with fiberoptic bronchoscopy, prevents creation of a false passage through lacerated mucosa.

Open globe injury may accompany head, neck, or other facial injury. Airway management in these patients must prevent increasing intraocular pressure to minimize the risk of vitreous extrusion. Preventing crying or struggling, coughing, or straining is paramount. Perform intubation under full muscle relaxation and deep sedation, if possible, considering associated injuries and the possibility of a full stomach.

Succinylcholine tends to increase intraocular pressure even in the absence of fasciculations, so always use a nondepolarizing relaxant.

Securing the Endotracheal Tube. Countless devices are on the market for securing endotracheal tubes in adults and neonates, but at present meticulous taping remains the most reliable means of stabilizing tubes in most infants and children (Fig. 21-6).

OROTRACHEAL TUBES. Divide three strips of adhesive tape (½ inch wide in infants, 1 inch wide after approximately age 1 year; approximately twice as long as the distance from just anterior to the ear to the corner of the mouth) in half lengthwise to the middle of the strip. Clean the face of blood, secretions, and oils and prepare the skin with benzoin. Apply the first piece of tape to the cheek so that it applies some traction on the corner of the mouth; the narrow upper half extends across the upper lip. Wrap the lower half around the tube beginning from below, pulling the tube into the crotch of the divided tape, and wrapping the tape several centimeters along the tube's length. Apply the second piece of tape similarly to the cheek, but with the lower half of the divided portion extending across the chin, and the upper half wrapped securely around the tube from above. Apply the final piece similarly to the first. Avoid the vermilion border of the lip, which is particularly vulnerable to injury and scarring. When properly secured, the tube should move little even with substantial traction.

NASOTRACHEAL TUBES. A similar approach also secures nasal tubes. Following the same tape and skin preparation, apply the first piece of tape so that the lower half crosses the skin below the nose and the upper half wraps around the tube from above, directing the tube toward the lip and away from nasal cartilage. Place the second piece so that the upper half extends across the nose, and the lower half wraps around the tube, *beginning from below.* Apply the final piece in the same way as the first. Take care to orient the tube toward the upper lip to prevent pressure injury to the borders of the nares.

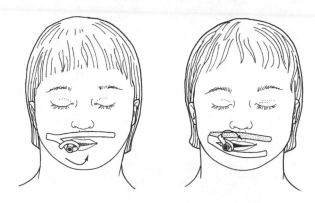

FIG. 21-6   Securing the endotracheal tube. See text for description of technique.

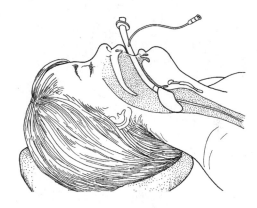

FIG. 21-7   The laryngeal mask airway surrounds the larynx and forms a seal to permit ventilation.

Laryngeal Mask Airway. The laryngeal mask airway (LMA) is a relatively new device for blind insertion into the pharynx to form a seal around the larynx.[30] It consists of a soft silicone rubber, spoon-shaped mask with an inflatable rim, connected at a 30-degree angle to a tube or shaft (Fig. 21-7). Although experience in pediatric patients is growing, there is very little in the emergency or critical care setting, so its potential remains uncertain.

In the patient with a very difficult airway, it may form a bridge between mask ventilation and intubation and, in some patients, may facilitate blind intubation or fiberoptic bronchoscopy.[31] It has also been effective in neonatal resuscitation.

It may be easier to insert when the larynx is anterior, a setting in which intubation is often difficult. Insertion, however, can produce coughing, gagging, and laryngospasm, as well as aspiration in patients with impaired protective reflexes. Cricoid pressure reportedly interferes with proper placement in some patients, so its use in the patient with a full stomach and impaired reflexes may be complicated. Uvular edema and posterior pharyngeal wall swelling can also occur.

Contraindications include limited mouth opening, inability to extend the neck, pharyngeal abnormality (including extreme tonsillar hypertrophy, hematoma, or abscess), airway obstruction at or below the larynx, poor chest compliance, and increased risk of regurgitation.

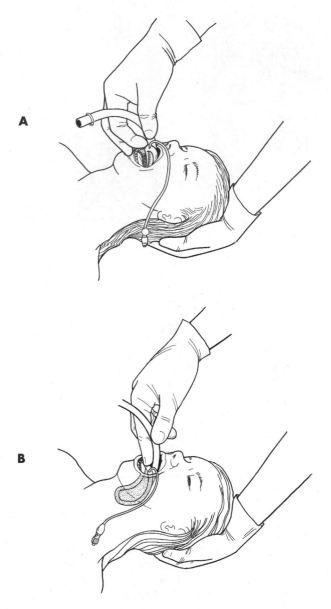

FIG. 21-8 **A,** Insert the laryngeal mask airway with the aperture facing anteriorly. **B,** Advance to the level of the upper esophageal sphincter, using the right index finger to maintain firm pressure on the cuff against the hard palate.

With the patient in the sniffing position (neck slightly flexed and head extended) and the rim of the LMA deflated, insert the mask into the mouth with the aperture facing anteriorly (Fig. 21-8, *A*). Advance the tip of the cuff posteriorly, with steady pressure on the hard palate, past the posterior aspect of the tongue, until encountering the resistance of the upper esophageal sphincter (Fig. 21-8, *B*). Then inflate the cuff; inflation typically causes the tube to move outward slightly and ensures that the longitudinal black line of the shaft is in the midline against the upper lip. Secure the tube with tape in much the same way as a standard endotracheal tube. Attach the universal connector on the shaft to a bag and mask or ventilator and begin positive-pressure ventilation. One can usually maintain a seal around the airway until peak pressures exceed 20 cm H_2O, after which the leak is likely to contribute to gastric distention.

SURGICAL APPROACHES. See Chapter 22.

REFERENCES

1. Airway management and ventilation. In *Advanced trauma life support, instructor's manual,* Chicago, 1993, Committee on Trauma, American College of Surgeons. pp 47-72.
2. Barrington KJ, Finer NN, Etches PC: Succinylcholine and atropine for premedication of the newborn infant before nasotracheal intubation: a randomized, controlled trial, *Crit Care Med* 17:1293, 1989.
3. Bhende M, et al: Validity of a disposable end-tidal CO_2 detector in verifying endotracheal tube placement in infants and children, *Ann Emerg Med* 21:142, 1992.
4. Birmingham PK, Cheney FW, Ward RJ: Esophageal intubation: a review of detection techniques, *Anesth Analg* 65:886, 1986.
5. Brady JP, Tooley WH: Cardiovascular and respiratory reflexes in the newborn, *Pediatr Clin North Am* 13:801, 1966.
6. Brown ACD, Sataloff RT: Special anesthetic techniques in head and neck surgery, *Otolaryngol Clin North Am* 14:587, 1981.
7. Burney RG, Winn R: Increased cerebrospinal fluid pressure during laryngoscopy and intubation for induction of anesthesia, *Anesth Analg Curr Res* 54:687, 1975.
8. Burstein CL, LoPinto FJ, Newman W: Electrocardiographic studies during endotracheal intubation. I. Effects during usual routine technics, *Anesthesiology* 11:224, 1950.
9. Cheney FW, Posner K, Caplan RA, et al: Standard of care and anesthesia liability, *JAMA* 261:1599, 1989.
10. Christianson L: Anesthesia for major craniofacial operations, *Int Anesth Clin* 23:117, 1985.
11. Cole WL, Stoelting VK: Oxygenation before intubation, *Anesth Analg Curr Res* 50:68, 1971.
12. Cordero L Jr, Hon EH: Neonatal bradycardia following nasopharyngeal stimulation, *J Pediatr* 78:441, 1971.
13. Coté CJ, Goudsouzian NG, Liu LMP, et al: Assessment of risk factors related to the acid aspiration syndrome in pediatric patients: gastric pH and residual volume, *Anesthesiology* 56:70, 1982.
14. Demers RR, Irwin RS: Pulmonary hygiene and artificial airway management, In Kirby RR, Smith RA, Desautels DA, editors: *Mechanical ventilation,* New York, 1985, Churchill Livingstone.
15. Denlinger JK, Ellison N, Ominsky AJ: Effects of intratracheal lidocaine on circulatory responses to tracheal intubation, *Anesthesiology* 41:409, 1974.
16. Durand M, Sangha B, Cabal LA, et al: Cardiopulmonary and intracranial pressure changes related to endotracheal suctioning in preterm infants, *Crit Care Med* 17:506, 1989.
17. Fanconi S, Duc G: Intratracheal suctioning in sick preterm infants: prevention of intracranial hypertension and cerebral hypoperfusion by muscle paralysis, *Pediatrics* 79:538, 1987.
18. Friesen RH, Honda AT, Thieme RE: Changes in anterior fontanel pressure in preterm neonates during tracheal intubation, *Anesth Analg* 66:874, 1987.
19. Hemmer D, Lee TS, Wright BD: Intubation of a child with a cervical spine injury with the aid of a fiberoptic bronchoscope, *Anaesth Intensive Care* 10:163, 1982.
20. Horellou MF, Mathe D, Feiss P: A hazard of nasotracheal intubation, *Anaesthesiology* 33:73, 1978.
21. Kelly MA, Finer NN: Nasotracheal intubation in the neonate: physiologic responses and effects of atropine and pancuronium, *J Pediatr* 105:303, 1984.
22. King BD, Harris LC Jr, Greifenstein FE, et al: Reflex circulatory responses to direct laryngoscopy and tracheal intubation performed during general anesthesia, *Anesthesiology* 12:556, 1951.
23. King BR, Baker MD, Breitman LE, et al: Endotracheal tube selection in children: a comparison of four methods, *Ann Emerg Med* 22:530-534, 1993.
24. Linko K, Paloheimo M, Tammisto T: Capnography for detection of accidental oesophageal inbutation, *Acta Anaesthesiol Scand* 27:199, 1983.
25. MacLeod BA, et al: Verification of endotracheal tube placement with colorimetric endtidal CO_2 detection, *Ann Emerg Med* 20:267, 1991.
26. Marshall TA, Deeder R, Pai S, et al: Physiologic changes associated with endotracheal intubation in preterm infants, *Crit Care Med* 12:501, 1984.

27. Minek EJ Jr, Clinton JE, Plummer D, et al: Fiberoptic intubation in the emergency department, *Ann Emerg Med* 19:359, 1990.

28. Ninan A, O'Donnell M, Hamilton K et al: Physiologic changes induced by endotracheal instillation and suctioning in critically ill preterm infants with and without sedation, *Am J Perinatol* 3:94, 1986.

29. Pang D, Wilberger JE: Spinal cord injury without radiologic abnormalities in children, *J Neurosurg* 57:114, 1982.

30. Paterson MD, Byrne PJ, Molesky MG, et al: Neonatal resuscitation using the laryngeal mask airway, *Anesthesiology* 80:1248-1253, 1994.

31. Pennant JH, White PF: The laryngeal mask airway, *Anesthesiology* 79:144-161, 1993.

32. Poulton TJ, James FM: Cough suppression by lidocaine, *Anesthesiology* 50:470, 1979.

33. Raju TNK, Vidyasagar D, Torres C, et al: Intracranial pressure during intubation and anesthesia in infants, *J Pediatr* 96:860, 1980.

34. Sakabe T, Maekawa T, Ishikawa T, et al: The effects of lidocaine on canine cerebral metabolism and circulation related to the electroencephalogram, *Anesthesiology* 40:433, 1974.

35. Sanders AB: Capnometry in emergency medicine, *Ann Emerg Med* 18:1287, 1989.

36. Shapiro HM, Wyte SR, Harris AB, et al: Acute intraoperative intracranial hypertension in neurosurgical patients: mechanical and pharmacologic factors, *Anesthesiology* 37:399, 1972.

37. Tintinalli JE, Claffey J: Complications of nasotracheal intubation, *Ann Emerg Med* 10:142, 1981.

38. Utting JE: Pitfalls in anaesthetic practice, *Br J Anaesth* 59:877, 1987.

39. Viegas O, Stoelting RK: Lidocaine in arterial blood after laryngotracheal administration, *Anesthesiology* 43:491, 1975.

40. Walls RM: Orotracheal intubation and potential cervical spine injury, *Ann Emerg Med* 16:373, 1987 (letter).

41. Watson CB: Fiberoptic bronchoscopy for anesthesia, *Anesthesiol Rev* 9:17, 1982.

42. Wells DG, Tredrea CR: Intubation of the patient with cervical spine injury, *Anaesth Intensive Care* 15:353, 1987 (letter).

43. White PF, Schlobohm RM, Pitts LH, et al: A randomized study of drugs for preventing increases in intracranial pressure during endotracheal suctioning. *Anesthesiology* 57:242, 1982.

44. Wycoff CC: Endotracheal intubation: effects on blood pressure and pulse rate, *Anesthesiology* 21:153, 1960.

45. Yaszemski MJ, Shepler TR: Sudden death from cord compression associated with atlanto-axial instability in rheumatoid arthritis: a case report, *Spine* 15:338, 1990.

46. Yealy DM, Cantees KK, Verdile VP, et al: Emergency airway management in trauma patients with a suspected cervical spine injury, *Anesth Analg* 68 (letter): 413, 1989.

22 The Surgical Airway

Charles M. Bower

In most pediatric airway emergencies there is partial rather than total airway obstruction. A rapid assessment of the clinical situation allows for appropriate intervention. If the child has *progressive* respiratory distress manifested by tachypnea, tachycardia, substernal and intercostal retractions, then emergency airway intervention is indicated. In most cases standard nasotracheal or orotracheal intubation with an endotracheal tube is preferable. Rarely are these standard techniques of intubation either not feasible or not advisable. In these circumstances surgical intervention or nonstandard intubation techniques are necessary.

Anatomy

Fig. 22-1 shows the surgical anatomy of the pediatric airway. The larynx includes the thyroid, cricoid, and arytenoid cartilages and surrounding soft tissue. Details can be found in any standard anatomy text.[15] In children the larynx is typically higher in the neck, and normal landmarks are often less distinct to palpation. With aging the larynx descends, and landmarks become more prominent. The inferior border of the larynx in infants is at approximately the level of the third or fourth cervical vertebra.[22] The superior aspect of the larynx is identifiable by palpating the hyoid bone. The hyoid is palpable very high in the neck by pinching its ends between two fingers. The thyroid cartilage is generally nondistinct and often the thyroid notch lies under the hyoid bone in a nonpalpable position.[27] The next most prominent bulge just below the indistinct thyroid cartilage is the cricoid cartilage. The cricothyroid membrane is a palpable indentation lying immediately superior to the cricoid bulge. The trachea below the cricoid, although often not distinct, is usually palpable down to the level of the sternal notch. Palpation of the sternal notch, the hyoid bone, the bilateral sternocleidomastoid muscles, and the mandibular arch can help locate the midline, and thus the larynx and trachea. Make sure that extrinsic masses or eccentric head positioning does not move the trachea from the midline.

The pediatric airway has a smaller diameter than that of adults. This leads to a proportionally much smaller cross-sectional area, and a larger resistance to airflow if edema, hematoma, or scar tissue partially occludes the laryngeal lumen of an infant.[27] The cricoid ring is the only area in the airway with a complete ring of cartilage and also is the location of the narrowest cross-sectional area of the upper airway in infants and young children. The respiratory mucosa in this region is delicate and loosely attached to the cartilaginous framework; therefore it more readily allows injury and resulting edema in this region to obstruct the airway markedly. The laryngeal cartilage in infants and young children is often malacic, or soft, making palpation of definite structures difficult, endoscopic visualization troublesome, and collapse of the upper airway with labored breathing more likely.[9,10]

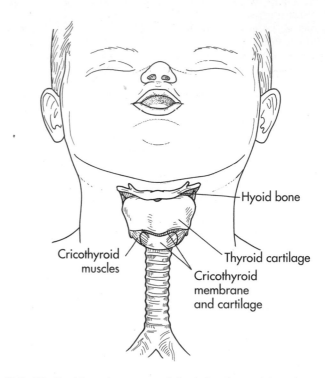

FIG. 22-1 Normal anatomy of the infant larynx. Note the position of the thyroid cartilage lying under the hyoid bone. The cricothyroid membrane attaches from the superior border of the cricoid to the thyroid cartilage.

Airway obstruction in infants may occur at locations other than the larynx. Upper airway obstruction may cause symptoms similar to those of lower airway problems; consider upper airway obstruction in all cases of stridor or wheezing (see Chapter 17).

Indications

Box 22-1 lists indications for establishment of a surgical airway. Surgical approaches to the airway or approaches requiring specialized equipment are indicated after failure to intubate the airway endotracheally.[25] In a few circumstances endotracheal intubation is difficult or impossible. Difficult intubation is more likely in patients with craniofacial and congenital laryngeal anomalies. Cervical spine fractures, cervical spine anomalies with potential for cervical spine injuries, and acute laryngeal injuries are all *relative* contraindications to endotracheal intubation, as inadvertent extension of the neck or intubation of a traumatized larynx may actually increase the extent of injury.[6,28] Pharyngeal and laryngeal burns can be severe enough to distort laryngeal anatomy and make intubation difficult. Subglottic and glottic stenosis as a late result of trauma may make intubation with an appropriate-size endotracheal tube impossible. This may also be true with congenital laryngeal stenosis, atresia, and extensive posterior cleft larynx.

Contraindications

Endotracheal intubation is the procedure of choice in all patients who do not have definite contraindications. Relative contraindications to surgical airway management include bleeding diatheses, unavailable or inadequate equipment, and adequate nonsurgical airway.

Techniques

If endotracheal intubation is unsuccessful or contraindicated, establish a surgical airway. Surgical approaches include percutaneous (needle) cricothyroidotomy, cricothyroidotomy, and tracheotomy. Of these cricothyroidotomy is probably the safest and quickest in an emergency, with percutaneous cricothyroidotomy a reasonable alternative, especially in children less than 5 years of age. Other alternate methods include the use of flexible or rigid bronchoscopes, percuta-neous catheter guided intubation, lighted stylets, or fiber-optic laryngoscopes. Which method to use depends on the availability of equipment and experience of the physician (see Chapter 21).

PERCUTANEOUS CRICOTHYROIDOTOMY

Percutaneous (needle) cricothyroidotomy provides an extremely rapid method of oxygen insufflation, by insertion of a needle directly into the trachea. Oxygen insufflation can maintain adequate oxygenation for a considerable period.[4] Although some authors advocate this method of management for a critical airway, others doubt the effectiveness of the procedure, because of its difficulty in infants and its inability to provide adequate ventilation.[2,12,13] Percutaneous cricothyroidotomy may be useful for older children and adults. However it can be extremely difficult to perform in infants and young children because of the softness of the cartilage and the mobility of the larynx and trachea.[19]

Contraindications/Complications

Violation of the cricothyroid membrane has resulted in subglottic stenosis and alteration of voice quality. Inappropriate insertion of the needle and positive-pressure ventilation can cause subcutaneous emphysema, pneumothorax, and pneumomediastinum.[24] Injury to the esophagus, great vessels, or nerves of the neck is possible if there is deviation from the midline on insertion of the needle.

Equipment

Box 22-2 lists the equipment needed for a percutaneous needle cricothyroidotomy.

Technique (Fig. 22-2)

Place the patient on a shoulder roll and extend the head, exposing the neck. Locate the cricothyroid membrane by palpating, first, the hyoid bone high in the neck; then, the thyroid cartilage; then the prominence of the cricoid cartilage. Stabilize the cricoid and thyroid cartilage between the thumb and finger of one hand and insert a 14- to 18-gauge intravenous catheter attached to a 3-ml syringe in the midline through the cricothyroid membrane immediately above the cricoid cartilage into the airway. Prevent lateral movement, which can cause injury to the great vessels or nerves of the neck. Aspirate air to indicate appropriate insertion into the trachea. Then direct the catheter inferiorly, remove the needle, and insert the catheter well into the trachea. Movement of air confirms the position. Attach the adapter from a 3-mm–internal diameter (ID) endotracheal tube (a 2.5-mm adapter) with a standard ventilatory circuit directly to the catheter for insufflation of oxygen. Alternatively attach a 3-ml syringe barrel to the catheter and an 8-mm ID endotracheal tube adapter to the syringe barrel.

Another option is to insert a 5-mm ID endotracheal tube directly into the barrel of the syringe and attach the tube to the ventilatory equipment. Insufflate oxygen to maintain the patient's breathing until there is time to create a more adequate airway by cricothyroidotomy or tracheotomy. When ventilating through a catheter, disconnect the bag from the endotracheal (ET) adapter to allow passive exhalation *if* airway obstruction from above is total.

BOX 22-2	**EQUIPMENT REQUIRED FOR PERCUTANEOUS (NEEDLE) CRICOTHYROIDOTOMY**

1. 18- to 14-Gauge intracath
2. 3-ml Syringe
3. Adapter from a 3-mm-ID endotracheal tube, adapter from 8-mm-ID endotracheal tube, or 5-mm-ID endotracheal tube
4. Oxygen delivery system

Another alternative to surgical cricothyroidotomy is to use the Seldinger technique of percutaneous insertion of an airway. After puncturing the cricothyroid membrane with a needle, insert a J-tipped guidewire into the trachea. Then pass successively larger dilators over the guidewire to make a channel into which to insert a small cuffed endotracheal tube or tracheotomy tube. Several percutaneous cricothyroidotomy kits are commercially available with prepackaged needles, J-wires, dilators, and appropriate instruments. Although some authors support the Seldinger technique for emergency airway management, others have found it more difficult and slower to perform than a traditional surgical approach and more prone to complications.

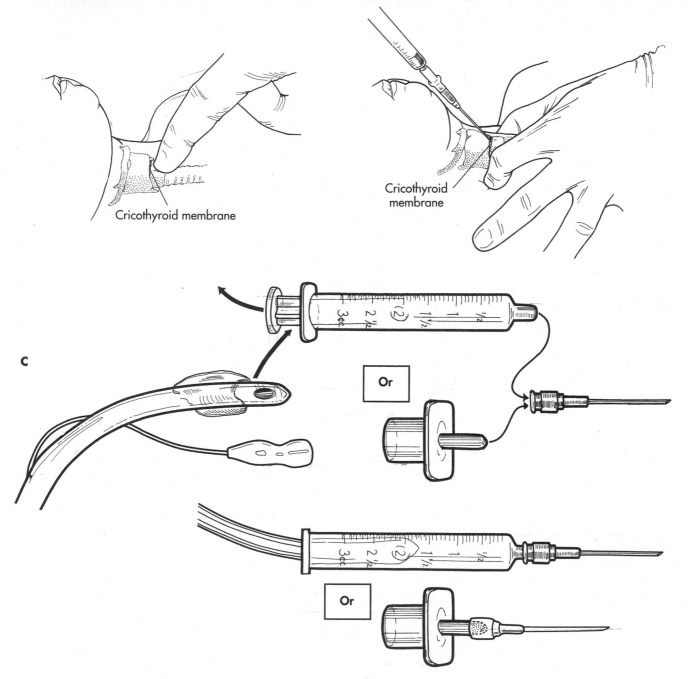

Cricothyroid membrane

Cricothyroid membrane

FIG. 22-2 Percutaneous, cricothyroidomy technique. **A,** Palpation of the cricothyroid membrane. **B,** Insertion of the catheter and aspiration of air. **C,** Equipment for attachment to oxygen delivery system.

Remarks

Percutaneous cricothyroidotomy may be difficult to perform but can provide *short-term* oxygenation in an emergency. Although the procedure can rapidly provide oxygenation, ventilation is usually inadequate. Place more than one needle if necessary. Jet ventilation via cricothyroidotomy may be tried in extreme circumstances, but high-pressure equipment is usually not available, and complications including subcutaneous emphysema and bilateral pneumothoraxes are common. Therefore do not perform jet ventilation via cricothyroidotomy in infants and young children. Use percutaneous cricothyroidotomy in emergencies when establishment of an immediate airway is essential and endotracheal intubation is impossible. Percutaneous cricothyroidotomy is an adjunct to maintain a patient who is in critical condition only until establishment of a more adequate airway.

SURGICAL CRICOTHYROIDOTOMY

A surgical cricothyroidotomy provides rapid access to the airway for maintenance of oxygenation and ventilation.[5,14,16,21,23] It is possible to perform the technique rapidly, and it is easier and has less potential for immediate complications than standard tracheotomy or percutaneous cricothyroidotomy.

Indications

Perform a cricothyroidotomy in cases of severe airway crisis or inability to intubate. Even in experienced hands, the establishment of an airway in an emergency can be difficult. The most experienced person available should perform the procedure.[16]

Contraindications/Complications

Violation of the cricothyroid membrane has resulted in subglottic stenosis and alteration of voice quality.[5,16] Subcutaneous emphysema, pneumomediastinum, pneumothorax, neurovascular injury, and damage of the esophagus and larynx can result from inappropriate technique.[3]

Equipment

Box 22-3 lists the equipment necessary for a cricothyroidotomy. The technique requires, at a minimum, a scalpel, a hemostat, and an endotracheal tube.

Technique (Fig. 22-3)

Place the patient on a shoulder roll and extend the neck, exposing the thyroid and cricoid cartilage. Locate the cricothyroid membrane by palpating first the hyoid bone high in the neck, next the thyroid cartilage, then the prominence of the cricoid cartilage. The cricothyroid membrane lies in the depression immediately above the cricoid cartilage. Anesthetize the skin with 1% lidocaine with or without epinephrine, if time allows. Stabilize the larynx between the finger and thumb of one hand and make a vertical incision overlying the thyroid and cricoid cartilages. Divide the strap muscles in the midline by blunt dissection with a hemostat, to expose the cricothyroid membrane. Make a horizontal incision through the cricothyroid membrane into the airway. Insert a tracheotomy tube, or endotracheal tube of appropriate caliber,

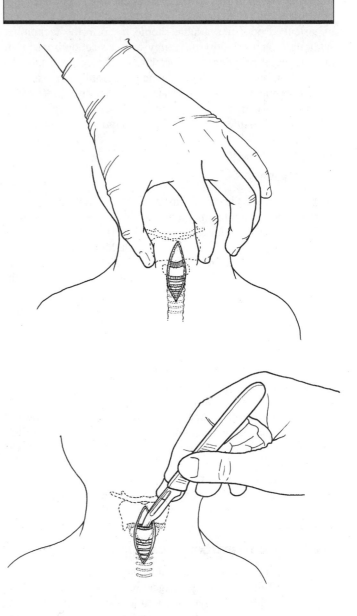

| BOX 22-3 | **EQUIPMENT REQUIRED FOR A SURGICAL CRICOTHYROIDOTOMY** |

1. Scalpel
2. Hemostat
3. Frazier tip or equivalent suction
4. Endotracheal tube or tracheotomy tube
5. Oxygen delivery system
6. Suction

FIG. 22-3   After a vertical or horizontal skin incision divide the strap muscles bluntly in the midline, and incise the cricothyroid membrane horizontally.

through the cricothyroid membrane and direct the tube inferiorly. Finally, connect the tracheotomy tube to a ventilator circuit and ventilate the patient. Subsequent conversion to a standard tracheotomy may prevent the complications of subglottic stenosis and voice change secondary to a cricothyroidotomy.

As an alternative, when surgical landmarks are more

obvious in older children and adults, make a horizontal stab incision with a 15 blade directly through the skin, muscle, and cricothyroid membrane into the tracheal lumen. Then use a hemostat to dilate the opening and insert an endotracheal tube.

Remarks

A cricothyroidotomy provides rapid access to the airway for maintenance of oxygenation and ventilation. The technique is easier and quicker than a standard tracheotomy but still may be quite difficult in infants and young children. The most experienced person available should perform the technique. Although even cricothyroidotomy may be suboptimal in an emergency, it remains the procedure of choice for establishment of an airway in a crisis. Since subglottic stenosis may be a complication of this procedure, cricothyroidotomy is indicated only in emergency circumstances. For prolonged ventilation, consider conversion to a standard tracheotomy.

TRACHEOTOMY
Indications

In patients with airway obstruction that is rapidly progressive, but not an acute emergency, standard tracheotomy is an option.[30] The technique, however, is extremely difficult to perform in an awake child even with local anesthetic and sedation.[26,31] Therefore, it is rarely indicated in the Emergency Department (ED). It is appropriate to intubate virtually all patients or otherwise maintain the airway; heavily sedate the patient or use a general anesthetic before attempting a tracheotomy. An urgent tracheotomy may be indicated in situations in which prolonged endotracheal intubation is not desirable such as in laryngeal trauma, cervical spine injury, or significant subglottic stenosis. The decision to perform a tracheotomy usually takes place after stabilization and placement of an endotracheal tube.

In this situation indications to perform a tracheotomy include prolonged ventilation, the need for pulmonary toilet, severe upper airway obstruction, and airway protection for upper airway injuries or inadequacy (i.e., craniofacial trauma, surgery, and patient inability to protect the airway). Individualize these treatment decisions depending on the status of the child, and the degree and duration of airway difficulty anticipated.

Contraindications/Complications

Immediate complications of tracheotomy include bleeding, bilateral pneumothorax, esophageal injury, subcutaneous emphysema, and hypoxia secondary to loss of respiratory drive. Late complications include accidental decannulation, mucous plugging, and erosion of the tracheal walls with brachiocephalic artery bleeding, pneumomediastinum, or tracheoesophageal fistula.[7]

Equipment

Tracheotomy tubes are available in a variety of styles and sizes. Adult and pediatric endotracheal tubes generally differ not only in their size, but in the presence of an inner cannula in the larger adult style tubes (Fig. 22-4). Most pediatric tracheotomy tubes consist of two parts, the tracheotomy tube itself and an obturator, which is only used to allow easy

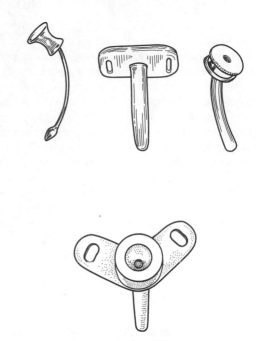

FIG. 22-4 Pediatric tracheotomy tubes are available in a variety of sizes and lengths. The obturator allows easy insertion, but remove it to allow for ventilation. Adult tracheotomy tubes are available in a variety of sizes and usually consist of an inner and an outer cannula. An obturator is also available to ease insertion, but remove it and place the inner cannula to allow for ventilation.

insertion of the tracheotomy tube. Secure the tracheotomy tubes with a tie around the neck. Frequent suctioning prevents buildup of debris in the tracheotomy tube, which may otherwise cause airway obstruction. In the event of airway obstruction remove the pediatric tracheotomy tube and insert a clean tube. Pediatric tracheotomy tubes have a variety of sizes as well as lengths. Match the exact length and diameter of tubes when the child requires a new tracheotomy tube.

Adult-style and some pediatric tracheotomy tubes consist of three parts, the tracheotomy tube proper, an inner cannula, and an obturator for use in insertion. After placement of the tracheotomy tube in the trachea using the obturator, remove the obturator and insert the inner cannula. In cases of obstruction, remove the inner cannula and replace it, leaving the body of the tracheotomy tube in position. It is rarely necessary to remove completely and replace an adult-style tracheotomy tube. Adult-style and some pediatric-style tubes are available in cuffed and uncuffed varieties. Inability to ventilate, with a large leak around the tracheotomy tube, may indicate a cuff malfunction. If this situation occurs, change the body of the tracheotomy tube.

Technique

To perform a tracheotomy, first place the patient on a shoulder roll with the head extended.[11,18,20] Make a vertical or horizontal incision low in the neck overlying the trachea midway between the sternal notch and the cricoid prominence. Divide the strap muscles in the midline and retract them laterally. On encountering the thyroid gland, as is often the case, either divide it or retract it for exposure of the trachea. Finally, enter the trachea with a vertical incision through three or four tracheal rings. Place stay sutures on either side of the incision in the trachea to help locate the trachea in case of early accidental decannulation. Insert an appropriate-sized tracheotomy tube into the trachea and secure it in place with ties around the neck.

Remarks

A tracheotomy is the best surgical option for maintaining an airway on a long-term basis, but it is difficult to perform in an emergency. The technique is an option in urgent situations if an adequate airway is not maintainable by other means and it is possible to sedate and anesthetize the patient adequately, but only an otolaryngologist or qualified surgeon should perform this procedure. Percutaneous tracheotomy using dilation often causes serious complications during emergency use that preclude recommendation.[1,8,29]

TECHNIQUE FOR CHANGING OR REINSERTING A TRACHEOTOMY TUBE INTRODUCTION

The most common serious complications of indwelling tracheotomy tubes are accidental decannulation and mucous plugging. Either may result in inability to ventilate a patient, with resulting asphyxia. These problems may be more common when using single-cannula pediatric tracheotomy tubes. In these children, a rapid change or reinsertion of the tracheotomy tube is essential to reestablish ventilation.

Indications

Change tracheotomy tubes in cases of airway obstruction with inability to ventilate through the tracheotomy tube after appropriate lavage and suctioning. Replace a tracheotomy tube that accidentally dislodges immediately as the tube site can close rapidly.

Complications

Inappropriate reinsertion may result in bleeding, formation of a false tract, or perforation of the trachea or esophagus, with resulting inability to ventilate and development of subcutaneous emphysema, pneumomediastinum, and pneumothorax.

Equipment

Box 22-4 lists the equipment necessary for a tracheotomy tube reinsertion or change. Have the appropriate style and size of tracheotomy tube as well as one size down available before beginning an elective change of the tracheotomy tube. A good light source, suction equipment, and ventilatory equipment are also important.

Technique (Fig. 22-5)

Place the patient on a shoulder roll with the head extended. If the old tracheotomy tube is in place, oxygenate the patient and lavage and suction. Check the new tracheotomy tube to make sure that the cuff works and that the obturator is in place. Next, cut the retaining ties around the neck while an assistant holds the child and the tracheotomy tube in place. Request that the assistant remove the old tracheotomy tube, then briefly examine the stoma. Insert the new tube, taking care to direct the curve of the tube downward toward the chest. Insertion of the tube should require little or no force. A water-soluble lubricant may facilitate insertion. If the tube

---

> **BOX 22-4**   **EQUIPMENT NEEDED FOR A TRACHEOTOMY CHANGE OR TUBE REINSERTION**
>
> 1. Tracheotomy tubes (same size and one size smaller)
> 2. Tracheotomy tube ties
> 3. Scissors
> 4. Shoulder roll (rolled towels)
> 5. Water-soluble lubricant
> 6. Suction

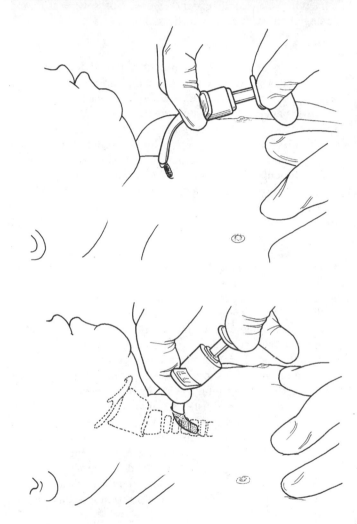

FIG. 22-5   Place the patient on a shoulder roll with the head extended. After removal of the old tube and inspection of the site, insert the new tracheotomy tube, curving the tube downward toward the chest.

does not go in, pull back ¼ inch and try to ease it in by turning the tube gently from side to side. If it is not possible to reinsert the tube with gentle force and turning side to side, try the next size smaller tube. This is often necessary if a considerable period has elapsed between dislodgment and reinsertion of the tracheotomy tube. Remove the obturator while the assistant helps hold the trach in place. Confirm appropriate placement by the presence of adequate ventilation. Finally, secure the tracheotomy tube in place with ties around the neck.

Changing and reinserting tracheotomy tubes are easy in most settings. However, take care not to force the tube in, as this can needlessly create a false passage. The use of a tube one or two sizes smaller may be necessary if the patient's decannulation has been lengthy. Have these tubes available at the bedside before electively changing a tracheotomy tube.

Rarely it is impossible to reinsert a tracheotomy tube in an emergency as a result of closure of the stoma, unavailability of an appropriate-sized tracheotomy tube, or other causes. In this situation insert a standard endotracheal tube into the tracheotomy stoma to establish an airway. If this is not possible, then attempt to intubate the patient orally or nasally. This will be possible except in cases of severe anatomic derangement such as subglottic stenosis.

Remarks

Appropriate training in and use of standard techniques of orotracheal and nasotracheal intubation are adequate to establish and maintain an airway in the vast majority of pediatric patients in respiratory distress. If they are available, adjuncts to tracheal intubation, such as a flexible broncho-scope, a Bullard laryngoscope, a lighted stylet, or retrograde passage of a catheter, can be helpful in establishing an airway under difficult circumstances. Rigid bronchoscopy with a small bronchoscope and Hopkins rod telescope can establish an airway in many situations and is an excellent choice if assessment of the airway is desirable or a distal tracheal lesion exists. If these techniques fail, or if the patient has contraindications to endotracheal intubation, such as a significant cervical spine injury or laryngeal trauma, then the establishment of a surgical airway may be a lifesaving option. A needle cricothyroidotomy is perhaps the quickest method of oxygenating the lungs, and it requires only equipment available in virtually any medical setting. However, it can be very difficult to perform in young children and it has the disadvantage of not allowing for adequate ventilation. If a few surgical supplies and experienced personnel are available, then performing a *cricothyroidotomy is the method of choice* for rapid establishment of an airway that will allow for both oxygenation and ventilation. An emergency tracheotomy is technically more difficult, requiring the expertise of a skilled surgeon, preferably in a relatively controlled environment. Finally, an understanding of the variety of sizes and styles of tracheotomy tubes available and a working knowledge of how to change or replace a tracheotomy tube can be lifesaving.

REFERENCES

1. Anderson HL, Bartlett RH: Elective tracheotomy for mechanical ventilation by the percutaneous technique, *Clin Chest Med* 12(3):555-560, 1991.
2. Attia RR, Battit GE, Murphy JD: Transtracheal ventilation, *JAMA* 234:1152, 1975.
3. Burkey B, Esclamado R, Morganroth M: The role of cricothyroidotomy in airway management, *Clin Chest Med* 12(3):561-571, 1991.
4. Coté C, Eavey R, Jones RD, et al: Cricothyroid membrane puncture: oxygenation and ventilation in a dog model using an intravenous catheter, *Crit Care Med* 16:615, 1988.
5. DeLaurier GA, Hawkins ML, Treat RC, et al: Acute airway management. Role of cricothyroidotomy, *Am Surg* 56(1):12-15, 1990.
6. Fuhrman GM, Stieg FH III, Buerk CA: Blunt laryngeal trauma: classification and management protocol, *J Trauma* 30(1):87-92, 1990.
7. Gianoli GH, Miller RH, Guarisco JL: Tracheotomy in the first year of life, *Ann Otol Rhinol Laryngol* 99(11):896-901, 1990.
8. Heffner JE: Percutaneous tracheotomy: novel technique or technical novelty? *Intens Care Med* 17(5):252-253, 1991.
9. Hilding AC, Hilding JA: Tolerance of the respiratory mucous membrane to trauma: surgical swabs and intratracheal tubes, *Ann Otol Rhinol Laryngol* 71:455, 1962.
10. Holinger PH, Kutnick SL, Schild JA, et al: Subglottic stenosis in infants and children, *Ann Otol Rhinol Laryngol* 85:591, 1976.
11. Hotaling AJ, Robbins WK, Madgy DN, et al: Pediatric tracheotomy: a review of technique, *Am J Otolaryngol* 13(2):115-119, 1992.
12. Jacobs HB: Emergency percutaneous transtracheal catheter and ventilator, *J Trauma* 12:50, 1972.
13. Jacoby JJ et al: Transtracheal resuscitation, *JAMA* 162:625, 1956.
14. Johnson DR, Dunlap A, McFeeley P, et al: Cricothyrotomy performed by prehospital personnel: a comparison of two techniques in a human cadaver model, *Am J Emerg Med* 11(3):207-209, 1993.
15. Lore JM: *An atlas of head and neck surgery,* ed 3, Philadelphia, 1988, WB Saunders.
16. McGill J, Clinton JE, Ruiz E: Cricothyrotomy in the emergency department, *Ann Emerg Med* 11:361, 1982.
17. Milner SM, Bennett JD: Emergency cricothyrotomy, *J Laryngol Otol* 105(11):883-885 1991.
18. Myers E, Stool S, Johnson J: Technique of tracheotomy. In Myers E, Stool S, Johnson J, editors: *Tracheotomy,* New York, 1985, Churchill Livingstone.
19. Oppenheimer P: Needle tracheotomy, *ORL Digest* 39:9, 1977.
20. Puhakka HJ, Kero P, Valli P, et al: Tracheotomy in pediatric patients, *Acta Paediatr* 81(3):231-234, 1992.
21. Salvino CK, Dries D, Gamelli R, et al: Emergency cricothyroidotomy in trauma victims, *J Trauma* 34(4):503-505, 1993.
22. Sasaki CT, Levin PA, Lautman MP, et al: Postnatal descent of the epiglottis in man, *Arch Otolaryngol* 103:169, 1977.
23. Seibert RW, Wetmore SJ: Airway obstruction in infants and children. In Suen JY, Wetmore SJ, editors: *Emergencies in otolaryngology,* New York, 1986, Churchill Livingstone.
24. Smith RB, Schaer WB, Pfaeffle H: Percutaneous transtracheal ventilation for anaesthesia and resuscitation: a review and report of complications, *Can Anaesth Soc J* 22:607-612, 1975.
25. Stauffer JL: Medical management of the airway, *Clin Chest Med* 12(3):449-482, 1991.
26. Stool SE, Eavey R: Tracheotomy. In Bluestone CD, Stool SE, Scheetz MD, editors: *Pediatric otolaryngology,* ed 2, Philadelphia; 1990, WB Saunders.
27. Tucker JA, Tucker GF: A clinical perspective on the development and anatomical aspects of the infant larynx and trachea. In Healy GB, McGill TJ, editors: *Laryngotracheal problems in the pediatric patient,* Springfield, Ill, 1979, Charles C Thomas.
28. Walls RM: Airway management in the blunt trauma patient: how important is the cervical spine? *Can J Surg* 35(1):27-30, 1992.
29. Wang MB, Berke GS, Ward PH, et al: Early experience with percutaneous tracheotomy. *Laryngoscope* 102(2):157-162, 1992.
30. Wenig BI, Applebaum EL: Indications for and techniques of tracheotomy, *Clin Chest Med* 12(3):545-553, 1991.
31. Wetmore RF, Handler SD, Potsic WP: Pediatric tracheotomy: experience during the past decade, *Ann Otol Rhinol Laryngol* 91:628, 1982.

PART V

OXYGEN DELIVERY TECHNIQUES

23 Oxygen Delivery

Daved van Stralen and Ronald M. Perkin

Goals of Oxygen Therapy

Of the two gas exchange aberrations (hypoxemia, hypercapnia) that occur during respiratory failure, hypoxemia is by far the more dangerous to the patient.[21] Usually it is also easier to correct. Initial administration of supplemental oxygen is a safe precaution in all critically ill and injured patients, even if there is no apparent hypoxemia.

Oxygen administration is intended to prevent or minimize end-organ dysfunction resulting from hypoxemia. However oxygen supplementation itself is only one aspect—and sometimes a minor one—of the preservation of adequate tissue function.[4,7]

There is no clinically useful measure of intracellular oxygen tension, so evidence of organ hypoxia must be based indirectly on organ function and oxygen delivery.[7] Since the brain, heart, kidneys, and respiratory muscles are the organs with the highest sustained oxygen demand, they are most profoundly affected by hypoxemia.[4] Tissue requirements for oxygen may also be increased in hypermetabolic states, such as fever, sepsis, and trauma.[6,7]

In general, a partial pressure of oxygen (Pao_2) of 60 mm Hg ensures adequate relief from hypoxemia. Little additional benefit is gained from further increases because of the functional characteristics of hemoglobin.[4] A saturation of 90% is achieved with a Pao_2 of 60 mm Hg (Fig. 23-1). This relationship assumes normally functioning hemoglobin and oxygen dissociation curves. In situations such as carbon monoxide poisoning, a reduction in available hemoglobin results in lower oxygen content and tissue oxygen delivery even with supranormal Pao_2. In acidosis or hyperthermia the oxygen dissociation curve shifts to the right, allowing greater unloading of oxygen at any given partial pressure of oxygen in the capillary. Improved delivery of oxygen to tissues thus occurs during acidosis or fever.[14]

The concept of oxygen delivery, given according to the following formula, is actually more important than Pao_2.[4,7] It encompasses not only Pao_2 but also cardiac output and hemoglobin concentration.

Oxygen delivery ≈ Cardiac output × Arterial oxygen content

Measurement of the arterial oxygen content is much more accurate, albeit more difficult, than measurement of Pao_2 because it takes into account the amount and status of hemoglobin.

The arterial oxygen content may be calculated by measuring the hemoglobin level and arterial oxygen saturation, while keeping in mind that 1 g of hemoglobin can combine maximally with 1.34 ml of oxygen. In addition the volume of total blood oxygen dissolved in the plasma (and dependent on Pao_2) may be calculated as $Pao_2 \times 0.003$ ml/mm Hg.

Arterial oxygen content (Cao_2) is expressed in units of milliliters per deciliter and may be calculated by the formula

$$Cao_2 = (Hemoglobin \times 1.34 \times \% \ Saturation) + (Pao_2 \times 0.003)$$

When oxygen content and delivery are assessed in this manner, it becomes apparent that altering the hemoglobin or cardiac output can have a more dramatic impact on oxygen delivery to the tissues than simply increasing Pao_2 (Fig. 23-2).[4]

Arterial oxygen tension (Pao_2) is determined by the inspired oxygen tension, the alveolar ventilation (V_A), and the distribution of ventilation and perfusion (V/Q).[4]

There are four major mechanisms of hypoxemia:
- Low inspired oxygen content (FIo_2)
- Alveolar hypoventilation
- V/Q mismatch, which varies from areas of perfusion with no ventilation (shunt) to areas of ventilation with no perfusion (dead space)
- Diffusion limitation across the alveolar capillary membrane

The method for increasing Pao_2 depends on the relative contributions of these mechanisms. An increase in the fractional inspired oxygen FIo_2, increase in V_A, or decrease in right-to-left shunt and/or V/Q mismatch may be required to increase Pao_2.[4]

Pure alveolar hypoventilation, most often seen in patients who take an overdose of drugs, results in systemic hypoxemia based on Pao_2.[4]

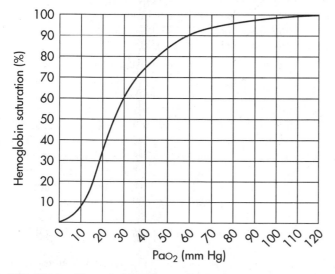

FIG. 23-1 The normal oxyhemoglobin dissociation curve. Near-maximal saturation of hemoglobin occurs at about a Pao_2 of 60 mm Hg; raising the Pao_2 above that point provides only a modest increase in saturation. Note, however, that a rapid fall-off in hemoglobin saturation (and thus oxygen content) occurs when Pao_2 drops below 40 mm Hg.

$$Pao_2 = FIo_2 \ (PB - 47) - Paco_2 \ /R$$

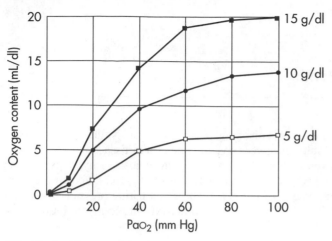

FIG. 23-2 Oxygen delivery to the tissues, reflected by blood oxygen content, can be more profoundly influenced by improving hemoglobin levels than by increasing oxygen tension (Pao_2). In patients with a hemoglobin level of 15 g/dl, adequate oxygen content can be attained with a Pao_2 between 40 and 60 mm Hg. Yet at this same Pao_2, oxygen content remains quite low in patients with lower hemoglobin levels. Furthermore, oxygen content does not increase markedly in anemic patients, even if the Pao_2 is raised to 100 mm Hg or higher.

$Paco_2$ signifies arterial carbon dioxide tension, $PB - 47$ represents barometric pressure minus water vapor pressure, and R is the respiratory quotient (usually 0.8).

Clinically hypoventilation results in hypoxemia with an elevated $Paco_2$. The calculated alveolar arterial-oxygen gradient $[(A - a) O_2$ gradient $= Pao_2 - Pao_2]$ or ratio (Pao_2 /Pao_2) is normal when the cause of hypoxemia is related to hypoventilation or low inspired oxygen concentration.

Both venous admixture and right-to-left shunt result in hypoxemia with normal to low levels of $Paco_2$ and an elevation in $(A - a) DO_2$. The main clinical difference is that the venous admixture type of V/Q mismatch responds more favorably to increases in FIo_2 than does right-to-left shunt.

Indications

Immediately administer 100% oxygen to all dyspneic, tachypneic, or cyanotic pediatric patients. The primary indication for oxygen therapy is the presence or risk of hypoxemia associated with disorders of the respiratory tract. Although diseases of the respiratory system are obvious indications for the use of supplemental oxygen, data from various settings indicate that it is also the initial therapy of choice in septic shock, trauma, and cardiogenic shock.[6] Hemodynamic monitoring and manipulation are useful; however, the goal of therapy should not be to normalize pressure readings, but to optimize oxygen delivery and reduce oxygen consumption.[2,6]

In addition, certain settings call for the administration of oxygen-enriched gases for the purpose of increasing alveolar and/or arterial oxygen tension above physiologic levels. For example, in smoke inhalation, maximal elevation of Pao_2 through the administration of 100% oxygen by nonrebreather mask enhances the elimination of carbon monoxide; in bronchopulmonary dysplasia supplemental oxygen can increase alveolar oxygen, relax the pulmonary artery bed, and reduce pulmonary artery hypertension.

Monitoring oxygen saturation through pulse oximetry has some limitations.[3] These are described in detail in Chapter 28.

Contraindications

There are few absolute contraindications to supplemental oxygen administration if properly done. In a patient with hypoxemia there is no contraindication; however, precautions in the administration are in order. Oxygen is a drug that has proper doses and routes of administration for maximum benefit, minimum toxicity, and reasonable cost-effectiveness.

Complications

Although slowing of the respiratory rate and worsening of hypercapnia after oxygen administration to patients with chronic obstructive pulmonary disease (COPD)[2] are well known, there are virtually no instances in which administration of oxygen for hypoxemia is contraindicated in pediatric patients. Respiratory depression with supplemental oxygen administration may occur in children with chronic lung disease and with chronic upper airway obstruction.[17]

Oxygen must be warmed and humidified. Cold air may decrease body temperature, increase oxygen consumption, and induce bronchospasm when administered to children.[8,13] Occasionally a cool, oxygen-enriched environment may be used to treat children with fever or upper airway obstruction caused by croup, but it should not be so cold that it induces shivering or bronchospasm.

Atmospheric gas is warmed and humidified en route to the alveoli. Alveolar gas normally possesses 100% relative humidity at 37° C. This translates to 44 mg water vapor per liter of gas.[16] Typical room air is 50% humidified at around 20° C, having 10 mg water vapor per liter. The difference in water and temperature is usually supplied by the upper airway, especially the nose.[16] Patients with respiratory distress, especially children, who may possess large adenoids, tend to do more mouth breathing. This is a less effective route for humidification and warming. Patients with endotracheal tubes lose this upper airway function entirely. Therefore complete warming and humidification are accomplished by the tracheobronchial tree. This stress acutely causes impairment of mucociliary activity and therefore secretion clearance. Secondary inflammation and possible infection result. Humidification and sometimes warming of therapeutic dry gas mixtures are necessary to prevent this.[16]

Humidification should be provided for all patients receiving oxygen. Warming should be added when an endotracheal tube is in place. Adequate warming is best assessed by a small thermometer placed just proximal to the endotracheal tube. A temperature of 32° to 37° C is optimal, although lesser values are temporarily acceptable in the patient with poorly controlled fever. Up to 39° C can be used to give a minor assist with rewarming a hypothermic patient. At 40° C and above, thermal tracheobronchitis may result.

Use of cool dry gas from unhumidified sources can contribute to temperature drop in infants less than 6 months of age. This is more significant in intubated patients when physiologic warming and humidification systems are bypassed. Intubated infants on a warming blanket can lose 0.031 C°/min, more when no warming blanket is used.[10] Use of a warming blanket, radiant warmer, and gas humidifier/

warmer reduces this temperature drop to 0.023 C°/min. In our experience with transports of 30 to 60 minutes children less than 10 kg lose 0.5 C° when intubated and lose no heat if not intubated.

Evaporative heat loss during hand ventilation causes this heat loss. Animal studies suggest that the normal heat content of the human is 0.89 cal/kg/C°. A 3-kg infant can lose 1 C° through evaporation of 4.3 ml water.[24] To counteract this heat loss infants use nonshivering thermogenesis through brown adipose metabolism. This causes metabolic acidosis if the infant is uncovered out of the thermoneutral zone (27° C).

In practice the major limitation on the amount and duration of oxygen therapy lies in the pulmonary toxicity of increased alveolar Po_2.[16] The rapidity of onset of pulmonary oxygen toxicity is clearly related to the duration of exposure as well as the level of oxygen delivered.[2] Administration of greater than 60% O_2 for more than 24 hours can be associated with alterations in pulmonary function and, if administered for more prolonged periods, can result in pulmonary oxygen toxicity.[2] On the other hand, inhalation of pure oxygen by human subjects under subatmospheric conditions equivalent to 35% O_2 at ambient pressure for extended periods has not been associated with clinical symptoms or laboratory evidence of pulmonary dysfunction. Consequently oxygen enrichment of inspired gas to $FIo_2 = 0.4$ for indefinite periods is generally considered "safe" with regard to pulmonary oxygen toxicity.

Although short-term oxygen administration is rarely detrimental to the pediatric patient, the means by which oxygen is administered may so agitate the child that respiratory distress and hypoxemia are worsened rather than improved. Therefore, although oxygen should be offered to any pediatric patient, the method of administration must be changed if it produces marked agitation.

Equipment/Techniques

There are various techniques for the administration of oxygen to infants and children. For newborns and small infants it is desirable to avoid a high flow rate because of its cooling effects. For these infants pediatric *nasal cannulas* (Fig. 23-3) work well when a moderate concentration of oxygen suffice. The cannulas also allow greater mobility and normalization of activity, interaction, and feeding[16] (Table 23-1).

The cannulas direct oxygen from a compressed, extracted, or liquid source into the nose at a rate of 0.5 to 5 L/min. When higher flows are used, nasal mucosal drying may occur. However, even with high O_2 flows, the FIo_2 only increases to approximately 0.40. Additionally, the FIo_2 may vary regardless of the O_2 flow. These variations occur because the FIo_2 depends on the patient's minute ventilation and inspiratory flow, which vary during inhalation. The greater the inspiratory flow, the lower the FIo_2, as more room air mixes with the fixed flow of oxygen. In addition there may be differences in the Pao_2 depending on whether the patient is breathing through the mouth or the nose.[16]

An alternative to the nasal cannula is the *face tent* (Fig. 23-4). This is a large trough that sits under the mandible and directs gas flow toward the mouth and nose. FIo_2 values similar to nasal cannula O_2 can be obtained, but about twice as much flow is required. Tents made of clear plastic that completely enclose the patient can deliver an FIo_2 equal to

Table 23-1   Oxygen Administration Techniques

Technique	Advantage	Disadvantage
Nasal cannula	Avoids high flow rate	Moderate oxygen concentrations FIo_2 varying with inspiratory flow rate May irritate nose FIo_2 decrease, from tent disruptions
Face tent	High flow rates for uncooperative infant or small child	Access to patient
Simple oxygen masks	Patient accessibility	FIo_2 varying with inspiratory flow rate
Venturi masks	Patient accessibility Constant flow rate Fixed dilution of gas	
Oxygen reservoir (nonbreathing mask)	Higher FIo_2 with respiratory flow rate	Resistance of valve that may fatigue infant or small child

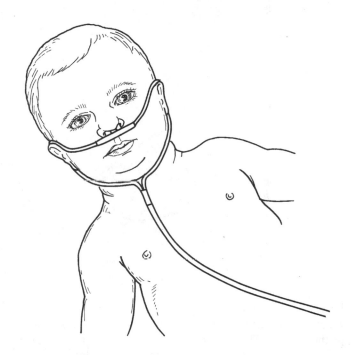

FIG. 23-3   Nasal prongs or cannula.

gas source if 10- to 15-L/min flows are used. They may occasionally be useful in the extremely uncooperative infant or small child. Unfortunately access to patient and intermittent FIo_2 decreases caused by tent disruption pose problems.[16]

Simple O_2 masks (Fig. 23-5) are soft, plastic masks placed over the patient's mouth and nose and maintained in position by an elastic strap around the back of the head or neck. One hundred percent O_2 can flow directly from a compressed or liquid source, or from an O_2 concentrator, into the mask at a fixed flow, or the O_2 can be diluted to various concentrations

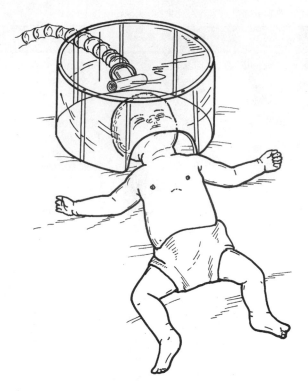

FIG. 23-4 Oxygen hood or face tent.

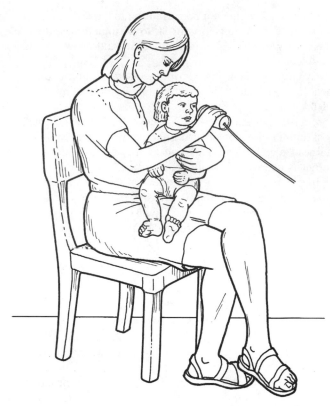

FIG. 23-6 Paper cup used for administering oxygen.

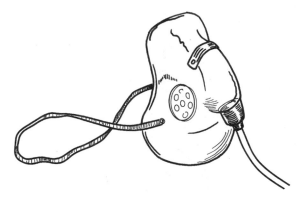

FIG. 23-5 Simple face mask.

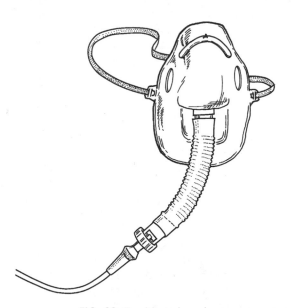

FIG. 23-7 Venturi mask.

by room air. As with nasal cannulas, the FIo_2 is variable because room air is drawn in through the holes on both sides of the mask.[16] The degree and duration of decrease depend on the minute ventilation, the inspiratory flow, and the tightness of the mask. The mask may be better tolerated by the child if it is held to the face by the parent rather than strapped around the head. If these measures fail, placing oxygen tubing through the bottom of a paper cup and instructing the parent to hold the cup close to the child's face may be accepted by the child (Fig. 23-6).

Venturi masks (Fig. 23-7) are constructed and worn in a fashion similar to those of the simple O_2 mask described previously. However, the barrel of the Venturi mask is designed to use the Bernoulli principle. The O_2 is delivered through a narrow jet surrounded by holes connecting to the atmosphere. The negative pressure generated by the flow of FIo_2 entrains a constant flow of air, giving a fixed dilution of gas delivered at high flows (40 L/min). An FIo_2 of 0.24, 0.26,

0.28, 0.30, or 0.35 can be delivered with high reliability despite variation in flow.[4] The advantage of these masks is that the FIo_2 of the gas inhaled by the patient does not exceed, and in most instances very closely approximates, that set by the Venturi.

Oxygen reservoir (nonbreathing or low dead space masks) (Fig. 23-8) were designed to circumvent the problem of having a small reservoir for delivered gas with the potential for dilution of the augmented FIo_2 by room air. The mask is similar to those described except that gas of FIo_2 up to 1 is

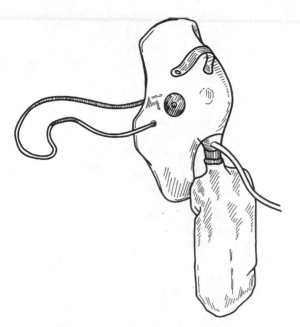

FIG. 23-8 Nonrebreathing mask.

delivered into a plastic reservoir that has a volume of approximately 1 L. The reservoir is connected to the mask through a one-way flap valve that opens during inhalation and closes during exhalation. This theoretically allows the patient to inhale 100% O_2 regardless of his or her minute ventilation or inspiratory flow pattern.[4] The valve often offers too much resistance to be effective with the weak inspiratory force of the infant, small child, or fatigued patient.

Oxygen delivery to the reservoir must exceed the patient's minute ventilation. If it does not, the reservoir collapses and the patient either inhales room air through a loosely fitted mask or suffocates if the mask fits tightly. In practice, face masks rarely fit tightly enough to prevent room air from entering them during inhalation. Because of this, these masks cannot reliably deliver gas with an FIo_2 greater than 0.7. *In addition, if the condition causing the hypoxemia is so severe that an FIo_2 greater than 0.6 is required, positive-pressure ventilation is generally needed immediately.*

Alternative Techniques

As part of the decision to administer oxygen, determine whether passive oxygen administration (such as with mask or cannula) is adequate or whether positive-pressure ventilation is required. Positive-pressure ventilation is needed if there is apnea, continued high work of breathing, altered mental status, respiratory failure, or persistent cyanosis despite a brief trial of high-concentration oxygen administration.[20] Positive pressure should be initiated with a bag and mask. If it is successful in improving the child's condition as judged by color, responsiveness, or pulse, continue positive-pressure ventilation for the duration of care with either mask or endotracheal tube. If endotracheal intubation can be achieved quickly, it may be preferable to positive-pressure ventilation by mask.

Continuous positive airway pressure (CPAP) can be given along with up to 100% oxygen by a reservoir mask that can be tightly applied.[12] Continuous flow systems are currently recommended, especially in pediatric patients, because demand systems impose an additional ventilation work load. CPAP is set with a partially occluding one-way valve on the expiratory side, and flow is adjusted to keep the reservoir bag full. Mask CPAP requires patient cooperation for good mask fit and prevention of gastric distention from aerophagia. Therefore, it is most useful in the larger child or adolescent. Typical values to help restore functional residual capacity with acute restrictive defects are 5 to 15 cm H_2O. Above 15 cm H_2O gastric distention is likely even without aerophagia, and good mask fit without patient discomfort becomes a major problem. Mask CPAP is most useful as a temporizing measure when avoidance of endotracheal intubation is desired.[23]

Excessive pressure by mask ventilation causes gastric distention and increases the risk of vomiting and aspiration.[1] If mask ventilation is chosen because of short transport time or difficulty with intubation, pass a nasogastric tube to decompress the stomach and decrease the risk of vomiting. The smaller nasogastric tube used in the pediatric patient permits an adequate mask-to-face seal during bag-mask ventilation.

OTHER METHODS TO IMPROVE ARTERIAL OXYGENATION
Hyperbaric Oxygen Therapy

Hyperbaric oxygen (HBO) therapy is the treatment of a patient entirely enclosed within a pressure vessel who is breathing oxygen (O_2) at a pressure greater than that at sea level (1 atmosphere absolute [ATA]).[25] There is a growing understanding of the mechanisms of action of HBO, and there are a number of disease states for which research has indicated possible therapeutic benefit (Box 23-1).[25]

Primary mechanisms of HBO action include a reduction in volume of gas-filled spaces and hyperoxygenation of all perfused tissue beds.[26] Hyperoxygenation of tissue results from a markedly increased arterial O_2 content, which is related principally to O_2 physically dissolving in plasma. The oxyhemoglobin dissociation curve is unchanged. The highest O_2 used in clinical practice is 3 ATA, and at this pressure arterial O_2 may reach 1900 to 2100 mm Hg. Dissolved O_2 can reach 6.8 volumes percent (6.8 ml O_2/100 ml blood).[25]

Carbon monoxide (CO) poisoning is currently cited as the best indication for the use of HBO treatment.[25,26] It has been established that HBO reduces blood concentrations of carboxyhemoglobin more rapidly than by breathing 100% oxygen at ambient pressure (carboxyhemoglobin half-life at room air: 5 hours, 20 minutes; carboxyhemoglobin half-life at 100% oxygen breathing: 90 minutes; carboxyhemoglobin half-life under HBO: 23 minutes). However, it may be difficult to achieve timely access to the chamber.

Supplemental oxygen inhalation is a cornerstone in the treatment of CO poisoning. Carboxyhemoglobin dissociation is hastened by an elevation in oxygen partial pressure. Although recent reports suggest that the mechanism of HBO may extend beyond its effect on COHgb, it is because of the reduction in COHgb half-life that HBO has been recommended and used to treat severe CO poisoning for more than 25 years. Controlled clinical studies are lacking, but a

> **BOX 23-1 CLINICAL USE OF HYPERBARIC OXYGEN**
>
> - Carbon monoxide poisoning
> - Air embolism
> - Decompression sickness
> - Compromised grafts and flaps
> - Radiation necrosis
> - Clostridial myonecrosis
> - Necrotizing infections
> - Refractory osteomyelitis
> - Compromised (refractory) cutaneous ulcers
> - Thermal burns
> - Crush/peripheral ischemia

number of reports describe a reversal of severe neurologic and cardiovascular depression temporally related to institution of HBO. The results of a relatively large retrospective study indicate that prompt administration of HBO can reduce mortality rate (13% when HBO is administered within 6 hours of patient discovery versus 30% if administered later).[25] HBO may also decrease the incidence of delayed neurologic sequelae by up to 40%.[25]

The inherent toxicity of O_2 must be addressed when HBO is used therapeutically. Because of careful administration the incidence of toxicity is remarkably low. However what must not be overlooked when considering the use of HBO is the ability of the clinical facility also to deliver proper medical care. The sophistication present in many of the hyperbaric chamber facilities today is largely analogous to that of an intensive care unit. Equipment is available for invasive cardiovascular monitoring, mechanical ventilation, cardiac pacing, and intravenous infusion. HBO should never be considered unless proper supportive medical care can be delivered.

INHALED GAS MIXTURES
Nitric Oxide

Regional constriction of the pulmonary vascular bed is a normal physiologic response. This protective reflex attempts to preserve the ideal ventilation-to-perfusion ratio (*V/Q*) between 1.0 and 0.8. *V/Q* mismatching is the most common cause of hypoxemia in the critically ill. Modulation of pulmonary vascular tone is a localized phenomenon and is independent of neural and humoral stimuli.[19] On occasion excessive pulmonary vasoconstriction may inadvertently contribute to a severe *V/Q* inequality that may lead to death of the patient. Adult respiratory distress syndrome, persistent pulmonary hypertension of the newborn, and pulmonary hypertension secondary to cardiac disease are but a few of these disorders.[19] In an important proportion of critically ill children these problems are present at admission or develop later; these children have high morbidity rates.

Various drugs have been used to reduce pulmonary vascular resistance. These include but are not limited to arachidonic acid metabolites, organic nitrates, organic nitrites, organic nitrocompounds, acetylcholine, calcium channel blockers, and magnesium sulfate.[18,19] The pharmacologic actions of these drugs vary but ultimately result in the decrease of intracellular (cytoplasmic) calcium, a decrease that causes smooth-muscle relaxation.

The major stumbling block preventing the use of these cytoplasmic calcium inhibitors as pulmonary vasodilators is the inability to achieve specific regional selectivity.[19] Associated with the attenuation of pulmonary vascular tension is a concomitant dilation of the systemic arterial vasculature—invariably leading to systemic hypotension and various other reported complications. Inhalation of nitric oxide (NO) gas may be the ideal solution to this problem because NO is inactivated before reaching the systemic circulation. NO gas has been shown to be a potent and rapid smooth-muscle relaxant.[18]

The importance of NO gas as a pulmonary vascular muscle relaxant rests on its characteristic of being delivered as a gas directly to the pulmonary vascular system, without affecting systemic vascular tone.[18] Like oxygen, NO gas can be administered via pulmonary airways.

Because NO gas is delivered from the alveolar side, it should selectively increase perfusion only to ventilated areas of the lung—normalizing the *V/Q* inequality. The result would be decreased FI_{O_2} requirement for many patients and consequent prevention of oxygen toxicity. If it is shown that inhaled NO gas relieves pulmonary vascular resistance only in ventilated areas of the lung, the prognosis for many intensive care patients suffering from hypoxemia or increased pulmonary hypertension may dramatically improve.[9,18] Morbidity secondary to these problems may also decrease significantly.

Helium-Oxygen Mixtures

In 1935 mixtures of helium and oxygen were introduced for use in the treatment of obstructive lesions of the larynx, trachea, and airways.

Helium is a biologically inert gas of low molecular weight whose density is one quarter that of ambient air. Compared to nitrogen-oxygen mixtures, helium-oxygen mixtures, because of their lower density, allow laminar flow conditions to persist at significantly higher flow rates.[11,16] For a given set of airway dimensions, turbulent flow that develops at high rates has a greater resistance than laminar flow. The substitution of helium for nitrogen enhances ventilation in patients with airway obstruction.[11,23]

Intravenous Oxygenation and CO_2 Removal Device

With the success of partial lung-bypass procedures in adults, interest in implantable devices capable of providing support of oxygenation and CO_2 removal has been renewed. An intravascular (venous) blood gas exchange device (IVOX) has been developed and tested in animals and humans to provide partial support of a failing respiratory system.

The IVOX is essentially a mechanical hollow fiber membrane oxygenator. Instead of taking the blood from the patient to the extracorporeal system and perfusing the oxygenator with gas, the IVOX accomplishes its tasks by having the patient's venous blood circulate around the fibers that form the oxygenator.[15] As a foreign body, the IVOX raises several safety and efficacy concerns that differ from those of traditional extracorporeal blood-oxygenator systems. The size of the gas transfer area (and effectiveness of blood contact) is a limiting factor in the ability of the device to exchange O_2 and CO_2. The largest device available is about one third as efficient as the simplest extracorporeal membrane oxygenator (see Chapter 27).

Remarks

In order for oxygen therapy to exercise a salutary effect on Pao_2, hypoxemia must be secondary to hypoventilation or the presence of low V/Q units within the lungs. Any true intrapulmonary right-to-left shunting (i.e., $V/Q = 0$) or extrapulmonary right-to-left shunting is unaffected by an elevation of alveolar oxygen tension (Pao_2).[5,22]

The 100% oxygen challenge further helps to separate cardiac from pulmonary causes. Administration of oxygen to the infant with true cyanotic heart disease does not affect his or her cyanosis, whereas the infant with pulmonary disease should show improvement not only by clinical observation but by measurement of pulse oximetry or arterial blood gas. Absolute standards for the degree of improvement necessary for definition of pulmonary cyanosis are difficult to establish for many reasons, including the possibility that some pulmonary disease may be superimposed on the cyanotic cardiac patient. In general any Pao_2 more than 100 makes true cyanotic congenital heart disease unlikely.[27]

In the child with congenital heart disease, evaluation of the response to supplemental oxygen helps differentiate cyanotic from noncyanotic lesions. A spun hematocrit can also contribute information. Chronic low oxygen tension stimulates erythropoietin production and an increase in red cell mass. These children have supranormal hematocrits compared to those of age-specific normal children.

The degree of "shunt effect" resulting from V/Q mismatching can then be expressed as a percentage of total pulmonary blood flow or shunt fraction (Qs/QT); this also is referred to as venous admixture or virtual shunt. When using this model, resulting Pao_2 values can be predicted in association with a given inspired oxygen concentration when a known amount of right-to-left shunting is occurring within the lungs (Fig. 23-9).[14,22] From the relationship of FIo_2 and Pao_2 for varying degrees of shunt, once shunt fraction achieves a certain level, increasing inspired oxygen concentration has little effect on the Pao_2 value. Thus with a shunt fraction in excess of 30% attainment of adequate arterial oxygenation (i.e., $Pao_2 > 60$ mm Hg) is not possible with an FIo_2 of 0.5 or less. If the shunt fraction exceeds 40%, adequate arterial oxygenation cannot be achieved under atmospheric conditions, even with maximal oxygen enrichment of inspired gas.[22]

The relationship of FIo_2 and Pao_2 can provide a general picture of the degree of abnormality in pulmonary function as it relates to oxygen transport. It also serves to indicate precarious situations in which small increments in shunt fraction result in hypoxemia refractory to oxygen therapy. From these relationships it is clear that the assessment of the oxygenation in a given patient must take into account the level of oxygen therapy required to generate a specific Pao_2 value. In situations characterized by extensive V/Q mismatching, such that the shunt effect of low V/Q units approximates 30% to 40% of pulmonary blood flow, mechanical means for improving V/Q matching (e.g., CPAP/PEEP) must be instituted.[12]

A final factor that places relative limits on the amount of oxygen delivered in a clinical setting of V/Q mismatching

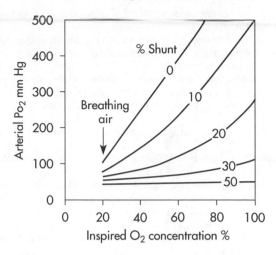

FIG. 23-9 Response of the arterial Po_2 to increased inspired oxygen concentrations in a lung with various amounts of shunt. Note that the Po_2 remains much below the normal level for 100% oxygen. Nevertheless useful gains in oxygenation occur even with severe degrees of shunting. (This diagram shows typical values only; changes in cardiac output, oxygen uptake, etc., affect the position of the lines.)

involves the phenomenon of alveolar nitrogen washout. With enrichment of the inspired oxygen concentration, alveolar nitrogen, an inert gas, is replaced over time by oxygen. Because oxygen is readily removed from alveoli by blood flow to the alveolar compartments, alveolar units with low levels of ventilation are at risk for having their gaseous contents completely absorbed. Therefore breathing high concentrations of oxygen can result in a loss of gas volume from low V/Q alveoli and, ultimately, alveoli collapse.[16,22] In this manner, the process of nitrogen washout can convert low V/Q units in the lung into totally atelectatic areas with $V/Q = 0$ (true intrapulmonary right-to-left shunt).[22] Obviously this can contribute further to the impairment in pulmonary oxygen exchange as well as to any preexisting loss of lung volume and associated decrease in lung compliance.

REFERENCES

1. Admani M, Yeh TF, Jain R, et al: Prevention of gastric inflation during mask ventilation in newborn infants, *Crit Care Med* 13:592-593, 1985.
2. Carlton TJ, Anthonisen NR: A guide for judicious use of oxygen in critical illness: steps to avoid or reduce cellular hypoxia—and improve outcome, *J Crit Illness* 7:1744-1757, 1992.
3. Curley FJ, Smyrnios NA: Routine monitoring of critically ill patients. *J Intensive Care Med* 5:153-174, 1990.
4. Dekich SE, Olsen GN: Techniques for administering oxygen effectively in the ICU, *J Crit Illness* 4:95-103, 1989.
5. Demling RH, Knox JB: Basic concepts of lung function and dysfunction: oxygenation, ventilation, and mechanics, *New Horizons* 1:362-370, 1993.
6. Edwards JD: Practical application of oxygen transport principles, *Crit Care Med* 18:S45, 1990.
7. Fahey JT, Lister G: Oxygen demand, delivery, and consumption. In Fuhrman BP, Zimmerman JJ, editors: *Pediatric critical care,* St. Louis, 1992, Mosby, pp 237-258.
8. Fireman P: The wheezing infant, *Pediatr Rev* 7:247-254, 1986.
9. Frostell CG, Blomquist H, Hedenstierna G, et al: Inhaled nitric oxide selectively reverses human hypoxic pulmonary vasoconstriction without causing systemic vasodilation, *Anesthesiology* 78:427-435, 1993.
10. Gauntlett I, Barnes J, Brown TCK, et al: Temperature maintenance in

infants undergoing anaesthesia and surgery, *Anaesth Intensive Care* 13:300-304, 1985.

11. Gluck EH, Onorato DJ, Castriotta R: Helium-oxygen mixtures in intubated patients with status asthmaticus and respiratory acidosis, *Chest* 98:693-698, 1990.

12. Habib DM, Perkin RM: Continuous distending pressure and assisted ventilation. In Levin DL, Morriss FC, editors: *Essentials of pediatric intensive care,* St. Louis, 1990, Quality Medical Publishing, pp. 897-910.

13. Hazinski TA: Bronchial hyperreactivity in infants, *Respir Care* 36:735-745, 1991.

14. Helfaer MA, Nichols DG, Rogers MC: Developmental physiology of the respiratory system. In Rogers MC, editor: *Textbook of pediatric intensive care,* Baltimore, 1992, Williams & Wilkens, pp. 104-133.

15. Lanigan LJ, Withington PS: Support when gas exchange fails: ECMO, $ECCO_2$ R and IVOX, *Clin Intensive Care* 2:210-216, 1991.

16. Martin LD, Rafferty JF, Walker LK, et al: Principles of respiratory support and mechanical ventilation. In Rogers MC, editor: *Textbook of pediatric intensive care,* Baltimore, 1992, Williams & Wilkens.

17. McColley SA, April MM, Carroll JL, et al: Respiratory compromise after adenotonsillectomy in children with obstructive sleep apnea, *Arch Otolarngeal Head Neck Surg* 118:940-943, 1992.

18. Miller CC, Miller JWR: Pulmonary vascular smooth-muscle regulation: The role of inhaled nitric oxide gas, *Respir Care* 37:1175-1185, 1992.

19. Perkin RM, Anas NG: Pulmonary hypertension in pediatric patients, *J Pediatr* 105:511-522, 1984.

20. Perkin RM, Anas NG: Acute respiratory failure. In Grossman M, Dieckman RA, editors: *Pediatric emergency medicine,* Philadelphia, 1991, JB Lippencott, pp. 84-88.

21. Schuster DP: A physiologic approach to initiating, maintaining, and withdrawing mechanical ventilating support during acute respiratory failure, *Am J Med* 88:268-277, 1990.

22. Shapiro BA, Harrison RA, Cane RD, et al: *Clinical application of blood gases,* ed 4, Chicago, 1989, Year Book Medical Publishers.

23. Stauffer JL: Medical management of the airway, *Clin Chest Med* 12:449-482, 1991.

24. Stevens ED, Fry FEJ: Cooling curves of fish, *Can J Zoo* 48:221-226, 1970.

25. Thom SR: Hyperbaric oxygen therapy, *J Intensive Care Med* 4:58-74, 1989.

26. Weaver LK: Hyperbaric treatment of respiratory emergencies, *Respir Care* 37:720-737, 1992.

27. Yabek SM: Neonatal cyanosis: reappraisal of response to 100% oxygen breathing *Am J Dis Child* 138:880-884, 1984.

PART VI

VENTILATION/OXYGENATION TECHNIQUES

24 Bag and Mask Ventilation

Raeford E. Brown, Jr.

The proper bag-valve-mask (BVM) ventilation of critically ill pediatric patients is extremely important, yet difficult to learn and retain without constant practice.

Indications

BVM ventilation is indicated for hypoventilation or airway obstruction and usually precedes endotracheal intubation.

Contraindications

BVM ventilation using positive pressure is relatively contraindicated in patients with congenital diaphragmatic hernia or tracheoesophageal fistula. In both of these circumstances direct positive pressure to the tracheobronchial tree through an endotracheal tube prevents respiratory embarrassment caused by BVM ventilation and air entrainment into the gastrointestinal (GI) tract.

Complications

Inadequate BVM ventilation may introduce air into the GI tract and produce ventilatory embarrassment or predispose to aspiration. In addition inappropriate placement of the mask may produce airway obstruction; failure to recognize abnormal pulmonary compliance may lead to continued hypoventilation, hypercapnia, and hypoxia.[1]

Equipment

The range of sizes of pediatric patients requires a variety of mask and ventilation circuit sizes. Clear, air-filled masks conform to the child's face when appropriately sized and ensure a tight seal, a view of the lips and tongue, and information regarding possibly regurgitated stomach contents. When properly applied, the mask should fit easily over the nose and rest in the dimple of the chin. If mask fit is correct, the person managing the airway should be able easily to introduce gas through a ventilating circuit into the airway without loss of gas into the atmosphere.

There are two types of circuits for BVM ventilation. The self-inflating circuit uses structural rigidity to reinflate after positive pressure is applied to the circuit. Because of this reinflating capability, the circuit draws fresh gas either from the atmosphere or, in the case of oxygen-supplemented ventilation, from available oxygen flow. Use a reservoir with the self-inflating circuit in order to deliver high fractional concentrations of inspired oxygen, such as is necessary for resuscitation. These circuits also have preset pop-off valves to protect the airway from excessive positive pressure. Occasionally, especially in cases of head malposition or very noncompliant lungs, these valves do not allow administration of enough pressure to the airway to ventilate the patient adequately.

Critical care and anesthesia practitioners also routinely use a second type of ventilating circuit, the anesthesia circuit. It is, in fact, a modification of the Mapleson A circuit (Fig. 24-1). In this configuration fresh gas flows into the circuit through a proximal fresh gas flow line. Exhaled gas from the patient fills the reservoir bag, and thus ventilation reintroduces the resulting mixture of fresh gas with alveolar and anatomic dead space gas to the patient. Either of these circuits is appropriate for the resuscitation of pediatric patients, and familiarity usually drives individual choice. However, although it is possible to use the self-inflating circuit to ventilate a patient without fresh gas flow, the Mapleson A circuit uses only fresh gas flow of oxygen and/or air. The Bain circuit, a modification of the Mapleson A, is also useful in the ventilation of pediatric patients (Fig. 24-2).

Technique

Position the body in the neutral or sniffing position (Figs. 24-3 and 24-4). Various maneuvers may be necessary to obtain this position depending on the size and age of the patient. For example, infants routinely require a shoulder roll to obtain a neutral position because of the large size of the occiput, whereas a large adolescent male may in fact require a head pillow to achieve a similar position. After the sniffing

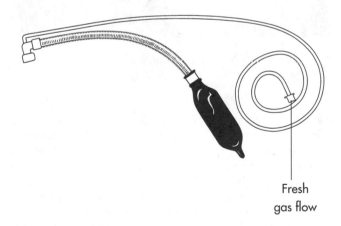

FIG. 24-1   Mapleson A circuit.

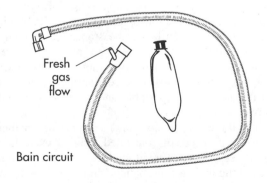

FIG. 24-2   Bain circuit.

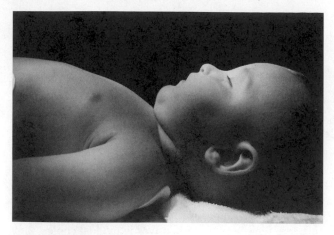

FIG. 24-3   Infant head malpositioned, producing airway obstruction.

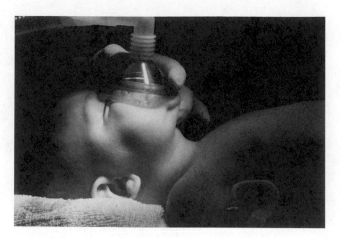

FIG. 24-5   Appropriate head position, mask placement, and hand placement for positive ventilation.

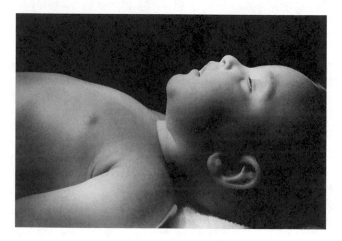

FIG. 24-4   Infant head appropriately positioned with shoulder roll, reducing airway obstruction.

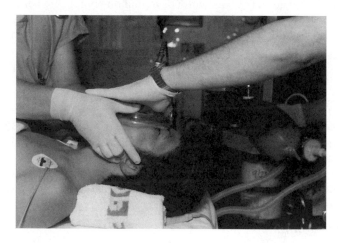

FIG. 24-6   Bag and mask ventilation using four hands.

position is obtained, apply a mask of proper size to the patient's face with fingers under the mandible to open the airway and thumb and first finger holding the mask firmly in position. Allow the patient to breathe spontaneously without assistance through an unobstructed airway, or assist ventilation by providing a positive-pressure breath as the patient inspires spontaneously, or control ventilation by providing positive-pressure breaths without any contribution from the patient (Fig. 24-5).

Assess the adequacy of bag and mask ventilation by chest rise with positive pressure and the presence of breath sounds bilaterally. Prevent inflation of the stomach. Recognize the difference between ventilating the stomach and raising the chest with adequate positive-pressure ventilation. It is easy to determine the adequacy of oxygenation by pulse oximetry. Rapidly assess the adequacy of ventilation, in patients with normal lungs, by using portable and/or disposable end-tidal CO_2 devices.[2]

Much of the resistance to proper ventilation, whether it be spontaneous, assisted, or controlled, originates in the upper airway and especially in relation to the tongue. In the supine position, in the unconscious patient, and especially in infants, the tongue rests on the posterior oropharynx and effectively

obstructs gas flow into the airway.[3] Adjuncts such as oral or nasopharyngeal airways or oropharyngeal mask airways may be useful in reducing the obstructive effect of the tongue. Patients who are semicomatose or partially anesthetized may attempt to breathe through a closed glottis. In this circumstance there are no audible breath sounds, and one notes a to-and-fro, seesaw motion of the chest and abdomen.

Occasionally adequate management of an airway in an emergency requires more than one set of hands. In these circumstances one resuscitator achieves correct head position, including jaw thrust, while the other provides positive-pressure ventilation (Fig. 24-6). This scenario usually occurs when patients are obese or have intraoral mass lesions. Infants, who have a large tongue relative to the size of their mouth, may require this four-handed ventilation technique to provide appropriate chest expansion and adequate oxygenation. In circumstances where two clinicians manage the airway, one routinely approaches the patient from the front, applying upward pressure with both hands at the angle of the jaw. This maneuver lifts the tongue off the posterior oropharynx and therefore clears the airway. The second clinician, approaching the patient from the head, provides bag-and-mask, mouth-to-mask, or occasionally mouth-to-mouth ventilation. Appropriate communication between the two clinicians managing the airway is extremely important to ensure the efficiency of the operation.

The unconscious patient and the conscious patient who requires assisted ventilation often have a full stomach at admission. Circumstances such as trauma, administration of narcotics, and stress reduce gastric emptying and increase the risk of regurgitation and aspiration in patients who do not have airway protection.[4] Two mechanisms can produce regurgitation and aspiration. Active regurgitation or vomiting occurs in conscious patients. Cricoid pressure, pressure applied to the neck to occlude the esophagus, does not preclude aspiration if the patient is actively vomiting. In fact patients who vomit actively may generate more than 100 mm Hg of intragastric pressure.[5] Cricoid pressure applied in this circumstance may result in esophageal rupture and mediastinitis. In the unconscious patient passive regurgitation is more common. As patients become hypoxemic and hypercapnic, gastroesophageal sphincter tone decreases, and gastric contents may slide up the esophagus and into the airway. With positive-pressure ventilation, gas passes into the stomach, promoting passive regurgitation. As the regurgitant volume reaches the oropharynx, positive-pressure ventilation carries this mixture into the airway, producing aspiration pneumonitis. Cricoid pressure is effective in reducing the probability of aspiration associated with positive-pressure ventilation in unconscious patients. Studies have demonstrated that cricoid pressure prevents aspiration in pediatric patients, including infants.

REFERENCES

1. Coté CJ, Ryan JF, Todres ID, et al: *A practice of anesthesia for infants and practice of anesthesiology,* ed 2, St. Louis, 1993, Mosby.
2. Coté CJ, Liu LM, Szyfelbein SK, et al: Intraoperative events diagnosed by expired carbon dioxide monitoring in children, *Can Anaesth Soc J* 33(3 pt 1):315-320, 1968.
3. Eckenhoff JE: Some anatomic considerations of the infant larynx influencing endotracheal anesthesia, *Anesthesiology* 12:401-410, 1951.
4. Roberts JT: *Fundamentals of tracheal intubation,* New York, 1983, Grune & Stratton.
5. Rogers MC, Tinker JH, Covino BG, et al: *Principals and practice of anesthesiology,* St. Louis, 1993, Mosby.

25 Conventional Mechanical Ventilation

Bradley P. Fuhrman, Lynn J. Hernan, and Michele C. Papo

Mechanical ventilation ensures adequate respiratory gas exchange in diverse settings. The versatility of the concept of "artificial respiration" has prompted the evolution of a complex array of techniques, as well as the proliferation of numerous abbreviations and acronyms. Though these techniques overlap in their applications, each confers some specific advantage in the appropriate situation, and each has specific limitations.

This chapter deals with the multiple variations of conventional positive-pressure ventilation and provides guidelines for effective respiratory support by these techniques.

Indications

Mechanical ventilation provides a means to support respiration when the patient is unable to breathe adequately without assistance, appears at risk of exhaustion, cannot maintain adequate lung expansion (or oxygenation) without support, cannot afford the energy expense of breathing, requires deep sedation or anesthesia, lacks adequate neural control of respiration, or lacks motivation to follow an essential respiratory therapeutic plan. Base the decision to use mechanical ventilation on a complete clinical picture and not on numeric values for oxygenation and carbon dioxide tension alone. Some children require assisted ventilation only briefly, such as for apnea after pharmacologic treatment of seizures. Bag and mask ventilation usually suffices in these situations, preventing the need for endotracheal intubation and mechanical ventilation.

Contraindications

There are no accepted absolute contraindications to mechanical ventilation. Unfortunately the process has advantages and disadvantages. Prevent barotrauma (volutrauma), even if less aggressive ventilator strategies result in hypercarbia. Other treatments (like extracorporeal membrane oxygenation) do not *supplant* mechanical ventilation.

Complications

Mechanical ventilation can disrupt lung architecture, promote pulmonary edema, and foster maldistribution of ventilation. In acute lung injury alveolar segments may differ substantially in compliance. Positive airway pressure (applied in the hope of expanding an atelectatic lung) may overdistend more compliant segments, thereby producing volutrauma. This may be manifested as pulmonary air leak (bronchopleural fistula) or as pulmonary interstitial emphysema (PIE). Pneumothoraces may compress the heart and impair cardiac output. Pneumomediastinum generally decompresses into the neck and rarely causes cardiac tamponade. PIE often creates an unanticipated alveolar dead space and wastes ventilation. It may also compress the pulmonary circulation and elevate pulmonary vascular resistance.

Positive airway pressure also has important direct negative effects on the circulation, affecting both cardiac activity and pulmonary circulation. It can impede ventricular filling, compress pulmonary circulation, and afterload reduce the left ventricle. The net result of these effects may be either adverse or beneficial.

Malposition of the endotracheal tube (e.g., right main stem bronchus intubation) may maldistribute ventilation and cause hypoxia and/or hypercarbia. It can also overdistend ventilated lung segments, causing volutrauma.

Nosocomial infection is also a common problem associated with prolonged endotracheal intubation.

Techniques

Principles of Mechanical Ventilation. The lungs expand during inspiration because the pressure drop from alveolus to pleural space (transalveolar pressure) rises.[5] During spontaneous breathing mechanical deformation of the thorax by the diaphragm and other muscles of respiration modulates this pressure drop over the respiratory cycle. Descent of the diaphragm depresses pleural pressure, raises transalveolar pressure, and inflates the lungs. In this process the lungs expand from their functional residual capacity to their peak inspiratory volume. Normally alveolar pressure approximates atmospheric pressure over most of the respiratory cycle.

During positive-pressure ventilation, whatever the technique, inspiration follows an increase in alveolar pressure above ambient and a consequent rise in transalveolar pressure. The inspiratory rise in lung volume is the result of this increase in alveolar pressure and, in turn, causes a rise in pleural pressure. Positive-pressure ventilation may, therefore, compress alveolar capillaries in inspiration. Positive-pressure inspiration predictably opposes systemic venous return[1] (Fig. 25-1).

Several factors determine the relation of airway pressure to lung volume over the respiratory cycle. The static pressure-volume relationship of the thorax defines the airway pressure required to support it (at any given volume) against its elastic recoil forces (Fig. 25-2). When there is no flow of air, as during simultaneous occlusion of both inspiratory and expiratory tubes of the ventilator, the airway pressure plateau reflects this pressure. During air flow, as during the inspiratory phase of the respiratory cycle, pressure drops from trachea to alveolus across resistance airways. This is measurable as the difference between tracheal inspiratory pressure and static (airway occlusion) pressure, which reflects simultaneous downstream (alveolar) pressure (Fig. 25-3).

Airway resistance and lung compliance together determine the time constant of every lung segment. The product of these two parameters for the whole lung determines its time constant, which in turn determines the time course of rise and fall of lung volume in response to ramp changes in airway pressure (inspiratory pressure and end-expiratory pressure) over the respiratory cycle (Fig. 25-4).

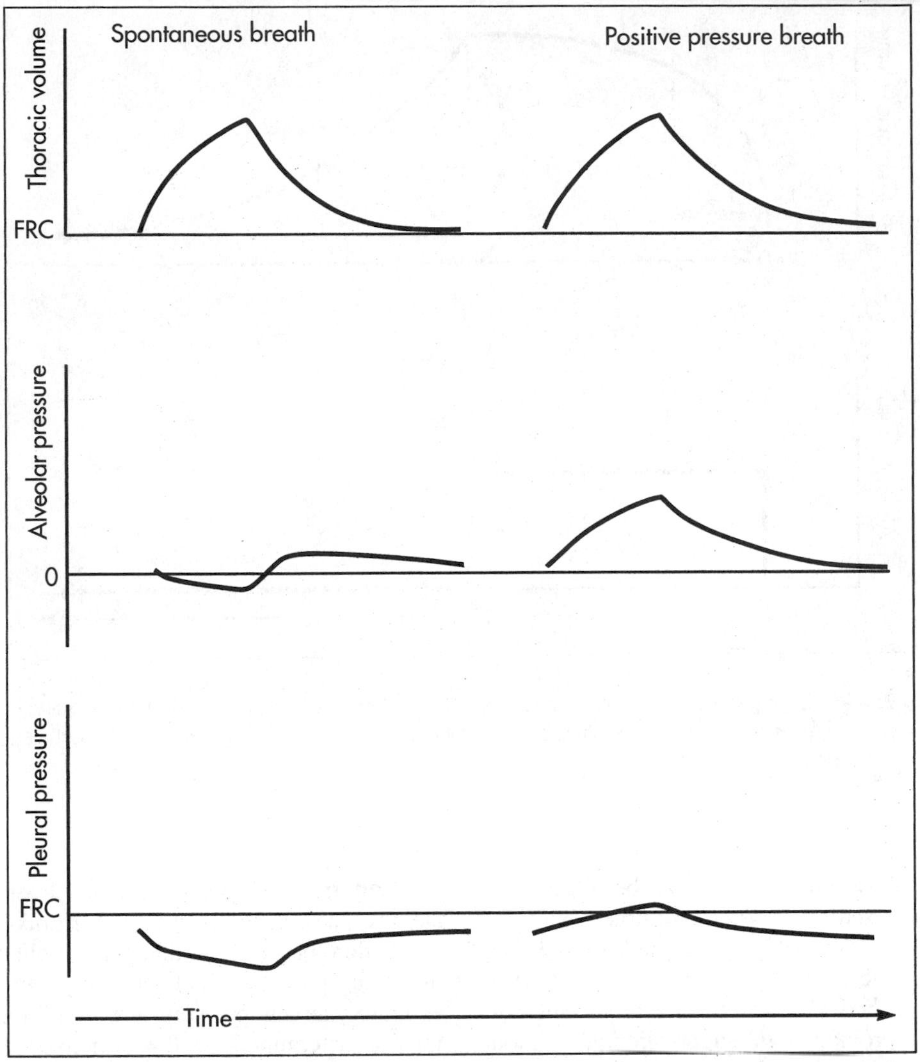

FIG. 25-1   Positive-pressure breaths raise pleural pressure and oppose systemic venous return.

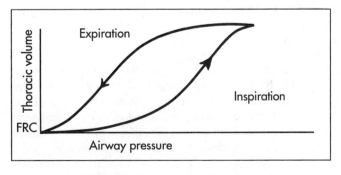

FIG. 25-2   Pressure-volume curve.

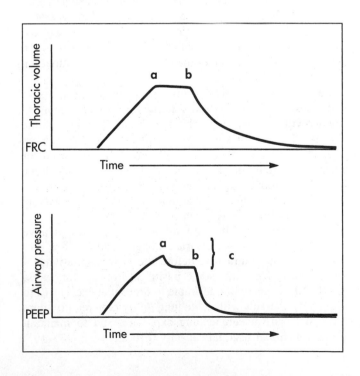

FIG. 25-3   Volume-regulated, time-cycled breath illustrating simultaneous occlusion of both inspiratory and expiratory ventilator ports (*time a*). This allows airway pressure to fall to a plateau value (*time b*) that approximates the alveolar pressure existent at (*a*). This decline (*c*) is an estimate of the pressure gradient across resistant airways during air flow.

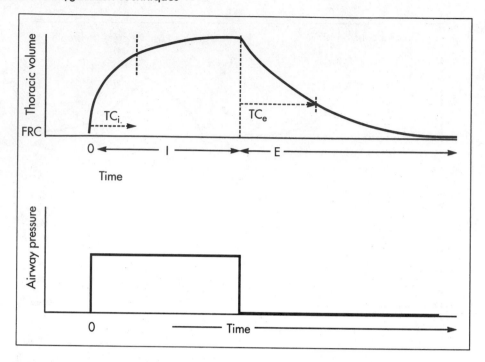

FIG. 25-4 During pressure ventilation the inspiratory time constant (TC_i) is the time required for lung volume to rise by about two thirds of the tidal volume. TC_e is the time required for exhalation of two thirds of the breath.

Initiation of Mechanical Ventilation. It can be difficult to select initial ventilator settings. When possible, select a respiratory rate that is roughly half the expected normal rate for age. For example, 20 breaths/min for infants, 15 breaths/min for young children, or 10 breaths/min for older children or adolescents usually provides total support for ventilation in children with *normal* lungs and normal carbon dioxide production when using conventional tidal volumes as described later. A more rapid rate is often necessary in the face of significant lung disease, when the patient is hypermetabolic (e.g., febrile), or when the therapeutic goal is hyperventilation. Likewise a lower rate often suffices when the patient's metabolism is slowed (e.g., hypothermia) or when ventilatory assistance, rather than total support of ventilation, is all that is necessary.

Gradually increase tidal volume or peak airway pressure until chest excursion appears normal to supernormal. In patients with normal lungs, this may require a tidal volume of 12 to 15 ml/kg, or a peak airway pressure of 20 to 25 cm H_2O. The presence of lung disease may produce a need for greater pressure to move adequate tidal volumes. If a volume of 12 ml/kg produces inordinately high airway pressures, it is generally appropriate to reduce tidal volume (or peak airway pressure) and increase respiratory rate accordingly.

Adjust inspiratory time to allow the chest to achieve plateau expansion before expiration begins and to allow it to achieve plateau contraction before the next inspiration occurs. In normal patients some positive end-expiratory pressure (PEEP) is generally desirable to prevent atelectasis (2 to 4 cm H_2O). Patients with acute lung injury may require more PEEP to ensure adequate lung expansion and to maintain normal functional residual capacity (FRC).

Categories of Conventional Positive-Pressure Ventilation. There are two primary forms of positive-pressure ventilation: pressure-regulated and volume-regulated ventilation. In pressure-regulated ventilation peak and end-expiratory airway pressures are "set." Lung volume rises and falls as determined by the principles outlined. In volume-regulated ventilation tidal volume, end-expiratory pressure and cycle times are "set," and inspiratory airway pressure follows passively.

In both of these forms of ventilation, timing within the respiratory cycle (duration of inspiration and expiration) is generally preset (time cycled). Recent modifications of these techniques include approaches that preclude time-cycled ventilation (e.g., pressure support ventilation).

Intermittent positive-pressure breathing (IPPB) is a technique whereby peak inspiratory pressure (or volume), inspiratory time, and expiratory time are preset without PEEP. Continuous positive-pressure breathing (CPPB) is similar to IPPB, but, because it entails the application of PEEP, positive airway pressure continues throughout the respiratory cycle. Ventilators can provide IPPB and CPPB in pressure-regulated or volume-regulated modes. Intermittent mandatory ventilation (IMV) is a volume-regulated technique designed to deliver a guaranteed (predetermined) number of preset breaths, while allowing spontaneous breathing that does not trigger further respiratory support. Pressure support ventilation (PSV) is a mode of pressure ventilation that precludes both time cycling and volume regulation, but that does support spontaneous breaths. Manufacturers have refined, combined, and intertwined these bare techniques to suit patient needs. The following discussion reviews each in its most distinct form.

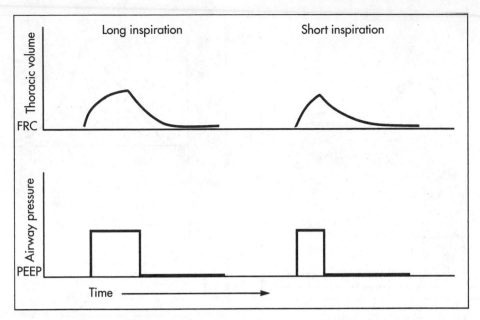

FIG. 25-5   Pressure-regulated ventilation. Lung volume rises until either the lung reaches its capacity (at that pressure) or proximal airway pressure time cycles to its expiratory value.

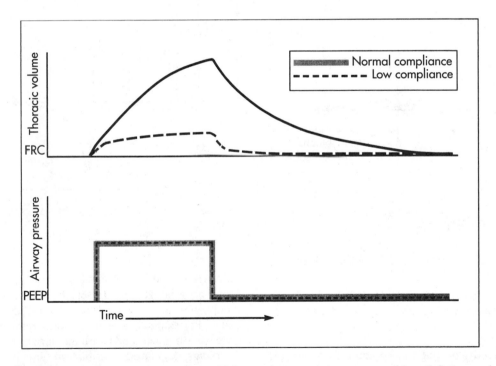

FIG. 25-6   Effect of lung compliance on lung volume and time course of lung inflation and deflation in pressure-regulated ventilation.

Pressure-Regulated Ventilation. The fundamental principle of pressure-regulated ventilation is that a ramp increase in airway pressure drives gas into the lungs. Lung volume rises logarithmically either until the lung reaches its capacity (at that pressure) or until proximal airway pressure time cycles to its expiratory value (Fig. 25-5). Passive expiration produces an exponential decline in lung volume determined by the time constant of the lung.

Lung compliance is an important determinant of end-inspiratory lung volume. It also plays a role in determining the time course of lung inflation and deflation during pressure ventilation (Fig. 25-6). In general the stiffer the lung, the less volume it accommodates at any given airway pressure, and the more rapidly it attains that volume (because of the shorter time constant).

Airway resistance is an important determinant of air flow

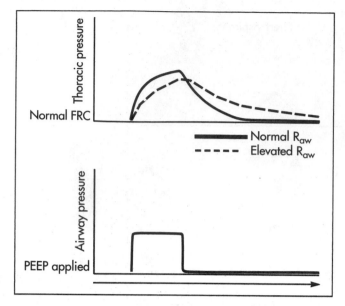

FIG. 25-7 Elevated airway resistance (R_{aw}) may limit tidal volume during pressure-regulated ventilation.

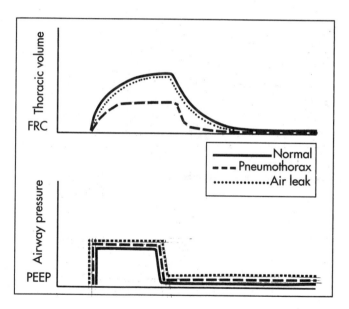

FIG. 25-8 Effect of pneumothorax on end-inspiratory lung volume in pressure-regulated ventilation.

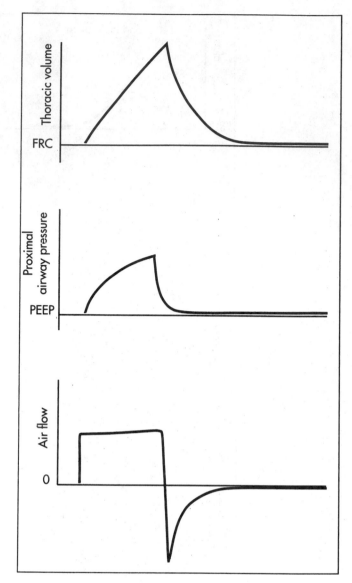

FIG. 25-9 Lung volume, airway pressure, and air flow during volume-regulated ventilation.

rate and consequently of pulmonary time constant (Fig. 25-7). Elevated airway resistance may so delay expiration that the lung fails to return (by the end of the respiratory cycle) to the volume that the applied PEEP would statically support. In that situation end-expiratory alveolar pressure exceeds the PEEP applied, a condition known as auto-PEEP.[4] High airway resistance may also prevent the lung from reaching its potential end-inspiratory volume by impeding inspiratory air flow. Together these factors may limit the size of the tidal volume during pressure ventilation (Fig. 25-7).

Pressure ventilation is advantageous in situations in which tracheal air leak allows some of the ventilator breath to be lost, because end-inspiratory lung volume is dependent on proximal peak airway pressure, not on the size of the breath delivered by the ventilator. During pressure ventilation, however, tidal volume is sensitive to changes in thoracic compliance and airway resistance (Fig. 25-8) for the reasons stated. For example, a pneumothorax reduces thorax compliance and diminishes tidal volume during pressure ventilation.

Volume-Regulated Ventilation. In its simplest form volume-regulated ventilation allows the physician to preset the tidal volume delivered by the ventilator. The physician also determines inspiratory and expiratory times. In general the inspiratory flow rate is fixed, lung volume rises linearly in inspiration, and airway pressure follows passively (Fig. 25-9). Determination of expiratory flow and lung volumes during volume-regulated ventilation is similar to that during pressure-regulated ventilation.

Lung compliance, therefore, determines the pressure required to support the lung at end-inspiratory volume, but not the size of the tidal breath. One may calculate compliance by dividing tidal volume by the pressure excursion from end-expiratory pressure to static end-inspiratory pressure (during

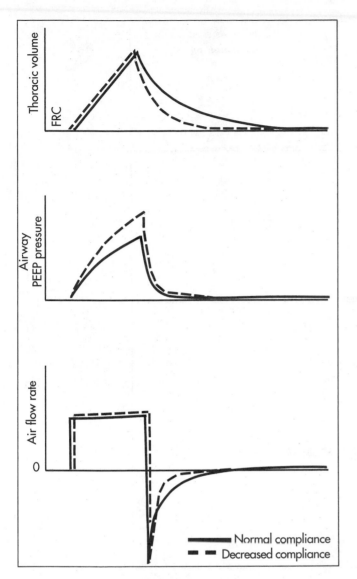

FIG. 25-10 Effect of areas of decreased lung compliance on airway pressure waveform during volume-regulated ventilation.

airway occlusion). Fig. 25-10 illustrates the effects of isolated differences in lung compliance on airway pressure waveforms.

Airway resistance is an important determinant of airway pressure during volume-regulated ventilation but, again, does not set tidal volume (Fig. 25-11). Nor does respiratory time constant determine tidal volume during volume ventilation. Airway resistance and time constant are important during expiration, just as they are in pressure-regulated ventilation. If air-trapping or auto-PEEP occurs, this "stacks" breaths, elevating both end-expiratory and end-inspiratory lung volumes, and consequently elevating peak inspiratory pressure (Fig. 25-12).

An important determinant of peak airway pressure during volume-regulated ventilation is inspiratory time, for inspiratory time and tidal volume determine the air flow rate. This in turn determines the pressure drop across resistance airways and influences proximal airway pressure (Fig. 25-13).

Volume-regulated ventilation is advantageous in the patient with rapidly changing lung compliance or airway

resistance, because tidal volume is largely guaranteed. On the other hand, consider alternative means of ventilation in the patient with unstable tracheal air leak, as the volume lost from the delivered breath diminishes the size of the patient's breath (Fig. 25-14).

During volume-regulated ventilation, the quantity of the patient's tidal volume is not synonymous with the volume delivered by the ventilator. Some volume is lost to expansion of tubing and humidifier. Calculate this lost volume as the pressure excursion (from PEEP to peak airway pressure) multiplied by circuit compliance (or compression volume). Calculate volumes lost to air leak (by subtraction) if accurate measures of inspiratory and expiratory tidal volume are available.

Intermittent Mandatory Ventilation. IMV is a mode of volume-regulated ventilation that allows the patient to inhale gas from the inspiratory limb of the ventilator circuit without triggering a controlled breath. The ventilator delivers a preset number of mandatory (regulated) breaths every minute (Fig. 25-15). During IMV mandatory breaths are volume regulated and obey the laws outlined for that form of mechanical ventilation. Spontaneous breaths are unassisted.

Developers of this mode of ventilation intended it as an aid to weaning from mechanical ventilation,[2] but it has become a common support mode for acute illness. During weaning it is possible to reduce the number of mandatory breaths smoothly without necessarily changing their characteristics. This promotes comfort during weaning.

Many patients do not, however, find IMV comfortable. The unanticipated arrival of a mandatory breath may surprise them. Or, because the mandatory breath differs in size or character from a spontaneous breath, the patient may resist the mandatory inspiration.

Pressure Support Ventilation. Pressure support ventilation (PSV) allows the physician to assist every breath by elevating proximal airway pressure above the preset PEEP for the duration of inspiration.[3] This augments transalveolar pressure, permitting the patient to inhale the quantity of breath he or she wants with less negative effort (negative pleural pressure). In effect PSV reduces work of breathing on a breath-by-breath basis (Fig. 25-16). Furthermore the patient is able to set the inspiratory time, expiratory time, respiratory frequency, and inspiratory flow rate during PSV. The physician merely selects and presets the amount of pressure support.

During PSV wean by gradually reducing the level of inspiratory pressure support.

Tailoring Ventilation to Patient Needs. In general monitor that which is not preset. It is therefore as important to measure tidal volume during pressure-regulated ventilation as it is to measure airway pressure during volume-regulated ventilation. This principle allows the physician to tailor the use of these devices to the real needs of the patient.

Supportive Care of the Mechanically Ventilated Patient. Agitation in mechanically ventilated patients may be a sign of hypoxemia, acidosis, reactive airway, discomfort, or anxiety. Although most children benefit from generous use of sedatives for prolonged mechanical ventilation, it is important to assess the cause of agitation before treating it reflexively with sedatives. Many patients also require the use of muscle relaxants to facilitate ventilation, especially those

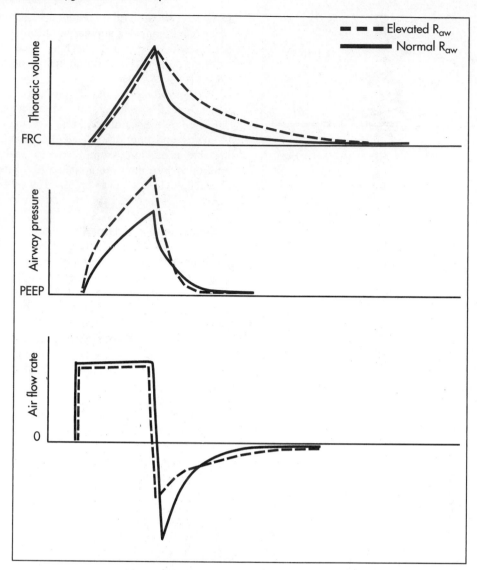

FIG. 25-11 Airway resistance affects airway pressure and the time course of exhalation in volume-regulated ventilation.

who have very severe lung disease. It is inappropriate to use muscle relaxants without sedation in conscious patients.

In addition good pulmonary toilet is necessary during mechanical ventilation with the frequency of suctioning determined by the character and volume of pulmonary secretions. Careful attention to the position of the endotracheal tube is also important, especially in infants, among whom a small movement of the tube may result in main stem bronchus intubation or extubation. General supportive care includes assurance of adequate oxygen-carrying capacity (hemoglobin), provision of nutrition as early in the course as feasible, and close observation for evidence of secondary infection. Chapter 28 discusses techniques for monitoring oxygenation and ventilation that may be appropriate for mechanical ventilation of children.

Weaning. It is appropriate to consider weaning from mechanical ventilation when the patient's condition is stable and when pulmonary disease begins to improve or the indication for assisted ventilation no longer exists. The process of weaning varies somewhat, depending on the mode of ventilation used. Generally it is appropriate to wean high levels of FIo_2 first to less toxic levels. If the patient has required elevated PEEP, it is also necessary to wean the PEEP to a more physiologic range (<5 cm H_2O) before discontinuing mechanical ventilation.

In volume-regulated ventilation modes most intensive care physicians wean by gradually reducing the number of ventilator-assisted breaths, allowing the patient progressively to assume a greater portion of the work of breathing. Providing a small amount of pressure support (e.g., 5 cm H_2O) may overcome the added work imposed by the resistance of breathing through a small-diameter endotracheal tube and thereby promote patient comfort as the mechanical ventilator rate declines.

In pressure-regulated modes it is necessary to reduce elevated peak inflation pressures as pulmonary compliance improves in order to prevent overdistention and volutrauma down to the range of 16 to 24 cm H_2O. Otherwise weaning in pressure-regulated modes is similar to weaning in volume-regulated modes.

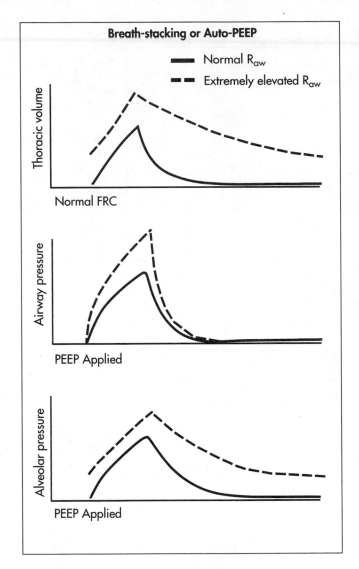

FIG. 25-12 Elevated airway resistance (R_{aw}) may cause "breath stacking" during volume-regulated ventilation.

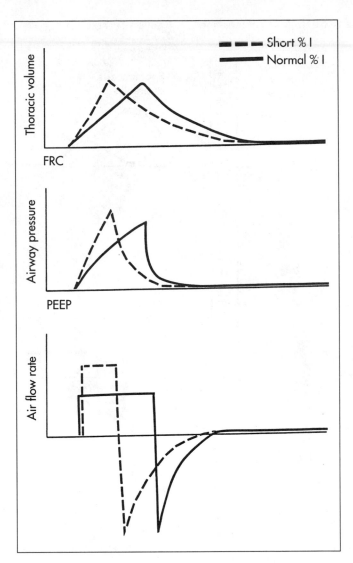

FIG. 25-13 Impact of inspiratory time on airway pressure in volume-regulated ventilation.

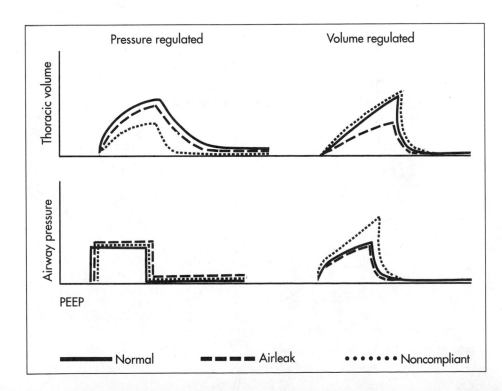

FIG. 25-14 Impact of tracheal air leak on thoracic volume and airway pressure in pressure-regulated and volume-regulated ventilation.

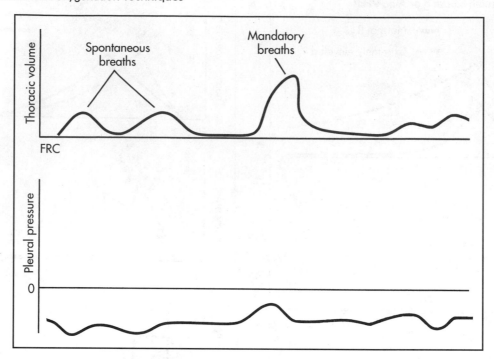

FIG. 25-15   Intermittent mandatory ventilation.

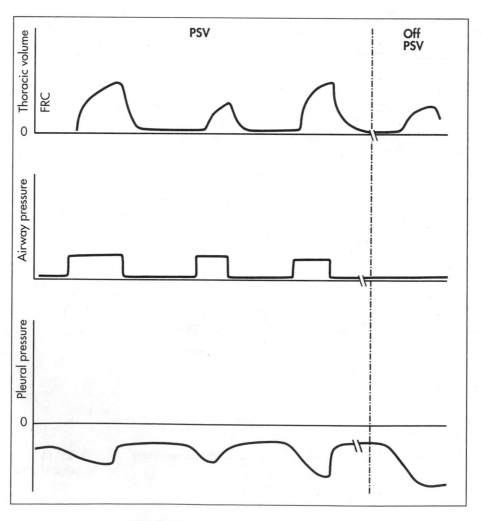

FIG. 25-16   Pressure support ventilation.

Patient comfort is a better indicator than arterial blood gases in assessing the adequacy of ventilation during weaning. Refer to Chapter 29 for a discussion of extubation criteria and technique.

Remarks

The best clues to guide changes in mechanical ventilation arise from observation and examination of the patient. Watch for symmetry and depth of chest rise, retractions and other evidence of distress, and breath stacking (incomplete exhalation before the next inspiration). Listen for wheezing, asymmetrically decreased breath sounds, and tracheal air leak.

Monitor what is not controllable. Periodically examine the ventilator to be sure it is doing what it is supposed to do. When there are technical questions, get help. A good hospital must always have technical support for its fleet of ventilators.

REFERENCES

1. Cassidy SS, Eschenbacher WL, Robertson CH Jr, et al: Cardiovascular effects of positive-pressure ventilation in normal subjects, *J Appl Physiol* 47:453-461, 1979.
2. Downs JB, et al: Intermittent mandatory ventilation: a new approach to weaning patients from mechanical ventilators, *Chest* 64:331, 1973.
3. MacIntyre NR: Respiratory function during pressure support ventilation, *Chest* 89:677, 1986.
4. Pepe PE, Marini JJ: Occult positive end-expiratory pressure in mechanical ventilated patients with airflow obstruction: the auto-PEEP effect, *Am Rev Respir Dis* 126(1):166-170, 1982.
5. Venkataraman ST, Orr RA: Mechanical ventilation and respiratory care. In Fuhrman BP, Zimmerman JJ, editors: *Pediatric critical care,* St. Louis, 1992, Mosby.

26 Alternative Ventilation

Mark J. Heulitt and Curtis B. Pickert

The primary goal of mechanical ventilatory support is to provide adequate gas exchange for a respiratory system that is incapable of independent gas exchange. Secondary goals of mechanical ventilation include supporting fatigued ventilatory muscles and retraining these muscles to facilitate weaning and extubation. Despite the clear success of conventional positive-pressure mechanical ventilatory support, in most children significant limitations remain. New modes of ventilation and adaptations of existing modes are sometimes lifesaving.

Alternative ventilatory techniques include the following categories: (1) ventilator modes and adjuncts to support patients with worsening acute respiratory failure (e.g., pressure control, high-frequency ventilation, constant flow ventilation, liquid ventilation, and nitric oxide); (2) ventilator modes to enhance weaning from mechanical ventilation (e.g., volume support); (3) ventilator modes used in lieu of endotracheal intubation (e.g., bi-level positive airway pressure [BiPAP]).

SUPPORT FOR WORSENING ACUTE RESPIRATORY FAILURE
Pressure Control Ventilation

In the ventilatory management of pediatric patients with adult respiratory distress syndrome (ARDS), the fundamental objectives are to provide adequate oxygenation and ventilation while limiting toxicity from barotrauma and increased inspired oxygen concentration.* Traditionally physicians have accomplished this by maintaining the inspired oxygen concentration (FIo_2) below 0.50 to 0.60, limiting peak inspiratory pressure (PIP) to <40 cm H_2O, and increasing the positive end-expiratory pressure (PEEP) to maintain a PaO_2 of greater than or equal to 60 mm Hg. Synchronized intermittent mandatory ventilation (SIMV) or volume-controlled ventilation has been the conventional means of providing this support via the mechanical ventilator. Recent reports cite the benefit of pressure-control ventilation (PCV), with or without inverse-ratio ventilation (IRV) in adults and children with ARDS.†

PCV uses a flow waveform characterized by a rapid upstroke with relatively high inspiratory flow rates, followed by a deceleration phase (Fig. 26-1). Compared to conventional SIMV or volume-controlled ventilation, the decelerating inspiratory flow waveform of PCV results in more uniform distribution of gas, therefore reducing overdistention of more compliant, healthy alveoli and improving ventilation to diseased alveoli. In theory, this would result in less ventilation-perfusion mismatch, less intrapulmonary shunt-

ing, and a decrease in dead space fraction. The pressure vs. time waveform is square, reflecting rapid attainment and maintenance of the PIP throughout the inspiratory phase of the cycle. The area under the pressure time curve (AUC) reflects the mean airway pressure (MAP), and the square waveform maximizes this value. This explains the observed phenomenon of a higher MAP in spite of a lower PIP and PEEP with PCV, as compared to the accelerating waveform of conventional volume ventilation. IRV further increases MAP by increasing the AUC and may allow aeration of diseased alveoli with prolonged time constants. Oxygenation and ventilation improve in spite of the use of lower inspired oxygen concentration and PIP.[37,59] However, plateau pressures are similar for similar tidal volumes.

Indications. There are no precise indications for the use of PCV in pediatric patients. Preliminary reports and experience suggest that it may provide an excellent alternative to conventional volume ventilation in patients with ARDS and other disease processes with diffuse alveolar edema, hypoxemia, and reduced lung compliance. In particular, patients requiring a PIP >35 cm H_2O or an FIo_2 >0.60 may benefit.

Contraindications. There are no absolute contraindications to the use of PCV. Because of differences in how this mode delivers gas, individualize its application and be familiar with potential adverse effects.

Complications. The elevation of MAP, which is intrinsic to the use of PCV with IRV, may adversely affect patients with unstable hemodynamics or low cardiac output. Generally, however, patients tolerate the mode well hemodynamically, and it has no concomitant adverse effects in patients with severe respiratory failure.[2,3]

Until recently, in younger patients requiring smaller tidal volumes, ventilators only administered PCV as an "assist-control" or "patient-triggered" mode. This created the potential for stacking of breaths and overdistention in the spontaneously breathing patient. As a result, patients receiving PCV or PCV-IRV have generally required sedation and neuromuscular blockade. The new generation of ventilators offers PCV with IMV and pressure-regulated volume control (PRVC); PRVC uses the same decelerating flow and square pressure waveforms while maintaining a preset tidal volume (Fig. 26-2). Before the development of PRVC, there was a risk of hypoventilation with PCV if the tidal volume decreased secondary to reduced compliance and staff did not recognize the change. For a given PIP, the tidal volume on PCV varies with changes in compliance, such as those caused by endotracheal tube obstruction, mucus plugging, reactive airway disease, or ARDS. Closely monitor expired tidal volume for such changes to prevent hypoventilation.

Currently only the Siemens Servo 300 ventilator supports PRVC. In this mode, the ventilator starts with four test breaths. For each of these breaths, the ventilator regulates the inspiratory pressure to a value based on the volume/pressure

---

*References 17, 27-29, 31, 33, 35, 36, 40, 42, 46, 47, 50, and 60.
†References 2, 3, 5, 6, 11, 26, 37, 44, 49, 52, and 59.

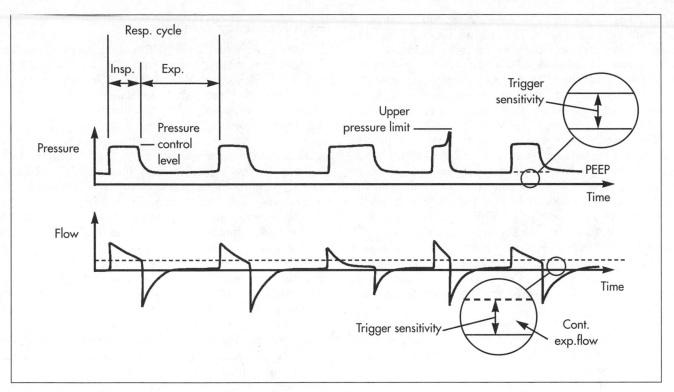

FIG. 26-1 Pressure and flow patterns of pressure-control ventilation. *Insp,* Inspiratory; *Exp,* expiratory.

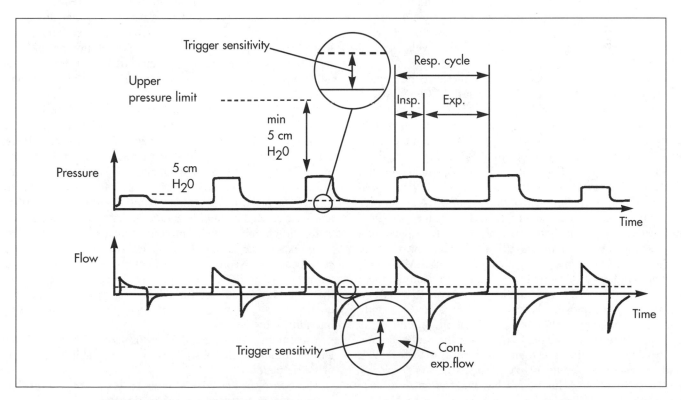

FIG. 26-2 Pressure and flow patterns of pressure-regulated volume control. *Resp,* Respiratory; *Insp,* inspiratory; *exp,* expiratory.

calculations for the previous breath compared to the preset target tidal/minute volume. The pressure for each breath can vary as much as 3 cm H_2O from the previous breath.

Equipment. Use any ventilator capable of administering PCV, PRVC, or volume control with decelerating flow. It is crucial that the medical, nursing, and respiratory staff familiarize themselves with the objectives for use of the mode and potential adverse effects.

Techniques. Before the transition to PCV, most patients will have initially undergone ventilation with a volume-regulated mode such as SIMV or volume control. Determine the preset PIP either by a desired tidal volume (adjust the PIP until the tidal volume is attained) or by establishing that the ventilator will not exceed a certain PIP, regardless of the tidal volume. PCV delivers the desired tidal volume at a lower PIP than SIMV. If IRV is used, the PIP required to deliver a certain tidal volume is even lower, since delivery occurs over a longer period of time. For a given PIP, changes in compliance result in changes in tidal volume. Monitor this closely.

Use a conventional inspiratory-to-expiratory time (I:E) ratio or an inverse ratio to increase the area under the pressure/time curve and maximize MAP for a given PIP. Typical ratios are 1:1, 2:1, or 3:1 (50%, 67%, or 75% inspiratory time, respectively).

In making the transition from SIMV to PCV with inversion of the I:E ratio, in some cases the patient does not have adequate time to expire gas received during inspiration. This results in increased end-expiratory pressure, known as "intrinsic" or "auto" PEEP.[30] Although formerly referred to as "inadvertent" PEEP, in this setting it is not unintentional and offers potential benefit to the patient by increasing alveolar recruitment or maintaining distention. The staff must monitor the patient's total PEEP (the sum of the "set" and the "auto" PEEP). Accomplish this by observing the pressure during an expiratory pause hold. If necessary, decrease the set PEEP somewhat to avoid potentially deleterious levels of total PEEP.

Alternatively, some clinicians prefer to reduce the inspiratory time as necessary to minimize "auto" PEEP and opt to raise MAP using "set" PEEP instead because the amount of "auto" PEEP is not necessarily static and may vary with changes in the underlying disease process. With either technique, it is important to monitor total PEEP.

Remarks. During PCV with reduced V_T (tidal volume) $Paco_2$ may increase.[53] The patient's $Paco_2$ should be allowed to rise with the pH maintained at or above 7.25. A buffer may be administered to the patient to maintain the pH. In a prospective study of pediatric patients with ARDS, we found a significant reduction in the PIP required to provide the designated tidal volume when changing from SIMV to PC with and without IRV (unpublished data). In addition, there was a consistent reduction in the dead space fraction and improved CO_2 removal. This resulted in a lower minute volume requirement, allowing a reduction in either the required PIP (and thus the tidal volume) or the ventilator rate. As in adults, just after the transition from SIMV to PCV, a mild, transient worsening of oxygenation occurs. Typically this lasts from 1 to 8 hours and has not warranted discontinuing PCV.

High-Frequency Ventilation

High-frequency ventilation (HFV) is a form of assisted mechanical ventilation using small tidal volumes and rapid respiratory rates to provide complete respiratory support. As in conventional mechanical ventilation, convective flow plays an important role in gas transport from the airway to the alveoli. However, other forms of gas transport assume a greater role in HFV. These mechanisms of gas transport include direct alveolar ventilation[21,22]; pendelluft[4] (i.e., varying rates of gas emptying from lung units); asymmetric velocity profiles[27] (i.e., gas molecules at the center of the airway move faster than those at the periphery to result in net convective transport); augmented dispersion[21] (i.e., gas dispersion and mixing increased by turbulence in the conducting airways); and molecular diffusion,[21,22] which represents the primary mechanism of gas mixing and exchange in terminal lung units. There are a number of different types of HFV. However, HFV in pediatric patients involves only high-frequency jet ventilation (HFJV) and high-frequency oscillatory ventilation (HFOV).

Indications. The indications for the use of either HFOV or HFJV in pediatric patients are similar. They include patients with barotrauma and respiratory failure that are unresponsive to conventional mechanical ventilation. Other uses include reduction in vascular pressure swings to control intracranial pressure in head trauma patients[32] and use in postoperative cardiac patients with ventricular dysfunction.[51]

Contraindications. Acute obstructive lung disease such as status asthmaticus is an absolute contraindication to the use of HFV. In status asthmaticus, generation of intrinsic PEEP occurs with associated pulmonary overdistention caused by decreased lung compliance and elevated airway resistance. HFV augments this overdistention because it requires much greater flow rates to achieve normocapnia. Larger flow rates cause higher driving pressures and outflow obstruction, with inadvertent trapping of gas in the lungs.[58] Both types of HFV have patient size restrictions because of limitations in available power. Limit HFOV to patients less than 35 to 40 kg and HFJV to patients less than 10 kg.

Complications. Similar complications occur with HFV as with other forms of positive-pressure ventilation. However, unlike with current modern conventional ventilators, there are more limitations to patient monitoring with HFV. For example, tidal volume is difficult to measure and airway pressure may not accurately reflect alveolar pressure. These limitations make the selection of initial settings and further adjustments largely empiric and based on clinical experience. Thus the clinician and respiratory care professionals must have experience in the use of HFV to reduce possible complications. Necrotizing tracheobronchitis has occurred with the use of HFV.[34] This problem appears to depend on the individual ventilator humidification system.[10] The frequency of this complication has decreased with improved humidification systems.

Equipment. At present, the Sensormedics 3100A (HFOV) and the Bunnell Life Pulse (HFJV) are available for HFV in pediatric patients.

The Sensormedics 3100A uses an oscillator design that incorporates a permanent magnet, a metal coil (attached to the piston), and a driver that controls the electric current to the coil. The driver alternates the polarity of the current. When the polarity is positive, it drives the piston forward (away from the magnet and toward the patient-inspiration). When polarity is negative, it drives the piston backward (toward the magnet and away from the patient-exhalation). The amount of power applied to the coil, the patient circuit pressure, and the piston centering pressure drive the piston a given distance in each direction.

The Bunnell Life Pulse High Frequency Jet Ventilator is a microprocessor-controlled high-frequency ventilator capable of delivering and monitoring between 240 and 660 humidified breaths per minute. The main components of the ventilator include a feedback control (used to control peak pressure and gas temperature), a patient box (contains the pressure transducer and the pinch valve), and a hi-lo jet tracheal tube. The Life Pulse also requires the addition of a conventional ventilator to provide fresh gas for the spontaneously breathing patient, to control PEEP, and to offer the low-rate intermittent mandatory ventilation breaths. Delivered tidal volumes are probably greater than the dead space.[23] The jet ventilator delivers the tidal volume via a small-bore catheter, which is part of the hi-lo jet tracheal tube. The opening and closing of a controlled valve delivers the flow of gas via this catheter. Because of the narrow orifice of the catheter, the ventilator produces a jet, entraining gas from around the catheter. Hence, the overall volume the subject receives exceeds the volume exiting from the catheter. Exhalation during HFJV is passive, produced by elastic recoil of the respiratory system.

Techniques. The technique used depends on the type of ventilator and the goal of the therapy.

SENSORMEDICS 3100A (HFOV). As with conventional ventilation, the goal of HFOV is to maintain oxygenation and ventilation. There are a total of seven controls for the Sensormedics 3100A: delta-P (power of oscillatory amplitude [PAW] measured proximal to the patient), MAP, FIo_2, frequency, inspiratory-expiratory (I:E) ratio (% I-time), bias flow, and piston centering. Adjust oxygenation with HFOV by changing FIo_2 and PAW (monitored by chest expansion seen on x-ray films). Adjust ventilation by changing the tidal volume (V_T) with changes in delta-P. Increases in power cause increases in V_T with an increase in delta-P. The range of settings for power is 0% to 100%. The relationship between delta-P and V_T is not linear in the high-power range of $\geq 60\%$. Thus for changes in V_T with power $> 60\%$, make changes in power, not in delta-P. Make adjustments in power in increments of 3% to 5%. The goal of HFOV is to minimize the V_T required to maintain ventilation in order to reduce barotrauma. In HFOV the endotracheal tube and the airways act as filters that decrease or attenuate the volume or pressure transmitted from the ventilator to the alveoli. The higher the frequency (Hz) and the smaller the endotracheal tube, the greater the effect of this filter and the attenuation of pressure (and volume) between the ventilator and the alveoli. An increase in rate increases attenuation and decreases alveolar V_T. Thus the higher the frequency, the lower the V_T with lower barotrauma.

Use HFOV with one of two strategies. In the high lung volume strategy, create alveolar recruitment using higher PAW. Use high PAW with increased amplitude (causing increased ventilation) and increased mean pressure (increased oxygenation). Initial settings include mean pressure settings at 1.5 to 3 cm H_2O above that on conventional ventilation, frequency 8 to 10 Hz in pediatric patients and 10 to 15 Hz in neonates, inspiratory time 33%, and power adjusted to maintain ventilation.

The other strategy for HFOV is the low PAW strategy for patients with preexisting air leak. In the low PAW strategy, use lower lung volumes. To use this method, the clinician must accept less optimal blood gas parameters. These values include Pao_2 45 to 60 mm Hg and $Paco_2$ 50 to 65 mm Hg. With lower PAW, lower frequency may be necessary (10 Hz). If it is necessary to increase PAW to maintain gas exchange, make these changes cautiously.

Optimal monitoring of the patient on HFOV includes arterial blood gases 1 hour after changes and every 4 to 8 hours thereafter; continuous transcutaneous CO_2 and pulse oximetry; and chest x-ray films after initial setup, daily, and anytime that the clinician suspects overinflation.

Weaning of HFOV usually begins with FIo_2 during the first 2 days, followed by weaning PAW. Increase the frequency to the maximum while weaning power. Convert to conventional mechanical ventilation settings ideally no greater than FIo_2 0.50 and PIP 35 cm H_2O.

LIFE PULSE (HFJV). Changing the operating characteristics such as MAP, frequency, and I:E ratio during HFJV affects a number of interrelated factors that can alter tidal volume and airway pressure and hence affect gas exchange. To initiate HFJV, reintubate the patient with a special hi-lo jet tracheal tube. The initial settings for HFJV depend on the indication for high-frequency ventilation. If $Paco_2$ is high, make maneuvers that increase minute ventilation first. These include increasing the PIP and the rate and decreasing the PEEP. If Pao_2 is low, increase conventional ventilator PEEP until the patient reaches the desired level of oxygenation. If hypoxemia persists and the chest x-ray film shows evidence of atelectasis, raise the conventional ventilator frequency to 10 breaths/min, or raise conventional ventilator PEEP further. If hypoxemia persists and the chest radiograph shows overdistention or air leak, reduce MAP by changing the conventional ventilator to continuous PAP and decrease HFV rate or PIP.

Accomplish weaning with the HFJV by reducing the HFJV PIP. Do this in increments of 1 to 2 cm H_2O. After reducing the PIP to 13 to 18 cm H_2O, increase conventional ventilator support, allowing the conventional breaths to interrupt the jet pulses. Consider a trial off HFJV when the HFJV PIP is less than 20 cm H_2O and the Fio_2 is less than 0.50.

Remarks. Some centers have used HFOV and HFJV in patients larger than those listed above, but there are no specific guidelines. High-frequency ventilation in pediatric patients is experimental. It is mandatory to limit its use to centers with experienced personnel. Survival rates are as high as 86% in ARDS with the use of HFOV in pediatric patients.[8]

Constant-Flow Ventilation

Constant flow ventilation (CFV) is a technique whereby the ventilator delivers a constant flow of fresh gas introduced into the mainstem bronchi[9,12] through a special catheter (Fig. 26-3) inserted through the endotracheal tube. The endotracheal tube is only for expiration. Gas transport appears to occur through turbulent mixing of gases in the airway and consequent augmented diffusion into the alveoli. In this way gas exchange occurs with lower pressure and volume due to a decrease in respiratory dead space.

Indications. The use and indications for CFV in pediatric patients are uncertain. In two studies in adults, CFV did not maintain normal levels of $Paco_2$, but did provide one third to one half the normal alveolar ventilation.[13,50] However, a new technique addresses this limitation with the delivery of fresh gas through a reverse thrust catheter and the combination of CFV and pressure control ventilation.[7]

Contraindications. This method of ventilatory support is experimental. Limit its use to controlled experimental protocols.

Complications. Since this method of ventilatory support requires a high flow of fresh gas, the entire system is under pressure and has the potential for rupture with air leak and loss of pressure. The loss of gas flow could result in loss of gas exchange with subsequent hypoxemia and hypercarbia.

Equipment. The combined use of CFV and pressure control ventilation has the greatest potential in pediatric patients. Equipment necessary includes a gas delivery system, a CFV catheter, and a ventilator (Fig. 26-4). With the reverse catheter, the gas exits from an annular narrow orifice in the direction away from the carina. The annular stream of gas follows the catheter outward (away from the carina), with a resulting low pressure zone that entrains air from the level of the carina. This, with the addition of pressure control ventilation, allows for the maintenance of adequate ventilation. This method results in the delivery of a continuous flow of fresh gas through the catheter to the carina. The expiratory valve of a conventional ventilator controls the respiratory rate and the I:E ratio. With the expiratory valve of the ventilator closed, all gas from the catheter flows into the lungs. The lungs exhale when the expiratory valve is open.

Techniques. Introduce a special catheter through the endotracheal tube, with the tip of the endotracheal tube placed at the level of the carina. Place the patient on a conventional mechanical ventilator in the pressure control mode. Begin gas flow through the CFV catheter. Increase the flow of gas through the catheter while decreasing the peak inspiratory pressure on the ventilator. Regulate gas exchange by adjusting the pressure control setting and CFV gas flow.

Remarks. The ability to maintain gas exchange with low peak inspiratory pressure is appealing. However, this method of ventilatory support has limited clinical application outside of research protocols at present.

Liquid Ventilation

Investigators have recently used liquid ventilation in animals with and without lung disease to improve lung function.[39,56,62] Perfluorocarbons instilled into the lungs alter surface tension, recruit and maintain functional residual capacity, and improve ventilation-perfusion matching. Perfluorocarbons have a high solubility for oxygen and CO_2 and a low surface tension. They eliminate the interfacial surface tension, improve distribution of pulmonary blood flow, and support physiologic gas exchange.

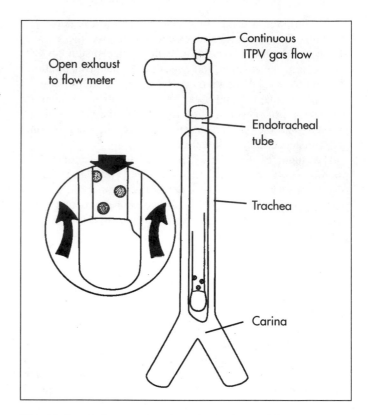

FIG. 26-3 Catheter and endotracheal tube and flow redirector used in CFV. *ITPV*, Intratracheal pulmonary ventilation.

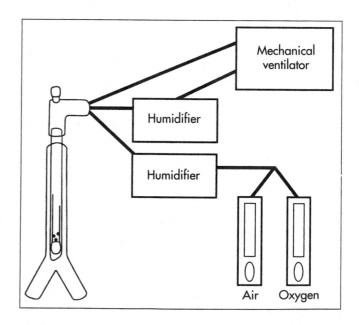

FIG. 26-4 Ventilator and catheter setup used in constant-flow ventilation.

Indications. The use of liquid ventilation at this time is experimental. Patients with surfactant-deficient lung disease and ARDS could potentially benefit from the improved oxygenation and compliance offered in this type of support.

Contraindications. Limit this method of ventilation to controlled experimental protocols by physicians experienced in its use.

Equipment. The equipment necessary for this type of ventilation is the perfluorocarbons and a mode of delivery. Currently the only available perfluorocarbon high in purity and medical grade is LiquiVent (Perflubron, perfluoro-octylbromide, Alliance Pharmaceutical Corp, San Diego, CA). Modes of delivery include by gravity[25] or in tandem with a conventional mechanical ventilator (perfluorocarbon–associated gas exchange [PAGE]).[24]

Techniques. There are two methods for the instillation of perfluorocarbons: tidal liquid breathing and PAGE. In tidal liquid breathing, the perfluorocarbon flows into the patient's lungs by gravity for a set cycle. In one study this method was used in human preterm neonates with V_T of 15 ml/kg of perfluorochemical delivered over 5 seconds.[25] Each V_T remained within the infant's lungs for 10 seconds and then drained by gravity, repeated at a rate of two or three liquid breaths per minute.

PAGE requires the instillation of perfluorocarbons in the lung at 30 ml/kg.[24,38] Gas ventilation with the conventional ventilator occurs after instillation of this volume. In PAGE the perfluorocarbons oxygenate in inspiration by pushing oxygen down the airway into the liquid-filled alveoli, where it forms bubbles. During exhalation CO_2 purges from the perfluorocarbons by the intrinsic elastic recoil of the bubbles, expelling gas from the lungs. Gas escapes before the liquid during exhalation as a result of its lower viscosity, density, and inertia.

Nitric Oxide

Patients with ARDS exhibit arterial hypoxemia caused by intrapulmonary shunting[8,15] with ventilation-perfusion mismatching. Acute pulmonary arterial hypertension causes vasoconstriction, and widespread occlusion of the pulmonary microvasculature causes intrapulmonary shunting.[55,61] The increased pulmonary arterial pressure is independent of changes in cardiac output and persists after the correction of systemic hypoxemia.[17,57] Pulmonary arterial hypertension can cause right ventricular dysfunction[57,63] with resultant pulmonary edema.[18,19,64] Infusing a vasodilator, with resultant reduction in pulmonary vascular resistance, reduces pulmonary edema. However, current vasodilators are not specific to the pulmonary vasculature and may cause concomitant systemic arterial hypotension, right ventricular ischemia, and heart failure.[55] Their diffuse effect on the pulmonary vasculature increases blood flow to areas with intrapulmonary shunting, causing ventilation-perfusion mismatching.[54] In contrast, in adult patients with ARDS, inhaled nitric oxide (NO), a potent vasodilator, decreases intrapulmonary shunting and improves arterial oxygenation while reducing the pulmonary artery pressure.[22,54,64] Improved arterial oxygenation is the result of a redistribution of pulmonary blood flow away from nonventilated regions of the lungs and toward ventilated regions, thus reducing ventilation-perfusion mismatching.

Indications. The use of inhaled NO is experimental. However, there is potential for its use in pediatric patients with ARDS or congenital heart disease with pulmonary hypertension. Currently it is appropriate to limit its use in pediatric patients with ARDS to patients who have failed maximal medical management, defined as persistent hypoxemia on toxic levels of support (Pao_2 <55 mm Hg with an FIo_2 $\geq$ 0.60 and PIP >40 cm H_2O).

Contraindications. There are no absolute contraindications to the use of NO. Limit NO use to controlled experimental protocols, monitoring both effect and toxicity.

Complications. NO is oxidized in the presence of oxygen to nitrogen dioxide (NO_2) The gas phase reaction of NO and O_2 is a slow reaction

$$K [NO]^2 [O_2] = 1 * 10^4 \text{ M}^{-2} \text{ s}^{-1}$$

The rate constant in aqueous solution is much faster

$$K = 1 * 10^6 \text{ M}^{-2} \text{ s}^{-1}$$

The rate of oxidation depends on the initial concentration of NO and the FIo_2. Concerns exist over the use of inhalational NO because exposure to NO_2 results in histologic evidence of lung injury; in one study exposure to 2 ppm NO_2 for 24 to 72 hours resulted in pulmonary changes consisting of loss of cilia, hypertrophy, and focal epithelial hyperplasia of the terminal bronchioles in rats.[30] Whether the degree of lung injury noted in animal studies is clinically relevant to humans is uncertain. Virtually all the NO that enters the patient's lungs is oxidized in the pulmonary and vascular tissue or in the blood.[16,29,43] In the blood NO reacts with oxyhemoglobin to form inorganic nitrate and methemoglobin. Inorganic nitrite is itself unstable in blood and reacts with hemoglobin to form methemoglobin and NO, which again form nitrate and methemoglobin. Monitor levels of methemoglobin while delivering NO.

Equipment. Inhalation circuits designed to deliver NO must ensure the accurate delivery of NO while maintaining low levels of NO_2. Conversion of NO to NO_2 is offset by minimizing the residence time of NO in the inhaled gas mixture. Accomplish this by delivering NO directly to the inspiratory circuit. The type of ventilator determines the delivery setup (Fig. 26-5). An important part of the system is the monitoring device. Two types of commercial systems are available for measuring NO and NO_2: the electrochemical cell and the chemical-luminescence system. In the electrochemical cell a chemical reaction that produces an electrical signal proportional to the gas concentration determines measurements. In the chemiluminescence system NO reacts with ozone (O_3) to produce an excited NO_2 form with subsequent light emission. Measurements of the emission intensity using a photomultiplier tube determine the concentration of sampled gases. Both systems have limitations. Humidity, pressure, the presence of other gases (e.g., oxygen, hydrogen, and carbon monoxide), gas flow, leaks and metal surfaces all influence the accuracy of measurements.

Techniques. All protocols for the use of NO in patients with ARDS are experimental. Protocols for the administration of NO usually begin at 20 ppm. Increase the rate of NO administration at 5- to 15-minute intervals to a maximum of 40 to 60 ppm. Define a positive response to NO as an increase in arterial oxygenation with the ability to wean ventilatory parameters to nontoxic levels (FIo_2 <0.60 and PIP <40 cm H_2O). Maintain the patient on the level of NO that results in a positive response for at least 12 hours before attempting to wean. After 12 hours decrease the NO by 2 ppm every 15 to 30 minutes until either a decrease in systemic oxygenation occurs or the patient's inhaled level of NO decreases to 2 to 6 ppm. Discontinue NO at this level. During the administration of NO, monitor methemoglobin

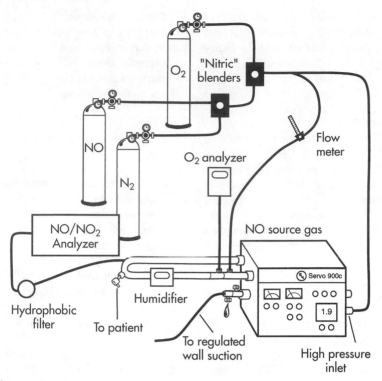

FIG. 26-5 Ventilator and monitor setup used in the delivery of NO.

every 6 hours when making changes in concentration and every 12 hours if NO level is stable.

Remarks. A recent study demonstrated an improvement in oxygenation in 14 of 16 pediatric patients with hypoxic respiratory failure.[1] In this study inhaled NO (20 ppm) improved Pao_2 from 61 ± 3 to 88 ± 6 mm Hg (p <0.0001), oxygenation index decreased from 35 ± 3 to 24 ± 2 (p <0.001), and intrapulmonary shunt fell from 42 ± 2% to 31 ± 2% (p <0.003). Although encouraging, this study is preliminary, and further work must define optimal dosing and potential toxicity.

Current monitoring systems were designed for industrial use. Development of medical systems to improve precision of dosing and prevention of toxicity is under way. In patients with ARDS, it may be appropriate to monitor delivered levels of NO as parts per billion rather than parts per million.

MODES TO ENCHANCE WEANING FROM MECHANICAL VENTILATION
Volume Support

Intubated patients with respiratory failure experience increased ventilatory work with spontaneous breathing because of increased airway resistance, decreased lung-thorax compliance, and asynchrony of the patient and the ventilator. The increased resistance and decreased compliance in ventilated patients causes ventilatory muscle dysfunction.[45] In volume support ventilation (VSV) as in pressure support ventilation (PSV), the work load on the ventilatory muscles during a VSV breath is more physiologic than an intermittent mandatory ventilation (IMV) breath because of the regular, more normal pressure-volume loads of VSV.[14,30,41] VSV is presently available only on the Siemens Servo 300 ventilator. Set the amount of support in VSV by selecting the desired

amount of tidal volume (V_T) for each spontaneous breath. When the patient triggers the ventilator, it maintains the preset volume as long as minimal inspiratory flow is occurring or until a preset breath cycle time limits it. This control over flow and volume by the patient causes improved patient comfort and patient-ventilator synchrony.[42] The advantage of this mode of ventilation over PSV is that VSV guarantees V_T with each breath.

Indications. Indications for the use of VSV are similar to those for PSV (see Chapter 25). Use low-level VSV (i.e., 3 to 6 cc/kg V_T) in a spontaneously breathing, ventilated pediatric patient to eliminate the pressure and work required for spontaneous air flow through an endotracheal tube. Use high-level VSV as an independent ventilatory support mode by applying the level of inspiratory tidal volume needed for adequate minute ventilation. To use VSV as a weaning tool in pediatric patients with poor pulmonary reserve, begin by setting the VSV level near VSV_{max}. Obtain VSV_{max} by setting the VSV level to produce tidal breaths equivalent to 10 to 12 cc/kg. Then decrease V_T in increments to maintain the patient's baseline respiratory rate and level of comfort.

Contraindications. There are no absolute contraindications to the use of VSV. Use it only in spontaneously breathing patients.

Complications. VSV is a new mode of ventilation. Complications are similar to those for PSV. Since VSV on the Siemens 300 ventilator is computer-regulated, it guarantees support volumes and increases inspiratory pressure with worsening compliance.

Equipment. VSV is presently only available on the Siemens Servo 300 ventilator.

Techniques. Use varying levels of VSV, depending on individual patient requirements. In-low level VSV (i.e., tidal volume 3 to 6 cc/kg), set the support level to offer enough

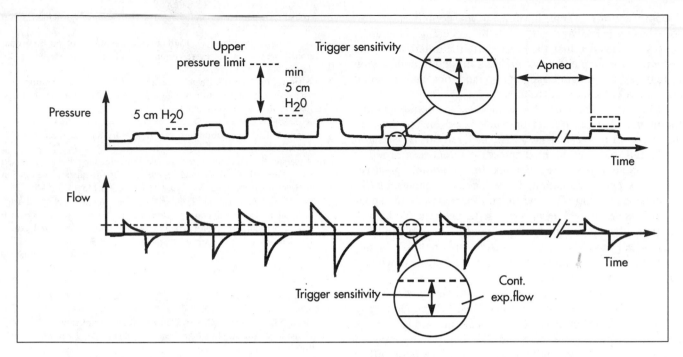

FIG. 26-6   Pressure and flow patterns of volume support ventilation. Exp, Expiratory.

support to overcome the patient's work associated with the resistance of an endotracheal tube; the support level varies according to the size of the endotracheal tube.[20] In high-level VSV, set the support level to serve as an independent ventilatory support mode. In this mode of ventilation, muscle loading may be more physiologic, with improved patient comfort and conditioning.[14]

After the desired level of volume support, expected spontaneous respiratory rate, and minute volume have been set, the ventilator delivers four test breaths at 5 cm H_2O (Fig. 26-6). For each of the following breaths, the ventilator regulates the inspiratory pressure to a value based on the pressure/volume calculation for the previous breath, compared to the preset tidal and minute volume. The pressure can change ±3 cm H_2O from one breath to the next. The ventilator terminates each inspiration when inspiratory flow has decreased to 5% of peak flow or after 80% of the set cycle time.

Remarks. VSV may offer a spontaneous breathing mode for a variety of patients. Since the patient can control both inspiration and expiration, patients with reactive airway disease may benefit from this mode. This mode may give patients with poor compliance the level of support necessary to support their gas exchange while still giving them full control over their respiratory cycle.

The new generation of ventilators such as the Siemens Servo 300 ventilator with flow triggering and a faster response time was found in animal experiments to reduce the work of breathing.[15,30] Further, the authors recently compared VSV to PSV in young lambs with and without an externally placed resistor.[30a] Work of breathing was similar without the external resistor for pressure support versus volume support. In contrast, with an external resistor to increase the work of breathing for the animal and to simulate the increased resistance pediatric patients face with certain disease processes and smaller endotracheal tubes, the work of breathing was considerably less for VSV as compared to PSV. This study illustrates some of the possible benefits of VSV in pediatric patients.

VENTILATOR MODES IN LIEU OF ENDOTRACHEAL INTUBATION
BiPAP

BiPAP is a pressure or time-cycled device to deliver preadjusted levels of inspiratory and expiratory pressure via a nasal mask or via a tracheostomy. BiPAP operates by delivering enough positive pressure to the airway so that it exceeds the resistance and elasticity of the respiratory system to inflate the lungs. The result of this delivery of positive pressure is to increase tidal volume and functional residual capacity (FRC).

Indications. Use BiPAP in patients who can breathe spontaneously, but who cannot meet their total respiratory requirements. Limit its use in the hospital to nonintubated patients or patients with a tracheostomy. Patients who could benefit from this type of support include patients with chronic airway obstruction, chronic lung disease, and respiratory hypoventilation caused by neuromuscular disease or congenital anomalies.

Contraindications. Do not use BiPAP in patients who require more than minimal ventilatory support, who have an air leak or cardiovascular instability, or who require FIO_2 of greater than 0.40. The manufacturer also lists apnea as a contraindication for use of BiPAP, although some clinicians have found it to be a suitable device (in the spontaneous/timed mode or timed mode) for temporary support of the neonate with an acute exacerbation of infantile apnea, such as that associated with otherwise mild respiratory syncytial virus infection.

Complications. There have been no complications reported using BiPAP as described in the preceding paragraphs. However, consider that there are certain limitations of the system. For example, the system has a limited humidification system and no integrated alarms or monitors, and it cannot maintain a constant tidal volume.

Equipment. The BiPAP system uses a continuous-flow circuit that delivers bilevel pressure based on the pressure support level and a baseline PEEP. Deliver BiPAP via nasal mask, full face mask, mouthpiece, or tracheostomy. The BiPAP system has three options for providing positive-pressure support ventilation. These include spontaneous (S), spontaneous/timed (S/T), and timed (T) modes. In the spontaneous mode all cycling in response to the patient's breathing pattern is between the baseline PEEP level and the clinician-selected inspiratory pressure support level. In this mode the unit only cycles to the inspiratory pressure when it senses the patient's breathing effort.

The second mode is the spontaneous/timed mode. In this mode, as in the spontaneous mode, BiPAP supports any breathing efforts initiated by the patient, along with a minimum breathing rate set by the clinician. While supported in this mode, if the patient fails to make an inspiratory effort within the interval set with the breathing rate, the unit delivers a breath based on the set pressure support level.

The third option is the timed mode, in which the ventilator delivers breaths such as those in the spontaneous mode, but control settings rather than patient effort determine cycling to both the inspiratory and expiratory pressure. In this mode the clinician sets the pressure support and PEEP levels, the number of breaths per minute, and the inspiratory time.

Techniques. Deliver BiPAP by placing an appropriately sized mask on the patient over the nasal bridge without gas flow or by attaching to the tracheostomy tube. Gradually increase the flow of oxygen and air through the nasal mask or tube. Begin with expiratory airway pressure at 2 cm H_2O, and initiate inspiratory flow with an inspiratory phase airway support pressure of 4 cm H_2O. Increase inspiratory flow in increments corresponding to 2 cm H_2O. Increase flow and delivered pressure while monitoring the patient closely for level of comfort and gas exchange. Adjust inspiratory flow to maximize patient comfort and gas exchange. When using the timed backup mode, set the backup rate at 2 breaths/min less than the estimated baseline respiratory rate, with a 30% inspiratory flow time.

Remarks. Experience with the use of BiPAP in pediatric patients has been limited. Recently a retrospective report of its use in pediatric patients with respiratory insufficiency demonstrated some efficacy.[48] Fifteen patients managed outside of the PICU escaped mechanical ventilation and major complications.

BiPAP offers a less invasive method of ventilatory support for patients with airway obstruction, chronic lung disease, and respiratory hypoventilation caused by neuromuscular disease or congenital anomalies.

REFERENCES

1. Abman S, Griebel JL, Parker DK, et al: Acute effects of inhaled nitric oxide in severe hypoxemic respiratory failure in pediatrics, *J Pediatr* 124:881-887, 1994.
2. Abraham E, Yoshihara G: Cardiorespiratory effects of pressure controlled inverse ratio ventilation in severe respiratory failure, *Chest* 96:1356-1359, 1989.
3. Abraham E, Yoshihara G: Cardiorespiratory effects of pressure controlled ventilation in severe respiratory failure, *Chest* 98:1445-1449, 1990.
4. Allen JL, Fredberg JF, Keefe JH, et al: Alveolar pressure magnitude and asynchrony during high-frequency oscillation of excised rabbit lungs, *Am Rev Respir* 132:343-349, 1985.
5. Al-Saady N, Bennett ED: Decelerating inspiratory flow waveform improves lung ventilation in severe respiratory failure, *Chest* 98:1445-1449, 1990.
6. Anderson JB: Ventilatory strategy in catastrophic lung disease: inversed ratio ventilation (IRV) and combined high-frequency ventilation (CHFV), *Acta Anaesthesiol Scand* 33 (suppl 90):145-148, 1989.
7. Aprigliano M, Kolobow T, Rossi N, et al: Intratracheal pulmonary ventilation and continuous positive-pressure ventilation in a sheep model of acute respiratory failure: a controlled randomized study, Extracorporeal life support organization Abstract Book, 1993, p. 12.
8. Arnold JH, Truog RD, Thompson JE, et al: High-frequency oscillatory ventilation in pediatric respiratory failure, *Crit Care Med* 21:272-278, 1993.
9. Asbaugh DG, Bigelow DB, Petty TL, et al: Acute respiratory distress in adults, *Lancet* 2:319-323, 1967.
10. Boros SJ, Mammel MC, Lewallen PK, et al: Necrotizing tracheobronchitis: a complication of high-frequency ventilation, *J Pediatr* 109:95-100, 1986.
11. Boysen PG, McGough E. Pressure-control and pressure-support ventilation: flow patterns, inspiratory time, and gas distribution, *Respir Care* 33(2):126-134, 1988.
12. Branson RD, Hurst JM, Davis K, editors: Alternate modes of ventilatory support. In *Problems in respiratory care*, vol 2, Philadelphia, 1989, Lippincott.
13. Breen PH, Sznajder JI, Morrison P: Constant flow ventilation in anesthetized patients: efficacy and safety, *Anesth Analg* 65:1161-1169, 1986.
14. Brochard L, Harf A, Lorino, et al: Inspiratory pressure support prevents diaphragmatic fatigue during weaning from mechanical ventilation, *Am Rev Resp Dis* 139:513-521, 1988.
15. Carmack J, Torres A, Anders M, et al: Comparison of inspiratory work of breathing in young lambs during flow-triggered and pressure-triggered ventilation, *Respir Care* 40:28-34, 1995.
16. Chiodi H, Mohler JG: Effects of exposure of blood hemoglobin to nitric oxide, *Environ Res* 37:355-363, 1985.
17. Davis SL, Furman DP, Costarino AT: Adult respiratory distress syndrome in children: associated disease, clinical course, and predictors of death, *J Pediatr* 123:35-45, 1993.
18. Debruin W, Notterman DA, Magid M, et al: Acute hypoxemia respiratory failure in infants and children: clinical and pathologic characteristics, *Crit Care Med* 20:1223-1234, 1992.
19. Erdmann AJ III, Vaughn TR Jr, Brigham KL, et al: Effects of increased vascular pressure on lung fluid balance in unaesthetized sheep, *Circ Res* 37:271-284, 1975.
20. Fiastro JF, Habib MP, Quan SF: Pressure support compensation for inspiratory work due to endotracheal tubes and demand CPAP, *Chest* 93:499-505, 1988.
21. Fredberg JJ: Augmented diffusion in the airways can support pulmonary gas exchange, *J Appl Physiol* 49:232-238, 1980.
22. Froese AB, Bryan AC: High-frequency ventilation, *Am Rev Respir Dis* 135:1363-1374, 1989.
23. Frouby JJ, Simonneau G, Benhamou D: Factors influencing pulmonary volumes and CO2 elimination during high-frequency jet ventilation, *Anesthesiology* 63:473-482, 1985.
24. Furham BP, Pacazan PR, DeFrancisis M: Perfluorocarbon associated gas exchange, *Crit Care Med* 19:712-723, 1991.
25. Greenspan JS, Wolfson MR, Rubenstein SD, et al: Liquid ventilation of human preterm neonates, *J Pediatr* 117:106-111, 1990.
26. Gurevitch MJ, VanDykes J, Young ES, et al: Improved oxygenation and lower peak airway pressure in adult respiratory distress syndrome, *Chest* 89:211-213, 1986.
27. Haselton FR, Scherer PW: Bronchial bifurcations and respiratory mass transport, *Science* 208:69-71, 1980.

28. Heulitt M, Anders M, Benham D: Acute respiratory distress syndrome in pediatric patients: redirecting therapy to reduce iatrogenic lung injury, *Respir Care* 40(1):74-85, 1995.

29. Heulitt MJ, Moss MM, Walker WM, et al: Morbidity and mortality in pediatric patients with respiratory failure, *Crit Care Med* 21:S156, 1993.

30. Heulitt MJ, Torres A, Anders M, et al: Comparison of work of breathing in ventilated spontaneous breathing lambs with and without bias flow, *Chest* 106(abstr):69S, 1994.

30a. Heulitt MJ, Torres A, Andres M, et al: Comparison of work breathing between volume support and pressure support in a young lamb with and without increased resistance, *Crit Care Med* 23:A226, 1995.

31. Hickling KG: Ventilatory management of ARDS: can it affect outcome? *Intensive Care Med* 16:219-226, 1990.

32. Hurst JM, Saul TG, Dehaven CB, et al: Use of high-frequency jet ventilation during mechanical hyperventilation to reduce intracranial pressure in patients with multiple organ system injury, *Neurosurgery* 15:530-534, 1984.

33. Kacmarek RM, Hess D: Pressure controlled inverse ration ventilation: panacea or auto-PEEP? *Respir Care* 35(10):945-948, 1990.

34. Kirpalani H, Higa T, Perlman M, et al: Diagnosis and therapy of necrotizing tracheobronchitis in ventilated neonates, *Crit Care Med* 13:772-779, 1985.

35. Kolobow T, Moretti M, Fumagalli R, et al: Adult respiratory distress syndrome following mechanical pulmonary ventilation at high peak inspiratory pressures (abstracted), *Am Rev Respir Dis* 131(suppl):A137, 1985.

36. Kolobow T, Moretti MP, Fumagalli R, et al: Severe impairment in lung function induced by high peak airway pressure during mechanical ventilation, *Am Rev Respir Dis* 135:312-315, 1987.

37. Lain DC, Di Benedetto R, Morris SL, et al: Pressure control inverse ratio ventilation as a method to reduce peak inspiratory pressure and provide adequate ventilation and oxygenation, *Chest* 95:1081-1088, 1989.

38. Leach CL, Fuhrmann BP, Morin FC, et al: Perfluorocarbon-gas exchange (partial liquid ventilation) in respiratory distress syndrome: a prospective, randomized, controlled study, *Crit Care Med* 21:1270-1278, 1993.

39. Lowe CA, Schaffer TH: Pulmonary vascular resistance in fluorocarbon-filled lung, *J Appl Physiol* 60:154-159, 1986.

40. Lyrene RK, Truog WE: Adult respiratory distress syndrome in a pediatric intensive care unit: predisposing conditions, clinical course, and outcome, *Pediatrics* 67:790-795, 1981.

41. MacIntyre NR: Respiratory function during pressure support ventilation, *Chest* 89:677-683, 1986.

42. MacIntyre NR, Leatherman NE: Ventilatory muscle loads and the frequency tidal volume pattern during inspiratory pressure assisted (pressure supported) ventilation, *Am Rev Respir Dis* 141(2):327-331, 1990.

43. Maeda N, Imaizumi K, Kon K et al: Effect of nitric oxide exposure on the red cell rheology: in relation to oxidative cross linking of membrane proteins, *J Jpn Soc Air Pollut* 19:283-291, 1984.

44. Marcy TW, Marini JJ: Inverse-ratio ventilation in ARDS: rationale and implementation, *Crit Care* (progress notes) 19:9-18, 1991.

45. Marini JJ: The physiologic determinants of ventilator dependence, *Respir Care* 31:271, 1986.

46. Montgomery AB, Stager MA, et al: Causes of mortality in patients with adult respiratory distress syndrome, *Am Rev Respir Dis* 132:485-489, 1985.

47. Nash G, Blennerhassett JB, Pontoppidan H: Pulmonary lesions associated with oxygen therapy and artificial ventilation, *New Engl J Med* 276(7):368-374, 1967.

48. Padman R, Lawless S, Von Nessen S: Use of BiPAP by nasal mask in the treatment of respiratory insufficiency in pediatric patients: preliminary investigation, *Pediatr Pulmonol* 17:119-123, 1994.

49. Paulson TE, Spear RM, Peterson BM: Improved survival using high-frequency pressure control ventilation with high PEEP in children with ARDS (abstract), Presented at the Pediatric Critical Care Colloquim, Philadelphia, March 27-31, 1993.

50. Perl A, Whitwarm JG, Chakrabati MF, et al: Continuous flow ventilation without respiratory movement in cat, dog, and human, *Br J Anaesthesiol* 58:544-550, 1986.

51. Pinsky MR, Matuschak GM, Bernardi M, et al: Hemodynamic effects of cardiac specific increases in intrathoracic pressure, *J Appl Physiol* 60:604, 1986.

52. Ralph DD, Robertson HT, Weaver LJ, et al: Distribution of ventilation and perfusion during positive end-expiratory pressure in adult respiratory distress syndrome, *Am Rev Respir Dis* 131:54-60, 1985.

53. Reynolds AM, Ryan DP, Doody DP: Permissive hypercapnia and pressure-controlled ventilation as treatment of severe adult respiratory distress syndrome in a pediatric burn patient, *Crit Care Med* 21(3):468-471, 1993.

54. Rossaint R, Falke KJ, Lopez BS, et al: Inhaled nitric oxide for the adult respiratory distress syndrome, *New Engl J Med* 328:399-405, 1993.

55. Royall JA, Matalon S: Pulmonary edema and ARDS. In Fuhrman BP, Zimmerman JJ, editors: *Pediatric critical care,* St. Louis, 1992, Mosby, pp 445-458.

56. Shaffer TH, Lowe CA, Bhutani VK, et al: Liquid ventilation: effects on pulmonary function in distressed meconium-stained lambs, *Pediatr Res* 18:47-52, 1984.

57. Sibbald WJ, Driedger AA, Myers ML, et al: Biventricular function in the adult respiratory distress syndrome, *Chest* 84:126-134, 1983.

58. Solway J, Rossing TH, Saari AF, et al: Expiratory flow limitations and dynamic pulmonary hyperinflation during high-frequency ventilation, *J Appl Physiol* 60:2071-2078, 1986.

59. Tharrat RS, Allen RP, Albertson TE: Pressure controlled–inverse ratio ventilation in severe adult respiratory failure, *Chest* 94:755-762, 1988.

60. Timmons OD, Dean JM, Vernon DD: Mortality rates and prognostic variables in children with adult respiratory distress syndrome, *J Pediatr* 119:896-899, 1991.

61. Tomashefski JF Jr, Davies P, Boggis C, et al: The pulmonary vascular lesion of the adult respiratory distress syndrome, *Am J Pathol* 112:112-126, 1977.

62. Tutuncu AS, Faithful S, Lachman B: Intratracheal perfluorocarbon administration combined with mechanical ventilation in experimental respiratory distress syndrome: dose-dependent improvement of gas exchange, *Crit Care Med* 21:962-969, 1993.

63. Vlahakes GJ, Turley K, Hoffman JI: The pathophysiology of failure in acute right ventricular hypertension: hemodynamic and biochemical correlations, *Circulation* 63:87-95, 1981.

64. Zapol WM, Snider MT: Pulmonary hypertension in severe acute respiratory failure, *N Engl J Med* 296:476-480, 1987.

27 Extracorporeal Oxygenation

Mark J. Heulitt

Despite many recent advances in intensive care medicine, acute lung injury or acute respiratory failure (ARF) remains a frequent life-threatening challenge to the pediatric intensive care specialist. Mortality rate among pediatric patients with ARF is in excess of 50%.[3,4,11,15,23] The mainstay of ARF therapy is conventional mechanical ventilation (CMV). The goal of CMV is to maintain adequate gas exchange while giving the lungs time to recover from the acute insult. Unfortunately too frequently CMV, in order to maintain gas exchange, exposes the patient to high inspiratory pressures and inspired oxygen, which increase the patient's morbidity and mortality rates. Recently extracorporeal life support (ECLS) has successfully supported some pediatric patients with acute respiratory failure who were unresponsive to CMV.

Indications

ECLS has successfully supported pediatric patients with adult respiratory distress syndrome (ARDS) and cardiac patients, as a bridge to transplantation or in the postoperative period. ECLS selection criteria for pediatric patients with ARF must include a way to identify patients with a high mortality risk whose disease process is most likely reversible. A high mortality risk accompanies failure to respond to maximum conventional medical management. The definition of failure of maximum conventional medical management is controversial. One definition is unresponsiveness to a trial of optimal positive end-expiratory pressure (PEEP),[18,22] pressure control ventilation,[13] and an optional trial of high-frequency ventilation. Failure of any of these therapies includes persistent hypoxemia ($Pao_2 < 55$ mm Hg) despite a FIo_2 of at least 0.60. Box 27-1 outlines indications or patient selection criteria for pediatric ECLS.

Contraindications

Patients with irreversible damage or a progressively fatal disease process are not candidates for pediatric ECLS.

Complications

Bleeding. Since patients supported with ECLS require systemic heparinization, the risk of bleeding is a potentially life-threatening complication of this therapy.[20] According to the Extracorporeal Life Support Organization (ELSO) registry of pediatric ECLS cases, 27% of patients had surgical site bleeding, 6% had significant gastrointestinal hemorrhage, and 5% had intracranial hemorrhage.[6] Surgical site bleeding includes bleeding from the cannula sites, chest tube insertion sites, and other sites with compromised skin integrity. It is usually possible to control this type of bleeding with local therapy, including pressure, electrocautery, topical agents, pressure dressings, and tightening of anticoagulant parameters. If bleeding is from a chest tube and continues despite the measures discussed, then reduce the amount of blood transfused by using a cell saver (Deknatel-Pleur-Evac 7000,

---

> **BOX 27-1 PEDIATRIC ECLS CRITERIA**
>
> **Conditions in which intubation is difficult or inappropriate**
>
> **Contraindications**
>
> Mechanical ventilation for < 10 days (or < 7 days of ventilation at a referral hospital)
>
> A lung biopsy result demonstrating extensive pulmonary fibrosis
>
> A history of cardiac arrest without clinical documentation of a normal neurologic examination result
>
> Any disease process considered progressively fatal
>
> Major burns
>
> **Relative contraindication**
>
> Septic shock
>
> Immunosuppression secondary to cancer therapy
>
> FIo_2 1 < 24 hours
>
> High ventilator settings: PIP* > 45 cm H_2O and FIo^2 > 0.60 for > 72 hours
>
> Fungal infection
>
> * *PIP*, Peak inspiratory pressure.

Fall River, MA) to collect blood draining from the chest tube. The blood bank should wash the chest tube drainage and return it to the patient. For this technique to be successful, the amount of bleeding must be large (750 ml/h) and continuous. Manage other bleeding complications such as major hemorrhage, even though life-threatening, with tightening of anticoagulant parameters, massive transfusions, and possibly surgical intervention while the patient is still on ECLS. It is rarely necessary to remove a patient from ECLS as a result of excessive bleeding.

Infection. Infection-related complications, such as culture-proven infections, have occurred in 20% of pediatric ECLS cases in the ELSO registry.[18] In a recent report of our experience at Arkansas Children's Hospital nosocomial infections were found in 23% of pediatric patients supported with ECLS.[19] Patients in whom nosocomial infections developed were supported for longer periods than those in whom they did not (mean 230 vs. 140 hours; $p < 0.01$). Bloodborne infections occurred most often while patients were cannulated; urinary tract and wound infections occurred more commonly after decannulation. Fungal organisms were isolated in 50% of nosocomial infections. Patients with fungal infections had a higher infection-related mortality rate. The mechanism by which nosocomial infections develop during ECLS is not well elucidated. Immune dysfunction caused by lymphopenia, neutropenia, alterations in T-cell populations, and activation of complement occurs in neonatal patients supported with ECLS.[1,2,24] These factors, along with the disruption of the

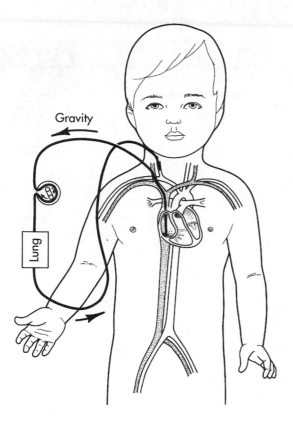

FIG. 27-1   Venoarterial extracorporeal life support.

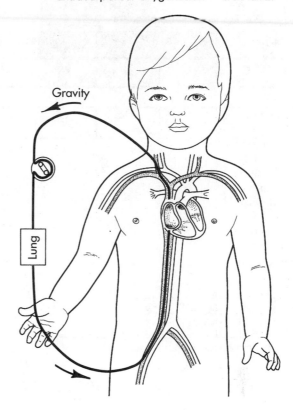

FIG. 27-2   Venovenous extracorporeal life support.

barrier protection supplied by the skin and the prolonged exposure to broad-spectrum antimicrobial agents, place patients at risk for nosocomial infections.

Mechanical Complications. Mechanical complications of ECLS include cannula malposition, clots in the circuit and membrane, oxygenator failure, tubing rupture, air in the circuit, pump malfunction, and host exchange malfunction. However, it is rare that one of these complications leads to patient instability.

Equipment

Figs. 27-1 through 27-3 show the components of the circuit for both venoarterial (VA) and venovenous (VV) ECLS. Desaturated venous blood drains from the right atrium by gravity to a reservoir. The pump advances blood to the membrane oxygenator, where gas exchange occurs. Oxygenated blood then flows through a heat exchanger, which rewarms it to body temperature and returns it to the patient. Following is a description of each of the individual components of the ECLS circuit.

Cannula. Blood drains from the patient via a venous cannula to the ECLS circuit and returns, oxygenated, to the patient via an arterial cannula. The size of the venous cannula determines the rate at which blood can drain from the right atrium. The size of the arterial cannula can limit flow by causing significant back-pressure in the circuit. Appropriate-sized cannulae can maximize blood flow and minimize resistance. Table 27-1 lists recommended cannula sizes for different sizes of pediatric patients.

Membrane Oxygenator. The membrane oxygenator consists of a silicone rubber membrane with a plastic screen wound in a spiral fashion around a polycarbonate spool. Gas

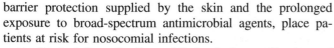

Table 27-1   Pediatric ECLS Cannulae

Weight (kg)	<8	8-12	12-20	20-35	35+
Venous (Fr)	12-16	16-20	20-24	21-24	>28
Arterial (Fr)	10-12	12-16	14-18	16-20	20+

flows through the interior of the envelope and blood flows between the turns in the membrane envelope. The pump setting controls blood flow to the membrane lung via a blood inlet located at the base of the membrane. A gas inlet located at the top of the membrane delivers gas to the membrane. This delivery system creates countercurrent gas and blood flow in the membrane. As blood flows past the membrane, the driving force for diffusion of oxygen into the blood is the pressure gradient between 100% oxygen in the ventilating gas and the oxygen tension in the venous blood. However despite the fact that there is a larger membrane pressure gradient for oxygen than for carbon dioxide, the rate of diffusion through the blood and the membrane per millimeter of mercury (mm/Hg) gradient is much greater for CO_2.

In the membrane lung oxygenation of the blood is a function of the membrane geometric characteristics, the thickness of the blood film on the screen, the membrane material, and its thickness. The FIo_2 of the sweep gas, the residence time of red cells in the gas exchange area, the hemoglobin concentration, and the inlet saturation also influence oxygenation of the blood in the membrane. Membrane function includes all of the factors mentioned, which together constitute rated flow[8] (Table 27-2). *Rated flow* is the amount of normal venous blood in liters that the membrane can raise from 75% to 95% oxyhemoglobin saturation per minute. The

Table 27-2 ECLS Circuit Components

Weight	<8 kg		8-12 kg		12-20 kg		20-35 kg		35+ kg	
Type of ECLS*	VA	VV	VA	VV	VA	VV	VA	VV	VA	VV
Oxygenator	800	1500	1500	2500	2500	3500	3500	4500	4500	4500
Surface area (m²)	0.8	1.5	1.5	2.5	2.5	3.5	3.5	4.5	4.5	4.5
Blood flow range of the membrane (L/min) rated flow)	1.2		1.8		1.8-4.5		4-5.5		5- 6.5	
Idle flow (ml/min)	150		300		500		500-900			
Gas flow range of the membrane (L/min)	2.4		4.5		7.5		10.5		13.5	
Circuit	1/4″		3/8″						1/2″	
Raceway	1/4″		3/8″				1/2″			

*ECLS, Extracorporal life support; VA, venoarterial; VV, venovenous.

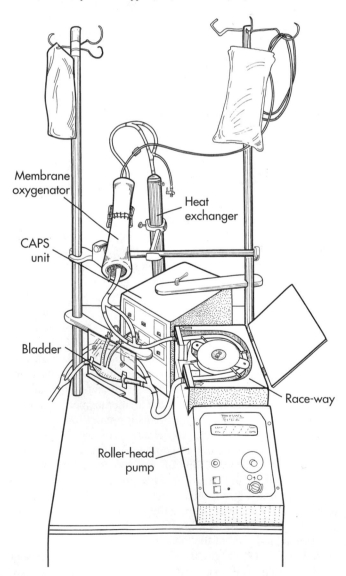

FIG. 27-3 Extracorporeal life support equipment. CAPS, Computerized perfusion system.

Labels: Membrane oxygenator; Heat exchanger; CAPS unit; Bladder; Race-way; Roller-head pump

size of the membrane chosen depends on the rate of ECLS flow and the type of cannulation. Membranes are available as 400, 600, 800, 1500, 2500, 3500, and 4500 sizes. Table 27-2 lists appropriate membrane size for the type of ECLS support and patient size.

Pump. ECLS support uses two types of pumps: the centrifugal pump and the roller head pump (positive displacement roller pump). Significant hemolysis occurs with use of the centrifugal pump in smaller patients with low flow rates.[21] This problem limits its use. Most ECLS centers use roller head pumps because they work in both small and large patients without complication. With the roller head pump compression of the raceway tubing produces displacement and forward flow of blood. The size of the tubing revolutions per minute (RPM) and the occlusion of the rollers against the pump tubing determine pump output. The pump's microprocessor calculates and displays pump flow in L/min on the basis of the size of the tubing and the RPMs.

Venous Reservoir

Blood returns from the right atrium by gravity to a 30 to 50-mL reservoir called a *bladder.* The bladder has numerous functions. It acts first as a bubble trap for free air introduced into the circuit. Second, it provides a large compliant vessel to monitor venous return. If venous return decreases, the bladder protects the right atrium from negative pressure by allowing the pump to pull against a larger volume in the bladder. An electronic device that functions as a servoregulator for the ECLS system monitors blood return to the bladder. The servoregulator alarms and stops the pump if venous flow decreases to prevent an increase in negative pressure in the bladder and circuit. If negative pressure increased unchecked, it would draw the gas out of solution, causing cavitation of the tubing and possible air embolism.

Circuit

The components of an ECLS circuit are the same for all modes of support. The tubing components of the circuit are

Table 27-3   Pediatric ECLS Parameters and Adjustments

Parameter	Desired value	Adjustments
Hematocrit	>40%	Infusion of packed red cells
Platelet count	>100,000	Infusion of platelets
(If bleeding is a problem)	>150,000	
Activated clotting time	200-230 sec	Adjustment of heparin infusion or, if evidence of excessive bleeding or abnormal clotting profiles, fresh-frozen plasma or cryoprecipitate
Svo_2	>70% < 80%	ECLS flow
		Sweep FIo_2
PCo_2	35-45 mm Hg	Sweep gas flow
Pao_2	>65 mm Hg	ECLS flow
		Sweep FIo_2
Pulse oximetry		ECLS flow
VA ECLS	>90%	Sweep FIo_2
VV ECLS	85%-90%	

ECLS, Extracorporeal life support; *Svo₂,* Percent saturation of oxygen in venous blood; *VA,* venoarterial; *VV,* venovenous.

available in manufactured tubing packs specially designed to meet each ECLS center's needs. The circuit is made of polyvinyl chloride (PVC) tubing, ¼ to ½ inch in diameter, and polycarbonate connectors. The tubing circuit must include essential entry ports, but these ports need to be limited to reduce the potential for blood loss and infection. Essential ports in the ECLS tubing circuit are (1) ports proximal to the bladder for blood sampling and intravenous (IV) fluid infusions, (2) ports after the pump head, but before the membrane, for setting pump occlusion and monitoring activated clotting time (ACT), and (3) ports after the membrane for pressure monitoring, blood sampling, and infusion of platelets. Also for monitoring venous saturation, add an in-line connection, a ¼ inch by ¼ inch connector with lock (Luer-Lok), for placement of an oxygen saturation catheter (e.g., the Oxymetrix 3, Abbott Critical Care Systems, Mountain View, CA). For temperature monitoring add a port for a temperature probe on the post–heat exchanger side of the arterial line. The sizes of the circuit and its components depend on the size of the patient and anticipated flow requirements. Table 27-3 outlines recommended circuit sizes for different sizes of pediatric patients.

The final component of the circuit tubing is the raceway tubing, which sits in the pathway of the roller head of the pump. Since each rotation of the roller head repeatedly compresses the raceway tubing, a resilient material is necessary for its construction. Materials include Supertygon (Norton Performance Plastics, Akron, OH) and Bypass 65 (American Bentley, Irvine, CA).

Heat Exchanger. The heat exchanger is a tube in a shell design with independent blood and water paths separated at each tube end by a pair of manifolds. A separate water bath heats the water in the heat exchanger. Water flows on the outside of the tubes in a direction countercurrent to the blood flow. Blood in the ECLS circuit preheat exchanger loses heat because of evaporation of water in the membrane lung. The purpose of the heat exchanger is to reheat the blood returning to the patient.

Techniques

The goal of ECLS support is to ensure adequate gas exchange and, in VA ECLS, also to support cardiac output. The ultimate goal of this therapy is to obtain adequate oxygen delivery to meet tissue oxygen needs. Systemic oxygen delivery is the product of cardiac output and arterial oxygen content. Important components of oxygen delivery include cardiac output, hemoglobin concentration, and hemoglobin saturation. The total cardiac output is the sum of the patient's own cardiac output and the bypass flow rate in VA ECLS and the patient's own cardiac output in VV ECLS. The rate of bypass flow and the function of the native lungs determine the hemoglobin saturation.

Types of ECLS Support. ECLS uses three distinct methods that depend on the cannulation site and amount of ventilatory support: VA, VV, and extracorporeal CO_2 removal ($ECCO_2$ R). The discussion that follows details the use of VA and VV ECLS only because of the lack of experience in the use of $ECCO_2$ R in pediatric patients.

VENOARTERIAL ECLS (VA ECLS). For venous drainage, in younger patients, place a cannula via the right internal jugular vein into the right atrium. In older pediatric patients use other venous sites, such as the inferior vena cava via the femoral vein or combined with the internal jugular vein, for venous drainage. After oxygenation in the ECLS circuit the blood returns to the patient through an arterial cannula in the carotid artery. Oxygenated blood can return to other arteries such as the femoral artery or sometimes directly to the aorta through an open sternotomy. This form of bypass has two functions: gas exchange in the membrane lung and hemodynamic support through delivery of flow and a pressure head into the arterial system.

The patient's size and requirements determine VA ECLS flow, which ranges from 100 to 140 ml/kg/min for infants to 80 to 100 ml/kg/min for young children, and 70 to 90 ml/kg/min for older children and adults. The combination of ECLS flow and cardiac output determines systemic perfusion. At the upper flow range, VA ECLS provides near-total cardiopulmonary support.

VENOVENOUS ECLS (VV ECLS). VA ECLS supports both gas exchange and cardiac output. VV ECLS supports only gas exchange. Thus, limit its use to patients with normal or near-normal cardiac function with severe respiratory failure. In VV ECLS blood drains from the venous circulation into the ECLS circuit, where gas exchange occurs in the membrane lung. After rewarming the blood returns to the venous circulation, where it mixes with more desaturated blood from the periphery. In younger infants drainage of the blood and its return occurs through a double-lumen cannula placed in the internal jugular vein.[5] This type of cannula is currently only available in sizes appropriate to smaller infants. In older patients cannulate at least two large veins, preferably the internal jugular vein and the femoral vein. The amount of gas exchange depends on the rate at which the membrane lung siphons blood, the size of the lung, and the flow rate and composition of the gas ventilating the membrane lung. Desirable flow rates vary with oxygen requirements but are generally 100 to 150 ml/kg/min. Increase drainage of blood by draining blood from two large veins and "Y-ing" this drainage back to the pump. Appropriate size of the membrane lung for a patient supported with VV ECLS is dependent on the patient's size (see Table 27-2). Also since oxygenated blood returning to the venous circulation and the pulmonary artery is not completely saturated as a result of recirculation, choose a membrane lung with a rated flow greater than the patient's expected cardiac output. After maximizing drainage, improve gas exchange further, if necessary, through increasing membrane surface area by placing two membrane lungs in parallel. Sometimes to improve oxygenation the membrane lung removes too much CO_2 and a marked respiratory alkalosis ensues. In order to decrease CO_2 removal, reduce the rate of gas flow ventilating the membrane lung (sweep gas). However, at very low sweep gas flows, the efficiency of the membrane lung falls with a reduction in oxygen transfer. In this situation ventilate the membrane lung with a gas containing CO_2 such as carbogen (95% O_2 and 5% CO_2). Titrate this gas to obtain the desired PCO_2 of 35 to 45 mm Hg.

Management of the Patient on ECLS

Cannulation. Perform cannulation at the bedside after anesthetizing the patient with a combination of an intravenous anesthetic, sedative, and neuromuscular blocking agent. After the surgeon has located the vessels for cannulation and just before insertion of the cannulae, administer beef lung heparin (100 units/kg) as a bolus. Initiate ECLS by unclamping the arterial line, clamping the bridge, and unclamping the venous line; then increase ECLS flow slowly. During the increase in ECLS flow it is common for the patient to have a transient decrease in arterial blood pressure as compliance changes in the membrane lung cause transient hypovolemia. This decrease in arterial blood pressure is usually responsive to volume infusion of 10 to 20 ml/kg of packed red blood cells (preferably) or plasmanate. Another cause of hypotension during the initiation of ECLS can be transient hypocalcemia, which responds to an infusion of calcium chloride 10 to 20 mg/kg.[16] After increasing ECLS flow to the desired level, decrease the patient's ventilator settings to "rest settings."

Maintenance on ECLS. The ECLS runs in pediatric and young adult patients are longer than those in neonatal patients with a reported range from 4 to 853 hours.[2,17] During the ECLS run maintain the ventilator on "rest settings" to reduce further barotrauma or oxygen toxicity. These settings are $FIO_2 < 0.60$, pressure control ventilation with peak inspiratory pressure 25 to 35 cm H_2O, frequency 6 to 20, and PEEP 8 to 12 cm H_2O. Maintenance of a patient on ECLS requires keeping physiologic parameters stable in the maintenance and weaning phases. In the maintenance phase keep the patient's condition stable until there is evidence of improvement in his or her physiologic status. Monitor and adjust as needed the hematocrit, platelet count, $S\bar{v}O_2$, PCO_2, activated clotting time, and mean arterial pressure as shown in Table 27-3. Use a constant infusion of heparin to maintain the patient's activated clotting time in the desired range. The dose of this infusion depends on the patient's weight, with a range between 20 to 60 U/kg/hour. Monitor oxygenation by measuring the mixed saturation, or $S\bar{v}O_2$, which is superior to arterial saturation because it more closely reflects oxygen consumption.[25] Maintain sedation with continuous infusions of midazolam (0.2 to 0.5 mg/kg/hour) and fentanyl (3 to 7 mg/kg/hour). During long runs greater than 1 week it may be necessary to increase these drugs or to change to other agents such as hydromorphone as a result of the development of tolerance. Use antibiotics only for proven infections. If culture results are negative or the patient has completed a course of antibiotics for a proven infection, then stop antibiotics. In addition provide total parenteral nutrition with lipid. Consider placing a transpyloric feeding tube in all patients before the initiation of ECLS, then start and advance enteral feeds as tolerated. Balance of intake and output is essential. Maintain output with diuretics (intermittent or continuous infusion) to promote urine excretion. Use hemofiltration in patients with renal insufficiency (decreased glomerular filtration rate).

Weaning from ECLS

Improvement in native lung function results in increased arterial oxygenation and improved static compliance or expired tidal volumes.[14] To wean from ECLS, first wean the FIO_2 on the membrane to 0.5 or less. After weaning the FIO_2, decrease the ECLS flow in 10- to 20-ml/min increments while maintaining the parameters in Table 27-4. Wean ECLS to *idle flow,* the minimum flow for a particular size of circuit and membrane. For example for an 800 membrane, idle flow is 150 ml/min (see Table 27-3). If the patient fails to wean secondary to hypercapnia, consider use of high-frequency oscillatory ventilation as a bridge off ECLS.[9] Persistent atelectasis can delay weaning of ECLS support and often warrants reinflation with bronchoscopy.[12]

Remarks

Because of the complex nature and long length of the ECMO run, the care of these patients requires a multidisciplinary approach. Routinely consult pharmacologic, nephrologic, and infectious disease staff in the care of these patients. With extracorporeal life support organization (ELSO) runs of 3 to 4 weeks and survival rates of 50% the care of these patients can be very difficult for even the most experienced ECMO professional. The key to a successful run is constant communication regarding the plan of care and regular updates on the

Table 27-4   Outcome of Pediatric ECLS

	Pediatric patients supported with ECLS 1986 - 1993		
	Survived (%)	Died (%)	Total
Diagnosis	**246 (48)**	**267 (52)**	**513**
Bacterial pneumonia	18 (47)	20 (53)	38
Viral pneumonia	78 (50)	78 (50)	156
Intrapulmonary hemorrhage	5 (62)	3 (38)	8
Aspiration	31 (58)	22 (44)	53
Pneumocystis	2 (29)	5 (71)	7
Acute respiratory distress syndrome	59 (43)	78 (57)	137
Other	53 (46)	61 (55)	114

Data from the Extracorporeal Life Support Organization (ELSO), Ann Arbor, Mich.

patient's condition with both the ECMO team and the family.

The use of ECLS in pediatric patients is complex, and, to date, its efficacy and impact on morbidity and mortality rates of ARDS remain unknown. There is no doubt that this technology has saved children's lives. Table 27-4 shows international pediatric pulmonary data regarding survival and diagnosis. Experience at Arkansas Children's Hospital is similar to that reported in the ELSO registry: since the inception of the program in January 1991, 19 pediatric and young adult patients with acute respiratory failure have undergone ECLS, with 11 (58%) surviving to hospital discharge.[10] Death is usually due to sepsis or multiple organ system failure. Follow-up data are available on all survivors, including both cerebral performance[7] and overall performance (Table 27-5) at hospital discharge. Ideally future research will help to determine who benefits from this technology.

Table 27-5   Discharge Pediatric Performance Categories

Preillness	Normal	Mild disability	Moderate disability	Severe disability	Brain death	Total pre- PCPC
Discharge pediatric cerebral performance categories (PCPC)						
Normal	7	2	1		8	18
Mild disability		1				1
Discharge pediatric overall performance categories (POPC)						
Normal	3	3		1	7	14
Mild disability		2	1		1	4
Moderate disability			1			1

REFERENCES

1. Brody Jl et al: Altered lymphocytes subsets during cardiopulmonary bypass, *Am J Clin Pathol* 87:626-628, 1987.
2. Darling EM et al: Complement activation during long-term extracorporeal membrane oxygenation in neonates, *J Extra-Corporeal Tech* 20:20-23, 1988.
3. Davis SL, Furman DP, Costarino AT: Adult respiratory distress syndrome in children: associated disease, clinical course, and predictors of death, *J Pediatr* 123:35-45, 1993.
4. Debruin W et al: Acute hypoxemia respiratory failure in infants and children: clinical and pathologic characteristics, *Crit Care Med* 20:1223-1234, 1992.
5. Durandy Y, Chevalier JY, Lecompte Y: Single-cannula veno-venous bypass for respiratory membrane lung support, *J Thorac Cardiovasc Surg* 99(3):404-409, 1990.
6. ECLS registry report of the Extracorporeal Life Support Organization. International Summary, April 1993.
7. Fiser DH: Assessing the outcome of pediatric intensive care, *J Pediatr* 121:68-74, 1992.
8. Galletti PM, Richardson PD, Snider MT: A standardized method for defining the overall gas transfer performance of artificial lungs, *Trans ASAIO* 18:359-368, 1972.
9. Heulitt MJ et al: High-frequency oscillatory ventilation as a bridge off ECLS for refractory hypercapnia in pediatric respiratory failure, Extracorporeal Life Support Organization (ELSO) meeting abstract book, 1993, p 40.
10. Heulitt MJ et al: Morbidity and mortality in pediatric patients with acute respiratory failure supported with extracorporeal life support. Extracorporeal Life Support Organization (ELSO) meeting abstract book, 1993, p 42.
11. Heulitt MJ et al: Morbidity and mortality in pediatric patients with respiratory failure, *Crit Care Med* 21(4):S156, 1993.
12. Karlson KH et al: Flexible fiberoptic bronchoscopy in children on extracorporeal membrane oxygenation, *Pediatr Pulmonol* 16:215-218, 1993.
13. Lain DC et al: Pressure control inverse ratio ventilation as a method to reduce peak inspiratory pressure and provide adequate ventilation and oxygenation, *Chest* 95:1081-1088, 1989.
14. Lortze A, Short BL, Taylor GA: Lung compliance as a measure of lung function in newborns with respiratory failure requiring extracorporeal membrane oxygenation, *Crit Care Med* 15:226-229, 1987.
15. Lyrene RK, Truog WE: Adult respiratory distress syndrome in a pediatric intensive care unit: predisposing conditions, clinical course, and outcome, *Pediatrics* 67:790-795, 1981.
16. Meliones JN, et al: Hemodynamic instability after the initiation of extracorporeal membrane oxygenation: role of ionized calcium, *Crit Care Med* 19:1247-1251, 1991.
17. Moller FW et al: Extracorporeal life support for pediatric respiratory failure, *Crit Care Med* 20:1112-1118, 1992.
18. Ralph DD et al: Distribution of ventilation and perfusion during positive end-expiratory pressure in the adult respiratory distress syndrome, *Am Rev Respir Dis* 131:54-60, 1985.
19. Schutze GE, Heulitt MJ: Infections during extracorporeal life support, *Clin Res* 40:838A, 1992.

20. Sell LL et al: Hemorrhagic complication of during extracorporeal membrane oxygenation: prevention and treatment, *J Pediatr Surg* 21:1087-1091, 1986.

21. Steinhorn RH et al: Hemolysis during long-term extracorporeal membrane oxygenation, *J Pediatr* 115:625-630, 1989.

22. Suter PM, Fairley HB, Isenberg MA: Optimum end-expiratory airway pressure in patients with acute respiratory failure, *N Engl J Med* 292:284-289, 1975.

23. Timmons OD, Dean JM, Vernon DD: Mortality rates and prognostic variables in children with adult respiratory distress syndrome, *J Pediatr* 119:896-899, 1991.

24. Zach TL et al: Leukopenia associated with extracorporeal membrane oxygenation in newborn infants, *J Pediatr* 116:440-444, 1990.

25. Zwischenberger JB et al: Does continuous monitoring of mixed venous oxygen saturation (Svo_2) accurately reflect (DO_2) and oxygen consumption (VO_2) following coronary artery bypass grafting (CABG)? *Surg Forum* 37:66-68, 1986.

28 Monitoring Oxygenation and Ventilation

Adalberto Torres, Jr.

Technologic advancements experienced in respiratory monitoring during the last 2 decades have created a number of viable noninvasive techniques for monitoring oxygenation and ventilation. Despite this progress, arterial blood gas (ABG) analysis remains the gold standard for assessing oxygenation and ventilation.

ARTERIAL BLOOD GASES
Percutaneous Arterial Puncture

Physicians routinely assess the child in respiratory distress with ABG analysis despite its shortcomings. Clinical correlation with ABG is imperative; obtaining an arterial sample of blood requires knowledge of fundamental anatomy and some technical experience.

Indications. The primary indication for arterial puncture is the evaluation of hypoxemia and/or hypercarbia in the child with respiratory distress. Although the institution of oxygen therapy does not require pretreatment assessment of arterial oxygen pressure (Pao_2), immediate ABG analysis may direct timely institution of other therapy (e.g., mechanical ventilation). ABG analysis during cardiopulmonary resuscitation (CPR) allows for the assessment of oxygenation and acid-base status, but experimental models have not demonstrated a correlation between ABG results and successful CPR.[153] Despite the widespread application of many of the highly advanced respiratory monitors available, the accuracy of these instruments often requires verification with ABGs.

Contraindications. Avoid performing arterial puncture through damaged skin (e.g., burn, infection) for infection control purposes. In patients with coagulopathies or in those receiving anticoagulation therapy, perform arterial puncture with extreme care because the risk of compression neuropathy secondary to hematoma formation is greater in this subgroup of patients.[106]

Complications. Complications of arterial puncture include local or systemic infection, exsanguination, and digital ischemia secondary to arterial spasm with or without fibrin deposition. These complications run a greater risk with arterial cannulation than following arterial puncture (see Chapter 33).

Equipment. All of the equipment required for performing an arterial puncture is readily available individually wrapped or as a prepackaged kit (Box 28-1). Prepackaged ABG syringes containing dry heparin allow for a smaller blood sample (0.5 to 1 ml) to be aspirated as a result of the reduced potential for heparin-related errors (see Techniques later in this section).

Although blood gas analyzers differ considerably, they similarly use three electrodes to measure pH, the partial pressure of carbon dioxide (Pco_2), and the partial pressure of oxygen (Po_2), and they have inlets to and outlets from the

---

> **BOX 28-1 EQUIPMENT FOR ARTERIAL PUNCTURE AND BLOOD SAMPLING**
>
> Iodophor or other sterilizing solution
> 1% lidocaine (without epinephrine)
> 1 ml syringe with 23- or 25-gauge needle
> Sterile gloves
> 2 × 2 cm sterile sponges
> Preheparinized 1-ml syringe with cap
> 21- or 23-gauge butterfly needle
> Plastic bag or cup with ice for storage

---

measuring chamber housing the electrode tips. Bedside blood gas analyzers may save valuable time in facilitating diagnostic and therapeutic decisions.[193] Some of these bedside blood gas chemistry instruments perform as well as laboratory-based instruments, but at least one instrument is inaccurate at Pao_2 values below 60 mm Hg.[127] Most instruments calculate values for base excess and for bicarbonate (HCO_3) and oxygen saturation; therefore interpret such values with caution.[24]

Regardless of the blood gas instrument used, the laboratory must ensure that the instrument is operating correctly, which requires a recent one- or two-point calibration of each electrode plus the measured response of a standard solution with known concentrations of pH, Pco_2, and Po_2.[78] Blood gas instruments vary in their degree of automation—from completely manual to fully automated. Modern blood gas analyzers are not only self-calibrating but are also self-cleaning, self-diagnostic for malfunction, relatively simple to operate, and require <200 μl of blood and <90 seconds for analysis.[163] Po_2 and Pco_2 levels in tonometered blood are known exactly; therefore this type of blood is best for assessing the accuracy of blood gas analyzers.[27] A fluorocarbon-containing emulsion is an excellent tracker of blood gas–analyzer proficiency with few differences.[79] The federal government has made proficiency testing programs mandatory for all laboratories since 1988.[32]

Technique. The initial step in arterial blood sampling is selection of site. Although the radial artery is commonly the site of choice, alternatives include femoral, brachial, ulnar, dorsalis pedis, and posterior tibial arteries (see Chapter 33). Assess collateral circulation before attempting puncture. Some physicians recommend performing a modified Allen's test (Fig. 28-1) to evaluate the adequacy of collateral circulation to the hand or foot, but this test does not guarantee that ischemia will not occur. The close proximity of nerves to the ulnar, brachial, posterior tibial, and dorsalis pedis arteries makes these sites less desirable than the radial and posterior tibial sites. Do not perform puncture of the superficial temporal artery because of the risk of cerebral emboli.

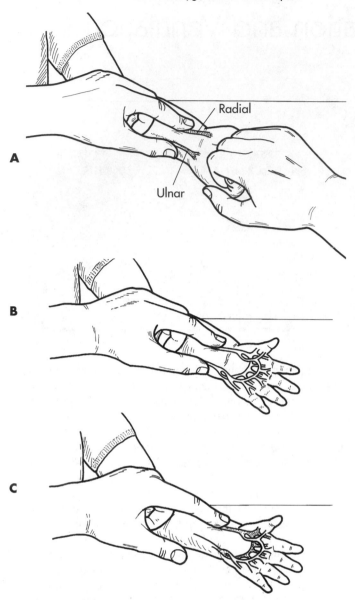

FIG. 28-1 The modified Allen's test. **A,** Close the child's hand with firm pressure while simultaneously occluding the ipsilateral radial and ulnar arteries with the index finger and thumb of your opposite hand. **B,** After a few seconds of allowing for an adequate reduction in blood volume within the hand, release the hand while maintaining point pressure on the radial and ulnar arteries. When performed properly, this hand should appear paler than the other hand. **C,** Release the pressure applied to the ulnar artery while maintaining point pressure on the radial artery. Reperfusion of the entire hand should occur within a few seconds if sufficient collateral circulation is present.

Prepare the skin overlying the pulse with iodophor or another sterilizing solution. Anesthetize the overlying skin with a small wheal of lidocaine (without epinephrine) placed with a 23-H or 25-gauge needle. Do not place a large wheal because doing so may obscure the pulse. After applying sterile gloves, localize the pulse with the nondominant hand while the dominant hand holds the preheparinized syringe. Puncture the skin through the wheal at a 15- to 90-degree angle to the plane of the arm. Apply gentle suction, if needed, to the syringe while advancing the needle. Apply suction while withdrawing the needle in case no blood flows during

Table 28-1 Potential Blood Gas Errors and Causes

Blood gas value errors	Cause(s)
$\uparrow P_{O_2}$	Air bubbles, pressurized injection into analyzer
$\uparrow P_{CO_2}$, $\downarrow$ pH	Stored at room temperature with delay in analysis ($\uparrow$ WBC and/or platelet count)
$\downarrow P_{CO_2}$	Excess heparin
$\downarrow P_{CO_2}$, $\downarrow P_{O_2}$, $\downarrow HCO_3$ with normal pH	Excess heparin

the first pass. If a couple of passes are unsuccessful, withdraw the needle to just below the dermis before changing direction. Consider removing and flushing the needle with heparinized saline to ensure patency before reattempting puncture. Transillumination or Doppler ultrasonography of the neonatal peripheral artery may aid in localizing the artery.[111] Apply firm pressure to the puncture site with sterile gauze or a sterile cotton ball for 5 to 10 minutes to avoid exsanguination and/or hematoma formation.

Proper handling of the blood sample is essential to avoid errors (Table 28-1). The P_{O_2} may be falsely elevated if the clinician does not expel all of the air from the sample.[110] If blood remains at room temperature for more than 20 minutes, the pH decreases as a result of a rise in P_{CO_2} secondary to leukocyte metabolism. Leukocytosis and/or thrombocytosis can significantly shorten the amount of storage time regardless of temperature.[83,166] Adding potassium chloride to the blood gas sample and storing it on ice prolongs the viability of the sample by several minutes, depending on the degree of leukocytosis.[145] Excessive heparin (i.e., 1000 U/ml of heparin filling more than the dead space of 1 ml syringe) falsely lowers the P_{CO_2} through a dilution effect.[71,93] However, a rising concentration of heparin results in a linear decrease in P_{CO_2}, P_{O_2}, HCO_3, and base excess with no change in pH, mimicking metabolic acidosis with respiratory compensation.[129,155] Pressurized injection of the blood sample into the analyzer may result in a falsely elevated P_{O_2}.[74] In addition, with elevated serum organic acid concentrations, the total CO_2 measured with the Kodak Ektachem 700 analyzer (Eastman Kodak Company, Rochester, NY) may be falsely raised.[146]

Regardless of the patient's body temperature, all blood gas instruments analyze and therefore report the pH, Pa_{O_2}, and Pa_{CO_2} of the blood at 37° C. This fact has generated a controversy regarding temperature correction of blood gas values to body temperature because a blood sample of given O_2 and CO_2 tensions manifests different gas tensions at various temperatures. Although a number of blood gas laboratories currently correct blood gases for body temperature, the effects of body temperature change in blood gases on organ function are not fully understood. The available technical and biologic data lead to the conclusion that "there is no clinical advantage to using values other than those at 37° C" (i.e., uncorrected values).[153] An excellent review and discussion of temperature correction of blood gas values is available.[4] Refer to Table 28-2 for normal pH and arterial blood gas values at various ages.

Table 28-2   Reference Arterial Blood Gas Values by Age*

Parameters	Newborn†	Neonate (<30 days)	Child and Adult
pH	7.25-7.40	7.35-7.40	7.35-7.45
PCO_2 (mm Hg)	35-41	35-41	35-45
PO_2 (mm Hg)	35-70	60-80	80-95
HCO_3 (mEq/L)	20-25	20-25	22-26

* FIO_2 and chronic disease influences these values and therefore their interpretation.

† The lower values correspond to the perinatal period.

Remarks. Because of the large number of potential causes for technical error, repeat the ABG if clinical correlation is lacking. Moreover, the activity and response of the child to the arterial puncture influences the level of oxygenation and ventilation. Therefore the clinician must consider these factors for accurate interpretation.

Sampling from Arterial Catheters

Rather than performing an arterial puncture for each gas determination, sampling from an indwelling arterial catheter minimizes the number of needlesticks the patient must endure (see Chapter 33 for indications for and the technique of insertion of arterial catheters). This section describes the technique for sampling blood from an indwelling arterial catheter. Recent adjustments in the sampling technique shift emphasis from minimizing the amount of the patient's blood sampled to minimizing the caretaker's exposure to blood.

Indications. The indications for ABG sampling from arterial catheters are similar to the indications listed for arterial puncture (see Percutaneous Arterial Puncture. Indications discussed in preceding paragraphs.

Contraindications. Do not schedule ABGs that do not result in an alteration of patient care. Repeated arterial blood sampling may create or worsen anemia and lead to an avoidable red blood cell transfusion.

Complications. The presence of an arterial catheter may result in a significant increase in the number of unnecessary ABGs drawn independent of the patient's clinical status, presence of a ventilator, use of pulse oximetry, or blood gas values.[124] The risks of repeated blood sampling for ABG analysis include significant blood loss, repeated caretaker exposure to potentially infectious blood, and the high cost of repeated ABG analysis (see Chapter 33 for complications of arterial catheterization).

Equipment. The standard supplies necessary to sample blood from an arterial catheter are the same as those necessary for an arterial puncture (Box 28-1). The major difference in equipment with this method is the T-connector, three-way stopcock, and pressure tubing/transducer apparatus attached to the arterial catheter (Fig. 28-2). Because of the large number of needlesticks that occur annually, the Food and Drug Administration strongly urges that needleless systems or recessed needle systems replace the use of hypodermic needles to gain access to intravenous lines.[58] Needleless syringes and other needleless accessories are now available for use in arterial blood sampling (Fig. 28-3).

Techniques. To minimize heparin-induced error, clamp the pressure tubing and clear the dead space volume by withdrawing 2 ml of heparinized saline/blood per ml of dead space volume from the T-connector or at the stopcock with one syringe.[141] Use a heparinized tuberculin syringe to aspirate a 0.2 to 0.5 ml sample of blood for analysis. After the air bubbles have been removed, place the sample syringe on ice or transfer it immediately to the laboratory for analysis. Flush the pressure tubing and arterial line with no more than 2 ml of heparinized saline until clear.

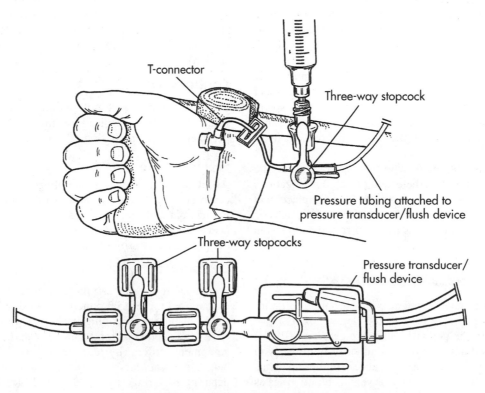

FIG. 28-2   A simple arterial catheter setup.

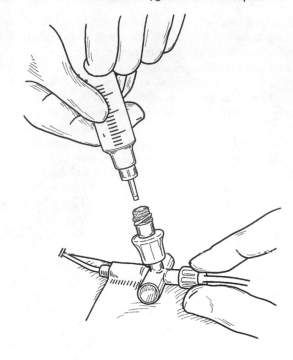

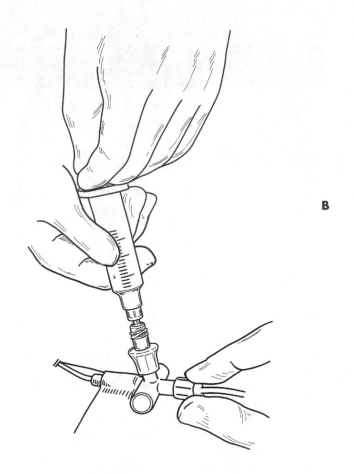

FIG. 28-3 **A,** A needleless syringe and stopcock hub for arterial sampling. The blunt tip of the syringe is available as a single unit. **B,** The hub accepts the blunt tip of the syringe without the use of excessive force.

To minimize the risk of emboli associated with retrograde flushing[28] and to decrease the amount of blood loss, use the 3-drop method of sampling. After clamping the T-connector and cleaning the injection port with povidone-iodine and alcohol, insert a 25-gauge needle from a heparinized 1 ml tuberculin syringe into the injection port. Allow three drops of blood mixed with flush to drip passively from the needle hub onto gauze for disposal. Attach the heparinized tuberculin syringe to the needle and aspirate the sample for analysis. It is not necessary to flush the line after unclamping the T-connector. Although the gas tensions are not significantly different between the 3-drop method and the conventional method of sampling,[183] the impact of flushing on "life span" or complications is not clear. However, the increased exposure to the patient's blood with the 3-drop method makes it less appealing.

Remarks. Despite the ease with which ABGs can be obtained with an arterial catheter in place, complications with these sampling techniques do occur. Plan for placement of an arterial catheter and for the frequency of ABG analysis on an individual basis and *not* as a part of routine admission procedures.

VENOUS AND CAPILLARY BLOOD GASES

A growing number of young patients with chronic respiratory diseases who are seen in the Emergency Department (ED) or who are admitted to the pediatric intensive care unit (PICU) require repeated evaluation of their ventilatory status early in their lives. Difficult or limited arterial access in these patients makes it reasonable to use capillary or venous blood gases as

assessment tools. Weigh the technical ease and low complication rate against the limitations of these sampling techniques.

Indications

As with many chronically ill infants, the heelstick or fingerstick technique is indicated for the evaluation of respiratory status whenever arterial access is difficult and the degree of oxygenation is not an issue (see Techniques later in this section).

Contraindications

Heelstick sampling is not optimal for blood gas analysis when the heel is bruised or inflamed or when there is peripheral vasoconstriction.

Complications

Avoid repeated heelstick sampling from the same site because repeated sampling causes inflammation and scarring. Bacteremia and osteomyelitis are reported complications of heelstick puncture, but their incidence is extremely low when the procedure is properly performed.[95,102]

Equipment

Venipuncture for gas sampling requires the same equipment as that used for arterial puncture (see Box 28-1). Use either a small, disposable warming pack or a warm cloth to "arterialize" the capillary blood sample. Capillary blood sampling equipment differs by the need for a 3-mm lancet and heparinized capillary tube rather than the butterfly needle and heparinized syringe used for arterial blood sampling.

Techniques

Prewarming the foot or finger for a few minutes enhances blood flow and promotes collection of an optimal sample. After adequately cleaning the sampling site and allowing it to dry, pierce the skin with a 3-mm lancet on the lateral or medial portion of the plantar surface of the heel. Blood should flow freely from the puncture site without squeezing the foot; squeezing may inhibit capillary filling or dilute the sample with serum or tissue fluid.[56] Perform another puncture of the same site if the blood does not flow freely. To avoid contaminating the sample with alcohol, wipe away the first drop of blood with gauze. Collect the following 0.2 to 0.3 ml of blood into a heparinized capillary tube; to minimize exposure to room air, place the tip of the tube deep into the drop of blood. In tubes supplied with a metal ball, pass a magnet over the capillary tube to aid in removal of air bubbles. Occlude the distal end of the tube with a small amount of wax before sample collection, and cap the proximal end after sampling until analysis. Venipuncture for gas analysis does not differ from the technique used in obtaining blood for chemical analysis.

Numerous studies have compared capillary and arterial blood gas values in neonates and infants. Several studies demonstrate good correlation between arterial and capillary pH and Pco_2 values but an inconsistent correlation with Po_2 values.* Capillary blood gas values may differ with age.[33] Appropriately obtained venous samples may be accurate in assessing acid-base status in well-perfused patients.[68,136]

Remarks

Despite the reported correlation that exists between arterial and capillary $Paco_2$ and pH, *all* capillary blood gas values may not correlate with their arterial counterparts.[44,150] Should capillary blood gas values be uninterpretable secondary to poor perfusion in an infant with respiratory distress, consider arterial puncture or placement of an arterial catheter. Confirm capillary or venous blood gas abnormalities with an ABG before instituting risky interventions such as intubation and mechanical ventilation.

PULSE OXIMETRY

The most widely accepted technologic advance in cardiorespiratory monitoring during the last 10 years is pulse oximetry. Because of its ease of operation and safety, pulse oximetry is rapidly becoming a standard part of continuous monitoring for ED evaluation and for monitoring outpatient procedures and surgery, as well as inpatients.

Indications

Hypoxemia often occurs without cyanosis. The primary clinical indication for pulse oximeter saturation (Spo_2) monitoring is the preclinical detection of hypoxemia.[158,172] The list of indications is constantly expanding (Box 28-2). The severely ill or injured child is at high risk for developing unrecognized hypoxemia during a prolonged diagnostic evaluation in the ED or radiology suite; therefore such patients should be monitored with pulse oximetry.[122,151]

> **BOX 28-2   INDICATIONS FOR PULSE OXIMETRY MONITORING**
>
> Perioperative and postoperative monitoring
> Pediatric and neonatal critical care
> Inpatient and outpatient oxygen therapy management
> Resuscitation monitoring (CPR, newborn)
> ED screening and therapy monitoring
> Transport of injured/sick child
> Peripheral circulation assessment (blood pressure, Allen's test)
> Intravascular volume assessment

Some physicians have also used pulse oximetry for evaluating the perfusion of injured limbs following open and closed reductions.[46,144] However, there are reports of compartment syndromes and significant lower limb vascular injuries with simultaneous limb Spo_2 values of at least 97%.[39,113] The automatic function of signal amplification as the pulse signal of the pulse oximeter decreases makes limb perfusion assessment a poor clinical application choice.[170]

Contraindications

There are no absolute contraindications to the application of pulse oximetry. Interpret pulse oximetry cautiously in children with chronic hypoxemia (e.g., cyanotic heart disease, pulmonary hypertension) because of the inaccuracy in these instruments with Spo_2 values below 70%.[160,161]

Complications

Major complications with pulse oximeters are rare. There are reports of superficial dermal injuries—including skin burns, skin erosion, and hyperpigmentation—resulting from prolonged probe application to one site during a low perfusion state,[34] a sensor cable in direct contact with skin during magnetic resonance imaging,[13] a disposable probe that had been damaged from repeated use,[120] and for no apparent reason.[18,135] Unless adequate safety tests have been performed, do not use probe sensors from one manufacturer with a pulse oximeter from a different manufacturer because doing so may result in a significant burn injury.[54,125]

Equipment

As of 1988, 29 manufacturers of pulse oximeters worldwide were producing more than 45 different models.[17] Few of these pulse oximeters have undergone testing in healthy and sick children.* The Nellcor N-100 and Ohmeda Biox 3700 pulse oximeters closely correlate with co-oximeter–measured saturations with precisions of ±4 regardless of age.[2,80,96] Spo_2 values with the Ohmeda Biox 3700 pulse oximeter are within 5% of co-oximeter–measured Sao_2 values in children with core temperatures as low as 31.3° C.[109] Pulse oximeter accuracy below an Spo_2 value of 70% is unreliable with most models.[62,149] Pulse oximeters come equipped with a plethysmographic signal display or a pulsatile signal display in addition to a heart rate display. When purchasing any brand of pulse oximeter, understand the method of calibration used because the population used for calibration (e.g., adult athletes) may not be an accurate representation of the patient

---

*References 50, 67, 73, 94, 116, and 189.

*References 23, 48, 52, 59, 61, 87, 121, 140, and 143.

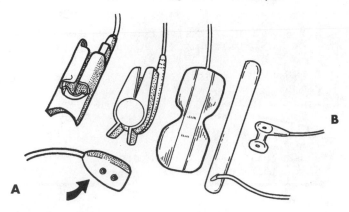

FIG. 28-4   Various pulse oximeter probes. **A,** The black probe (arrow) is a reflectance oximeter probe that is applied to the skin of the forehead or chest with an adhesive ring. **B,** The other probes wrap around or clip onto a digit or earlobe (ear oximeter probe not pictured).

population. A variety of pulse oximeter probes come in sizes suitable for patients of almost any size (Fig. 28-4). A prototype reflectance pulse oximeter sensor that uses four wavelengths of light yields accurate Spo_2 readings on the forehead or cheek.[169]

The advent of microprocessors and light-emitting diodes (LEDs) propelled pulse oximetry into clinical practice by the late 1970s. Pulse oximetry takes advantage of the reflective and absorbance properties of the four hemoglobin (Hgb) species (oxyhemoglobin [HbO_2], reduced Hgb, methemoglobin [metHb], and carboxyhemoglobin [COHb]). The extinction coefficient, a measure of absorbance, varies over the spectrum of light wavelength for each of the four species of Hgb (Fig. 28-5). By using four wavelengths of light to identify the four species of Hgb, co-oximeters provide the *fractional* percentage of Hgb saturation of the total Hgb content. Using an LED, the pulse oximeter delivers light at two wavelengths (660 and 940 nm) through tissue with an arterial pulse to a photodiode. Because of the similar extinction coefficients of metHb and HbO_2 in the 660 nm range and the lack of light absorbance of COHb in the 940 nm range (see Fig. 28-5), pulse oximeters do not detect COHb or metHb accurately. Therefore the pulse oximeter is only capable of providing the percentage of *functional* hemoglobin saturation (i.e., the fraction of HbO_2 to Hgb available for saturation [reduced Hgb]). If there is suspicion of a dyshemoglobinemia, obtain a co-oximeter Sao_2 because it provides a more accurate representation of oxygen *content* (see Techniques later in the following paragraphs).

Techniques

Attach the pulse oximeter probe to a digit on the foot or toe. The size and activity of the patient dictates which probe and site to use. Monitor neonates weighing less than 3 kg with the probe across the palm or the anterior part of the foot.[81] Because of the presence of right-to-left shunting in many neonates during the first day of life, obtain Spo_2 measurements from the right hand because this site provides a better index of brain oxygenation than does the foot or left hand.[49,117] Long response times related to probe site (toe vs. right index finger) and therefore circulation time may delay

therapeutic interventions.[37] Extensive burns involving the limbs and head limit the potential sites for placement of oximeter probes, but Spo_2 readings with a tongue probe in paralyzed, intubated patients are comparable to peripheral Spo_2 values.[43,88] Check proper sensor application routinely as part of the evaluation of the child with a low Spo_2 value.[69,159]

Evaluation of the signal quality is essential in interpreting pulse oximeter readings. The presence of an arterial plethysmograph with a dicrotic notch ensures a good pulse and therefore the best Spo_2 value.[190] Interpretation of Spo_2 values from pulse oximeters without a plethysmographic display requires correlation of the heart rate display of the oximeter with a pulse obtained either by manual count or with a cardiorespiratory monitor. Although this correlation indicates accuracy for some pulse oximeters, it may not hold true for *all* pulse oximeters.[152] Hypotension, vascular disease, and vasopressor therapy may create inaccuracies through their effects on signal quality.[175] Excessive sensor motion,[11,100,101,186] bright environmental lighting,[3,8,40,137] and intravenous dyes[156] may adversely affect the accuracy of a pulse oximeter by impeding signal transmission. Meconium-stained skin absorbs more red than infrared light, which gives a falsely low Spo_2 value.[89] Jaundice does not affect the latest generation of pulse oximeters.[15,179] The two wavelengths of light used do not distinguish COHb from HbO_2 or reduced Hgb. This phenomenon results in erroneously high Spo_2 readings contrary to the co-oximeter–measured blood saturations in patients with high COHb concentrations.[10] Significant levels of MetHb cause Spo_2 readings that overestimate the fractional HbO_2 and underestimate the Pao_2 (Table 28-3).[181] Spo_2 readings may be inaccurate during sickle cell crisis, but this fact has yet to be firmly established.[90] Fetal Hbg levels up to 100% do not cause clinically significant errors in Spo_2.[142] Dopamine infusions in infants also reportedly can disrupt the correlation between arterial HbO_2 saturation (Sao_2) and Spo_2 values despite normoperfusion ($r = 0.75$, $p < 0.00005$).[53] Theoretically, Spo_2 readings may underestimate Sao_2 during peripheral vasoconstriction because of reverse venous pulsation. Reference values for Spo_2 at high altitudes are now available.[16,105,171]

Interpretation requires not only an understanding of the technical principles with which pulse oximetry works but also a working understanding of the physiology of gas exchange. For example, a leftward shift of the hemoglobin dissociation curve secondary to alkalosis, hypothermia, or a decrease in 2,3-diphosphoglycerate (as seen following a large transfusion of red blood cells) results in a lower Pao_2 for a given Sao_2. This scenario may translate into a Pao_2 of 50 mm Hg when a Spo_2 of >90% is present. Correlation with ABG Sao_2 (by co-oximeter) is necessary for conditions in which there are alterations in the hemoglobin dissociation curve.

The degree of hyperoxemia is not discernible at Spo_2 values of 99% to 100%. Pulse oximeters reliably avoid hyperoxemia (Pao_2 80 to 90 mm Hg) in neonates (premature or otherwise) who are receiving supplemental oxygen by maintaining $Spo_2 \leq 95\%$.[26,138] Lowering the cutoff point for hyperoxemia to 92% increases the sensitivity for detecting hyperoxemia but also reduces the specificity significantly,

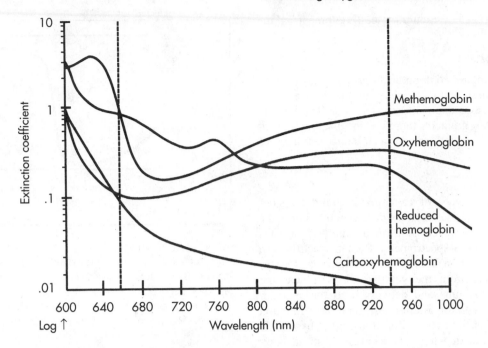

FIG. 28-5 Extinction coefficients of the four species of hemoglobin. The dashed lines represent the two common wavelengths of light used for pulse oximetry (see text).

(Redrawn with permission from Wukitsch MW, et al, *J Clin Monit* 4:290, 1988.)

Table 28-3 The Relationship of Functional Sao_2 (i.e., Spo_2), Fractional Sao_2, and Pao_2 in Methemoglobinemia

Time after admission	Flo^2	Pao_2 (mm Hg)	Spo_2 (%)	Sao_2 (%, CO-OX)	Fract metHb (%, CO-OX)
0	0.4	155	63	43.7	54.8
4 h	0.35	102	81	66.1	30.2
8 h	0.3	104	85	74.1	22.6
16 h	0.3	110	89	82.2	15.2
24 h	0.21	100	95	93.1	5.8

Modified from Watcha M, Connor MT, Hing AV: Pulse oximetry in methemoglobinemia, *Am J Dis Child* 143:845, 1989.

BOX 28-3 **HISTORICAL AND CLINICAL CONDITIONS THAT AFFECT PULSE OXIMETRY RELIABILITY**

Chronic hypoxemia (Spo_2 70%)
Hypotensive states
Vasoactive agents or intravenous dye administration
Thick, meconium-stained skin
Methemoglobinemia
Carbon monoxide poisoning
Hypothermia, alkalosis (leftward shift of HbO_2 dissociation curve)

---

which makes pulse oximetry less reliable for detecting hypoxemia.[5]

Remarks

Pulse oximetry clearly has the advantage of aiding in the preclinical detection of hypoxemia,[21,42] but whether these instruments are cost-effective or improve patient outcome is unknown.[130] Despite the widespread acceptance of this technology, avoid being lulled into a false sense of security, because acceptable Spo_2 readings may occur in the presence of true clinical hypoxemia or even asystole.[47] Always obtain an ABG to confirm or relieve clinical suspicions. The reliability of any pulse oximeter is questionable during certain historical or clinical conditions (Box 28-3).

CAPNOGRAPHY

Capnography is the continuous, real-time, graphic display of Pco_2 measured in exhaled gas (i.e., end-tidal Pco_2). The monitoring of end-tidal Pco_2 ($Petco_2$) is currently standard care for intubated patients during surgery. $Petco_2$ monitoring is also rapidly gaining acceptance as a ventilatory monitoring technique outside of the surgical suite. Practice settings ranging from the ED and PICU to conventional dental offices have used $Petco_2$.[85]

Indications

$Petco_2$ monitoring may aid in the establishment of tracheal intubation and in ventilator management of the intubated infant or child. $Petco_2$ monitoring prevents extreme hypocapnia (<20 mm Hg) in the intubated, head-injured patient during mechanical ventilation and transport.[108] Besides being a rapid and accurate indicator of successful intubation during emergency situations, $Petco_2$ correlates closely with cardiac output[184] and has been indicative of successful CPR in both animal[76,154,176] and adult human studies.* There are reports of nonintubated patients being adequately monitored

---

*References 12, 60, 70, 99, 128, and 178.

with a sidestream $P_{et}co_2$ monitor (see Equipment in the following paragraphs).[25,104]

Contraindications

There are no absolute contraindications to using $P_{et}co_2$ monitors. In children with severe pulmonary disease or cyanotic heart disease, large differences exist between the Pa_{co_2} and the $P_{et}co_2$ gradient; therefore in this subgroup of patients $P_{et}co_2$ does not provide a reliable estimate of Pa_{co_2}.[103]

Equipment

There are two main types of capnograph monitors: sidestream and mainstream. The classic sidestream monitor is the mass spectrometer. However, sidestream analysis of CO_2 may be a product of mass spectrometry, Raman spectroscopy, or infrared light absorption. The sidestream monitor aspirates gas at a preset rate from the ventilator circuit near the patient's endotracheal tube and delivers it to the analyzer located within the monitor. Mainstream analyzers function by assessing infrared light absorption transmitted by a LED to a photodiode, both of which are located on an analyzer that is attached directly to the patient's endotracheal tube. Disadvantages of sidestream $P_{et}co_2$ analyzers as compared to mainstream analyzers include slower response times (2 to 3 seconds as compared to less than 0.5 seconds with most mainstream monitors) and decreased accuracy from sampling catheter obstruction or sample catheter turbulence of gas that is distorting the proximal and distal ends of the expired CO_2 sample. The primary disadvantage of the mainstream $P_{et}co_2$ monitors is their limited application to the intubated subject. Technical refinements made in mainstream analyzer probes have resulted in the addition of very little dead space and/or weight to the neonate's or infant's ventilator circuit.

$P_{et}co_2$ monitors are now available as separate units combined with a pulse oximeter or as part of a cardiorespiratory monitor. Simple, pocket-size devices that confirm the presence of CO_2 by a color change are useful during the transport of the intubated child or immediately following intubation to confirm proper endotracheal tube placement.[12,20,84,148]

Techniques

To use the simple, colorimetric device, attach the unit to the endotracheal tube following intubation; allow six breaths to wash the CO_2 from the esophagus before reading the color change. If the tube is correctly positioned in the trachea, the color will be yellow with exhalation ($P_{et}co_2$ 2% to 5% or 15 to 38 mm Hg) and purple with inhalation ($P_{et}co_2$ 0.03% to 0.05% or 4 mm Hg). An intermediate tan color ($P_{et}co_2$ 0.5% to 2% or 4 to 15 mm Hg) may result from an esophageal intubation or from low pulmonary blood flow. During effective CPR, the color is usually tan or yellow; a change to bright yellow may indicate the return of spontaneous circulation. Conversely, a purple color during CPR may indicate an esophageal intubation or that CPR is ineffective.

To use the more complex capnograph, attach the sampling catheter or mainstream analyzer directly to the proximal end of the endotracheal tube. For nonintubated subjects, place the sampling catheter inside a dental mouth hook, in one of the prongs of a nasal O_2 catheter, or shield it inside a catheter placed in the nose or pharynx.[185]

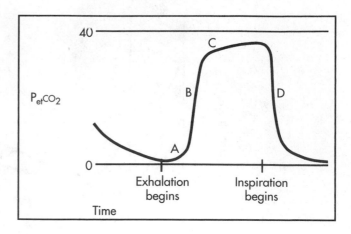

FIG 28-6 A normal capnogram. Segment A represents the beginning of exhalation, when pure dead space gas is exhaled. Segment B represents exhaled dead space gas mixed with alveolar gas. Segment C represents pure alveolar gas during the latter portion of exhalation. Note the slight rise in the slope of segment C. Segment D represents the initiation of inspiration with a sudden fall in P_{co_2}.

There is only one normal capnogram (Fig. 28-6), and any variation from the normal pattern indicates an abnormality. Several distinct capnogram patterns are encountered.[168] A sudden drop of $P_{et}co_2$ to a near-zero value (Fig. 28-7, A) indicates that the analyzer is no longer sensing the presence of CO_2 in the exhaled gas and indicates a potentially disastrous event such as esophageal intubation, complete airway disconnection, or a totally obstructed endotracheal tube. An exponential decrease in $P_{et}co_2$ over a short period (Fig. 28-7, B) represents a dramatic increase in physiologic dead space ventilation and a significant widening of the difference between Pa_{co_2} and $P_{et}co_2$ (Pa-etco$_2$). This phenomenon includes events such as sudden hypotension, circulatory arrest, and massive pulmonary embolism. A poor plateau (Fig. 28-7, C) occurs with the incomplete emptying seen with partial endotracheal tube obstruction or bronchospasm. This pattern also occurs with the small tidal volumes used during mechanical ventilation of neonates and infants. However, this problem is often correctable by placing the tip of the sampling catheter at the distal rather than the proximal end of the endotracheal tube.[7,115] Poor plateaus may occur with high respiratory frequencies when the total delay time of the instrument exceeds the respiratory cycle time.[157] A gradual rise in both the baseline and $P_{et}co_2$ (Fig. 28-7, D) suggests rebreathing of expiratory gases. This rebreathing may be secondary to a ventilator valve malfunction or inadequate flow during manual bag ventilation. A biphasic waveform (Fig. 28-7, E) may indicate a right main stem bronchial intubation or some pathophysiologic cause for a unilateral hypoventilation of one lung, such as unilateral bronchial stenosis or compression of an entire lung.[72] A notched plateau (Fig. 28-7, F) may be the first signal that spontaneous ventilation is returning in a patient who is recovering from or receiving inadequate amounts of neuromuscular blockade. Cardiogenic oscillations (Fig. 28-7, G) occur at the end of expiration or in early inspiration. The cause of this pattern is not fully understood but is of little

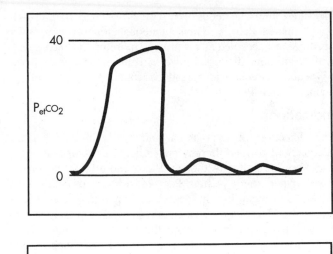

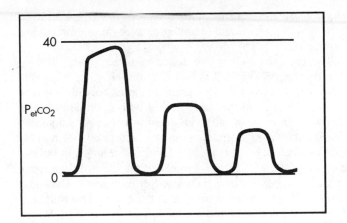

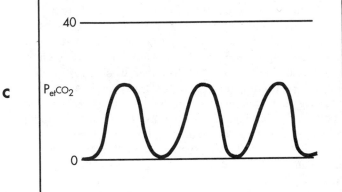

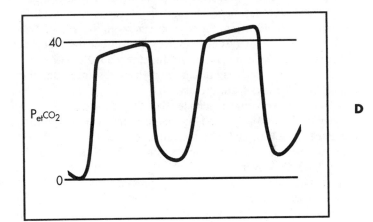

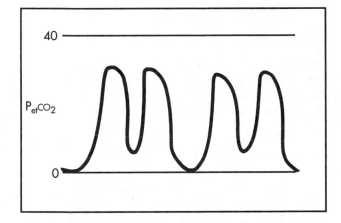

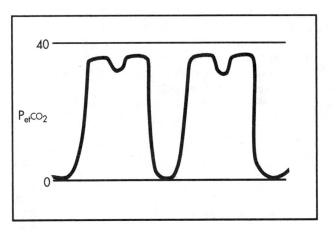

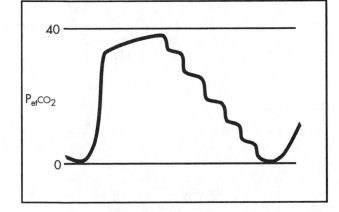

FIG. 28-7   Various capnogram patterns (see text).

physiologic consequence. Other sources describe additional capnograph patterns and their significance during mechanical ventilation.[31,35,45,167]

The typical Pa-etco₂ difference in patients without lung disease (i.e., V_D/V_T*<0.3) is 0 to 5 mm Hg (i.e., Paco₂ 0 to 5 mm Hg > Petco₂).[132] This gradient varies not only between patients but also in the same patient with multiple measurements.[119] In mechanically ventilated infants with pulmonary disease, the Pa-etco₂ gradient may be as large as ± 12 mm Hg (95% confidence interval).[57,77] Dynamic changes in pulmonary blood flow,[192] lung volume, and the ratio of dead space to tidal volume influence Pa-etco₂ difference.[118] These dynamic changes are often present in the child with respiratory failure, which makes the estimation of Paco₂ from Petco₂ inaccurate.[51] High metabolic rates, small lung volumes, and high breathing frequencies seen in children may lead to greater fluctuations in Paco₂ and result in Petco₂ that is *higher* than Paco₂.[123] Other factors that affect the Pa-etco₂ difference include air leaks around the endotracheal tube, fresh gas flows that may dilute the measured sample, and the sampling distance from the alveoli.[6]

There is growing evidence that the Pa-etco₂ gradient correlates with V_D/V_T and the alveolar-arterial oxygen difference (A-aDO₂) and may therefore serve as an indicator of the efficiency of ventilatory support in respiratory failure.[182,191] However, attempts at improving alveolar recruitment with positive end-expiratory pressure (PEEP) therapy guided with Pa-etco₂ monitoring have met with limited success in adult clinical studies.[22,86,126]

Certain medications affect the Pa-etco₂ gradient. In one adult human study, Petco₂ still retained its accurate predictive value of successful resuscitation despite a significant drop in Petco₂ during CPR because of epinephrine administration.[30] Experimentally, the administration of sodium bicarbonate (NaHCO₃) increases the excretion of CO₂ and therefore adversely affects the correlation of Petco₂ with perfusion during CPR for approximately 5 minutes following administration.[65]

Remarks

Petco₂ monitoring is useful in rapidly detecting adverse events that may occur during and after intubation.[41] Capnography also facilitates the safe transport of the critically ill, intubated child. Understanding the change in Pa-etco₂ gradient with changing intrapulmonary dynamics to optimize ventilator therapy is the most important role that Petco₂ monitoring may play in the future. The complex relationship between tidal volume, duration of expiration, alveolar dead space, and ventilation inequalities is not well delineated. Whether Petco₂ monitoring affects patient outcome (e.g., less time on the ventilator and therefore less risk of nosocomial infection or adverse events) or is cost-effective (e.g., reduces the number of blood gases drawn) is unknown.

TRANSCUTANEOUS MONITORS

In the early 1970s, German investigators demonstrated that a polarographic Clark electrode placed on the skin of a neonate

measured transcutaneous Po₂ (Ptco₂) values that closely approximated Pao₂.[173] Transcutaneous monitors have since become well accepted as respiratory monitors for the neonate with respiratory distress. However, transcutaneous monitors have not received widespread acceptability outside of the neonatal intensive care unit.

Indications

The detection of hypoxemia and the evaluation of the adequacy of oxygen therapy are indications shared by Ptco₂ and Spo₂ monitors. Although Ptco₂ monitoring underestimates hyperoxemia at high Pao₂ tensions, it provides more information regarding the degree of hyperoxemia than does Spo₂.[114,149] Despite the association between the incidence of retinopathy of prematurity and the duration of exposure to Ptco₂ levels of ≥ 80 mm Hg, continuous Ptco₂ monitoring to prevent the occurrence of Ptco₂ values ≥ 70 mm Hg has not been effective in reducing the incidence or severity of retinopathy of prematurity in infants at greatest risk (i.e., those weighing <1100 g).[9,66] Because Ptco₂ values are more sensitive to changes in blood flow than to changes in blood pressure, a useful application for Ptco₂ monitoring is in assessing the viability of surgical skin flaps and autografts.[1,75,91] Neonatal units often use transcutaneous monitors for monitoring ventilation and/or oxygenation *trends* during respiratory illnesses such as croup[64] or for evaluating pulmonary function in children with cystic fibrosis[139] or asthma.[38,55,177,187]

Contraindications

Avoid Ptco₂ monitoring in patients with hypothermia because of the increased risk of skin burns.

Complications

The primary risk from prolonged application of a Ptco₂ heated electrode is skin burns. To avoid this problem, keep the temperature of the electrode at ≤44° C and change electrode sites every 4 hours.[188]

Equipment

Transcutaneous Ptco₂ sensors are heated, polarographic oxygen electrodes that are essentially the same as the ones used in conventional blood gas analyzers. Disposable adhesive rings allow direct sensor attachment to the patient's skin. Transcutaneous CO₂ (Ptcco₂) electrodes are either miniaturized Severinghaus electrodes or infrared capnometers. Both types come equipped with a heating element and temperature sensor similar to the Ptco₂ electrode. Electrodes capable of measuring both Ptco₂ and Ptcco₂ simultaneously are also available, but the combined electrode may have reduced performance compared to a single electrode.[97] One- and/or two-point calibrations are necessary between uses.

Techniques

By heating the stratum corneum layer of the skin to ≥44° C, the sensor melts the lipid component of this layer from solid to liquid, which allows tissue O₂ and CO₂ to diffuse to the surface for detection. Therefore place the sensor on skin that has very little subcutaneous fat, ample capillary blood flow, and a thin epidermis, such as the chest and lateral sides of the abdomen. Sensors placed on the trunk are also less likely to

---

*V_D, Physiologic dead space to V_T, tidal volume ratio.

Table 28-4   The Ptco$_2$ Index (Ptco$_2$/Pao$_2$)

Age groups	Ptco$_2$ index	Reference
Premature infants	1.14	*J Perinat Med* 1:183, 1973
		Med Biol Eng Comput 13:436, 1975
Term newborns	1.00	*Birth Defects Original Article*
		Series XV:286, 1979
Children	0.84	*Crit Care Med* 10:765, 1982
Adults	0.79	*Crit Care Med* 9:706, 1981
Older adults	0.70	*J Clin Monit* 1:130, 1985

Modified from Barker, SJ, Tremper KK: Transcutaneous oxygen tension: a physiological variable for monitoring oxygen tension, *J Clin Monit* 1:130, 1985.

be affected by vasoconstriction seen during low perfusion states. It may be necessary to wait 10 to 20 minutes after initial attachment to allow for adequate heating and gas diffusion. Most manufacturers recommend calibration of the sensor before each site change every 4 hours. Unlike Ptco$_2$, Ptcco$_2$ monitoring depends less on heating the skin and has good correlation between Paco$_2$ values and Ptcco$_2$ values measured at 42° C.[82]

Ptco$_2$ is a measure of tissue Po$_2$, not of Pao$_2$. The ratio of Ptco$_2$ to Pao$_2$, known as the Ptco$_2$ index, varies with age (Table 28-4). The best correlation between Ptco$_2$ and Pao$_2$ occurs during the neonatal period and thus has popularity in neonatal medicine. Besides a decreasing index with age, any condition that decreases skin perfusion (e.g., hypotension, hypovolemia, hypothermia) results in a smaller-than-usual index for a patient of a given age.[48] Air bubbles trapped under the membrane, air leaks under loose adhesive, high electrode temperature, and the immediate reading of the Ptco$_2$ after applying the electrode result in an erroneously high Ptco$_2$ index.[133] Ptco$_2$ readings during polycythemic and hyperviscous states are valid.[180] Cautiously interpret Ptco$_2$ values in infants with bronchopulmonary dysplasia because of the significant reduction in correlation with Pao$_2$ in this subgroup of patients.[143,147]

Similar to Ptco$_2$ values, Ptcco$_2$ values represent the CO$_2$ tension at the surface of the skin; they do not represent Paco$_2$. Ptcco$_2$ values exceed Paco$_2$ values at every age, but there is an increase in Pa-tcco$_2$ difference with increasing electrode temperature.[36,57] Use calibration factors to compensate for the increased CO$_2$ solubility and/or tissue production with increased electrode temperature.[131] Unfortunately, a significantly different correlation between Ptcco$_2$ and Paco$_2$ values exists in the presence of hypotension and/or acidosis, which makes the application of a calibration factor less reliable.[19,29,77,107] In critically ill neonates with severe lung disease, Ptcco$_2$ monitoring is better than Petco$_2$ monitoring because of its increased accuracy.[115]

Remarks

Despite the availability of transcutaneous monitors for more than 20 years, Ptco$_2$ monitoring is not as well accepted as pulse oximetry outside of neonatal intensive care units. The inability to predict Pao$_2$ from a given Ptco$_2$ and a slow response time as compared to pulse oximetry has significantly hindered widespread acceptance of transcutaneous

monitoring into areas such as the ED or PICU.[63,133,188] Ptco$_2$ monitors in older children and adults represent the degree of cutaneous blood flow more accurately than the adequacy of oxygenation and may therefore be a useful indicator of the successful resuscitation of shock. One possible advantage to transcutaneous monitors is the potential for a reduction in cost[134] and in the number of ABGs drawn.[14] However, if those using the instrument consider the monitor to be unreliable, they will draw ABGs to establish the accuracy or validity of abnormal values and therefore increase the total number of blood gases drawn.[92]

INTRAARTERIAL AND EXTRAARTERIAL BEDSIDE BLOOD GAS MONITORS

Technologic advances in blood gas monitors now make it possible to *continuously* monitor pH, Pco$_2$, and Pao$_2$ at the bedside without phlebotomy. Some adult ICUs now use this new, optode technology, and it will be available soon for use in PICUs.

Indications

The indications for continuous blood gas and pH monitoring are to ensure adequacy of oxygenation and ventilation in patients with cardiorespiratory disease. However, reserve this technology for patients who will require *repeated* ABG measurements for more than 2 days in a setting such as the PICU. It is still unclear which patients are most likely to benefit from this monitoring technique.

Contraindications

Avoid placing an indwelling arterial catheter through damaged skin (e.g., burn, infection) for infection control purposes. There is no increased risk of thrombosis, vessel trauma, or infection in clinical trials, but the length of these studies has generally been <96 hours.[164,194]

Equipment

There are two basic models of bedside blood gas monitors: the extraarterial sensor system (Fig. 28-8) and the intraarterial probe system. Both methods use fiberoptic technology that indicates a variation in the analyte (i.e., blood gases and pH) by changes in the color of a reversible reagent and by the intensity of fluorescent light reflected back by the reagent. Despite the need for placing the indwelling probe through a 20-gauge catheter, its small size (approximately 0.62 mm) permits the aspiration of blood and does not alter the arterial waveform or accuracy of the blood pressure reading.[134] The display module updates the blood gas values every 6 to 30 seconds. Set high and low alarm limits to provide visual and auditory indications when the patient exceeds preset values. The response time for a significant change in blood values to trigger the alarm is <30 seconds. It is necessary to perform two-point calibration with tonometered gases.

Techniques

A properly functioning arterial catheter, mean arterial pressures >40 mm Hg, no evidence of vasospasm, and Pao$_2$ levels in the range of 60 to 150 mm Hg are necessary to ensure clinically reliable measurements of intraarterial blood gases and pH in critically ill adults.[162] Attach the indwelling

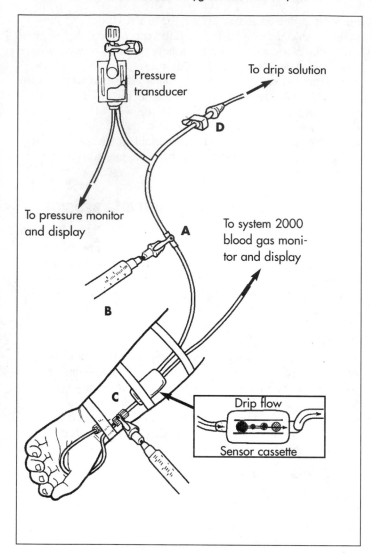

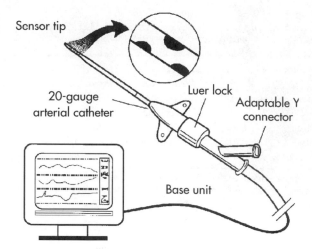

FIG. 28-9 Components of the continuous intraarterial blood gas monitoring system.

(Redrawn with permission from Zimmerman JL, Dellinger RP, *Crit Care Med* 21:495, 1993.)

FIG. 28-8 An extraarterial bedside blood gas sensor system (the CDI 2000, CDI-3M Healthcare, Tustin, Calif.). The inset depicts a longitudinal section through the sensor cassette showing the three optodes (pH, Pco_2, Po_2) and the thermistor. **A,** An "upstream" stopcock to allow function of the aspirating reservoir. **B,** A syringe representing the aspirating reservoir; other devices may also be used (e.g., needleless syringe and hub). **C,** A stopcock available for obtaining blood samples. **D,** A fast flush mechanism, often in series or parallel with the pressure transducer.

(Redrawn with permission from Shapiro BA, et al, *Crit Care Med* 21:487, 1993.)

sensor with the Luer-Lok to a previously placed arterial catheter. The sensor tip of the indwelling analyzer protrudes distal to the arterial cannula (Fig. 28-9), and the side-window arrangement of the analyte chamber found with a new system allows for rotation of the sensor when vessel-wall interaction causes any inaccuracy.[92] Minimal electrode drift after 24 hours of use occurs with the fluorescent optode sensors. After arterial blood flows into the sensor cassette, the extraarterial sensor requires a period of 2 minutes to provide an accurate reading. The extraarterial blood gas system provides blood gas readings every 3 minutes rather than continuously, which is still more rapid than conventional blood sampling and analysis.[165] To date there have been no clinical trials of the

extraarterial blood gas monitors with arterial cannulae smaller than 20 gauge.

Early intraarterial blood gas systems used miniaturized Clark electrodes instead of fluorescent optode sensors. These early systems were subject to large amounts of electrode drift, which made them unreliable as well as limited in measuring only a single blood gas (Pao_2).[98] Fluorescent optode systems have performed much better than the early electrochemical sensor systems in vitro and in vivo, but during adverse conditions such as hypothermia, they have not fared well.[112]

Remarks

Some of the obvious benefits of intravascular blood gas monitoring include a reduction in patient blood loss, diminished exposure of health-care workers to possibly infected blood, and a decrease in turnaround time, which facilitates weaning or therapy in a time-efficient manner. Some of the issues that remain to be answered include reliability during periods of hemodynamic instability, effects of vasoactive agents on accuracy, accuracy in pediatric patients, and cost-effectiveness in an age of relatively inexpensive and noninvasive measures of oxygenation and ventilation.[174] It is unclear whether intravascular blood gas monitoring will become an accepted technique in PICUs. New technologies for monitoring the adequacy of oxygenation and ventilation continue to emerge, and clinicians must evaluate their cost-effectiveness and their impact on outcome.

REFERENCES

1. Achauer BM, Black KS, Beran AV: Transcutaneous Po_2 monitoring of flap circulation following surgery, *Birth Defects: Original Article Series* XV:517-522, 1979.
2. Al Khudhairi D, et al: Evaluation of a pulse oximeter during profound hypothermia: an assessment of the Biox 3700 during induction of hypothermia before cardiac surgery in paediatric patients, *Int J Clin Monit Comput* 7:217-222, 1990.
3. Amar D, et al: Fluorescent light interferes with pulse oximetry, *J Clin Monit* 5(2):135-137, 1989.

4. Ashwood ER, Kost G, Kenny M: Temperature correction of blood-gas and pH measurements, *Clin Chem* 29(11):1877-1885, 1983.

5. Bachkert P, et al: Is pulse oximetry reliable in detecting hyperoxemia in the neonate? *Adv Exp Med Biol* 220:165-169, 1987.

6. Badgwell JM, Heavner JE: End-tidal carbon dioxide pressure in neonates and infants measured by aspiration and flow-through capnography, *J Clin Monit* 7(4):285-288, 1991.

7. Badgwell JM, et al: End-tidal Pco_2 measurements sampled at the distal end of the endotracheal tube in infants and children, *Anesth Analg* 66:959-964, 1987.

8. Bagshaw ONT, et al: Oximetry in cyanotic heart disease (letter), *Lancet* 20(2):254-255, 1992.

9. Bancalari E, et al: Influence of transcutaneous oxygen monitoring on the incidence of retinopathy of prematurity, *Pediatrics* 79:663-669, 1987.

10. Barker SJ, Tremper KK: The effect of carbon monoxide inhalation on pulse oximetry and transcutaneous Po_2, *Anesthesiology* 66:677-679, 1987.

11. Barrington KJ, Finer NN, Ryan CA: Evaluation of pulse oximetry as a continuous monitoring technique in the neonatal intensive care unit, *Crit Care Med* 16(11):1147-1153, 1988.

12. Barton CW, Callahan ML: Successful prediction by capnometry of resuscitation from cardiac arrest, *Ann Emerg Med* 17:393, 1988.

13. Bashein G, Syrovy G: Burns associated with pulse oximetry during magnetic resonance imaging, *Anesthesiology* 75:382-383, 1991.

14. Beachy P, Whitfield JM: The effect of transcutaneous Po_2 monitoring on the frequency of arterial blood gas analysis in the newborn with respiratory distress, *Crit Care Med* 9:584-586, 1981.

15. Beall SN, Moorthy SS: Jaundice, oximetry, and spurious hemoglobin desaturation, *Anesth Analg* 68:806-807, 1989.

16. Bergqvist G: Oxygen saturation in newborns at altitude (letter), *Am J Dis Child* 146(10):1134, 1992.

17. Berlin S et al: Pulse oximetry: a technology that needs direction, *Respir Care* 33:243-244, 1988.

18. Bethune DW, Baliga N: Skin injury with a pulse oximeter, *Br J Anaesth* 69(6):665, 1992.

19. Bhat R, et al: Simultaneous tissue pH and transcutaneous carbon dioxide monitoring in critically ill neonates, *Crit Care Med* 9:744-749, 1981.

20. Bhende MS, et al: Utility of an end-tidal carbon dioxide detector during stabilization and transport of critically ill children, *Pediatrics* 89:1042-1044, 1992.

21. Bierman MI, Stein KL, Snyder JV: Pulse oximetry in the postoperative care of cardiac surgical patients, *Chest* 102(5):1367-1370, 1992.

22. Blanch L, et al: Effect of PEEP on the arterial minus end-tidal carbon dioxide gradient, *Chest* 92:451-454, 1987.

23. Boxer RA, et al: Non-invasive pulse oximetry in children with cyanotic congenital heart disease, *Crit Care Med* 15:1062-1064, 1987.

24. Breuer HWM, et al: Oxygen saturation calculation procedures: a critical analysis of six equations for the determination of oxygen saturation, *Intensive Care Med* 15:385-389, 1989.

25. Brodsky J, Brock-Utne JG: End-tidal CO_2 monitoring for patients receiving epidural opiates, *J Cardiothorac Vasc Anesth* 5:102-103, 1991.

26. Bucher HU, et al: Hyperoxemia in newborn infants: detection by pulse oximetry, *Pediatrics* 84:226-230, 1989.

27. Burnett RW, et al: IFCC document Stage 3, Draft 1, dated 1989 02. An approved IFCC recommendation. IFCC method (1988) for tonometry of blood: reference materials for Pco_2 and Po_2, *Clin Chim Acta* 185:S17-24, 1989.

28. Butt WW, et al: Complications resulting from use of arterial catheters: retrograde flow and rapid elevation in blood pressure, *Pediatrics* 76:250-254, 1985.

29. Cabal LA, et al: Factors affecting heated transcutaneous Po_2 and unheated transcutaneous Pco_2 in preterm infants, *Crit Care Med* 9:298-304, 1981.

30. Callaham M, Barton C, Matthay M: Effect of epinephrine on the ability of end-tidal carbon dioxide readings to predict initial resuscitation from cardiac arrest, *Crit Care Med* 20:337-343, 1992.

31. Carlon GC, et al: Capnography in mechanically ventilated patients, *Crit Care Med* 16:550-556, 1988.

32. Casaburi R: The impact of new federal regulations on the blood gas laboratory (letter), *Chest* 101:4-5, 1992.

33. Chantarojanasiri T, et al: Arterialized capillary blood gases and acid-base studies in normal Thai children, *J Med Assoc Thai* 72(S1):57-60, 1989.

34. Chemello PD, Nelson SR, Wolford LM: Finger injury resulting from pulse oximetry during orthognathic surgery, *Oral Surg Oral Med Oral Pathol* 69:161-163, 1990.

35. Chen PP, Gin T: Spurious end-tidal CO_2 diagnosed by capnogram, *Anaesthesia* 47(10):910-911, 1992.

36. Cheriyan G, et al: Transcutaneous estimation of arterial carbon dioxide in intensive care: which electrode temperature? *Arch Dis Child* 61:652-656, 1986.

37. Clark JS, et al: Noninvasive assessment of blood gases, *Am Rev Respir Dis* 145:220-232, 1992.

38. Clarke JR, Reese A, Silverman M: Comparison of the squeeze technique and transcutaneous oxygen tension for measuring the response to bronchial challenge in normal and wheezy infants, *Pediatr Pulmonol* 15(4):244-250, 1993.

39. Clay NR, Dent CM: Limitations of pulse oximetry to assess limb vascularity, *J Bone Joint Surg Br* 73(2):344, 1991.

40. Costarino AT, Davis DA, Keon TP: Falsely normal saturation reading with the pulse oximeter, *Anesthesiology* 67:830-831, 1987.

41. Coté CJ, et al: Intraoperative events diagnosed by expired carbon dioxide monitoring in children, *Can Anaesth Soc J* 33(3):315-320, 1986.

42. Coté CJ, et al: A single-blind study of pulse oximetry in children, *Anesthesiology* 68:184-188, 1988.

43. Coté CJ, et al: Tongue oximetry in children with extensive thermal injury: comparison with peripheral oximetry, *Can J Anaesth* 39(5, part 1):454-457, 1992.

44. Cowtney SE, et al: Capillary blood gases in the neonate, *Am J Dis Child* 144:168-172, 1990.

45. Curley MAQ, Thompson JE: End-tidal CO_2 monitoring in critically ill infants and children, *Crit Care Neonatal Update* 16(4):397-403, 1990.

46. David HG: Pulse oximetry in closed limb fractures, *Ann R. Coll Surg Engl* 73(5):283-284, 1991.

47. Dawalibi L, Rozario C, Van den Bergh AA: Pulse oximetry in pulseless patients, *Anaesthesia* 46(11)990-991, 1991.

48. Deckardt R, Steward DJ: Noninvasive arterial hemoglobin oxygen saturation versus transcutaneous oxygen tension monitoring in the preterm infant, *Crit Care Med* 12:935-939, 1984.

49. Dimich I, et al: Evaluation of oxygen saturation monitoring by pulse oximetry in neonates in the delivery room, *Can J Anaesth* 38(8):985-988, 1991.

50. Duc GV, Cumarasamy N: Digital arteriolar oxygen tension as a guide to oxygen therapy of the newborn, *Biol Neonate* 24:134-137, 1974.

51. Dumpit FM, Brady JP: A simple technique for measuring alveolar CO_2 in infants, *J Appl Physiol* 45(4):648-650, 1978.

52. Durand M, Ramanathan R: Pulse oximetry for continuous oxygen monitoring in sick newborn infants, *J Pediatr* 109:1052-1056, 1986.

53. Dziedzic K, Vidyasagar D: Pulse oximetry in neonatal intensive care, *Clin Perinatol* 16:177-197, 1989.

54. ECRI problem reporting system: Different manufacturers' patient probes and pulse oximeters, *Health Devices* 19(7):244-245, 1990.

55. Eber E, Varga EM, Zach MS: Cold air challenge of airway reactivity in children: a correlation of transcutaneously measured oxygen tension and conventional lung functions, *Pediatr Pulmonol* 10(4):273-277, 1991.

56. Engle WA, Rescorla FJ: Vascular access and blood sampling techniques in infants and children. In Roberts JR, Hedges JR, editors: *Clinical procedures in emergency medicine,* ed 2, Philadelphia, 1991, WB Saunders.

57. Epstein MF, et al: Estimation of $Paco_2$ by two noninvasive methods in the critically ill newborn infant, *J Pediatr* 106:282-286, 1985.

58. FDA safety alert: Needlestick and other risks from hypodermic needles on secondary IV administration sets, piggyback, and intermittent IV, *CDRH,* HFZ-250, Rockville, Md 20857.

59. Fait CD, et al: Pulse oximetry in critically ill children, *J Clin Monit* 1:232-235, 1985.

60. Falk JL, Rackow EC, Weil MH: End-tidal carbon dioxide concentration during cardiopulmonary resuscitation, *N Engl J Med* 318(10):607-611, 1988.

61. Fanconi S: Reliability of pulse oximetry in hypoxic infants, *J Pediatr* 112:424-427, 1988.

62. Fanconi S: Pulse oximetry for hypoxemia: a warning to users and manufacturers, *Intensive Care Med* 15:540-542, 1989.

63. Fanconi S, et al: Pulse oximetry in pediatric intensive care: comparison with measured saturations and transcutaneous oxygen tension, *J Pediatr* 107:362-366, 1985.

64. Fanconi S, et al: Transcutaneous carbon dioxide pressure for monitoring patients with severe croup, *J Pediatr* 117(5):701-705, 1990.

65. Federiuk CS, Sanders AB: Artificial perfusion during cardiac arrest. In Roberts JR, Hedges JR, editors: *Clinical procedures in emergency medicine,* ed 2, Philadelphia, 1991, WB Saunders.

66. Flynn JT, et al: A cohort study of transcutaneous oxygen tension and the incidence and severity of retinopathy of prematurity, *N Engl J Med* 326:1050-1054, 1992.

67. Folger GM, Kouri P, Sabbah HN: Arterialized capillary blood sampling in the neonate: a reappraisal, *Heart Lung* 9:521-526, 1980.

68. Gambino SR, Thiede WH: Comparisons of pH in human arterial, venous, and capillary blood, *Am J Clin Pathol* 32:298-300, 1959.

69. Gardosi JA, Damianou D, Schram CM: Inappropriate sensor application in pulse oximetry, *Lancet* 340(8824):920, 1992.

70. Garnett AR et al: End-tidal carbon dioxide monitoring during cardiopulmonary resuscitation, *JAMA* 257:512-515, 1987.

71. Gayed AM, Marino ME, Dolansli EA: Comparison of the effects of dry and liquid heparin on neonatal arterial blood gases, *Am J Perinatol* 9(3):159-161, 1992.

72. Gilbert D, Benumof JL: Biphasic carbon dioxide elimination waveform with right mainstem bronchial intubation, *Anesth Analg* 69:829-832, 1989.

73. Glasgow JFT, Flynn DM, Swyer PR: A comparison of descending aortic and arterialized capillary blood in the sick newborn, *Can Med Assoc J* 106:660-662, 1972.

74. Gosling P, Dickson G: Syringe injection pressure: a neglected factor in blood Po_2 determination, *Ann Clin Biochem* 27:147-151, 1990.

75. Greenhalgh DG, Warden GD: Transcutaneous oxygen and carbon dioxide measurements for determination of skin graft "take," *J Burn Care Rehabil* 13:334-339, 1992.

76. Gudipati CV, et al: Expired carbon dioxide: a noninvasive monitor of cardiopulmonary resuscitation, *Circulation* 77:234-239, 1988.

77. Hand IL, et al: Discrepancies between transcutaneous and end-tidal carbon dioxide monitoring in the critically ill neonate with respiratory distress syndrome, *Crit Care Med* 17:556-559, 1989.

78. Hansen JE: Arterial blood gases, *Clin Chest Med* 10(2):227-237, 1989.

79. Hansen JE, et al: Comparison of blood gas analyzer biases in measuring tonometered blood and a fluorocarbon-containing, proficiency-testing material, *Am Rev Respir Dis* 140:403-409, 1989.

80. Hay WW, Brockway JM, Eyzaguirre M: Neonatal pulse oximetry: accuracy and reliability, *Pediatrics* 83(5):717-722, 1989.

81. Hay WW, Thilo E, Curlander JB: Pulse oximetry in neonatal medicine, *Clin Perinatol* 18(3):441-472, 1991.

82. Herrell N, et al: Optimal temperature for the measurement of transcutaneous carbon dioxide tension in the neonate, *J Pediatr* 97:114-117, 1980.

83. Hess CE, et al: Pseudohypoxemia secondary to leukemia and thrombocytosis, *N Engl J Med* 301:361-363, 1979.

84. Higgins D, Forrest ETS, Lloyd-Thomas A: Colorimetric end-tidal carbon dioxide monitoring during transfer of intubated children, *Intensive Care Med* 17:63-64, 1991.

85. Iwasaki J, et al: An investigation of capnography and pulse oximetry as monitors of pediatric patients sedated for dental treatment, *Pediatr Dent* 11(2):111-117, 1989.

86. Jardin F, et al: Inability to titrate PEEP in patients with acute respiratory failure using end-tidal carbon dioxide measurements, *Anesthesiology* 62:530-533, 1985.

87. Jennis MS, Peabody JL: Pulse oximetry: an alternative method for the assessment of oxygenation in newborn infants, *Pediatrics* 79:524-528, 1987.

88. Jobes DR, Nicolson SC: Monitoring of arterial hemoglobin oxygen saturation using a tongue sensor, *Anesth Analg* 67:186-188, 1988.

89. Johnson N, et al: The effect of meconium on neonatal and fetal reflectance pulse oximetry, *J Perinat Med* 18(5):351-355, 1990.

90. Keifer JC, et al: Pulse oximetry inaccuracy with sickle cell hemoglobin: is it due to a different absorption spectra? *Resp Care* 34:1019-1020, 1989.

91. Keller HP, Klaye P, Hockerts T: Transcutaneous Po_2 measurements on skin transplants, *Birth Defects: Original Article Series* XV:511-516, 1979.

92. Kilbride HW, Meenstein GB: Continuous transcutaneous oxygen monitoring in acutely ill preterm infants, *Crit Care Med* 12:121-124, 1984.

93. Kirshon B, Moise KJ: Effect of heparin on umbilical arterial blood gases, *J Reprod Med* 34(4):267-269, 1989.

94. Koch G, Wendel H: Comparison of pH, carbon dioxide tension, standard bicarbonate and oxygen tension in capillary blood and in arterial blood during the neonatal period, *Acta Paediatr Scand* 56:10-16, 1967.

95. Lauer BA, Altenburger KM: Outbreak of staphylococcal infections following heel puncture for blood sampling, *Am J Dis Child* 135:277-278, 1981.

96. Lebecque P, et al: Pulse oximetry versus measured arterial oxygen saturation: a comparison of the Nellcor N100 and the Biox III, *Pediatr Pulmonol* 10:132-135, 1991.

97. Lee HK, Broadhurst E, Helms P: Evaluation of two combined oxygen and carbon dioxide transcutaneous sensors, *Arch Dis Child* 64(2):279-282, 1989.

98. Lemus JF, et al: Continuous intra-arterial oxygen monitoring: accuracy and reliability in the surgical intensive care unit, *Am Surg* 58(12):740-742, 1992.

99. Lepilin MG, et al: End-tidal carbon dioxide as a noninvasive monitor of circulatory status during cardiopulmonary resuscitation: a preliminary clinical study, *Crit Care Med* 15:958-959, 1987.

100. Levene S, McKenzie SA: Pulse oximetry in children, *Lancet* 1:415, 1988.

101. Levene S, Lear GH, McKenzie SA: Comparison of pulse oximeters in healthy sleeping infants, *Respir Med* 83(3):233-235, 1989.

102. Lilien LD, et al: Neonatal osteomyelitis of the calcaneus: complication of heel puncture, *J Pediatr* 88:478-480, 1976.

103. Lindahl SGE, Yates AP, Hatch DJ: Relationship between invasive and noninvasive measurements of gas exchange in anesthetized infants and children, *Anesthesiology* 66:168-175, 1987.

104. Liu S, Lee T, Bongard F: Accuracy of capnography in nonintubated surgical patients, *Chest* 102:1512-1515, 1992.

105. Lozano JM, et al: Pulse oximetry reference values at high altitude, *Arch Dis Child* 67(3):299-301, 1992.

106. Luce EA, et al: Compression neuropathy following brachial arterial puncture in anticoagulated patients, *J Trauma* 16:717-721, 1976.

107. Luz G, et al: Discrepancies between transcutaneous and end-tidal carbon dioxide monitoring in the critically ill neonate with respiratory distress syndrome, *Crit Care Med* 18(9):1050, 1990.

108. Mackersie RC, Karagianes TG: Use of end-tidal carbon dioxide tension for monitoring induced hypocapnia in head-injured patients, *Crit Care Med* 18(7):764-765, 1990.

109. Macnab JA, Baker-Brown G, Anderson EE: Oximetry in children recovering from deep hypothermia for cardiac surgery, *Crit Care Med* 18(10):1066-1069, 1990.

110. Madiedo G, Sciacca R, Hause L: Air bubbles and temperatures effect on blood gas analysis, *J Clin Pathol* 33:864-867, 1980.

111. Maher JJ, Dougherty JM: Radial artery cannulation guided by Doppler ultrasound, *Am J Emerg Med* 7:260-262, 1989.

112. Mark JB, et al: Continuous arterial and venous blood gas monitoring during cardiopulmonary bypass, *J Thorac Cardiovasc Surg* 102:431-439, 1991.

113. Mars M, Hadley GP: Pulse oximetry in the assessment of limb perfusion, *S Afr Med J* 82(6):486, 1992.

114. Marsden D, et al: Transcutaneous oxygen and carbon dioxide monitoring in intensive care, *Arch Dis Child* 60:1158-1161, 1985.

115. McEvedy BAB, et al: End-tidal, transcutaneous, and arterial Pco_2 measurements in critically ill neonates: a comparative study, *Anesthesiology* 69:112-116, 1988.

116. McLain BI, Evans J, Dear PRF: Comparison of capillary and arterial blood gas measurements in neonates, *Arch Dis Child* 63:743-747, 1988.

117. Meier-Stauss P, et al: Pulse oximetry used for documenting oxygen saturation and right-to-left shunting immediately after birth, *Eur J Pediatr* 149:851-855, 1990.

118. Meny RG, Bhat AM, Aranas E: Mass spectrometer monitoring of expired carbon dioxide in critically ill neonates, *Crit Care Med* 13(12):1064-1066, 1985.

119. Meredith KS, Monaco FJ: Evaluation of a mainstream capnometer and end-tidal carbon dioxide monitoring in mechanically ventilated infants, *Pediatr Pulmonol* 9:254-259, 1990.

120. Mills GH, Ralph SJ: Burns due to pulse oximetry, *Anaesthesia* 47:276-277, 1992.

121. Mok J, et al: Evaluation of noninvasive measurements of oxygenation in stable infants, *Crit Care Med* 14:960-963, 1986.

122. Moore FA, Haenel JB: Advances in oxygen monitoring of trauma patients, *Med Instrum* 22(3):135-142, 1988.

123. Moorthy SS, Losasso AM, Wilcox J: End-tidal Pco_2 greater than $Paco_2$, *Crit Care Med* 12:534-535, 1984.

124. Maukkassa FF, et al: ABGs and arterial lines: the relationship to unnecessarily drawn arterial blood gas samples, *J Trauma* 30(9):1087-1095, 1990.

125. Murphy KG, Secunda JA, Rockoff MA: Severe burns from a pulse oximeter, *Anesthesiology* 73:350-352, 1990.

126. Murray IP, et al: Titration of PEEP by the arterial minus end-tidal carbon dioxide gradient, *Chest* 85:100-104, 1984.

127. Nicolson SC, et al: Evaluation of a user-operated patient-side blood gas and chemistry monitor in children undergoing cardiac surgery, *J Cardiothorac Anesth* 3(6):741-744, 1989.

128. Omato JP, et al: Relationship between cardiac output and the end-tidal carbon dioxide tension, *Ann Emerg Med* 19:1104-1106, 1990.

129. Ordog G, Wasserberger J, Balasubramaniam S: Effect of heparin on arterial blood gases, *Ann Emerg Med* 14:233-238, 1985.

130. Orkin DJ: Practice standards: the midas touch or the emperor's new clothes? *Anesthesiology* 70(4):567-571, 1989.

131. Palmisano BW, Severinghaus JW: Transcutaneous Pco_2 and Po_2: a multicenter study of accuracy, *J Clin Monit* 6(3):189-195, 1990.

132. Pascucci RC, Schena JA, Thompson JE: Comparison of a sidestream and mainstream capnometer in infants, *Crit Care Med* 17:560-562, 1989.

133. Peabody JL, Emery JR: Noninvasive monitoring of blood gases in the newborn, *Clin Perinatol* 12:147-160, 1985.

134. Peavey KJ, Hall MW: Transcutaneous oxygen monitoring: economic impact on neonatal care, *Pediatrics* 75:1065-1067, 1985.

135. Pettersen B, Kongsgaard U, Aune H: Skin injury in an infant with pulse oximetry, *Br J Anaesth* 69:204-205, 1992.

136. Phillips B, Peretz DI: A comparison of central venous and arterial blood gas values in the critically ill, *Ann Intern Med* 70:745-749, 1969.

137. Poets CF, Seidenberg J, Von der Hardt H: Failure of pulse oximeter to detect sensor detachment, *Lancet* 341(8839):244, 1993.

138. Poets CF, et al: Reliability of a pulse oximeter in the detection of hyperoxemia, *J Pediatr* 122:87-90, 1993.

139. Pradal U, Braggion C, Mastella G: Transcutaneous blood gas analysis during sleep and exercise in cystic fibrosis, *Pediatr Pulmonol* 8(3):162-167, 1990.

140. Praud JP, et al: Accuracy of two-wavelength pulse oximetry in neonates and infants, *Pediatr Pulmonol* 6:180-182, 1989.

141. Preusser BA, et al: Quantifying the minimum discard sample required for accurate arterial blood gases, *Nurs Res* 38(5):276-279; 1989.

142. Rajadurai VS, et al: Effect of fetal haemoglobin on the accuracy of pulse oximetry in preterm infants, *J Paediatr Child Health* 28:43-46, 1992.

143. Ramanathan R, Durand M, Larrazabal C: Pulse oximetry in very low birth weight infants with acute and chronic disease, *Pediatrics* 79:612-617, 1987.

144. Ray SA, Ivory JP, Beavis JP: Use of pulse oximetry during manipulation of supracondylar fractures of the humerus, *Injury* 21(2):103-104, 1991.

145. Rello J, et al: False hypoxemia induced by leukocytosis (letter), *Crit Care Med* 17(9):970, 1989.

146. Rifai N, et al: Organic acids interfere in the measurement of carbon dioxide concentration by the Kodak Ektachem 700, *Ann Clin Biochem* 29:105-108, 1992.

147. Rome, ES, et al: Limitations of transcutaneous Po_2 and Pco_2 monitoring in infants with bronchopulmonary dysplasia, *Pediatrics* 74:217-220, 1984.

148. Rosenberg M, Block CS: A simple, disposable end-tidal carbon dioxide detector, *Anesth Prog* 38:24-26, 1991.

149. Russell RIR, Helms PJ: Comparative accuracy of pulse oximetry and transcutaneous oxygen in assessing arterial saturation in pediatric intensive care, *Crit Care Med* 18:725-727, 1990.

150. Saili A, Dutta AK, Sarna MS: Reliability of capillary blood gas estimation in neonates, *Indian Pediatr* 29(5):567-570, 1992.

151. Salvo I, et al: Pulse oximetry in MRI units (letter), *J Clin Anesth* 2:65-66, 1990.

152. Salyer JW, Lewis DD: Pulse oximetry: application in the pediatric and neonatal critical care unit, *AACN Clin Issues Crit Care Nurs* 1(2):339-347, 1990.

153. Sanders AB, Ewy GA, Taft TV: Resuscitation and arterial blood gas abnormalities during prolonged cardiopulmonary resuscitation, *Ann Emerg Med* 13:676-679, 1984.

154. Sanders AB, et al: Expired Pco_2 as a prognostic indicator of successful resuscitation from cardiac arrest, *Ann Emerg Med* 14:948-952, 1985.

155. Scheinhorn D, Angelillo V: Heparin sodium and arterial blood gas analysis, *Chest* 73:244-245, 1978.

156. Scheller M, Unger RJ, Kelner MJ: Effects of intravenously administered dyes on pulse oximeter readings, *Anesthesiology* 65:550-552, 1986.

157. Schena J, Thompson J, Crone RK: Mechanical influences on the capnogram, *Crit Care Med* 12:672-674, 1984.

158. Sendak MJ, Harris AP, Donham RT: Use of pulse oximetry to assess arterial oxygen saturation during newborn resuscitation, *Crit Care Med* 14(8):739-740, 1986.

159. Serpell MG: Children's fingers and spurious pulse oximetry, *Anaesthesia* 46(8):702-703, 1991.

160. Severinghaus JW, Naifeh KH: Accuracy of response of six pulse oximeters to profound hypoxia, *Anesthesiology* 67:551-558, 1987.

161. Severinghaus JW, Naifeh KH, Koh SO: Errors in 14 pulse oximeters during profound hypoxia, *J Clin Monit* 5:72-81, 1989.

162. Shapiro BA, Cane RD: Progress in the development of a fluorescent intravascular blood gas system in man (letter), *J Clin Monit* 7(2):212, 1991.

163. Shapiro BA, et al: *Clinical application of blood gases,* ed 4, Chicago, 1989, Year Book Medical.

164. Shapiro BA, et al: Preliminary evaluation of an intra-arterial blood gas system in dogs and humans, *Crit Care Med* 17(5):455-460, 1989.

165. Shapiro BA, et al: Clinical performance of a blood gas monitor: a prospective, multicenter trial, *Crit Care Med* 21:487-494, 1993.

166. Shohat M, et al: Determination of blood gases in children with extreme leukocytosis, *Crit Care Med* 16:787-788, 1988.

167. Skoog RE: Capnography in the postanesthesia care unit, *J Post Anesth Nurs* 4(3):147-155, 1989.

168. Swedlow DB: Capnometry and capnography: the anesthesia disaster early warning system, *Semin Anesth* 5:194-205, 1986.

169. Takatani S, et al: Experimental and clinical evaluation of a noninvasive reflectance pulse oximeter sensor, *J Clin Monit* 8(4):257-266, 1992.

170. Temper KK, Barker SJ: Pulse oximetry, *Anesthesiology* 70:98-108, 1989.

171. Thilo EH, et al: Oxygen saturation by pulse oximetry in healthy infants at an altitude of 1610 m (5280 ft): what is normal? *Am J Dis Child* 145(10):1137-1140, 1991.

172. Thomson KD, Inoue T, Payne JP: The use of pulse oximetry in post-operative hypoxaemia in patients after propofol induction of anaesthesia, *Int J Clin Monit Comput* 6:7-10, 1989.

173. Tobin MJ: Respiratory monitoring in the intensive care unit, *Am Rev Respir Dis* 138:1625-1642, 1988.

174. Tremper KK: The optode: next generation in blood gas measurement, *Crit Care Med* 17:481-482, 1989.

175. Tremper KK, et al: Accuracy of a pulse oximeter in the critically ill adult: effect of temperature and hemodynamics, *Anesthesiology* 63:A175, 1985.

176. Trevino RP, et al: End-tidal CO_2 as a guide to successful cardiopulmonary resuscitation: a preliminary report, *Crit Care Med* 13:910-911, 1985.

177. van Brockhoven P: Comparison of FEV1 and transcutaneous oxygen tension in the measurement of airway responsiveness to methacholine, *Pediatr Pulmonol* 11(3):254-258, 1991.

178. Varon AJ, Morrina J, Civetta JM: Clinical utility of a colorimetric end-tidal CO_2 detector in cardiopulmonary resuscitation and emergency intubation, *J Clin Monit* 7:289-293, 1991.

179. Veyckemans F, et al: Hyperbilirubinemia does not interfere with hemoglobin saturation measured by pulse oximetry, *Anesthesiology* 70:118-122, 1989.

180. Waffarn F, Tolle CD, Huxtable RF: Effects of polycythemia and hyperviscosity on cutaneous blood flow and transcutaneous P_{O_2} and P_{CO_2} in the neonate, *Pediatrics* 74:389-394, 1984.

181. Watcha M, Connor MT, Hing AV: Pulse oximetry in methemoglobinemia, *AJDC* 143:845-847, 1989.

182. Watkins AMC, Weindling AM: Monitoring of end-tidal CO_2 in neonatal intensive care, *Arch Dis Child* 62:837-839, 1987.

183. Weibley RE, Riggs D: Evaluation of an improved sampling method for blood gas analysis from indwelling arterial catheters, *Crit Care Med* 17(8):803-805, 1989.

184. Weil MH, et al: Cardiac output and end-tidal carbon dioxide, *Crit Care Med* 13:907-909, 1985.

185. Weingarten M: Respiratory monitoring of carbon dioxide and oxygen: a ten-year perspective. *J Clin Monit* 6(3):217-225, 1990.

186. Wilson S: Conscious sedation and pulse oximetry: false alarms? *Pediatr Dent* 12(4):228-232, 1990.

187. Wilts M, et al: Measurement of bronchial responsiveness in young children: comparison of transcutaneous oxygen tension and functional residual capacity during induced bronchoconstriction and bronchodilatation, *Pediatr Pulmonol* 12(3):181-185, 1992.

188. Winberley PD, et al: International Federation of Clinical Chemistry (IFCC) Scientific Division Committee on pH, blood gases and electrolytes: guidelines for transcutaneous P_{O_2} and P_{CO_2} measurement, *Ann Biol Clin* 48:39-43, 1990.

189. Winquist RA, Stamm SJ: Arterialized capillary sampling using histamine iontophoresis, *J Pediatr* 76:455-458, 1970.

190. Wukitsch MW, et al: Pulse oximetry: analysis of theory, technology, and practice, *J Clin Monit* 4:290-301, 1988.

191. Yamanaka MK, Sue DY: Comparison of arterial-end-tidal P_{CO_2} difference and dead space/tidal volume ratio in respiratory failure, *Chest* 92(5):832-835, 1987.

192. Yogasakaran BS: Misleading capnography in primary pulmonary hypertension, *J Cardiothorac Vasc Anesth* 6(3):385-386, 1992.

193. Zaloga GP, et al: Bedside blood gas and electrolyte monitoring in critically ill patients, *Crit Care Med* 17(9):920-925, 1989.

194. Zimmerman JL, Dellinger RP: Initial evaluation of a new intra-arterial blood gas system in humans, *Crit Care Med* 21:495-500, 1993.

29 Management of Endotracheal Extubation

Bonnie C. Desselle and Gregory L. Stidham

Endotracheal extubation is the culmination of a successful course of airway protection and/or mechanical ventilation therapy. However the success of an extubation depends on several factors in addition to the recovery of pulmonary function, including the clinician's ability to assess accurately the patient's readiness for extubation, the correct handling of the actual extubation procedure, and the prompt identification and treatment of several potential postextubation complications.

Indications and Contraindications

Preextubation Assessment

PREDICTING READINESS FOR EXTUBATION. Several investigators have examined the potential use of easily measurable parameters as predictors of successful extubation in mechanically ventilated adults.* Table 29-1 summarizes some of these. Unfortunately investigators have conducted considerably fewer studies in pediatric patients. Shimada et al.[23] have shown that a crying vital capacity of greater than 15 ml/kg and a maximal negative inspiratory force of less than −45 cm H_2O in infants are associated with successful extubation. Finally there is one time-honored clinical test of muscle reserve, particularly useful in patients who have undergone neuromuscular blockade, which is unique in its simplicity. The ability to raise the head from a pillow for 5 seconds or more virtually ensures adequate muscle strength for normal ventilation.

Postextubation subglottic edema represents a potential complication independent of inadequate respiratory muscle reserve. A good test to identify patients at risk for postextubation croup and upper airway obstruction is the "endotracheal tube cuff leak." One performs this test by allowing the airway pressure to increase passively with a manometer in place until an air leak is audible. An air leak at 20 to 30 cm H_2O pressure is associated with a minimal probability of postextubation airway obstructive symptoms.[1,10,13,22,25] The absence of an air leak does not predict an extubation failure, though it does indicate a greater chance that difficulties will occur.

WEANING TRIALS. After weaning a patient to minimal ventilatory support ($FIo_2 < 0.50$, PEEP < 2 to 5 cm H_2O, rate ≤6/min with adequate oxygenation and ventilation and minimal work of breathing, consider the patient's pulmonary reserve adequate for extubation. Although historically many have considered a trial of continuous positive airway pressure (CPAP) alone without positive-pressure support the final trial of extubation readiness, there are more recent counterarguments to this step. The increased airway resistance imposed by breathing through the narrow endotracheal tube produces significantly increased work of breathing. This

increased work may be especially significant in the infant, for whom CPAP trials may be particularly misleading as indicators of extubation readiness.[18] Several studies have suggested that extubation of infants from rates of 6 or less without a CPAP trial is safe and advantageous.[16,17]

VISUALIZATION. Some have advocated visualization of the supraglottic airway as a way of assessing this anatomic feature for extubation readiness.[3] With adequate sedation visualize the child's larynx with a laryngoscope and examine the airway for aryepiglottic, epiglottic, and vocal cord swelling. This procedure may be particularly useful in children with acute epiglottitis,[12] in whom reduction of epiglottic swelling with reappearance of the normal epiglottic curvature virtually guarantees successful extubation. Others however argue that this is an unnecessary precaution with acute epiglottitis[4] and that other guidelines (such as time since defervescence, reappearance of air leak, and arbitrary duration of intubation) are sufficient.

LEVEL OF CONSCIOUSNESS. Neurologically injured or impaired patients present additional challenges. Children who are recovering from impaired consciousness often have varying levels of consciousness, with waxing and waning of their ability to protect their airway. To ensure that these patients are truly candidates for extubation the physician and nursing staff must evaluate both cough and gag reflexes every several hours for at least 24 hours before anticipated extubation to ensure that these protective reflexes are consistently present.

Complications

Upper Airway Compromise. Close monitoring of patients after extubation is crucial to the early recognition and treatment of potential complications. Routine monitoring of heart and respiratory rates, pulse oximetry, and occasionally transcutaneous carbon dioxide monitoring give clues to respiratory deterioration.

Simple clinical monitoring of air exchange and retractions may be the most helpful in observing for upper airway obstruction secondary to subglottic edema. Treat this complication, the most common complication after extubation, with racemic epinephrine and steroids. Patients in whom serious subglottic edema develops generally have symptoms within the first 2 hours after extubation, and their obstruction generally peaks at 8 to 12 hours. Patients who have no symptoms in the first 2 hours generally do not experience severe obstruction. Especially in high-risk patients the early use of aerosolized racemic epinephrine, even *before* the onset of symptoms, may be more important than even prophylactic treatments undertaken before extubation.

The use of an inhaled gas mixture of helium and oxygen (usually 60%:40%) may represent an important temporizing measure in patients with moderately severe subglottic edema. Because density of helium is much lower than that of nitrogen, the resistance to flow of this gas mixture is much

---

*References 7, 9, 20, 21, 24, 26, 27, and 29.

Table 29-1 Predictors of Successful Extubation in Intubated Adult Patients*

Oxygenation	Ventilatory mechanics	Respiratory muscle strength	Ventilatory demand	Ventilatory reserve
$Pao_2/FIo_2 > 200$	Vital capacity > 10–15 ml/kg	Negative inspiratory force < −30 mm Hg	Minute ventilation <10 l/min $Paco_2 \leq 40$	Mandatory voluntary ventilation > 2x minute ventilation for $Paco_2 \leq 40$
Alveolar-arterial Po_2 gradient < 350 mm Hg $Pao_2 > 60$ with $FIo_2 < 0.35$	Tidal volume >5 ml/lg		Vd/Vt < 0.6	

*Pao_2, Partial pressure of oxygen in arterial blood; FIo_2, fractional concentration of oxygen in inspired gas; Po_2, partial pressure of oxygen; $Paco_2$, partial pressure of carbon dioxide in arterial blood; Vd/Vt, dead space/tidal volume.

less than that of the usual oxygen/nitrogen mixture. This approach has helped to prevent the additional trauma of reintubation in patients who are approaching failure from upper airway obstruction,[14,15] but in no way obviates the need for careful clinical monitoring and prompt reintubation when the patient is progressing toward respiratory failure.

Reintubate patients in whom the extubation attempt is unsuccessful as a result of upper airway obstruction with a tube at least 0.5 mm smaller than the previous tube. Plan a second attempt at extubation in 24 to 48 hours, after institution of steroids and tissue dehydration strategies described in Preextubation Procedure. At this point, consider otolaryngologic consultation in light of the increased likelihood of other anatomic lesions and of prior underlying airway narrowing. Laryngoscopy and bronchoscopy at the time of reattempted extubation may reveal tracheal stenosis, granulomas, webs, or dislocated arytenoid cartilage.[2,28] Vocal cord ulcerations and motion abnormalities may also be present, though these problems usually resolve without intervention. Vocal cord paresis may be particularly problematic, however, because of its association with marked increased risk of aspiration. Prior knowledge that paresis exists may help to reduce this risk.

Atelectasis. Less dramatic than postextubation croup is the relatively common complication of atelectasis after extubation. This complication may be due to interference with mucociliary clearance during and immediately after extubation, in combination with the resolving underlying lung disease. Right upper lobe involvement is most common. This observation may reflect the occasional high (tracheal) orifice of the right upper lobe bronchus, which mucosal edema may partially occlude if the endotracheal tube has intermittently caused irritation to the orifice. The clinicain should anticipate atelectasis and look for it clinically and/or radiographically after extubation. Treat atelectasis with chest physiotherapy concentrating on the involved portions of lung.

Equipment and Technique

Preextubation Preparation

STEROIDS. Although some controversy concerning the use of steroid treatment before extubation still exists, a number of well-designed, controlled studies suggest its efficacy.[5,6,8,11] These studies have all shown the effectiveness of various doses of different steroids for various lengths of time before the planned time of extubation. Some intensivists use dexamethasone (0.25 mg/kg/dose intravenously) in patients in whom the endotracheal tube leak test has identified as at high risk for postextubation upper airway obstruction, and in those with significant risk factors (traumatic intubation, prolonged or multiple intubations, cervical or laryngeal surgical procedures, etc.). Begin steroid treatment approximately 24 hours before planned extubation and continue it into the first 24 hours after extubation.

TISSUE DEHYDRATION. In addition to steroid pretreatment consider a variation of an approach originally proposed by Otherson[19] in the pretreatment of high-risk patients. Within approximately 18 hours of the anticipated time of extubation, administer two doses of intravenous 25% albumin (0.5 to 1 g/kg) over 10 to 15 minutes simultaneously with furosemide (1 mg/kg) in an effort to reduce tissue edema and promote diuresis of mobilized extravascular fluid. Fluid restriction before extubation helps to promote tissue dehydration, ideally also facilitating reduction of subglottic edema. Although no one has conducted rigorous controlled trials on any of these regimens, Otherson's experience with historical predictors has suggested this approach to be helpful in high-risk patients.

Extubation Procedure

On extubation patients are at unusual risk for vomiting and potential aspiration. The prior presence of the endotracheal tube may temporarily impair the adequacy of laryngeal reflexes and vocal cord function. The tendency to swallow air, particularly in younger children, during periods of respiratory distress may also contribute to the risk of vomiting and aspiration. Consequently, maintain NPO status for 4 to 6 hours before extubation and evacuate stomach contents with a nasogastric tube.

Preparation for extubation necessarily must also include preparation for possible reintubation, including ensuring the availability of necessary medications and equipment, such as sedating and paralyzing agents, suction with a Yankauer suction probe, laryngoscope, and appropriate sizes of endotracheal tubes.

The actual procedure for extubation is the following: (1) Place the patient in a semi-erect position; (2) carefully suction the endotracheal tube, as well as the nasal and oral passages; (3) hyperoxygenate the patient with 100% oxygen for several minutes using manual bag ventilation; (4) deflate the endotracheal tube cuff, if present; (5) instruct older and cooperative patients to cough as the tube is removed, or remove the tube while delivering positive pressure; (6) encourage deep breathing and coughing immediately after tube removal.

REFERENCES

1. Adderley RJ, Mullins GC: When to extubate the croup patient: the "leak" test, *Can J Anesth* 34(3):304-306, 1987.
2. Alessi DM, Hanson DG, Berci G: Bedside videolaryngoscopic assessment of intubation-induced injury, *Ann R Coll Surg Engl* 72:353-356, 1990.
3. Benjamin B: Prolonged intubation injuries of the larynx: endoscopic diagnosis, classification, and treatment, *Ann Otol Rhin Laryngol* 160 (suppl):1-15, 1993.
4. Butt W, Shann F, Walker C, et al: Acute epiglottitis: a different approach to management, *Crit Care Med* 16(1):43-47, 1988.
5. Couser RJ, Ferrara TB, Falde B, et al: Effectiveness of dexamethasone in preventing extubation failure in preterm infants at increased risk for airway edema, *J Pediatr* 121(4):591-596, 1992.
6. Damon JY, Rauss A, Dreyfuss D et al: Evaluation of risk factors for laryngeal edema after tracheal extubation in adults and its prevention by dexamethasone, *Anesthesiology* 77(2):245-251, 1992.
7. Feeley TW, Hedley-White J: Weaning from controlled ventilation and supplemental oxygen, *N Engl J Med* 292:903-906, 1975.
8. Ferrara TB, Georgieff MK, Ebert J et al: Routine use of dexamethasone for the prevention of post-extubation respiratory distress, *J Perinatol* 9(30):287-290, 1989.
9. Fiastro JF, Habib MP, Shon BY et al: Comparison of standard weaning parameters and the mechanical work of breathing in mechanically ventilated patients, *Chest* 94:232-238, 1988.
10. Fisher MM, Raper RF: The "cuff-leak" test for extubation, *Anaesthesia* 47(1):10-12, 1992.
11. Freezer N, Butt W, Phelan P: Steroids in croup: do they increase the incidence of successful extubation? *Anaesth Intensive Care* 18(2):224-228, 1990.
12. Gonzalez C, Reilly JS, Kenna MA et al: Duration of intubation in children with acute epiglottitis, *Otolaryngol Head Neck Surg* 95(4):477-481, 1986.
13. Kemper KH, Benson MS, Bishop MJ: Predictors of post-extubation stridor in pediatric trauma patients, *Crit Care Med* 19(3):304-306, 1991.
14. Kemper KJ, Izenberg S, Marvin JA et al: Treatment of post-extubation stridor in a pediatric patient with burns: the role of heliox, *J Burn Care Rehabil* 11(4):337-339, 1990.
15. Kemper KJ, Ritz RH, Benson MS et al: Helium-oxygen mixture in the treatment of post-extubation stridor in pediatric trauma patients, *Crit Care Med* 19(3):356-359, 1991.
16. Kim EH: Successful extubation of newborn infants without pre-extubation trial of continuous positive airway pressure, *J Perinatol* 9(1):72-76, 1986.
17. Kim EH, Boutwell WC: Successful direct extubation of very low birth weight infants from low intermittent mandatory ventilation rate, *Pediatrics* 80(3):409-414, 1987.
18. LaSouef PN, England SJ, Bryan AC: Total resistance of the respiratory system in preterm infants with and without an endotracheal tube, *J Pediatr* 104(1):108-111, 1984.
19. Otherson HB: Intubation injuries of the trachea in children: management and prevention, *Ann Surg* 189:601-606, 1979.
20. Pierson DJ: Weaning from mechanical ventilation in acute respiratory failure: concepts, indications, and techniques, *Respir Care* 28:646-662, 1983.
21. Sahn SA, Lakshminarayan S: Bedside criteria for discontinuation of mechanical ventilation, *Chest* 63:1002-1005, 1973.
22. Seid AB, Godin MS, Pransy SM et al: The prognostic value of endotracheal tube air leak following tracheal surgery in children, *Arch Otolaryngol Head Neck Surg* 118(4):448-449, 1992.
23. Shimada Y, Yoshiya I, Tnaka K et al: Crying vital capacity and maximal inspiratory pressure as clinical indicators of readiness for weaning of infants less than a year of age, *Anesthesiology* 51:456-459, 1979.
24. Tahvanaienen J, Salmenpera M, Kikki P: Extubation criteria after weaning from intermittent mandatory ventilation and continuous positive airway pressure, *Crit Care Med* 11:702-707, 1983.
25. Tamburro RF, Bugnitz MC: Tracheal airleak as a predictor of post-extubation stridor in the paediatric intensive care unit, *Clin Intern Care* 4:52-55, 1993.
26. Tobin MK: Respiratory parameters for successful weaning, *J Crit Illness* 5:819-837, 1990.
27. Tobin MK, Skorodin M, Alex CG: Weaning from mechanical ventilation. In Taylor RW, Shoemaker, editors: *Critical care: state of the art*, Fullerton, Calif, 1991, Society of Critical Care Medicine.
28. Tolley NS, Cheesman TD, Morgan D et al: Dislocated arytenoid: an intubation-induced injury, *Ann R Coll Surg Engl* 72:353-356, 1990.
29. Yang KI, Tobin MJ: A prospective study of indexes predicting the outcome of trials of weaning from mechanical ventilation, *N Engl J Med* 5:819-837, 1991.

PART VII

VASCULAR ACCESS AND HEMODYNAMIC MONITORING

30 Peripheral Vascular Access

Patricia A. Webster and Mary R. Salassi-Scotter

Since the institution of modern intravenous therapy over 50 years ago, peripheral vascular access has been a challenge in the pediatric patient.[33] Until the late 1960s venesection or surgical venous cutdown was the most reliable method of establishing vascular access in the infant or small child.[6] However, continued improvement in catheter size and type and simplified percutaneous techniques have made peripheral, percutaneously placed catheters the vascular access method of choice.

Indications

Indications for placing peripheral venous catheters include replacement of fluids, administration of blood products, correction of electrolyte abnormalities, administration of medications, parenteral nutrition when enteral nutrition is inadequate or contraindicated, and blood sampling for diagnostic tests.[4,12,23,24,27]

Following established protocols for emergency access situations can decrease the time needed to establish intravenous access.[1,4,9,24] Attempt large-bore peripheral, percutaneously placed catheters first, then try more invasive methods. In an emergency, the cutdown has its greatest utility. The success rate for emergency cutdown is 81%, although the cutdown is seldom completed before vascular access is achieved by other means. The cutdown however remains a useful technique because it is more stable than an intraosseous line and is therefore more useful postresuscitation.[9]

In nonemergencies, use the cutdown only when all other methods of obtaining percutaneous venous access have failed, including percutaneously placed central venous lines.[30] Nonemergency indications for the cutdown include extreme obesity, intravenous (IV) drug abuse, burns or scars over peripheral veins,[26] and cases in which it is no longer possible to cannulate peripheral veins percutaneously because of frequent previous catheter placement.

Peripherally inserted central catheters, or PICC lines, are long-term IV access devices for peripheral insertion; either use them peripherally or advance into the central circulation.[3,11] These lines may be particularly useful for the prolonged (>3 weeks) delivery of chemotherapy, total parenteral nutrition, and hyperosmolar or other vessel-irritating fluids in the absence of other central venous access.[2,5] Other indications for PICC lines include previous multiple unsuccessful peripheral IV attempts or an existing need for vascular access without surgical risk.[11] This chapter only addresses the peripheral use of these lines. However, the clinical indications for the line, type of therapy, and level and expertise of the practitioner dictate whether to thread the PICC lines centrally or peripherally.[2]

Contraindications

There are few, if any, true contraindications to the use of peripheral venous catheters, percutaneous or cutdown.[12] Relative contraindications include cellulitis overlying the vein,[26] proximal vein injury, and unstable fractures proximal to the IV site.[25] Consider the possibility of proximal vein occlusion or disruption in the presence of severe abdominal trauma or severe pelvic fracture.[18] Avoid deep venous punctures or cutdowns in children with uncorrected coagulopathies and placement of catheters in the neck veins of small infants with respiratory distress or intracranial abnormality.[23]

Complications

Peripheral venous catheterization may result in both local and systemic complications, as shown in Table 30-1. Severe complications are rare, especially with appropriate insertion technique and care of the catheter. The most common complications in pediatric patients are phlebitis and IV infiltration. In addition air or catheter embolus may occur,[25] as well as hematoma formation.[32] Injury to adjacent structures (arteries, tendons, nerves) or to the vein itself may occur during attempts at catheterization or cutdown. Infectious complications are infrequent but more likely to occur with a cutdown than with a percutaneously placed catheter. The risk of infection diminishes with removal if catheters placed by cutdown are removed within 24 hours of placement.[18] It is possible to decrease the incidence of wound-or catheter-associated infection with the use of a topical antibiotic ointment.[16] Rarely compartment syndrome may occur, especially if extravasation entails the use of a deep intravenous catheter and infusion pump.

Equipment

Catheters for peripheral venous access include butterfly needles, over-the-needle catheters, and through-the-needle catheters. The primary use of butterfly needles is as venipuncture devices for blood sampling. They are relatively easy to place but infiltrate easily; therefore do not use them for long-term access or for infusion of fluids at fast rates or large volumes.[4] Through-the-needle catheters are somewhat more difficult to place, and it is best to place them in large veins. Over-the-needle catheters have the greatest versatility and are appropriate for placement in large or small veins. Steel needles result in fewer infectious complications, but plastic catheters last three times as long as they do.[12]

Intravenous catheters are made in a variety of sizes and materials. Nonstick (Teflon) and polyvinylchloride (PVC) catheters are stiff and may damage the vein intima, predisposing to thrombophlebitis. Use these catheters for short-term therapy. Silicone catheters are more flexible and more difficult to place. The composition of most catheters is polyurethane. These catheters have the advantages of intermediate flexibility, ease of placement, and good tensile strength with thin walls. They are also nonthrombogenic and nonhemolytic.[3] A new catheter design is now available that retracts the needle into a sheath to prevent needle punctures.

Needles and peripheral catheters are available in diameters

Table 30-1 Complications Associated With Peripheral Vascular Access

Complications	Contributing factors	Prevention strategies
Localized		
Phlebitis/inflammation	Vein intima injury secondary to cannula movement; chemical irritation from medications; hyperosmolar fluids; duration of therapy > 72 hours.	Use of a short extension set at the hub decreases catheter manipulation/movement during tubing changes,[27] check site every 1-2 hours; change site PRN and every 48-72 hours.[7,12]
Site infection	Cutaneous colonization of the insertion site; contamination of the catheter hub; moisture under the site dressing and prolonged catheterization.[13]	Thorough site preparation with aseptic technique; maintain dry, occlusive sterile dressings at site; change peripheral catheters every 48-72 hours.[7,13]
Infiltration and subsequent tissue injury or necrosis	Infiltration is more likely with steele needles, with high flow rates, with larger needle gauges, with antibiotic administration, highly concentrated dextrose solutions,[17] and with the use of small veins,[3] particularly in the infant who has limited extravascular tissue and is unable to communicate pain[17]; necrosis is more common with the extravasation of hyperosmolar solutions, certain medications, and calcium; accidental arterial infusion and arteriospasm may also result in necrosis and lower extremity ischemia with greater saphenous use.[12]	Use smallest possible gauge of catheter in largest possible site; dilute medications and hyperosmolar fluids appropriately; observe IV sites carefully in small infants and children.
Hematoma and bleeding	Hemorrhage is more common with coagulopathies and puncture of deep vessels, or laceration of adjacent arteries.[23]	Careful siting of IVs in patients with known coagulopathies; remove tourniquets before removing needles; apply direct pressure after IV removal.
Pressure necrosis, peripheral nerve palsy, compromised peripheral circulation, positional deformities[12]	Risk is increased with prolonged restriction of movement restraints that are too tight, and delays in recognition of infiltrations in restrained extremities.	Avoid encircling extremities with tape; pad all joints; complete frequent circulation and neurovascular checks to all restrained extremities.
Systemic		
Thrombosis	More likely with puncture of deep veins.[23]	Use proper catheter sizes to prevent vein intima injury; change catheter sites frequently; flush deep vein lines with heparinized solutions PRN.
Pulmonary thromboembolism	Clot embolization caused by forceful flushing of obstructed lines or manipulation of clotted sites.	Prevent forceful flushing of obstructed lines.
Air embolism	Improper flushing or tubing or change.	Flush all needles/catheters and tubing before starting IVs.
Catheter fragment embolism[4]	Results from defective product or inadvertent slicing/breaking of IV catheters during insertion or manipulation.	Flush catheters to ensure patency before use; leave stylets/catheters assembled as a unit; never reinsert stylets in catheters.[27]
Fluid overload/electrolyte imbalance	Improper flushing/monitoring of infusions and large fluid volume use during resuscitation increases the risk of fluid imbalance and inadvertent heparinization.[12]	Risk is minimized with the use of infusion pumps, volume control chambers, and/or microdrip tubing.[4,27]

ranging from 12- to 27-gauge with lengths from ½ to 3 inches. Use the smallest possible catheter that will deliver the solution or medications at the prescribed rate (Table 30-2). Small cannulae ease insertion and may decrease phlebitis and risk of infiltration by increasing blood flow around the catheter, thus decreasing direct contact of the catheter with the vein.[27] However, flow rates are proportional to catheter length and diameter. Use the shortest and largest catheter possible to achieve maximum volume administration rates.

PICC lines are soft, pliable, biocompatible silicone catheters that may remain in place for up to 6 months. They are typically antithrombogenic and radiopaque[15] and are available in catheter sizes of 16- to 23-gauge with lengths of 33.5 to 60 cm and corresponding needle sizes of 13 to 20 gauge. Most catheters are available in a complete kit that includes break-away needles or sheaths and guidewires. A variety of brands are available in both single and double lumens.[3]

In addition to the catheter, assemble the following supplies: a padded board for restraint, adhesive tape, warm compresses, alcohol or povidone-iodine preparation pads, sterile

Table 30-2   Recommended Intravenous Needle/Catheter Sizes for Pediatric Patients

Age range	Weight (kg)	Appropriate IV Needle/Catheter Sizes (gauge)
Newborn - 6 months	3.5-8	22 to 27
6+ months - 3 years	8-15	21 to 24
3+ - 8 years	15-28	20 to 23
8+ - 12 years	28-45	18 to 22
> 12 years	> 45.0	16 to 22

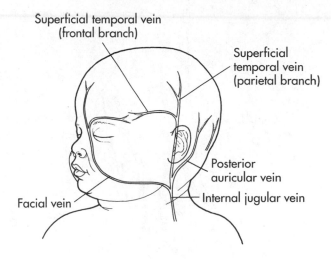

FIG. 30-1   Superficial scalp veins.

BOX 30-1   EQUIPMENT FOR VENESECTION

Tourniquet
Sterile skin preparation solution
Sterile gloves
1% Lidocaine
Saline solution for flush
IV catheters (various sizes) or tubing
Antibiotic ointment and dressing
Venesection tray
   Sterile drapes
   Sterile 4 × 4s
   Needles and syringes
   Scalpel with Nos 10 and 11 blades
   Curved Kelley hemostat
   Iris scissors
   Vein introducer or hemostat
   3-0 and 4-0 silk suture
   Needle holder

---

occlusive transparent dressing or adhesive bandage (Band-Aid) 3 to 5 ml of normal saline solution in a syringe to flush the catheter, gloves, tourniquet, safety razor, IV solution connected to primed IV tubing, a short (3 to 5 inch) extension tubing or stopcock, scissors, transilluminator (optional), and IV infusion pump.

Other recommended supplies and equipment for PICC insertion include sterile gloves, gowns and drapes, masks, forceps or tweezers (nontoothed), sterile 4 × 4s or 2 × 2s, tourniquet,[3] povidone-iodine and alcohol swab sticks, transparent occlusive dressings, 5- to 10-ml syringes with needles, IV extension tubing, catheter kits in appropriate sizes and lengths, tape measure, and sterile scissors.[2]

Preassemble the equipment to perform a cutdown on a sterilized tray, thus ensuring rapid availability of the necessary equipment (Box 30-1). An adequate light source is invaluable to successful percutaneous or cutdown catheter placement. An assistant wearing sterile gloves and gown is helpful when performing a cutdown.

Technique

Selection of Site. When choosing the location for catheter placement in a pediatric patient, consider the child's age, development, mobility, and hand dominance. Also consider the patient's hydration status, diagnosis, rate and volume of proposed therapy, and complicating factors of existing medical conditions (i.e., presence of scars, inflammation, edema, or local injury). During emergencies choose the largest and most accessible veins distant from resuscitative efforts.[4,12,27] Choose peripheral catheter sites above the diaphragm during cardiopulmonary resuscitation (CPR). The most commonly used IV sites in children are the superficial veins of the scalp (Fig. 30-1), hand, arm (Fig. 30-2), leg and foot (Fig. 30-3). In general begin distally and work proximally. When common sites are unavailable, next consider the external jugular site (see Chapter 31), then the deep brachial site, before selecting the cutdown approach.

There are several possible locations to perform peripheral venous cutdown. The saphenous vein at the ankle is the most commonly chosen site, but cutdown is possible at the distal[28] or proximal cephalic vein, the basilic vein, and the brachial vein as well as less commonly used locations, such as the facial vein[34] or thyroid vein.[29]

The distal saphenous vein is an ideal site for cutdown because of its consistent location, separation from important structures, and distance from other resuscitative measures. The distal cephalic vein or "intern's vein" at the wrist is analogous to the saphenous vein and is also easily accessible. It is possible to establish access here with the same rapidity as that of the distal saphenous cutdown.[28]

The antecubital sites in either extremity afford the primary choices for PICC lines for threading peripherally. Most clinicians insert these catheters into either the median basilic or cephalic vein (Fig. 30-4).[8,15] The cephalic vein follows a less straight path and may also have a higher rate of phlebitis, so the preferred vein may be the basilic.[8] Alternative placement sites in infants and children also include the external jugular, internal jugular, subclavian, and femoral veins.[5] However these sites, generally used for central access,[4] may have either higher associated risks or rates of complications.

Peripheral Venipuncture Technique. Gather and prepare all equipment; check the patency of the catheter and flush air from the needle/catheter with a small amount of sterile saline solution, then disconnect the syringe.[4,12,27] Flushing the needle/catheter decreases the risk of air and catheter fragment emboli. Next carefully assess for potential IV sites and

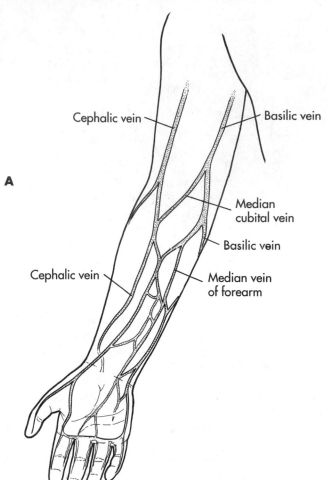

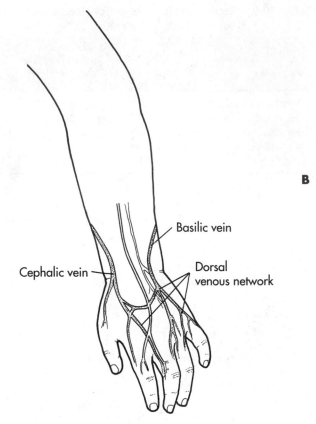

FIG. 30-2 **A** and **B** Veins of the hand and forearm.

select an appropriate vessel. Transillumination, warm compresses (not to exceed 40° C), gentle tapping or massaging, and dependent positioning below the level of the heart may facilitate identification of veins at vasoconstricted sites.[12,27]

Topical nitroglycerine also increases vein visualization because of venodilation.[31] Administer an antipyretic to febrile children first, if possible, as veins may become more fragile with fever.[27] Position and restrain the patient and/or the extremity as appropriate,[4] stabilizing the selected site on a padded board before venipuncture.[27] If necessary prepare the site by shaving, then clean the skin with an appropriate antiseptic.[4] Infants and children with sensitive skin may not tolerate iodine preparations, and alcohol skin preparations may be preferable.[27] Apply a tourniquet proximal to the vein as close as possible to the venipuncture site.[4,12] A rubber band makes an adequate tourniquet for scalp veins.[4] Use a tourniquet for the minimum amount of time possible. The tourniquet should prevent venous return but not arterial blood inflow. Wear protective gloves to prevent skin contact with the patient's blood. Select a straight segment of the vein and stretch the skin taut to stabilize and distend it.[4,12,27] Areas where veins converge provide greater stability.[12]

Introduce the needle/catheter through the skin and slowly advance into the vein until a flash of blood appears in the catheter hub. When placing butterfly needles, introduce the needle with the bevel up; when placing over-the-needle catheters, introduce the needle with the bevel down.[4] Puncturing the skin with an 18-gauge needle before venipuncture assists in preventing damage to the catheter when using 22-gauge or larger catheters.[4,12] Puncture the skin ¼ inch below the vein at a 20- to 30-degree angle, then adjust the angle to 10 to 15 degrees before piercing the vein.[23,27] With very small vessels and patients with poor perfusion the "blood flash" in the hub may be minimal and delayed. Wait momentarily to determine whether venipuncture has been successful.[12] For over-the-needle catheters slowly advance the stylet a few millimeters after obtaining a flash of blood, then hold it stable while advancing the catheter into the vein.[4] On encountering resistance, momentarily stop advancing the catheter, as the vein may be in spasm. Gently removing the tourniquet and instilling a small amount of flush solution may distend the vein and facilitate catheter placement.[12] Removing the tourniquet before manipulating the needle/catheter decreases the risk of injuring veins and causing hematomas.[23,27]

This cannulation technique works well for common IV sites. An alternative peripheral site to consider before cutdown is the deep brachial site. This is especially useful in the older child and adolescent. The technique is blind. First palpate the brachial artery medial to the biceps. At the flexor crease, introduce an over-the-needle catheter (18-gauge, 2½-inch needle usually best) at a 30-degree angle at a point half the patient's finger breadth medial to arterial pulse. Advance *slowly* and withdraw if arterialized blood appears (brachial

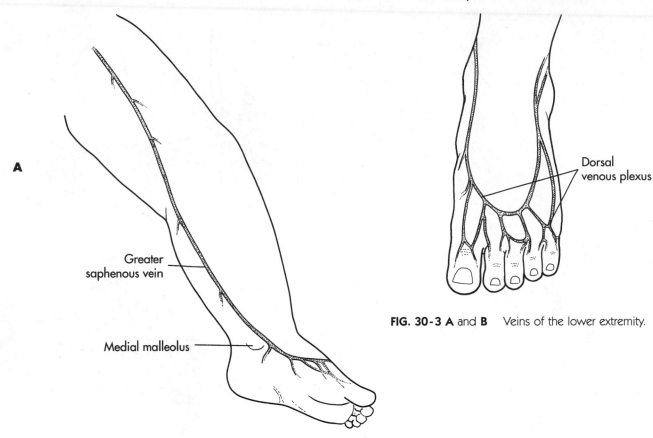

A

Greater
saphenous vein

Medial malleolus

B

Dorsal
venous plexus

FIG. 30-3 A and **B** Veins of the lower extremity.

artery) or if the patient complains of hand paresthesias (median nerve). A controlled entry and minor repositioning of the angle of the catheter improve success and minimize injury to artery and nerve. Variability in anatomic arrangement of vessels also causes some failures. After successful cannulation stabilize the catheter and attach a primed IV extension set to the catheter hub. Flush the catheter gently with saline solution from a prefilled syringe to confirm IV placement.[12] If the catheter does not flush easily, try rotating or pulling it back slightly as the bevel may have lodged against the vein intima.[27] Remove gloves and secure the catheter with tape.[4,27] After securing the catheter also secure the IV tubing to prevent tension on the catheter.[27] Dress the catheter, using sterile technique, and allow for visualization of the catheter insertion site. Do not tape over the insertion site. Clear biocclusive dressings allow for monitoring of the skin around the site.[12] Recheck the patency of the catheter again after taping. Disconnect the syringe, attach the primed IV tubing to the hub of the extension set, and regulate the infusion rate.[4,27] Infusion pumps are useful for ensuring an appropriate rate of flow. Alarms may not identify infiltrations, however, and careful observation of the IV site is still necessary.[17]

Cutdown Technique. The technique for placing catheters by venous cutdown has evolved over the past several years. Description of the classic technique at the distal saphenous vein follows, along with variations. Immobilize the leg completely and secure it to a padded board. Identify the site. Prepare the skin with a sterile skin preparation solution and drape with sterile towels. Infiltrate the skin overlying the vein with 1% lidocaine, taking care to prevent inadvertent punc-

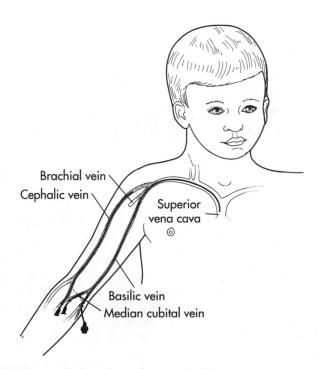

Brachial vein

Cephalic vein

Superior
vena cava

Basilic vein

Median cubital vein

FIG. 30-4 Choice of sites for peripherally inserted central catheters.

ture of the vein. Identify the medial malleolus and, using a No. 10 scalpel blade, make a transverse incision through the dermis one patient's fingers breadth superior and one patient's fingers breadth anterior to the medial malleolus ex-

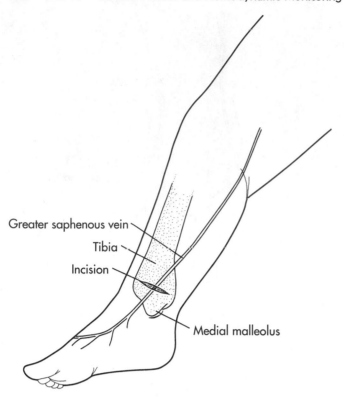

FIG. 30-5 Landmarks for distal greater saphenous vein cutdown.

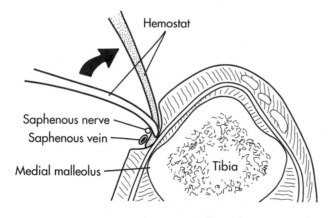

FIG. 30-6 Saphenous vein isolation.

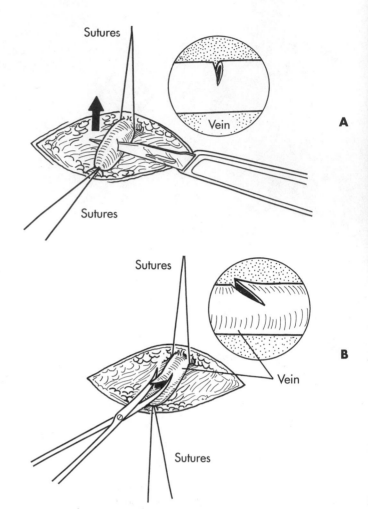

FIG. 30-7 A and **B** Venotomy using a scalpel or iris scissors.

tending to the anterior border of the tibia (Fig. 30-5). Using a curved hemostat with the point held down, scrape the surface of the tibia from the anterior to the posterior edges of the wound, picking up the tissues on the point of the hemostat (Fig. 30-6).[19] Open the hemostat wide. The vein should stand out against the silver background of the hemostat.

This method isolates the vein more rapidly than traditional methods that attempt to identify the vein and then dissect it away from the periosteum.[26] Pass a loop of 3-0 silk suture under the vein and cut the loop, dividing the suture into two lengths, leaving both sutures long enough to provide traction on the vein. Use the distal suture to ligate the vein, thus ensuring a bloodless field. Then place traction on the proximal suture to stabilize the vein, but do not ligate the vein. Make a venotomy either by cutting a wedge shape in the vein

with iris scissors or by transecting the upper one-third to one-half of the vein with the No. 11 scalpel blade turned upward (Fig. 30-7). With a vein introducer or a hemostat hold the venotomy site open and advance the catheter into the vessel 5 to 6 cm (Fig. 30-8). Use a catheter one size larger than the vessel itself. Flush the catheter with saline solution or advance with a twisting motion to facilitate placement. In the older child who requires short-term rapid fluid replacement, an option is to place a length of sterile IV tubing that is beveled and rounded at one end directly into the vein. Tie the proximal suture around the vein and the catheter to prevent the extravasation of blood or IV fluids from the venotomy. Do not occlude the catheter with the suture. Close the wound with 4-0 silk and place another suture through the skin to secure the catheter. Last apply an antibiotic ointment and dressing.

The classic technique of cutdown placement has the disadvantage of ligating the vein, thus making it useless for future cannulations. Several variations on the traditional technique preserve vein function and speed achievement of access. It is now more common to use these techniques than the classic method. In the minicutdown technique place an over-the-needle catheter into the vein under direct visualization. Surrounding adventitia supports the vein. No venotomy or vein ligation is necessary. If oozing occurs, close the subcutaneous tissue over the vein. It is possible to use the vein repeatedly with this technique, but lack of a venotomy

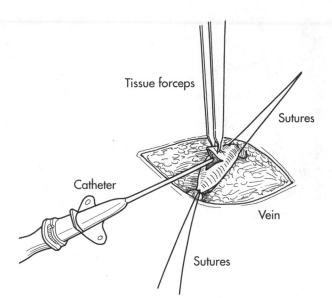

FIG. 30-8 Catheter placement.

limits the size of the catheter.[22] Another option is to place larger catheters by a technique described by Schockley that introduces a catheter over a guidewire. Place sutures around the vein to facilitate catheter placement but do not ligate the vein. Make a 1- to 2-mm venotomy and advance a guidewire-dilator-catheter apparatus as a unit into the vein, thus effecting successive dilation of the vein. Remove the guidewire and dilator.[20] Alternately, place the catheter into the vein through a stab wound distal to the skin incision. This may decrease the likelihood of infection and is an option with either the traditional technique or the mini-cutdown technique.[25]

Although the landmarks for other locations differ, the technique for the cutdown remains the same. When performing a basilic vein cutdown, divide the upper arm into thirds; the basilic vein lies in the groove between the biceps and the triceps muscles in the middle of the distal third portion of the upper arm (Fig. 30-9). Make a short transverse incision on the anteromedial surface of the arm in the middle of the distal third part of the upper arm from the biceps to the triceps. Locate the vein in the superficial fat above the muscle fascia and the brachial artery.[21,26] Prevent injury to the median cutaneous nerve, which has a variable course around the basilic vein.[14] It is also acceptable to center the incision over a palpable brachial artery with the basilic vein superficial and medial to the pulse.

The distal cephalic vein or "intern's vein" runs along the lateral surface of the radius (Fig. 30-10). Make an incision one fingers breadth proximal to the dorsal tubercle of the radius. Extend the incision dorsally along the radial aspect of the wrist. Avoid the volar aspect of the wrist to prevent injury to the radial artery.[28]

The proximal cephalic vein on the lateral upper arm is also easily accessible. Make a transverse incision 2 cm proximal to the distal flexor crease of the upper arm, centered between the lateral epicondyle and the biceps tendon (see Fig. 30-9). Prevent injury to the lateral cutaneous nerve, which lies deep to the vein.[14]

One can use the external jugular and facial veins for peripheral cutdowns, but it is more common to use these locations for the insertion of soft silastic central venous catheters. Approach the external jugular through a short transverse incision directly over the vein. Compression over the soft tissues above the clavicle or positioning the head down helps the vein to fill. The facial vein is deep to the external jugular and anterior to the internal jugular (Fig. 30-11). Retract the sternocleidomastoid muscle laterally or split it longitudinally to locate the vein.[10]

PICC Line Insertion Technique. Thread the PICC line via an initial venipuncture made with an introducing needle. Advance either with or without the use of a stylet. Catheters without stylets cause the least vein damage, but are more difficult to advance. Flexible wires, rather than more rigid stylets, are preferable because they cause less damage to the vein intima.[2] The use of stylets or guidewires during insertion may also result in catheter breakage unless removal is cautious.[11]

Several types and brands of catheters are available and thus the manufacturer's recommendations dicate the exact insertion technique.[8] The following summarizes the two general techniques for PICC line placement.

Gather needed equipment and assemble it on a sterile field.[2,11] Select and locate the vein, then position and restrain the patient as necessary. Premedication or sedation may be helpful in decreasing anxiety and the possibility of venospasm. For antecubital sites position the child supine with the extremity extending 90 degrees from the trunk and the head turned toward the chosen limb. A rolled towel under the elbow facilitates access to the antecubital area.[8] For antecubital sites it is necessary to apply a tourniquet firmly around the upper arm near the axilla.[2]

Wash hands and apply sterile gown, gloves, mask, and cap. Using a sterile tape measure, measure the distance from insertion to proposed termination site.[2,11] Then cut the catheter to the desired length. Flush the catheter with sterile saline solution to expel air and help lubricate the stylet wire.[11] Retract the stylet 1 to 2 cm proximal to the distal end of the catheter, then bend the stylet wire over the catheter hub to prevent migration of the stylet. For antecubital sites place a solid drape under the arm, then prepare the insertion site from mid upper arm to mid lower arm. Finally apply a fenestrated drape over the site.[2] Anesthetize the area overlying the venipuncture site.[4] A 1- to 2-hour application of eutectic mixture of local anesthetics (EMLA) cream before the start of the procedure produces good local anesthesia without producing venospasm (see also Chapter 15).

Don new sterile gloves, then, using a breakaway introducer needle, perform the venipuncture. After successful venipuncture insert the catheter through the introducer needle and slowly advance 2 to 3 inches. Use a sterile 4 × 4 to release the tourniquet and continue to advance the catheter to the predetermined length.[2] If using a stylet, ensure that it remains well within the lumen of the catheter during advancement. Advancing the catheter slowly, with a slight twisting motion, reduces damage to the vein intima.[8] Once the catheter is in place, apply thumb pressure to the vein 1 to 2 inches above the insertion site and slowly remove the introducer needle. After removing the breakaway needle from the site, snap the needle wings together and peel the needle away from the catheter.[2] With the needle removed, secure the catheter temporarily and remove the stylet wire if

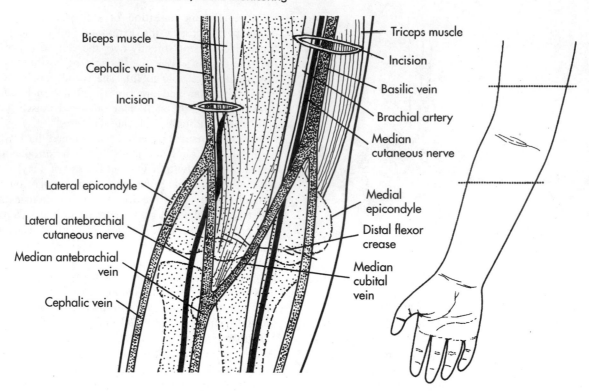

FIG. 30-9 Landmarks for basilic and proximal cephalic vein cutdowns.

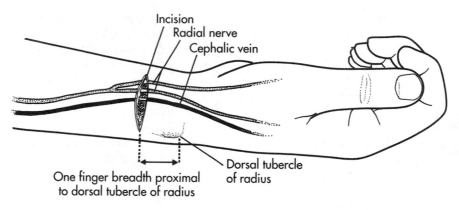

FIG. 30-10 Landmarks for distal cephalic vein cutdown.

applicable. Attach a primed extension set to the hub of the catheter, flush gently, and aspirate to see whether blood returns; then radiographically confirm the placement of centrally located catheters.[2,5,8]

For the Seldinger variation the same basic technique applies, but use a guidewire to place an introducing sheath to help in threading the catheter. After cannulation of the vein with a needle or over-the-needle catheter, thread the straight end of the guidewire into the introducing needle or IV catheter and advance 5 to 10 cm into the vein before removing the introducing needle. Stop advancing the wire on encountering resistance. Making a nick in the skin and subcutaneous tissues with a scalpel blade may be helpful before threading the introducer sheath over the wire.[8] Thread

the sheath/introducer assembly over the guidewire, and once it is in place, remove the guidewire. With the catheter in place remove the introducing sheath, typically by pulling it apart. Flush the catheter with heparinized saline solution after confirming blood return by aspirating the catheter.[4,8,11]

Secure the catheter with bandages (Steri-Strips) or sutures, being careful to prevent placing tension on the catheter hub.[11] Because of the long length and very small lumen of the catheter blood return may be minimal or, on occasion, absent. If there is no blood flow from the catheter, monitor the line very carefully. If any other problems occur with the infusion, assume that the catheter is not in the vessel and remove it.

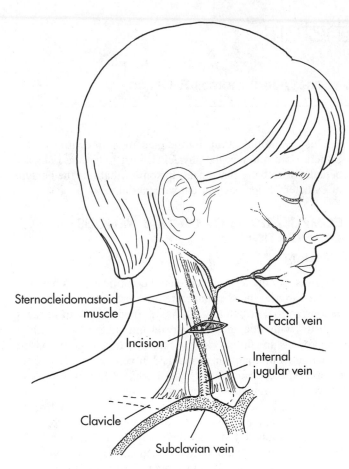

FIG. 30-11   Landmarks for facial vein cutdown.

Sternocleidomastoid muscle

Incision

Facial vein

Internal jugular vein

Clavicle

Subclavian vein

REFERENCES

1. Arrighi DA et al: Prospective randomized trial of rapid venous access for patients in hypovolemic shock, *Ann Emerg Med* 18:927-930, 1989.
2. Brown JM: Peripherally inserted central catheters use in home care, *J Intravenous Nurs* 12:144-150, 1989.
3. Camp-Sorrell D: Advanced central venous access: selection, catheters, devices, and nursing management, *J Intravenous Nurs* 13:361-370, 1990.
4. Chameides L, editor: *Textbook of pediatric advanced life support,* Dallas, 1990, American Heart Association.
5. Dolcourt JS, Bose CL: Percutaneous insertion of silastic venous catheters in newborn infants with birth weights of 510-3920 grams, *Pediatrics* 78:245-247, 1986.
6. Filston HC, Johnson DG: Percutaneous venous cannulation in neonates and infants: a method for catheter insertion without "cut-down," *Pediatrics* 48:896-901, 1971.
7. Giuffrida DJ et al: Central vs. peripheral venous catheters in critically ill patients, *Chest* 90:806-809, 1986.
8. Goodwin ML: The Seldinger method for PICC insertion, *J Intravenous Nurs* 12:238-243, 1989.
9. Kanter RK et al: Pediatric emergency intravenous access, *Am J Dis Child* 140:132-134, 1986.
10. Kosloske AM, Klein MD: Techniques of central venous access for long term parenteral nutrition in infants, *Surg Gynecol Obstet* 154:395-399, 1982.
11. Loughran SC, Edwards S, McClure S: Peripherally inserted central catheters. Guidewire versus nonguidewire use: a comparative study, *J Intravenous Nurs* 15:152-159, 1992.
12. Macdonald MG, Eichelberger MR: Peripheral intravenous (IV) line placement. In Fletcher MA, MacDonald MG, editors: *Atlas of procedures in neonatology,* ed 2, Philadelphia, 1993, JB Lippincott.
13. Maki DG, Ringer M: Evaluation of dressing regimens for prevention of infection with peripheral intravenous catheters, *JAMA* 258:2396-2403, 1987.
14. McIntosh BB, Dulchavsky SA: Peripheral vascular cutdown, *Crit Care Clin* 8:807-818, 1992.
15. Meares C: PICC and MLC lines: options worth exploring, *Nurs 92* 22:52-55, 1992.
16. Moran JM, Atwood RP, Rowe MI: A clinical and bacteriologic study of infections associated with venous cutdowns, *N Engl J Med* 272:554-560, 1965.
17. Phelps SJ, Helms RA: Risk factors affecting infiltration in peripheral venous line in infants, *J Pediatr* 111:384-389, 1987.
18. Posner MC, Moore EE: Distal greater saphenous vein cutdown: technique of choice for rapid volume resuscitation, *J Emerg Med* 3:395-399, 1985.
19. Randolph J: Technique for insertion of plastic catheter into saphenous vein, *Pediatrics* 24:631-635, 1959.
20. Schockley LW, Butzier DJ: A modified wire-guided technique for venous cutdown access, *Ann Emerg Med* 19:393-395, 1990.
21. Scranton PE: *Practical techniques in venipuncture,* Baltimore, 1977, Williams & Wilkins.
22. Shiu MH: A method for conservation of veins in the surgical cutdown, *Surg Gynecol Obstet* 134:315-316, 1972.
23. Short BL: Venipuncture. In Fletcher MA, MacDonald MG, editors: *Atlas of procedures in neonatology,* ed 2, Philadelphia, 1993, JB Lippincott.
24. Silverman BK, editor: Vascular access. In *Advanced pediatric life support,* Elk Grove Village, Ill, 1989, American Academy of Pediatrics.
25. Simon RR, Brenner BE, editors: *Emergency procedures and techniques,* Baltimore, 1987, Williams & Wilkins.
26. Simon RR, Hoffman JR, Smith M: Modified new approaches for rapid intravenous access, *Ann Emerg Med* 16:44-49, 1987.
27. Summerfield AL: Inserting intravascular (IV) catheters. In Smith DP, editor: *Comprehensive child and family nursing skills,* St. Louis, 1991, Mosby.
28. Talan DA, Simon RR, Hoffman JR: Cephalic vein cutdown at the wrist: comparison to the standard saphenous vein ankle cutdown, *Ann Emerg Med* 17:38-42, 1988.
29. Toufanian A, Knight P: The middle thyroid vein: an alternate route for central venous catheter insertion, *J Pediatr Surg* 18:156-157, 1983.
30. Turner CS: Vascular access. In Ashcraft KW, Holder TM, editors: *Pediatric surgery,* Philadelphia, 1993, WB Saunders.
31. Vaksmann G, Rey C, Breviere G-M et al: Nitroglycerine ointment as an aid to venous cannulation in children. *J Pediatr* 111:89-91, 1987.
32. Wax PM, Talan DA: Advances in cutdown techniques, *Emerg Med Clin North Am* 7:65-82, 1989.
33. Zimmerman JJ, Strauss RH: History and current application of intravenous therapy in children, *Pediatr Emerg Care* 5:120-127, 1989.
34. Zumbo GL, Mullin MJ, Nelson TG: Catheter placement in infants needing total parenteral nutrition utilizing common facial vein, *Arch Surg* 102:71-73, 1971.

31 Central Venous Catheters

Edward G. Fernandez, Michael F. Sweeney, and Thomas P. Green

Central venous catheters play an important role in the management of critically ill and injured patients, serving both as reliable vascular access and the site of venous pressure monitoring.[12,15] Improvement in catheter technology and insertion techniques have made the use of central venous catheters safer and more practical.

Intensivists usually insert central venous catheters in large veins such as the internal or external jugular, the subclavian, and the common femoral. Other options include the axillary and antecubital veins. This chapter reviews indications for the use of these catheters, techniques commonly used for catheter placement, and common complications. The review includes only catheters with a tip that reaches the central or intrathoracic venous system. Chapter 30 addresses peripheral catheters.

INDICATIONS

A central venous catheter is indicated in a pediatric patient for monitoring of central venous pressures or central venous blood sampling[12,15]; administration of drugs or concentrated solutions, including parenteral alimentation that may only infuse into the central circulation[5]; plasmapheresis, exchange transfusion, or dialysis[8]; and venous access not possible with peripheral intravenous catheters.[12]

In critically ill or injured patients, several of these indications frequently exist simultaneously, and in Emergency Departments and pediatric intensive care units (PICUs) the placement of central venous catheters has become commonplace. In these settings, catheters also provide a tempting measure of expediency and convenience. Staff often perform routine blood sampling through these catheters, and in the presence of multiple lumen catheters, medical personnel spend less time on intravenous line placement. However, these catheters have a significant rate of complications. For maximum benefit and minimal risk, restrict catheter placement to patients who meet one or more of the accepted indications.

CONTRAINDICATIONS

Do not insert these catheters through infected skin. Avoid placement of catheters in sites that are not easily compressable in patients with bleeding diatheses. Hypercoagulable states predispose to catheter-related thrombotic problems. In patients with intraabdominal catastrophes and/or abdominal trauma, femoral catheters are usually inadvisable.[9] Do not place upper body lines in close proximity to existing subcutaneous foreign bodies such as ventriculoperitoneal shunts. Avoid bilateral internal jugular lines when increased intracranial pressure exists. Expect that bacteria will soon colonize deep venous catheters placed in patients with bacteremia.[17]

Most contraindications for the placement of central venous catheters are relative; the physician must judge the risks and benefits of catheter placement. In some situations the benefits of catheter placement warrant substantial risk.

COMPLICATIONS OF CENTRAL VENOUS CANNULATION
Bleeding

The most common insertion-related complication is bleeding due to arterial needle puncture or perforation of a deep venous/arterial structure.[21,24] This is more likely to occur in patients with coagulopathy or thrombocytopenia.[24] Large hematomas in the neck can cause airway compromise. Bleeding from a jugular or subclavian vein can enter into the pleural space, causing a hemothorax. Bleeding into the pericardium may cause tamponade.

Bleeding is easier to prevent than to treat. Normalize the patient's coagulation status and platelet count before attempted cannulation, if possible. Adequate sedation and local anesthesia prevent patient motion and decrease the probability of inadvertent needle movement. Good patient positioning will provide the highest likelihood of successful cannulation on the first needle pass.

Once bleeding begins, direct compression is the best immediate treatment. Unfortunately, local hematoma formation may compress or distort the venous anatomy, rendering further attempts at the same site more difficult.

Pneumothorax

Needle puncture of the lung during internal jugular or subclavian vein cannulation may lead to pneumothorax. Always look for this complication in the x-ray study performed to check catheter position.

Less common complications include various nerve injuries, chylothorax, embolic phenomena, and catheter fragmentation.[21] Arrhythmias are usually benign and simple to manage by repositioning the offending foreign body.[1,21]

Catheter Thrombosis

Suspect catheter thrombosis when there is a dampened wave form on the monitor, difficulty in drawing blood, or infusion failure. It may be necessary to exclude thrombosis of the vessel by Doppler ultrasound, dye studies, or standard ultrasound using micro-air bubble normal saline for contrast. It is best to manage catheter lumen thrombosis in the early stages before complete occlusion. Instill 1 ml of a solution of urokinase (5000 U/ml) and allow to dwell inside each lumen of a catheter for 4 hours.[11] If unsuccessful, then use 2 ml (10,000 U) for 4 hours. If still unsuccessful, try a continuous infusion of urokinase, 200 U/kg/hour/lumen for 12 to 24 hours.[3,11] For residual thrombosis, repeat the infusion for another 24 hours. An alternative to urokinase is hydrochloric acid (0.1 N, 0.2 to 0.5 ml) instilled per lumen and allowed to dwell for 20 minutes.[7] Some physicians have also used tissue plasminogen activator in adults for this purpose.[2] Alternatively, change the catheter over a wire. In this way a longer catheter may bypass a site of thrombosis. Some also recommend low-dose heparin and/or warfarin therapy for thrombosis prevention.[4]

Infection

Risks of infection associated with femoral catheters are similar to those at subclavian or jugular sites.[25] There is the same risk of infection per day, and the chance of infection does not increase with the age of the catheter.[26] Detect local infection by the presence of erythema, induration, and discharge at the site of insertion.[27] Diagnose catheter infection by a positive blood culture drawn through the catheter or a positive catheter tip culture with a simultaneous negative peripheral blood culture.[25] Confirm catheter sepsis in a symptomatic patient with positive peripheral and catheter blood cultures.[25]

The most effective management of an infected catheter is to remove it.[17,18] Antibiotic treatment may be indicated, depending on the patient's clinical status and immune competence. If indications for central venous access are still present, infection of a new catheter will be less likely with administration of systemic antibiotics for 24 to 48 hours before reinsertion of a central catheter.[17] An attempt to sterilize the catheter with antibiotic therapy may be successful.[18] This is not advisable in fungal sepsis, where studies support removal of the catheter.[6] After an infected catheter has been changed over a wire, fungi often recolonize it within 48 hours.[17] Prophylactic changing of a catheter every 48 hours to 1 week is ineffective in preventing infection.[17]

Perforation

Erosion of a vessel by a catheter may lead to ascites, pleural effusions, pericardial effusion, and possibly pericardial tamponade.[1,21,24] It is best to avoid this complication by keeping catheters away from vascular wall pressure points. Inability to freely aspirate blood from the tip lumen is a valuable warning sign. A small migration of short (5 cm), multi-lumen catheters might allow the proximal port to withdraw outside the vessel. Evaluate periodic chest x-ray films for mediastinal widening, catheters lying against vessel walls, and pleural effusions. Sudden, unexplained hemodynamic and respiratory compromise or a fall in hematocrit may be signs of catheter-related complications.

EQUIPMENT

The usual composition of venous catheters is silicone polymer (silastic) or one of the plastics (polyethylene, polyvinylchloride, polyurethane). Silastic catheters are soft, relatively nonthrombogenic, and amenable to long-term use.[5] However, withdrawal of blood from small silastic catheters can be problematic. Polymeric plastic catheters offer advantages for hemodynamic monitoring.[9]

Table 31-1 details varieties of catheter size, lumen number, and catheter lengths commonly available. The usual length of catheters available is from 5 to 50 cm. The number of lumens

Table 31-1 Catheters for Central Venous Placement*

Size (French)	Inside diameter (mm)	Lengths available (cm)	Number of lumens
3	20	5 - 50	1
4	18	5 - 50	1-3
5	16	5 - 50	1-3
7	12	8 - 20	1-3
10.5		12, 15	2
11		13, 20	2

*The lengths available and number of lumens are a general guide to catheters that are commercially available. Special-use catheters with different sizes and specifications are also available, or manufacturers can produce them on special order.

Table 31-2 Central Venous Catheter Use in Pediatric Patients*

Weight (kg)	Age (years)	Catheter size (French)
<5	0 - 0.5	3, 4
>5	0.5 - 1.5	5, 7
>15	5 - adult	5 - 11

*Catheter sizes represent those most commonly used for central venous catheters for infusion and pressure monitoring. Larger catheters may be necessary even in the smallest patients, for specific indications such as dialysis.

varies from one to four. External circumference sizes range from 3 to 13 French. Heparin, antibiotic, or antiseptic impregnated catheters are now available.[13] The type of catheter chosen should take into account existing and anticipated indications.

Patient size and the site of catheter insertion are additional important determinants of the choice of a catheter. Table 31-2 displays the common relationships between patient age and catheter choice. Insert the catheter the distance from insertion site to acceptable tip position as estimated externally, usually with the aid of a tape measure.

TECHNIQUE
Patient Preparation

Proper patient positioning, adequate sedation, and excellent analgesia are essential for successful pediatric line placement. Use a sedative anxiolytic agent (e.g., benzodiazepine). Midazolam is often an excellent choice because of its amnesic properties and short elimination half-life. Consider narcotics, but the safest analgesia is with local anesthetic. An anticholinergic to control upper airway secretions is advisable with heavy sedation. Anesthetics such as ketamine and propofol can be very effective choices, but use only with precautions appropriate for any general anesthetic (see Chapter 13).

For the administration of heavy sedation or anesthesia, anticipate the occurrence of respiratory depression. Use these drugs only if management of a compromised airway or respiratory arrest can expeditiously occur. Ensure availability of oxygen and equipment necessary for airway management and positive-pressure ventilation. Routinely monitor vital signs, including pulse oximetry.

Use local anesthesia with 1% lidocaine in all patients. A topical anesthetic cream (EMLA) that contains a eutectic mixture of 2.5% lidocaine and 2.5% prilocaine is now available, and, when applied at least 1 hour before the attempt, provides excellent cutaneous analgesia.[20] However, it does not anesthetize subcutaneous tissue.

Positioning of the patient is often the difference between a successful and unsuccessful attempt. The proper position varies according to the site (see individual placement sites below). Clean the skin with an iodine, chlorhexidine, or alcohol containing prep solution. Allow to dry for maximum antimicrobial effect.[10,16]

Venous Catheter Placement

Guidewire Technique. Most intensivists insert central venous catheters using the modified Seldinger technique, which involves inserting a flexible guidewire through an initial needle cannulation[22] (Figs. 31-1 through 31-3). Use a short bevel needle attached to a non-Luer lock syringe. Line up the bevel with the marking on the syringe so that it is clear at all times the direction in which the bevel is pointing. Maintain slight negative pressure on the plunger during insertion and withdrawal. The needle often transfixes the vein and enters the lumen during withdrawal. After blood freely flows into the barrel of the syringe, steady the needle with one hand while removing the syringe, and insert the wire through the needle into the vein with the other (see Fig. 31-1). Use the J end of the wire first. The purpose of this curve is to facilitate wire passage via the main venous channel. If the J tip does not pass, use the straight end of the wire. In either case, the wire should pass freely without resistance or snagging. If the wire does not pass freely, it may be necessary to withdraw it and make minor adjustments in the needle position. If wire withdrawal meets with significant resistance, remove the needle and guidewire together. Failure to do so may cut the wire, leaving a fragment inside the vein.

If suspicion of intraarterial placement exists, insert a small catheter over the wire and measure pressure following wire removal. If the pressure is arterial, remove the catheter and apply direct pressure until hematoma formation ceases.

After free passage of the wire for an appropriate distance, withdraw the needle over the wire, taking care not to change the wire position. Make a small stab incision along the wire at the point of skin insertion with a No. 11 scalpel blade, taking care not to cut the wire. Hold the blade parallel to the skin and insert above the wire. Pass a dilator, if needed, over the wire into the vein to ease passage of the catheter. Hold the dilator close to the skin and insert it a short distance into the vein with a rotatory motion. After removing the dilator, pass the catheter over the wire and into the vein. Using a sterile gauze to handle the catheter often facilitates catheter manipulation while preserving asepsis. Ensure that the end of the wire is visible outside the catheter before the tip of the catheter enters the skin to prevent loss of the guidewire into the patient during passage of the catheter (see Fig. 31-2).

When it is desirable to reposition the catheter after placement, such as in pulmonary artery catheterization, place a sheath over the dilator and into the vein. After removal of the dilator, place the catheter through the sheath.

After intravenous placement of the catheter, check each

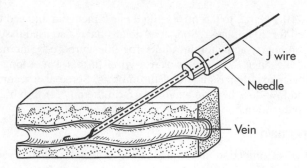

FIG. 31-1   Introduction of wire through needle.

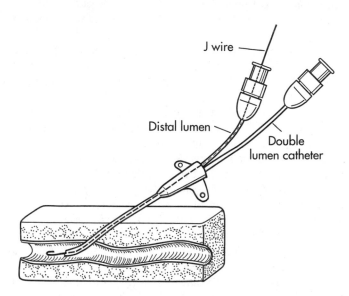

FIG. 31-2   Catheter placement over wire.

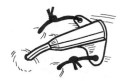

Suture when tied
Pulls catheter into vein

FIG. 31-3   Suture placement.

lumen to ensure that it is possible to aspirate blood and flush saline freely. Fix the catheter to the skin with skin sutures, which should keep the catheter in position as shown in Fig. 31-3. Apply antimicrobial ointment and a sterile dressing to all skin puncture sites. Perform an x-ray study if needed to confirm the desired catheter position and check for insertion-related complications.

Venous Cutdown. Fig. 31-4 details three variations of the cutdown technique. In each technique, make an incision over the site of anticipated venous entry, retract the subcutaneous tissues, and expose the vein.[23] Place circumferential ligatures around the vein above and below the anticipated insertion site. In the classic technique (see Fig. 31-4, *A*), after tying the distal ligature, make a small nick in the vein and pass the

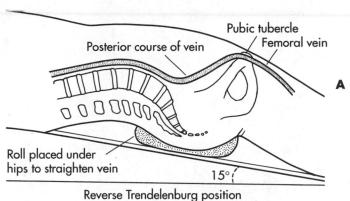

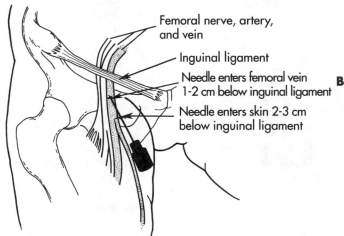

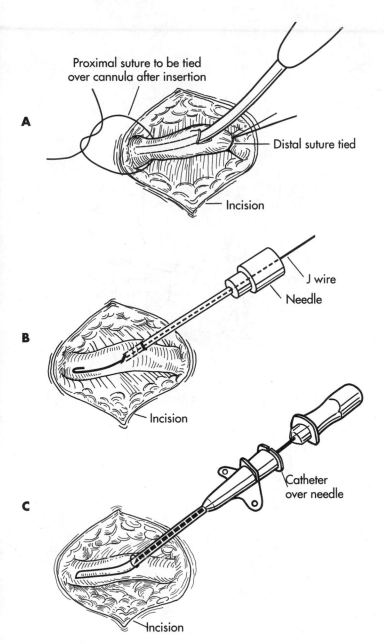

FIG. 31-5 A, Position: supine; negative Trendelenburg; limb straight; hip joint position of ease; roll of cloth under hip to extend and straighten vein. **B,** Anatomy of femoral triangle. Note: (1) Right femoral vein is easier to cannulate than left due to a straighter path to the inferior vena cava. (2) Low femoral catheter. Measure from site of insertion to umbilicus, with some leeway for the downward path of the vein. (3) High femoral catheter. Measure from site of insertion to xiphisternum. (4) In infants, vein is 5 to 6 mm medial to arterial pulse. (5) In adolescents, vein is 10 to 15 mm medial to arterial pulse.

FIG. 31-4 A, Classical method. Make a nick between distal and peripheral ligatures and introduce the catheter. Tie both ligatures, tieing the peripheral ligature over the cannula. **B,** Seldinger technique. **C,** Catheter over needle.

Sites for Central Venous Acess

Common Femoral Venous Catheterization. Fig. 31-5 depicts the anatomy and positioning for common femoral venous catheterization. Place the patient in slight reverse Trendelenburg position with an appropriate-size roll under the hips.[14]

Subclavian or Proximal Axillary Venous Catheterization. Fig. 31-6 shows features of subclavian vein catheterization. Patient movement during placement substantially increases the risk of complication. Young patients usually require heavy sedation. Place the patient supine and in an allowable Trendelenburg position. Turn the face toward the opposite side and maintain neck extension by a transverse or longitudinal shoulder roll.

Internal Jugular Vein Catheterization. Positioning of the patient for internal jugular cannulation is very similar to that used for the subclavian vein. The right side is preferable because of the straight course to the right atrium, the absence of the thoracic duct, and the lower pleural dome on the right side.

catheter through the hole.[19] Depending on the size of the vein, considerable skill may be necessary to provide a large enough venotomy without transecting the vein. After successful catheter placement, tie down the proximal suture, secure the catheter, and close the wound.

Alternatives to this classic technique avoid the venisection and are often easier to master. After controlling the vein with ligatures, insert a needle or standard intravenous catheter under direct vision (see Fig. 31-4, *B* and *C*). Then pass a wire an appropriate distance through the needle/catheter. Proceed with central venous placement over the guidewire as previously discussed. Remove the ligatures, secure the catheter, and close the wound. Ligation of the vein may not be necessary with this technique.

200

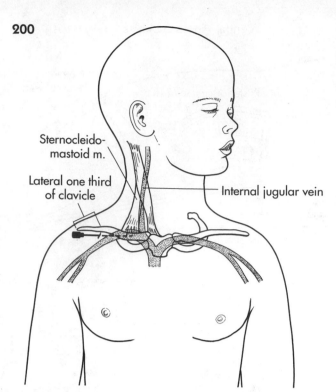

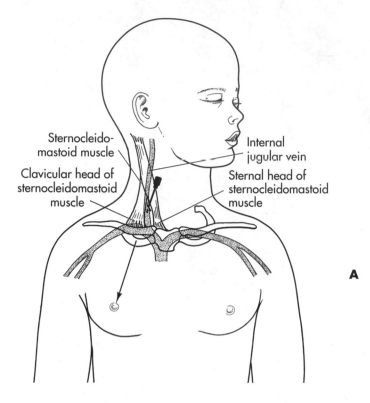

FIG. 31-6 Subclavian venous cannulation. Position: supine; Trendelenburg; face turned toward opposite side; neck extended, using roll under the ipsilateral shoulder. Note: (1) Inject local anesthesia up to periosteum of clavicle. (2) Enter skin below lateral two thirds of clavicle and aim needle at suprasternal notch; needle touches lower end of clavicle and rides below clavicle into the vein. (3) Position curve of J wire open inferiorly. (4) Turn neck to same side while passing wire to prevent wire passage up ipsilateral internal jugular. (5) Catheter insertion from site of insertion to angle of Louis. (6) Auscultation of chest and chest x-ray to detect pneumothorax after cannulation. (7) Left subclavian may be easier to cannulate than right.

FIG. 31-7 For legend see opposite page.

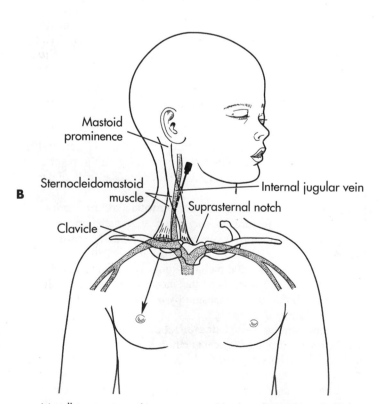

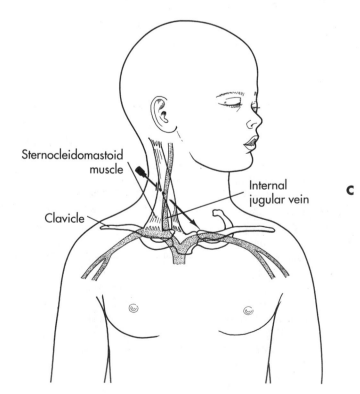

Needle entry into skin at anterior border of muscle at half the distance between mastoid prominence and suprasternal notch

Fig. 31-7 details three approaches to the internal jugular vein. The middle approach is preferred because it combines ease of placement with very low risk of insertion-related complications.

External Jugular Vein Catheterization. Position the patient the same as for internal jugular cannulation. Fig. 31-8 shows the anatomic landmarks. Because the route to the right atrium is tortuous, the use of a J-wire is especially helpful. Success rates in pediatric patients are lower with this site (approximately 70%).[23] The right side is preferable with this approach.

Antecubital Venous Catheterization. Large, visible, palpable veins are present in the antecubital fossa and can be used for central venous catheter placement (see Chapter 30 for antecubital anatomy). However, use of the cephalic vein is likely to result in an inability to pass the catheter into the proximal axillary vein.

Sites for Venous Cutdowns. The long saphenous, antecubital, and common or superficial femoral veins are the vessels that are commonly used when a cutdown is necessary.[19,23] Fig. 31-9 shows the relevant anatomy of the saphenous and antecubital sites. Chapter 30 depicts anatomy of peripheral locations.

Positioning of the Central Catheter Tip. Confirm central venous catheter tip position with an x-ray study as soon as is reasonable. The tip should not intrude against a venous wall or the right atrium because these positions are associated with a high incidence of perforation.[21] Ideally position catheters entering the superior or vena cava just above the superior vena cava–right atrial junction (Fig. 31-10). Position inferior vena cava catheters just below the junction of the right atrium and the inferior vena cava.

Choice of Central Venous Catheter Sites

A working knowledge of several techniques and the facility to place catheters at several possible sites will give the intensivist or emergency medicine physician the skills to deal with the problems and particular circumstances presented by most patients.

In most PICUs the femoral and internal jugular veins are the most frequently used sites. Femoral catheterization is convenient, safe, and relatively easy to perform. The arterial

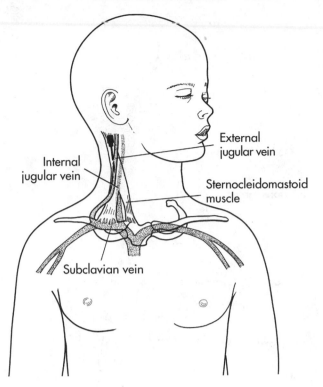

FIG. 31-8   External jugular cannulation.

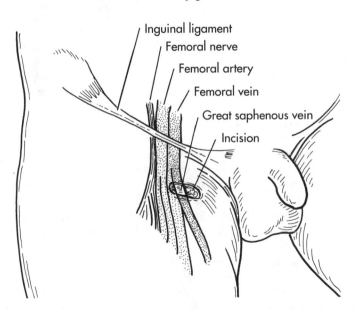

FIG. 31-9   Cutdown of saphenous vein at groin. Note: Incision extends laterally from point where scrotum/labial folds meet thigh to just below pubic tubercle/outer portion of mons; superficial dissection exposes the vein.

FIG. 31-7   **A,** Internal jugular cannulation (low approach) is most common. Position same as for subclavian, with needle entry at apex of triangle formed by heads of the sternocleidomastoid; aim needle toward ipsilateral nipple. **B,** Internal jugular cannulation (anterior approach). Position same as for subclavian, with needle entry halfway along anterior border of sternocleidomastoid; aim needle toward ipsilateral nipple. **C,** Internal jugular cannulation (posterior approach) is rare. Position same as for subclavian; needle enters along posterior border of sternocleidomastoid two thirds of the way to clavicle; aim toward suprasternal notch. Note: (1) Do not compress skin to try to move carotid artery away from vein because this can distort venous anatomy. (2) Using a finder needle to find the vein before using the introducer needle is not usually helpful in pediatric practice. (3) Valsava maneuver during needling and catheter passage can prevent air embolism. (4) To determine the length of catheter for insertion, measure from site of insertion to angle of Louis.

pulsations serve as a landmark for the vein.[6] In case of bleeding, the neck of the femur and pelvis serve as hard surfaces to aid direct pressure. In addition, the femoral area is remote from movement during cardiopulmonary resuscitation. With good nursing care, the femoral site has no higher incidence of complications than other sites, even with long-term use.[25]

Since the internal jugular vein is the largest vein of those available for percutaneous access, many physicians prefer this site. In terms of insertion safety, this vein has somewhat

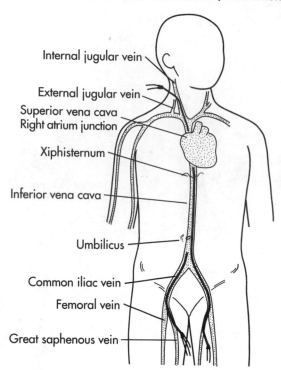

FIG. 31-10 Placement of central venous catheters. Note: (1) Short femoral catheter. Tip of catheter should reach lower inferior vena cava (IVC) below the origin of the renal veins. Measure from site of insertion to the umbilicus and allow some margin for the posterior course of the catheter. (2) Long femoral catheter. Tip of catheter should reach IVC–right atrial (RA) junction. Measure from site of insertion to xiphisternum. (3) Neck catheters. Tip of catheter should reach just above superior vena cava-RA junction. Measure from site of insertion to angle of Louis.

more risk than the femoral insertion site, but less risk than the subclavian.[24] Subclavian catheters allow the best level of comfort and mobility for the patient. Insertion-related complications remain a concern.[21,24] The risk of insertion-related complications is very low in the antecubital fossa. However, movement of the arm can cause migration of the catheter and irritation of the vessel wall and predispose to perforation, thrombosis, and phlebitis.

Cutdowns are usually indicated when percutaneous attempts have failed, in severe dehydration and exsanguination when veins constrict and collapse, and in patients whose venous anatomy is abnormal. However, cutdowns are more susceptible to infection and require a certain degree of surgical expertise.

REFERENCES

1. Agarwal KC, Ali Khan MA, Falls A, et al: Cardiac perforation from central venous catheterization: survival after cardiac tamponade in an infant, *Pediatrics* 73:333-338, 1984.
2. Atkinson JB, Bagnall HA, Gomperts E, et al: Investigational use of tissue plasminogen activator (t-PA) for occluded central venous catheters, *J Parenter Enter Nutr* 14:310-311, 1990.
3. Bagnall HA, Gomperts E, Atkinson JB, et al: Continous infusion of low dose urokinase in the treatment of central venous catheter thrombosis in infants and children, *Pediatrics* 83:963-966, 1989.
4. Bern MM, Lokich JJ, Wallach SR, et al: Very low doses of warfarin can prevent thrombosis in central venous catheters, *Ann Intern Med* 112:423-428, 1990.
5. Broviac JW, Cole JJ, Scribner BH: A silicone rubber atrial catheter for prolonged parenteral alimentation, *Surg Gynecol Obstet* 136:602, 1973.
6. Dato VM, Dajani AS; et al: Candidemia in children with central venous catheters: role of catheter removal and amphotericin B therapy, *Pediatr Infect Dis J* 9:309-314, May 1990.
7. Duffy LF, Kerzner B, Gebus V, et al: Treatment of central venous catheter occlusions with hydrocloric acid, *J Pediatr* 1002-1004, June 1989.
8. Dunea G, Domenico L, Guennenson P, et al: A survey of permanent double-lumen catheters in hemodialysis patients, *ASAIO Trans* 37(3):M276-277, July-Sept 1991.
9. Fuhrman BP, Zimmerman JJ, et al: *Pediatric critical care*, St. Louis, 1992, Mosby.
10. Gilliam DL, Nelson CL: Comparison of a one-step idophor skin prep versus traditional preparation in total joint surgery, *Clin Orthop* 250:258-260, 1990.
11. Haire WD, Leibermann RP, Lund GB, et al: Obstructed central venous catheters: restoring function with a 12-hour infusion of low-dose urokinase, *Cancer* 66:2279-2285, 1990.
12. Hickman RO, Buckner CD, Cligt RA, et al: A modified right atrial catheter for access to the venous system in marrow transplant recipients, *Surg Gynecol Obstet* 148:871, 1979.
13. Kamal GD, Pfaller MA, Rempe LE, et al: Reduced intravascular catheter infection by antibiotic bonding, *JAMA* 265:2364-2368, 1991.
14. Kanter RK, Gorton JM, Palmieri K, et al: Anatomy of femoral vessels in infants and guidelines for venous catheterization, *Pediatrics* 83:1020-1022, 1989.
15. Kaye W, et al: Invasive monitoring techniques: arterial cannulation, bedside pulmonary artery catheterization and arterial puncture, *Heart Lung* 12:395, 1983.
16. Mackenzie I, et al: Preoperative skin preparation and surgical outcome, *J Hosp Infect* 11 (suppl B):27-32, 1988.
17. Olson ME, Lam K, Bodey GP, et al: Evaluation of strategies for central venous catheter replacement, *Crit Care Med* 20:797-804, 1992.
18. Prince A, Heller B, Levy J, Heird W, et al: Management of fever in patients with central venous catheters, *Pediatr Inf Dis* 5:20-24, 1986.
19. Randolph J, et al: Technique for insertion of a plastic catheter into the saphenous vein, *Pediatrics* 631-635, 1959.
20. Sakamoto M, Kano T, Sadanaga M, et al: Dermal patch anaesthesia; comparison of 10% lignocaine gel with absorption promotor and EMAL cream, *Anaesthesia* 48(5):390-392, 1993.
21. Scott WL: Complications associated with central venous catheters, *Chest* 94:1221-1224, 1988.
22. Seldinger SI, et al: Catheter replacement of the needle in percutaneous arteriography, *Acta Radiol* 39:368, 1953.
23. Simon RR, Hoffman JR, Smith M, et al: Modified new approaches for rapid intravenous access, *Ann Emerg Med* 16:44-49, 1987.
24. Smith-Wright DL, Green TP, Lock JE, et al: Complications of vascular catheterization in critically ill children, *Crit Care Med* 12:1015-1017, 1984.
25. Stenzel JP, Green TP, Fuhrman BP, et al: Percutaneous femoral venous catheterizations: a prospective study of complications, *J Pediatr* 114:411-415, 1989.
26. Stenzel JP, Green TP, Fuhrman BP, et al: Percutaneous central venous catheterization in a pediatric intensive care unit: a survival analysis of complications, *Crit Care Med* 17:984-988, 1989.
27. Williams JF, Seneff MG, Friedman BC, et al: Use of femoral venous catheters in critically ill adults: prospective study, *Crit Care Med* 19:550-553, 1991.

32 Pulmonary Artery Catheterization

Luis O. Toro-Figueroa and Daniel L. Levin

SWAN-GANZ CATHETERS

Since the development of the balloon-tipped, flow-directed pulmonary artery catheter by Swan and Ganz[14,17,37,38] 23 years ago, its design and use have evolved, driven by both clinical experience and development of new technologies. Clinical application, however, has not followed properly performed prospective studies. At the same time, technologic development has integrated multiple functions into a single catheter offering even more uses that have not been proven effective.

The following blood pressures are measurable directly through flow-directed pulmonary artery catheterization of the right side of the heart: (1) central venous pressure (CVP) or right atrial blood pressure (RAP), (2) right ventricular blood pressure (RVP), (3) pulmonary arterial blood pressure (PAP), and (4) pulmonary arterial occlusion pressure (PAOP), or wedge pressure. See Table 32-1 for normal blood pressure values.

PAOP indirectly reflects left ventricular end-diastolic pressure (LVEDP) except in the conditions listed in Box 32-1. It only reflects left ventricular end-diastolic pressure during diastole when the mitral valve is open and there is free communication among the left ventricle, left atrium, pulmonary veins, pulmonary capillaries, and pulmonary arteries. LVEDP does not always accurately reflect left-sided heart preload. Left ventricular end-diastolic volume (LVEDV) correlates best with preload of the left side of the heart and LVEDP is only one of its major determinants.[30] LVEDV depends on the juxtacardiac pressure and ventricular compliance as well. These two variables can cause shifts in the left ventricular pressure-volume curve independent of changes in the LVEDP.[26] When any of the conditions that result in poor correlation between PAOP and LVEDV exist, two-dimensional echocardiography can provide left ventricular end-diastolic dimensions (LVEDDs), which may correlate better with LVEDV.[30]

Indications

The indications for Swan-Ganz catheterization are (1) to guide treatment of shock and low cardiac output states that are unresponsive to initial fluid, inotropic, and/or vasodilator therapy; (2) to assess and manage the cardiopulmonary interactions in patients treated with high intrathoracic pressure to maintain alveolar recruitment (e.g., partial end-expiratory pressure [PEEP] greater than 15 cm H_2O in patients with acute respiratory distress syndrome [ARDS]); (3) to monitor and treat pulmonary arterial hypertension; and (4) to assist in the perioperative surveillance and treatment of complex patients (e.g., complex heart defect repair, polytrauma, liver transplantation) who are at risk for development of shocklike states, cardiopulmonary instability, or systemic inflammatory response syndrome (SIRS).

Table 32-1 Pulmonary Artery Catheter–Measured Blood Pressures and Saturations

Normal blood pressure values*	Normal blood saturation	
CVP or RAP mean 3 mm Hg	Right atrium	75%
RVP Systolic 30 mm Hg	Right ventricle	75%
Mean 10 mm Hg	Pulmonary artery	75%
Diastolic 3 mm Hg	PAOP	> 90%
PAP Systolic 30 mm Hg		
Mean 20 mm Hg		
Diastolic 10 mm Hg		
PAOP mean 8 mm Hg		

*CVP, Central venous pressure; RAP, right atrial blood pressure; RVP, right ventricular blood pressure; PAP, pulmonary arterial blood pressure; PAOP, pulmonary artery occlusion pressure.

BOX 32-1 CONDITIONS IN WHICH PAOP DOES NOT REFLECT LVEDP

- Pulmonary venous obstruction
- Decreased left ventricular compliance
- Increased pulmonary vascular resistance
- Increased mean airway pressure
- Cardiac valvar disease
- Overwedging
- Eccentric balloon occlusion
- Erroneous transducer height

Contraindications

There are no known absolute contraindications to Swan-Ganz catheterization. Some of the following are relative contraindications: (1) cardiopulmonary instability with rapidly changing vital signs (near-arrest state), (2) cardiac arrhythmias or ventricular irritability that direct catheter stimulation of the endocardium may worsen, (3) intracardiac shunting (which renders thermodilution technique inaccurate as a result of loss of indicator), and/or (4) tricuspid or pulmonary valve insufficiency (which prevents flow-directed catheter forward movement, making placement difficult, and makes the thermodilution technique inaccurate through loss of indicator).

Complications

There are no data from prospective studies on complications in children. Pollack, Reed, Holbrook, et al.[28] in 1980, reported a retrospective analysis of 22 bedside catheterizations in 19 patients ranging from 2 days to 19 years, with 42% weighing less than 15 kg. The entire procedure took less than 1 hour in more than half of the patients; the longest lasted 4 hours. Catheters were in place an average of 2.2 days, with a range of 30 minutes to 8 days. Catheter malposition (two), dislodgment (two), and balloon rupture (one) caused the removal of five catheters within the first 24 hours after placement. Complications of vascular access included a pneumothorax from an internal jugular approach and bleeding from a femoral cutdown site. Fourteen patients experienced ectopic beats during catheter manipulation. Failure to "wedge" occurred in 9 of 22 catheterizations within 24 hours after placement (4 malpositions in the pulmonary artery, 3 balloon ruptures, 2 dislodgments into the right ventricle). Three patients experienced spontaneous "wedging" and one experienced hypotension during balloon inflation.

The following is a composite list of complications reported in the medical literature in adult age patients: catheter migration; arrhythmias,[9,34] including premature atrial or ventricular depolarizations,[9] ventricular tachycardia,[9] complete heart block,[39] and right bundle branch block[9,39]; bacteremia[9,25]; pulmonary embolus[9,10]; thrombosis[35] (subclavian vein)[9]; valvar perforation (pulmonic)[9]; thrombocytopenia[12]; "wedge" pressure errors[24,29]; microbial colonization[27]; pneumothorax[34]; failure to "wedge"[40]; inadvertent arterial catheterization; balloon rupture; "overwedging"; pulmonary hemorrhage; pulmonary artery false aneurysm; intravascular[35] or intracardiac knot formation; pulmonary infarction; pulmonary artery perforation; interobserver variability in measurements; and air embolism, including paradoxic central nervous system (CNS) air embolization.

Equipment

Currently there are many commercially available balloon-tipped, flow-directed pulmonary artery catheters. At least three major manufacturers offer an assortment of catheters to meet most clinical needs. One offers more than 25 variations.

Both four- and five-channel catheters are in common use; the four-channel is the most popular pediatric and adult catheter. It is available in 5-Fr and 7-Fr diameters; the five-channel configuration is only available in 7 Fr. The four-channel catheter usually contains (1) a flotation and occlusion balloon lumen, (2) a right atrial blood pressure proximal lumen, (3) a pulmonary arterial blood pressure and pulmonary arterial occlusion pressure distal lumen, and (4) a distally placed thermodilution sensor for cardiac output measurement.

In general in the standard flow-directed pulmonary artery catheter distance between the proximal (injectate) lumen in the right atrium and the distal tip in the pulmonary artery varies; 10-, 15-, 20-, and 30-cm distances are standard. Special-order catheters with shorter distances between distal and proximal ports are available for pediatric use. In 1986 Bourland determined in 61 pediatric patients, ages 0 to 165 months, the distance from the right atrial lumen to the distal catheter tip when properly positioned in the pulmonary artery[2] (Fig. 32-1). To date there are no independent studies validating these findings, but they provide a sensible guide in determining proximal lumen distance when ordering customized catheters.

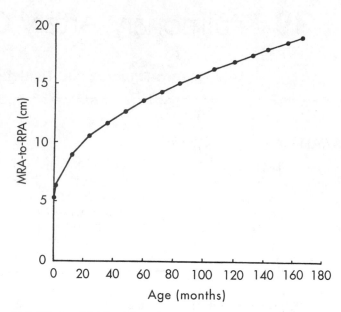

FIG. 32-1 Middle right atrium (*MRA*) to right pulmonary artery (*RPA*) versus age as a predictor of CVP port position. MRA to RPA = 1.504 + 0.156 × length − 0.117 × SSSP. *SSSP*, distance from the suprasternal notch to suprapubis.

(From Bourland LM: *Crit Care Med* 14:974-976, 1986.)

Adding to the complexity of choosing from the many catheters available is the assortment of technologic options available for the fifth channel. Some of these options are a fiberoptic continuous mixed venous oxygen saturation sensor, an extra right atrial infusion port, a right ventricular pressure measurement lumen, a transluminal ventricular endocardial pacing wire,[3,32,33] and the right ventricular and pulmonary artery electrodes to sense intracardiac R waves in conjunction with a rapid-response thermistor to detect beat-to-beat blood temperature changes. This allows direct measurement of ejection fraction and end-systolic, end-diastolic, and stroke volumes of the right ventricle.[7] No studies have validated these options for pediatric application even though they are commercially available and some centers use them clinically in children.

Choosing the appropriate catheter for a particular patient with a specific disease process is a potentially complex and difficult decision. However, use of 5 Fr catheters for children less than 15-kg body weight and 7 Fr for those greater than 15 kg has been a practical approach in choosing an appropriate size of flow-directed pulmonary artery catheter. In choosing the distance between right atrial and pulmonary artery lumens, refer to Fig. 32-1 or use the following arbitrary guidelines: 10 cm for children less than 2 years of age, 15 cm for children 2 to 7 years of age, and 20 cm for children 8 to 15 years of age.

A percutaneous introducer kit is useful for obtaining vascular access for ease of both catheterization and future repositioning. There are various kits available commercially. They usually contain the following: povidone-iodine swab sticks, a fenestrated drape, 1% lidocaine with a 3-ml syringe and a 25-gauge needle, a 22-gauge search needle to locate the vein, an 18-gauge thin-wall needle and/or an 18-gauge over-the-needle catheter, a 0.035-inch diameter/45-cm length J spring guidewire, gauze pads, a scalpel, an appropriate-size

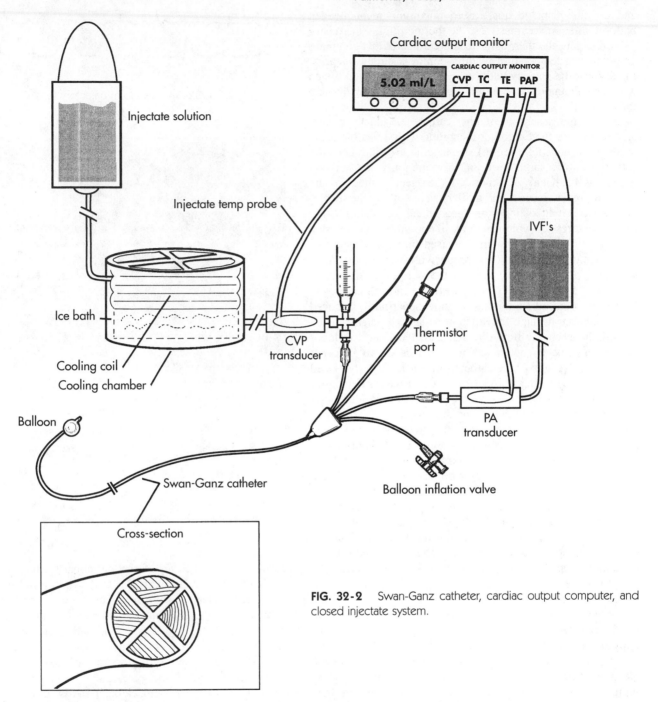

Cardiac output monitor

Injectate solution

Injectate temp probe

Ice bath

Cooling coil
Cooling chamber

CVP transducer

Thermistor port

PA transducer

Balloon

Swan-Ganz catheter

Balloon inflation valve

IVF's

CARDIAC OUTPUT MONITOR
CVP TC TE PAP

5.02 ml/L

Cross-section

FIG. 32-2   Swan-Ganz catheter, cardiac output computer, and closed injectate system.

sheath dilator assembly, an appropriate-size hemostasis valve with sideport, a catheter sleeve, povidone-iodine ointment, a straight cutting needle with 4-0 silk suture, and obturator.

Compatible pressure transducers are necessary to interface between the catheter and the oscilloscope monitor in order to measure and record the relevant pressures. Display electrocardiographic (ECG) and pulmonary artery pressure waveforms continuously at minimum precaution. A self-contained computer that calculates the area under the thermodilution curve and provides a visual display of the cardiac output is now available as a component of the patient's cardiac monitor. Some of these electronic devices display additional functions such as continuous mixed venous saturation or right ventricular ejection fraction and end-systolic, end-diastolic, and stroke volumes.

When using iced injectate for thermodilution, a means of cooling the injectate fluid to 0° C is necessary. It may be in the form of a few 20-ml vials of normal saline solution in an ice container or a commercially available closed injectate system (Fig. 32-2).[42] Sterile carbon dioxide for balloon inflation is an option to minimize the risk of air embolization in the event of balloon rupture.

CATHETER INSERTION
Technique

Test the catheter before insertion; first check the balloon integrity by attaching a syringe and injecting the appropriate volume (0.5 ml for a 5 Fr and 1.5 ml for a 7 Fr) of air or sterile carbon dioxide. Because of the risk of balloon rupture and air embolism do not exceed maximum recommended balloon inflation volumes. Test the thermodilution thermistor by connecting the thermistor to the cardiac output computer or module; a temperature reading confirms circuit integrity. Finally test the patency and integrity of each infusion lumen with a small amount of the fluid that will be infusing through the catheter.

During the insertion of the catheter maintain aseptic technique. Use the Seldinger technique with a flexible polyurethane or nonstick (Teflon) sheath dilator to introduce the catheter into a large vein, most commonly the internal jugular, subclavian, or femoral. Other access sites are the external jugular, basilic, and axillary veins. Avoid the subclavian approach in patients on mechanical ventilators using high pressures or volumes and, if possible, the internal jugular vein in patients with increased intracranial pressure (see Chapter 31 for details of proper vascular access). After securing vascular access, remove the introducer and attach the hemostasis valve with side port to the indwelling sheath. Infuse a solution containing 1 unit heparin/ml balanced saline solution through the sideport to keep it patent.

Initially insert the flow-directed catheter a short distance through a catheter contamination shield or sleeve[17]; do not extend the sleeve over the catheter until it is properly placed in the pulmonary artery (PA). Connect transducers to monitor CVP and PAP continuously via a 30-ml flow-interrupter device, high-pressure tubing, and stopcocks to the proximal and distal ports, respectively. Place the transducer at the level of the left atrium and secure it to prevent accidental movement. Fluid-fill all connections and check to be sure they are airtight in order to prevent air embolization. Accomplish the transducer calibration procedure, including zeroing, electronically, according to the monitor manufacturer's specifications. Confirm mechanical calibration by holding the tip of the catheter 27 inches above the transducer; the PAP should read 20 mm Hg. Finally before insertion wiggle the catheter to demonstrate an appropriate waveform amplitude on the monitor screen.

Flotation of the Swan-Ganz catheter through the right side of the heart requires adequate blood flow to maneuver the tip of the catheter into the pulmonary artery. Bedside fluoroscopy may greatly facilitate flow-directed catheterization. During flotation continuous visual inspection of pressure and electrocardiogram waveforms and digital readouts is of paramount importance. Changes in pressure and waveform illustrate the catheter's trajectory. Deflate the catheter when introducing it through the hemostasis valve, sheath, and vena cava. When respiratory fluctuations representing intrathoracic positioning appear in the pressure waveform tracing, slowly inflate the balloon with the prescribed volume of gas and advance it into the right ventricle. As the catheter advances, observe the step-up in systolic and mean blood pressures, as well as the increase in the amplitude of the waveform (Fig. 32-3). In the absence of arrhythmias continue to float the tip of the catheter into the main pulmonary artery.

On entering the pulmonary artery, observe widening and rounding of the waveform together with a dicrotic notch corresponding to closure of the pulmonary valve. Also note the increase in the diastolic pressure. Continue to advance the tip of the catheter to the pulmonary artery occlusion position,

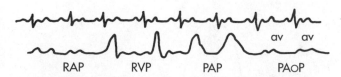

FIG. 32-3 Waveform trajectory to PAOP.

BOX 32-2 **PAOP RELIABILITY CRITERIA**

- A PAOP equal to or less than the pulmonary artery diastolic blood pressure (PADP).

- Presence of a and v waves in the PAOP waveform.

- The PAOP waveform appears and disappears quickly with balloon inflation and deflation.

- Free flow of blood indicates distal lumen patency during PAOP.

- Less respiratory variability during PAOP than during PAP.

- The PAOP oxygen tension 10 mm Hg greater than the PAP oxygen tension.[23]

- Catheter tip below the left atrium (West's zone III) on the lateral chest roentgenogram.

- Zero and calibrate transducers at least every 8 hours.

- Transducers, lines, stopcocks, and catheter lumens are air- and clot-free.

---

verified by dampening of the pulmonary artery waveform tracing into a waveform similar to the right atrial waveform. The pressure and waveform reflect those of the left atrium. Then deflate the balloon; the tracing should represent the pulmonary artery waveform. Optimally do not inflate the balloon for more than two respiratory cycles. To corroborate the reliability of the PAOP pressures and waveform, refer to Box 32-2 and Fig. 32-3.

After clinically verifying catheter position, secure it with a clamp or tape and pull the sleeve over the catheter to protect it from contamination. Obtain anteroposterior and lateral chest roentgenograms to confirm proper position. The lateral chest roentgenogram assists in determining whether the catheter tip is in West's zone III (below the left atrium). Only zone III (pulmonary artery pressure [Pa] > pulmonary venous pressure [PV] > alveolar pressure [P_A]) provides an open communicating vessel between the distal lumen (PA) of the Swan-Ganz catheter and the left atrium (LA). Remember however that both intrathoracic pressure and patient position affect the three physiologic (not anatomic) zones described by West (Fig. 32-4). Use continuous PA pressure and waveform monitoring to detect catheter tip migration and/or wedging. Simultaneous display and/or hard copy of electrocardiogram and PAOP is useful in assessing PAOP during phasic breathing.

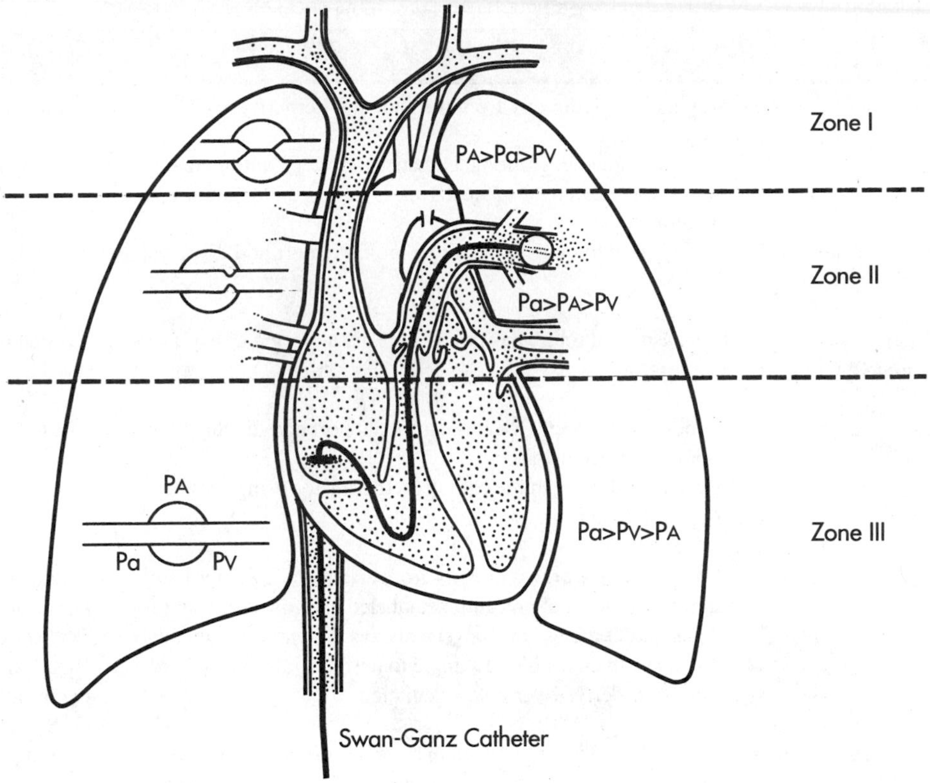

FIG. 32-4 Swan-Ganz catheter tip position in relation to West's zones.

THERMODILUTION CARDIAC OUTPUT MEASUREMENT

The thermodilution catheter for measuring cardiac output incorporates a thermistor in the distal tip of the Swan-Ganz catheter and it has become the method of choice for measuring cardiac output in both pediatric[4,11,13] and adult critically ill patients. It makes available direct and derived information about cardiopulmonary performance at the bedside[5,28] to assist in the management of patients with shock, ARDS, SIRS, or multiple organ system failure (MOSF) and those who have undergone cardiothoracic surgery. Information measured and derived from pressures and thermodilution guides therapeutic interventions, such as fluid, inotropic, and vasodilator therapy and mean airway pressure management. Thermodilution has several advantages over the dye indicator dilution method, including reproducibility, absence of deleterious cardiopulmonary effects, accuracy over a wide range of cardiac output, easy detection, nontoxic indicator, and simplicity.

The thermodilution method with iced injectate requires placement of several vials of injectate solution in an ice bath for a period of 40 minutes to achieve 0° C. Usually one vial serves as a site to monitor the injectate temperature while rapidly drawing fluid from another into a syringe just before injection. Do not place prefilled syringes in the ice bath because of the potential for bacterial contamination of the injectate fluid. Manufacturer-specific computation constants to compensate for different catheter sizes, temperatures, and volumes for injectate when computing the cardiac output are given in product inserts. To obtain accurate and reproducible

thermodilution-measured cardiac outputs, observe the conditions outlined in Box 32-3. Refer to Table 32-2 for normal values for hemodynamic and oxygenation measurements and derived variables.

To determine cardiac output using the thermodilution method, inject a known amount of solution (usually at 0° C to 4° C although it can be at room temperature) rapidly into the right atrium; the injectate mixes with blood in the right atrium and ventricle during forward flow and a change in temperature of blood is detected by the thermistor at the distal tip of the catheter. The cardiac output computer then uses the time-temperature curve generated by the thermistor and, using a modified Stewart-Hamilton equation, electronically integrates the area under the curve, which is inversely proportional to cardiac output. The computer displays the cardiac output in liters per minute as a digital readout, and some models display the time-temperature curve for inspection and assessment as well. The time-temperature curve is similar to the dye dilution curve. It starts with a rapid upstroke (injectate rapid response) and has a smooth prolonged downslope until it reaches baseline. In high cardiac output states, because of rapid mixing and transit of the injectate, the downslope is sharper, making the area under the curve smaller. In low cardiac states the mixing and transit times diminish; therefore the slope of the curve is more gradual and less acute, making the area under the curve much larger. For pediatric patients compute the cardiac index by dividing the cardiac output by the child's body surface area.

Table 32-2 Normal Values for Hemodynamic and Oxygenation Measurements and Derived Variables[6,16,20,32,36]

Directly measured variables	Source	Value
Core temperature Heart rate (HR)	Preferably measured directly from the patient; alternatively obtained from the monitor	Normal range by age
Systolic, mean, and diastolic arterial pressure (SAP, MAP, DAP)	Obtained from indwelling arterial catheter (monitor), automated blood pressure device, or manually measured with a manual pressure manometer	Normal range by age
Central venous pressure or mean right atrial pressure (CVP or MRAP)	Directly measured through Swan-Ganz proximal port and displayed on the monitor	Mean 3 mm Hg
Systolic, mean, diastolic pulmonary artery pressure (SPAP, MPAP, and DPAP)	Directly measured through the Swan-Ganz distal port and displayed on the monitor	Normal range by age
Pulmonary artery occlusion (wedge) pressure (PAOP)	Directly measured through Swan-Ganz distal port and displayed on monitor during occlusion	Mean 8 mm Hg
Cardiac output (CO)	Directly measured through the catheter's thermistor using the thermodilution method: $CO = HR \times SV$	Normal = 4-8 L/min
Arterial blood gases	Arterial blood sample drawn directly from an arterial catheter using standard technique and precautions, labeled carefully, and sent for blood gas and hemoglobin analysis; always drawn simultaneously with the mixed venous blood sample to perform intrapulmonary shunt or other derived-variable calculation	pH range 7.35-7.45 P_{CO_2} range 35-45 mm Hg T_{CO_2} range 23-29 mmol/L H_{CO_3} range 18-24 mmol/L P_{O_2} range 80-95 mm Hg O_2 Sat range 96%-100%
Mixed venous blood gas (MVBG) and pH	Mixed venous blood sample drawn in a similar fashion; a mixed venous hemoglobin sample necessary since the results of the two samples can differ significantly	pH range 7.28-7.42 mm Hg P_{CO_2} range 38-52 mm Hg T_{CO_2} range 24-30 mmol/L H_{CO_3} range 22-28 mmol/L P_{O_2} range 37-42 mm Hg O_2 Sat range 60%-80%

Derived Variables	**Source**	**Value**
Cardiac index (CI)	Reflects the capacity of the ventricle to mobilize a given volume (liters) over a period (minute) indexed to the subject's body surface area (M^2): $CI = CO/BSA$	Normal = 3.3-6 L/min/m^2
Stroke volume (SV)	The amount of blood pumped by the ventricle during one contraction: $SV = (CO/HR)(1000$ ml/L$)$	Normal = 60-100 ml/beat
Stroke volume index or Stroke index (SVI or SI)	Stroke volume indexed to the patient's body surface area: $SVI (SI) = CI/HR$ or $SVI (SI) = SV/BSA$	Normal = 33-47 ml/beat/m^2
Systemic vascular resistance index (SVRI)	The resistance against which the left ventricle has to work to eject its volume; resistance equal to pressure difference across a circuit divided by the flow or cardiac output across that circuit; indexed by substituting cardiac index for cardiac output; clinically represents the ventricular afterload across the systemic circulation: $SVRI = \dfrac{(MAP - CVP) \times 80}{CI}$	Converted from Wood's units to units of force, by a factor of 80: Normal = 800-1600 dyne-sec/cm^5/m^2
Pulmonary vascular resistance index (PVRI)	Represents right ventricular afterload across the pulmonary circuit: $PVRI = \dfrac{(MPAP - PAOP) \times 80}{CI}$	Normal = < 250 dyne-sec/cm^5/m^2
Stroke work and stroke work index (SW and SWI)	Represents the external work during a single ventricular contraction; average pressure generated by the ventricle (MAP − VEDP) multiplied by stroke volume and conversion factor for converting pressure into work (0.0136): $SW = SV (MAP - VEDP) \times 0.0136$	Normal = 45 to 75 g-m/m^2/beat
	PAO reflects left ventricular end diastolic pressure; alternatively value indexed with the BSA: $LVSWI = SVI (MAP - PAOP) \times 0.0136$	Normal = 50-62 g-m/m^2/beat
	For the right ventricle average pressure generated by the ventricle: MPAP − CVP (MRAP) $RVSWI = SVI (MPAP - MRAP) \times 0.0136$	Normal = 5-10 g-m/m^2/beat

Table 32-2 Normal Values for Hemodynamic and Oxygenation Measurements and Derived Variables—cont'd

Directly measured variables	Source	Value
Oxygen delivery index (DO_2I)	The measure of global oxygen delivery to the tissue beds, dependent on adequate oxygenation, hemoglobin concentration, and cardiac output: $DO_2I = (CaO_2)(CI)(10)$ CaO_2 = Arterial oxygen content = $(1.34)(aHb)(O_2 \text{ Sat}) + (0.003)(PaO_2)$	Normal = 570-670 $ml/min/m^2$
Oxygen consumption index (VO_2I)	Represents the amount of oxygen consumed globally by the tissues: $VO_2I = (CaO_2 - C\bar{v}O_2)(CI)$ $C\bar{v}O_2$ = Mixed venous oxygen content $= (1.34)(m\bar{v}Hb)(O_2Sat) + (0.003)(P\bar{v}O_2)$	Normal = 120-200 $ml/min/m^2$
Arteriovenous oxygen content difference [$C(a-v)DO_2$ or $avDO_2$]	Average amount of oxygen extracted per unit of blood volume; for stable oxygen consumption inversely related to cardiac output: $avDO_2 = CaO_2 - C\bar{v}O_2$	Normal = 3-5.5 ml/dl
Extraction ratio or oxygen utilization ratio (O_2 Extr or OUR)	Amount of delivered oxygen consumed by the tissues: $OUR = \dfrac{CaO_2 - C\bar{v}O_2}{CaO_2}$	Normal = 0.24-0.28
Venoarterial admixture or intrapulmonary shunt fraction ($\dot{Q}s/\dot{Q}t$)	Fraction of cardiac output not oxygenated during passage through the lungs, resulting in right to left shunting: $\dot{Q}s/\dot{Q}t = \dfrac{CCO_2 - CaO_2}{CCO_2 - C\bar{v}O_2}$ CCO_2 = Pulmonary end capillary O_2 content = $(1.34)(aHb)(1.0$ for O_2 Sat$) + (0.003)(P_AO_2)$ $P_AO_2 = (FIO_2)(P_B - P_{H_2O}) - (PaCO_2/R)$ R = Respiratory quotient = 0.8	Normal ≤ 5%
Coronary artery perfusion pressure (CAPP)	Represents the coronary artery perfusion pressure during diastole: $CAPP = DAP - PAOP$	Normal (adults) = > 40 mm Hg

---

BOX 32-3 **CONDITIONS CONDUCTIVE TO ACCURATE AND REPRODUCIBLE THERMODILUTION MEASURED CARDIAC OUTPUT**

- Proper mixing of injectate and blood.

- Temperature of the injectate must be preserved.

- Duration of the injection less than 2 seconds.

- Injection lumen must not contain any medications.

- Appropriate distance between injection site and thermistor.

- Accurate determination of the volume and temperature of the injectate.

- Absence of tricuspid, pulmonary insufficiency, or intracardiac mixing occurs.

- Relatively steady state as reflected by the heart rate and systemic arterial blood pressure.

- Perform cardiac output measurements in triplicate determinations within minutes of each other.

- Each value must be within 10% to 15% of each other.

Interpretation

Eisenberg, Jaffe, Shuster, et al.,[8] in 1984, prospectively evaluated 103 catheterizations in which they asked physicians to predict the range of hemodynamic variables and plan for therapy. They predicted PAOP correctly 30% of the time and cardiac output, CVP, and systemic vascular resistance correctly approximately 50% of the time. Swan-Ganz catheterization altered therapy in 58% of the cases and suggested the addition of unanticipated therapy in 30%. They concluded that Swan-Ganz catheterization is therefore indicated and useful.

Iberti, Fischer, Leibowitz, et al.,[19] in 1990, conducted a study of physicians' understanding of the concepts and application of the data they measured and derived through Swan-Ganz catheterization. Multiple-choice examination of 496 physicians in 13 medical centers resulted in a mean test score of 20.7 (67%), with a standard deviation of 5.4 and a range of 6 to 31 (19% to 31%). They concluded that physician understanding of the device is extremely variable, leading to erroneous diagnostic and therapeutic interventions, and that credentialing policies should ensure individual competency. This study highlights the need for critical scrutiny of the indications for catheterization in relation to the disease process, the interpretation of the data directly measured, or the derived parameters in the context of the clinical state of the patient, and the meticulous adherence to the technique and criteria that ensure the accuracy, reliability, and reproducibility of this procedure. The process of evalu-

> **BOX 32-4 CONDITIONS THAT ACCOMPANY ELEVATED PADP**
>
> - Increased pulmonary blood flow
>
> - Increased pulmonary vascular resistance
>
> - Increased pulmonary venous blood pressure

ation, intervention, and interpretation of the Swan-Ganz measured and derived data is not a static one. It requires constant reevaluation of the physiologic changes caused by a specific therapeutic intervention in the context of the disease process and prior responses to similar interventions.

The left atrial pressure (LAP), approximated by PAOP, is usually within 4 mm Hg of the pulmonary artery diastolic pressure (PADP) except when one of the conditions listed in Box 32-1 is present. Therefore when PAOP and PADP are within 4 mm Hg, pulmonary artery occlusion is not necessary. Box 32-4 lists the conditions that may be present with elevated PADP. In the presence of normal pulmonary artery pressure PAOP also reflects pulmonary hydrostatic pressure.

Maintenance

The clinical care of the flow-directed pulmonary artery catheter is similar to that of a central venous catheter. Always adhere to aseptic technique when handling the catheter. The sleeve prevents contamination during repositioning of the catheter.

Persistent occlusion waveform indicates a wedged catheter tip and requires immediate repositioning to prevent complications. To prevent balloon rupture in this situation, switch the balloon lumen lock to the open position, disconnect the syringe, and allow the balloon to deflate spontaneously. Air aspiration with a syringe can cause balloon rupture, and blood return from the balloon lumen indicates that balloon rupture has occurred. Consider replacing or removing the catheter, whichever is clinically indicated; lock the port and do not use it. Pulmonary infarction, fictitiously elevated PAOP, and pulmonary artery rupture can result from exceeding the recommended balloon volume capacity.

Discontinuation

The guidelines for removal of a Swan-Ganz catheter are (1) resolution of the initial indication for catheterization, (2) lack of frequent therapeutic intervention as a result of the steady state of the patient, (3) development of thrombus formation attributable to the catheter, (4) refractory arrhythmias secondary to direct stimulation by the catheter, (5) pulmonary embolism with distribution related to catheter position, and/or (6) colonization, bacteremia, and/or sepsis that does not respond to appropriate antibiotic therapy through the suspected port(s). Always deflate the balloon when withdrawing or removing the catheter. When discontinuing the catheter in postoperative open heart repair patients, it may be useful to record pressures and waveforms and draw blood gases while pulling the catheter tip through the different vessels and cardiac chambers. Refer to Table 32-1 for normal

intracardiac pressures and saturations. Mixing in the right atrium is incomplete; therefore the venous saturations along the jet streams from the coronary sinus, the superior vena cava, and the inferior vena cava decrease, in that order.

CONTINUOUS MIXED OXYGEN SATURATION MONITORING

Continuous mixed venous saturation measurement is possible through reflectance spectrophotometry, which uses multiple wavelengths of light, reflected through red blood cells as they flow by, to measure deoxyhemoglobin and oxyhemoglobin to determine mixed venous blood oxygen saturation (Svo_2).[22] The fiberoptic filaments reside in a lumen of a flow-directed pulmonary artery catheter with one transmitting and one detecting fiberoptic filament exposed to the pulmonary blood flow distally. Two advantages of fiberoptic catheters are that they provide a measure of adequacy of signal and they display the reflected light intensity.[31] The light intensity warns of catheter tip migration and validates the displayed Svo_2. There is however controversy over the clinical efficacy of continuous Svo_2 monitoring.[15] When hemoglobin concentration, arterial oxygen saturation, and oxygen consumption are stable, continuous mixed venous oxygen saturation properly reflects cardiac output.[21,41] To date there are no prospective randomized studies in adult or pediatric patients that clearly validate this technology. Theoretical advantages provided by continuous Svo_2 are that it facilitates anticipatory monitoring of clinical changes and it provides "real-time" capacity to evaluate therapeutic interventions.[1] The theoretic disadvantages are that cardiac output correlates poorly with Svo_2 in many clinical entities, especially in those in which there is dissociation between oxygen delivery and oxygen consumption; that a critical Svo_2 level for specific organ dysfunction(s) is not known; and that the accuracy of the technology itself is uncertain. Rouby et al.[39] in 1990 demonstrated that the three-wavelength system is more accurate than the two-wavelength system, with or without a second detecting fiberoptic filament, when hematocrit is stable.

Indications

There are no established indications for continuous Svo_2 in children. However some of the indications proposed for adult patients apply to pediatric patients. The proposed indications for use in adults include disease entities that may affect the oxygen transport and delivery system (e.g., shock and other low cardiac output states), conditions associated with abnormal oxygen transport or delivery (e.g., cardiac surgery,[18] posttransplantation, MOSF, SIRS, high mean airway pressure, or pentobarbital coma), and disease entities entailing impaired oxygen use (e.g., sepsis or ARDS).

Contraindications

There are no known contraindications to continuous Svo_2 monitoring. Always analyze the risks versus benefits as described for Swan-Ganz catheterization.

Complications

The risk of complications from continuous Svo_2 is similar to that of flow-directed pulmonary artery catheters. One theoretical concern is the possibility that clinicians may implement therapeutic interventions based on inaccurately obtained data obtained from "numbers" rather than physiologic applicability or pertinence to a pathophysiologic process.

Equipment

Presently there are a few options in Svo_2 catheters and monitors. The five-lumen catheters usually are available in sizes 7.5 Fr and 8.5 Fr and the four-lumen catheters in 5.5-Fr size. There is a single-lumen 4-Fr thermodilution catheter available with only a cardiac output thermistor. As previously discussed, they may emit two to three wavelengths; the three-wavelength technology is the most accurate to date.

Technique

Most monitoring devices require calibration before insertion and verification in vivo. Usually recalibration is not necessary if the measured sample value is within 4% of the monitored Svo_2 value. Conduct continuing surveillance for catheter tip migration or wedging, looking for a decreasing PAP waveform that may simulate a PAOP waveform, an increased or high value for Svo_2, or a diminished light intensity as displayed by the monitor. Appropriate placement of the catheter tip is paramount for accurate results.

Remarks

The determinants of Svo_2 are arterial oxygen saturation, cardiac output, hemoglobin concentration, and oxygen consumption. The physiologic range for the Svo_2 is 65% to 80%. A fall in Svo_2 usually implies a decrease in arterial oxygen saturation or cardiac output, development of relative anemia, or an increase in oxygen consumption. An increase in Svo_2 may be difficult to interpret. Pathologic and nonpathologic conditions that may impair oxygen consumption (e.g., sepsis or anesthesia), increased oxygen delivery (e.g., early hypermetabolic compensated septic shock, cirrhosis, or inotropic and/or vasoactive therapy), and/or therapeutic interventions that lead to high Pao_2 are responsible for an increase in Svo_2.

There is a need for validation studies of use of the technique in pediatric patients.

REFERENCES

1. Birman H, Haq A, Hew E et al: Continuous monitoring of mixed venous oxygen saturation in hemodynamically unstable patients, *Chest* 86:753-755, 1984.
2. Bourland LM: Allometric determination of the distance from the central venous pressure port to wedge position of balloon-tip catheters in pediatric patients, *Crit Care Med* 14:974-976, 1986.
3. Colardyn F, Vandenbogaerde J, De Niel C, et al: Ventricular pacing via a Swan-Ganz catheter: a new mode of pacemaker therapy, *Acta Cardiol* 41:233-229, 1986.
4. Colgan FJ, Stewart S: An assessment of cardiac output by thermodilution in infants and children following cardiac surgery, *Crit Care Med* 5:220-225, 1977.
5. Dalen JE: Bedside hemodynamic monitoring, *N Engl J Med* 301(21):1176-1178, 1979.
6. Dean JM, Wetzel RC, Rogers MC: Arterial blood gas derived variables as estimates of intrapulmonary shunt in critically ill children, *Crit Care Med* 13(12):1029-1033, 1985.
7. Dhainault JF, Burnet F, Monsallier JF et al: Bedside evaluation of right ventricular performance using a rapid computerized thermodilution method, *Crit Care Med* 15(2):148-152, 1987.
8. Eisenberg PR, Jaffe AS, Shuster DP: Clinical evaluation compared to pulmonary artery catheterization in the hemodynamic assessment of critically ill patients, *Crit Care Med* 12:549-553, 1984.
9. Elliott CG, Zimmerman GA, Clemmer TP: Complications of pulmonary artery catheterization in the care of critically ill patients, *Chest* 76:647-652, 1979.
10. Fairfax WR, Thomas F, Orme JF: Pulmonary artery catheter occlusion as an indication of pulmonary embolus, *Chest* 86:270-271, 1984.
11. Fanconi S, Burger R: Measurement of cardiac output in children, *Intens Care World* 9(1):8-12, 1992.
12. Feinberg BI, LaMantia KR, Addonizio P et al: Pulmonary artery catheter-associated thrombocytopenia: Effect of heparin coating, *Mt Sinai J Med* 54:147-149, 1987.
13. Freed MD, Keane JF: Cardiac output measured by thermodilution in infants and children, *J Pediatr* 92:39-42, 1978.
14. Ganz WW, Forrester JS, Chonette D et al: A new flow-directed catheter technique for measurement of pulmonary artery and capillary wedge pressure without fluoroscopy, *Am J Cardiol* 25:96, 1970.
15. Gettienger A: Mixed venous saturation: the puzzle is still incomplete, *Chest* 94(4):786-787, 1990.
16. Grabenkort W: A cardiopulmonary physiologic profile for use with the Swan-Ganz catheter, *Resident Staff Physician* 29(7):80-85, 1983.
17. Heard SO, Davis RF, Sherertz RJ et al: Influence of sterile protective sleeves on the sterility of pulmonary artery catheters, *Crit Care Med* 15(5):499-502, 1987.
18. Hecker BR, Brown DL, Wilson D: A comparison of two pulmonary artery mixed venous catheters during changing conditions of cardiac surgery, *J Cardiothoracic Anesthesia* 3:269-275, 1989.
19. Iberti TJ, Fischer EP, Leibowitz AB et al: A multicenter study of physicians' knowledge of the pulmonary artery catheter, *JAMA* 264(22):2928-2932, 1990.
20. Kandel G, Aberman A: Mixed venous oxygen saturation, *Arch Intern Med* 143:1400-1402, 1983.
21. Krovetz LJ, McLoughlin TG, Mitchell MB et al: Hemodynamic findings in normal children, *Pediatr Res* 1:122-130, 1967.
22. Martin WE, Cheny PW, Johnson CC et al: Continuous monitoring of mixed venous oxygen saturation in man, *Anesth Analg* 52:784-793, 1973.
23. Morris AH, Chapman RH: Wedge pressure confirmatin by aspiration of pulmonary capillary blood, *Crit Care Med* 13(9):756-759, 1985.
24. Morris AH, Chapman RH, Gardner RM: Frequency of wedge pressure errors in the ICU, *Crit Care Med* 13(9):705-708, 1985.
25. Myers ML, Austin TW, Sibbald WJ: Pulmonary artery catheter infections: a prospective study, *Ann Surg* 201(2):237-241, 1985.
26. Nadeau S, Noble WH: Misinterpretation of pressure measurements from the pulmonary artery catheter, *Can Anaesth Soc J* 33(3):352-363, 1986.
27. Nelson LD, Martinez OV, Anderson HB: Incidence of microbial colonization in open versus closed delivery systems for thermodilution injectate, *Crit Care Med* 14(4):291-293, 1986.
28. Pollack MM, Reed TP, Holbrook PR et al: Bedside pulmonary artery catheterization in pediatrics, *J Pediatr* 96(2):274-276, 1980.
29. Quintana E, Sanchez JM, Serra C et al: Erroneous interpretation of pulmonary capillary wedge pressure in massive pulmonary embolism, *Crit Care Med* 11(12):933-935, 1983.
30. Raper R, Sibbald WJ: Misled by the Wedge? The Swan-Ganz catheter and left ventricular preload, *Chest* 89(3):427-434, 1986.
31. Rouby JJ, Poète P, Bodin L et al: Three mixed venous saturation catheters in patients with circulatory shock and respiratory failure, *Chest* 98(4):954-958, 1990.
32. Ruiz BC, Tucker WK, Kirby RR: Laboratory report: a program for calculation of intrapulmonary shunts, blood-gas and acid-base values with a programmable calculator, *Anesthesiology* 42(1):88-95, 1975.
33. Simoos ML, Demey HE, Bossaert LL et al: The paceport catheter: a new pacemaker system introduced through a Swan-Ganz catheter, *Cathet Cardiovasc Diagn* 15(1):66-70, 1988.
34. Sise MJ, Hollingsworth P, Brimm JE et al: Complications of the flow-directed pulmonary-artery catheter: a prospective analysis in 219 patients, *Crit Care Med* 9(4):315-318, 1981.
35. Smith-Wright DL, Green TP, Lock JE et al: Complications of vascular catheterization in critically ill children, *Crit Care Med* 12(12):1015-1017, 1984.

36. Stopfkuchen H: Hemodynamic monitoring in childhood, *Intens Care Med* 15 (suppl 1):527-531, 1989.
37. Swan HJC, Ganz W: Use of balloon flotation catheters in critically ill patients, *Surg Clin North Am* 55(3):501-520, 1975.
38. Swan HJC, Ganz W, Forrester J et al: Catheterization of the heart in man with use of a flow-directed balloon-tipped catheter, *N Engl J Med* 283(9):447-451, 1970.
39. Thomson IR, Dalton BC, Lappas DG et al: Right bundle-branch block and complete heart block caused by the Swan-Ganz catheter, *Anesthesiology* 51(4):359-362, 1979.
40. Traeger SM: Failure to wedge and pulmonary hypertension during pulmonary artery catheterization: a sign of totally occlusive pulmonary embolism, *Crit Care Med* 13(7):544-547, 1985.
41. Vaughn S, Puri VK: Cardiac output changes and continuous mixed venous oxygen saturation measurement in the critically ill, *Crit Care Med* 16:495-498, 1988.
42. Yonkman CA, Hamory BH: Sterility and efficiency of two methods of cardiac output determination: closed loop and capped syringe method, *Heart Lung* 17(2):121-128, 1988.

33 Arterial Catheterization

Curt M. Steinhart

INDICATIONS

Indwelling arterial catheters allow performance of a number of important functions with relative safety and substantial reliability.[9,14,21] Continuous monitoring of systemic arterial blood pressure, including systolic, diastolic, and mean pressures is crucial in the care of the critically ill or injured pediatric patient. Changes in blood pressure often indicate important hemodynamic alterations that reflect vital delivery of oxygen and nutrients to numerous vascular beds. Monitoring systemic arterial blood pressure allows for careful monitoring and titration of various therapeutic interventions, including intravenous fluids, intravascular volume expanders, blood products, and vasoactive agents (e.g., catecholamines, inotropes, and vasodilators).

Placement of indwelling systemic arterial catheters allows ready access for arterial blood gas sampling. After properly placing the catheter, staff can draw samples of systemic arterial blood without pain even at frequent intervals. This allows arterial blood gas analysis free from the effects of respiratory changes induced by crying in the infant and small child.

In the critically ill pediatric population, venipuncture for frequent laboratory analysis can be both painful to the patient and progressively challenging to the phlebotomist confronted with a diminishing source of suitable veins. Sampling from an indwelling arterial catheter allows ease in blood letting and saves peripheral veins for future placement of intravenous catheters. Similarly, it is possible to use arterial catheters to withdraw blood during exchange transfusion.

Pediatric intensive care units (PICUs) commonly use removal of plasma ultrafiltrate via continuous arteriovenous hemofiltration (CAVH) for renal insufficiency and for clearance of certain substances and toxins. With CAVH blood moves via an arterial catheter from the arterial circulation across the membrane filter and returns via a venous catheter.

CONTRAINDICATIONS

There are very few contraindications to arterial catheterization. An absolute contraindication is the likelihood of abnormal perfusion distal to the potential cannulation site. Consider using the Allen Test before radial artery cannulation[17,21] to verify adequate collateral flow through the ulnar artery. However, some authors believe that the Allen Test is superfluous because neither does a normal test guarantee adequate collateral flow nor does an abnormal test absolutely preclude safe placement.[17,20]

As with all catheters, do not place arterial catheters through areas with skin infection or in any vessel where concern about distal flow exists. (This circumstance occurs when considering femoral artery cannulation following cardiac catheterization.)

COMPLICATIONS

Despite the relative safety and desirability of having arterial access, complications from arterial lines, although uncommon, may be catastrophic. Thrombus formation at the catheter site may completely occlude the cannulated vessel, rendering distal sites completely ischemic.[4,10,11] In the femoral artery this can result in total leg ischemia, gangrene, and amputation. Although not as disastrous as complete occlusion of an artery, distal embolic problems are more frequent. Major distal embolization may result in loss of distal structures such as feet, toes, hands, and fingers.[10,11] On a more limited basis, embolization may render distal parts of fingers and toes ischemic, leading to eventual autoamputation. In addition, there are reports of cerebral infarction with temporal artery cannulation.[2,15]

Infections associated with arterial catheters are very infrequent and of less concern than with venous catheters. Nonetheless, infectious arterial phlebitis (arteritis) and aneurysm formation do occur and may lead to disseminated infection and septicemia.[6-8,13,19] The high rate of arterial blood flow relative to venous flow appears to be the major reason that arterial catheters are infrequently infected. In most PICUs arterial line fluids are routinely changed every 24 or 48 hours, a practice that somewhat limits the number of violations into the intraflow system. However, staff frequently must interrupt arterial lines for arterial blood sampling. Whether by "drip technique" or via a stopcock withdrawal, sampling does involve interruption of line integrity. Despite these interruptions, infectious complications remain uncommon.[1,8]

Arteriovenous fistulas may develop, particularly with prolonged use of an arterial catheter in a single site. Connections with adjacent veins may develop and require surgical repair.

Finally, a major hazard of any arterial catheter is separation of any component of the system with exsanguination. Secure connections to stopcocks and tubing tightly, or rapid blood loss can occur. To avoid or reduce the incidence of complications, remove functioning catheters when the indication for placement is no longer present.

EQUIPMENT

See Box 33-1.

TECHNIQUE
Placement

Percutaneous Insertion. A number of techniques are available for arterial cannulation, all of which require successful arterial puncture. The most common method uses a catheter over-a-needle. After selection of the site, skin preparation, and, if needed, local anesthesia, puncture the skin and

---

BOX 33-1 EQUIPMENT

Site preparation

1. Tape
2. Armboard — several sizes
3. Benzoin
4. Iodine solution/swabs
5. Iodine ointment
6. Gloves
7. Xylocaine, 1% or 2%

Additional items for arteriotomy/cutdown

8. Sterile towels for draping
9. Sterile mask, gloves, and gown
10. Procedure lamp

Maintenance

1. Infusion pump or pressure infuser
2. Saline solution—0.45% or 0.9%
3. Heparin—add 1 to 2 U/ml of fluid
4. Flush device/flow controller—3 ml/hr

Monitoring

1. Pressure transducer
2. Transducer cable
3. Monitor with pressure module

Cannulation

1. Catheters 20, 22, and 24 gauge
2. Catheter with guidewire kit—2.5, 3.0 Fr.
3. Guidewires—0.015-0.018-0.021-inch diameter
4. Suture—4.0 silk or nylon
5. Syringes
6. T-connector

Additional items for arteriotomy/cutdown

7. Procedure tray—sterile
   a. Scalpel handle
   b. Scalpel blades—Nos. 11 and 15
   c. Scissors—small
   d. Forceps—straight and curved—small
   e. Retractors—small, skin
   f. Needle holder
   g. Hemostats (three)—mosquito size
   h. Right angle hemostat
   i. Sterile gauze sponges

---

direct the catheter toward the underlying artery. Watch for flashback of blood while continuously advancing the catheter and stylet (direct technique) (Fig. 33-1). When flashback occurs, insert the catheter a bit further before removing the stylet. If blood returns rapidly, attach a syringe with flush solution, aspirate the line, and, if rapid blood return is still present, advance the catheter while flushing gently. Advance the catheter to its hub so that as much catheter as possible is below the skin to make the line more secure and to minimize chances for dislodgement. Securely affix the catheter with tape and Benzoin or sutures. Should there be no flashback despite inserting the entire catheter (transfixation technique),

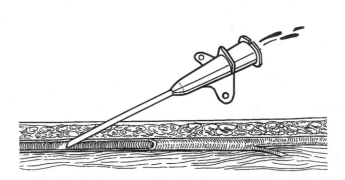

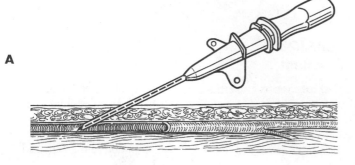

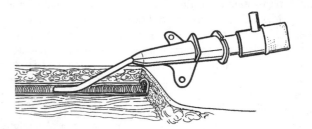

FIG. 33-1 Direct percutaneous technique. **A** and **B,** Direct the catheter and needle toward the artery until flashback of blood is visible. **C,** Withdraw the needle and insert the catheter its entire length into the artery.

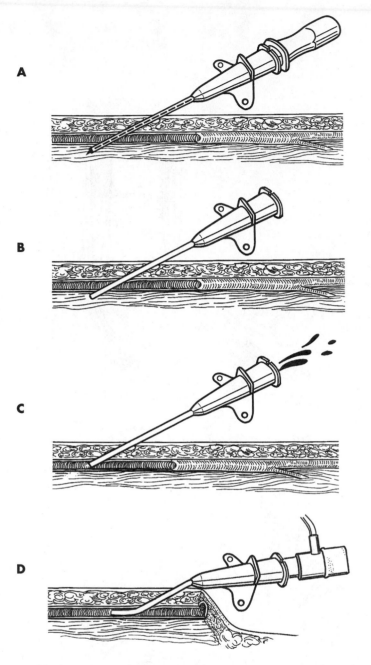

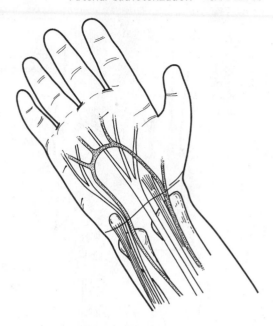

FIG. 33-3   Radial artery anatomy.

FIG. 33-2   Transfixation percutaneous technique. Pass the catheter and needle through the artery (**A**). Remove the needle (**B**) and slowly withdraw the catheter until flashback of blood is visible (**C**). Insert the catheter its entire length into the artery (**D**).

remove the stylet and slowly withdraw the catheter while observing for rapid blood return (Fig. 33-2). When rapid blood return occurs, use the procedure previously described and attach a flush solution, aspirating to ensure proper placement, and then advance while flushing gently. If no rapid blood return occurs either during catheter insertion or withdrawal, repeat the procedure from the point of skin puncture. Alternatively, withdraw the catheter to a point just below the skin surface, very carefully rethread the stylet, and proceed again with catheter advancement, looking for flashback as above. Rethread the stylet cautiously, since shearing of the catheter can occur.

Use the standard technique described previously for placement of catheters in the radial (Fig. 33-3), dorsalis pedis (Fig. 33-4), posterior tibial[16] (Fig. 33-5), brachial, or temporal arteries. Use the standard technique for femoral artery cannulation as well (Fig. 33-6); however, the depth of the femoral artery, leg movement, and likelihood of dislodgement often require a longer catheter. Use a longer catheter for the axillary artery.[3,5]

When a longer catheter is necessary, use a guidewire. A number of commercially available products provide a puncture needle, guidewire, and catheter that slides over the guidewire. To place arterial catheters over guidewires, prepare the skin and prepare a sterile field. Give local anesthesia and slowly advance a needle attached to an aspirating syringe toward the artery while gently, but continuously, aspirating. When blood flows rapidly into the syringe, detach the syringe from the needle and carefully advance the guidewire through the needle. After inserting a sufficient length of guidewire to exit the needle and enter the artery, retrieve the needle from the distal end of the guidewire, feed the catheter over the guidewire, and push the catheter through the skin and subcutaneous tissue into the artery. When the catheter is fully inserted, withdraw the guidewire, attach a flush solution to the catheter, aspirate to ensure proper position, and flush with heparinized saline solution to clear blood from the catheter. Secure the line with sutures and apply a sterile dressing.

On the basis of experience and personal preference, a combination of the two techniques may be used. One combination uses a commercially available catheter supplied with a short, attached guidewire. With this arrangement, place the catheter through the skin and direct it toward the artery. When flashback of blood occurs, advance the short guidewire into the artery and then insert the catheter over the guidewire before removing both the needle and the guidewire. An alternate method with the guidewire technique is to place a short catheter into the artery using the percutaneous method previously described, and then thread a guidewire through

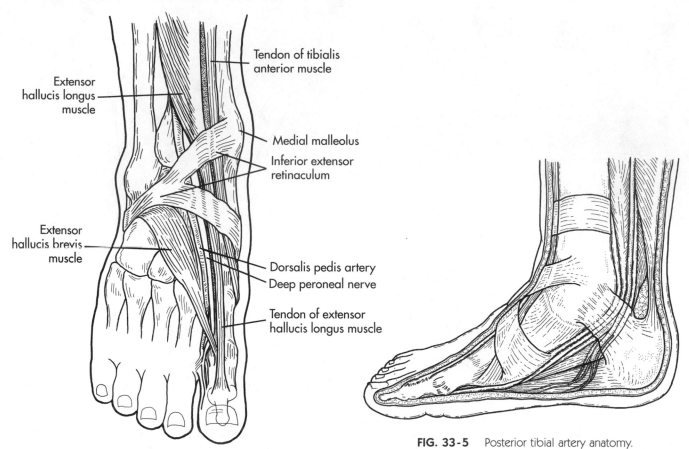

Extensor hallucis longus muscle

Tendon of tibialis anterior muscle

Medial malleolus

Inferior extensor retinaculum

Extensor hallucis brevis muscle

Dorsalis pedis artery

Deep peroneal nerve

Tendon of extensor hallucis longus muscle

FIG. 33-4 Dorsalis pedis artery anatomy.

FIG. 33-5 Posterior tibial artery anatomy.

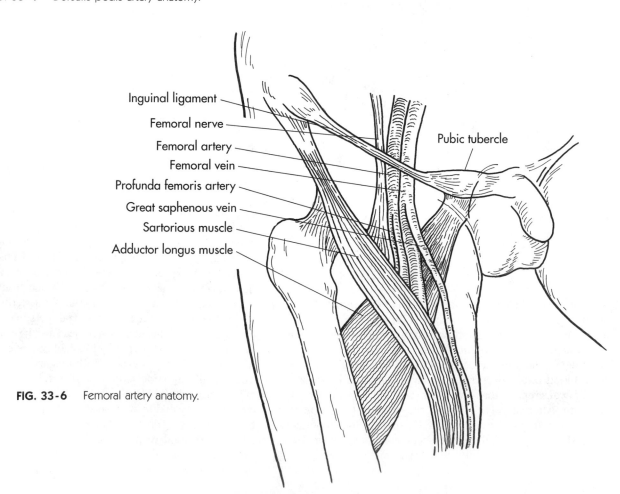

Inguinal ligament

Femoral nerve

Femoral artery

Femoral vein

Profunda femoris artery

Great saphenous vein

Sartorious muscle

Adductor longus muscle

Pubic tubercle

FIG. 33-6 Femoral artery anatomy.

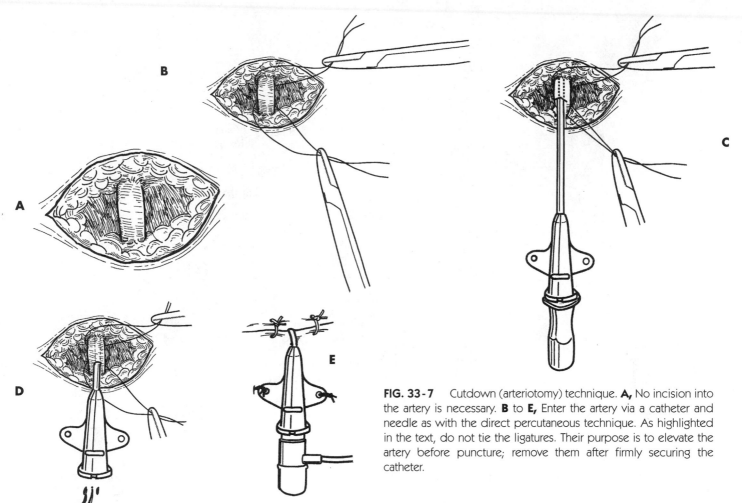

FIG. 33-7 Cutdown (arteriotomy) technique. **A,** No incision into the artery is necessary. **B** to **E,** Enter the artery via a catheter and needle as with the direct percutaneous technique. As highlighted in the text, do not tie the ligatures. Their purpose is to elevate the artery before puncture; remove them after firmly securing the catheter.

the catheter. Without disturbing the guidewire, remove the short catheter and replace it by threading a longer catheter over the wire. The advantages of this technique are (1) it is not necessary to thread the guidewire through the needle, but rather through a properly placed catheter; (2) it is easier to determine proper position in the artery and to avoid inadvertent placement of the guidewire outside the artery; and (3) it is easier to establish a small catheter initially, particularly in the small infant or in the child who is uncooperative and moving.

Finally, advances in Doppler technology have led to the development of devices that can help the operator locate the artery.[12] To use these devices, attach the blunt end of a disposable needle to a Doppler device, which sends a signal to the operator regarding the proximity of the arterial pulse. After puncturing the artery, use one of the techniques described previously to cannulate the artery and to secure the catheter in place.

Arteriotomy. Placement of an arterial catheter via cutdown (arteriotomy) technique is similar to the percutaneous technique, but visualize the vessel to be cannulated directly. Following sterile preparation and draping, inject 1% lidocaine subcutaneously. For the radial artery, make a 1-cm incision perpendicular to the long axis of the forearm 1 to 2 cm proximal to the wrist directly over the course of the artery. Using small mosquito hemostats, bluntly dissect the

subcutaneous tissue. Maintain tissue separation in a direction parallel to the artery. After visualizing the artery, exercise care in "freeing" it from surrounding tissues, avoiding unnecessary trauma that might result in bleeding, hematoma formation, or tearing of the artery (Fig. 33-7). After isolating the artery, place ligatures around it at the proximal and distal ends. *Do not tie either ligature.* They are strictly for stabilization before cannulation.

To insert the catheter, pull gently on the distal ligature to elevate the artery slightly. Under direct observation, puncture the artery only far enough to ensure that the catheter is within the vessel. Avoid creating a false channel. Although there should be blood return visible in the stylet, arterial spasm or slight occlusion may hinder rapid return. When the catheter is clearly within the arterial lumen, remove the stylet and carefully thread the catheter to its entire length. As with percutaneous placement, attaching a T-connector and syringe containing heparinized flush solution greatly eases this process. After completely threading the catheter, secure it to the skin with sutures. Next, carefully remove the ligatures and close the wound. Apply a sterile dressing and further secure the catheter with adhesive tape. Attach the appropriate connections as with percutaneous catheter placement.

For sites other than the radial artery, the technique is similar, although the anatomy differs. When possible, avoid dorsalis pedis arteriotomy in favor of posterior tibial arteri-

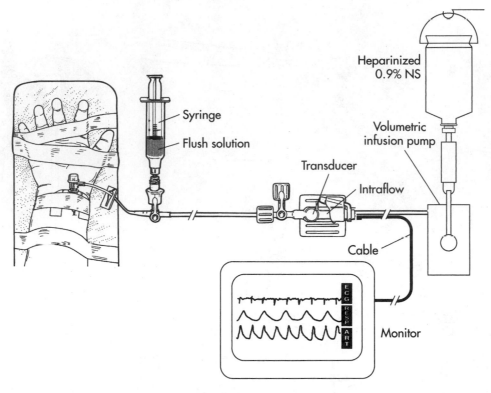

FIG. 33-8 Arterial line setup. This diagram illustrates the setup for an arterial catheter from the insertion site to the monitor and includes stopcock sites and the intraflow infusion site. *NS,* Normal saline.

otomy to avoid damage to tendons (see Fig. 33-4 and 33-5). To access the femoral artery by arteriotomy, carefully perform a dissection of the femoral triangle using an incision 1.5 to 2 cm below the inguinal ligament (see Fig. 33-6).

Maintenance and Sampling

Maintain arterial catheter patency using a continuous infusion of heparinized solution containing 1 U of heparin added to each milliliter of 0.9% normal saline. For older children, use 2 U of heparin per milliliter of 0.9% normal saline. Administer the solution through an intraflow system by volumetric infusion pump at a rate of 1 to 3 ml/hour (Fig. 33-8). Change the solution and tubing to the intraflow every 24 to 48 hours.

Accomplish sampling by either the drip or stopcock technique. The drip method may be easier under most circumstances, but when removing large volumes of blood at one time (greater than 4 ml) or when measuring prothrombin/partial thromboplastin times, the stopcock technique may prove more useful.

To use the drip technique, place several gauze sponges under the flashport of the T-connector (Fig. 33-9). Cleanse the flashport with povidone iodine. After the povidone iodine has dried, occlude the T-connector with the clamp. Puncture the flashport with a small-gauge needle (No. 21, 23, or 25) and allow 6 drops of blood to drip onto the gauze sponges. Collect blood by allowing it to drip into microtubes or via a blood gas syringe that provides very gentle aspiration. After obtaining all needed samples, remove the needle from the flashport, release the clamp from the T-connector, and gently flush 0.2 to 0.4 ml of heparinized solution at the nearest

stopcock to clear blood from the flashport. Using this technique wastes little blood; it is unnecessary to return diluted blood.

Alternatively, remove blood from the stopcock nearest the arterial catheter (Fig. 33-10) by first aspirating an aliquot

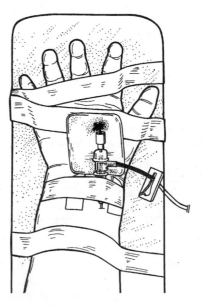

FIG. 33-9 Drip technique. This diagram illustrates the needle placed through the T-connector flashport. The gauze sponges placed below the flashport prevent blood from soiling the area. Note proper taping to secure the wrist.

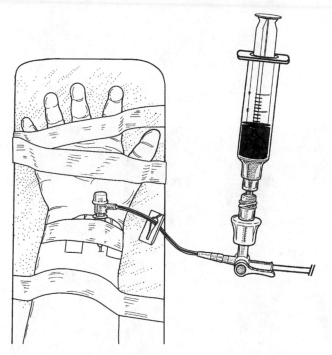

FIG. 33-10 Stopcock technique. This diagram illustrates sampling via a syringe at the nearest stopcock. Close the stopcock to the infusion tubing to avoid sampling dilution.

(usually 3 ml) of fluid containing blood into a "discard" syringe. Then draw the predetermined amount of blood into a sampling syringe (or syringes). Using the stopcock port, flush the stopcock and T-connector with 1 ml of heparinized flush solution. Although blood-containing fluid in the discard syringe may be returned through the arterial catheter before the line is cleared with heparinized flush solution, this practice may increase the potential for distal embolic phenomena. Some PICUs choose to return the blood via a peripheral or central vein, whereas others simply discard the solution. Some centers use only the stopcock technique, since the drip technique heightens concern about infection of personnel from exposure to blood.

REMARKS

Become familiar with a variety of techniques before developing a preference. The following tips are location-specific:

Radial artery: Immobilize the forearm, wrist, and hand using an armboard and tape; place the wrist in moderate extension and maintain the position with a gauze roll; maintain the thumb in moderate abduction with tape. Proper positioning brings the radial artery close to the surface and keeps it parallel to the long axis of the forearm.

Dorsalis pedis: Enter the vessel as distal as possible and remain parallel to the long axis of the foot; distal puncture avoids the inferior extensor retinaculum, which diffuses the pulse and makes precise location of the artery more difficult.

Posterior tibial: Insert the catheter parallel and lateral to the Achilles tendon (tendo calcaneus) using a steep angle. For young infants, access the medial or lateral plantar arteries below the bifurcation of the posterior tibial artery at angles of 45 and 20 degrees to the tendo calcaneus, respectively.

Femoral artery: Place the lower extremities in the 45-degree frogleg position to form a 90-degree angle between the two extremities; proper positioning allows the femoral vessels to align along a line connecting the knee with the umbilicus. Perform skin puncture 1 to 2 cm below the inguinal ligament.[18]

Axillary artery: Abduct the upper arm to an angle between 90 and 135 degrees from the trunk and rotate slightly externally; puncture the artery high in the axilla. Verify that the tip is at least 2 cm from the origin of the right common carotid artery.

Brachial artery: Avoid brachial artery cannulation, if possible, due to poor collateral flow.

Temporal artery: Retrograde emboli into the carotid artery and intracranial vessels can occur; avoid this approach unless the benefit clearly outweighs the risk.

REFERENCES

1. Adams JM, Speer ME, Rudolph AJ: Bacterial colonization of radial artery catheters, *Pediatrics* 65:94-97, 1980.
2. Bull MN, Schreiner RL, Garg BP, et al: Neurologic complications following temporal artery catheterization, *J Pediatr* 96:1071-1073, 1980.
3. Cantwell GP, Holzman BH, Caceres MJ: Percutaneous catheterization of the axillary artery in the pediatric patient, *Crit Care Med* 18:880-881, 1990.
4. Chang C, Dughi J, Shitabata P, et al: Air embolism and the radial arterial line, *Crit Care Med* 16:141-143, 1988.
5. deAngelis J: Axillary arterial monitoring, *Crit Care Med* 4:205-206, 1976.
6. Ducharme FM, Gauthier M, Lacroix J, et al: Incidence of infection related to arterial catheterization in children: a prospective study, *Crit Care Med* 16:272-276, 1988.
7. Falk, PS, Scuderi PE, Sherertz RJ, et al: Infected radial artery pseudoaneurysms occurring after percutaneous cannulation, *Chest* 101:490-495, 1992.
8. Furfaro S, Gauthier M, Lacroix J, et al: Arterial catheter-related infections in children, *Am J Dis Child* 145:1037-1043, 1991.
9. Gardner RM, Schwartz R, Wong HC, et al: Percutaneous indwelling radial-artery catheters for monitoring cardiovascular function, *N Engl J Med* 290:1227-1231, 1974.
10. Hack WWM, Vos A, Okken A: Incidence of forearm and hand ischemia related to radial artery cannulation in newborn infants, *Intensive Care Med* 16:50-53, 1990.
11. Hack WWM, Vos A, van der Les J, et al: Incidence and duration of total occlusion of the radial artery in newborn infants after catheter removal, *Eur J Pediatr* 149:275-277, 1990.
12. Maher JJ, Dougherty JM: Radial artery cannulation guided by Doppler ultrasound, *Am J Emerg Med* 7:260-262, 1989.
13. McEllistrem RF, O'Toole DP, Keane P: Post-cannulation radial artery aneurysm—a rare complication, *Can J Anaesth* 37:907-909, 1990.
14. Miyasaka K, Edmonds JF, Conn AW: Complications of radial artery lines in the pediatric patient, *Can Anaesth Soc J* 23:9-14, 1976.
15. Prian GW, Wright GB, Rumack CM, et al: Apparent cerebral embolization after temporal artery catheterization, *J Pediatr* 93:115-118, 1978.
16. Rawle P: Cannulation of the posterior tibial artery, *Anaesthesia* 45:589-590, 1990.
17. Slogoff S, Keats AS, Arlund C: On the safety of radial artery cannulation, *Anesthesiology* 59:42-47, 1983.
18. Soderstrom CA, Wasserman DH, Durham CM, et al: Superiority of the femoral artery for monitoring, *Am J Surg* 144:309-312, 1982.
19. Swanson E, Freiberg A, Salter DR: Radial artery infections and aneurysms after catheterization, *J Hand Surg* 15A:166-171.
20. Thomson SR, Hirshberg A: Allen's text re-examined, *Crit Care Med* 16:915 (letter), 1988.
21. Toro-Figueroa LO, Yeakel K: Arterial catheters. In Levin DL, Morriss FC, editors: *Essentials of pediatric intensive care*, St. Louis, 1990, Quality Medical Publishing.

34 Intraosseous Infusion

Debra H. Fiser

Establishing vascular access quickly in critically ill infants and toddlers is often very difficult even for experienced practitioners. The technique of intraosseous infusion (IOI) offers a simplified alternative for short-term, emergency vascular access.

IOI takes advantage of the vascular drainage system in long bones where the marrow sinusoids drain into medullary venous channels (Fig. 34-1). Nutrient and emissary veins direct this flow into the systemic venous circulation. Absorption of fluids and most drugs infused into the marrow cavity is rapid and complete.[18,45] However, because of the replacement of the red marrow with less vascular yellow marrow in older children, the technique may not be as useful for children over the age of 5 years.[64]

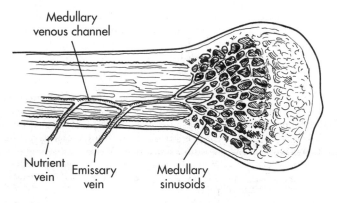

FIG. 34-1 Marrow sinusoids drain into medullary venous channels; nutrient and emissary veins direct this flow into the systemic venous circulation.

INDICATIONS

Use IOI for life-threatening situations in which it is impossible to obtain rapid emergency vascular access conventionally. These situations most often include cardiopulmonary arrest, shock, burns, and life-threatening status epilepticus.[14]

In addition to administration of blood products and fluids into the marrow cavity, IOI of pharmacologic agents is also possible (Box 34-1). In fact, studies have demonstrated that only a few medications delivered by this route produce subtherapeutic levels using standard intravenous doses; among these are chloramphenicol, vancomycin, and tobramycin.[20]

The clinical laboratory can also analyze marrow aspirated before infusion for blood chemistries, $Paco_2$, pH and hemoglobin.[2,5,37] It may be useful to culture the marrow as an alternative to peripheral blood culture or to use marrow for type and crossmatch as well.[2,37]

BOX 34-1 MEDICATIONS ADMINISTERED BY IOI

Ampicillin[31,42]	Insulin[28,29,58]
Atracurium[23]	Isoproterenol[52]
Atropine[19,23,31,44,52,59]	Levarterenol[39]
Calcium chloride[36]	Lidocaine[23,59]
Calcium gluconate[1]	Local anesthetics[26,27]
Cefotaxime[20,42]	Lorazepam[21]
Ceftriaxone*[42]	Morphine[28,29]
Dexamethasone[59]	Naloxone[23]
Dextrose[16,35,36]	Pancuronium[30,52]
Diazepam[6,30,31,53]	Penicillin[13,55]
Diazoxide[59]	Phenobarbital[4,6,30,52]
Digitalis[41,55,39]	Phenytoin[52,63]
Dobutamine[3]	Propranolol[25]
Dopamine[3,35,65]	Sodium thiopental[23,39,46]
Ephedrine[51]	Sodium
Epinephrine[36,50,51,65]	bicarbonate[11,16,19,31,36,52,53,56,65]
Gentamicin[42]	Succinylcholine[23,31,55,57]
Heparin[55,59]	Sulfonamides[55]

*Use larger dose for IOI because of protein binding.

CONTRAINDICATIONS

There are only a few contraindications to IOI.[30,33] Avoid IOI with an ipsilateral fractured extremity because of the risk of extravasation. Likewise, following penetration of the cortex of the bone during an unsuccessful IOI attempt, abandon that side for future attempts in preference to the opposite side. Other contraindications include osteopetrosis and osteogenesis imperfecta. Avoid introducing the needle through an area of cellulitis or infected burn to prevent infectious complications such as osteomyelitis.[30,33]

Avoid prolonged placement of the IOI needle because the risk of complications increases with increasing duration of use.[60] Remove the needle as soon as possible, usually within 2 hours of placement. As a rule, it is easier to obtain conventional vascular access after using IOI for fluid and pharmacologic resuscitation, which often returns the patient to a state of circulatory stability.

Because of the theoretic risk of fat embolism, weigh the risks and benefits before using IOI in children known to have a right-to-left intracardiac shunt.[54]

COMPLICATIONS

Complications related to the procedure are rare, particularly with correct technique. The most frequent, and potentially serious, problem encountered is extravasation of fluid. Causes of extravasation include incomplete cortex penetration with the needle, penetration through the posterior cortex, extravasation through a bony defect (fracture or previous IOI puncture site), and extravasation through a nutrient vessel foramen.[47] The risk of extravasation increases with prolonged infusion[60] and with infusion under pressure.[15,60] The complications of extravasation, particularly the risk of skin necrosis, may increase with infusion of catecholamines.[9] There are several recent reports of compartment syndrome following IOI extravasation that required fasciotomy or even amputation of the extremity.* Several of these cases occurred in association with prolonged infusion.

Infectious complications, including localized cellulitis, subcutaneous abscesses, and osteomyelitis (less than 1%) also occur in rare instances.[40,48] Risk for infection increases when using IOI in a bacteremic patient, when infusing hypertonic solutions, and when the needle remains in situ for an extended time.[48]

To date, numerous clinical and experimental studies have failed to identify any lasting detrimental effects on the bone, growth plate, or marrow elements.† However, fractures have occurred in an infant related to needle insertion.[24] Some transient changes in the peripheral blood smear also occur, including decreased cellularity,[43] a decrease in circulating monocytes along with an increase in basophils and nucleated red blood cells,[49] the presence of circulating blasts in peripheral blood,[22] increased numbers of burr cells and schistocytes,[49] and polychromasia.[49]

EQUIPMENT

Box 34-2 lists the necessary supplies for IOI. A number of types of IOI needles are presently available on the market. Needles with a handle to grip are ideal. Some products have an adjustable-length shaft to decrease the risk of penetrating the posterior aspect of the cortex. Other products resemble a screw with sideports. This design enhances the stability of the needle during infusion. Another design has side ports to enhance flow rates, especially if the distal needle orifice is lodged against the posterior cortex. Due to the increased risk of fractures, avoid 15-gauge needles in young infants.[10]

BOX 34-2   **EQUIPMENT AND SUPPLIES FOR IOI**
Bone marrow or IOI needle with stylet, 15- to 18-gauge
Restraints
Sandbag or other support for knee
Skin preparation solution (alcohol or iodine)
Local anesthetic, needle, and syringe (optional)
10-ml syringe
Heparinized saline flush solution (1 U of heparin per milliliter)
Infusion fluid
T-connector or stopcock (optional)
Intravenous infusion set (optional)
Pressure bag (optional)
4 × 4 gauze and tape

---

*References 8, 15, 34, 47, 60, and 66.

†References 1, 7, 11, 12, 17, 19, 61, 62, and 65.

TECHNIQUE

The most popular location for IOI insertion is the proximal tibia. After assembling the necessary supplies and equipment, restrain the extremity with a small sandbag in the popliteal fossa for support to optimize positioning and to minimize the risk of fractures.[32,38] Cleanse the skin aseptically with iodine or alcohol. Rarely will it be necessary to use local anesthetic in a patient who requires IOI because of the level of obtundation; however, infiltrate the area, including the periosteum, liberally with a local anesthetic for patients who are conscious.

As illustrated in Fig. 34-2, identify the insertion point in the midline on the medial flat surface of the anterior tibia, 1 to 3 cm (2 fingers breadth) below the tibial tuberosity.[3,33] For young infants, the insertion point is at the level of the tibial tuberosity to avoid the midshaft region and its associated risk of fracture (Fig. 34-3).[32]

Advance the needle, using firm pressure and a screwing motion or a back-and-forth rotary motion at an angle of 60 to 90 degrees away from the epiphyseal plate.[48] At the point of cortex penetration, resistance decreases. The needle stands upright without support. Remove the stylet, attach a syringe to the needle, and attempt to aspirate marrow to confirm placement. If it is not possible to aspirate marrow, confirm placement by noting lack of resistance to the infusion of 5 to 10 ml of crystalloid solution. Flushing the needle with heparinized saline solution may help to prevent clotting in the needle. Inject drugs and fluids directly or use a T-connector or stopcock setup; alternatively, assemble an intravenous infusion set for slower infusion or add a pressure bag for more rapid infusion. With pressure infusion at 300 mm Hg, it is possible to achieve flows in the range of 41 ml/min.[51] Tape gauze pads in place to stabilize the apparatus without obscuring visualization of the site. Alternatively, clamp a hemostat to the base of the needle at the level of the skin and tape the hemostat firmly to the extremity.

Observe the site every 5 to 10 minutes during infusion for evidence of extravasation; monitor distal pulses as well.[8,60] Evidence of extravasation should prompt careful evaluation to detect compartment syndrome (see also Chapter 37).

After stabilizing the patient hemodynamically, obtain conventional vascular access as soon as possible and discontinue the IOI. After removing the needle, hold manual pressure for 5 minutes and then apply a sterile dressing. If there will be a delay of more than an hour in obtaining conventional access, radiographic confirmation of placement of the IOI needle is ideal.[34,60] Some authors recommend follow-up x-ray films in any patient who has had IOI attempted or performed to rule out occult fracture.[32]

Alternative sites for consideration if the proximal tibia approach is unacceptable or fails include the distal femur, distal tibia, and anterior superior iliac spine. When using the distal femur, insert the needle 2 to 3 cm proximal to the external condyle in the midline (Fig. 34-4) and direct it superiorly at an angle of 75 to 80 degrees.[18] Another possibility is the distal tibia. In this location, insert the needle perpendicularly just proximal to the middle malleolus and posterior to the saphenous vein (Fig. 34-5).[19] The anterior superior iliac spine is also readily identifiable and accessible for IOI in older children (Fig. 34-6). The relative efficacy,

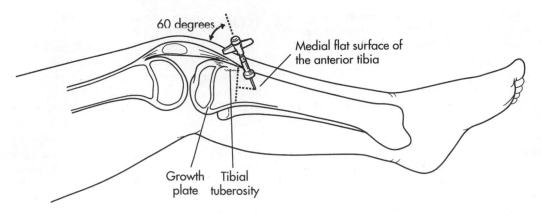

FIG. 34-2 Standard anterior tibial approach. The insertion point is in the midline on the medial flat surface of the anterior tibia, 1 to 3 cm (2 fingers breadth) below the tibial tuberosity.

FIG. 34-3 Anterior tibial approach for young infants. The insertion point is at the level of the tibial tuberosity.

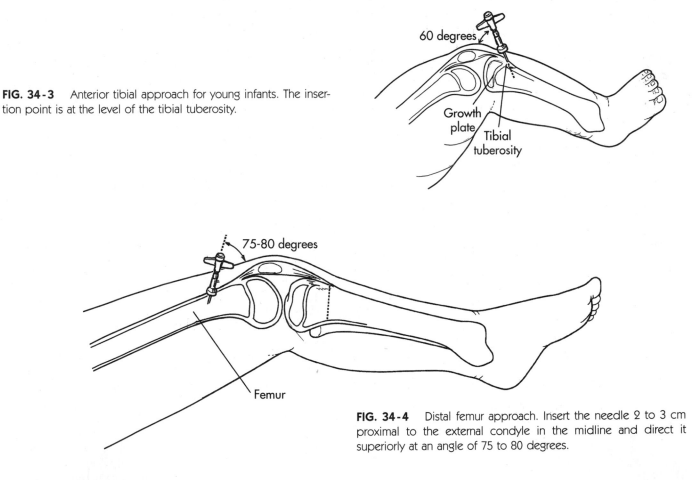

FIG. 34-4 Distal femur approach. Insert the needle 2 to 3 cm proximal to the external condyle in the midline and direct it superiorly at an angle of 75 to 80 degrees.

FIG. 34-5 Distal tibia approach. Insert the needle perpendicularly just proximal to the middle malleolus and posterior to the saphenous vein.

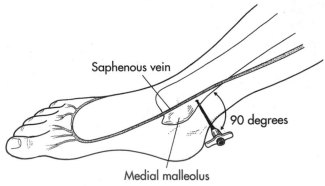

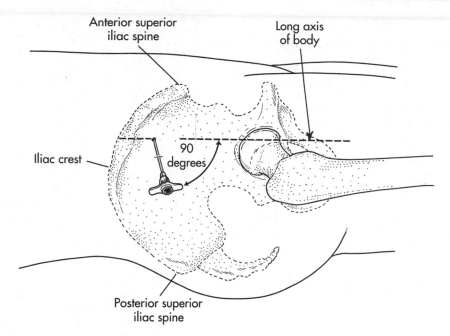

FIG. 34-6   Anterior superior iliac spine approach. Insert the needle at an angle of 90 degrees to the long axis of the body.

safety, and feasibility of these sites are unknown. Avoid use of the sternum with its associated risk of mediastinitis.[16]

REMARKS

Not withstanding the rare severe complication associated with this procedure, IOI can be lifesaving when rapid conventional vascular access is impossible. It is usually possible to avoid the most important complications by using appropriate technique and carefully monitoring the site for signs of extravasation.

REFERENCES

1. Arbeiter HI, Greengard J: Tibial bone marrow infusions in infancy, *J Pediatr* 25:1-12, 1944.
2. Baldwin ST, Johnston C: Intraosseous infusion: a technique whose time has returned, *Alabama Med* 56:29-31, 1987.
3. Berg RA: Emergency infusion of catecholamines into bone marrow, *Am J Dis Child* 138:810-811, 1984.
4. Brickman K, Rega P, Choo M, et al: Comparison of serum phenobarbital levels after single versus multiple attempts at intraosseous infusion, *Ann Emerg Med* 19:31-33, 1990.
5. Brickman K, Rega P, Guinness M: A comparative study of intraosseous, intravenous and intra-arterial pH changes during hypoventilation in dogs, *Ann Emerg Med* 16 (abstr):510, 1987.
6. Brickman KR, Rega P, Guinness M: A comparative study of intraosseous versus peripheral intravenous infusion of diazepam and phenobarbital in dogs, *Ann Emerg Med* 16:1141-1144, 1987.
7. Brickman KR, Rega P, Koltz M, et al: Analysis of growth plate abnormalities following intraosseous infusion through the proximal tibial epiphysis in pigs, *Ann Emerg Med* 17:121-123, 1988.
8. Burke T, Kehl DK: Intraosseous infusion in infants, *J Bone Joint Surg* 75:428-429, 1993.
9. Christensen DW, Vernon DD, Banner W Jr, et al: Skin necrosis complicating intraosseous infusion, *Pediatr Emerg Care* 7:289-290, 1991.
10. Crane RG: Where are the fractures and needles? (letter)? *Ann Emerg Med* 19:731, 1990.
11. Dedrick DK, Mase C, Ranger W, et al: The effects of intraosseous infusion on the growth plate in a nestling rabbit model, *Ann Emerg Med* 21:494-497, 1992.
12. Dubick MA, Pfeiffer JW, Clifford CB, et al: Comparison of intraosseous and intravenous delivery of hypertonic saline/dextran in anesthestized, euvolemic pigs, *Ann Emerg Med* 21:498-503, 1992.
13. Elston JT, Jaynes RV, Kaump DH, et al: Intraosseous infusion in infants, *Am J Clin Pathol* 17:143-150, 1947.
14. Fiser DH: Intraosseous infusion, *N Engl J Med* 32:1579-1581, 1990.
15. Galpin RD, Kronick JB, Willis RB, et al; Bilateral lower extremity compartment syndromes secondary to intraosseous fluid resuscitation, *J Pediatr Orthop* 11:773-776, 1991.
16. Glaeser PW, Losek JD: Emergency intraosseous infusions in children, *Am J Emerg Med* 4:34-36, 1986.
17. Heinild S, Sondergaard T, Tudrad F: Bone marrow infusion in childhood: experiences from a thousand infusions, *J Pediatr* 30:400-412, 1947.
18. Hodge D, Delgado-Paredes C, Fleisher G: Intraosseous infusion flow rates in hypovolemic "pediatric" dogs, *Ann Emerg Med* 16:305-307, 1987.
19. Iserson KV: Intraosseous infusions in adults, *J Emerg Med* 7:587-591, 1989.
20. Jaimovich DG, Kumar A, Francom S: Evaluation of intraosseous vs intravenous antibiotic levels in a porcine model, *Am J Dis Child* 145:946-949, 1991.
21. Jim KF, Lathers CM, Farris VL, et al: Suppression of pentylenetetrazol-elicited seizure activity by intraosseous lorazepam in pigs, *Epilepsia* 30:480-486, 1989.
22. Joffe M: Blasts in the peripheral blood with intraosseous infusion, *Pediatr Emerg Care* 6:106-107, 1990.
23. Katan BS, Olshaker JS, Dickerson SE: Intraosseous infusion of muscle relaxants, *Am J Emerg Med* 6:353-354, 1988.
24. La Fleche FR, Milzman DP: Where are the fractures and needles? (reply), *Ann Emerg Med* 19:731, 1990.
25. Lathers CM, Jim KF, Spivey WH: A comparison of intraosseous and intravenous routes of administration for antiseizure agents, *Epilepsia* 30:472-479, 1989.
26. Lilienthal B: Cardiovascular responses to intraosseous injections of prilocaine containing vasoconstrictors, *Oral Surg* 42:552-558, 1976.
27. Lilienthal B, Reynolds AK: Cardiovascular responses to intraosseous injections containing catecholamines, *Oral Surg* 40:574-583, 1975.

28. Macht DI: Studies on intraosseous injections of epinephrine, *Am J Physiol* 38:269-272, 1943.

29. Macht DI. Absorption of drugs through the bone marrow, *Proc Soc Exp Biol Med* 47:299-305, 1941.

30. Manley L, Haley K, Dick M: Intraosseous infusion: rapid vascular access for critically ill or injured infants and children, *J Emerg Nurs* 14:63-69, 1988.

31. McNamara RM, Spivey WH, Unger HD, et al: Emergency applications of intraosseous infusion, *J Emerg Med* 5:97-101, 1987.

32. Melker RJ, Miller G, Gearen P, et al: Complications of intraosseous infusion (letter), *Ann Emerg Med* 19:731-732, 1990.

33. Miner WF, Corneli HM, Bolte RG, et al: Prehospital use of intraosseous infusion by paramedics, *Pediatr Emerg Care* 5:5-7, 1989.

34. Moscati R: Compartment syndrome with resultant amputation following intraosseous infusion (letter), *Am J Emerg Med* 8:470-471, 1990.

35. Neish SR, Macon MG, Moore JWM, et al: Intraosseous infusion of hypertonic glucose and dopamine, *Am J Dis Child* 142:878-880, 1988.

36. Orlowski JP, Porembka DT, Gallagher JM, et al: Comparison study of intraosseous, central intravenous, and peripheral intravenous infusions of emergency drugs, *Am J Dis Child* 144:112-117, 1990.

37. Orlowski JP, Porembka DT, Gallagher JM, et al: The bone marrow as a source of laboratory studies, *Ann Emerg Med* 18:1348-1351, 1989.

38. Parrish GA, Turkewitz D, Skiendzielewski JJ: Intraosseous infusions in the emergency department, *Am J Emerg Med* 4:59-63, 1986.

39. Pillar S: Re-emphasis on bone marrow as a medium for administration of fluid, *N Engl J Med* 251:846-851, 1954.

40. Platt SL, Notterman DA, Winchester P: Fungal osteomyelitis and sepsis from intraosseous infusion, *Pediatr Emerg Med* 9:149-150, 1993.

41. Pollack CV, Pender ES: Intraosseous administration of digoxin: same-dose comparison with intravenous administration in the dog model, *J Miss State Med Assoc* 32:335-338, 1991.

42. Pollack CV, Pender ES, Woodall BN, et al: Intraosseous administration of antibiotics: same-dose comparison with intravenous administration in the weaning pig, *Ann Emerg Med* 20:772-776, 1991.

43. Pollack CV, Pender ES, Woodall BN, et al: Long-term local effects of intraosseous infusion on tibial bone marrow in the weanling pig model, *Am J Emerg Med* 10:27-31, 1992.

44. Prete MR, Hannan CV, Burkle FM: Plasma atropine concentrations via the intravenous, endotracheal, and intraosseous routes of administration, *Am J Emerg Med* 5:101-104, 1987.

45. Redmond AD, Plunkett PK: Intraosseous infusion, *Arch Emerg Med* 3:231-233, 1986.

46. Reisman HA, Tainsky IA: The bone marrow as an alternate route for transfusion in pediatrics, *Am J Dis Child* 68:253-256, 1944.

47. Ribeiro JA, Price CT, Knapp DR: Compartment syndrome of the lower extremity after intraosseous infusion of fluid, *J Bone Joint Surg* 75A:430-433, 1993.

48. Rosetti VA, Thompson BM, Miller J, et al: Intraosseous infusion: an alternative route of pediatric intravascular access, *Ann Emerg Med* 14:885-888, 1985.

49. Ross SP, McMannis SI, Kowal-Vern A, et al: Effect of intraosseous saline infusion on hematologic parameters, *Ann Emerg Med* 20:243-245, 1991.

50. Sapien R, Stein H, Padbury JF, et al: Intraosseous versus intravenous epinephrine infusions in lambs: pharmacokinetics and pharmacodynamics, *Pediatr Emerg Care* 8:179-183, 1992.

51. Shoor PM, Berryhill RE, Benumof JL: Intraosseous infusion: pressure-flow relationship and pharmacokinetics, *J Trauma* 19:772-774, 1979.

52. Smith RJ, Keseg DP, Manley LK, et al: Intraosseous infusions by prehospital personnel in critically ill pediatric patients, *Ann Emerg Med* 17:491-495, 1988.

53. Spivey WH, Lathers CM, Malone DR, et al: Comparison of intraosseous, central, and peripheral routes of sodium bicarbonate administration during CPR in pigs, *Ann Emerg Med* 14:1135-1140, 1985.

54. Stewart FC, Kain ZN: Intraosseous infusion: elective use in pediatric anesthesia, *Anesth Analg* 75:626-629, 1992.

55. Tarrow AB, Turkel H, Thompson MS: Infusions via the bone marrow and biopsy of the bone and bone marrow, *Anesthesiology* 13:501-509, 1952.

56. Thompson BM, Rossetti V, Miller J, et al: Intraosseous administration of sodium bicarbonate: an effective means of pH normalization in the canine model, *Ann Emerg Med* 13 (abstr):405, 1984.

57. Tobias JD, Nichols DG: Intraosseous succinylcholine for orotracheal intubation, *Pediatr Emerg Care* 6:108-109, 1990.

58. Tocantins LM, O'Neill JF, Price AH: Infusions of blood and other fluids via bone marrow in traumatic shock and other forms of peripheral circulatory failure, *Ann Surg* 114:1085-1092, 1941.

59. Valdes MM: Intraosseous fluid administration in emergencies, *Lancet* 1:1235-1236, 1977.

60. Vidal R, Kissoon N, Gayle M: Compartment syndrome following intraosseous infusion, *Pediatrics* 91:1201-1202, 1993.

61. Vinsel PJ, Moore GP, O'Hair KC: Comparison of intraosseous versus intravenous loading of phenytoin in pigs and effect on bone marrow, *Am J Emerg Med* 8:181-183, 1990.

62. Wallden L: On injuries of bone and bone marrow after intraosseous injections: an experimental investigation, *Acta Chir Scand* 96:152-162, 1947.

63. Walsh-Kelly CM, Berens RJ, Glaeser PW, et al: Intraosseous infusion of phenytoin, *Am J Emerg Med* 4:523-524, 1986.

64. Warwick R, Williams PL: *Gray's anatomy*, Edinburgh, 1973, Longman, p. 49.

65. Woodall BN, Pender ES, Pollack SV, et al: Intraosseous infusion of resuscitative fluids and drugs: long-term effect on linear bone growth in pigs, *South Med J* 85:820-824, 1991.

66. Wright R, Reynolds SL, Nachtsheim B: Compartment syndrome secondary to prolonged intraosseous infusion, *Pediatr Emerg Care* 10:157-159, 1994.

35 Pressure Transduction in the Pediatric Intensive Care Unit

M. Michele Moss

Measurement of intravascular pressures is a cornerstone of patient assessment in the pediatric intensive care unit (PICU). Intraarterial, central venous, and pulmonary arterial pressures provide crucial information about the hemodynamic status of the patient. Although many techniques exist for measuring systemic arterial pressure, fluid-filled, strain gauge transduction systems are the most commonly used for continuous readout of intravascular and intracardiac pressures. These systems allow transformation of intravascular pressure into an electrical signal for recording on an oscilloscope, digital display, recording paper, or in a computer. Despite differences in the characteristics of the hemodynamic pressures of interest, all fluid-filled systems have the same basic components—transducer, amplifier, recording device, and catheter with tubing and stopcocks.

Three components comprise hemodynamic pressures.[2] The *static*, or *residual* pressure is the pressure inside the fluid-filled vascular structure (vessel or heart) and is the pressure of interest. The static pressure varies with the contraction of the heart, giving the characteristic pressure tracings of the monitored vessel or cardiac chamber. The kinetic energy of the moving fluid, in this case blood, imparts *dynamic* pressure. High blood flow aimed directly at the catheter tip produces the dynamic pressure. Hence, dynamic pressure artifact is greater with arterial catheters, especially with those in femoral or other central arteries, than with venous catheters. It is possible to minimize, but not completely eliminate, dynamic pressure artifact from the system by changing the direction of the catheter or applying a damping device. *Hydrostatic* pressure results from the effect of gravity producing a pressure difference from one end of the system to the other (i.e., from the tip of the catheter to the air-reference port of the transducer). Careful positioning of the transducer at the same level as the tip of the catheter eliminates hydrostatic pressure.

Indications

The indication for invasive intravascular pressure monitoring is a need for frequent and rapid assessment of pressures in a patient with either variability of the pressures or the potential for variability due to the disease process or therapeutic interventions. Chapters pertaining to each type of catheter discuss the specific indications for their insertion (see Chapters 31 to 33).

Contraindications

Chapters 31 to 33 also discuss the specific contraindications for insertion of each.

Complications

Electrical Hazard. Because of the proximity of the electric current to the fluid-filled monitoring system and hence to the patient, the potential for electric shock exists.[2] Cardiac arrhythmias and twitching of the skeletal muscle can occur with electric leak to the patient. Close assessment by biomedical technicians of new and older monitoring equipment can detect electric leakage. Adequate grounding of the equipment with a three-pronged plug can prevent harm to the patient. The third prong serves as the ground. The presence of 60-cycle interference on the electrocardiogram trace from a monitor may indicate poor grounding. If present, the biomedical technicians should evaluate both the equipment and the ground before any further patient use.

Equipment

Transducers. Transducers enable conversion of biophysical events, in this case intravascular pressure changes, to electronic signals for recording and examination. The strain gauge, the most common type of transducer used for pressure measurement, evolved from the principle of the Wheatstone bridge. In a Wheatstone bridge a voltage change occurs when there is alteration in the resistance to the flow of current in the wires. The change in resistance occurs when the applied pressure changes the length and width of the wires in the gauge. The change in pressure is proportional to the change in voltage produced.

Fig. 35-1 depicts the traditional domed pressure transducer with the fluid-filled dome connected to the intravascular catheter by way of fluid-filled tubing.[2,4] Because fluid is not compressible, the vasculature transmits the pressure wave to the transducer with little distortion. A flexible metal membrane transmits the change in intravascular pressure to the strain gauge wires, producing a change in voltage and generating an electrical output signal. Because of the durability and stability of this transducer, it is useful in clinical and research settings. A disposable pressure transducer is available that houses a pressure-sensor chip with a transverse voltage strain gauge (Fig. 35-2). The chip, mounted on a backplate and covered with a dome, allows fluid to flow through it as part of the catheter flush system. Although this transducer is also stable, it is part of the flush system and therefore is disposable.

Many other types of pressure transducers are available.[4] It is possible to miniaturize strain gauge transducers by using semiconductors rather than wires. These transducers are then small enough for mounting on catheter tips. These transducer-tipped catheters, such as the Millar catheter, are

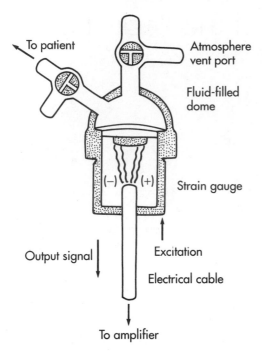

FIG. 35-1 Fluid-filled domed transducer with strain gauge. Pressure applied to the dome causes a change in resistance in the wires of the Wheatstone bridge in the strain gauge. These changes cause generation of an electrical signal.

useful for short-term pressure evaluation such as during cardiac catheterization. Optical methods of pressure measurement are also adaptable to catheter technology. Fiberoptic catheters exist that have a flexible membrane at the catheter tip. When the membrane moves, presumably from a change in pressure, it alters reflection of an internal source of light. That alteration in the flux of light transmits to an external phototube, which generates an electrical signal in proportion to the pressure change. It is common to use this technology for monitoring of intracranial pressure. Because of the inflexibility of the optical fibers, this technique is not useful intravascularly. Servo and piezoelectric manometers are also available. Because of the shorter useful life and extreme expense of many of these techniques, they are not amenable to daily clinical use.

Amplifiers and Recording Devices. Because the voltage produced by the strain gauge is fairly low in relation to the amount of voltage required to produce a visual display on a monitor, it is necessary to amplify the signal. Modern amplifiers are able to increase the electrical signal, as well as filter out environmental noise. Important requirements of a good amplification system include easy operation by medical personnel, low distortion of signal despite amplification and filtering, and stable calibration.[2,4]

Display devices include oscilloscopes, digital readouts, hard-copy recordings, and computer storage. Most monitoring systems have both oscilloscopes and continuous digital readout, as well as the ability to interface with other storage systems. Continuous visualization of the pressure tracing on the oscilloscope is important for adequate interpretation of the quality of the pressure measurement by medical caretak-

ers. It is easy to visualize numeric readings of the hemodynamic pressures with accompanying digital readout displays. Most systems can project mean pressure, as well as systolic and diastolic pressures. Sometimes strip chart recorders interface with the monitor system to provide direct recording of the pressure, thus allowing specific interpretation of the pressures such as at end-expiration. Correlation of the hemodynamic pressure with other physiologic occurrences such as arrhythmias or changing intracranial pressure can occur with direct recording.

Catheter and Tubing System. The intravascular catheter and connecting tubing form the fluid-filled part of the monitoring system. Saline or other intravenous fluid flows through the system at a given rate, usually only a few milliliters per hour. For older, domed-type transducers, the fluid is static in the dome itself, whereas in the newer disposable transducers the fluid flows past the strain gauge. Do not use rapid flow rates or frequent changes in the flow rate because they can disrupt the zero reference. The fluid usually contains heparin to discourage clotting at the tip of the catheter. It is also possible to infuse vasodilators to prevent spasm, particularly in the small peripheral arteries.[3]

Although the fluid filling the system does not distort the transmitted pressure wave, characteristics of the catheter and tubing may alter the pressure wave before it reaches the transducer. The transducer responds to the altered pressure wave, giving a distorted pressure reading. Some of the factors affecting the quality of pressure wave are the length, diameter, and stiffness of the catheter and connecting tubing, as well as the presence of air bubbles or blood clots within the catheter or tubing.

Each catheter and tubing system has a specific *resonant frequency* based on the characteristics of the catheter and tubing. Resonant frequency refers to the frequency at which oscillations in the system reach their maximum amplitude.[2] These oscillations, which are caused by reverberations from the tubing system itself, are separate from the frequency of the pulse. If the system has a resonant frequency near that of the pressure waveform, a higher pressure, "overshoot," occurs. Many amplifiers are able to "filter" out this overshoot within a certain range, but the range can be exceeded. Overshoot affects systemic arterial pressure traces more than venous pressure traces.

Techniques

Transducer Position. Positioning of the transducer next to the patient is crucial for accurate, meaningful pressure measurement to eliminate the effect of hydrostatic pressure. For pediatric patients, place the pressure transducers next to the patient and secure either to rolled towels under the transducers or to the bed itself. Ensure that the transducer with its air-reference port is level with the tip of the catheter inside the vascular system. For central venous and pulmonary arterial catheters, the best location for the transducers is at the phlebostatic axis, a point located at the fourth intercostal space in the midaxillary line.[5] (Fig. 35-3) This most closely approximates the tip of catheters inside the heart or pulmonary arteries. For arterial catheters, place the transducer either at the level of the catheter in the artery or at the phlebostatic axis. If placed at the latter location, the pressure

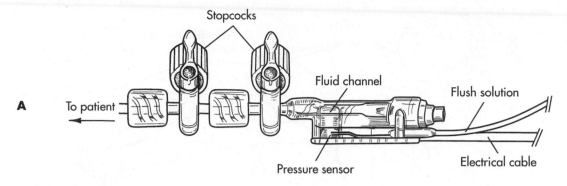

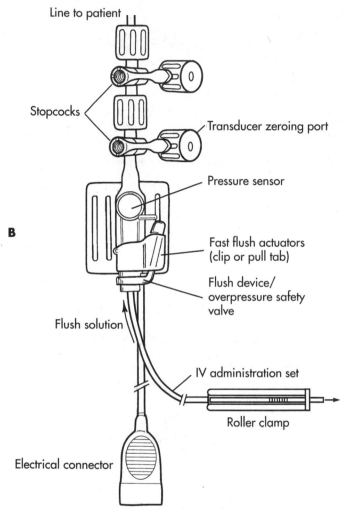

FIG. 35-2   A, Disposable flow through pressure transducer showing position of the pressure sensor in fluid channel. **B,** Disposable pressure transducer in the flow-through system showing relationship to the electrical cable and the fluid system.

to zero either directly by adjusting the "zero" knob on the monitor or in newer monitors through internal calibration by the monitor. Perform this zero reference at least twice a day or more frequently, depending on environmental changes.

Calibration of the transducer is different from the zero reference. To calibrate a transducer, deliver a known pressure either internally by the monitor system or externally using a mercury manometer. If the reading does not equal the known pressure, adjust the monitor accordingly. Because external calibration remains the standard for accuracy, calibrate the monitor at least daily or any time concern about the validity of a pressure measurement exists.

Interpretation. In addition to the pressure measurement itself, the contour of the physiologic pressure wave yields important information about the hemodynamic status of the patient. Evaluation of the pressure wave also enables assessment of the quality of the monitoring system, allowing accurate interpretation of the information generated. An example of this is when a pressure wave loses its expected contour; the cause may be air bubbles in the tubing.

Fig. 35-4 shows the systemic arterial pressure trace. The trace reflects events in both systole and diastole. During systole the aortic valve opens while the left ventricle is contracting, allowing rapid ejection of blood into the aorta. This generates a rapid upstroke on the pressure trace. Runoff of blood into the peripheral arteries then occurs, and the pressure trace falls. When the aortic valve closes, a small increase occurs in the aortic pressure, causing a small dip on the downslope of the pressure trace called the dicrotic notch. During diastole no further ejection from the left ventricle occurs, and the flow of blood continues into the peripheral arteries. The lowest point on the trace before the onset of systolic ejection is the diastolic pressure.

Observation of the pressure trace frequently shows variations in the beat-to-beat arterial pressure. Many of these changes in pressure are physiologic, such as the change in systolic pressure with normal spontaneous respiration. However, wide swings in the systolic pressure with inspiration,

most closely reflects aortic root pressure.[2] For convenience and consistency, many intensive care units place all intravascular pressure transducers at the phlebostatic axis.

Zero Reference and Calibration. Because all pressure measurements are in reference to atmospheric pressure, check this relationship, termed the *zero reference,* frequently. Perform this check by opening the system to atmospheric pressure, termed *opening to air,* by turning the stopcock in the system off to the patient and on to atmosphere. The pressure should read zero. However, the "weight of the air," the temperature of the air and fluid, and other environmental factors may cause drift away from zero. Correct the system

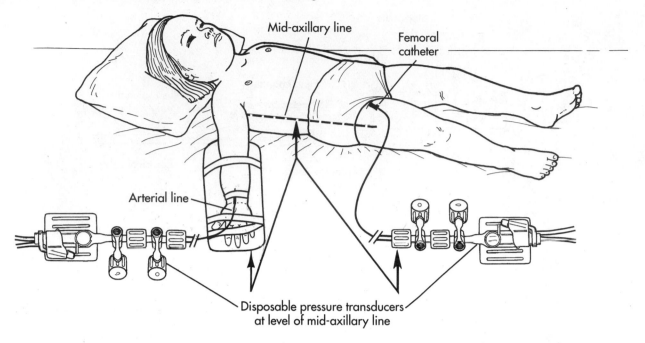

FIG. 35-3 Phlebostatic axis in a small child showing determination of the midchest position. Position the transducers at the level of the phlebostatic axis.

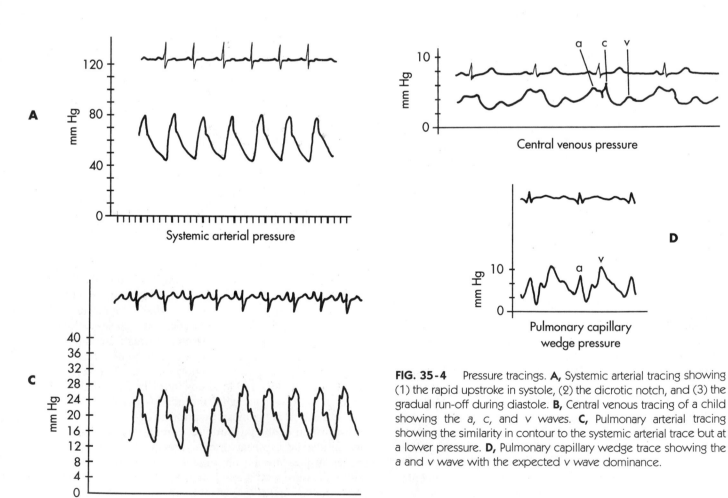

FIG. 35-4 Pressure tracings. **A,** Systemic arterial tracing showing (1) the rapid upstroke in systole, (2) the dicrotic notch, and (3) the gradual run-off during diastole. **B,** Central venous tracing of a child showing the a, c, and v waves. **C,** Pulmonary arterial tracing showing the similarity in contour to the systemic arterial trace but at a lower pressure. **D,** Pulmonary capillary wedge trace showing the a and v wave with the expected v wave dominance.

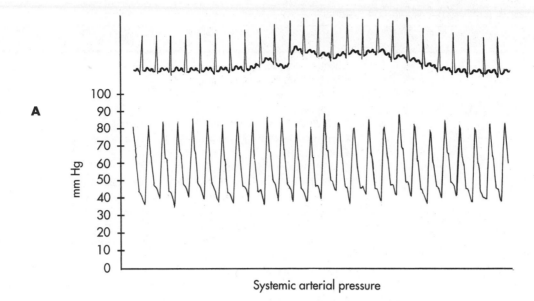

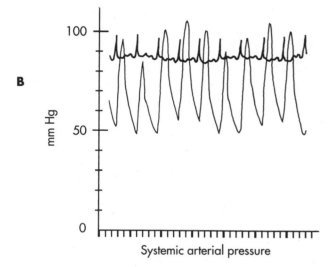

FIG. 35-5 Variations in the systemic arterial tracing caused by hemodynamic abnormalities. **A,** Widened pulse pressure as seen in an infant with a large patent ductus arteriosus. **B,** Pulsus paradoxus in a patient with status asthmaticus showing marked variation in systolic pressure.

pulsus paradoxus, may indicate cardiac tamponade, severe status asthmaticus with high intrathoracic pressures, and intravascular volume depletion in a patient with wide variations in intrathoracic pressure as with mechanical ventilation (Fig. 35-5, *B*).

Other pressure information generated by the systemic arterial pressure includes the pulse pressure and the mean arterial pressure (MAP). The pulse pressure is the difference between the systolic and diastolic pressure. A widened pulse pressure reflects a large stroke volume, whereas a narrow pulse pressure reflects a limited stroke volume. In children the pulse pressure widens in conditions causing a rapid run-off of blood after left ventricular ejection, including the following: patent ductus arteriosus, presence of a surgically created aortopulmonary arterial shunt (i.e., the Blalock-Taussig shunt), aortic insufficiency, and marked lowering of the systemic vascular resistance as in sepsis (see Fig. 35-5). Conditions associated with a narrow pulse pressure include severe aortic stenosis, cardiac tamponade, and poor cardiac contractility associated with an increase in systemic vascular resistance.

The MAP reflects both the cardiac output and the systemic vascular resistance. Newer monitoring systems electronically calculate the MAP and display the reading with the systolic and diastolic pressures. The MAP increases and decreases with changes in cardiac output and vascular tone of the patient.

The central venous pressure (CVP) reflects events that occur in the right atrium and, to some extent, the right ventricle. The CVP trace consists of the following: an *a wave* that occurs during atrial systole, a *c wave* that reflects the onset of ventricular filling (rarely seen in children because of the normally rapid heart rates), and a *v wave* that occurs during ventricular and atrial filling (see Fig. 35-4). In right atrial and CVP tracings, the *a wave* is dominant, usually 1 to 2 mm Hg greater than the *v wave*. Decreased right ventricular compliance results in an increase in the *a wave*. A *"cannon a wave"* occurs during atrioventricular dissociation when the atrium contracts against a closed tricuspid valve, causing a marked increase in atrial pressure, sometimes as high as 15 mm Hg. *V wave* dominance can occur with insufficiency of the tricuspid valve.

The Swan-Ganz catheter allows visualization of pulmonary arterial and capillary wedge pressures. The pulmonary

Table 35-1 Troubleshooting Pressure Monitoring Systems

Problem	Solution
No wave form	Check power supply
	Check all connections including:
	Tubing connections
	Stopcocks
	Electrical connection from transducer to monitor
	Check transducer by tapping gently to determine its responsiveness
	Check cables
	Check pressure range setting
	Check that catheter is still in vascular space by withdrawing blood
Dampened waveform	Check for air bubbles or clots in the system
	Check for kinks in the tubing or partly occluded stopcock
	Vascular spasm especially arterial—flush gently or add papaverine to system
	Too small a catheter—consider replacing with a larger diameter catheter
Reading too high	Check balance and calibration
	Check location of transducer
	Check that stopcocks are completely open
	Check for a too-rapid flow through transducer
	Evaluate tracing for the presence of overshoot artifact
Reading too low	Check balance and calibration
	Check location of transducer
	Check for loose connections
Artifact	Consider catheter whip
	Check for patient movement
	Check for electrical interference—if present have system evaluated immediately by biomedical personnel
Waveform drifting	Check cable for kinking, compression, or poor connection
	Consider change in temperature of fluids
Unable to flush line	Check stopcocks and tubing for kinks or obstructions
	Check for blood return to determine if catheter is in vessel

Adapted from VanRiper J, VanRiper S: Fluid-filled monitoring systems. In Darovic GO, editor: *Hemodynamic monitoring,* ed 4, Philadelphia, 1987, WB Saunders.

arterial waveform is similar to the systemic arterial waveform, but, in children, is about one third to one fourth of the systolic pressure (see Fig. 35-4). The pulmonary capillary wedge tracing reflects events in the left atrium and left ventricle. Like the CVP, the pulmonary capillary wedge trace consists of the *a, c,* and *v waves* (see Fig. 35-4). However, the *v wave* is the dominant wave on the left side of the heart. The *v wave* may be increased in conditions that increase left atrial volume, such as mitral regurgitation and left to right shunt lesions. The *a wave* may become the dominant wave with diminished left ventricle compliance, especially with obstruction to left ventricular outflow, such as aortic stenosis and coarctation of the aorta.

Remarks

To maximize accuracy of pressure measurements using a fluid-filled system, consider the following (Fig. 35-6):[2,5]

1. Avoid soft, compliant tubing and catheters that are compressible and therefore able to absorb energy from the transmitted pressure wave. An attenuated waveform with a factitiously decreased pressure results from an overly compliant system.
2. Avoid excess tubing because the longer the tubing, the closer the resonant frequency of the system to the physiologic range and resonance. Limit tubing to no more than 4 feet from the catheter tip to the transducer.
3. Use as large a diameter catheter as is safely possible to transmit a more accurate pressure wave. In theory, small-diameter catheters could result in loss of energy from the pressure wave and an attenuated pressure trace.
4. Keep the system free of air bubbles and blood clots. Introduction of air that is compressible into the noncompressible fluid-filled system results in loss of energy and therefore dampening of the pressure wave. The presence of clot at the tip of the catheter prevents complete transmission of the pressure wave, also causing a dampened pressure wave.
5. Catheter whip caused by movement of the catheter with cardiac contraction is most common with pulmonary artery catheters.[1] This motion artifact also causes the pressures to be inaccurate. High-frequency filters in the amplification system can minimize this artifact. Repositioning of the catheter may also be helpful.

See also Table 35-1 for troubleshooting of the fluid-filled strain gauge pressure monitoring system.

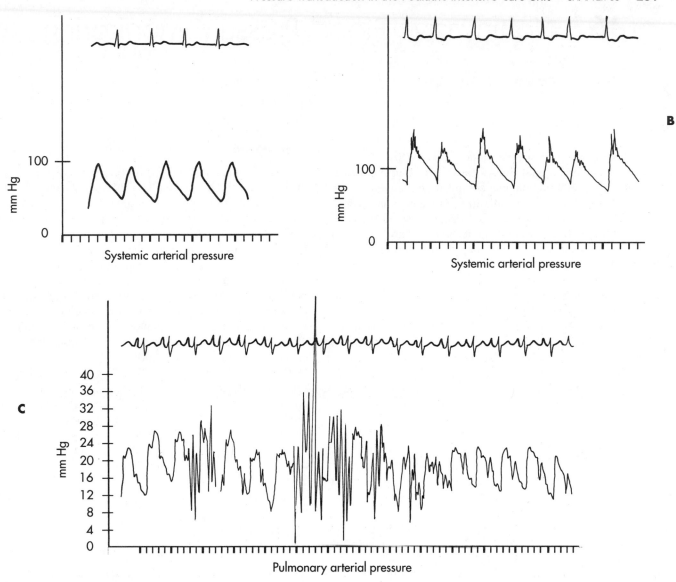

FIG. 35-6   Variations in pressure tracings caused by the monitoring system. **A,** Arterial pressure waveform that is overdamped with loss of the dicrotic notch as seen with blood clots or air bubbles in system. **B,** Arterial pressure waveform with overshoot of systolic pressure due to overshoot. Note the peaked appearance with vibrations of the systolic portion of the contour. **C,** Pulmonary arterial pressure waveform showing catheter whip. Note the marked vibrations of the pressure throughout the cardiac cycle, not just with systole. Improve this by repositioning the catheter.

REFERENCES

1. Amin DK, Shah PK, Swan HJC: The Swan-Ganz catheter: techniques for avoiding common errors, *J Crit Illness* 8(11):1263-1271, 1993.
2. Daily EK, Schroeder JS: *Techniques in bedside hemodynamic monitoring,* ed 4, St. Louis, 1989, Mosby.
3. Heulitt MJ: Double-blind, randomized, controlled trial of papaverine-containing infusions to prevent failure of arterial catheters in pediatric patients, *Crit Care Med* 21(6):825-829, 1993.
4. Milnor WR: *Hemodynamics,* ed 2, Baltimore, 1989, Williams & Wilkins.
5. VanRiper S, VanRiper J: Arterial pressure monitoring. In Darovic GO, editor: *Hemodynamic monitoring: invasive and noninvasive clinical applications,* Philadelphia, 1987, WB Saunders.

36 Noninvasive Blood Pressure Monitoring

Edward J. Truemper

Noninvasive systemic arterial blood pressure (SABP) is one of the most common vital signs measured in clinical practice. The medical literature contains compiled normative data for infants and children and standardized procedures using several widely accepted methods.[48,49] Pediatric applications of noninvasive SABP measurement techniques have included large-scale screening in healthy subjects to determine factors that influence the amplitude of SABP such as age and body habitus and to identify antecedent factors for future risk of hypertension in adulthood and inclusion in routine annual physical examinations.*

All widely used noninvasive SABP recording methods indirectly record blood pressure by applying counterpressure to an artery. An occlusive, inflatable cuff fitted circumferentially around a limb supplies external pressure. These systems inflate the cuff pneumatically, either manually or automatically, until cuff pressure occludes blood flow in the artery under examination. As the external cuff pressure gradually falls, characteristic changes in arterial wall motion and blood flow that one can monitor by a variety of methods occur. Depending on the recording technique and sampling algorithm, these changes can indicate the points where the occluding cuff pressure approximates the true systolic, diastolic, or mean arterial pressure.

Regardless of the instrument employed, studies have validated almost all noninvasive blood pressure methods in normotensive patients of all ages. Instrumentation is either manual or automated, based on the extent of observer participation, in the inflation-deflation cycle and the detection algorithm for selection of arterial pressures. The most common noninvasive method is the auscultatory sphygmomanometry technique, which is the gold standard for noninvasive methods. Automated instruments using either oscillometric or Doppler technologies have largely supplanted the auscultatory method in most patient care areas because of their ease of use and ability to automate repeated measurements at a preset time interval.

Many clinical arenas, including transport, Emergency Department (ED), operating rooms, and intensive care units, care for large numbers of patients who can experience rapid changes in SABP. The developers of noninvasive instrumentation intended its use for measuring SABP in patients with stable hemodynamic characteristics. There have been no systematic investigations of application of noninvasive instruments to record blood pressure in potentially unstable pediatric patients who exhibit either hypertension or hypotension. Therefore the degree of error in noninvasive SABP compared to that of "true" SABP remains largely unknown or varies widely in these clinical circumstances; use it cautiously under these conditions.

*References 3, 5, 11, 24, 25, 27, 29, 35, 48, 49, 51, and 60-63.

Indications

Current recommendations for routine noninvasive screening of SABP in children (ages 3 to 20 years)[48] include annual assessment of blood pressure in the office setting as part of a general physical examination. If the physician documents a moderately elevated blood pressure on the initial recording above the 90th percentile for age, rather than label the child as "hypertensive," he or she should make repeated measurements and appraise the patient for potential confounding physiologic and mechanical factors. Perform repeated blood pressure recordings over two to three office visits if elevation is moderate on the first encounter. Under these circumstances avoid blood drawing and other examinations that can increase blood pressure transiently.[5]

Many EDs use noninvasive SABP as part of the initial and serial hemodynamic assessments to help determine hemodynamic response to treatment. If severe hypertension is present, evaluate the child subsequently for an organic cause and initiate treatment to prevent end-organ damage.[48] In hypotensive patients the auscultatory and most automated noninvasive techniques either fail to detect or overestimate SABP. In situations characterized by cardiovascular instability use intraarterial access for direct SABP measurement when feasible.

Contraindications

Frequent cuff inflation leads to impedance of venous return, reduction in limb blood flow, and venous distention.[39,56] These characteristics can potentially retard healing or potentiate ischemia in the damaged extremity. Therefore avoid cuff inflation in clinical conditions characterized by high metabolic activity in the limb or vascular insufficiency such as vascular trauma, surgical wounds, burns, fractures, local deep infections (i.e., osteomyelitis, gangrene, cellulitis), vascular embolism, or thrombosis. In most emergencies intraarterial access is difficult to obtain in the first minutes of resuscitation. Under these circumstances one can use noninvasive SABP monitoring to titrate intravenous cardiotonic agents and fluids. Do not use noninvasive SABP monitoring routinely to titrate continuous infusions of cardiotonic, pressor, or afterload reduction agents for the purpose of improving cardiac output or manipulating blood pressure for extended periods unless arterial cannulation is not feasible.

Complications

Noninvasive SABP monitoring has caused ulnar palsies with frequent cuff inflation over short periods.[4] Also, since hypotension is a late finding in shock, clinical management that is based solely on normalization of blood pressure can lead to undertreatment and potentiation of secondary damage.

Equipment

All noninvasive devices consist of six major components, (1) a pneumatic bladder, (2) inflation apparatus, (3) deflation apparatus, (4) pressure sensor and monitor, (5) signal detector, and (6) manual or electronic algorithm for pressure determination. Bladder and cuff dimensions are very important in the correct measurement of blood pressure regardless of the noninvasive technique used.* Use a nondistensible cuff to prevent dispersion of bladder pressure from the limb. All devices include a method of securing the cuff to the extremity with either self-fastening synthetic fiber (Velcro) or other adhesive strips.

Standard recommendations for bladder length and width have undergone considerable modification over the past 20 years. The most accepted bladder length is at least 90% or more of the circumference of the upper arm.[48] In some children the bladder may completely surround the arm with variable overlap. However there are no reports of measurement error in this circumstance, and some investigators consider it to improve accuracy.[53,59] Bladder width is ideally 120% of the diameter of the upper arm.[12,20,41,42] This results in a bladder width of approximately 38% of extremity circumference. Significantly wider cuffs underestimate the systolic pressure, whereas cuffs narrower than the recommended standard overestimate the systolic and diastolic pressures.[12,37] Since the current limited number of mass-produced cuff sizes cannot accommodate small incremental changes in arm circumference, a range of 33% to 43% (38% ± 5%) of extremity length for cuff bladder width is acceptable.[35] Another method, based on the Minneapolis Children's Blood Pressure Study, uses midpoint arm circumference determined by measuring the distance from the acromion to the olecranon.[35]

Because there are more than 40 manufacturers of noninvasive SABP instrumentation, it is impossible to give individual recommendations for cuff and bladder dimensions since components currently are not standardized. Also do not use tables based on cuff size relative to age since arm dimensions vary considerably with age.[44] Table 36-1 lists commonly available blood pressure cuff dimensions based on cuff type. Each institution should establish acceptable ranges for cuff and bladder dimensions relative to arm size for its noninvasive SABP recorders, and medical personnel should be instructed in their use.

The inflation and deflation system typically includes nondistensible tubing for the transmission of inflation gas and a manually or electronically controlled pressurization-exhaust system. The biomedical department should examine systems periodically for gas leaks and seal them if gas loss occurs at >1 mm Hg.

The auscultatory sphygmomanometry method employs either a mercury or an aneroid manometer for pressure detection and a stethoscope for detection of Korotkoff sounds. The mercury manometer consists of a graduated mercury-filled column mounted vertically. Examine the manometer to ensure that the mercury meniscus rests at the zero level. If the meniscus is below zero, add mercury to reach

*References 1, 21, 23, 26, 31, 33, 36, 37, 42, and 53.

Table 36-1   Suggested Cuff Bladder Dimensions*

Midpoint upper arm circumference† (cm)	Bladder width 33-43% of arm circumference (cm)	Bladder length ≥90% of arm circumference (cm)
14-18	6	16
19-24	8	22
25-30	10	27
31-39	13	35
40-52	17	47

* See text for discussion.
† Measured at the mid-point of the circumference between the olecranon and the acromion

this level. In addition, the column air vent and filter should be free of dust, which can interfere with column ventilation and affect the response time of mercury column rise during pressurization and venting.[10] The hospital biomedical department should examine mercury manometer systems annually.

Aneroid manometers measure pressure by means of a metal bellows that transmits cuff pressure by a mechanical gauge to an indicator needle. Perform calibration at least annually or monthly if the device receives heavy use. The calibration procedure employs a Y connection interposed between the cuff bladder apparatus and aneroid and mercury manometers. Make adjustments at several pressures to ensure scale accuracy in the anticipated SABP range.

Automated systems employing either Doppler, oscillometric, or infrasound detection require considerations for cuff and bladder dimensions similar to those for manual methods. Base calibration and instrument checks on the manufacturer's recommendation are published in the system's operating manual provided with each instrument.

Techniques

Manual Methods

AUSCULTATION SPHYGMOMANOMETRY. To determine systolic and diastolic blood pressure in infants and children with the auscultation sphygmomanometry technique, pay close attention to the myriad of physiologic and mechanical variables that can affect recordings. The most important factor is the choice of an appropriate size of cuff and bladder. Table 36-1 lists recommended cuff-bladder dimensions. Pay particular attention to suitable cuff size in the obese child, who is at increased risk of spuriously high SABP recordings. Room temperature, level of activity, time of day, time of year, prior physical activity, blood sampling, and noninvasive examinations all affect blood pressure to a variable degree.[12,13,44,45,50,57] In infants crying, feeding, or nonnutritive sucking can variably increase SABP. In order to prevent erroneous measurements, adjust the environment to reduce the child's anxiety before the study. For children capable of comprehending the examination, demonstrating the technique on the examiner often is sufficiently calming to obtain a reliable pressure.

Wrap the cuff snugly around the arm with the bladder fitted over the brachial artery. Seat ambulatory patients comfortably for several minutes with their legs uncrossed before the study. Extend the arm on a comfortable flat

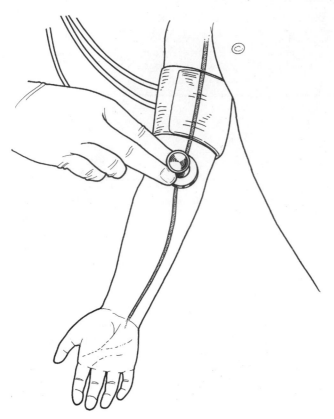

FIG. 36-1 Illustration of the auscultatory sphygmomanometer technique in relation to the arterial pulse pressure wave.

surface at the level of the heart to maintain hydrostatic equivalence. If using a mercury manometer, place the mercury column at the examiner's eye level to prevent observer error from parallax. Position the aneroid manometer at eye level as well, with the indicator face parallel to the examiner's face for similar reasons. Initially perform inflation rapidly, palpating the distal pulse. Inflate the cuff to 20 mm Hg over the pressure point where loss of arterial pulsations initially occurs. Using the cessation of arterial sounds as the indicator of full arterial compression can lead to erroneously low interpretation of the systolic blood pressure (BP) that is due to the phenomenon termed the *auscultatory gap*. The auscultatory gap results from venous overdistention caused by slow cuff inflation and low flow. Korotkoff sounds disappear between their first appearance and their reappearance at a pressure as much as 20 mm Hg lower than the true systolic pressure. In cooperative patients repetitive clinching and releasing of the fist before cuff inflation increases limb blood flow. This, coupled with rapid cuff inflation, prevents the auscultatory gap.

After inflating the cuff to peak pressure, place the bell of the stethoscope over the brachial artery in the antecubital fossa (Fig. 36-1). Do not use the diaphragm for auscultation, especially in children, since its dimensions preclude an adequate seal, limiting sound transmission.[44,45] Also the stethoscope bell is superior in detecting the low frequencies of the Korotkoff sounds. Next deflate the cuff at a rate of 2 to 3 mm Hg/heartbeat. The initial Korotkoff sound is a clear tapping sound that corresponds to the systolic pressure. With

further cuff deflation the tapping signs convert to low-amplitude murmurs defined as the second Korotkoff sound. As the occluding pressure continues to fall, the murmurs become sharper and higher in amplitude, indicating the third Korotkoff sound. Further cuff deflation produces a sudden change in the audible frequency characterized by low-pitched sounds, the fourth Korotkoff sound. In infants and children below the age of 13 years the fourth Korotkoff sound is the indicator of diastolic pressure.[48] With further pressure release the muffled sounds gradually fade until the audible signal disappears. The point of cessation of audible signals is the fifth Korotkoff sound, the indicator of diastolic blood pressure in adults and children older than 13 years of age.[48] Occasionally audible sounds continue until the manometer reaches zero. As little as 10 mm Hg of external pressure by the stethoscope can produce arterial compression.[30]

One commonly employed diversion from this technique is repetitive inflation-deflation in the range of the systolic or diastolic pressure that does not allow full cuff deflation in order to determine more precisely the systolic or diastolic pressure. Avoid this maneuver since it can create venous engorgement and artificially inflate both pressures. To compare serial values over time properly, include the position of the patient during the study, limb examined, cuff size, recording technique or instrument, and systolic and diastolic pressures (example: BP = 110/65, supine, right arm, infant cuff, auscultation).[48] If the pressure difference between the fourth and fifth Korotkoff sounds is more than 10 mm Hg, then record both pressures (i.e., BP = 110/65/50). If the recorded blood pressure is significantly different from previous measurements, seek mechanical or physiologic reasons for the discrepancy. If the blood pressure is above the normotensive range, perform at least two measurements and average them since the first recording is frequently highest in serial measurements. Wait at least 1 to 2 minutes before the next study to allow for regression of limb venous congestion. In cooperative patients raising the arm vertically facilitates venous drainage before the next study.

In patients with severe hypotension and increased systemic vascular resistance the auscultatory method often fails to measure blood pressure accurately because of the extremely low audible frequency and inability to identify characteristic Korotkoff sounds.[8] An additional confounding variable is some examiners' preference for certain numbers during the course of multiple patient examinations.[35] Frequent cuff reinflation produces venous overdistention, which can either minimize Korotkoff sounds or spuriously increase systolic blood pressure.

RANDOM-ZERO SPHYGMOMANOMETRY. Use of the random-zero sphygmomanometer is similar in method to standard sphygmomanometry except for insertion of a mechanical device between the mercury reservoir and column.[31,47] The purpose of this adaptation is to eliminate "digit preference," a common source of error encountered with the traditional auscultatory method.[35] Initially spin a wheel that randomly raises the column between 0 and 60 mm Hg. Then perform the inflation-deflation cycle and detect Korotkoff sounds in a manner identical to the standard auscultatory method. At the completion of the study adjust the pressures by subtracting the value of the zero offset from the systolic and diastolic pressures. This method offers the advantage of

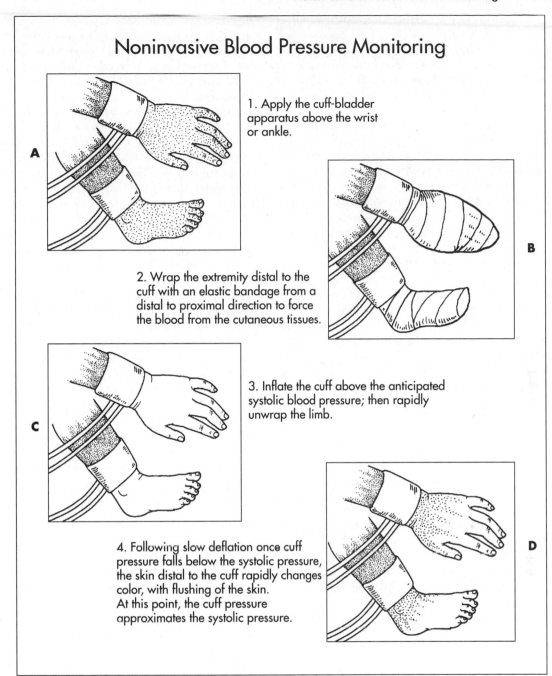

Noninvasive Blood Pressure Monitoring

A

1. Apply the cuff-bladder apparatus above the wrist or ankle.

2. Wrap the extremity distal to the cuff with an elastic bandage from a distal to proximal direction to force the blood from the cutaneous tissues.

B

C

3. Inflate the cuff above the anticipated systolic blood pressure; then rapidly unwrap the limb.

4. Following slow deflation once cuff pressure falls below the systolic pressure, the skin distal to the cuff rapidly changes color, with flushing of the skin. At this point, the cuff pressure approximates the systolic pressure.

D

FIG. 36-2   A to **D,** Illustration of the events necessary to perform SABP measurements by the flush method. See text for details.

preventing the examiner from predetermining the systolic and diastolic pressures.[31,47] In children this method is disadvantageous since it is necessary to inflate the cuff to 60 mm Hg above cessation of the brachial pulse, which can be uncomfortable and raise the child's stress level. Alleviate this problem by employing a smaller device that randomizes the zero offset between 0 and 30 mm Hg, thereby reducing the peak inflation pressure by one-half. Comparisons of serial measurements of standard auscultation, Doppler (Arteriosonde 1216), infrasound (Physiometrics SR-2), and random-zero sphygmomanometry (Gelman-Hawksley) devices in adolescents revealed that the random-zero mea-

surements were closest to those produced by the standard mercury manometry method of the three systems.[2]

FLUSH METHOD. The examiner may choose to substitute the flush method for the auscultatory method when Korotkoff sounds are too faint, such as in small infants or patients experiencing hypotension.* Place the patient in a supine or recumbent position. Apply the cuff-bladder apparatus above the wrist or ankle (Fig. 36-2, *A*). Wrap the extremity distal to the cuff tightly with an elastic bandage from a distal to proximal direction to force the blood from the cutaneous

*References 2, 17, 22, 31, 38, and 58.

tissues (Fig. 36-2, *B*). Once wrapping is completed, inflate the cuff above the anticipated systolic blood pressure and then rapidly unwrap the limb (Fig. 36-2, *C*). During deflation once the cuff pressure falls below the systolic pressure, the skin distal to the cuff rapidly flushes (Fig. 36-2, *D*). At this point the cuff pressure approximates the systolic pressure.[22,38]

In most studies comparisons of arm and leg measurements yield equivalent SABP results.[22,38,55] In one infant study leg measurements of systolic blood pressure were variably higher than measurements performed on the ipsilateral arm.[17] Advantages include approximation of systolic pressure when other methods fail to detect blood pressure. Disadvantages include no diastolic pressure recording; variable underestimation of systolic pressure; inability to determine skin flushing in subjects manifesting severe anemia, cutaneous hypothermia, or vasoconstriction; and the cumbersome nature of the technique in emergencies, when frequent measurements are invariably necessary. In small infants the technique cannot detect systolic pressures below 20 mm Hg.[24] Most pediatric intensive care units (PICUs) have discontinued use of this technique in favor of the manual Doppler or automated method.

PALPATORY METHOD. The technical considerations in the palpatory method are analogous to those in the sphygmomanometry method. Place two fingers over the distal brachial artery. Patient positioning, cuff placement, and the inflation and deflation cycle occur in a manner identical to that used in the auscultatory method. After first noting pulsations during the deflation phase, record the corresponding cuff pressure as the systolic pressure. Advantages of this method include ease of use, lack of expense, and clinically acceptable systolic pressure measurements in normotensive children.[16] Disadvantages include possible methodological errors in pressure recording similar to those factors identified with the sphygmomanometry technique, inability to obtain diastolic pressure, and significant underestimation of systolic pressure by as much as 60 mm Hg in patients manifesting hypotension and increased vascular resistance.[8]

DOPPLER. When appropriate equipment is available, the manual Doppler technique is superior to the flush or palpatory method since it provides a closer approximation of the intraarterial systolic pressure and is easier to use in emergencies. This technique employs the Doppler principle in determining systolic blood pressure by measuring the Doppler shift of an ultrasonic beam reflected from the arterial wall or red blood cells. Place the small piezoelectric transducer capable of transmitting and receiving sound over the artery distal to the cuff-bladder apparatus. The sounds correspond to the Doppler shift frequency, which changes during compression of the artery. Perform the inflation-deflation cycle similarly to other manual methods. With the cuff inflated to a suprasystolic pressure, blood flow in the compressed artery is absent; therefore no shift in Doppler frequency is audible. With cuff deflation the first audible signal approximates the "true" systolic pressure. Further cuff deflation does not produce significantly different Doppler shift signals in the audible range that can demarcate diastolic pressure. Thus do not use the manual Doppler method to determine diastolic pressure.[47,54] Validation studies of one manual Doppler instrument (Pedisphyg system) in normotensive children demonstrated more accuracy than that produced by automated infrasound and other Doppler devices.[54]

Although use of manual Doppler instruments is easier for serial measurements than other manual techniques one drawback is their inability to provide diastolic blood pressure measurements.

Automated Systems. Systems that either partially or totally automate the inflation-deflation cycle and include observer-independent algorithms for detection of systolic, diastolic, and mean arterial pressure have largely replaced manual methods of SABP measurement in most emergency settings because of the removal of observer bias and reduced manual effort required to obtain serial measurements. Mechanical factors that affect SABP determination, such as relations of cuff-bladder geometric characteristics to limb dimensions, also apply to automated systems.

OSCILLOMETRY. The oscillometric method is the most widely used noninvasive SABP monitoring technique, largely supplanting the auscultatory method in most hospitals because of its ease of use and capacity to determine systolic, diastolic, and mean arterial pressures and heart rate automatically at preset intervals.* In addition, most comprehensive bedside monitoring systems in modern ICUs have recently incorporated oscillatory SABP recording.

The basic principles involve measuring the vibratory oscillations within the occluding cuff when occluding pressure occurs.[40] Modern oscillometric instruments use the following algorithm in some form: Cuff inflation occurs to suprasystolic level, followed by release of cuff pressure in small gradients. With the appearance of pulsations indicating pulsatile blood flow within the compressed artery, record systolic pressure. With decreasing occlusion pressure, pulsation strength continues to increase and eventually peaks: the point of the mean pressure. Further cuff deflation produces a variable plateau followed by a gradual decline in pulse oscillation amplitude. Diastolic pressure is at the point where oscillation amplitude initially declines.

Early oscillometric instruments could only determine mean blood pressure.[28,34,43,46] Software and hardware system improvements employed in most current bedside ICU monitors can measure systolic, diastolic, and mean arterial pressure. In all currently manufactured systems cuff inflation is automatic at a variable user-defined interval as frequently as once a minute. Cuff deflation occurs in a stepwise fashion at 2- to 7-mm Hg gradients, depending on the system algorithm.

Previous studies have demonstrated good correlation compared to that of other noninvasive and direct intraarterial instruments with clinically acceptable variation (<5 to 15 mm Hg) in premature and full-term infants, children, and adults with SABP in the normotensive range.[6,9,15,19,52] At the physiologic extremes above and below the normotensive range, correlation diminishes, and significant variation from intraarterial values in individual patients can occur. Some oscillometric systems are incapable of measuring systolic blood pressure >210 mm Hg or underestimate systolic blood pressure in patients manifesting severe hypertension.[32] In hypotensive premature infants and adults these systems

---

* References 6, 9, 15, 16, 18, 19, 32, and 40.

variably overestimate blood pressure, sometimes reporting SABP in the normotensive range.[7,14] Oscillometry yields erroneous SABP values in patients who have atrial or ventricular arrhythmias.[7] In these circumstances use instruments that incorporate the oscillometric method with caution.

Take care to limit cuff inflation to once every 5 minutes to prevent venous engorgement in the limb. Oscillometry SABP monitoring of the lower limb is common, especially in neonates and pediatric patients, as a matter of convenience. No published data currently compare intraarterial values to lower limb values from either the thigh or the calf.

DOPPLER. Some ultrasound devices automatically detect changes in Doppler shift frequencies during sequential cuff deflation. Automated Doppler systems incorporate a transducer within the cuff, positioned over the artery. In the manual Doppler method the observer cannot detect subtle audible frequency shifts after identifying an audible signal. With cuff deflation below systolic pressure the vessel opens and closes, producing intermittent signals during vessel patency. With progressive deflation toward the diastolic pressure the opening and closing phases approach each other until they merge, indicating the diastolic pressure. The automated Doppler method can detect these Doppler shift changes and record them graphically for the determination of systolic and diastolic pressures.

A variety of commercial Doppler instruments have been available for more than 20 years. Comparisons of the accuracy of Doppler instruments to that of direct arterial measurements have shown variable results. The Arteriosonde 1210 and 1216 instruments have shown considerable scatter of as much as 50 mm Hg for systolic and diastolic pressures relative to intraarterial pressure.[47] On the other hand the Parks Ultrasonic Doppler Flow detector demonstrated very small scatter and a high degree of correlation ($r = 0.99$) for systolic pressure compared to those of directly measured systolic pressure.[47]

As with other indirect SABP detection methods, pay particular attention to cuff dimensions. Disadvantages include audible artifact from the cuff deflation with sensor incorporation into the cuff or motion artifact, as in the case of an active infant.

INFRASOUND. The infrasound method uses a microphone transducer that detects changes in subaudible frequencies generated by the motion of the arterial wall during cuff deflation as indicators of systolic and diastolic pressures.

The Infrasound 3000 system inflates the cuff manually and deflates it automatically at a linear rate of 3 mm Hg/sec.[57] The Physiometrics instrument employs a rigid cuff with an inflatable bladder into which the patient inserts an arm. Cuff inflation and deflation occur automatically, and it processes signals electronically and transfers them by recording pen to a circular paper disk. In the case of the Infrasonics device, the rigid cuff leads to underestimation of both systolic and diastolic pressure since the bladder is too large relative to arm circumference.[2,61] Two comparative studies in a pediatric population aged 5 to 17 years revealed that in younger children (age <7 years) it underestimated systolic and diastolic blood pressures by an average of 1 to 7 mm Hg, whereas in older children it overestimated both pressures by 2 to 5 mm Hg. There is limited experience with both instruments other than in ambulatory patients.[2,57,61]

Remarks

If Korotkoff sounds are too faint to determine reliably the systolic and diastolic points, raise the arm for 1 to 2 minutes to relieve venous congestion and increase sound amplification.

With pulsus alternans automated methods are unable to rectify the bidimensional pulsations electronically. The auscultatory method can detect the difference in systolic pressure pulsations with gradual cuff inflation, holding it for several seconds near the systolic pressure. In the ambulatory subject allowing the legs to dangle from a seated position accentuates the difference in amplitude since this results in decreased venous return.

In patients experiencing hypotension frequently the auscultatory method fails to detect Korotkoff sounds since they fall below the audible range. Substitution of either the palpatory or Doppler method can give an approximation of the systolic pressure in these circumstances.

Predetermine bladder widths for specific arm length ranges and record them on each cuff for each instrument type in the patient care area. This prevents inadvertent use of too-large or too-small bladder, regardless of the technique.

If the arm is extremely large in circumference, so that the largest arm cuff fails to meet recommendations for cuff length, substitution of a thigh cuff provides adequate compression of the brachial artery.

REFERENCES

1. Alexander H, Cohhen ML, Steinfeld L: Criteria in the choice of an occluding cuff for the indirect measurement of blood pressure, *Med Biol Eng Comput* 15:2-10, 1977.
2. Barker WF, Hediger ML, Kataz SH et al: Concurrent validity studies of blood pressure instrumentation: The Philadelphia Blood Pressure Project, *Hypertension* 6:85-91, 1984.
3. Baron AE, Freyer B, Fixler DE: Longitudinal blood pressure in blacks, whites, and Mexican Americans during adolescence and early adulthood, *Am J Epidemiol* 123:809-817, 1986.
4. Betts EK: Hazard of automated noninvasive blood pressure monitoring, *Anesthesiology* 55:717-723, 1981.
5. Blood pressure of youths 12-17 years: United States vital and health statistics: series 11. Data from the National Health Survey, No 163. DHEW Pub No (HRA) 77-1645, Washington, DC, 1977, US Government Printing Office.
6. Borow KM, Newburger JW: Noninvasive estimation of central aortic pressure oscillometric method for analyzing systemic artery pulsatile blood flow: comparative study of indirect systolic, diastolic, and mean brachial artery pressure with simultaneous direct ascending aortic pressure measurements, *Am Heart J* 103:879-886, 1982.
7. Carmella JP, Desmonts JM: Fiabilite du monitorage oscillometrique automatique e la pression arterielle: influence de l'hypotension et des du rythme, *Arch Mal Coeur* 79:1794-1799, 1986.
8. Cohn JN: Blood pressure measurement in shock, *JAMA* 199:118-124, 1971.
9. Colan SD, Fujii A, Borow KM et al: Noninvasive determination of systolic, diastolic, and end-systolic blood pressure in neonates, infants, and young children: comparison with central aortic pressure measurements, *Am J Cardiol* 52:867-870, 1983.
10. Conceicao S, Ward MK, Kerr DNS: Defects in sphygmomanometers: an important source of error in blood pressure recording, *Br Med J* 1:886-888, 1976.
11. Cornoni-Huntley J, Harlan WR, Leaverton PE: Blood pressure in adolescence: the United States health examination survey, *Hypertension* 1:566-571, 1979.
12. Day R: Blood pressure determinations in children, *J Pediatr* 14:148-155, 1939.

13. de Swiet M, Fayers P, Shinebourne EA: Systolic blood pressure in a population of infants in the first year of life: the Brompton Study, *Pediatrics* 65:1028-1035, 1980.

14. Diprose GK, Evans DH, Archer LNJ et al: Dinemap fails to detect hypotension in very low birth weight infants, *Arch Dis Child* 61:771-773, 1986.

15. Ellison RC, Gamble WJ, Taft DS: A device for the automated measurement of blood pressure in epidemiologic studies, *Am J Epidemiol* 120:542-549, 1984.

16. Elseed AM, Shinnebourne EA, Joseph MC: Assessment of techniques for measurement of blood pressure in infants and children, *Arch Dis Child* 48:932-938, 1973.

17. Forfar JO, Kibel MA: Blood pressure in the newborn estimated by the flush method, *Arch Dis Child* 31:126-130, 1956.

18. Forster FK, Turney D: Oscillometric determination of diastolic, mean, and systolic blood pressure: a numerical model, *J Bioeng* 108:359-364, 1986.

19. Frieson RH, Lichtor JL: Indirect measurement of blood pressure in neonates and infants utilizing an automated noninvasive oscillometric monitor, *Anesth Analg* 60:742-745, 1981.

20. Frohlich ED, Grim C, Labarthe DR et al: Recommendations for human blood pressure determination by sphygmomanometers: report of a special task force appointed by the steering committee, American Heart Association, *Circulation* 77:502A-514A, 1988.

21. Geddes LA, Whistler SJ: The error in indirect blood pressure measurement with the incorrect size of cuff, *Am Heart J* 96:4-8, 1978.

22. Goldring D, Wohltman H: Flush method for blood pressure determinations in newborn infants, *J Pediatr* 40:285-289, 1952.

23. Hansen RL, Stickler GB: The "non-hypertension" or "small-cuff" syndrome, *Clin Pediatr* 5:579-580, 1966.

24. Higgins MW, Hinton PC, Keller JB: Weight and obesity as predictors of blood pressure and hypertension. In Loggie JMH, Horan MJ, Gruskin AB et al, editors: *NHLBI workshop on juvenile hypertension,* New York, 1984, Biomedical Publishers.

25. Higgins MW, Keller JB, Metzner HL et al: Studies of blood pressure in Tecumseh, Michigan. II. Antecedents in children of high blood pressure in young adults, *Hypertension* 2 (suppl I): I117-I123, 1980.

26. Karvonen MT, Telivuo LJ, Jarvinen EJK: Sphygmomanometer cuff size and the accuracy of indirect measurement of blood pressure, *Am J Cardiol* 38:688-693, 1964.

27. Kilcoyne MM, Richter RW, Alsup PA: Adolescent hypertension. 1. Detection and prevalence, *Circulation* 50:758-764, 1974.

28. Kimble KJ, Darnall RA, Yelderman M, et al: An automated oscillometric technique for estimating mean arterial pressure in critically ill newborns, *Anesthesiology* 54:423-425, 1981.

29. Lauer R, Clarke W: Immediate and long-term prognostic significance of childhood blood pressure levels. In Lauer R, Shekelle RB, editors: *Childhood prevention of atherosclerosis and hypertension,* New York, 1980, Raven Press.

30. Londe S, Klitzner TS, Moss AJ: Effects of pressure exerted on the stethoscope head on auscultatory blood pressure. In Loggie JMH, Horan MJ, Gruskin AB et al, editors: *NHLBI workshop on juvenile hypertension,* New York, 1984, Biomedical Publishers.

31. Long M, Dunlop JR, Holland WW: Blood pressure recording in children, *Arch Dis Child* 46:636-640, 1971.

32. Loubser PG: Comparison of intra-arterial and automated oscillometric blood pressure measurements methods in postoperative hypertensive patients, *Med Instrum* 20:255-259, 1986.

33. Lunn LG, Jones MD: The effect of cuff width on systolic blood pressure measurements in neonates, *J Pediatr* 91:963-966, 1977.

34. Mauck GW, Smith CR, Geddes LA et al: The meaning of the point of maximum oscillations in cuff pressure in the indirect measurement of blood pressure, Part II. *Transasme* 102:28-33, 1980.

35. McGarvey ST, Zinner SH: Epidemiology of blood pressure in the first two years of life. In Loggie JMH, editor: *Pediatric and adolescent hypertension,* Cambridge, 1992, Blackwell Scientific Publications.

36. Moss AJ: Indirect methods of blood pressure measurement, *Pediatr Clin North Am* 25:3-14, 1978.

37. Moss AJ, Adams FH: Auscultatory and intra-arterial pressure: a comparison in children with special reference to cuff width, *Pediatrics* 66:1094-1097, 1965.

38. Moss AJ, Liebling W, Austin WO et al: An evaluation of the flush method for determining blood pressures in infants, *Pediatrics* 20:53-61, 1957.

39. Paulas DA: Noninvasive blood pressure measurement, *Med Instrum* 15:91-97, 1981.

40. Pessenhofer H: Single cuff comparison of two methods for indirect measurement of arterial blood pressure: standard auscultatory method versus automated oscillometric method, *Basic Rev Cardiol* 81:101-109, 1986.

41. Park MK, Guntheroth WG: Direct blood pressure measurements in brachial and femoral arteries in children, *Circulation* 41:231-237, 1970.

42. Park MK, Kawabori I, Guntheroth WG: Need for an improved standard for blood pressure cuff size, *Clin Pediatr* 15:784-787, 1976.

43. Posey JA, Geddes LA, Williams H et al: The meaning of maximum oscillations in cuff pressure in the direct measurement of blood pressure, Part I. *Cardiovasc Res Cent Bull* 8:15-25, 1969.

44. Prineas RJ, Gillum RF, Horibe H et al: The Minneapolis Children's Blood Pressure Study: the standards of measurement of children's blood pressure, *Hypertension* 2(suppl I): I-18-24, 1980.

45. Prineas RJ, Jacobs D: Quality of Korotkoff sounds: bell vs diaphragm, cubital fossa vs. brachial artery, *Prev Med* 12:715-719, 1983.

46. Ramsey M III: Noninvasive automatic determination of mean arterial pressure, *Med Biol Eng Comput* 17:11-18, 1979.

47. Reder RF, Dimich I, Cohen ML et al: Evaluating indirect blood pressure of three systems in infants and children, *Pediatrics* 62:326-330, 1978.

48. Report of the Second Task Force on Blood Pressure Control in Children, 1987, *Pediatrics* 79:1-25, 1987.

49. Report of the Task Force on Blood Pressure Control in Children, *Pediatrics* 59:797-820, 1977.

50. Richardson DW, Honour AJ, Fenton GW et al: Variation in arterial pressure throughout the day and night, *Clin Sci* 26:445-460, 1964.

51. Schachter J, Kuller LH, Perfetti C: Blood pressure during the first five years of life: relation to ethnic group (black or white) and to parental hypertension, *Am J Epidemiol* 119:451-553, 1984.

52. Silas JH, Barker AT, Ramsay LE: Clinical evaluation of Dinamap 845 automated blood pressure recorder, *Br Heart J* 43:202-205, 1980.

53. Steinfeld L, Alexander H, Cohen ML: Updating sphygmomanometry, *Am J Cardiol* 33:107-110, 1973.

54. Steinfeld L, Dimich I, Reder R: Sphygmomanometry in the pediatric patient, *J Pediatr* 92:934-938, 1978.

55. Sullivan MP, Kobayashi M: Evaluation of the flush technique for the determination of blood pressure in infancy, *Pediatrics* 15:84-87, 1955.

56. Sy WP: Ulnar nerve palsy possibly related to use of automatically cycled blood pressure cuff, *Anesth Analg* 60:687-691, 1981.

57. van der Berg BJ: Comparisons of blood pressure measurements by ausulation and physiometric infrasound recording techniques, *Hypertension* 2(suppl I): I-8-I-17, 1980.

58. Virnig NL, Reynolds JW: Reliability of flush blood pressure measurements in the sick newborn infant, *J Pediatr* 84:594-598, 1974.

59. Voors AW: Cuff bladder size in a blood pressure survey of children, *Am J Epidemiol* 101:489-494, 1975.

60. Voors AW, Foster TA, Freichs RR: Studies of blood pressure in children, ages 5-14 years in a totally biracial community—the Bogalusa heart study, *Circulation* 54:319-327, 1976.

61. Voors AW, Webber LS, Frerichs RR et al: Body weight and body mass as determinants of basal blood pressure in children: the Bogalusa heart Study, *Am J Epidemiol* 106:101-108, 1977.

62. Zinner SH, Levy PS, Kass EH: Familial aggregation of blood pressure in childhood, *N Engl J Med* 284:401-409, 1971.

63. Zinner SH, Rosner B, Oh WO et al: Significance of blood pressure in infancy, *Hypertension* 7:411-416, 1985.

37 Peripheral Extravasation Injury

James D. Marshall

The peripheral intravenous administration of fluids and drugs constitutes commonplace yet hazardous therapy in modern medical care. Extravasation is the unintentional instillation or leakage of agents into the perivascular and subcutaneous spaces during their administration.[22] It is easy to misplace or displace cannulation devices. Despite correct preparation and administration of infused substances through an apparently patent cannulated vessel, intimal inflammation with luminal narrowing similar to phlebitis[48] may cause local pressure increases and eventual extravasation of infusate at the cannulation site.[62] Injury to the local integument and proximal structures can result if the agent or carrier fluid is directly cytotoxic or if innocuous agents create adverse local conditions such as elevated tissue pressure and ischemia.[14,28,80,104] The spectrum of injury extends from brief minimal discomfort through extensive necrosis and may add significantly to the morbidity and cost of treatment.[65]

The causative agents of this iatrogenic disease are diverse (Table 37-1). Extravasated irritant drugs produce local pain and inflammation, whereas vesicant drugs cause blistering or frank ulceration,[22] although volume of injectate, depth of administration, and local tissue factors greatly influence any resulting injury.[54] Rudolph and Larson[86] have proposed a useful clinical division of the vesicant category: (1) agents that do not bind tissue nucleic acids but cause immediate tissue damage before local inactivation or redistribution and (2) agents that bind tissue deoxyribonucleic acid (DNA), causing both immediate damage and, with local retention of active drug, prolonged vesicant effects.

The diagnosis of extravasation is clinical, though certain drugs (radiopharmaceuticals,[13] contrast agents,[2,90] $CaCl_2$[42] ethylenediamine tetraacetic acid (EDTA),[88] and anthracyclines)[19,27,32,33,38] may be detectable when retained in the subcutaneous tissue. Symptoms include local pain, burning sensations and other paresthesias, and pressure at the site; signs are erythema, immediate swelling with extravasated infusate and later swelling in reactive tissue edema, induration, slowing of infusion rate, and failure to aspirate blood from the catheter.[22] Induration that persists at anthracycline extravasation sites for more than 24 hours may be an indicator of impending necrosis and ulceration.[49] Infusion pump pressure alarms are unreliable, as advanced extravasation may be present before the alarms activate.[65,66] Certain conditions may mimic extravasation and require timely intervention, although extravasation has apparently not occurred (Table 37-1). Severe extravasations occur in patients unable to sense or complain of symptoms.[45,66]

Relatively cytotoxic, voluminous, or deep extravasations or those that severely disrupt local vasculature may result in an acute compartment syndrome (CS), defined as a condition in which increased pressure within a limited space (compartment) compromises the circulation and function of the tissues within that space.[56,70] Virtually any group of muscle bellies, nerves, and associated vasculature tightly enveloped by fascia and bone is at some risk, including the compartments of the forearm, hand, leg, and foot. The earliest signs of CS are sensory: diminished two-point discrimination (>1 cm)[41] and 256 cps vibratory sensation[79] in the distal distribution of involved peripheral sensory nerves. Symptoms of weakness, severe resting pain increased by passive stretch of involved musculature, tenseness of overlying skin, and distal pulselessness (caution: pulses may be present even in severe CS)[40] are variably present.

A certain number of extravasations occur in every institution, and children seem to be at increased risk.[49] Most require some therapy. Some controllable factors predispose infusions to failure, and many institutions implement operator guidelines to help prevent extravasation (Box 37-1). Fig. 37-1 outlines an algorithm for initial management, which is based on the available literature. Although true "antidotes" are rare, specific medical interventions may contain and/or chemically neutralize an extravasated noxious drug, disperse the drug or solution through the tissues for rapid systemic absorption, or reverse the pharmacologic effects locally (see Table 37-1). Most medical therapy has evolved from reason and limited, often contradictory case series. Antidotes are mostly unproven, though many have passed the test of time.[86]

Obtain appropriate professional consultation soon after the injury for both initial and long-term management to reduce morbidity.[86] Necrotic ulcers resulting from extravasation appear within 14 to 21 days of the event,[22,49] tend to be indolent and painful, and may expand over weeks if the offending drug (i.e., adriamycin) remains potent at the site.[38] Surgery for full-thickness necrotic lesions and radiation injuries requires extensive débridement to prepare the ulcer bed for skin graft or flap coverage.[60,83] Timing and staging of surgery are debatable, but surgery seems indicated if significant prolonged pain or full-thickness ulceration occurs.[49,60,63] Special patient information and education are critical as physicians frequently monitor and treat these injuries on an outpatient basis[49] and they are a source of much litigation.[86]

Extravasations that result in clinical CS require emergency attention. Intracompartmental pressure (IP) approaching mean arterial blood pressure within 30 mm Hg compromises perfusion and may cause widespread necrosis if persistent.[51] It is possible to measure IP accurately with a variety of devices percutaneously inserted into afflicted muscle bellies.[70] The Stryker STIC handheld monitoring device, which uses a fluid-filled sterile needle inserted percutaneously into any compartment, is useful for rapid, repeated diagnostic evaluations for CS. The Camino fiber-optic device (Fig. 37-2) provides continuous digital IP information without fluid injection and is appropriate for borderline CS requiring longer monitoring.[23,93] Each objective measurement of intracompartmental

Table 37-1 Causes and Medical Therapy

Agent	Therapy
Antineoplastic irritants	
Carmustine/BCNU[54,22]	$NaHCO_3$ 8.4%[a] 5ml IL[b,6,54,66]
Cyclophosphamide[22]	
Dacarbazine/DTIC[22,54]	
Streptozocin[22]	
Teniposide[22]	
Thiotepa[54,22]	
Antineoplastic vesicants	
Actinomycin D[22,54, note 7]	Na thiosulfate 10%, 4 ml in 6 ml sterile water IL[22,54]
Anthracyclines[9,22,82,99, notes 3 and 7]	
Daunorubicin[11,22,54,105, note 6]	$NaHCO_3$ 8.4% 5 ml IL + dexamethasone 4 mg IL[54,66]
	Desamethasone 4 mg IL[22,54]
Doxorubicin[11,22,54,86,95,105, note 6]	Hydrocortisone 50-200 mg IL + hydrocortisone 1% cream topical BID[6,22,25,66,105]
	$NaHCO_3$ 8.4% 5 ml IL + dexamethasone 4 mg IL[54,66,108] or hydrocortisone 100 mg IL[95]
	DMSO 90%[note 4] + vitamin E 10% q12h × 48h topically[22,64]
	DMSO 50%-99% q2-6h × 3-14 days topically, optional immediate dexamethasone or hydrocortisone IL[61,76]
	IL infiltration with Na thiosulfate 2%, then after 3-5 minutes, hydrocortisone 50mg/ml; betamethasone/garamycin ointment topically q12h × 2d, then q24 until lesion healed beneath tight elastic bandage[98]
Chromomycin A3[54]	
Cisplatinum[22,36]	
Carboplatin[69*]	
Epirubicin[15]	
Fluorouracil[22]	
Ifosfamide[69*]	
Mechlorethamine[54, note 6]	Na thiosulfate 10%, 4 ml in 6 ml sterile water IL[7]
Methotrexate[99]	
Mithramycin[22,54]	Na edetate (EDTA) 150 mg/ml, 1 ml IL[54,66]
Mitomycin C[1,54,57]	DMSO 90%-99% (or 90% + vitamin E 10%) 1-2 ml BID-QID × 2-7 days topically to site of extravasation[1,64]
	Na thiosulfate 10% 4 ml in 6 ml sterile water IL[7,22,54]
Mitozantrone[22,78]	
Mustine[22]	Na thiosulfate 25%, 1.6 ml in 3 ml sterile water for injection, IL[22]
Streptozocin[54]	
Vinblastine[22,54]	$NaHCO_3$ 8.4% 5 ml IL[54,66]
	Hyaluronidase 150 U/ml, 1 ml IL[54] + heat[66, note 5]
Vincristine[22,54]	Hydrocortisone 25-50 mg/ml of extravasate IL[66]
	$NaHCO_3$ 8.4% 5 ml IL[54,66]
	Hyaluronidase 150 U IL + heat[54,66, note 5]
Vindesine[22]	Hyaluronidase 150 U IL + heat[66]
Ischemia-inducing agents	
Dobutamine[52]	
Dopamine[14,92,99]	Phentolamine 5-10 mg IL[66,92]
	Phentolamine 0.1-0.2 mg/kg max 10 mg IL[7, 8]
	Phentolamine (1 mg/ml NS) 0.5 mg IL to cover injured area[21]
	Nitroglycerin 2% topically to extravasation site[29,102]
Epinephrine[67,68,99]	Phentolamine 1-10 mg IL[66,30]
	Phentolamine 0.1-0.2 mg/kg max 10 mg IL[7,8]
	Phentolamine; 2 mg + 2% lidocaine as digital nerve block injection[67]; infiltrated along the course of digital arteries and directly into site[68]
Metaraminol[99]	Phentolamine 5-10 mg IL[66]
	Phentolamine 0.1-0.2 mg/kg max 10 mg IL[7,8]
Norepinephrine[39,47]	Phentolamine 10-15 mg IL[66,107]
	Phentolamine 0.1-0.2 mg/kg max 10 mg IL[7,8]
Vasopressin[74]	Guanethidine 10 mg/10 ml NS + heparin 1000 U/ml intraarterial distal to tourniquet; tourniquet slowly released after 10 minutes (one case).[24]

Table 37-1   Causes and Medical Therapy—cont'd

Agent	Therapy
Physicochemical irritants and vesicants	
Acylovir[84]	
Ampicillin[14]	
Aminophylline[105]	Hyaluronidase[6] 15 U/ml NS, 0.2 ml × 5 doses IL[66,105]
Amphotericin B[75]	
Arginine hydrochloride[5,12]	
Blood products (RBCs, albumin)[14]	
Calcium solutions	Hyaluronidase 15 U/ml NS, 0.2 ml × 5 doses IL[66,105]
	Hyaluronidase 150 U/1000 ml NS IL, volume sufficient to make skin
	Overlying extravasation tense but not blanched, up to 60 minutes postextravasation[49,50]
Chloride[42,50,99]	
Gluconate[50,99]	
Gluceptate[104]	
Disodium EDTA	
Carbenicillin[14]	
Cephalothin[14]	
Chloramphenicol[14]	
Contrast agents[16,17,18,34,54,63,72,73]	
Dextrose ≥ 10% solutions[104]	Hyaluronidase 15 U/ml NS × 5 doses IL[66,105]
Diazepam[99]	Hyaluronidase 15 U/ml NS × 5 doses IL[66,105]
Dilantin[20,46,81, note 8]	
Fluorescein[35]	
Gentamicin[14]	
Hypertonic saline[60]	
Indanyl sodium[14]	
Lipid emulsion[14,43]	
Maintenance IV fluids[14]	
Nafcillin[14,97,106]	
Oxacillin[14]	Hyaluronidase 15 U/ml NS × 5 doses IL[66,105]
PN solutions[14]	
Potassium solutions[50]	Hyaluronidase 15 U/ml NS × 5 doses IL[66,105]
Sodium bicarbonate[39]	
Streptokinase[10]	Hyaluronidase 15 U/ml NS × 5 doses IL[66,105]
Tetracycline[99]	
Thiopental[39,99]	
Urea[39]	
Radioactive Agents	
Iodine-131-iodocholesterol[13]	
Miscellaneous agents (theoretical)[91]	Monitoring of site, application of warm compresses[53]

Notes:

1. NaHCO$_3$ 8.4% is itself cytotoxic as a result of high pKa. Although its use is suggested frequently in the extravasation injury literature, may be contraindicated.

2. "Intralesional": surrounding the extravasation in multiple puncture sites, from intradermal to subcutaneous, using 25- to 30-gauge needles; occasional authors[82] recommend antidote injection through the infiltrated catheter before removal.

3. Cold (ice) applied locally 20 min. q6h × 72 hours is recommended by some authors as sole therapy for anthracycline extravasation to limit dispersion of the drug[58,59,87]

4. DMSO 50% is the maximum available concentration for commercial purposes. Greater concentrations are available for research proposes only.[85] Side effect of DMSO is local blistering with prolonged application.[76]

5. Dry heat should be applied to extravasation site when hyaluronidase used for drugs in this category, to help disperse enzyme (and extravasate) through the tissues for faster systemic absorption.[55]

6. Meclorethamine,[50] daunorubicin,[50] and doxorubicin[86,100] may cause a transient "flare phenomenon" that shows immediate redness and swelling along the path of the vein, lasts usually 1-2 h (up to 24 h), and is not associated with extravasation.

7. A "radiation-recall" effect, wherein areas that have received radiation in the past could undergo tissue damage and even ulceration when the patient receives various systemic anthracyclines[31,86] or actinomycin D,[54] may rarely occur and does not apparently result from extravasation.

8. "Purple glove syndrome" may result from phenytoin administration into forearm and hand veins although extravasation cannot be documented.[20,46,81]

* Denotes drugs or drug studies that were determined to be vesicants in animal models, but are included because of their potential toxicity in humans. *BCNU*, carmustine; *DTTC*, dacarbazine; *IL*, intralesional; *BID*, twice daily; *DMSO*, dimethyl sulfoxide; *NAHCO$_3$*, sodium bicarbonate; *NS*, normal saline; *PN*, parenteral nutrition; *QID*, four times daily; *RBC*, red blood cell.

BOX 37-1 EXTRAVASATION PREVENTION GUIDELINES[22]

1. Staff

Experienced in techniques of drug preparation
Sound knowledge of properties and side effects of drug
Acquainted with a protocol for management of extravasation injuries
Working in quiet environment

2. Administration

Veins

Vein preference sequence: large forearm > dorsal hand > wrist > antecubital fossa[54]
Away from joints, in areas of deep soft tissue[95]
Avoidance of obstructed veins
　Draining of areas of SVC syndrome, surgical obstruction,[66,54] peripheral vascular disease, radiation sites[55]
Minimization of attempts at venipuncture
Venodilation of small veins 5-10 minutes before cannulation
　Local heat
　Topical glyceryl trinitrate paste
Maintained venodilation if necessary: topical GTN (Nitrobid) q8h[103]

Cannulae

Short-term infusions via 21-gauge "butterfly" set
Long-term infusions via small-gauge flexible synthetic (e.g., Teflon) catheter
Prolonged infusions most safely delivered via centrally placed catheter.
Implanted venous access devices
　Monitored for needle/port and catheter continuum[4,26,101]
Patency assessed by free flow of NS or D_5W, and easy blood return

Delivery systems

Volumetric cassette pumps ($\leq$ 20 lbs/in^2) or free flow infusion[66]
Avoidance of manual "push" infusions and high-pressure pumps[65]

Monitoring

Patient instruction to alert staff for burning or stinging sensation
Frequent visual site assessment through clear, minimal dressings

3. Drugs

Appropriate dilution of drug[54]
Infusion over shortest period consistent with patient's venous capacity[55]
Vesicants given first sequence[94] or last[54]
Minimum 10 ml NS or D_5W flush after drug infusion to dilute local drug concentration
Removal of cannula and application of pressure to site after drug infusion

---

SVC, Superior vena cava; *GTN,* glyceryl trinitrate; *NS,* normal saline; D_5W, 5% dextrose in water.

---

pressure should be correlated with concurrent mean arterial blood pressure and a repeated physical examination. It is essential that systemic oxygen delivery and venous drainage are optimized at the site of injury.[37,71,96] Surgical release of selected compartmental envelopes (skin, fascia, epimysium) with debridement dramatically reduces IP and thus promotes perfusion, although wound infection and prolonged healing may severely compromise an already desperately ill patient.[40,77,89] The outcome of extravasation injury is generally excellent with only temporary loss of a cannulation site,[58] but reports of di-

sasters exist, including median and ulnar neuropathy,[10] limb shortening,[44] disabling joint stiffness, and amputation.[99] Physical therapy aimed at early mobilization and return to normal activity reduces long-term morbidity.[82] A multidisciplinary team approach is beneficial.

Administration of drugs and fluids through peripheral veins is relatively simple and safe if one anticipates the potential infusate toxicity and technical hazard of the procedure. Thoughtful and rapid management of extravasations reduces ultimate injury.

Stop infusion
↓
Disconnect tubing from cannula
↓
Attempt to aspirate extravasated drug through cannula
↓
Give antidote intralesionally as indicated
↓
Remove cannula and tape
↓
Apply topical ointments if indicated
↓
Mark extravasation border with indelible ink and photograph
↓
Thermal therapy
    Ice packs (anthracyclines) 20 min q6h × 3 days
    Dry heat (vinca alkaloids and other agents) as tolerated
↓
Completely evaluate extremity

Surface injury only
↓
Elevate extremity
(at least 24 hours)
↓
Apply loose dressing
↓
Frequent reevaluation

Definite or high risk for
compartment syndrome
↓
Place extremity at heart level
↓
Remove all constricting wraps
↓
Frequent physical examination;
consider intramuscular pressure
monitoring

Consult appropriate medical/surgical specialties
    Pharmacology
    Plastic surgery (débridement, grafting)
    Orthopedic surgery (release procedures)
    Physical therapy (splinting, range-of-motion exercise)
↓
Document incident
    Time/date, drug concentration and volume, appearance, description and
    photo, names of staff involved in incident, instructions given to patient
↓
Advise patient
    Significance of etiologic agent
    Seriousness of injury and immediate therapy required
    Follow up required
    Expectations of injury progress and healing

FIG. 37-1   Initial management algorithm.

Digital monitor

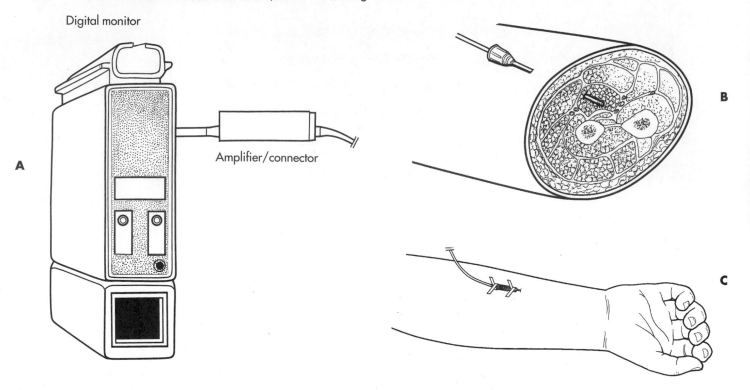

FIG. 37-2, A to C Camino fiber-optic device for long-term intracompartmental pressure monitoring. After inserting the probe intramuscularly, combine continuous pressure readouts with repeated physical examinations to warn of impending ischemic conditions and to help determine the required extent of therapy.

REFERENCES

1. Alberts DS, Dorr RT: Case report: topical DMSO for mitomycin-C-induced skin ulceration, *Oncol Nurs Forum* 18(4):693-695, 1991.
2. Aquino S, Villanueva-Meyer J: Uptake of Tc-99m MDP in soft tissues related to radiographic contrast media extravasation, *Clin Nuclear Med* 17(12):974, 1992.
3. Awbrey BJ, Sienkiewicz PS, Mankin HJ: Chronic exercise induced compartment pressure elevation measured with a miniaturized fluid pressure monitor: a laboratory and clinical study, *Am J Sports Med* 16(6):610-615, 1988.
4. Bach F et al: Cytostatic extravasation: a serious complication of long-term venous access, *Cancer* 68(3):538-539, 1991.
5. Baker GL, Franklin JD: Management of arginine monohydrochloride extravasation in the forearm, *South Med J* 84(3):381-384, 1991.
6. Barlock AL, Howser DM, Hubbard SM: Nursing management of adriamycin extravasation, *Am J Nurs* Jan:94-96, 1979.
7. Beason R: Antineoplastic vesicant extravasation, *J Intrav Nurs* 13(2):111-114, 1990.
8. Benitz WE, Tatro DS: *The pediatric drug handbook*, ed 2, St. Louis, 1988, Mosby.
9. Bhawan J, Petry J, Rybak ME: Histologic changes induced in skin by extravasation of doxorubicin (adriamycin), *J Cutaneous Pathol* 16(3):158-163, 1989.
10. Blankenship JC: Median and ulnar neuropathy after streptokinase infusion, *Heart Lung* 20(3):221-223, 1991.
11. Bowers DG, Lynch JB: Adriamycin extravasation, *Plast Reconstr Surg* 61:86-92, 1978.
12. Bowlby NA, Elanjien SI: Necrosis caused by extravasation of arginine hydrochloride, *Ann Pharmacother* 26(2):263-264, 1992 (letter).
13. Breen SL, Driedger AA: Radiation injury from interstitial injection of iodine-131-iodocholesterol, *J Nuclear Med* 32(5) 892, 1991 (letter).
14. Brown A, Hoelzer D, Piercy S: Skin necrosis from extravasation of intravenous fluids in children, *Plast Reconstr Surg* 64:145-150, 1979.
15. Cassidy J, Rankin EM: Hypersensitivity reaction to epirubicin, *Med Oncol Tumor Pharmacother* 6(4):297-298, 1989.
16. Cohan RH et al: Extravasation of nonionic radiologic contrast media: efficacy of conservative treatment, *Radiology* 176(1):65-67, 1990.
17. Cohan RH et al: Extravascular extravasation of radiographic contrast media: effects of conventional and low-osmolar agents in the rat thigh, *Invest Radiol* 25(5):504-510, 1990.
18. Cohan RH et al: Extravascular toxicity of two magnetic resonance contrast agents: preliminary experience in the rat, *Invest Radiol* 26(3):224-226, 1991.
19. Cohen FJ, Manganaro J, Bezozo RC: Identification of involved tissue during surgical treatment of doxorubicin-induced extravasation injury, *J Hand Surg* 8(1):43-45, 1983.
20. Comer JB: Extravasation from intravenous phenytoin, *Am J Intrav Nurs Clin Nutr* January:23-29. 1984.
21. Cooper BE: High dose phentolamine for extravasation of pressors, *Clin Pharm* 8(10):689, 1989 (letter).
22. Cox K et al: The management of toxic drug extravasation: guidelines drawn up for the Clinical Oncological Society of Australia, *Med J Aust* 148:185-189, 1988.
23. Crenshaw AG et al: A new "transducer-tipped" fiber optic catheter for measuring intramuscular pressures, *J Orthop Res* 8:464-468, 1990.
24. Crocker MC: Intravascular guanethidine in the treatment of estravasated vasopressin, *N Engl J Med* 304(23):1430, 1981.
25. Cullen ML: Current interventions for doxorubicin extravasation, *Oncol Nurs Forum* 9(1):52-53, 1982.
26. Curran CF, Luce JK: Extravasation of doxorubicin from vascular access devices, *Select Cancer Ther* 6(2):103-107, 1990.
27. Dahlstrom KK, Chenoufi HL, Daugaard S: Flourescence microscopic demonstration and demarcation of doxorubicin extravasation: experimental and clinical studies, *Cancer* 65(8):1722-1726, 1990.
28. Daniel RK, Williams HB: The free transfer of skin flaps by microvascular anastomoses, *Plast Reconstr Surg* 52(1):16-31, 1973.
29. Denkler KA, Cohen BE: Reversal of dopamine extravasation injury with topical nitroglycerin ointment, *Plast Reconstr Surg* 84(5):811-813, 1989.
30. Deshmukh N, Tolland JT: Treatment of accidental epinephrine injection in a finger, *J Emerg Med* 7(4):408, 1989 (letter).
31. Donaldson SS, Glick JM, Wilbur JR: Adriamycin activating a recall phenomenon after radiation therapy, *Ann Intern Med* 81(3):407-408, 1974.

32. Dorr RT et al: High levels doxorubicin in the tissues of a patient experiencing extravasation during a 4-day infusion, *Cancer* 64(12):2462-2464, 1989.

33. Duray PH, Cuono CB, Madri JA: Demonstration of cutaneous doxorubicin extravasation by rhodamine-filtered flourescence microscopy, *J Surg Oncol* 31(1):21-25, 1986.

34. Elam EA et al: Cutaneous ulceration due to contrast extravasation: experimental assessment of injury and potential antidotes, *Invest Radiol* 26(1):13-16, 1991.

35. Elman MJ et al: Skin necrosis following fluorescein extravasation: a survey of the Macula Society, *Retina* 7(2):89-93, 1987.

36. Fields S et al: Local soft tissue toxicity following cisplatin extravasation, *J Natl Cancer Inst* 82(20):1649-1650, 1990 (letter).

37. Garfin SR et al: Quantification of intracompartmental pressure and volume under plaster casts, *J Bone Joint Surg* 63-A(3):449-453, 1981.

38. Garnick M et al: Persistence of anthracycline levels following dermal and subcutaneous adriamycin extravasation, *Proc Am Assoc Cancer Res Am Soc Clin Oncol* 22:173, 1981, (abstract).

39. Gaze NR: Tissue necrosis caused by commonly used intravenous infusions, *Lancet* 2:417, 1978.

40. Gelberman RH et al: Decompression of forearm compartment syndromes, *Clin Orthop* 134:225-229, 1978.

41. Gelberman RH et al: Compartment syndromes of the forearm: diagnosis and treatment, *Clin Orthop* 161:252-261, 1981.

42. Goldminz D et al: Calcinosis cutis following extravasation of calcium chloride, *Arch Dermatol* 124(6):922-925, 1988.

43. Graber R, Laufman H: Massive subcutaneous necrosis after extravasation of intravenous infusion of fat emulsion, *Am J Surg* 107:878-880, 1964.

44. Guy RL et al: Limb shortening secondary to complications of vascular cannulae in the neonatal period, *Skeletal Radiol* 19(6):423-425, 1990.

45. Handler EG: Superficial compartment syndrome of the foot after infiltration of intravenous fluid, *Arch Phys Med Rehab* 71(1):58-59, 1990.

46. Hanna DR: Purple glove syndrome: a complication of intravenous phenytoin, *J Neurosci Nurs* 24(6):340-345, 1992.

47. Hardy SB, Hamilton JM: Treatment of tissue necrosis following intravenous use of norepinephrine, *Plast Reconstr Surg* 20(5):360-365, 1957.

48. Hecker JF: Failure of intravenous infusions from extravasations and phlebitis, *Anesth Intens Care* 17(4): 433-439, 1989.

49. Heckler FR: Current thoughts on extravasation injuries, *Clin Plastic Surg* 16(3):557-563, 1989.

50. Heckler FR, McGraw J: Calcium related cutaneous necrosis, *Surg Forum* 27:553-555, 1976.

51. Heppenstall RB et al: The compartment syndrome: an experimental and clinical study of muscular energy metabolism using phosphorous NMR spectroscopy, *Clin Orthop* 226:138-155, 1988.

52. Hoff JV, Beatty PA, Wade JL: Dermal necrosis from dobutamine, *N Engl J Med* 300(3):1280, 1979.

53. Hoop B: The infiltrated radiopharmaceutical injection: risk considerations, *J Nuclear Med* 32(5):890-891, 1991 (editorial).

54. Ignoffo RJ, Friedman MA: Therapy of local toxicities caused by extravasation of cancer chemotherapeutic drugs, *Cancer Treat Rev* 7:17-27, 1980.

55. Jameson J, O'Donnell J: Guidelines for extravasation of intravenous drugs, *Infusion* 7:157-165, 1983.

56. Jobe MT: Volkman's contracture and compartment syndromes. In Crenshaw AH, editor: *Campbell's operative orthopaedics*, ed 8, vol 5, St Louis, 1992, Mosby.

57. Khanna AK et al: Mitomycin C extravasation ulcers, *J Surg Oncol* 28(2):108-110, 1985.

58. Larson DL: Treatment of tissue necrosis by antitumor agents, *Cancer* 49(9):1796-1799, 1982.

59. Larson DL: What is the appropriate management of tissue extravasation by antitumor agents? *Plast Reconstr Surg* 75(3):397-405, 1985.

60. Larson DL: Alterations in wound healing secondary to infusion injury, *Clin Plast Surg* 17(3):509-517, 1990.

61. Lawrence HJ et al: Topical dimethylsulfoxide may prevent tissue damage from anthracycline extravasation, *Cancer Chemother Pharmacol* 23(5):316-318, 1989.

62. Lewis GBH, Hecker JF: Radiological examination of failure of intravenous infusions, *Br J Surg* 78(4):500-501, 1991.

63. Loth TS, Eversmann WW Jr: Extravasation injuries in the upper extremity, *Clin Ortho* 272:248-254, 1991.

64. Ludwig CU et al: Prevention of cytotoxic induced skin ulcers with dimethylsulfoxide (DMSO) and alpha-tocopherole, *Eur J Cancer Clin Oncol* 23(3):327-329, 1987.

65. Lynch DJ, Key JC, White RR: Management and prevention of infiltration and extravation injury, *Surg Clin North Am* 59(5):939-949, 1979.

66. MacCara ME: Extravasation: a hazard of intravenous therapy, *Drug Intell Clin Pharm* 17:713-717, 1983.

67. Maguire WM et al: Epinephrine-induced vasospasm reversed by phentolamine digital block, *Am J Emerg Med* 8(1):46-47, 1990.

68. Markovchick V, Burkhart KK: The reversal of the ischemic effects of epinephrine on a finger with local injections of phentolamine, *J Emerg Med* 9(5):323-324, 1991.

69. Marnocha RS, Hutson PR: Intradermal carboplatin and isfosfamide estravasation in the mouse, *Cancer* 70(4):850-853, 1992.

70. Matsen FA: *Compartment syndromes,* New York, 1980, Grune & Stratton.

71. Matsen FA, Krugmire RB, King RV: Increased tissue pressure and its effects on muscle oxygenation in level and elevated human limbs, *Clin Orthop* 144:311, 1979.

72. McAlister WH, Kissane JM: Comparison of soft tissue effects of conventional ionic, low osmolar ionic, and nonionic iodine containing contrast material in experimental animals, *Pediatr Radiol* 20(3):170-174, 1990.

73. McAlister WH, McAlister VI, Kissane JM: The effect of Gd-dimeglumine on subcutaneous tissues: a study with rats, *Am J Neuroradiol* 11(2):325-327, 1990.

74. Mogan GR, Wormser GP, Gottfried EB: Infected gangrene: a serious complication of peripheral vasopressin administration, *Am J Gastroenterol* 73:426-429, 1980.

75. Olson C, McCoy LK: Amphotericin B extravasation: a case report, *Natl Intravenous Ther Assn* 8(4):299-300, 1985.

76. Olver IN et al: A prospective study of topical dimethyl sulfoxide for treating anthracycline extravasation, *J Clin Oncol* 6(11):1732-1735, 1988.

77. Patman RD, Thompson JE, Persson AV: Use and technic of fasciotomy as an adjunct to limb salvage, *South Med J* 66(10):1108-1116, 1973.

78. Peters FT, Beijnen JH, ten Bokkel Huinink WW: Mitoxantrone extravasation injury, *Cancer Treat Rep.* 71(10):992-993, 1987 (letter).

79. Philips JH et al: Vibratory sensory testing in acute compartment syndromes: a clinical and experimental study, *Plast Reconstr Surg* 79(5):796-301, 1987.

80. Pond GD, Dorr RT, McAleese KA: Skin ulceration from extravasation of low-osmolality contrast medium: a complication of automation, *Am J Roentgen* 158(4):915-916, 1992 (letter).

81. Rao VK, Feldman PD, Dibbel DG: Extravasation injury to the hand by intravenous phenytoin: report of three cases, *J Neurosurg* 68(6):967-969, 1988.

82. Reilly JJ, Neifeld JP, Rosenberg SA: Clinical course and management of accidental adriamycin extravasation, *Cancer* 40:2053-2053, 1977.

83. Reinisch JF, Puckett CL: Management of radiation wounds, *Surg Clin North Am* 64(4):795-802, 1984.

84. Robbins MS, Stromquist C, Tan LH: Acyclovir pH: possible cause of extravasation injury, *Ann Pharmacother* 27(2):238, 1993.

85. Rospond RM, Engel LM: Dimethyl sulfoxide for treating anthracycline extravasation, *Clin Pharm* 12(8):560-561, 1993.

86. Rudolph R, Larson DL: Etiology and treatment of chemotherapeutic agent extravasation injuries: a review, *J Clin Oncol* 5(7):1116-1126, 1987.

87. Scarim SK: Treatment of doxorubicin extravasations, *DICP* 23(5):386-387, 1989.

88. Schumacher HR Jr et al: Calcinosis at the site of leakage from extravasation of calcium disodium edetate intravenous chelator therapy in a child with lead poisoning, *Clin Orthop* 219:221-225, 1987.

89. Schwartz JT et al: Acute compartment syndrome of the thigh, a spectrum of injury, *J Bone Joint Surg* 71-A(3):392-400, 1989.

90. Shaeffer J et al: Early detection of extravasation of radiographic contrast medium: work in progress, *Radiology* 184(1):141-144, 1992.

91. Shapiro B, Pillay M, Cox PH: Dosimetric consequences of interstitial extravasation following IV administration of a radiopharmaceutical, *Eur J Nucl Med* 12(10):522-523, 1987.

92. Siwy BK, Sadove AM: Acute management of dopamine infiltration injury with Regitine, *Plast Reconst Surg* 80(4):610-612, 1987.

93. Skjeldal S et al: Acute compartment syndrome: for how long can muscle tolerate increased tissue pressure? *Eur J Surg* 158:437-438, 1992.

94. Stuart MS: Sequence of administering vesicant cytotoxic drugs, *Oncol Nurs Forum* 9:53, 1982.

95. Swartz AJ: Chemotherapy extravasation management. Part I. Doxorubicin, *Cancer Nurs* 2:405-407, 1979.

96. Szabo RM, Gelberman RH: Peripheral nerve compression—etiology, critical pressure threshold, and clinical assessment, *Orthopedics* 7:1461, 1984.

97. Tilden SJ et al: Cutaneous necrosis associated with intravenous nafcillin therapy, *Am J Dis Child* 134:1046-1048, 1980.

98. Tsavaris NB et al: Prevention of tissue necrosis due to accidental extravasation of cytostatic drugs by a conservative approach, *Cancer Chemother Pharmacol* 30(4):330-333, 1992.

99. Upton J, Mulliken J, Murray J: Major intravenous extravasation injuries, *Am J Surg* 137:497-506, 1979.

100. Vogelzang M: "Adriamycin flare": a skin reaction resembling extravasation, *Cancer Treat Rep* 63(11-12):2067-2069, 1979.

101. Wickham RS: Advances in venous access devices and nursing management strategies, *Nurs Clin North Am* 25(2):345-364, 1990.

102. Wong AF, McCulloch LM, Sola A: Treatment of peripheral tissue ischemia with topical nitroglycerin ointment in neonates, *J Pediatr* 121(6):980-983, 1992.

103. Wright A, Hecker JF, Lewis GB: Use of transdermal glyceryl trinitrate to reduce failure of intravenous infusion due to phlebitis and extravasation, *Lancet* 2(8465):1148-1150, 1985.

104. Yosowitz P et al: Peripheral infiltration necrosis, *Ann Surg* 182:553-556, 1975.

105. Zenk KE: Management of intravenous extrvasations, *Infusion* 5:77-79, 1981.

106. Zenk KE, Dungy CI, Greene GR: Nafcillin extravasation injury: use of hyaluronidase as an antidote, *Am J Dis Child* 135:1113-1114, 1981.

107. Zucker G: Use of phentolamine to prevent necrosis due to levarterenol, *JAMA* 163(16):1477-1479, 1957.

108. Zweig JI, Kabakow B: An apparently effective countermeasure for doxorubicin extravasation, *JAMA* 239(20):2116, 1978 (letter).

Part VIII

NONVASCULAR ACCESS TECHNIQUES

38 Alternatives to Conventional Drug Administration

F. Keith Battan

Timely access for drug and fluid administration is essential to pediatric emergency and critical care. However, achieving intravascular access in seriously ill children is often impossible or significantly delayed.[8] The younger the child, the lower the success rates in achieving intravenous (IV) access.[10,15] Although the intraosseous (IO) route is excellent for rapid vascular access in critical situations, it is inappropriate for nonresuscitation scenarios. Fortunately there are numerous alternative routes for drug administration in children who do not require conventional vascular cannulation.

Administering fluids before the advent of IV therapy involved nonvascular means. This was first described by Arnaldo Cantani (1837-1893), who performed hypodermoclysis (i.e., subcutaneous infusion of saline solution).[9] Rectal and intraperitoneal fluid administration was practiced in the early 1900s, in an era during which mortality from summertime diarrhea approached 50%.[1] Sagittal sinus infusions in children with open fontanelles were also described.[9] None of these nonvascular techniques achieved much success in volume resuscitation, and drug delivery was rarely described in the early literature.

Nonvascular means of delivering drugs to central circulation are receiving increasing attention in recent years. Many of the nonvascular routes are transmucosal entry sites that share many features such as absorption, pharmacokinetics, and safety. Nonvascular routes of access for delivery of medications include endotracheal (ET), inhaled, intracardiac (IC), intramuscular (IM), intranasal (IN), sublingual (SL), oral (PO), subcutaneous (SC), and rectal (PR).[2,3,5-7,12-14,16-20]

The choice of which nonvascular site to use for a given clinical scenario is based on several factors relating to safety and efficacy, including: (1) drug absorption; (2) feasibility, given the child's age, cooperation, and degree of illness (e.g., SL transmucosal administration isn't possible in obtunded, uncooperative, or uncoordinated children); (3) pharmacokinetics of a drug for a given site (e.g., orally administered benzodiazepines are substantially degraded during first-pass hepatic metabolism, leading to delayed time to onset, lower bioavailability, and lower serum levels); and (4) safety of administration (e.g., oral drugs can be aspirated by a child whose protective airway reflexes are blunted).

For all advanced life support (ALS) medications, IV is the most efficacious and preferred route of administration.[15] IV is the gold standard for all drug delivery methods because of predictable and rapid onset, titratability, and known pharmacokinetics. However, the pain and risks of IV delivery may be much higher than that of other routes.

Eutectic mixture of local anesthetics (EMLA) is an example of a *topical drug* that has important value in Emergency Department (ED) or intensive care unit care of children. *Transcutaneous drugs* have systemic absorption, whereas most topical drugs have limited effect on the skin, eye, or other surface and do not penetrate into the vascular system.

Endotracheal tubes are very important conduits for delivering ALS medications such as epinephrine, atropine, and lidocaine when no vascular access has been established.

Inhalation medications are ubiquitous in pediatrics, not only for inhaled β_2 agents and ipratropium, but also for antibiotics and nitrous oxide. Action specific to or absorption through the respiratory tract is attained quickly and reliably with excellent safety.

IC delivery of medication, principally epinephrine, is a means-of-last-resort intervention for patients *in extremis,* when no other form of delivery (e.g. IV, IO, or ET) is possible. Complications are varied and serious, and this route is rarely indicated.

IM injection has the principal advantage of ease of administration. Depot preparations can be delivered intramuscularly for long-acting deposition. A disadvantage is painful administration.

Intranasal administration of sedative agents such as midazolam (Versed) is common (Table 38-1). Painful injections are obviated, onset is rapid and reliable, and short duration of action makes this drug and this method very amenable to ED use. Table 38-1 compares kinetic and clinical differences of various methods for midazolam administration.

SL administration is based on the rich vascular plexus of the oral mucosa. A variety of medications can be given, including sedatives, antihypertensives, and ALS medications such as epinephrine, naloxone, and atropine. Onset of action isn't as rapid as the IV route, but faster than IM.

PO delivery of agents such as steroids, antibiotics, and activated charcoal is common in all critical-care areas. Children with altered mental status or those who are critically ill are not candidates for this mode of drug delivery.

Table 38-1 Midazolam Kinetics vs. Method of Administration

Route	Dose (mg/kg)	Bioavailability (%)	T_{MAX} (min)	Elim $T_{1/2}$ (min)
IV	0.05-0.3	[100]	40+/−30	50-126
IM	0.1-0.33	90	30	
PO	0.5-0.75	41	51	90-150
PR	0.3		16	106+/−29
IN	0.2-0.3	51	11+/−2	41

The doses listed above are to illustrate kinetics and do not represent recommended clinical doses.

Table 38-2 Advantages and Disadvantages of Nonvascular Access Methods

Nonvascular access route	Advantages	Disadvantages	Examples
Endotracheal	Administration of epinephrine, lidocaine, naloxone and atropine possible through endotracheal tube	Limited number of drugs available to be administered No fluid resuscitation possible	Epinephrine Atropine
Intranasal	Ease of administration Favorable pharmacokinetics	Some agents (e.g., midazolam) have a burning sensation with intranasal administration	Midazolam Fentanyl
Sublingual	Onset faster than intramuscular Patient acceptance	Requires child's cooperation for transmucosal delivery SL vein hard to cannulate	Nifedipine Naloxone
Oral	Ease of administration Patient acceptance	Delayed onset Requires normal mental status First-pass hepatic metabolism, poor titratability	Antibiotics Chloral hydrate
Rectal	Higher serum levels compared to oral Ease of administration	Limited drugs amendable to PR route	Acetaminophen Diazepam
Subcutaneous	Sustained release possible Ease of administration	Slow onset Small volumes of drug	Heparin Morphine
Inhalation	Favorable pharmacokinetics Ease of administration	Limited use with respiratory failure	Albuterol Nitrous oxide
Intracardiac	Direct delivery into central circulation	Risk for multiple major complications Painful delivery	Epinephrine
Intramuscular	Ease of administration	Unsuitable for repeated administrations	Narcotics Ceftriaxone
Topical, transcutaneous	Painless Ease of administration	Limited drug possibilities	EMLA Nitroglycerin

Subcutaneous routes are ideal for drugs when immediate onset of action is not important and sustained release may be desirable. Examples include heparin, insulin, epinephrine, and antibiotics.

Topical drugs (nitroglycerin, scopolamine, and EMLA) have delayed onset compared to IV, poor titratability, and unsuitability for repeated administration.

PR administration is ideal when the oral route for medications isn't available; proper rectal delivery avoids hepatic first-pass metabolism and achieves higher serum levels. It can be used for anticonvulsants, antipyretics, and antiemetics.

Table 38-2 summarizes the relative advantages and disadvantages of the various nonvascular access methods.

REFERENCES

1. Blackfan KD, Maxey KF: The intraperitoneal injection of saline solution, *Am J Dis Child* 15:19, 1981.
2. DeBoer AG, DeLeede LGJ, Breinmer DD: Drug absorption by sublingual and rectal routes, *Br J Anesth* 56-69, 1984.
3. Diamant MJ, et al: The use of midazolam for sedation of infants and children, *Am J Radiol* 150(2):377-378, 1988.
4. Hussain AA: Mechanism of nasal absorption of drugs, *Prog Clin Biol Res* 292:261-272, 1989.
5. Kanto J, Alloned H: Pharmacokinetics and the sedative effect of midazolam, *Int J Clin Pharmacol Ther Toxicol* 21:460-463, 1983.
6. Lam TK, Ng KW, Chan YS: Use of midazolam in children, *Lancet* 2(8610):565, 1988.
7. Mathews HML, Carson IW, Lyons SM, et al: A pharmacokinetic study of midazolam in pediatric patients undergoing cardiac surgery, *Br J Anaesth* 61:302-307, 1988.
8. Mayer TA: Emergency vascular access: old solutions to an old problem, Editorial, *Am J Emerg Med* 4(1):98-101, 1986.
9. Miller R, Leno T: Advances in pediatric emergency department procedures, *Emerg Med Clin North Am* 9(3):639-654, 1991.
10. Orlowski JB: My kingdom for an intravenous line, *Am J Dis Child* 138:803, 1984.
11. Proceedings of the International Symposium on the uses of midazolam and flumazenil in intensive care, *Resuscitation* 16(suppl):S1-106, 1988.
12. Raeder JC, et al: Prolonged elimination of midazolam after intramuscular administration, *Acta Anaesthiol Scand* 1988.
13. Raybould D, Bradshaw EG: Premedication for day care surgery. A study of oral midazolam, *Anesthesia* 42:591-595, 1987.
14. Rita L, Seleny FL, Mazurek A, et al: Intramuscular midazolam for pediatric preanesthetic sedation: a double-blind controlled study with morphine, *Anesthesiology* 63:528-531, 1985.
15. Rosetti V, et al: Difficulty and delay in intravenous access in pediatric arrests, *Ann Emerg Med* 13:406, 1984.
16. Saarnivaara L, Lindgren L, Klemola UM: Comparison of chloral hydrate and midazolam by mouth as premedicants in children undergoing otolaryngological surgery, *Br J Anaesth* 61:390-396, 1988.
17. Saint-Maurice D, Meistelman C, Rey E, et al: The pharmacokinetics of rectal midazolam for premedication in children, *Anesthesiology* 65:536-538, 1986.
18. Sandler ES, et al: Midazolam versus fentanyl as premedication for painful procedures in children with cancer, *Pediatrics* 89:631-634, 1992.
19. Sievers TD, et al: Midazolam for conscious sedation during pediatric oncology procedures: safety and recovery parameters, *Pediatrics* 88:1172-1179, 1991.
20. Taylor MB, Vine PR, Hatch DJ: Intramuscular midazolam premedication in small children, *Anaesthesia* 41:21-26, 1986.
21. Wright SW, et al: Midazolam use in the emergency department, *Am J Emerg Med* 8:97-100, 1990.

39 Endotracheal Drug Administration

Joan Bothner

The absorptive properties of the lung have been recognized since 1857, when Claude Bernard reported on the use of intrapulmonary curare.[1] Not until endotracheal intubation, performed to ensure a patent airway and to optimize oxygenation and ventilation, did the use of emergency drugs via the endotracheal route become a simple alternative delivery method.

Redding, Asuncion, and Pearson[17] introduced the endotracheal route of epinephrine administration in a canine model. Administration of epinephrine via the intracardiac and intravenous routes was clearly superior, but endotracheal epinephrine diluted in 10 ml of saline or water was also found to be effective.

Subsequent investigators have examined the efficacy of the endotracheal administration of several other emergency drugs, including atropine, lidocaine, naloxone, diazepam, midazolam, and bretylium. Nearly all studies have been carried out on animal models, with significant differences in methodology, making the results difficult to extrapolate to the pediatric population.

There are documented cases of clinical responsiveness to endotracheally administered epinephrine in the pediatric literature, mostly in the setting of perinatal asphyxia and bradycardia. However, Quinton, O'Byrne, and Aitkenhead[14] demonstrated poor clinical response of endotracheal administration in human adult victims of asystolic arrest when they compared endotracheal to intravenous epinephrine administration.[14]

Multiple animal studies have clearly shown that the endotracheal dose needs to be substantially larger than an intravenous dose of epinephrine. Roberts, Greenberg, Knaub, et al.[18] demonstrated blood levels to be ten times lower with endotracheal epinephrine compared to intravenous epinephrine in anesthetized dogs. However, plasma levels remained elevated after endotracheal administration. Ralston, Tacker, Showen, et al.[15] studied epinephrine in pulseless electrical activity in dogs and found median effective endotracheal doses to be 14 µg/kg intravenously and 130 µg/kg endotracheally. Hornchen, Schuttler, Stoeckel, et al.[9] demonstrated similar effects using adolescent pigs, with effective epinephrine doses of 10 µg/kg intravenously and 100 µg/kg endotracheally.

Endotracheally administered epinephrine produces a lower peak plasma level than intravenously administered epinephrine, but time to attaining maximum levels is similar. However, endotracheally administered drug has a marked increase in duration of plasma level elevation, ascribed to a "depot effect." This depot effect, due possibly to vasoconstriction after drug administration and ventilation/perfusion mismatch, leads to a fourfold increase in duration of sustained epinephrine plasma level after endotracheal administration. The bioavailability of endotracheally administered epinephrine in dogs is 80% to 85%.[7]

Methods of administration and techniques to deliver more drug into the lower airway have also been developed and evaluated. Redding, Asuncion, and Pearson[17] found undiluted epinephrine to be ineffective, and Ralston, Tacker, Showen, et al.[15] and Hornchen, Schuttler, Stoeckel, et al.[9] both used epinephrine diluted in 10 ml of normal saline.[9] Mace[12] demonstrated that increased volume of diluent significantly increased lidocaine plasma levels after endotracheal administration.

Choice of diluent has also been investigated. Greenberg, Baskin, Kaplan, et al.[4] demonstrated less effect on Po_2 with endotracheal saline versus sterile water in anesthetized dogs. Hahnel, Lindner, Schurmann, et al.[8] have published the only study done in humans and demonstrated significantly higher plasma lidocaine levels and less impairment of Pao_2 using sterile water as the diluent vs. normal saline. Thus normal saline may be better for endotracheal administration of all emergency drugs except lidocaine, for which the diluent of choice is sterile water. Volumes of 25 ml cause no detectable change in respiratory status or significant change in arterial blood gas values of adult human patients in a canine arrest model.[6] Optimal volume in the pediatric patient is not known, but per dose volumes greater than 1 ml/kg should be used cautiously to avert problems with gas exchange.

Evaluations of techniques of drug delivery have led to several recommendations. Greenberg and Spivey[6] demonstrated the benefit of positive-pressure ventilation after endotracheal administration of Dionisil to dogs. Mace[12] demonstrated higher plasma lidocaine levels after administration of undiluted lidocaine either through a catheter or followed by a bolus of normal saline vs. instillation directly into the endotracheal tube. Dilution with an equal volume of normal saline, however, led to the highest plasma levels.

There have been no studies demonstrating therapeutic drug levels after endotracheal administration of atropine. Elam[3] demonstrated equal effectiveness of intravenous and endotracheal atropine in ameliorating bradycardia in dogs. Howard and Bingham[10] demonstrated that endotracheal atropine, in a dose double that of the intravenous dose, achieved similar levels of tachycardia and time of onset in anesthetized pediatric patients. The optimal endotracheal dose of atropine is unknown. The duration of action is extended fourfold after endotracheal administration.

Lidocaine is well absorbed endotracheally, with most studies using doses of 2 to 3 mg/kg. Dilution with at least an equal volume of sterile water attains the highest serum levels. Onset of action is slightly longer than with intravenous administration, with duration of action extended twofold. Current recommended endotracheal dose in pediatric patients is 3 mg/kg.[21] There are no data on repeated endotracheal doses. Bretylium has not been demonstrated to achieve adequate serum levels after endotracheal administration.[13]

Naloxone administered endotracheally reverses morphine-

Table 39-1 Endotracheal Drugs

Drugs	Indications	Dose	Remarks
Epinephrine (1:1000) (1 mg/ml)	Asystole Bradycardia Ventricular tachycardia Ventricular fibrillation PEA	0.1 mg/kg	Repeat q3-5 min Dilute with normal saline
Atropine (0.1 mg/ml)	Bradycardia	0.02 mg/kg	Optimal ET dose unknown; consider 2 × IV dose in normal saline
Lidocaine (10 mg/ml) (1%) (20 mg/ml) (2%)	Ventricular tachycardia Ventricular fibrillation	2-3 mg/kg	IV if possible Dilute with sterile water in normal saline
Naloxone (1 mg/ml)	Opiate-induced respiratory depression Altered level of consciousness	0.1 mg/kg IV	Optimal ET dose unknown; consider 2- to 4-mg total dose

PEA, Pulseless electrical activity; *ET,* endotracheal; *IV,* intravenous.

induced respiratory depression in rabbits; and successful resuscitation of a heroin-overdosed patient has been reported.[5,20] The pharmocokinetics of endotracheal naloxone appear very similar to those of intravenous administration. Optimum dosing is not known, and the current intravenous dose is recommended.

Endotracheally administered diazepam has been demonstrated to achieve high serum levels in animal studies, but concerns regarding adverse effects on lung tissue preclude its use.[19] Rectal administration is easier, safer, and probably similarly efficacious for status epilepticus.[2]

Indications

The indication for endotracheal emergency drug administration is a life-threatening condition requiring immediate therapy when intravenous or intraosseus access is not available. Drugs that may be administered endotracheally in pediatric patients include epinephrine, atropine, lidocaine, and naloxone. Epinephrine is indicated for bradycardia with cardiorespiratory compromise, pulseless electrical activity, asystole, unstable ventricular tachycardia, and ventricular fibrillation. Atropine may also be indicated for unstable bradycardia. Lidocaine is indicated for ventricular fibrillation or for ventricular tachycardia. Naloxone is indicated for opiate-induced respiratory depression.

Contraindications

There are no absolute contraindications to endotracheal drug administration, although there are important contraindications to the drugs themselves. The effect of pulmonary diseases such as pneumonia, atelectasis, pulmonary edema, and cystic fibrosis on the efficacy of endotracheally administered emergency drugs is not known. Endotracheal naloxone is relatively contraindicated in newborn infants of opiate-addicted mothers because of possible precipitation of withdrawal seizures.

Complications

Theoretic complications of endotracheal epinephrine administration include prolonged tachycardia, hypertension, and arrythymias due to the depot effect and more sustained duration of action of endotracheal drugs, although these effects have not been demonstrated in pediatric patients. Detrimental histologic effects on lung tissue have not been seen. The extent of impairment of gas exchange after endotracheal drug administration in humans is not known.[11] The complications are otherwise related only to the drug itself, not to the method of administration.

Equipment

Equipment for endotracheal administration of emergency drugs includes only an appropriate-sized endotracheal tube, a small feeding tube or catheter, sterile saline, sterile water, and a bagging device to provide ventilation.

Technique

Dilute all drugs in at least 2 ml of sterile normal saline; recommended volumes are 5 to 10 ml in small infants, and 10 to 20 ml in older children and adults,[11] or 1 ml/kg total volume. Dilute lidocaine in sterile water and all other endotracheal drugs in normal saline. Insert a small feeding tube or catheter into the properly placed endotracheal tube until resistance is met, and attach the syringe containing the medication to the catheter. Instill the medication into the tube, flush the catheter with air, and follow with several rapid insufflations.

Remarks

Dilution and reaching the distal airway are essential to attaining adequate levels of emergency drugs after endotracheal administration. Current dosing guidelines are based primarily on animal studies; data in the pediatric population are virtually nonexistent. Table 39-1 summarizes endotracheal drugs, indications, and doses.

REFERENCES

1. Bernard C: *Lecons sur les effects des substances toxiques et medicamenteuses,* Paris, 1857, JB Baillìer, p 286.
2. Dieckmann RA: Rectal diazepam for prehospital pediatric status epilepticus, *Ann Emerg Med* 23:216-224, 1994.
3. Elam JO: The intrapulmonary route for CPR drugs. In Safar P, editor: *Advances in cardiopulmonary resuscitation,* New York, 1977, Springer-Verlag, p 132.

4. Greenberg MI, Baskin SI, Kaplan AM, et al: Effects of endotracheal administered distilled water and normal saline on the arterial blood gases of dogs, *Ann Emerg Med* 11(11):600-604, 1982.

5. Greenberg MI, Roberts JR, Baskin SI: Endotracheal naloxone reversal of morphine-induced respiratory depression in rabbits, *Ann Emerg Med* 9(6):289-292, 1980.

6. Greenberg MI, Spivey WH: Comparison of deep and shallow endotracheal administration of dionosil in dogs and effect of manual hyperventilation, *Ann Emerg Med* 14(3):209-212, 1985.

7. Hahnel J, Lindner KH, Ahnefeld FW: Endobronchial administration of emergency drugs, *Resuscitation* 17:261-272, 1989.

8. Hahnel JH, Lindner KH, Schurmann C, et al: Plasma lidocaine levels and Pao₂ with endobronchial administration: dilution with normal saline or distilled water? *Ann Emerg Med* 19(11):1314-1317, 1990.

9. Hornchen U, Schuttler J, Stoeckel H, et al: Endobronchial instillation of epinephrine during cardiopulmonary resuscitation, *Crit Care Med* 15:1037-1039, 1987.

10. Howard RF, Bingham RM: Endotracheal compared with intravenous administration of atropine, *Arch Dis Child* 65:449-450, 1990.

11. Johnston C: Endotracheal drug delivery, *Pediatr Emerg Care* 8(2)94-96, 1992.

12. Mace SE: Effect of technique of administration on plasma lidocaine levels, *Ann Emerg Med* 15(5):552-556, 1986.

13. Murphy KM, Caplen SM, Nowak RM, et al: Endotracheal bretylium tosylate in a canine model, *Ann Emerg Med* 13(2):87-91, 1984.

14. Quinton DN, O'Byrne G, Aitkenhead AR: Comparison of endotracheal and peripheral intravenous adrenaline in cardiac arrest, *Lancet* 1(8537):828-829, 1987.

15. Ralston SH, Tacker WA, Showen L, et al: Endotracheal versus intravenous epinephrine during electromechanical dissociation with CPR in dogs, *Ann Emerg Med* 14(11):1044-1048, 1985.

16. Ralston SH, Voorhees WD, Babbs CF: Intrapulmonary epinephrine during prolonged cardiopulmonary resuscitation: improved regional blood flow and resuscitation in dogs, *Ann Emerg Med* 13(2):79-86, 1984.

17. Redding JS, Asuncion JS, Pearson JW: Effective routes of drug administration during cardiac arrest, *Anesth Analg* 46:253-258, 1967.

18. Roberts JR, Greenberg MI, Knaub MA, et al: Blood levels following intravenous and endotracheal epinephrine administration, *J Am Coll Emerg Phys* 8:53-56, 1979.

19. Rusli M, Spivey WH, Bonner H, et al: Endotracheal diazepam: absorption and pulmonary pathologic effects, *Ann Emerg Med* 16(3).314-318, 1987.

20. Tandberg D, Abercrombie D: Treatment of heroin overdose with endotracheal naloxone, *Ann Emerg Med* 11(8):443-445, 1982.

21. Zaritsky A: Pediatric resuscitation pharmacology, *Ann Emerg Med* 22(2):445-455, 1993.

40 Intranasal Drug Administration

F. Keith Battan

Several classes of systemic medications can be delivered intranasally to achieve systemic effects, including sedatives such as midazolam and synthetic opioids such as sufentanil, corticosteroids, anticholinergics, and hormones.* Conventional intranasal (IN) drugs used for topical treatment (e.g., vasoconstrictors or steroids) are not associated with appreciable systemic effects. Advantages of IN delivery include ease of administration, the avoidance of a painful injection, and rapid and reliable onset of action.[2,39] Pharmacokinetics of drugs delivered in this manner are favorable to Emergency Department and critical-care use and are also well suited to clinical circumstances in which rapid drug effects are needed for infants and young children and more painful delivery methods are unwarranted.[6]

Characteristics of pharmacologic agents amenable to IN delivery include low molecular weight, high lipophilicity, and lack of vasoactive properties.[3,12,29,30] Transmucosal nasal delivery allows systemic absorption without exposure to the gastrointestinal tract,[13] where many biologic substances are degraded rapidly,[9] mainly through first-pass hepatic metabolism.[16] However, for some medications there may be a first-pass degradation effect occurring at the nasal mucosa level caused by a defensive enzymatic barrier contained within the nasal epithelium.[12,29] The clinical effects of this process are largely unknown at present.[7]

The vascular supply of the nasal mucosa is rich,[4] absorption of appropriate drugs into the central circulation is rapid,[30] titratability is good, and the resultant pharmacokinetics approach those achieved during intravenous (IV) administration.† For drugs that have high first-pass hepatic metabolism like the benzodiazepines, IN administration results in much higher systemic bioavailability compared to oral or some forms of rectal use.[20,26,28,34,38] Compared to IN administration, sublingual administration has pharmacokinetics close to oral delivery and therefore more blunted effects. In an animal model, IN epinephrine (after pretreatment with phentolamine to decrease local vasoconstriction) had effects on cerebral perfusion pressure and resuscitation rates similar to those with IV use.[4] These properties allow repeated doses of sedative agents to be given, facilitating *titration* of the sedative to the desired level of consciousness.[34]

Indications

IN delivery of medications is indicated when IV access is either unavailable or unnecessary for the intended procedure. An example would be the use of IN midazolam for a minor surgical procedure when IV access isn't warranted or for optimal titration of sedative dosing.[2,17,25,27,33] IN administration is also indicated for local nasal conditions, primarily allergic rhinitis, in which vasoconstrictors and topical steroids are sometimes necessary.

Contraindications

Contraindications are those for the agent used. Adverse effects from the medications described for IN use are uncommon, except for discomfort associated with a fluid volume in the nose and occasionally a burning sensation.

Complications

Complications are again those of the agent used (e.g., decreased chest wall compliance with sufentanil).[1] There is potential for inadvertent swallowing (resulting in oral kinetics), gagging, or even aspiration following inappropriately rapid IN delivery of the medication. Burning and lacrimation on instillation of midazolam are described.[15,18,36] Septal perforation with long-term use of IN steroids is possible. The long-term effect of IN vasoconstrictors on rhinitis has not been well studied in children, although rebound effects on withdrawal of the agent (rhinitis medicamentosus) are well-known problems associated with overuse of nasal vasoconstrictors.

Equipment

The only equipment needed is a small needleless syringe (usually a 1-ml tuberculosis syringe) for the instillation of the medication into the nares. Atomizers or sprayers can also be used for IN delivery.

Technique

Position the child supine with the head back, so that the nares are nearly horizontal. Slight Trendelenburg positioning may be helpful (Fig. 40-1). Ask the parent to hold the patient during this phase if desired. Drop the medication slowly into either nare, allowing time for transmucosal absorption. Wait for the agent to become effective, given its IN kinetics. Use monitoring techniques appropriate for the administered agent.

Atomizers or sprayers for administration of topical vasoconstrictors or steroids are best activated by the child himself while he is upright.

Remarks

Because there is no need for set-up time for IN delivery, IN medications can be administered very quickly. If the child is observed to sputter, cough, or swallow during IN administration, the drug is being given too quickly. Use the most concentrated formulation of the drug to minimize volume.

*References 3, 5, 7, 8, 10, 11, 15, 19, 22, 23, 31, 32, and 37.
†References 4, 12, 14, 21, 32, and 35.

255

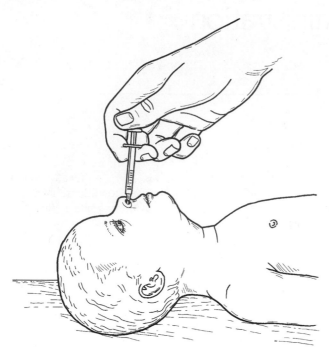

FIG. 40-1 Intranasal drug administration.

REFERENCES

1. Abrams R, Morrison JE, Villasevor A et al: Safety and effectiveness of intranasal administration of sedative medications (ketamine, midazolam, or sufentanil) for urgent brief pediatric dental procedures, *Anesth Prog* 40:63-66; 1993.

2. Battan FK, Harley JR: A randomized controlled trial of intranasal midazolam as sedation for laceration repair, *Pediatr Emerg Care* 2(abstr):222, 1990.

3. Biddle C, Gilliland C: Transdermal and transmucosal administration of pain-relieving and anxiolytic drugs: a primer for the critical care practitioner, *Heart Lung* 21(2):115-124, 1992.

4. Bleske BE, Warren EW, Rice TL, et al: Comparison of intravenous and intranasal administration of epinephrine during CPR in a canine model, *Ann Emerg Med* 21:1125-1130, 1992.

5. Chien YW, Chang SF: Intranasal drug delivery for systemic medications, *Crit Rev Ther Drug Carrier Syst* 4(2):167-194, 1987.

6. Diamant MJ, et al: The use of midazolam for sedation of infants and children, *Am J Radiol* 150(2):377-387, 1988.

7. Gizurarson S: Animal models for intranasal drug delivery studies, *Acta Pharm Nord* 2(2):105-122, 1990.

8. Gizurarson S, Bechgaard E: Intranasal administration of insulin to humans, *Diabetes Res Clin Pract* 12(2):71-84, 1991.

9. Henderson JM, Brodsky DA, Fisher DM, et al.: Preinduction of anesthesia in pediatric patients with nasally administered sufentanil, *Anesthesiology* 65:536-538, 1988.

10. Hermens WA: Delivery of hormones: some new concepts, *Pharm Weekly Sci* 14(4A):253-257, 1992.

11. Homan RV: Transnasal butorphanol, *Am Fam Physician* 49(1):188-192, 1994.

12. Hussain AA: Mechanism of nasal absorption of drugs, *Prog Clin Biol Res* 292:261-272, 1989.

13. Jaimovich DG, Osborne JS, Shadino CL: Comparison of intravenous and endotracheal administration of midazolam and the effect on pulmonary function and histology in the lamb model, *Ann Emerg Med* 21:480-485, 1992.

14. Kanto J, Alloned H: Pharmacokinetics and the sedative effect of midazolam, *Int J Clin Pharmacol Ther Toxicol* 21:460-463, 1983.

15. Karl HW, Rosenberger JL, Larch MG, et al: Transmucosal administration of midazolam for premedication of pediatric patients, *Anesthesiology* 78:855-891, 1993.

16. Lam TK, Ng KW, Chan YS: Use of midazolam in children, *Lancet* 2(8610):565, 1988.

17. Latson LA, Cheatam JP, Gumbiner CH, et al: Midazolam nose drops for outpatient echocardiography sedation in infants, *Am Heart J* 121:209-211, 1991.

18. Lugo RA, et al: Complications of intranasal midazolam, *Pediatrics* 92(4):638 (letter), 1993.

19. Mabry RL: Intranasal corticosteroids and cromolyn, *Am J Otolaryngol* 14(5):295-300, 1993.

20. Malinovsky J, et al: Plasma concentrations of midazolam after intravenous, nasal, or rectal administration in children, *Br J Anaesth* 70:617-620, 1993.

21. Mathews HML, Carson, IW, Lyons SM, et al: A pharmacokinetic study of midazolam in paediatric patients undergoing cardiac surgery, *Br J Anaesth* 61:302-307, 1988.

22. Meltzer EO: Intranasal anticholinergic therapy of rhinorrhea, *J Allergy Clin Immunol* 90(6 pt 2):1055-1064, 1992.

23. Mygind N, Borum P: Intranasal ipratropium: literature abstracts and comments, *Rhinology* (suppl) 9:37-44, 1989.

24. Pontiroli AE, Calderara A, Pozza G: Intranasal drug delivery: potential advantages and limitations from a clinical pharmacokinetic perspective, *Clin Pharmacokinetics* 17(5):299-307, 1989.

25. Proceedings of the International Symposium on the uses of midazolam and flumazenil in intensive care, *Resuscitation* 16(suppl):S1-106, 1988.

26. Raeder JC, et al: Prolonged elimination of midazolam after intramuscular administration, *Acta Anaesthiol Scand* 32(6):464-466, 1988.

27. Rosario M, Alves I, Luis AS: Intranasal midazolam for sedation in upper endoscopy, *Gastroenterology* 98(abstr):A-10, 1990.

28. Saarnivaara L, Lindgren L, Klemola UM: Comparison of chloral hydrate and midazolam by mouth as premedicants in children undergoing otolaryngological surgery, *Br J Anaesth* 61:390-396, 1988.

29. Sarker MA: Drug metabolism in the nasal mucosa, *Pharm Res* 9(1):1-9, 1992.

30. Schipper NG, Verhoef JC, Merkus FW: The nasal mucociliary clearance: relevance to nasal drug delivery, *Pharm Res* 8(7):807-814, 1991.

31. Slover R, et al: Use of intranasal midazolam in preschool children, *Anesth Analg* 70(abstr):5377, 1990.

32. Spector SL: Ocular, nasal and oral cromolyn sodium in the management of nonasthmatic allergic problems, *Allergy Proc* 10(3):191-254, 1989.

33. Theroux MC, West DW, Corddry DH, et al: Efficacy of intranasal midazolam in facilitating suturing of lacerations in preschool children in the emergency department, *Pediatrics* 91:624-627, 1993.

34. Walbergh EJ, Wills RJ, Eckert J, et al: Plasma concentrations of midazolam in children following intranasal administration, *Anesthesiology* 71:A1066, 1989.

35. Walbergh EJ, Eckert J: Pharmacokinetics of intravenous and intranasal midazolam in children, *Anesthesiology* 74:233-235, 1991.

36. Wilton NCT, et al: Preanesthetic sedation of preschool children using intranasal midazolam, *Anesthesiology* 69:972-975, 1988.

37. Wilton NCT, Leigh J, Rosen D, et al: Preanesthetic sedation of preschool children using intranasal midazolam, *Anesthesiology* 69:962-975, 1988.

38. Wong L, McQueen KD: Midazolam routes of administration, *DICP* 25(5):476-477, 1991.

39. Yealy, et al: Intranasal midazolam as a sedative for children during laceration repair, *Am J Emerg Med* 10:584-587, 1992.

41 Oral Drug Administration

Joan Bothner

Oral drug administration is well-accepted, effective and safe. It is the optimal route of administration for a wide variety of medications. However, applicability of the oral route in the emergency or critical-care setting is limited as a result of delayed onset of action, erratic absorption, inability to titrate effect, and time lag to reach therapeutic levels.

Indications

A common indication for oral medication in the Emergency Department (ED) or intensive care unit (ICU) is the need for sedation for frightening or painful procedures. Oral transmucosal fentanyl citrate has been shown to be safe and effective as premedication for anesthesia and surgery.[11] Doses are 15 to 20 µg/kg. Peak concentrations are reached within 20 to 25 minutes of administration and decrease rapidly.[5,12] Lind, Marcus, Meers, et al.[4] studied oral transmucosal fentanyl in the ED administered as a solution and found that 60% of patients became drowsy or sedated within 30 minutes of administration. Side effects included nausea, dizziness, and dry mouth in 20% to 40% of patients. There were no significant changes in vital signs or oxygen saturation.

Ketamine is well accepted orally and provides rapid sedation with few side effects.[2,13] It provides sedation, amnesia, and analgesia. Bioavailability is 16%, compared to 93% intramuscularly or intravenously, and peak plasma levels are one fifth as high. Sedation occurs within 15 to 20 minutes, respiratory function is well maintained, and emergence phenomena are rare after oral administration.[3] Dosage range is from 3 to 6 mg/kg, although 10 mg/kg is probably safe and effective.[13]

Midazolam is also effective as a preanesthetic medication and sedative in pediatric patients. Bioavailability after oral administration is 15% to 25% as a result of incomplete absorption and extensive first-pass metabolism.[7] Doses of 0.5 to 0.75 mg/kg achieve sedation within 20 to 30 minutes of administration and appear to have no significant respiratory or cardiovascular side effects.[1,3,6]

Fever control is a common indication for oral medication in the ED or ICU. Acetaminophen and ibuprofen are both effective and achieve peak levels within 30 to 45 minutes of administration.

Gastric decontamination after toxic ingestion is an indication for oral activated charcoal. Activated charcoal is very effective in preventing absorption of ingested substances if given within 1 hour of ingestion but does not bind elementary metals, some pesticides, iron, cyanide, or alcohols. Activated charcoal is contraindicated after ingestion of a corrosive agent because of lack of efficacy and obscuration of endoscopy. Usual dose is 1 g/kg. Palatability may be improved by mixing with cherry syrup, sweetened drinks, and chocolate, which do not reduce efficacy.[8] Other oral agents that may be indicated after toxic ingestions include N-acetylcysteine after acetaminophen overdose and polyethylene glycol–electrolyte lavage solutions for whole bowel irrigation.

Asthma is a common presenting complaint to the ED. A recent metaanalysis of steroid therapy concluded that the oral and intravenous routes are equally efficacious in the initial treatment of acute asthma.[9] Treatment with oral prednisone at a dose of 2 mg/kg decreases hospitalization rate, compared to placebo.[10] Consider oral prednisone in any moderate or severe asthma patient who is not vomiting and is not in severe respiratory distress.

Contraindications

Oral medication is contraindicated in any patient who cannot protect his or her airway because of altered level of consciousness. Other contraindications include severe respiratory distress; inadequate gag or cough; emesis; gastrointestinal obstruction; cardiovascular instability; and ingestion of a substance capable of inducing neurologic, respiratory, or cardiac depression. The major contraindication is a requirement for more rapid or better-controlled drug administration.

Complications

Complications of oral administration of drugs are few. They include emesis, as well as aspiration with resultant laryngospasm or aspiration pneumonia. Complications are associated with the drug themselves; therefore all children should be monitored in a manner appropriate to the expected level of neurologic and cardiopulmonary depression.

Equipment

Equipment necessary for oral drug administration is minimal. For small children and infants, use disposable plastic syringes to instill medication into the mouth with minimal spillage and spitting. Flavored syrups are readily accepted and are useful for disguising bitter-tasting preparations and for dissolving crushed tablets. Crush tablets between two spoons or with a mortar and pestal. Acetaminophen elixir is an excellent vehicle for midazolam administration (15 to 20 mg/kg). Older infants and children will drink medication from a plastic cup. Small infants will suck medication from a nipple. Administration of medication via nasogastric tube is not routinely recommended, except for activated charcoal.

Techniques

Administration of oral medication via syringe is an easy route for small infants and young children. Gently restrain the child with the parent's help. Place the syringe along the buccal surface of the mouth, and slowly instill the medication, holding the chin extended and the mouth closed, and allowing the child time to swallow (Fig. 41-1).

For a small infant, place the medication in an empty

Table 41-1 Nonvascular Access: Oral Drug Therapy in the ED and ICU

Drug	Dose	Onset	Duration
		Sedation/Analgesia	
Midazolam	0.5-0.75 mg/kg	20-30 minutes	60 minutes
Ketamine	3-6 mg/kg	20-30 minutes	60 minutes
Chloral hydrate	25-50 mg/kg	45-60 minutes	60-120 minutes
Fentanyl	15-20 µg/kg	15-30 minutes	75-120 minutes
		Asthma	
Prednisone	2 mg/kg	4 hours	Biologic half-life 18-36 hours
		Antipyretics	
Acetaminophen	15-20 mg/kg	15-60 minutes	2-4 hours
Ibuprofen	10 mg/kg	1 hour	6-8 hours
		Other Drugs	
Activated charcoal	1 g/kg	Immediate	Repeat as indicated
Polyethylene glycol electrolyte solution	20 ml/hour	Immediate	Nasogastric infusion; use until rectal effusate is clear
Dextrose oral gel, 40%	25 g of gel = 10 g dextrose	2-5 minutes	10-20 minutes

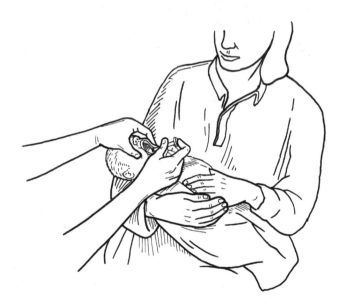

FIG. 41-1 Drug administration with syringe.

nipple and place the nipple into the infant's mouth. Do not dilute oral medication in large amounts of liquids such as formula or juice.

Remarks

Many agents available as IV solutions are bitter tasting and contain significant amounts of alcohol. Substituting tablet forms, which are then crushed and mixed in flavored syrups, is a viable and well-accepted alternative. Proper placement into the mouth will avoid tongue thrusting and spitting the medication out. When administering activated charcoal to a cooperative patient, adding a flavoring agent may avoid the need for nasogastric tube placement and is not likely to decrease efficacy significantly.

Table 41-1 summarizes common oral drugs for use in the ED or ICU.

REFERENCES

1. Feld LH, Negus JB, White PF: Oral midazolam preanesthetic medication in pediatric outpatients, *Anesthesiology* 78:831-834, 1990.
2. Gutstein HB, Johnson KL, Heard MB: Oral ketamine preanesthetic medication in children, *Anesthesiology* 76:28-33, 1992.
3. Lin YC, Moynihan RJ, Hackel A: A comparison of oral midazolam, oral ketamine, and oral midazolam combined with ketamine as preanesthetic medication for pediatric outpatients, *Anesthesiology* 79:A1177, 1993.
4. Lind, GH, Marcus MA, Mears SL, et al: Oral transmucosal fentanyl citrate for analgesia and sedation in the emergency department, *Ann Emerg Med* 20:1117-1120, 1991.
5. McEvoy GK, editor: *American Hospital Formulary drug information*, Bethesda, Md, 1994, American Society of Hospital Pharmacists.
6. Ogden A, Kennedy L. Glass N: Oral midazolam vs oral ketamine for sedation of children with cancer for painful procedures (meeting abstract), *Proc Annu Meet Am Soc Clin Oncol* 12:A1503, 1993.
7. Payne K, Mattheyse FJ, Liebenberg B, et al: The pharmacokinetics of midazolam in pediatric patients, *Eur J Clin Pharmacol* 37:267-272, 1989.
8. Rodgers GC, Matyunas NJ: Gastrointestinal decontamination for acute poisoning, *Pediatr Clin North Am* 33:261-285, 1986.
9. Rowe BH, Keller JL, Oxman AD: Effectiveness of steroid therapy in acute exacerbation of asthma, *Am J Emerg Med* 10:301-310, 1992.
10. Scarfone RJ, Fuchs SM, Nager AL, et al: Controlled trial of oral prednisone in the emergency department treatment of children with acute asthma, *Pediatrics* 92:513-518, 1993.
11. Stanley TH, Hague BH, Mock DL, et al: Oral transmucosal fentanyl citrate (lollipop) medication in human volunteers, *Anesth Analg* 69:21-27, 1989.
12. Streisand JB, Varvel JR, Stanski DR, et al: Adsorption and bioavailability of oral transmucosal fentanyl citrate, *Anesthesiology* 75:223-229, 1991.
13. Tobias JD, Phipps S, Smith B, et al: Oral ketamine premedication to alleviate the distress of invasive procedures in pediatric oncology patients, *Pediatrics* 90:537-541, 1992.

42 Sublingual Drug Administration

Kathryn D. Clark

The rich vascular plexus of the oral mucosa lends itself to drug delivery through simple absorption and direct injection. Increasing numbers of sublingual (SL) drugs are being investigated. Nitroglycerin, nifedipine, captopril, benzodiazepines (including lorazepam), opioids, and buprenorphine are effective by SL transmucosal administration.[2-4,8] Epinephrine, atropine, naloxone, and lidocaine have been given by SL injection (Tables 42-1 and 42-2).[6,10,11]

Anatomy and Physiology

The oral mucosa consists of an epithelium; a basement membrane; a lamina propria; and a submucosa, which contains the blood vessels. Drugs must permeate through these four layers. Passage across these layers is predominantly by first-order simple diffusion. As a consequence, rapid absorption and good bioavailability exist for low-molecular-weight lipophilic drugs. Once passage through to the submucosa is complete, drugs are absorbed into the systemic circulation through the rich mucosal network of systemic veins and lymphatics. This avoids first-pass hepatic metabolism, which may substantially reduce serum levels of certain medications.[5,7]

The inferior surface of the tongue is covered by a mucous membrane through which the sublingual venous plexus can be seen. The SL artery and vein course on either side of the frenulum. SL injection is made into the venous plexus and therefore into the systemic circulation.

Indications

The sublingual mucosa offers a convenient and accessible area for transmucosal drug administration. SL drug delivery may be preferred over oral delivery in patients with swallowing difficulties. Drug delivery may be rapidly stopped by removal of the medication from the oral cavity. For certain medications such as nitroglycerin, in which first-pass metabolism results in inactivation, SL delivery is the method of choice. SL transmucosal absorption has been shown to be more rapid than oral administration (nitroglycerin), similar to oral administration (benzodiazepines), or slower than oral administration (nifedipine).[8]

In life-threatening situations such as cardiac arrest without intravenous (IV) access, SL injection is an option for delivery of medications. However, other delivery methods such as intraosseous infusion are preferred. Studies show SL injection to provide rapid absorption, with an onset of action intermediate between IV and intramuscular administration.[12] Pharmacokinetics for SL injection of epinephrine have been described showing onset of physiologic effects 35 seconds longer than with IV administration and with a more prolonged duration of response.[9,12]

Table 42-1 Drugs for Sublingual Transmucosal Absorption

Drug	Adult dose	Extrapolated pediatric dose
Nitroglycerin	0.4 mg	Unknown
Nifedipine	10-20 mg	0.25-0.5 mg/kg[1,2]
Captopril	25 mg	0.15-2 mg/kg
Lorazepam	2 mg (4 mg max)	0.1 mg/kg
Buprenorphine	0.4-0.8 mg	2-6 μg/kg[3]

[1]Not approved by the Food and Drug Administration for children.
[2]Studies were conducted with adults, using standard adult doses; hence standard pediatric doses are given. Equivalent PO/SL doses were used in the studies.
[3]Has only been used in children ages 2 to 12 years old.

Table 42-2 Drugs for Sublingual Injection

Drug	Dose
Epinephrine	0.01 mg/kg
Naloxone	0.1 mg/kg
Atropine	0.02 mg/kg (min. 0.1 mg)
Lidocaine	1 mg/kg

Contraindications

SL injection is painful. Avoid in the conscious patient or in a patient with other possible vascular access. The contraindications for SL transmucosal drug administration relate predominantly to the drugs themselves.

Complications

Patient cooperation is key in the transmucosal SL administration of medication in pediatrics. The patient must hold the medication under the tongue, without swallowing prematurely; otherwise kinetics of drug delivery will approach kinetics of oral administration.

SL injection may lead to complications such as aspiration or obstruction caused by bleeding or upper airway swelling.[9] SL injection of epinephrine may cause vasoconstriction with necrosis of sublingual and lingual tissues[11]; thus injection of SL epinephrine should be reserved for instances when other methods of administration are impossible.

If SL administration is being used without IV access, rapid fluid administration will not be possible in case of complications requiring intravenous fluids.

Equipment/Techniques

For transmucosal SL absorption, place pills under the tongue, to one side of the frenulum, where they dissolve. For some

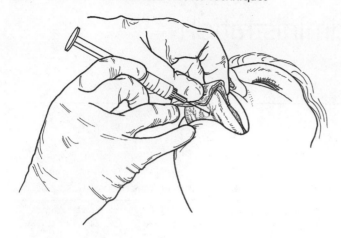

FIG. 42-1 Sublingual injection.

medications (e.g., nifedipine) it is possible to remove the encapsulated solution with a syringe and administer this solution SL.

Perform SL injection 1 to 2 cm lateral to the midline of the sublingual tissues.[11] Insert the needle into the ventral surface of the tongue. Avoid the two veins on either side of the midline. With the patient lying supine, pick up the tip of his or her tongue in a gauze swab and draw it out of the patient's mouth. Insert the needle directed posteriorly (vertically downwards) as shown in Fig. 42-1. Volumes of up to 2 ml may be injected.[1]

Remarks

Recent studies indicate that nifedipine is more effective following oral rather than sublingual administration.[8] The optimal method of nifedipine administration is to have the patient bite, completely masticate, and then swallow the contents. Alternatively, the 0.34-ml solution of nifedipine in

the capsule may be removed with a syringe and squirted into the patient's mouth.

Other SL medications under investigation are predominantly for adults. Oral and SL dose recommendations currently are similar. Whether these doses are appropriate in children requires further evaluation.

REFERENCES

1. Bullough, J: Intraglossal injections in unconscious patients, *Lancet* 1(7011):80-81, 1958.
2. Dessi-Fulgheri P, Bandiera F, Rubattu S, et al: Comparison of sublingual and oral captopril in hypertension, *Clin Exper Hypertension* 19(2-3):593-597, 1987.
3. Gong L, Middleton RK: Sublingual administration of opioids, *Ann Pharmacother* 26(12):1525-1527, 1992.
4. Greenblatt DJ, Divoll M, Harmatz JS, et al: Pharmacokinetic comparison of sublingual lorazepam with intravenous, intramuscular and oral lorazepam, *J Pharm Sci* 71:248-252, 1982.
5. Harris D, Robinson JR: Drug delivery via the mucous membranes of the oral cavity, *J Pharm Sci* 81(1):1-10, 1992.
6. Maio RF, Gaukel B, Freeman B: Intralingual naloxone injection for narcotic-induced respiratory depression, *Ann Emerg Med* 16:572-573, 1987.
7. Meyer J Squieer CA, Gerson SJ: *The structure and function of oral mucosa*, Oxford, 1984, Pergamon.
8. Motwani JG, Lipworth BJ: Clinical pharmacokinetics of drugs administered buccally and sublingually, *Clin Pharmacokinetics* 21(2):83-94, 1991.
9. Nichols WA: Intralingual injection site for emergency stimulant drugs, *Oral Surg* 32:677-684, 1971.
10. Ordog GJ, Wasserberger J, Jones J, et al: Efficacy of absorption of sublingual and intravenous Cardio-Green, *Ann Emerg Med* 13:426-428, 1984.
11. Rothrock SG, Green SM, et al: Successful resuscitation from cardiac arrest using sublingual injection for medication delivery, *Ann Emerg Med* 22(4):751-753, 1993.
12. Sklar E, Schwartz M: The ventral surface of the tongue: an emergency site of injection, *Oral Surg* 19:28-31, 1965.

43 Inhalation

Kathryn D. Clark

Inhalation therapy is a simple procedure to initiate with few complications or contraindications, and it has the benefit of rapid onset of drug action. Goals of inhalation therapy include mobilization of bronchial secretions, relief of bronchospasm and edema, and administration of antibiotic or prophylactic agents.[7] Therefore inhalation therapy is used for delivery of β-adrenergics, steroids, racemic epinephrine, and anticholinergics in the treatment of asthma or croup and for the delivery of antibiotics or antivirals in the treatment of cystic fibrosis, respiratory syncytial virus, or *Pneumocystis carinii*.[15] In addition, inhaled anesthetics such as nitrous oxide may be used for conscious sedation in the Emergency Department (ED) or intensive care unit. Nitric oxide acts as a specific pulmonary vasodilator; thus it is used to treat persistent pulmonary hypertension in the neonate and in adult respiratory distress syndrome (see Chapter 23).[4]

Anatomy and Physiology

Several factors play a role in the passage of inhaled medication through the upper to the lower, smaller airways. The larger or faster a particle, the more likely it is to contact the upper airway and not proceed beyond. Long, slow breathing enhances gravitational deposition, the means of medication delivery to the small airways.[2] Droplet size is also an important consideration. Depth of penetration into the respiratory tract increases as droplet size decreases. Airway size and obstruction within the airways as in bronchoconstriction, inflammation, and mucous plugging affect delivery of medication.

Indications

Use inhalation therapy when drug action specific to or absorption through the respiratory tract is desired. Inhalation therapy maximizes pulmonary effects, with a minimum of extrapulmonary side effects.[3,12] In the treatment of asthma, aerosols have a more rapid onset of action, fewer side effects, and similar duration of action as compared with oral β-agonists.[14] Table 43-1 summarizes common drugs and doses for inhalation therapy.

Contraindications

The contraindication to inhalation therapy is lack of cooperation. Contraindications to a specific medication may be myriad. For example, do not use nitrous oxide in patients unable to protect their airways or in patients with middle-ear disease, head injury, bowel obstruction, or pneumothorax because of rapid diffusion of nitrogen and expansion of these gas-filled areas.[5] Extreme tachycardia, propensity for arrhythmia, and hypertension may be relative contraindications for use of β-agonists in the asthmatic patient.[14]

Complications

Complications of inhalation therapy are rare. Inconsistent delivery of medication may result from mechanical failure of the delivery system (e.g., loss of medication within the tubing or lack of patient cooperation). Nosocomial infection may occur because the nebulizer may become contaminated with microorganisms. Follow cleaning guidelines for the specific nebulizer or use disposable equipment.[16] Most complications are due to the side effects of medication, particularly tremor and tachycardia with β-agonists[12] or extensive sedation or nausea with nitrous oxide.[5,6,9]

Equipment

Aerosolized drug therapy for spontaneously breathing patients can be delivered via metered-dose inhaler (MDI) or small-volume nebulizer (SVN).

Nebulization requires a medication cup (nebulizer), compressed gas source (oxygen or room air), oxygen tubing, tee piece, mask, mouthpiece or tubing, saline, and medication (Fig. 43-1 shows equipment setup). Most modern ventilators have in-line medication nebulizers. An adaptor must be used to attach the nebulizer to the ventilator circuit.

Use of an MDI requires the MDI canister and spacer with or without a mask (Fig. 43-2).

A small-particle aerosol generator is used to administer the antiviral drug ribavirin. From a large reservoir, the nebulized ribivarin flows into a drying chamber where the water evaporates, leaving only the molecular ribavirin to pass into the patient's airways.[16] Special filters should be used to

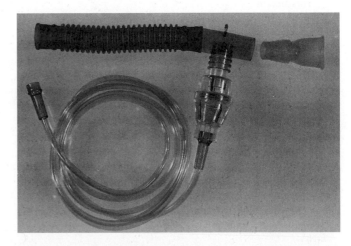

FIG. 43-1 Small-volume nebulizer. An updraft nebulizer includes a medication cup and oxygen tubing attached to a tee piece with reservoir. A mouthpiece, as pictured, or mask is inserted into one end of the tee piece.

Table 43-1 Drugs effective by inhalation

Medications	Dose	Side Effects
β agonists		Palpitation Tachycardia Tremor
Albuterol	MDI: two puffs q5min (max. 12) NEB: 0.5% solution, 0.03 ml/mg (max. 1 ml) Continuous NEB: 0.5 mg/kg/hr (max. 15 mg/hour)	
Metaproterenol	MDI: two puffs NEB: 5% 0.01 ml/kg (max. 0.3 ml)	
Terbutaline	MDI: 2 puffs q5min (max. 12) NEB: 0.1 mg/kg max. 2.5 mg[*]	
Anticholinergics		Thickening of secretions Hypertension Decreased gastrointestinal- motility
Atropine	0.05 mg/kg (max. 2.5 mg)	
Ipratropium bromide	MDI: 2 puffs qid NEB: 250 μg/dose	
Corticosteroids		Oropharyngeal candidiasis Dysphonia
Beclomethasone Betamethasone Triamcinolone	2 puffs each nostril tid (not recommended <6 years of age)	
Cromolyn sodium	MDI: 2 puffs bid-qid NEB: 20 mg/2 ml amp; 1 amp bid-qid	
Racemic epinephrine	0.05 ml/kg per dose of 2.25% solution (max. 0.5 ml)	Tachyarrhythmias Headache Nausea Palpitations
Anesthetics		
N_2O (nitrous oxide)	30%-50%	Restlessness Vomiting Nausea
Antivirals		
Ribavirin	6 g in 300 ml sterile water delivered 12-18 hr/day	Worsening respiratory status Arrhythmia
Antibiotics		
Aminoglycosides[†‡]		
Gentamicin	2 mg/kg in 10 ml NS	
Kanamicin	250 mg[‡]	
Tobramicin	[†]	
Penicillin S		
Carbenicillin	[†]	
Amoxicillin	[†]	
Pentamidine	300 mg in 6 ml sterile water q4 weeks via Respirgard II nebulizer reservoir[‡§]	Bronchospasm Bad taste Dizziness
Antifungals		
Nystatin	[†]	
Amphotericin B	[†]	
Mucolytics		
Acetylcysteine	3-5 ml 20% solution[‡]	
Under investigation		
Amiloride		
Furosemide		
Surfactant		
DNAse		
Ciprofloxacin		

[*]Not approved by Food and Drug Administration.
[†]Varying experimental dosages.
[‡]Doses obtained from adult studies.
[§]A special nebulizer is required to avoid exhalation of the drug into the work atmosphere.

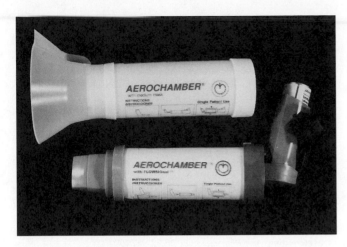

FIG. 43-2   A metered-dose inhaler is most effectively used with a spacer, with or without a mask.

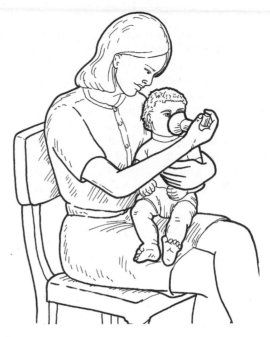

FIG. 43-3   An MDI with spaces and mask can be used in children as young as age 6 months for delivery of bronchodilators.

protect the ventilator because ribavirin has been reported to precipitate in the valves and circuits.

Technique

Metered-dose inhaler. In an MDI the active drug is suspended in a fluorocarbon propellant, and on activation a metered dose of fluid is released. Most of the aerosol spray impacts in the oropharynx. To use an MDI, (1) stand up; (2) hold the inhaler with mouthpiece downward; (3) shake the inhaler and remove the cap; (4) hold the inhaler upright and breathe out fully; (5) close lips around the mouthpiece of the inhaler; (6) activate the inhaler while inspiring slowly and deeply; (7) hold breath for 10 seconds; (8) if dose is to be repeated, wait about 1 minute. Spacers, extension tubes interposed between the MDI and mouth (Fig. 43-3), allow slowing of the aerosol spray, reducing oropharyngeal deposition and enhancing penetration to smaller airways. Spacers eliminate the need for synchronization of canister activation and inhalation and improve the drug delivery.[1,10] The medication dose is discharged into the spacing device and then inhaled. In patients having difficulty using spacers (i.e., children less than 1 year of age), use a spacer with a mask. Place the mask on the face, covering the mouth and nose. Spray one puff from the MDI and hold the mask firmly to the face while the patient inhales at least six times.

Nebulization. Measure medication and diluent into the cup. Attach tee piece to the top of the nebulizer. Insert the mouthpiece into one end of the tee piece and place a short length of aerosol tubing on the opposite end of the tee piece to act as a reservoir (to increase amount of inhaled medications). For use with mask replace tee piece with mask. Establish oxygen flow at 5 to 6 L/min. Allow the patient to position the mask, mouthpiece, or tubing for blow-by until medication is finished. For blow-by, occlude one end of the tee piece; do not attach the mask.

A severe asthmatic may require continuous aerosols.[13] To administer, refill the SVN medication cups before completion or use a large-volume nebulizer (LVN). Place medication and saline into the LVN. Mix desired dose of medication with enough normal saline to make 80 ml of total fluid. This will be approximately 4 hours of solution. The recommended

dose is 0.5 mg/kg/hour of albuterol. Adjust flow to 8 to 10 L/min to obtain 20 ml/hr of medication delivery. Reassess patient frequently.

For ventilated patients, therapy may be delivered via an SVN connected in-line to the ventilatory circuit or by using an Embu bag. To attach SVN in-line, place medication and saline into nebulizer. Secure nebulizer and place tee piece with nebulizer in-line with ventilator. Adapters depend on the actual ventilator used. Ventilator settings need to be adjusted to compensate for added flow from the in-line nebulizer system.

To deliver medication with an Embu bag, attach SVN to tee piece. On one end of tee piece, attach aerosol tubing and positive end-expiratory pressure (PEEP) valve, which will connect to the endotracheal tube. On the opposite end of the tee piece, attach an adapter and an Embu bag with pressure monitor. Adjust flow to 5 L/min. With bagging, medication is delivered to the patient. Pressures may be adjusted with PEEP valve.

The lung deposition of aerosolized drugs delivered to intubated infants is only about one twentieth of that in nonintubated adults and one tenth of that in intubated adults. The implication is that higher dosages are needed when aerosolized drugs are delivered to an intubated infant to achieve a dose equivalent to that received by nonintubated patients.[16]

Remarks

There may be a trade-off between a calm child vs. effective medication delivery. Parental involvement, such as administration of medication while the patient is in the parent's lap, may decrease agitation; however, crying may actually improve medication delivery due to the child's deeper, more frequent breaths. Most small children tolerate blow-by better than mask use, but more medication is lost to the atmosphere with blow-by.

No significant difference has been demonstrated between nebulizers and MDIs used with a spacer in the ED.[10,11] The youngest age of subjects included in these studies was 6.

When possible, efficacy should be objectively evaluated. Peak flow rates may be measured in cooperative patients, before and after treatment. Usually patients 5 to 6 years and older are able to cooperate. Instruct the patient to (1) take a few slow, moderately deep breaths, (2) breathe in as far possible, (3) hold breath while placing mouthpiece in mouth beyond teeth, (4) seal lips tightly around the mouthpiece, (5) blow out as hard and fast as possible, and (6) repeat at least two times.

There is a learning curve involved with the use of peak flow meters; thus they may prove more useful over time such as for home monitoring.

REFERENCES

1. Canny GJ, Levison H: Aerosols—therapeutic use and delivery in childhood asthma, *Ann Allergy* 60:11-20, 1988.
2. Clarke SW: Aerosols as a way of treating patients, *Eur J Respir Dis* 69:525-533, 1986.
3. Dahl AR, Bond JA, Pedridov-Fisher J, et al: Effects of the respiratory tract on inhaled materials, *Toxicol Appl Pharmacol* 93:484-492, 1988.
4. Frostell C, Fratacci MD, Wain JC, et al: Inhaled nitric oxide: a selective pulmonary vasodilator reversing hypoxic pulmonary vasoconstriction, *Circulation* 83:2038-2047, 1991.
5. Gamis AS, Knapp JF, Glenski JA, et al: Nitrous oxide analgesia in a pediatric emergency department, *Ann Emerg Med* 18:177-181, 1989.
6. Hallonsten, AL: Sedation by the use of inhalation agents in dental care, *Acta Anaesthesiol Scand* 88:31-35, 1988.
7. Hill LS: The inhaled route of drug administration in the therapy of asthma, *Br J Clin Pract* 42:313-315, 1988.
8. Idris AH, McDermott MF, Ranicci KC, et al: Emergency department treatment of severe asthma, *Chest* 103:665-672, 1993.
9. Jastak JT: Nitrous oxide in dental practice, *Int Anesthesiol Clin* 27:92-97, 1989.
10. Kerem E, Levison H, Schuh S, et al: Efficacy of albuterol administered by nebulizer versus spacer device in children with acute asthma, *J Pediatr* 123:313-317, 1993.
11. Kisch GL, Paloucek FP: Metered dose inhalers and nebulizers in the acute setting, *Ann Pharmacother* 26:92-95, 1992.
12. Nathan RA. B2-agonist therapy; oral vs inhaled delivery, *J Asthma* 29:49-54, 1992.
13. Papo MC, Frank J, Thompson AE, et al: A prospective, randomized study of continuous versus intermittent nebulized albuterol for severe status asthmaticus in children, *Crit Care Med* 21:1479-1486, 1993.
14. Popa V: Beta-adrenergic drugs, *Clin Chest Med* 7:313-329, 1986.
15. Stout SA, Derendorf H: Local treatment of respiratory infections with antibiotics, *Drug Intell Clin Pharm* 21:322-329, 1987.
16. Whitaker KB: Aerosolized drug therapy. In *Comprehensive perinatal and pediatric respiratory care,* Albany, 1992, Delmar Publishers, pp 200-208.

44 Topical Delivery

John R. Williams

The topical administration of medication originated in ancient Greece, but it is only during the 20th century that the skin has been used as an effective method of drug delivery.[2] Like parenteral injections, transcutaneous delivery avoids the first-pass metabolism seen with many oral pharmaceuticals. Topical administration can have either a local or a systemic effect, depending on the condition being treated and the drug being used. The use of dimethylsulfoxide as a topical vehicle for systemic delivery of lipid-soluble drugs may provide for expansion of transcutaneous drugs in the future.

Topical absorption depends on penetration of the outermost layer of the skin, the stratum corneum (also known as the horny layer). This layer acts not only as a barrier to the penetration of substances, but in certain circumstances it may also function as a drug reservoir. Factors that influence skin penetration include (1) hydration, (2) temperature, (3) inflammation, (4) age-related changes in lipid composition and thickness of the stratum corneum, and (5) lipid solubility and molecular weight of the drug and the vehicle.[2,7,9]

Indications

Topical medications are indicated for the treatment of certain dermatologic disorders, for the treatment of systemic illnesses that respond to the available transdermal drug delivery systems, and for local anesthesia. A full discussion of topical agents used for local anesthesia is found in Part III of this text. Table 44-1 contains a list of frequently administered topical agents.

Contraindications

The only absolute contraindication is known hypersensitivity to the medication or the topical vehicle. The use of high-potency topical fluorinated steroids is not recommended in pediatrics, except under the supervision of a dermatologist. Use only low-potency topical steroids (e.g., 1% hydrocortisone) on the face, scrotum, vulva, and diaper area. Remember that topical steroids can have both local and systemic adverse effects.[3,9]

Complications

Adverse reactions to cutaneous preparations include allergic and irritant contact dermatitis, occlusion folliculitis, alopecia, and systemic side effects of the individual drug if it is absorbed in excess.[7]

Technique

Hospital personnel applying topical agents should either wear gloves or use an applicator device to avoid excess exposure to the drug.[5] Scrubbing the skin with harsh detergents and soaps makes the stratum corneum more permeable and therefore increases absorption as well. Plastic occlusive dressings enhance skin penetration by increasing the hydration and the temperature of the skin.[2,3,9]

Remarks

The stratum corneum barrier is thinnest, and often most penetrable, in sites such as the face, scrotum, and vulva. It can be disrupted by disease, trauma, burns, and toxins. If the barrier is disrupted, absorption will obviously be affected.[2,7,9]

Nitroglycerin ointment placed on the dorsum of the hand has been reported to be an effective aid in the placement of intravenous catheters in adults. To date, pediatric reports have generally been less favorable, and even unfavorable in neonates.[1,4,6,8]

REFERENCES

1. Guran P, Beal G, Brion N, et al: Topical nitroglycerin as an aid to insertion of peripheral venous catheters in neonates, *J Pediatr* 115:1025, 1989.
2. Kligman AM: Skin permeability: dermatologic aspects of transdermal drug delivery, *Am Heart J* 108:200-206, 1984.
3. Lucky AW: Principles of the use of glucocorticosteroids in the growing child, *Pediatr Dermatol* 1:226-235, 1984.
4. Maynard EC, Oh W: Topical nitroglycerin ointment as an aid to insertion of peripheral venous catheters in neonates, *J Pediatr* 114:474-476, 1989.
5. Perry AG, Potter PA: *Clinical nursing skills and techniques,* ed 2, St. Louis, 1990, Mosby, pp 495-498.
6. Roberge RJ, Kelly M, Evans TC, et al: Facilitated intravenous access through local application of nitroglycerin ointment, *Ann Emerg Med* 16:546-549, 1987.
7. Sheretz EF: Pharmacology. Part I. Topical therapy in dermatology, *J Am Acad Dermatol* 21:108-114, 1989.
8. Vaksmann G, Rey C, Breviere GM, et al: Nitroglycerin ointment as aid to venous cannulation in children, *J Pediatr* 111:89-91, 1987.
9. Weston WL, Lane AT: *Color textbook of pediatric dermatology,* St. Louis, 1991, Mosby, pp 255-271.

Table 44-1 Commonly Used Topical Agents

Local effect	Systemic effect (transdermal continuous release preparations)
Antibiotics	Nitroglycerin
Antifungals	Clonidine
Corticosteroids	Scopolamine
Lubricants	Estradiol
Topical anesthetics	

45 Subcutaneous and Intradermal Delivery

F. Keith Battan

The subcutaneous (SC) injection of medication was first reported almost 150 years ago in Western Europe.[3] Today both SC and intradermal (ID) injections comprise a substantial percentage of all parenterally administered drugs. SC injections provide a systemic effect that avoids the first-pass metabolism seen with many pharmaceuticals given orally. ID injections provide a local effect.

Indications

Medications that are frequently given by the SC and ID routes are listed in Table 45-1. A comparison of absorption patterns of SC and intramuscular injections shows that SC absorption is usually slower, with more sustained release of medication into the circulation. Factors affecting SC and ID absorption include the local blood flow and the capillary surface area to the injection site, along with the solubility of the injected substance. Local blood flow can be affected by exercise, temperature, edema, impaired circulation, and drug-induced phenomena such as vasoconstriction.[2,5]

Contraindications

SC delivery is inappropriate for medications that are irritating and are nonwater soluble. Irritating substances can cause pain, necrosis, and even sloughing of tissue.[5,7]

Complications

Complications from SC and ID drug delivery include infection, sterile abscess formation, and lipodystrophy. Sterile abscesses result from the injection of either an irritating or nonsoluble substance or too great a volume for the tissue site selected. Lipodystrophy, frequently seen in diabetics, results from repeated same-site injections.[5,7,8]

Equipment

The equipment needed for SC and ID injections includes an antiseptic swab, syringe, needle, and medication.[4,7] A syringe size of 1 to 2 ml is adequate for SC injections since the maximum volume to be given is 0.5 ml in pediatrics and 1 ml in adults. Needle selection ranges from 3/8 to 5/8 inch in length, and 30 to 25 gauge in diameter, depending on the depth of the SC tissue. For ID injections a syringe size of 1 ml is usually adequate. Needle length varies from 1/4 to 1/2 inch and from 30 to 25 gauge in diameter.

Technique

The most common sites for SC injection are the lateral aspect of the upper arms, the anterior aspect of the thighs, and the abdomen in the area extending from the costal margins to the iliac crests (Fig. 45-1). The injection sites should be clear of skin lesions, inflammatory lesions, and bony prominences.

Clean the injection site with an antiseptic swab and allow the area to dry completely. This will prevent possible injec-

Table 45-1 Commonly Administered SC and ID Drugs in a Pediatric Emergency Department

Subcutaneous	Intradermal
Insulin	Local anesthesia
Heparin	Tuberculin tests
Epinephrine	
Terbutaline	
Certain vaccines	

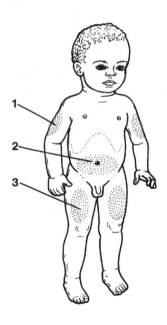

FIG. 45-1 Common sites for subcutaneous injections. *1,* Lateral aspect of upper arms; *2,* abdomen from costal margins to iliac crests; *3,* anterior thighs.

tion of an irritating antiseptic solution into the SC tissue. Insert the needle in a quick, dartlike motion at a 45- to 90-degree angle, depending on the patient's available SC tissue. Aspirate the plunger to rule out inadvertent vascular placement. If blood appears in the syringe, remove the entire setup, discard, and select a new site for injection. If there is no blood return with aspiration, inject the medication slowly. Finish the procedure by removing the needle and discarding the setup. Massaging of the injection site after completion of the procedure may enhance absorption and relieve pain.[4,7,12]

Place intradermal injections just below the epidermis into the dermis of the skin and cause a bleb to form (Fig. 45-2). After cleansing the injection site with an antiseptic swab, insert the needle at a 15-degree angle to the skin, with the bevel pointing upward. Inject the medication slowly and

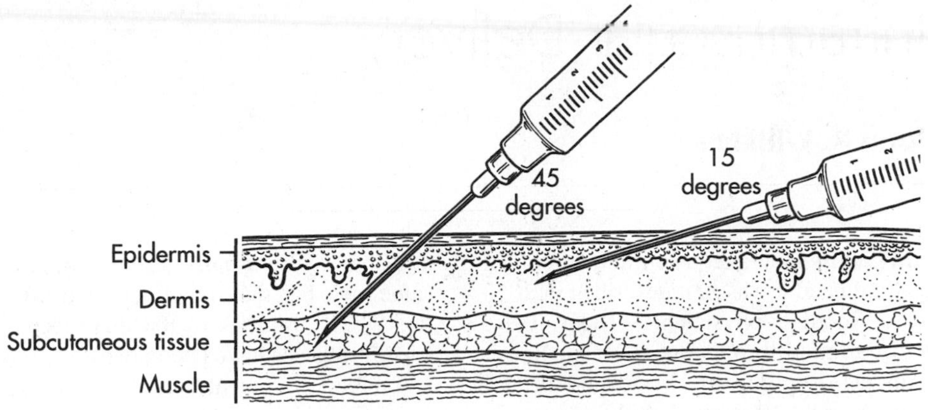

FIG. 45-2   Subcutaneous (left) and intradermal (right) injections in relation to the histology of the skin.

watch for bleb formation to occur, signifying a true ID injection. Finish the procedure by removing the needle and discarding the setup. The ID site should not be massaged after the injection because the injected medication may diffuse into the tissue or back through the needle site. Place tuberculin tests on the ventral surface of the forearm and allergy tests either on the back or upper chest.[4]

Remarks

Patients requiring routine SC medications must rotate their injection sites frequently to avoid complications.[7,8,12] Subcutaneous injections of heparin are usually given only in the abdomen and are not massaged after the injection because of the possibility of a bleeding complication.[4]

In the treatment of asthma, inhaled β_2-agonists have proven to be as effective as SC epinephrine and terbutaline. Because acrosol therapy is noninvasive and has fewer reported adverse effects, it is used before SC sympathomimetics, except in children who are totally unable to cooperate with inhalational therapy.[1,6,9-11]

Adequate restraint is always essential for the prevention of complications during parenteral injections in uncooperative children.

REFERENCES

1. Becker AB, Nelson NA, Simous FE: Inhaled salbutamol (albuterol) vs injected epinephrine in the treatment of acute asthma in children, *J Pediatr* 102:465-469, 1983.
2. Gilman AG, Rall TW, Niew AS, et al: *Goodman and Gilman's The pharmacologica I basis of therapeutics,* ed 8, Elmsford, NY, 1990, Pergamon Press, pp 5-10.
3. Howard-Jones N: The origins of hypodermic medication, *Sci Am* 224:96-102, 1971.
4. Kozier B, Erb G, Olivieri R: *Fundamentals of nursing, concepts, process, and practice,* ed 4, Redwood City, Calif, 1991, Addison Wesley, pp 1277-1279.
5. Newton DW, Newton M: Route, site, and technique: three key decisions in giving parenteral medication, *Nursing '79* 9:18-25, 1979.
6. Noseda A, Yernault JC: Sympathomimetics in acute severe asthma: inhaled or parenteral, nebulizer or spacer? *Eur Respir J* 2:377-381, 1989.
7. Perry AG, Potter PA: *Clinical nursing skills and techniques,* ed 2, St. Louis, 1990, Mosby, pp 495-498.
8. Pitel M: The subcutaneous injection, *Am J Nurs* 71:76-79, 1971.
9. Ruddy RM, Kolski G, Scarpa N, et al: Aerosolized metaproterenol compared to subcutaneous epinephrine in the emergency treatment of acute childhood asthma, *Pediatr Pulmonol* 2:230-236, 1986.
10. Spiteri MA, Millar AB, Pavia D, et al: Subcutaneous adrenaline versus terbutaline in the treatment of acute severe asthma, *Thorax* 43:19-23, 1988.
11. Uden DL, Goetz DR, Kohen DP, et al: Comparison of nebulized terbutaline and subcutaneous epinephrine in the treatment of acute asthma, *Ann Emerg Med* 14:229-232, 1985.
12. Wong D: *Whaley and Wong's Essentials of pediatric nursing,* ed 4, St. Louis, 1993, Mosby, p 680.

46 Intramuscular Delivery

John R. Williams

The intramuscular (IM) and subcutaneous administration of medication by syringe and needle was first described in 1853 by Alexander Wood, a Scottish physician.[13] Today, these procedures continue to be found throughout all of medicine. In pediatrics the use of IM drug delivery has experienced a marked increase during the past 10 years, largely because of favorable reports concerning the outpatient antibiotic treatment of febrile infants (age greater than 28 days), febrile children with sickle cell hemoglobinopathies, and children with serious infection.[1,19,20] Despite this recent upswing in frequency, many physicians are unaware of proper site and equipment selection, as well as possible pain and other complications resulting from IM drug administration.[16]

Indications

The parenteral delivery of medication by the IM route is advantageous when intravenous access has not been obtained either because of difficulty in placement or lack of ongoing need, to avoid the subcutaneous injection of a potentially irritating substance, or for the deposition of a long-acting substance such as benzathine penicillin G. Drug absorption from IM placement depends on the blood flow and the capillary surface area through the region of injection, as well as the solubility of the preparation. Aqueous solutions, are more rapidly absorbed than oily solutions or suspensions because of their greater solubility.[10]

Contraindications

Contraindications to IM drug delivery include (1) known allergy to the medication or the suspensory vehicle, (2) circulatory failure to the injection site, (3) patient coagulopathy, (4) recent repeated use of area for IM administration, and (5) dorsogluteal sites in children less than 3 years of age. A relative contraindication is that drug doses cannot be titrated with IM injections. If additional medication is likely to be needed, consider the intravenous route.

Complications

Reported incidence of complications from IM injections range from 0.4% in a hospitalized adult population to 9% in a questionnaire survey of pediatric nurses.[2,11] Complications that include nerve injury, muscular injury, and abscess formation have been reported.

The risk of nerve injury is determined primarily by the exact site of drug injection (intraneuronal injection or drug deposition into the tissue surrounding the neuron), the neurotoxic potential of drug, and the quantity of drug injected.[7] Nerve injury to the sciatic, radial, superior gluteal, inferior gluteal, posterior femoral cutaneous, pudendal, median, ulnar, and axillary nerves has been reported.* Muscular fibrosis

and contracture usually result from repeated injections in the same site, but they have occurred after only a single injection.[2,3,17,18] Injuries to the quadriceps, deltoid, gluteal, and triceps muscles have been noted.[3,17,18] Abscesses, both sterile and infectious, can also occur at the site of injection. Abscess formation is believed to take place secondary to drug injection subcutaneously or to injection of a large volume into a small muscle mass, causing ischemia and necrosis.[2,3,16]

Other complications in the literature include cellulitis, osteomyelitis, septic hip, transverse myelitis, gangrene, tissue necrosis, and local atrophy.[2-4,16,22-24] One way in which tissue necrosis can occur is vasospasm induced by injection directly into a blood vessel.

Equipment

The equipment needed for an IM injection includes an antiseptic swab, the medication, a syringe, and a needle. Determine syringe size based on the volume of medication to be given. Maximum volumes for single injection sites are 0.5 ml for premature and small infants, 1 ml for older infants and toddlers, 2 ml for school-age children, and 3 ml in adolescents and adults. The larger the volume to be injected, the larger the muscle mass needed.[16,24]

Needle size depends on the quantity and viscosity of medication and the patient's muscle mass and depth of subcutaneous tissue. The needle must be of sufficient length to pass through the subcutaneous tissue and deposit the medication intramuscularly. The needle length for infants, small children, and any child with decreased subcutaneous tissue and/or muscle mass is 1 inch. Needle selection for older children and adolescents depends on patient size and depth of overlying subcutaneous tissue. Use the smallest-diameter needle (largest-gauge) that still allows free flow of the injectate.[2,3,12,16,24]

Technique

To ensure IM delivery of medication, displace the overlying skin and subcutaneous tissue and then grasp the muscle between thumb and index finger to isolate and stabilize the muscle.[16,24] The antiseptic solution should be dry before needle insertion to prevent placement of an irritating substance subcutaneously. Perform needle insertion quickly, in a single, dartlike motion. Aspirate back on the plunger to check for inadvertent intraarterial or intravenous placement. If blood is aspirated, remove the needle, discard the syringe and medication, and prepare a new setup. Inject the medication slowly over 3 to 5 seconds to allow the muscle to accommodate to the volume of the injectate with less pressure and therefore less pain. Perform needle removal quickly and discard the setup.[14,15,24]

The *vastus lateralis* muscle is the preferred IM injection site for infants and small children and is acceptable for all ages (Fig. 46-1).[3,8,21,24] Advantages include no nearby major

---

*References 2, 3, 5, 6, 8, 9, 15, 16, and 21.

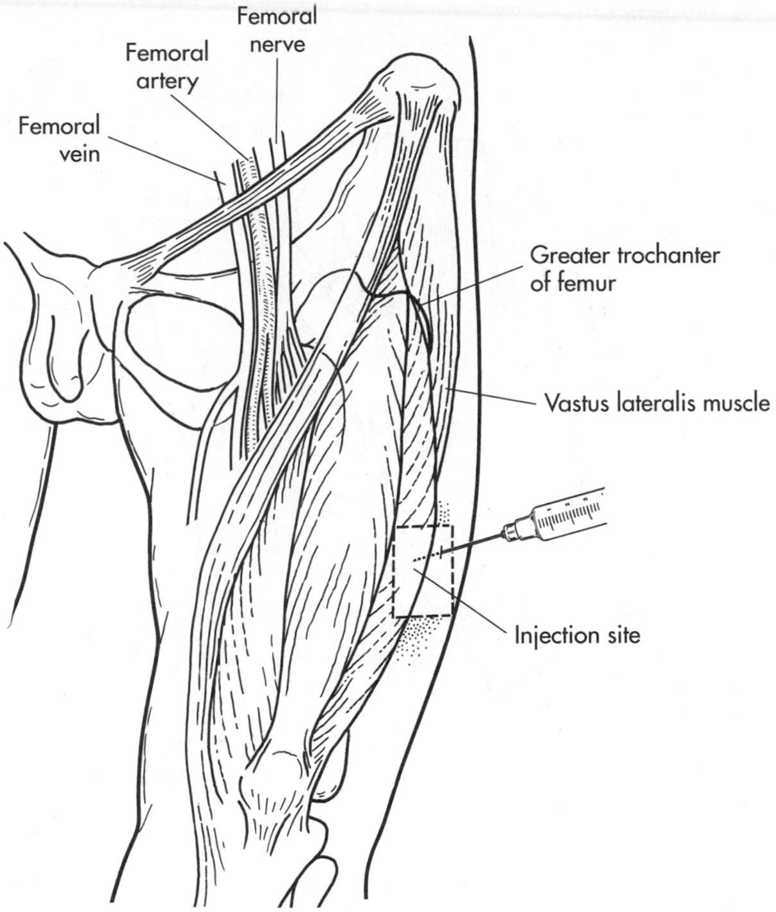

FIG. 46-1 Vastus lateralis injection site.

nerves or vascular structures and a large, easily accessible muscle. To locate the injection site, divide the distance between the greater trochanter of the femur and the knee into thirds. Select the middle third of the muscle belly along the anterior, lateral aspect of the thigh, and insert the needle inferiorly toward the knee at a 45-degree angle with the long axis of the leg.[3,14,16,24]

The *ventrogluteal* site involves the gluteus medius and the gluteus minimus muscles (Fig. 46-2). Advantages of this site include no nearby major vascular structures or nerves and less overlying subcutaneous tissue than seen with the dorsogluteal site. It can be used in all age groups. The injection site is located by placing the palm of the hand over the greater trochanter (right palm on left hip, left palm on right hip) and the index finger on the anterior superior iliac spine. Extend the middle finger posteriorly along the iliac crest, forming a triangle. Inject in the center of the triangle by inserting the needle almost perpendicular to the site with 10 to 15 degrees' angulation toward the iliac crest.[3,14,24]

The *dorsogluteal* site involves injections into the gluteus maximus muscle. Its usage has decreased because of the known risk of sciatic nerve damage and the variability in the depth of the overlying subcutaneous tissue between patients.* This site is contraindicated in children less than 3

years of age and in nonambulatory patients because the gluteal muscles only develop with locomotion.[3,14,16,24] If used, determine the injection site by drawing an imaginary line between the greater trochanter and the posterior superior iliac spine. Inject slightly lateral and superior to the midpoint of this line by inserting the needle at a 90-degree angle to the surface on which the patient is lying prone.[3,14,24]

The *deltoid* muscle is a frequent site for IM administration, but its small size and the potential for axillary and radial nerve injury limit its usefulness. The deltoid site can be used beginning in adolescence if injected volumes are limited to 1 ml. The injection site is 2 to 3 cm below the acromion process at the midpoint of the lateral aspect of the arm. Insert the needle almost perpendicular to the arm, with 10 to 15 degrees of angulation toward the acromion process. Be aware that the axillary nerve lies beneath the deltoid muscle and that the radial nerve has a superficial location, beginning at the proximal aspect of the middle third of the humerus.[2,3,16,24]

Remarks

Adequate restraint is always essential for the prevention of complications. When withdrawing medication from a glass ampule, use a filter to avoid drawing up glass particles.[24]

Tracking irritating substances through the subcutaneous tissue can be avoided by the Z-tract method. The Z-tract method consists of distracting the overlying skin and subcu-

---

*References 5, 6, 8, 9, 15, and 21.

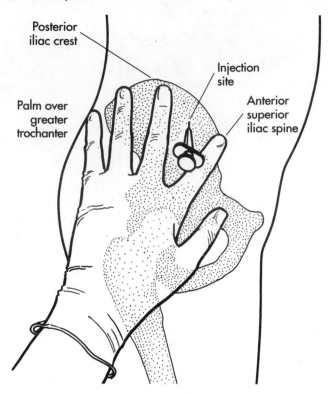

FIG. 46-2 Ventrogluteal injection site (see text for details).

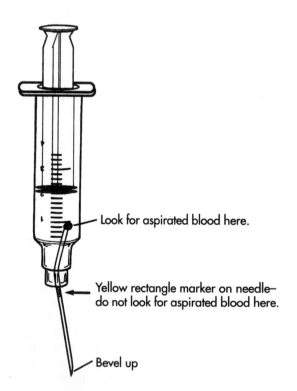

Look for aspirated blood here.

Yellow rectangle marker on needle—
do not look for aspirated blood here.

Bevel up

FIG. 46-3 Tubex cartridge for administration of IM benzathine penicillin.

taneous tissue to one side of the injection site. The retracted tissue is released on withdrawal of the needle, allowing the return to its normal position and preventing any leakage back into the subcutaneous tissue.[14,24]

Take special care when administering IM benzathine penicillin. Because of its viscosity, it is often difficult to see

aspirated blood at the hub of the syringe. Wyeth Laboratories has developed a TUBEX cartridge that allows aspirated blood from inadvertent intravascular placement to be seen more easily. At the base of the needle there is a yellow rectangle. The blood visualization area of the glass cartridge is found by drawing an imaginary line from this yellow rectangle to the shoulder of the cartridge. Any aspirated blood appears at this visualization area because the needle is bent inside the cartridge as shown in Fig. 46-3. If the injection is given with the needle bevel facing upward, the yellow rectangle should be visible.

REFERENCES

1. Baskin MN, O'Rourke EJ, Fleisher GR: Outpatient treatment of febrile infants 28-89 days of age with intramuscular administration of ceftriaxone, *J Pediatr* 120:22-27, 1992.
2. Beecroft PC, Redick S: Possible complications of intramuscular injections on the pediatric unit, *Pediatr Nurs* 15:333-336, 1989.
3. Bergeson PS, Singer SA, Kaplan AM: Intramuscular injections in children, *Pediatrics* 70:944-948, 1982.
4. Buchta RM: Atrophy after parenteral injection, *Am J Dis Child* 130:900, 1976.
5. Combes MA, Clark WK, Gregory CF, et al: Sciatic nerve injury in infants: recognition and prevention of impairment resulting from intragluteal injections, *JAMA* 173:1336-1339, 1960.
6. Curtis PH, Tucker HJ: Sciatic palsy in premature infants, *JAMA* 174:1586-1588, 1960.
7. Gentili F, Hudson AR, Hunter D: Clinical and experimental aspects of injection injuries of peripheral nerves, *Can J Neurol Sci* 7:143-151, 1980.
8. Gilles FH, French JH: Postinjection sciatic nerve palsies in infants and children, *J Pediatr* 58:195-204, 1961.
9. Gilles FH, Matson DD: Sciatic nerve injury following misplaced gluteal injection, *J Pediatr* 76:247-254, 1970.
10. Gilman AG, Rall TW, Nies AS, et al: *Goodman and Gilman's The*

pharmacological basis of therapeutics, ed 8, Elmsford, NY, 1990, Pergamon Press, pp 5-10.

11. Greenblatt DJ, Allen MD: Intramuscular-site complications, *JAMA* 240:542-544, 1978.

12. Hick JF, Charboneau JW, Brakke DM, et al: Optimum needle length for diphtheria-tetanus-pertussis inoculation of infants, *Pediatrics* 84:136-137, 1989.

13. Howard-Jones N: The origins of hypodermic medication, *Sci Am* 224:96-102, 1971.

14. Kozier B, Erb G, Olivieri R: *Fundamentals of nursing concepts, process and practice,* ed 4, Redwood City, Calif, 1991, Addison Wesley, pp 1279-1284.

15. Lachman E: Applied anatomy of intragluteal injections, *Am Surg* 29:236-241, 1963.

16. Losek JD, Gyuro J: Pediatric intramuscular injections: do you know the procedure and complications? *Pediatr Emerg Care* 8:79-81, 1992.

17. McCloskey JR, Chung SM: Quadriceps contracture as a result of multiple intramuscular injection, *Am J Dis Child* 131:416-417, 1977.

18. Norman MG, Temple AR, Murphy JV: Infantile quadriceps-femoris contracture resulting from intramuscular injections, *New Engl J Med* 282:964-966, 1970.

19. Powel KR, Mawhorter SD: Outpatient treatment of serious infections in infants and children with ceftriaxone, *J Pediatr* 110:898-901, 1987.

20. Rogers ZR, Morrison RA, Vedro DA, et al: Outpatient management of febrile illness in infants and young children with sickle cell anemia, *J Pediatr* 117:736-739, 1990.

21. Silber DL: Injection technique in infants, *JAMA* 249:1007, 1983.

22. Talbert JL, Haslam RH, Haller JA: Gangrene of the foot following intramuscular injection in the lateral thigh: a case report with recommendations for prevention, *J Pediatr* 70:110-114, 1967.

23. Weir MR, Fearnow RG: Transverse myelitis and penicillin, *Pediatrics* 71:988, 1983.

24. Wong D: *Whaley and Wong's Essentials of pediatric nursing,* ed 4, St. Louis, 1993, Mosby, pp 675-680.

47 Intracardiac Injections

Carol A. Ledwith

Intracardiac injection is a rare pediatric procedure. Current understanding of intracardiac injection is based exclusively on experience with adult patients.

Indications

Cardiac arrest (asystole, pulseless electrical activity, ventricular fibrillation, and pulseless ventricular tachycardia) is the only condition that warrants consideration of intracardiac administration of medications.[1-3,6,8]

Consider intracardiac administration of resuscitation medications in pediatric patients only if peripheral and central intravenous, endotracheal, and intraosseous routes are all inaccessible. Several authors[3,6,8] have recommended intracardiac injection as the route of choice for adult patients in cardiac arrest who do not have central venous access, but this is not recommended for pediatric patients. None of the authors[3,6,8] who advocate intracardiac injection in the absence of central venous access has presented data substantiating the theoretic advantage (i.e., injection of resuscitation medications closer to the site of action) of intracardiac injection over peripheral venous, endotracheal, or intraosseous routes. The Pediatric Advanced Life Support course does not include intracardiac injection in access recommendations.

Epinephrine is the only resuscitation medication with a history of extensive use by the intracardiac route,[1,3,6,8] although lidocaine, calcium, and sodium bicarbonate have all been administered by this route in adults.[1,6,8,9] Intracardiac administration of epinephrine offers no pharmacokinetic advantage over central venous administration.[9,10] The half-life of epinephrine has been reported to be about 2 minutes after an intravenous bolus.[4]

Contraindications

Intracardiac injection of resuscitation medications is a procedure of last resort. There are no absolute contraindications, except availability of another route.

Complications

The most important complication of intracardiac injection is that there must be interruption of cardiac compressions.[6,7,9,12] Other possible complications include inadvertent injection into the myocardium[9,12]; hemopericardium[2,6,9]; pericardial effusion[2,8]; cardiac tamponade[6,8]; pneumothorax[2,5,6,8,9]; coronary artery and ventricular laceration[4,6,8,9]; and injection into the left ventricle, aorta, or other surrounding structures.[11]

Equipment

Equipment includes a 22-gauge, 2.5-inch spinal needle attached to a syringe. As time is of the essence, do not attach an electrocardiogram lead to the needle. Aspiration of blood confirms entry into the ventricular lumen.

Technique

Two different techniques, the parasternal-intercostal (Fig. 47-1) and the subxiphoid (Fig. 47-2) approaches, have been successfully used in adults,[1,5,6] and both have been reported to have few serious complications in large series. Both techniques allow direct access to the right ventricle. Davison, Barresi, Parker, et al.[2] prospectively evaluated 53 patients who received 147 intracardiac injections, all but one of which were subxiphoid. No cardiac tamponade was observed, although 6 of 17 echocardiograms revealed pericardial effusion, and 8 of 28 autopsies revealed hemopericardium. No autopsies revealed coronary artery or ventricular lacerations. In the largest series available, from 1990, Jespersen, Granborg, Hanson, et al.[6] report 542 intracardiac injections given to 247 patients, all by the parasternal approach. Cardiac massage was not interrupted for more than 20 seconds, pneumothorax was reported in 11 of 80 patients, and hemopericardium was reported in 3. Coronary artery and myocardial injury were not found. Hao-Hui[5] reported fewer complications when the parasternal injection site was just to the left of the sternum.

The subxiphoid approach has been adopted as the standard in pediatrics, although neither approach has been evaluated in pediatric patients for efficacy or safety. Several authors[3,5,6,8] have recommended the parasternal as the preferable approach in adults.

For the subxiphoid approach, enter the skin just below the tip of the xiphoid, between the edge of the xiphoid and the xiphoid-costal angle. Point the needle at a 45-degree angle while aiming toward the left scapula and aspirate while advancing. For the parasternal approach, enter the skin

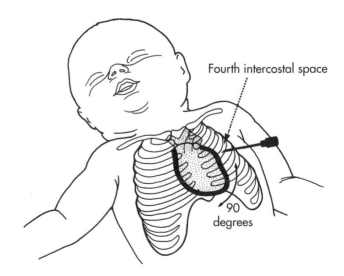

FIG. 47-1 Parasternal intracardiac injection. Enter the fourth intercostal space, over the fifth rib, within 1 cm of the sternal border, perpendicular to the skin.

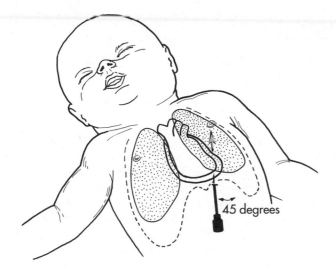

45 degrees

FIG. 47-2   Subxiphoid intracardiac injection. Enter the left costoxiphoid angle, aiming toward the left scapula, at a 45-degree angle to the skin.

perpendicularly in the fourth intercostal space, over the rib, just to the left of the sternal border. The injection site must be just next to (i.e., within 1 cm of) the sternal border. Inject when free flow of blood is obtained.

Remarks

Reserve consideration of intracardiac injection of resuscitation medications for the patient in cardiac arrest with no possible alternative access route.

REFERENCES

1. Amey BD, Harrison EE, Straub EJ, et al: Paramedic use of intracardiac medications in prehospital sudden cardiac death, *J Am College Emerg Phys* 7(4):130-134, 1978.
2. Davison R, Barresi V, Parker M, et al: Intracardiac injections during cardiopulmonary resuscitation: a low-risk procedure, *JAMA* 244 (10):1110-1111, 1980.
3. Eldor J: A new proposal of CPR based on coronary perfusion pressure, *Resuscitation* 23(1):71-76, 1992.
4. FitzGerald GA, Barnes P, Hamilton CA, et al: Circulating adrenaline and blood pressure: the metabolic effects and kinetics of infused adrenaline in man, *Eur Clin Invest* 10:401-406, 1980.
5. Hao-Hui C: Closed-chest intracardiac injection, *Resuscitation* 9(1):103-106, 1981.
6. Jespersen HF, Granborg J, Hanson U, et al: Feasibility of intracardiac injection of drugs during cardiac arrest, *Eur Heart J* 11:269-274, 1990.
7. Keszler H, Carroll GC: Intracardiac injections during resuscitation, *JAMA* 246(2):123, 1981.
8. Pedersen A, Jespersen H, Torp-Pedersen C: The place of intracardiac injections in the treatment of cardiac arrest, *Drugs* 42(6):915-918, 1991.
9. Pentel P, Benowitz N: Pharmacokinetic and pharmacodynamic considerations in drug therapy of cardiac emergencies, *Clin Pharmacokinetics* 9:273-308, 1984.
10. Redding JS, Asuncion JS, Pearson JW: Effective routes of drug administration during cardiac arrest, *Anesth Analg* 46:253-257, 1967.
11. Sabin HI, Khunti K, Coghill SB, et al: Accuracy of intracardiac injections determined by a post-mortem study, *Lancet* 2(8358):1054-1055, 1983.
12. Yakitis RW: Intracardiac injections during resuscitation, *JAMA* 246(2):123, 1981.

48 Rectal Drug Administration

Joan Bothner

Rectal drug administration has long been used as an alternative to oral drug therapy. It is safe and practical and is now a well-accepted route for delivering anticonvulsants, nonnarcotic and narcotic analgesics, antipyretics, antiemetics, and preanesthetic agents. An important advantage of rectal drug therapy is the partial avoidance of hepatic first-pass metabolism. The upper rectum is drained via the superior hemorrhoidal vein, which drains into the portal vein and subsequently into the liver. The lower rectum and anus are drained by the middle and inferior rectal veins, which empty into the inferior vena cava via the internal iliac vein and then into the systemic circulation (Fig 48-1). Placement of drugs too proximally into the rectum may lead to hepatic microsomal metabolism and decreased serum levels. This has been demonstrated with lidocaine and propranolol and has been hypothesized with diazepam. Other factors in determining peak serum levels include migration distance in the rectum and absorption rate. The migration of drugs in suppository bases is limited to the rectal area; spread of enemas is throughout the colon. By using solutions rather than suppositories, the processes of drug release and dissolution into rectal fluid are avoided, both of which are affected by length of time of exposure and presence of feces.[11]

Indications

The emergency management of seizures is a common indication for rectal drug administration because intravenous access is often difficult in the seizing pediatric patient. The agent studied most completely in this setting is diazepam. The intravenous solution is probably superior to suppository forms in rate of absorption and bioavailability. The serum concentration of diazepam necessary to stop seizure activity is not precisely known, although levels attained after rectal administration are in the range thought to be therapeutic. Efficacy of rectal diazepam is approximately 80% in stopping seizure activity. Time of onset is 5 to 10 minutes, and duration of action is estimated to be 30 minutes. Efficacy of rectal diazepam is increased if given during the first 15 minutes of seizure activity. Side effects are minimal, and respiratory depression is rare. Recommended dosing is 0.5 mg/kg.[2,7] Data on rectal administration of lorazepam are limited, but this agent appears effective at a dose of 0.05 mg/kg. Carbamazepine and phenobarbital are also well absorbed rectally, but delayed onset of action makes them unsuitable in status epilepticus. Rectal valproic acid syrup has been reported as efficacious in pediatric status epilepticus, but again data are limited.[11]

The pediatric patient can be easily sedated for a necessary procedure without intravenous access. Rectal midazolam is a safe, effective agent for sedation and anxiolysis, and has been best studied as a premedication for anesthesia induction. Absorption is rapid, and peak levels are reached within 15 to 30 minutes. Bioavailability has ranged from 18% to 52% after rectal administration. Elimination half-life is short, reducing the risk of prolonged sedative effect.[5,11] Rectal midazolam does not significantly affect heart rate, blood pressure, or oxygen saturation over a wide dosage range, but appropriate monitoring is necessary. Spear, Yaster, Berkowitz, et al.[8] found a dose of 1 mg/kg as a premedication for general anesthesia to be optimal. All children given this dose were awake and cooperative 90 minutes after administration. De Jong and Verburg[1] found that response of children to intravenous catheter placement was similar in children given 0.5 mg/kg midazolam rectally and those given 0.15 mg/kg intramuscularly. Paradoxic reactions to rectal midazolam have been demonstrated to increase with doses higher than 0.35 mg/kg.[6]

Ketamine given rectally is also well absorbed, is devoid of local irritant effect, and has unique sedative, amnesic, anesthetic, and analgesic properties. Van der Bijl, Roelofse, and Stander[10] compared rectally administered midazolam (0.3 mg/kg) to ketamine (5 mg/kg) as preanesthetic agents and found both to be effective.[10] Midazolam had marginal advantages as far as mask acceptance, anxiolysis, sedation, and adverse reactions. Rectal thiopental has been shown to be superior to intramuscular meperidine, promethazine, and chlorpromazine for pediatric sedation but had a 25% failure rate and needs further evaluation.[4] Rectal diazepam, as discussed above, is also useful for sedation. Morphine is well absorbed rectally, but there is considerable variability in onset and effect, and this drug has not been evaluated in the acute management of pain in the pediatric patient.

Rectal administration of perforated nifedipine capsules has been shown to be effective in the management of acute severe hypertension in eight of nine children, with onset within 10 minutes and duration of effect greater than 3 hours.[9] Nifedipine suppositories have been demonstrated to be effective in adults. Further work may lead to the rectal route becoming an alternative mode of administration, thereby increasing the applicability of this agent to young infants.

Rectal administration of antipyretics is indicated in patients with nausea or vomiting or who are otherwise unable to take oral medications. Acetaminophen is well absorbed rectally, although peak levels are attained more slowly than after oral administration.[3,12]

Table 48-1 lists drugs, doses, and time to onset of commonly used rectal agents.

Contraindications

Contraindications to rectal drug administration are limited. Avoid this route of therapy in the severely immunocompromised or neutropenic patient because of possible introduction of gut bacteria and resultant bacteremia. Patients with extremely rapid gut transit times or voluminous diarrhea may not absorb the drug.

Table 48-1   Nonvascular Access: Rectally Administered Drugs

Sedation		
Drug	**Dose**	**Onset**
Midazolam	0.5 mg/kg	15-30 minutes
Ketamine	5.0 mg/kg	20-30 minutes
Thiopental	25 mg/kg	15-30 minutes
Chloral hydrate	50 mg/kg	30-60 minutes
Anticonvulsants		
Diazepam	0.5 mg/kg	5-10 minutes
Lorazepam	0.05 mg/kg	20-30 minutes
Valproic acid	20-40 mg/kg	Slow: peak 1-4 hours, variable
Antipyretics		
Acetaminophen	15-20 mg/kg	30-45 minutes
Antihypertensives		
Nifedipine	0.2-0.5 mg/kg	10 minutes

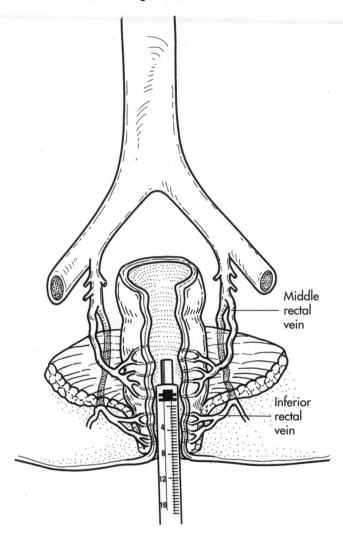

FIG. 48-1   Venous drainage of the middle and inferior rectum and syringe insertion.

Complications

Complications of rectal drug administration include rectal mucosal inflammation and rectal irritation, although this has not been addressed in most studies. Diazepam may cause local irritation. Rectal ulcers and stenosis have been linked to long-term use of suppositories containing aspirin, caffeine, and ergotamine.[11] Other possible complications include rectal trauma, bowel perforation, inappropriate placement, expulsion of the drug, and incomplete absorption because of the presence of feces in the rectal vault. Cardiopulmonary depression is rare, but monitor all patients on the basis of the drug delivered.

Equipment

Equipment varies with method of administration. Multiple authors have used lubricated 5 or 8 French feeding tubes or red rubber catheters attached to a plastic syringe. Bulb-syringe–type rectal tubes with blunt tips are also effective but not universally available. Intravenous catheters attached to syringes and lubricated, 1-ml tuberulin-type syringes are also effective. A cardiorespiratory monitor, pulse oximeter, and resuscitation equipment and drugs are required with drugs associated with cardiopulmonary depression. Sterile aqueous-soluble lubricating jelly has been used in most studies for facilitating insertion of the injection device. Its effect on drug absorption has not been evaluated.

Technique

There are two alternate techniques. In the first, lubricate a red rubber catheter or a 5 to 8 French feeding tube with a water-soluble lubricating jelly, and insert the tube 4 to 5 cm into the rectum. Attach a syringe containing the appropriate dose of the medication to be given, undiluted, and instill the medication. Follow instillation with injection of 1 cc of air to clear the tubing, and withdraw the tube.

An alternative technique uses a lubricated, 1-ml disposable tuberculin-type syringe. Draw the appropriate drug dose into the lubricated syringe. Insert the needleless syringe directly into the rectum to the end of the syringe, inject the medication, and remove the syringe. This technique instills the medication 4 to 5 cm into the rectum (Fig. 48-1), does not require flushing after instillation, and may be preferable because of ease and universal availability of disposable 1-ml plastic syringes.

Remarks

Accurate pediatric weights in emergency settings are often unavailable, and overestimation and resultant overdosing of these agents can have significant adverse effects. Consider a length-based method of weight and drug calculation. Taping the buttocks together after drug administration may decrease the incidence of drug leakage or expulsion. Older children may not like rectal drug administration.

REFERENCES

1. De Jong PC, Verburg MP: Comparison of rectal to intramuscular administration of midazolam and atropine for premedication of children, *Acta Anaesthesiol Scand* 32:485-489, 1988.
2. Dieckmann RA: Rectal diazepam for prehospital pediatric status epilepticus, *Ann Emerg Med* 23:216-224, 1994.
3. McEvoy GK, editor: *American Hospital Formulary Service Drug Information,* Bethesda, Md, 1994, American Society of Hospital Pharmacists.

4. O'Brien JF, Falk JL, Carey BE, et al: Rectal thiopental compared with intramuscular meperidine, promethazine and chlorpromazine for pediatric sedation, *Ann Emerg Med* 20:644-647, 1991.

5. Payne K, Mattheyse FJ, Liebenberg D, et al: The pharmacokinetics of midazolam in paediatric patients, *Eur J Clin Pharmacol* 37:267-272, 1989.

6. Roelofse JA, Stegmann DH, Hartshorne J, et al: Paradoxical reactions to rectal midazolam as premedication in children, *Int J Oral Maxillofacial Surg* 19:2-6, 1990.

7. Siegler RS: The administration of rectal diazepam for acute management of seizures, *J Emerg Med* 8:155-159, 1990.

8. Spear RM, Yaster M, Berkowitz ID, et al: Preinduction of anesthesia in children with rectally administered midazolam, *Anesthesiology* 74:670-674, 1991.

9. Uchiyama M, Sakai K: Rectal administration of perforated nifedipine capsules in acute severe hypertension in children, *BJCP* 46:100-101, 1992.

10. van der Bijl P, Roelofse JA, Stander IA: Rectal ketamine and midazolam for premedication in pediatric dentistry, *J Oral Maxillofacial Surg* 49:1050-1054, 1991.

11. van Hoogdalem EJ, de Boer AG, Breimer DD: Pharmacokinetics of rectal drug administration, Part I, *Clin Pharmacokinetics* 21:11-26, 1991.

12. van Hoogdalem EJ, de Boer AG, Breimer DD: Pharmacokinetics of rectal drug administration. Part II. Clinical applications of peripherally acting drugs, and conclusions, *Clin Pharmacokinetics* 21:110-128, 1991.

CARDIOPULMONARY RESUSCITATION

49 Epidemiology of Cardiac Arrest

Michael Tunik

Pediatric cardiopulmonary arrest (CPA) is rare, and outcome is dismal. The common causes are summarized in Box 49-1. Table 49-1 lists the major published pediatric CPA series. The most frequent etiologies in children are sudden infant death syndrome (SIDS), multiple trauma (motor vehicle–related, falls, child abuse), and respiratory failure. Other less frequent causes include hypovolemic and septic shock, burns, and infectious diseases. The causes of CPA in infants are SIDS, upper and lower airway obstruction, drowning, infectious disease (septic shock), trauma, and meningitis. In older children injuries predominate. There is an increasing frequency of penetrating trauma deaths from firearm injuries, especially among poor, inner city, adolescent males. The frequency of pediatric CPA vs. adult CPA is approximately 1:25.[1]

The survival rate of children suffering *respiratory arrest* alone is from 44% to 84%. Many of these children survive neurologically intact after simple measures of airway opening, ventilation, and oxygenation. However, when true *cardiac arrest* or CPA occurs outcome is extremely poor. The most common rhythm in pediatric CPA is asystole (70% to 90%).* Survival from pediatric asystole is rare, and most pediatric survivors suffer severe neurologic impairment. Ventricular tachycardia or fibrillation is a relatively

---

> **BOX 49-1 MAJOR CAUSES OF PEDIATRIC CARDIOPULMONARY ARREST**
>
> **Upper airway obstruction**
>
> Croup*
> Foreign body obstruction*
> Supraglottitis
> Angioedema
> Trauma (blunt and penetrating)
> Abscess, bacterial infection
>
> **Lower airway disease**
>
> Drowning*
> Inhalation injury*
> Asthma*
> Pneumonia*
> Bronchiolitis*
> Bronchopulmonary
>   dysplasia
> Chest trauma
> Foreign body obstruction
>
> **Neurologic**
>
> Head trauma*
> CNS infection*
> Botulism
>
> **Neurologic (cont'd)**
>
> Cervical spine trauma
> Increased intracervical
>   pressure
> Ventriculoperitoneal
>   shunt obstruction
>
> **Cardiovascular**
>
> Hypovolemic shock*
> Septic shock*
> Congenital heart defect
> Cardiogenic shock
> Dysrhythmias
> Myocarditis
> Pericardial effusion
> Status epilepticus
>
> **Other**
>
> Sudden infant death
>   syndrome*
> Burns*
> Intoxications

---

*References 3, 5-7, 10, 12, 15, and 16.

*Leading cause.

Table 49-1 Published Reviews of Pediatric Cardiopulmonary Arrest

Year	Author	Number of cases	Location	Arrest type	Initial ECG rhythm noted?	Outcome data (type of arrest and survival [%])
1982	Friesen, Duncan, Tweed, et al.[5]	66	E,H	C	Yes 34/66	C = 11%
1983	Eisenberg, Bergner, Hallstrom, et al.[3]	119	P	C	Yes 103/119	C = 7%
1983	Lewis, Minter, Eshelman, et al.[8]	105	E,H	R & C	No	R = 75% C = 18%
1984	Torphy, Minter, Thompson, et al.[15]	91	E	C	Yes	C = 5.4%
1984	Ludwig, Kettrick, and Parker[9]	130	E,H	R & C	No	?R & C = 55%
1984	Rosenberg[12]	26	E	C	Yes	C = 15%
1984	Wark and Overton[17]	41	H	C	No	C = 42%
1986	O'Rourke[11]	34	E	C	No	C = 21%
1986	Gillis, Dickson, Rieder, et al.[6]	42	H	R & C	Yes	R = 44% C = 9%

Continued.

Table 49-1 Published Reviews of Pediatric Cardiopulmonary Arrest—cont'd

Year	Author	Number of cases	Location	Arrest type	Initial ECG rhythm noted?	Outcome data (type of arrest and survival [%])
1986	Nichols, Kettrick, Swedlow, et al.[10]	47	E,H	C & ?R	Yes	R = 50% C = 10%
1987	Zaritsky, Nadkarni, Getson, et al.[16]	113	E,H	R & C	No	R = 67% C = 9%
1987	Fiser and Wrape[4]	41	E,H	R & C	No	R & C = 22%
1990	Thompson, Bonner, Lower, et al.[14]	95	E	R & C	No	R = 84% C = 4.3%
1991	Goetting and Paradis[7]	40	H	C	No	C = 40%
1995	Dieckmann and Vardis[2]	65	P	C	Yes	C = 3%

E, Emergency Department; *H,* hospital; *P,* prehospital; *C,* cardiac; *R,* respiratory.

infrequent cardiac rhythm in pediatric CPA (3% to 20%), and the overall survival rate of children is about 35%, significantly better than the survival rate with asystole, and may be associated with good neurologic outcome. Occurrence rates and outcome from pulseless electrical activity in children are unknown.

No national denominator of pediatric CPA is currently available. Current information is extracted from a limited number of published articles on pediatric CPA that vary greatly in study design, clinical setting, definitions of CPA, and outcome. A national core data set is imperative to standardize definitions of key variables such as age, sex, presenting rhythm, site of CPA, etiology, prehospital care, pharmacologic and other therapy, including intubation, defibrillation, and vascular access, as well as objective short- and long-term neurologic outcome.

REFERENCES

1. DeBard ML: Cardiopulmonary resuscitation: analysis of six years' experience and review of the literature, *Ann Emerg Med* 10:408-416, 1981.
2. Dieckmann RA, Vardis R: High-dose epinephrine in pediatric out-of-hospital cardiopulmonary arrest, *Pediatrics* 95:901-913, 1995.
3. Eisenberg M, Bergner L, Hallstrom A, et al: Epidemiology of cardiac arrest and resuscitation in children, *Ann Emerg Med* 12:672-674, 1983.
4. Fiser DH, Wrape V: Outcome of cardiopulmonary resuscitation in children, *Pediatr Emerg Care* 3:235-238, 1987.
5. Friesen RM, Duncan P, Tweed WA, et al: Appraisal of pediatric cardiopulmonary resuscitation, *Can Med Assoc J* 126:1055-1058, 1982.
6. Gillis J, Dickson D, Rieder M, et al: Results of inpatient pediatric resuscitation, *Crit Care Med* 469-471, 1986.
7. Goetting MG, Paradis NA: High-dose epinephrine improves outcome from pediatric cardiac arrest, *Ann Emerg Med* 20:22-26, 1991.
8. Lewis JK, Minter M, Eshelman SJ, et al: Outcome of pediatric resuscitation, *Ann Emerg Med* 12:297-299, 1983.
9. Ludwig S, Kettrick RG, Parker M: Pediatric cardiopulmonary resuscitation, *Clin Pediatr* 23:71-75, 1984.
10. Nichols DG, Kettrick RG, Swedlow DB, et al: Factors influencing outcome of cardiopulmonary resuscitation, *Pediatr Emerg Care* 2:1-5, 1986.
11. O'Rourke PP: Outcome of children who are apneic and pulseless in the emergency room, *Crit Care Med* 14:466-468, 1986.
12. Rosenberg NM: Pediatric cardiopulmonary arrest in the emergency department, *Am J Emerg Med* 2:497-499, 1984.
13. Seidel JS, Henderson DP, editors: *Emergency medical services for children: a report to the nation*, Washington, DC, 1991, National Center for Education in Maternal and Child Health.
14. Thompson JE, Bonner B, Lower G: Pediatric cardiopulmonary arrests in rural populations, *Pediatrics* 86:302-306, 1990.
15. Torphy DE, Minter MG, Thompson BM: Cardiorespiratory arrest and resuscitation in children, *Am J Dis Child* 138:1099-1102, 1984.
16. Zaritsky A, Nadkarni V, Getson P, et al: CPR in children, *Ann Emerg Med* 1107-1111, 1987.
17. Wark H, Overton JH: A pediatric "cardiac arrest" survey, *Br J Anaesth* 56:1271-1274, 1984.

50 Organization of the Resuscitation

Morton E. Salomon

The outcome of pediatric cardiopulmonary arrest (CPA) is usually poor, with mortality or severe morbidity in almost every patient.[9-11] Interventions must be prompt, and reperfusion must be achieved within 15 to 20 minutes for good neurologic outcome.[8]

Maintaining organization, leadership, and calm during a resuscitation effort (code) minimizes duplication of effort, incomplete performance of procedures, and disjointed management, but can be more difficult than the medical decision-making. A resuscitation that proceeds as a well-run team effort can optimize the care of the patient and may even improve outcome.[4]

THE RESUSCITATION TEAM

A team approach, with participants adhering to their team assignments, produces a more thorough and efficient code. Team work also reduces anxiety and bolsters self-confidence.[7]

Table 50-1 lists the members of an ideal resuscitation team. Having eight to ten people participate in the resuscitation is not always possible. On the other hand, in large teaching hospitals there can be too many responders, which adds to the chaos in the resuscitation room. Restrict the team to a maximum of ten responders.

Team Leader

The role of the team leader is outlined in Box 50-1. The team leader directs and coordinates all of the team's actions and must be the only person in charge. The leader's first task is to declare authority, as soon as possible, in a manner that leaves no doubt who is in charge. Only the team leader gives orders during the resuscitation. Other team members contribute to the resuscitation management by making suggestions to the leader.

Once the resuscitation team is assembled, the team leader assigns roles and designates someone to communicate with the patient's family and primary physician. The leader is responsible for overall patient assessment, but can delegate specific parameters. During the course of resuscitation, the leader ensures effective performance of both advanced life support (ALS) and basic life support (BLS). The leader decides when to interrupt chest compressions to check a pulse and must ensure that interruptions do not exceed 30 seconds.

The leader directs all patient management and reassesses effectiveness by reviewing ventilation, oxygenation, perfusion, and cardiac rhythm. The leader provides periodic updates and plans to the other team members. In this way team members can anticipate their duties and make contributions to the management.[4,7] The leader is also in charge of problem solving. If the resuscitation effort is not effective, the leader must review the steps already taken, determine

> **BOX 50-1 ROLE OF THE TEAM LEADER**
>
> Asserts leadership
> Assigns roles
> Directs patient assessment
> Oversees performance of basic life support (BLS)
> Limits duration of BLS interruptions
> Makes all management decisions
> Takes suggestions from team members
> Performs constant reassessment
> Oversees problem solving
> Communicates progress/plans to team members
> Ensures team safety
> Controls crowd
> Terminates cardiopulmonary resuscitation
> Oversees postresuscitation care
> Arranges patient admission or transfer
> Arranges debriefing session
> Reviews accuracy of chart documentation
> Speaks with family
> Fills out death certificate and notifies medical examiner

whether procedures were done correctly, and decide on new interventions.

The leader is also responsible for team safety, particularly when it comes to needlesticks and defibrillation. Another responsibility is crowd control. If the leader is unable to attend to this task, he or she must assign it to someone else. The leader must also ensure that other patients in the Emergency Department (ED) or on the hospital ward are not neglected during the resuscitation. Finally, the leader makes the decision to terminate resuscitation efforts, whenever it is clear that the situation is hopeless. It is advisable to seek agreement of the team before making this decision.[1,4,7]

If the resuscitation is unsuccessful, the leader must contact the medical examiner, when appropriate, and fill out the death certificate. If the patient survives, the leader must oversee the postresuscitation care and arrange for the patient's admission. No matter what the outcome, the leader should speak to the family at the end of the code and arrange for a team debriefing.

Clearly the leader has a broad range of responsibilities and must avoid becoming involved in any time-consuming procedures. Attempting procedures distracts from the leadership role. However, if the resuscitation team is small, she or he may need to perform procedures.

Airway

The principal concern of the airway team member is airway management, which is particularly critical to the child's

Table 50-1 Members of the Resuscitation Team

No. of Persons	Assignment	Desired professional training	Tasks
1	Team leader	Senior MD	See Box 50-1
1	Airway	MD/nurse anesthetist/ respiratory therapist/ paramedic	Ventilation/intubation/C-spine protection Monitors O_2Sat and ETCO$_2$
1	Chest compression	RN/EMT	Closed cardiac massage
2	Extremities	MD/RN/paramedic	Pulses, IV, IO, venous cutdown, ECG leads, blood samples, administers drugs
1	Crash cart	RN	Draws up and administers medications and IV solutions
1	Record keeper	RN	Documents interventions and patient responses, keeps dosing intervals
1	Circulator	RN	Brings additional equipment, takes VS, assists procedures
1	Family liaison	Chaplain/social worker/ psychiatric RN	Stays with family, contacts primary physician
1	Crowd control	RN/security officer	Keeps room clear of bystanders

RN, Registered nurse; *EMT,* emergency medical technician; *ETCO$_2$,* end tidal CO_2; *IV,* intravenous line; *IO,* intraosseus line; *ECG,* electrocardiograph; *VS,* vital signs.

outcome. Begin bag-mask (BVM) ventilation immediately and then perform intubation as quickly as possible. Once the endotracheal tube is secure, keep an experienced person at the patient's head to continue ventilation and oxygenation and monitor their effectiveness.

If trauma is involved, the intubator must carry out proper cervical spine management. A second team member provides jaw thrust and in-line immobilization while the intubator provides BVM ventilation and/or intubation.

Chest Compression

Chest compression is most effective when the job is rotated frequently, thereby preventing fatigue and monotony. If defibrillation or cardioversion is required, this is best performed by another team member such as the circulating nurse, thereby reducing the length of time cardiac message is interrupted.

Extremities

Assign two team members to the extremities because there are so many functions to perform and because access is so difficult to achieve in infants and young children. The extremity team members provide the team leader with assessment data, particularly pulse monitoring. As soon as patient assessment is complete, vascular access is attempted. If an intravenous (IV) site is not visible, one team member must insert an intraosseous (IO) line; a physician may consider a venous cutdown. These team members must also apply electrocardiogram leads, obtain arterial blood samples, and administer drugs as ordered by the team leader. If only one person is available for assignment to the extremities, the crash cart/medication coordinator can perform drug administration.

Crash/Medication Coordinator

In the hospital setting the keeper of the crash cart is usually a nurse. This team member dispenses equipment from the crash cart, draws up medications as ordered by the team leader, mixes IV solutions, and drips and administers IV or IO drugs if needed. He or she takes orders from the team

leader only. In pediatric resuscitations the medication/crash cart nurse must be familiar with pediatric dosing and able to confirm the accuracy of the doses being ordered.[7] Before handing over medication for administration, the medication nurse repeats the name of the drug and the dosage ordered. Once the drug is given, the team member administering it reports the name and dosage to the record keeper.

Record Keeper

The record keeper or recorder is usually, but not necessarily, another nurse. This member stands in a position to observe and hear everything. The recorder is the keeper of the code record and documents medications and all other interventions and the patient's response. The recorder also plays the key role of reminding the team leader of dosing intervals.

Circulator

The circulator (or helper) nurse is a multipurpose team member. Her or his principal role is to bring additional equipment to the resuscitation as needed. The circulator also takes vital signs and temperature and assists other team members with procedures. If necessary, the helper nurse can also assist with crowd control.

Family Liaison

Liaison with the family is often overlooked during a resuscitation effort. Ideally a staff member should stay with the family throughout the resuscitation. This job can be assigned to a chaplain, social worker, or a psychiatric nurse, if available. But a medical professional must obtain history from the family and provide periodic updates during the course of the resuscitation effort. This team member must also attempt to contact the patient's primary physician. If the patient dies, the family liaison person must stay with them to help with their grieving and to facilitate viewing of the body.

Crowd Control

In the out-of-hospital setting or a large urban hospital, crowd control can be critical to the efficient performance of cardiopulmonary resuscitation (CPR). Under circumstances in

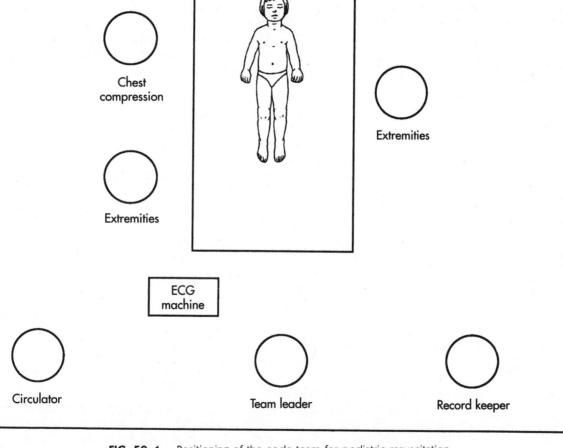

FIG. 50-1   Positioning of the code team for pediatric resuscitation.

which police or media accompany the patient to the hospital, a large number of family members turn up, or too many responders come to the code, assertive crowd control is imperative. In this situation, place a member of the hospital security staff at the door of the resuscitation room. This allows other team members to concentrate their efforts on the patient. Sometimes the family may stay with the child.

Positioning of the Code Team

Position code team members strategically around the patient in a manner that allows them to perform their functions efficiently. This depends in part on the physical layout of the resuscitation room. Fig. 50-1 suggests one possible arrangement of the team in a pediatric resuscitation. Unlike an adult code, during which the team leader can position himself or herself at the upper thorax, a pediatric resuscitation requires that the leader step away from the patient to allow other team members greater access to the small body. Accomplish this by having the leader stand at the foot of the stretcher with an umbrella view of all team members and the patient's monitor. The recorder must also have a good view of the entire work effort. Place the medication nurse and crash cart near the head of the patient so that airway and intubation equipment can be readily passed to the airway team member.[4]

PHASES OF RESUSCITATION

Seven sequential phases of resuscitation have been identified[4] and are listed in Box 50-2. Abbreviated versions are also applicable to out-of-hospital and inpatient resuscitations.

Anticipation Phase

The ED frequently has the luxury of being forewarned of an impending resuscitation by the emergency medical services (EMS) system emergency medical technicians (EMTs). Key consultants can be alerted, and the resuscitation team gathered. The leader must assert her leadership and assign roles to the other team members. As the members learn their assignments, they begin preparing their equipment, while the leader remains in contact with the EMTs treating the patient en route. Once all preparations are completed, the team members should position themselves around the stretcher as discussed above.[2,4]

Entry Phase

On arrival at the ED, EMTs should find an orderly and quiet resuscitation room that is fully equipped and has a stretcher ready to receive their patient. The first communication during patient entry comes from an EMT who reports the patient's history, most recent vital signs, response to care, and key clinical findings directly to the leader.

If CPA occurs in the in-hospital setting, there can be no anticipation phase, and the resuscitation effort starts with the discovery of the patient in CPA. The first person on the scene must call for help and then begin one-person CPR. The second person on the scene brings a crash cart and defibrillator to the bedside, places a backboard under the patient, and assists the first rescuer with CPR.[7] BLS continues until the code team is assembled and ALS can be undertaken.

Resuscitation Phase

The leader must conduct the code in a decisive and unflappable manner. The resuscitation room must be quiet, and only one voice heard giving orders. If an order is not understood, the team member must request clarification or repetition.

If the resuscitation is unsuccessful, the team leader should ask for suggestions before terminating the code. For emotional and ethical reasons, it is usually best not to terminate a code until all reasonable interventions have been tried and all team members agree that the situation is hopeless.[2,4]

Maintenance Phase

If effective spontaneous circulation is reestablished, the code enters the maintenance phase, during which the team stabilizes vital signs, secures access and airway, and anticipates

---

BOX 50-2 **PHASES OF RESUSCITATION**

1. Anticipation
2. Entry
3. Resuscitation
4. Maintenance
5. Family/physician notification
6. Transfer of patient
7. Critique

---

further problems. This is a very vulnerable period for the patient because the team's anxiety may dissipate, and attention wander. The leader must ensure adequate observation and interventions while releasing some team members for other duties.[4]

Family Notification

It is the responsibility of the leader to update the patient's family of the child's status. If another physician has been performing family liaison during resuscitation effort, communication responsibility might be better delegated to that physician. If the patient has been resuscitated successfully, the family should be informed of the child's condition, anticipated disposition, and possible prognosis. If the patient has died, this information should be articulated directly and clearly, without euphemisms. The physician then stays with the family, allowing them to express their grief. At the appropriate moment the physician should raise the issues of autopsy and organ donation with the family. Encourage the family to view and touch the body before it is sent to the morgue, but forewarn them about the tubes and catheters that will remain in place before autopsy. Finally, the resuscitation team must take responsibility for arranging follow up for the family, including communication of autopsy results.[4]

Transfer Phase

If the patient survives, responsibility for the care of that patient remains with the resuscitation team until another medical team—generally from the intensive care unit (ICU)—takes over. A complete record of resuscitation must accompany the patient to the ICU.[4]

Debriefing Phase

A debriefing is necessary after every resuscitation as soon as possible after the event. During the debriefing, review the pathophysiology of the arrest, the interventions that were made, and the reasoning behind the medical management. Discuss what was done right, as well as what was done poorly. Review reasons for terminating the code. Give team members an opportunity to express their observations and conclusions. In addition to reviewing the medical aspects of the code, the debriefing sessions should allow team members to express their emotions and grief.[2,4] In many death situations, a formal critical incident stress debriefing may be needed.

A video recorder mounted in a strategic location in the resuscitation room can provide an innovative and insightful adjunct to postresuscitation debriefing.[13] Video allows a more accurate and detailed view of the team's management than chart notes. The presence of the video camera also probably encourages better and more professional performance on the part of the resuscitation team. During the debriefing session, the resuscitation team sits down to review the video together; a senior staff member is usually present to lead the discussion. The video is especially effective in uncovering problems with the layout of equipment, positioning of the team, ineffective leadership, errors in BLS technique, and difficulties with crowd control. To avoid problems with litigation, the video can be protected from discovery by the hospital risk management or quality improvement sections of a state's health code.[13]

REFERENCES

1. American Heart Association: Subcommittee on Emergency Cardiac Care: *Advanced cardiac life support,* ed 2, Chapter 16: Putting it all together: resuscitation of the patient, 1987, American Heart Association.
2. American Heart Association: Emergency Cardiac Care Committee and Subcommittees: Guidelines for cardiopulmonary resuscitation and emergency cardiac care: recommendations of the 1992 National Conference, *JAMA* 268:2171-2302, 1992.
3. Baranowski AP, Mathias J, Harris M: Proposed reference chart in paediatric resuscitation, *BMJ* (letter) 297(6659):133-134, 1988.
4. Burkle FM, Rice MM: Code organization, *Am J Emerg Med* 5:235-239, 1987.
5. Dieckmann RA, Vardis R: High-dose epinephrine in pediatric out-of-hospital cardiopulmonary arrest, *Pediatrics* 95:901-913, 1995.
6. Sisenberg M, Bergner L, Hallstrom A, et al: Epidemiology of cardiac arrest and resuscitation in children, *Ann Emerg Med* 12:672-674, 1983.
7. Ellstrom K, Della Bella L: Understanding your role during a code, *Nursing* 90:37-42, May 1990.
8. Hanashiro PK, Wilson JR: Cardiopulmonary resuscitation: a current perspective, *Med Clin North Am* 70(4):729-747, July 1986.
9. Lewis JK, Minter MG, Eshelman SJ, et al: Outcome of pediatric resuscitation, *Ann Emerg Med* 12:297-299, 1983.
10. Lewis JM: Pediatric arrest card, *Ann Emerg Med* 14 (letter):372-373, 1985.
11. Ludwig S, Kettrick RG, Parker M: Pediatric cardiopulmonary resuscitation: a review of 130 cases, *Clin Pediatr* 23:71-75, 1984.
12. Zaritsky A, Nadkarni V, Getson P, et al: CPR in children, *Ann Emerg Med* 1107-1111, 1987.
13. Weston CFM, Richmond P, McCabe MJ, et al: Video recording of cardiac arrest management: an aid to training and audit, *Resuscitation* 24:13-15, 1992.

51 Selection of Drugs and Equipment

Robert Luten and George Foltin

Historically cards, charts, and computer printouts have been recommended to help selection of drugs and equipment, based on the child's age or weight. Formulas have also been suggested to aid in selection of equipment.[1,2] However, some of the formulas not only have been shown to be marginal in accuracy,[8] but require a specific age or weight for calculation. Estimation of weight, by even experienced clinicians, is usually inaccurate.[8]

A recent concept for dosing and sizing derives from a patient's length, which can be easily measured in urgent situations.[3,5,7,8] Length not only is directly related to a patient's weight, but also has been shown to be an accurate predictor of certain equipment sizes, more accurate than patient age/weight-based charts, commonly used formulas,[6,8] or other anthropomorphic parameters used to determine equipment sizes.

Table 51-1 gives length measurements that correspond to frequently used pediatric equipment. After a single length measurement in an emergency one can then use this chart to select accurate-sized equipment. Table 51-2 compares different methods of achieving accurate drug doses and equipment sizes.

Two commercial products use length for drug dose determination. The *First Five Minutes* tape uses a length measure-

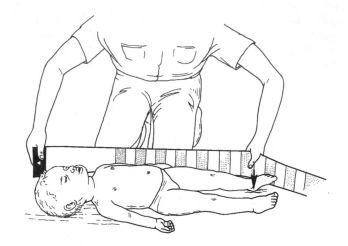

FIG. 51-1 Color-coded Broselow tape used to assess pediatric drug doses and equipment.

ment combined with a body habitus determination and provides a reference book with doses based on weight.[3] Drug doses and equipment can be also assessed directly and read from a tape using the color-coded Broselow tape[4,7] (Fig. 51-1).

Table 51-1 Length-Based Equipment Chart*

Item	Length (cm)						
	58-70	70-85	85-95	95-107	107-124	124-138	138-155
ET Tube size (mm)	3.5	4.0	4.5	5.0	5.5	6.0	6.5
Lip-tip length (mm)	10.5	12.0	13.5	15.0	16.5	18.0	19.5
Laryngoscope	1 Straight	1 Straight	2 Straight or curved	2 Straight or curved	2 Straight or curved	2-3 Straight or curved	3 Straight or curved
Suction catheter	8 F	8-10 F	10 F	10 F	10 F	10 F	12 F
Stylet	6 F	6 F	6 F	6 F	14 F	14 F	14 F
Oral airway	Infant/small child	Small child	Child	Child	Child/small adult	Child/small adult	Medium adult
Bag-valve mask	Infant	Child	Child	Child	Child	Child/adult	Adult
O$_2$ mask	Newborn	Pediatric	Pediatric	Pediatric	Adult	Adult	Adult
Vascular access catheter/butterfly	22-24/23-25, intraosseous	20-22/23-25, intraosseous	18-22/21-23, intraosseous	18-22/21-23, intraosseous	18-20/21-23	18-20/21-22	16-20/18-21
Nasogastric tube	5-8 F	8-10 F	10 F	10-12 F	12-14 F	14-18 F	18 F
Urinary catheter	5-8 F	8-10 F	10 F	10-12 F	10-12 F	12 F	12 F
Chest tube	12-12 F	16-20 F	20-24 F	20-24 F	24-32 F	28-32 F	32-40 F
Blood pressure cuff	Newborn, infant	Infant, child	Child	Child	Child	Child/adult	Adult

Adapted from Luten RC, Wears RL, Broselow J, et al: Length-based endotracheal tube sizing for pediatric resuscitation, *Ann Emerg Med* 21:900-904, 1992.
*Directions for use: 1. Measure patient length with centimeter tape. 2. Using measured length in centimeters, assess appropriate equipment and drug dose column. 3. Read sizes and doses off tape.

Table 51-2 Comparison of Various Drug/Equipment Aids

| | Steps | Accuracy | | Comments |
		Drug dosage	Equipment selections	
Weight/age-based methods				

Memory	3	Poor, inconsistent	Poor, inconsistent	Three steps:
				1. Recollection of dose
				2. Weight estimation
				3. Calculation
				   Associated with
				   anxiety and error

Dosage/equipment/cards	2	Vary according to accuracy of weight estimation Decimal error 1/10 or 10 × dose	Only as accurate as formulas, which may be unreliable since weight and age are unknown and must be estimated	Associated with moderate anxiety and error
Precalculated, equipment cards or computer printouts	1	Vary according to accuracy of weight estimation	Only as accurate as formulas, which may be unreliable since weight and age are unknown and must be estimated	Associated with mild to moderate anxiety and error
Length-based methods				
Length-based equipment chart	2	N/A	Minimal anxiety and error	Two steps: 1. Measure 2. Access chart
First 5 minutes	2 +	High accuracy	Moderate accuracy	Three steps: 1. Measurement 2. Determination of habitus 3. Reference to a book
Broselow tape	1	High accuracy		Minimal anxiety and error Measure and read directly from tape

All weight based methods depend on an accurate body weight estimation. Formulas for predicting equipment sizes also depend on weight or age estimation. Even with accurate age or weight the formulas are less accurate than length. Length provides the most accurate, least anxiety-producing, and most rapid method of determining drug dosages and equipment sizes.

REFERENCES

1. Chameides L: *Textbook of pediatric advanced life support,* American Heart Association, 1988.
2. Fleisher GR, Ludwig S: *Textbook of pediatric emergency medicine,* ed 3, Baltimore, 1993, Williams & Wilkens.
3. Garland JS, Kishaba RG, Nelson DB, et al: A rapid and accurate method of estimating body weight, *Am J Emerg Med* 4(5):390-393, 1986.
4. Hinkle AJ: A rapid and reliable method for selecting endotracheal tube size in children, *Anesth Analg,* 1988 (abstract).
5. Hughes G, Spoudeas H, Kovar IZ et al: Tape measure to aid prescription in pediatric resuscitation, *Arch Emerg Med* 7:21-27, 1990.
6. Keep, PJ, Manford ML: Endotracheal tube sizes for children, *Anesthesia* 29:181, 1974.
7. Lubitz DS, et al: A rapid method for estimating weight and resuscitation drug dosages from length in the pediatric age group, *Ann Emerg Med* 17:576, 1988.
8. Luten RC, Wears RL, Broselow J, et al: Length-based endotracheal tube sizing for pediatric resuscitation, *Ann Emerg Med* 21:900-904, 1992.

George Foltin

CIRCULATORY SUPPORT
Assessing Pulselessness

During cardiopulmonary resuscitation (CPR), once an airway is secured and oxygenation and ventilations are established (see Parts IV, V, and VI), assess the need for cardiac compression. For the infant less than 1 year of age palpate the pulse at either the brachial or the femoral location (Figs. 52-1 and 52-2). For the infant and child older than 1 year of age check the carotid pulse (Fig. 52-3).

Checking for precordial activity can be misleading. A child can have adequate pulses but undetectable precordial impulses. The American Heart Association (AHA) 1992 guidelines for lay rescuers suggest not even checking for pulse in a child without respirations but rather assuming that such a child is pulseless and requires compressions.[8]

Chest Compressions

Chest compressions consist of regular, timed pressure applied to the chest wall that result in core circulation of blood to vital organs for a short period until spontaneous circulation can be restored. Controversy exists over the exact mechanism by which chest compressions result in blood flow. One theory is that direct compression of the ventricles results in blood flow through the lungs and body.[4] The other theory holds that pressure differences created between the thorax and extrathoracic circulatory system cause movement of blood.[6]

Perform compressions on a hard surface for optimal performance. Assure compression and relaxation phases are of equal duration. The chest must be allowed to return completely to the original position, but keep a hand on the patient. Table 52-1 provides the appropriate depth and rates of compressions for the different age groups. Techniques of chest compression vary by age in the pediatric population.

Techniques

For the newborn and the small infant deliver chest compressions to the lower third of the sternum by the following methods:

1. Wrap both hands around the chest with thumbs next to each other on the anterior chest wall and the fingers intertwined in the back to serve as a hard surface. Place the thumbs over the lower third of the sternum, one finger breadth below the intermammary line. The position lifts the infant's shoulders with the head tilted back slightly into a neutral position that allows patency of the airway (Fig. 52-4).

2. For one-handed compression identify the appropriate landmark for compression by placing the index, middle, and ring fingers on the chest with the index finger at the intermammary line. Lift the index finger off the chest and perform compressions with the middle and ring fingers to compress

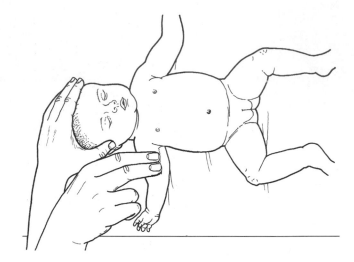

FIG. 52-1 Palpating brachial pulse in infant.

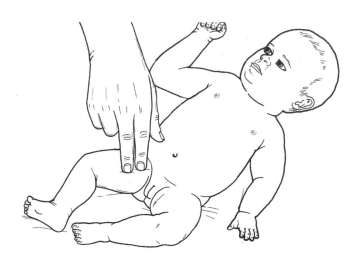

FIG. 52-2 Palpating femoral artery in infant.

the lower third of the baby's sternum. The other hand can be positioned behind the baby's back to provide a hard surface and to lift the baby's shoulders. Tilt the head back slightly, to provide a position for a patent airway; or grasp the forehead, placing the patient in an optimal position to establish an airway (Figs. 52-5 and 52-6).

3. When carrying the baby and performing CPR, the forearm provides a hard surface that allows effective compressions. The hand, open palm up, supports the neck and head. Keep the head and body at the same level even when lifting the child to provide ventilation (Fig. 52-7). Many out-of-hospital providers transport patients on a rigid backboard when providing ventilation and compression rather than using this technique.

Table 52-1   Basic Life Support in Children

Age	Breathing rate	Compression rate/min	Depth	Hand placement for compression
Less than 1 year	20/min	100-120	0.5-1 inch	Two or three fingers at midsternum, one finger below nipple line, or two thumbs at midsternum with hands encircling chest
1-7 years	15/min	80-100	1-1.5 inches	Three fingers or heel of one hand, two fingers above xiphoid
Over 7 years	12/min	80-100	1.5-2 inches	Heel of both hands with body pressure, two fingers above xiphoid

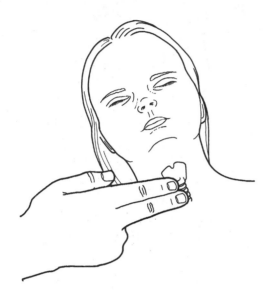

FIG. 52-3   Checking carotid pulse in child older than 1 year of age.

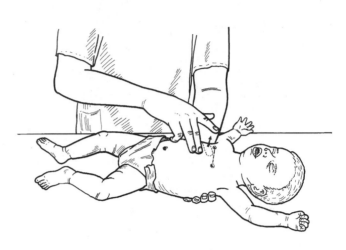

FIG. 52-5   Closed chest massage, sternum–two-finger, one-handed. One hand is placed behind baby's back while closed chest massage is performed with the other hand.

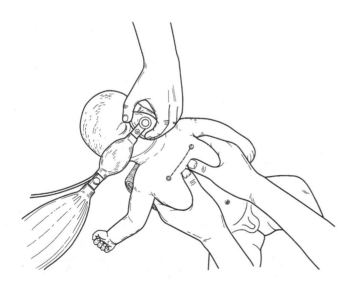

FIG. 52-4   Closed chest massage, two-handed.

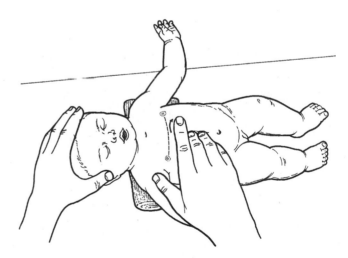

FIG. 52-6   Closed chest massage, sternum–two-finger. One-hand grasps forehead while closed chest massage is performed with the other hand.

4. To obtain the proper hand position for effective compressions in the child, trace the lower margin of the victim's rib cage, using the hand nearer the feet, to the midline. Place the middle finger on the lower sternal notch, the index finger next to the middle finger, and then the heel of the hand next to the index finger. Lift the fingers off the victim while performing CPR (Fig. 52-8).

For all of the techniques described for chest compression, allot 1 to 1.5 seconds every five compressions to interpose ventilation (see Chapter 24). After the first minute of CPR check for a pulse and then do so every 5 minutes.

Other models for compression during CPR include the use of interposed abdominal compressions,[5] high-frequency (rapid manual) CPR, and open chest compressions,[2] although none of these techniques has proved beneficial to survival in pediatric cardiopulmonary arrest (CPA).

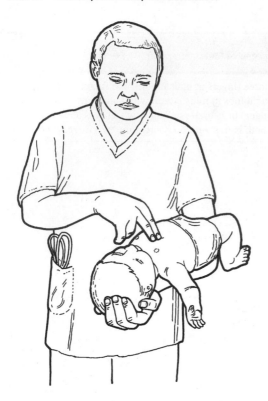

FIG. 52-7 Closed chest massage is performed while holding infant on forearm.

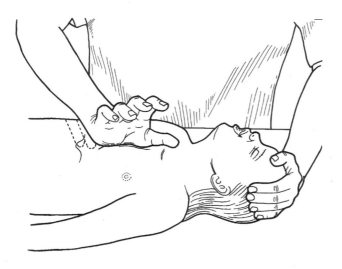

FIG. 52-8 Proper hand position for performance of closed chest massage.

PEDIATRIC DEFIBRILLATION/CARDIOVERSION

Defibrillation (an asynchronous depolarization of the myocardium) is intended to convert ventricular fibrillation or pulseless ventricular tachycardia to sinus rhythm (also see Chapter 57 for indications for cardioversion). Open the airway and perform assisted bag-mask ventilation with 100% oxygen and cardiac compressions during preparation for defibrillation.

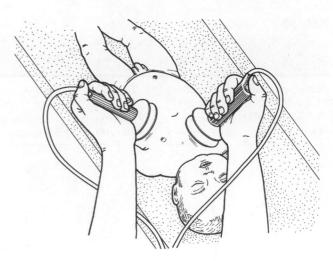

FIG. 52-9 Paddle placement for pediatric defibrillation. One 24 cm² paddle is placed on right upper chest, and the second on left chest over apex of heart lateral to left nipple.

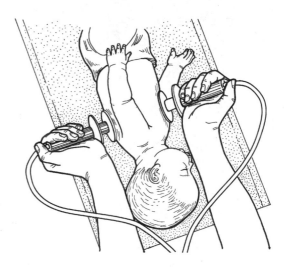

FIG. 52-10 Alternate approach to paddle placement for pediatric defibrillation. One 80 cm² paddle is placed over left anterior chest wall, and the second over left posterior chest wall.

Paddle Size

Defibrillation/cardioversion paddles are available in two sizes, 8 × 10 cm, or 80 cm² (for adults and children greater than 10 kg or 1 year of age) and smaller pediatric paddles 4 × 6 cm, or 24 cm² (for infants less than 1 year of age or less than 10 kg). The larger surface area contact possible with the 8- to 10-cm paddles decreases impedance and maximizes current flow.[1] The paddle must be in complete contact with the chest wall, and the two electrode paddles and electrical contact media must be separated to prevent electrical bridging. Use the largest paddle size that achieves full contact with the chest wall.

Contact Media

Use electrically conductive media (salt-containing electrode paste or cream) to maximize current flow and minimize resistance. Never use paddles without an electrically conductive media, and do not use alcohol pads.[1,7]

Paddle Position

Apply one 24-cm[2] paddle to the right upper chest, and the second to the left chest over the apex of the heart lateral to the left nipple (Fig. 52-9). Apply firm pressure to ensure uniform contact of the entire paddle surface to the chest wall. If pediatric paddles are not available, an alternate approach for small infants is 8 × 10 cm or 80 cm[2] paddles: one applied over the left anterior chest wall and the second over the left posterior chest wall. Roll the infant onto the right side, if possible, for this paddle placement[3] (Fig. 52-10).

REFERENCES

1. Atkins DL, Sirna S, Kieso R, et al: Pediatric defibrillation: importance of paddle size in determining transthoracic impedance, *Pediatrics* 82:914-918, 1988.
2. Fleisher, Sagy M, Swedlow DB et al: Open verses closed-chest cardiac compression in a canine model of pediatric cardiopulmonary resuscitation, *Am J Emerg Med* 3:305-310, 1985.
3. Kerber RE, Jensen SR, Grayzel J, et al: Elective cardioversion: influence of influence of paddle electrode location and size on success rates and energy requirements, *N Engl J Med* 305:658-662, 1981.
4. Kouwenhoven WB, Jude JR, Knickerbocker, CG: Closed-chest cardiac massage, *JAMA* 73:1064-1067, 1960.
5. Mateer JR, Stuevan HA, Thompson BM et al: Prehospital IAC-CPR verses standard CPR, *Am J Emerg Med* 3:143-146, 1985.
6. Rudikoff MT, Maughan WL, Effron M, et al: Mechanism of blood flow during cardiopulmonary resuscitation, *Circulation* 61:258-265, 1980.
7. Sirna SJ, Ferguson DW, Charbonnier F et al: Factors affecting transthoracic impedance during electrical cardioversion, *Am J Cardiol* 62:1048-1052, 1988.
8. Dieckmann RA, Vardis R: High-dose epinephrine in pediatric out-of-hospital cardiopulmonary arrest, *Pediatrics* 95:901-913, 1995.

53 Medications

Mariann Manno

Pediatric cardiopulmonary resuscitation (CPR) is a series of interventions aimed at restoring and supporting vital functions. Since pediatric cardiopulmonary arrest (CPA) is most often related to hypoxia-ischemia, first manage the airway and breathing. After the airway is secured, ventilation is adequate, and effective chest compressions have commenced, begin fluids and medications.

There are few effective medications in pediatric resuscitation. Asystole is the rhythm present in the overwhelming majority of pediatric arrests and reflects profound hypoxia-ischemia. Primary resuscitation medications are oxygen and epinephrine. Atropine, bicarbonate, calcium, and glucose have limited roles and have unproven benefit.

Less frequently used medications include antiarrhythmic drugs (lidocaine, bretylium), catecholamines to support blood pressure after reperfusion (e.g., dopamine, dobutamine, and epinephrine), and calcium to treat specific electrolyte abnormalities (e.g., hyperkalemia).

Epinephrine

Epinephrine is the premier drug in pediatric cardiac arrest and acts primarily through alpha-adrenergic stimulation. The primary alpha effects are aortic vasoconstriction, increased aortic diastolic blood pressure, and increased coronary perfusion. Although previous authors have suggested a beneficial epinephrine effect on inotropy and chronotrophy through beta-adrenergic stimulation, these effects are unproven.

The indications for epinephrine in CPA are asystole and pulseless electrical activity (PEA). Epinephrine is also indicated to convert fine ventricular fibrillation to a coarser pattern for easier electrical defibrillation, but epinephrine follows defibrillation in the initial resuscitation sequence for ventricular fibrillation.

The optimal dose of epinephrine in pediatric CPA remains unknown. Work done by Redding and Pearson (1963) suggested that a dose of 1 mg was effective for the return of spontaneous circulation in 10-kg dogs. This was adopted as the standard dose for humans and the traditional pediatric dose of 0.01 mg/kg was extrapolated from the 1-mg/kg adult dose. Several studies have evaluated use of standard (SDE) and high-dose epinephrine (HDE). Two studies compared rates of return of spontaneous circulation, successful resuscitation, and discharge from the hospital in adults who were randomized to receive either SDE or HDE. No improvement in outcome from HDE was found in either study group.[6]

One pediatric study compared patients who received 2 standard doses (0.01 mg/kg) of epinephrine followed by high-dose epinephrine (0.2 mg/kg) with a historical control group who received only standard-dose epinephrine. The HDE group had a higher rate of return of spontaneous circulation and better outcome than the group of historic controls.[3,4] However a 4-year study by Dieckmann in San Francisco reviewed 65 pediatric medical CPA patients and found no difference in outcome between SDE and HDE groups.[2] In light of the controversy the American Heart Association (1992) revised guidelines for pediatric advanced life support and currently recommends 0.01 mg/kg (1:10,000) for the initial dose of epinephrine in all forms of CPA. Second and subsequent doses should be at least 0 to 0.1 mg/kg (1:1000) and may be as high as 0.2 mg/kg (1:1000) administered at 3- to 5-minute intervals. If repeated doses are required, use a continuous infusion of 20 µg/kg/min.[5]

Epinephrine may be administered by the intravenous (IV), intraosseous (IO), and endotracheal (ET) routes. The recommended initial ET dose is 0.1 mg/kg (1:1000 solution, diluted), or 10 times the initial IV dose.

Sodium Bicarbonate

The indications for sodium bicarbonate are unclear. A documented severe metabolic acidosis or presumed acidosis after prolonged arrest may be a relative indication if the child is well ventilated. Hyperkalemia is an absolute indication. When given for metabolic acidosis bicarbonate combines with the hydrogen ion to produce water and carbon dioxide. In an underventilated patient worsening acidosis may develop if the patient is unable to eliminate excess carbon dioxide. Rapid elevation in serum carbon dioxide tension worsens intracellular acidosis, which in turn may depress myocardial function. Other complications of bicarbonate include hypernatremia and hyperosmolar states, especially in the very young infant. The recommended dose of bicarbonate is 1 mEq/kg by the IV or IO route. Bicarbonate is irritating to the airways and destroys lung surfactant and should never be administered by ET. In infants less than 6 months of age administer 0.5 mEq/kg/dose to reduce the osmotic load of the drug. Since bicarbonate precipitates with calcium in intravenous lines and inactivates catecholamines, give only by direct intravenous administration and flush the IV line before administering other drugs.

Atropine

Atropine is a parasympatholytic agent that has both peripheral and central effects, but its actions in cardiac standstill are not established. Atropine acts peripherally as a vagolytic agent accelerating the sinus and atrial pacemakers and increasing atrioventricular (AV) conduction. At low doses atropine acts centrally to stimulate the vagal medullary nucleus, causing bradycardia. Atropine is indicated for symptomatic bradycardia and bradycardia with AV block. Like epinephrine it can be administered by the IV, IO, and ET routes. Recommended doses are 0.02 mg/kg IV, IO, or ET, which can be repeated every 5 to 10 minutes. The minimum recommended dose of atropine to prevent paradoxic bradycardia is 0.1 mg. The maximum total dose is 1 mg in a child and 2 mg in an adolescent.

Table 53-1   Resuscitation Medications in Children

Drug	Dose	Route	Indications	Comments
Epinephrine (1:10000=0.1 mg/ml) (1:1000 = 1.0 mg/ml)	SDE: 0.01 mg/kg HDE: 0.1 to 0.2 mg/kg ETT: 0.1 mg/kg	IV IO ETT	Asystole PEA V Fib, pulseless V tach before defibrillation	Decreased effect if acidosis severe Dilute with saline for ET administration to 5-10 ml (infants) and 10-20 ml (children)
Atropine (0.1 mg/ml)	0.02 mg/kg Minimum: 0.1 mg Maximum: 2 mg	IV IO ETT	Symptomatic bradycardia Heart block	Evaluate hypoxia as cause of bradycardia
Sodium bicarbonate (8.4% = 1 mEq/ml) (4.2% = 0.5 mEq/ml)	1-2 mEq/kg 0.5 mEq/kg (neonates)	IV IO	Metabolic acidosis Prolonged arrest Hyperkalemia	Precipitates with Ca Inactivates catechols Monitor ventilation
Glucose (1 g/kg = 4 ml D25)	1 g/kg: 4 ml/kg D25	IV IO	Symptomatic (coma, seizures) hypoglycemia	
Lidocaine (1% = 10 mg/ml) (2% = 20 mg/ml)	1 mg/kg	IV IO ETT	Ventricular arrhythmias	Dilute with water for ETT administration to 5-10 ml (infants) or 10-20 ml (children)
Adenosine (3 mg/ml)	0.1 mg/kg	IV	Supraventricular tachycardia	*Rapid* IV push then *rapid* IV flush
Bretylium (50 mg/ml)	5 mg/kg initially 10 mg/kg afterwards; maximum: 30 mg/kg	IV IO	Ventricular arrhythmias May cause hypotension	Use with caution with digitalis
Calcium chloride (10% = 100 mg/ml)	20 mg/kg or 2 ml/kg	IV IO	Hyperkalemia Hypermagnesemia Hypocalcemia Ca channel blocker overdose	Not indicated for PEA or asystole
Dopamine (200 mg/5 ml)	Low: 2-5 µg/kg/min Mod: 5-20 µg/kg/min High: >20 µg/kg/min	IV IO	Poor renal perfusion Shock	Need adequate volume resuscitation Titrate for effect
Dobutamine (25 mg/ml)	1-15 µg/kg/min	IV IO	Cardiogenic shock	Need adequate volume resuscitation Peripheral vasodilation
Epinephrine (1:1000 = 1 mg/ml)	0.05-0.3 µg/kg/min	IV IO	Hypotension Bradycardia	Need adequate volume resuscitation Titrate for response
Naloxone (1 mg/ml)	0.1 mg/kg/dose	IV IM IO ETT	Narcotic overdose	Repeat q3-5 min as needed Caution

SDE, Standard-dose epinephrine; *HDE,* high-dose epinephrine; *ETT,* endotracheal tube; *IV,* intravenous; *IO,* intraosseous; *IM,* intramuscular; *PEA,* pulseless electrical activity; *V fib,* ventricular fibrillation; *V tach,* ventricular tachycardia; D_{25}, 25% dextrose.

Lidocaine and bretyllium are both drugs for ventricular fibrillation and pulseless ventricular tachycardia. They act to suppress ventricular ectopy and increase the fibrillation threshold. The dose of lidocaine is 1 mg/kg IV or IO, and 3 mg/kg by endotracheal route. Bretyllium is a second-line antiarrhythmic after lidocaine at an initial dose of 5 mg/kg. If unsuccessful, use 10 mg/kg to a total of 30 mg/kg.

Table 53-1 summarizes all of the common drugs for CPA pharmacotherapy.

REFERENCES

1. Brown C et al: Comparison of standard dose epinephrine in cardiac arrest outside the hospital, *N Engl J Med* 327:1051-1055, 1992.
2. Dieckmann RA, Vardis R: Failure of high dose epinephrine to improve outcome from pediatric out-of-hospital cardiopulmonary arrest.
3. Goetting M et al: High dose epinephrine in refractory pediatric cardiac arrest, *Crit Care Med* 17:1258-1262, 1989.
4. Goetting M et al: High dose epinephrine improves outcome from pediatric cardiac arrest, *Ann Emerg Med* 20:22-26, 1991.
5. Pediatric ALS and neonatal resuscitation, *JAMA* 268:2262-2281, 1992.
6. Stiell I, et al: High dose epinephrine in adult cardiac arrest, 327:1045-1050, 1992.
7. Callahan M, Madsen CD, Barton CW, et al: A randomized clinical trial of high-dose epinephrine and norepinephrine vs. standard-dose epinephrine in prehospital cardiac arrest, *JAMA* 268:2667-2672, 1992.

CARDIOVASCULAR TECHNIQUES

54 Cardiac Monitoring

Carolyn A. Altman

Indications

Emergency Department (ED) and pediatric intensive care unit (PICU) patients are often at risk for disturbances in heart rate and rhythm, making reliable and accurate cardiac monitoring essential. Cardiac monitors provide information on beat to beat heart rate, bradyarrhythmias and tachyarrhythmias, conduction disturbances, and heart rate trends.

Contraindications

There are no contraindications to the use of cardiac monitors.

Complications

If unrecognized, artifact may yield dangerously misleading data. For example, disconnected or loose wires and electrodes may cause an electrical signal that mimicks asystole or ventricular fibrillation. Observers may misdiagnose tachycardia if the tachometer counts T *and* R waves ("double counting"). Regular, rhythmic interference (e.g., from ventilators, chest physical therapy) may also falsely suggest tachycardia. Misinterpretation of rhythm disturbances is also possible if true P waves are not visible as a result of lead placement perpendicular to the P wave axis, if 60-cycles/sec noise obscures atrial activity, or if an inappropriately high filter or sensitivity setting "eliminates" the atrial signal. It is also possible to miss pulseless electrical activity, if the patient's pulse and blood pressure do not correlate regularly with the electrical activity displayed on the monitor.

Meticulous attention to skin care as well as selection and rotation of electrode sites usually prevent the skin breakdown or infection that may otherwise accompany chronic cardiac monitoring.

Equipment

Necessary equipment to perform satisfactory cardiac monitoring includes a cardiac monitor conforming to the standards of the American Heart Association,[3] preferably with memory capability for later recall and evaluation of rate and rhythm disturbances. The ability to display multiple leads simultaneously can assist in the identification of arrhythmias and the exclusion of artifact (Fig. 54-1).

Color-coded cables and lead wires (24 inches or less in length) improve the likelihood of quickly connecting the patient correctly to the monitor. Disposable adhesive electrodes are both convenient and comfortable for the patient. A recorder allows analysis and documentation with hard copy.

Technique

Turn on the monitor's power. Follow the manufacturer's instructions to set age-appropriate rate alarms (see Table 55-1). Inspect the lead wires for any dirt, corrosion, or damage that might interfere with signal transmission. To ensure good contact, *snap* the lead wires into the cables.

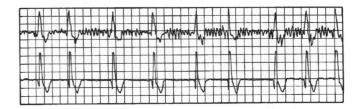

FIG. 54-1 Artifact. Simultaneous display of several leads can assist in the identification of artifact as in this patient receiving vibratory chest physical therapy. Although the top strip may initially suggest an extremely rapid atrial flutter, the bottom tracing displays the true sinus rhythm.

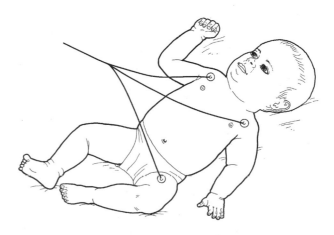

FIG. 54-2 Lead placement. Place electrodes on the shoulders or lateral chest, with the ground on the lower abdomen or upper thigh. Select stable locations yielding a strip free of artifact, with visible P waves and R waves that trigger the tachometer.[1]

Select two sites for electrodes on the lateral chest or shoulders and one site on the lower abdomen or upper leg (Fig. 54-2). Choose areas without bony prominences where the skin is smooth and flat. To prevent skin breakdown and infection, do not place electrodes on bruised or excoriated areas. To prepare the skin for electrode application first cut or shave away as much hair as possible. To remove the dirt, oils, and dead skin cells that increase skin resistance and decrease signal transmission, wash the sites with water and a nonlotion soap. Next, to remove substances that might increase impedance or decrease electrode adhesion, wipe the sites with alcohol and then dry thoroughly. Mildly abrade the electrode sites with gauze, a washcloth, or a manufacturer's electrocardiography (ECG) preparation pad. One to five strokes can amply reduce skin resistance.[2]

Before applying the electrodes to the patient, snap or connect the electrode patches to the lead wires. Then apply the electrodes to the patient by pressing around the periphery of the patches. Pressure directly on the center (over the electrode gel cup) may cause gel dispersement or air trapping, which interferes with signal transmission. To prevent electrical interference and creation of artifact, keep the lead wires clear of other machines surrounding the patient. Prepare new skin sites and apply fresh, moist electrodes every 24 to 48 hours.

Remarks

In order to provide useful and valid data, corroborate and correlate the information provided by the cardiac monitor with the patient's clinical condition.

REFERENCES

1. Chameides L, editor: *Textbook of pediatric advanced life support,* Dallas, 1988, American Heart Association.
2. Clochesy J, Cifani L, Howe K: Electrode site preparation techniques: a follow-up study, *Heart Lung* 20:27-30, 1991.
3. Mirvis D et al: Instrumentation and practice standards for electrocardiographic monitoring in special care units: a report for health care professionals by a task force on clinical cardiology, American Heart Association, *Circulation* 79:464-471, 1989.

55 Electrocardiography: Performance and Interpretation

Indications

Although cardiac monitors display essential information on heart rate and rhythm, there are many circumstances when a full, 15-lead electrocardiogram (ECG) may supply additional invaluable diagnostic data. Electrocardiography may identify patients at risk for rhythm disturbances, such as those with Wolff-Parkinson-White or long QT syndrome. Accurate diagnosis of an arrhythmia in progress may depend on the examination of a full ECG for the presence and axis of P waves, and the axis and morphologic features of the QRS complex. Also ECGs are used to screen for the presence of atrial enlargement, ventricular hypertrophy, or cardiac malposition in patients with a suspected cardiac abnormality.

In addition ECGs are a necessary part of the evaluation for myocardial ischemia, pericarditis, various drug effects or toxicities, severe electrolyte abnormalities, and other metabolic disturbances.

Contraindications

There are no contraindications to use of electrocardiography.

Complications

Faulty interpretation may arise when artifact is not detected. Improper lead placement, interference (i.e., from muscle movement, ventilators, or 60-cycle/sec noise), or poor connections between the patient and the cardiography all yield potentially misleading data.

Equipment

Equipment necessary for performing the ECG includes the cardiograph, color-coded and letter-coded lead wires, electrodes, and standard ECG paper. Modern cardiographs evolved from the string galvanometer adapted for ECG recording by Einthoven in 1913 and are based on the premise that an electrical current creates a magnetic field.[4] The potential difference between two electrodes causes current flow. An amplifier first augments the signals several times and a coil suspended between the two poles of a permanent magnet transmits this current. The current flow in the coil creates a magnetic field that interacts with the permanent magnet's magnetic field, causing the coil to rotate. The ECG writing stylus attaches to the coil and moves with coil rotation. It is important that cardiographs have adequate frequency response to reproduce the most rapid waves in the ECG signal faithfully (e.g., ventricular depolarization). The American Heart Association recommends a frequency response for cardiographs of 0.5 to 100 cycles/sec.[4] The most comfortable, convenient electrodes are the disposable self-adhesive electrodes available in many pediatric centers.

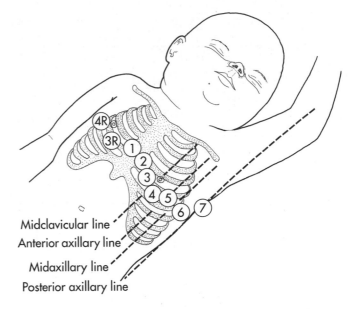

FIG. 55-1 Precordial lead placement: proper placement of precordial electrodes. Lead V_1, Fourth intercostal space, right parasternum; lead V_2, fourth intercostal space, left parasternum; lead V_4, fifth intercostal space, left midclavicular line; lead V_{4R}, fifth intercostal space, right midclavicular line; lead V_5, parallels V_4, in anterior axillary line; lead V_6, parallels V_4, in midaxillary line. In addition, leads V_{3R} and V_7 may be placed as illustrated.

Technique

Turn on the cardiograph. Examine the electrodes and leads for corrosion, damage, or dirt that might interfere with signal transmission. Place the patient in a supine position, relaxed and quiet. Anxiety or motion may create muscle tremor and movement artifact.

Select the electrode sites: Place leads on the right arm, left arm, and left leg to obtain the bipolar leads (I, II, III) and unipolar leads (aVR, aVL, aVF). Fig. 55-1 demonstrates the proper placement of the pediatric precordial leads V_{1-7} and V_{3R-4R}.

Prepare the electrode sites by first shaving any areas of thick hair. Next rub the sites with gauze or a manufacturer's ECG preparation pad. One to five strokes can amply reduce skin resistance.[1] Apply the adhesive electrodes, then clip on the leads. Cardiographs record on standardized paper that has light lines 1 mm apart and heavy lines 5 mm apart. To record the ECG first select a scale that permits clear visualization of P and T waves, without overlapping of the QRS complexes. In standard scale, 1 mV = 10 mm deflection = 10 small boxes (Fig. 55-2). Record the ECG at 25 mm/sec. At this standard paper speed, each large box = 0.2 second and each small box

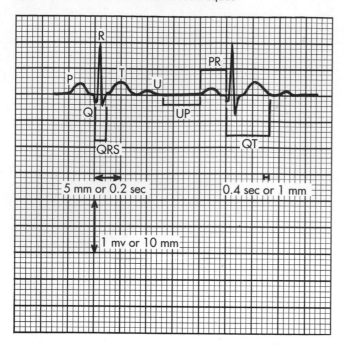

FIG. 55-2 The normal ECG waveforms and measurements on standard ECG paper.

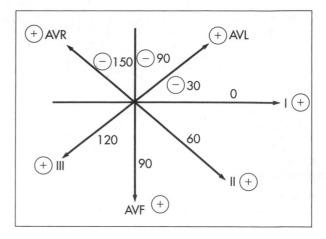

FIG. 55-3 Frontal plane QRS axis.

= 0.04 second (Fig. 55-2). Obtain a rhythm strip composed of leads II, V_1, and V_6.

Interpretation

The following section on ECG interpretation derives largely from Garson's classic text on the subject.[4]

Normal ECG Findings. Fig. 55-2 depicts the normal ECG waveform and intervals.

P WAVES. P waves reflect atrial depolarization. The normal duration is 0.03 to 0.09 second for children 3 years old or less; and 0.05 to 0.1 second for those over 3 years of age. The P wave amplitude should not exceed 2.5 mm. The P wave in V_1 may be biphasic normally.

QRS. QRS complexes reflect ventricular depolarization. The normal duration in Lead V_5 is 0.09 second or less if the child is less than 4 years, and 0.1 second or less for ages 4 to 16. The amplitude of the QRS varies with age (Table 55-1). At minimum the R + S should be more than 5 mm in the limb leads and more than 8 mm in the chest leads.

A Q wave may appear normally in any lead except the right chest leads or a VR. The normal Q wave amplitude varies with age (Table 55-1). However, a Q wave more than 0.03 second in duration is always abnormal.

T WAVES. T waves reflect ventricular repolarization. Electrical polarity usually follows the QRS, with the exception that between the ages of 2 days and adolescence the T wave is normally inverted in the right precordial leads.

U WAVES. U waves reflect Purkinje cell repolarization.

PR INTERVALS. PR intervals encompass the atrial depolarization and repolarization that occurs before the beginning of ventricular depolarization. Measure the interval from the beginning of the P wave to the beginning of the QRS. Normally the PR interval is ≈ 0.12 second in lead II, but does vary with age (Table 55-1).

TP (OR UP IF U WAVE) INTERVAL. No electrical activity occurs during the TP interval so it is the true isoelectric baseline. If the P wave is not buried in the T wave, use this interval as the baseline of all amplitude measurements (i.e., P wave and QRS height or ST segment changes).

QT INTERVALS. QT intervals reflect the total time for ventricular depolarization and repolarization, from the beginning of the QRS to the end of the T wave. Include the U wave in the interval if it measures 50% or more of the T wave amplitude. Correct for heart rate: QTc = measured QT (sec) ÷ (square root of the preceding RR interval). The QTc should be less than or equal to 0.45 second until 6 months of age, and 0.44 second or less in older children.[2]

Axis. Axis refers to the direction of the mean vector of cardiac electrical forces during a specific interval. Fig. 55-3 demonstrates the lead axis in the frontal plane.

FRONTAL PLANE QRS AXIS. To estimate the direction of this axis first determine the most isoelectric (sum of positive and negative forces ≈ 0) QRS complex in the frontal plane. The frontal plane QRS axis is directed toward one of the two perpendiculars to the lead with the isoelectric QRS. The axis is in the vicinity of that perpendicular that points in the same direction as the frontal plane lead with the maximum net positive deflection (Fig. 55-4). The normal frontal plane QRS axis changes with age (Table 55-1). Diagnose "axis deviation" if the axis falls outside the normal sector (Fig. 55-4).

FRONTAL PLANE P WAVE AXIS. This axis is useful in determining the site of origin of atrial depolarization (Fig. 55-5). A P wave originating in the high right atrium suggests sinus rhythm.

Heart Rate. Estimate the heart rate on the ECG by counting the number of large (0.2 second) boxes between two successive R waves (Fig. 55-6). Or calculate the exact heart rate.

$$HR = 60 \div (RR \text{ interval, seconds})$$

Chamber Enlargement and Hypertrophy. Assessment of chamber enlargement or hypertrophy by ECG interpretation carries only a 60% to 70% positive predictive value in pediatrics.[3,8]

RIGHT VENTRICULAR HYPERTROPHY. Diagnose right ventricular hypertrophy (RVH) by the following criteria:

1. QR pattern in the right chest leads. This finding quite reliably predicts RVH.

Table 55-1   Summary of Normal Values

Age group	Heart rate* (beats/min)	Frontal plane QRS vector (degrees)	PR Interval (sec)	Q† III (mm)‡	Q† V6 (mm)	RV1 (mm)*	SV1 (mm)	R/S V1	RV6 (mm)	SV6 (mm)	R/S V6	SV1† + RV6 (mm)	R† + S V4 (mm)
Less than 1 day	93-154 (123)	+59 to −163 (137)	0.08-0.16 (0.11)	4.5	2	5-26 (14)	0-23 (8)	0.01-U (2.2)§	0-11 (4)	0-9.5 (3)	0.1-U (2.0)	28	52.5
1-2 days	91-159 (123)	+64 to −161 (134)	0.08-0.14 (0.11)	6.5	2.5	5-27 (14)	0-21 (9)	0.1-U (2.0)	0-12 (4.5)	0-9.5 (3)	0.1-U (2.5)	29	52
3-6 days	91-166 (129)	+77 to −163 (132)	0.07-0.14 (0.10)	5.5	3	3-24 (13)	0-17 (7)	0.2-U (2.7)	0.5-12 (5)	0-10 (3.5)	0.1-U (2.2)	24.5	49
1-3 weeks	107-182 (148)	+65 to +161 (110)	0.07-0.14 (0.10)	6	3	3-21 (11)	0-11 (4)	1.0-U (2.9)	2.5-16.5 (7.5)	0-10 (3.5)	0.1-U (3.3)	21	49
1-2 months	121-179 (149)	+31 to +113 (74)	0.07-0.13 (0.10)	7.5	3	3-18 (10)	0-12 (5)	0.3-U (2.3)	5-21.5 (11.5)	0-6.5 (3)	0.2-U (4.8)	29	53.5
3-5 months	106-186 (141)	+7 to +104 (60)	0.07-0.15 (0.11)	6.5	3	3-20 (10)	0-17 (6)	0.1-U (2.3)	6.5-22.5 (13)	0-10 (3)	0.2-U (6.2)	32	61.5
6-11 months	109-169 (134)	+6 to +99 (56)	0.07-16 (0.11)	8.5	3	1.5-20 (9.5)	0.5-18 (4)	0.1-3.9 (1.6)	6-22.5 (12.5)	0-7 (2)	0.2-U (7.6)	32	53
1-2 years	89-151 (119)	+7 to +101 (55)	0.08-0.15 (0.11)	6	3	2.5-17 (9)	0.5-21 (8)	0.05-4.3 (1.4)	6-22.5 (13)	0-6.5 (2)	0.3-U (9.3)	39	49.5
3-4 years	73-137 (108)	+6 to +104 (55)	0.09-0.16 (0.12)	5	3.5	1-18 (8)	0.2-21 (10)	0.3-2.8 (0.9)	8-24.5 (15)	0-5 (1.5)	0.6-U (10.8)	42	53.5
5-7 years	65-133 (100)	+11 to +143 (65)	0.09-0.16 (0.12)	4	4.5	0.5-14 (7)	0.3-24 (12)	0.02-2.0 (0.7)	8.5-26.5 (16)	0-4 (1)	0.9-U (11.5)	47	54
8-11 years	62-130 (91)	+9 to +114 (61)	0.09-0.17 (0.13)	3	3	0-12 (5.5)	0.3-25 (12)	0-1.8 (0.5)	9-25.5 (16)	0-4 (1)	1.5-U (14.3)	45.5	53
12-15 years	60-119 (85)	+11 to +130 (59)	0.09-0.18 (0.14)	3	3	0-10 (4)	0.3-21 (11)	0-1.7 (0.5)	6.5-23 (14)	0-4 (1)	1.4-U (14.7)	41	50

*2%-98% mean.
†98th percentile.
‡ mm at normal standardization.
§ Undefined (S wave may equal zero).
From Garson A: *The electrocardiogram in infants and children: a systematic approach,* Philadelphia, 1983, Lea & Febiger.

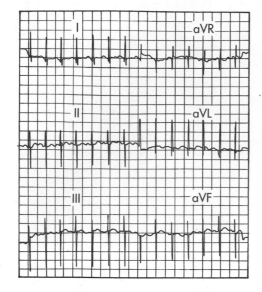

A

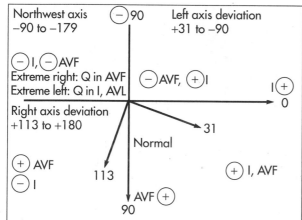

B

FIG. 55-4 Frontal plane QRS determination. **A,** The frontal plane leads of a sample ECG of a 2-month-old. The QRS complex in lead aVR is the closest to being isoelectric (approximately six boxes above and six boxes below the baseline). Lead aVR's vector points to −150. Therefore the frontal plane axis is directed either in the vicinity of the perpendicular −60 or +120. Lead aVL, with a vector at −30, has the maximum net positive deflection (four boxes below baseline and 15 above). Consequently the frontal plane axis points to this same direction: the perpendicular at −60. According to Table 55-1, the normal axis for a 2-month-old falls between +31 and +113. Therefore this patient has left axis deviation. **B,** The normal and abnormal axes for a 2-month-old, which illustrate that the polarity of leads I and AVF may be used as a rough guideline for placing the axis in a particular quadrant.

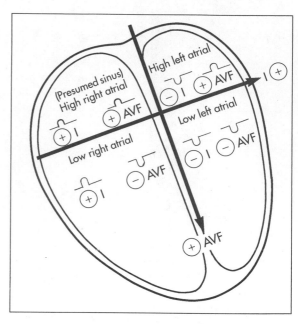

FIG. 55-5 Atrial frontal plane QRS axis. The axis may be determined by inspecting the P wave polarity in leads I and AVF. The frontal plane P wave axis is directed from the site of origin of the P wave to the AV node. AV, atrioventricular.

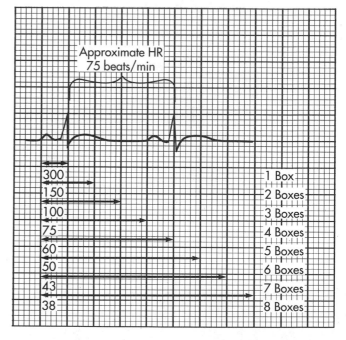

FIG. 55-6 Heart rate may be estimated by counting out the number of large boxes in an RR interval as shown here.

2. T wave changes:
   a. An upright T wave in right chest leads between 1 week of age and adolescence (must first rule out a reciprocal change of left ventricular hypertrophy).
   b. T wave inversion with an upright convexity in terminal portion is a strain pattern indicative of severe RVH.
   c. In the presence of other ECG RVH signs, an inverted T wave in aVF indicates severe RVH.

3. R wave amplitude in V_1 exceeding the normal for age (Table 55-1) is a more specific, less sensitive sign of RVH.
4. S wave amplitude in V_6 exceeding the normal for age (Table 55-1) is a more sensitive, less specific sign.
5. R/S ratio in V_1 exceeding the normal for age (Table 55-1) is evidence for RVH, but is more reliable in presence of a deep S in V_6.

6. RsR' in V_1 correlates well with mild RVH if the R' is greater than 10 mm in patients less than 1 year, or R' is more than 15 mm in those 1 year or older. Otherwise if the QRS duration is normal, an RsR' pattern is normal.

7. Right axis deviation in patients older than 3 months also correlates with RVH.

LEFT VENTRICULAR HYPERTROPHY. The ECG diagnosis of left ventricular hypertrophy (LVH) is correct only 50% of the time. Criteria include the following:

1. T wave inversion in left chest leads with upright convexity in the terminal portion is the most reliable sign of LVH. This indicates "LVH with strain." ST depression often is present.

2. Excessive amplitude of the R wave in V_6 or S wave in V_1 (Table 55-1) is a relatively poor predictor of LVH in the presence of normal T waves.

3. The sum of the amplitudes of the R wave in V_6 and S wave in V_1 exceeding normal for age (Table 55-1) correlates with LVH.

4. Abnormally deep Q waves in II, III, aVF, and V_6 (Table 55-1) are nonspecific signs of LVH.

BIVENTRICULAR HYPERTROPHY. Criteria for the diagnosis of biventricular hypertrophy (BVH) include the following:

1. If the tracing meets voltage criteria for either LVH or RVH, BVH exists if the other ventricle generates more than the mean normal voltage (Table 55-1).

2. R + S wave amplitude in midprecordial leads excessive for age (Table 55-1) is consistent with BVH.

RIGHT ATRIAL ENLARGEMENT. If the P wave amplitude of a patient in sinus rhythm exceeds 2.5 mm in any lead, diagnose right atrial enlargement (RAE).

LEFT ATRIAL ENLARGEMENT. Diagnostic criteria for left atrial enlargement (LAE) include the following:

1. A late (after first 0.04 second), large (more than 1 mm deep, more than .04 second), or negative deflection in the P wave in V_1 indicates LAE.

2. An abnormally wide P wave (more than 0.9 second in children less than 3 years; or more than 0.1 second in those 3 years or older) suggests LAE, but this is not a sensitive test.

Conduction Disturbances. Criteria for the diagnosis of common conduction disturbances follow.

RIGHT BUNDLE BRANCH BLOCK. RBBB is a conduction abnormality associated with delayed right ventricular activation (Fig. 55-7). Diagnose RBBB if all of the following are present on the ECG:

1. QRS duration prolonged for age, with RsR' pattern in right chest leads

2. Normal initial (during first 0.04 second) forces

3. A terminal conduction delay directed anteriorly and to the right (width of R' in V_1 usually twice width of RS, and S in V_6 twice width of R)

LEFT BUNDLE BRANCH BLOCK. LBBB is a conduction abnormality associated with a delay in left ventricular activation (Fig. 55-7). Diagnose LBBB if all of the following are present on ECG:

1. QRS duration prolonged for age, with aberrancy of entire QRS complex;

2. Absent normal initial forces in leads reflecting the left ventricle (absent Q in I, aVL, V_6); and

3. Notched, slurred QRS complexes pointing leftward and posterior (tall notched R wave in V_6, along with QS or small R/deep S in V_1).

INTERVENTRICULAR CONDUCTION DELAY. Interventricular conduction delay (IVCD) signifies a nonspecific delay in ventricular activation. Diagnose IVCD if the QRS is prolonged for age, but without the features of LBBB or RBBB.

WOLFF-PARKINSON-WHITE. In the Wolff-Parkinson-White (WPW) abnormality a bundle of Kent (or accessory muscle connection) allows preexcitation of the ventricle and provides the anatomic substrate for supraventricular tachycardia (SVT) (Fig. 55-8). Diagnostic criteria include the following.

1. A PR interval short for age is usually present, as activation from the atrium to the ventricle occurs rapidly through the accessory connection. The PR interval is not necessarily short in all leads.

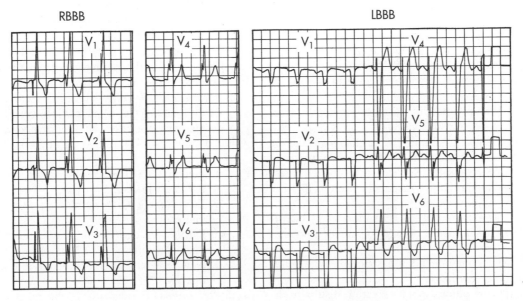

FIG. 55-7 Bundle branch block. Leads V_1-V_6 in right and left bundle branch block patterns.

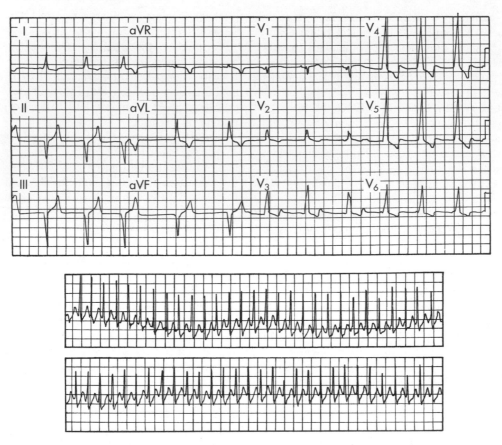

FIG. 55-8 WPW and SVT. *Top panel:* The short PR interval and delta wave diagnostic for WPW are seen on the ECG in normal sinus rhythm. Note also the absence of a Q wave in lead V6, as well as left axis deviation. *Bottom panel:* The same patient in supraventricular tachycardia. P waves are not seen during SVT. *WPW,* Wolff-Parkinson-White syndrome; *SVT,* supraventricular tachycardia.

2. A delta wave may be present as an initial slurring of the QRS complex (may resemble LBBB). The delta wave is not necessarily present in all leads.
3. Absence of a Q wave in V_6 or left axis deviation often occurs and may be a helpful clue when the delta wave is subtle.

LONG QTC. A congenital or acquired prolongation of the corrected QT interval may place a patient at risk for ventricular arrhythmias and sudden death (Fig. 55-9).

1. A QTc measured at greater than 0.45 second in children under 6 months of age, or greater than 0.44 second in older children is abnormally prolonged.[3]
2. T waves are often inverted, biphasic, or variable in size and shape in patients with long QTc.

ST and T Wave Changes. ST and T wave changes occur in a variety of circumstances found in a critical care setting.

SECONDARY T WAVE CHANGES. Secondary T wave changes result from primary abnormalities of depolarization: that is, RBBB, hypertrophy, preexcitation.

FUNCTIONAL T WAVE CHANGES. Functional T wave changes result from the influence of the sympathetic nervous system.

1. Inverted T waves may occur in association with fear, anxiety, or hyperventilation.
2. With early repolarization J point elevation results from elimination of the ST segment.

PRIMARY T WAVE CHANGES

1. *Ischemia.* Ischemic T wave changes may occur in patients with anomalous left coronary artery, severe aortic/pulmonary stenosis, or Kawasaki disease. They may also be present in stressed neonates. Findings include the following:
   a. Peaked, prolonged, flattened, or inverted T waves.
   b. ST depression may occur with ischemia. If ischemic ST changes are present in the left chest leads, the T waves are flat or upright. (In LVH with strain ST depression may be present with inverted T waves.)
2. *Myocarditis.* Seventy percent of children with myocarditis have ECG changes.[7] However a normal ECG result does not rule out severe myocardial damage.[5] Common ECG findings in myocarditis include the following:
   a. Flat, inverted T waves are present, particularly in the left chest leads.
   b. Low-voltage QRS complexes result from myocardial edema.
   c. Diffuse ST depression occurs secondary to subendocardial injury.
   d. New Q waves, accompanied by ST elevation, occur rarely.
3. *Pericarditis.* Pericarditis is the most common pathologic cause of ST elevation in children. The QRS

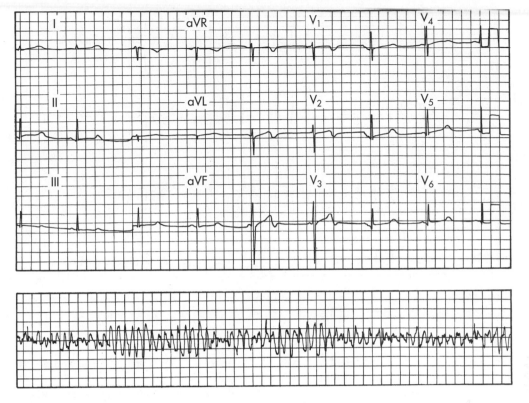

FIG. 55-9 Long QTC. *Top panel:* A long QTc is seen on this ECG during sinus rhythm. These patients are at risk for torsade de pointes, a multiform ventricular tachycardia depicted in the bottom panel.

complex is not affected. Four stages evolve on the ECG (Fig. 55-10):

a. Stage I: ST elevation in II, aVF, V_3-V_6 with reciprocal ST depression in aVR, V_1 probably results from subepicardial myocarditis. (Neonates may show right chest lead ST elevation.) To distinguish pericarditis from infarction, note that ST elevation generally occurs in only a *few* leads in infarction and is accompanied by T wave inversion.

b. Stage II: The ST segments normalize and T waves flatten.

c. Stage III: The T waves invert in the same leads where ST elevation occurred.

d. Stage IV: The ECG result normalizes with resolution of pericarditis.

4. *Infarction.* Children with Kawasaki disease, anomalous left coronary artery, or severe neonatal stress are at risk for myocardial infarction. Note the following sequence on ECG:

a. "Hyperacute" T waves: These peaked, tall T waves are rarely observed, as they occur only in the first minutes after infarction.

b. ST elevation then develops in the region overlying the infarction. ST depression in the reciprocal leads may also occur (Fig. 55-11).

c. Abnormally wide Q waves develop because normal muscle opposite the infarction faces unopposed, electrically inert muscle. Q waves appear hours to days after ST changes occur.

Other causes of abnormal Q waves (without infarction) include the following:

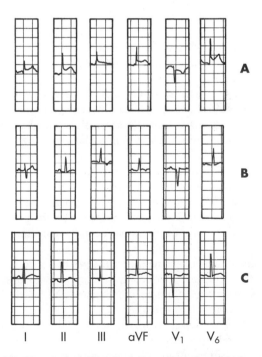

FIG. 55-10 Pericarditis. Evolution of pericarditis in a 12-year-old. **A,** ST elevation, with upright T waves in all leads except V_1. The ST/T ratios in leads I and V_6 are 0.42 and 0.33, respectively. Since these are greater than 0.25, pericarditis is suggested. **B,** The ST elevation is resolving and is replaced with T wave inversion in leads III and aV$_F$. This electrocardiogram was taken 4 days after the first. **C,** Two weeks later, the ST-T wave changes are resolved but there is a Q wave in lead III wider than on previous tracings. This could indicate a small area of old inferior myocardial infarction.

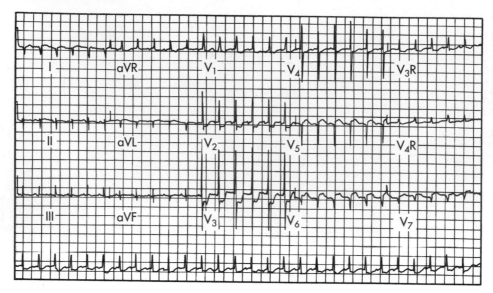

FIG. 55-11 Infarction. Abnormal Q waves accompanied by ST elevation in the left chest leads suggests a lateral infarction. Note the reciprocal ST depression in the right chest leads.

1. Ventricular abnormalities such as RVH, LVH with strain, ventricular inversion, and hypertrophic cardiomyopathy may all have Q waves.
2. Pneumothorax or other lung diseases cause Q waves by malposition of the heart in the chest.
3. Replacement of cardiac muscle by noncardiac tissue (prosthetic material, cardiac tumors, etc.) may cause abnormal Q waves.
4. Conduction abnormalities: Q waves may occur on ECGs with WPW or LBBB patterns.
5. Intracranial hemorrhage: A QS pattern in V_1 and V_2 may occur.

PRIMARY ST CHANGES. Primary ST changes may result from myocardial infarction, pericarditis, cor pulmonale, head injury, electrolyte disturbances, use of digitalis, pneumothorax, pneumopericardium, early ventricular repolarization, or normal atrial repolarization.

Metabolic Abnormalities and Systemic Perturbations.
Metabolic abnormalities and systemic perturbations that may affect the ECG often occur in the critical care setting.

HYPERKALEMIA. ECG changes correlate with the potassium level. The following progression occurs with increasing levels:
1. Peaked T waves are neither sensitive nor specific.
2. IVCD occurs as conduction velocity diminishes. The QRS complexes often become bizarre and ST elevation often accompanies them.
3. Prolonged P waves are indicative of significant intra-atrial conduction delay.
4. During "sinoventricular" conduction the P waves disappear.
5. Arrhythmias generally correlate with the highest potassium levels and may include atrioventricular (AV) block, ventricular tachycardia, and ventricular fibrillation.

HYPOXIA AND ACIDOSIS
1. Hypoxia and acidosis cause changes on the ECG similar to those seen with hyperkalemia.

2. AV block, atrial arrhythmias, and ventricular arrhythmias are all possible.

HYPOKALEMIA AND HYPOMAGNESEMIA. Hypokalemia and hypomagnesemia cause similar changes.
1. T wave amplitudes decrease, and U wave amplitudes increase.
2. ST depression may occur.
3. A measurably long QTc may occur, secondary to the broadening of the T and U waves.
4. Arrhythmias are rare; however, digoxin increases the potential for arrhythmias.

HYPERCALCEMIA. ECG findings in hypercalcemia include the following:
1. A decrease in sinus rate may occur, and sinus arrest is possible.
2. The QT interval may be short, secondary to a shortening of the ST segment.
3. Arrhythmias are uncommon. Digoxin increases the risk of ventricular arrhythmias and AV block.

HYPOCALCEMIA. ECG findings in hypocalcemia include the following:
1. The QTc interval may be prolonged.
2. Arrhythmias are rare, but AV block may occur.

HYPERMAGNESEMIA. Hypermagnesemia may rarely cause a prolongation of the PR interval or IVCD.

CENTRAL NERVOUS SYSTEM INJURY. ECG changes are present in 75% of patients with central nervous system injury.[6] Possible changes are as follows:
1. A prolonged QTc is the most common abnormality.
2. T waves may become notched and bizarre, flattened, or inverted with ST depression.
3. The U wave may be prominent.
4. Any tachyarrhythmia or bradyarrhythmia is possible.
5. The J or Osborne wave, an extra deflection between the QRS and the ST segment, may occur.

HYPOTHERMIA. Possible findings on the ECGs of hypothermic patients include the following:
1. J or Osborne waves may be present.

Table 55-2   Rhythm Interpretation

Rhythm	Rate and variability	P Wave	QRS	Comment
Sinus	Normal for age Regular	Precedes each QRS P wave upright in I, aVF	Normal, RBBB, LBBB, IVCD, RR interval varies ≤ 0.08 sec	Normal
Sinus arrhythmia	Normal for age Irregular	Precedes each QRS Structure and axis as NSR	Same as NSR RR varies > 0.08 each with respiration	Normal variant
Sinus tachycardia	Above normal for age (but not usually >220-230) Gradual increase, decrease Regular	Precedes each QRS Morphology and axis as NSR	Same as during NSR Minor variations in RR intervals	Seen in states requiring increased cardiac output (i.e., sepsis, fever), CHF, myocarditis, fear; or after treatment with vasodilators, sympathomimetics
Premature ventricular contractions (Fig. 55-12)	Normal for age Irregular *Often* with compensatory pause after QRS	No P wave before abnormal QRS Examine preceding T waves for hidden P waves	Premature, abnormal QRS Wider or *different* from QRS during NSR	Common causes: Mechanical (i.e., CVL), hypoxia, hypoglycemia, ↓ or ↑K, ↑Ca, drug toxicity, CHD, myocarditis; found also in up to 2% of normal children
Premature atrial contractions (Fig. 55-13)	Normal for age Irregular *Usually* no compensatory pause	P wave occurs > 0.08 seconds before next expected P wave Examine preceding T waves for hidden P waves		Common Causes: mechanical (i.e., CVL), hypoglycemia, hypoxia, ↑Ca, ↓K, enlarged atria, sympathomimetic drugs, or digoxin toxicity Seen in 13% of normal children
First-degree AV block	Normal for age Regular	Prolonged PR interval for age Same morphology, axis as in NSR	Same as during NSR	Associated with stretched atria Seen in 8% of sleeping normal children
Second-degree AV block (intermittent failure of AV conduction) (Fig. 55-14)	Normal for age Irregular	Mobitz type I: (Wenkebach) Progressive PR lengthening until P not conducted	Progressive RR shortening until QRS dropped	Vagal tone influential; seen in 11% of sleeping, normal children
		Mobitz type II: Intermittent loss of AV conduction; no change in PR	RR unchanging, except for dropped QRS	Uncommon May progress to complete AV block
Third-degree AV block (complete AV block) (Fig. 55-15)	Junctional or ventricular escape rate slower than NSR for age Usually regular	P waves present that should conduct (>0.4 seconds after QRS or beyond T wave), but do not	RR unchanged by any preceding P waves	Can be congenital or acquired (from surgery, infection) May develop over time in certain CHD
Supraventricular tachycardia (Fig. 55-8)	Usually ≈ 240 beats/min; in infants, rates as high as 320 beats/min; RR unvarying; starts and stops abruptly	May not see P waves Look for different axis or structure from NSR	QRS of normal structure in >90%; wide QRS must first rule out VT; look for delta wave of WPW in NSR	46% Have predisposing factors: drugs, fever, sepsis, WPW
Atrial flutter (Fig. 55-16)	Atrial rate 280-450 BPM; ventricular rate depends on AV conduction ratio; variable, rhythm irregular	Look in II, III, aVF, or V$_1$ for flutter waves with sawtooth or picket fence appearance	Usually as in NSR; aberrated conduction occasionally seen	At risk: normal infants with frequent PACs; older children with atrial surgery or chronic atrial dilatation

Continued.

Table 55-2 Rhythm Interpretation*—cont'd

Rhythm	Rate and variability	P Wave	QRS	Comment
Atrial fibrillation (Fig. 55-17)	Irregularly irregular 2° = extremely variable AV conduction	Bizarre, chaotic atrial depolarizations	Rare to see identical RR intervals on one rhythm strip	Usually with abnormal heart or WPW, at least of adolescent age
Ventricular tachycardia (Fig. 55-12)	Average ≈ 195 beats/min (range: 120-400 beats/min)	May be dissociated from ventricle, retrograde, or not visible	Wider or *different* from normal sinus rhythm; look for fusion complexes, sinus capture beats Structure usually similar to patient's single PVCs	Associated with myocardial injury; long QTc; ventilatory, temperature, or electrolyte abnormalities; acidosis; or certain antiarrhythmic, sympathomimetic, recreational, or oral decongestant agents
Accelerated ventricular rhythm	Rate not higher than normal for age in NSR Regular	May be dissociated, retrograde, or not visible	Wide or *different* QRS, of similar structure to patient's single PVCs	Benign
Electromechanical dissociation	Electrical heart rate without pulse			Can be associated with hypoxia, pneumothorax, severe acidosis, hypovolemia
Ventricular fibrillation (Fig. 55-18)	No pulse No organized electrical activity	None	Low-amplitude, rapid, irregular depolarizations without identifiable QRS	Associated with hypoxia, chest trauma, long QTc, hypothermia, severe myocardial hypertrophy, and WPW

NSR, normal sinus rhythm; *CHF*, congestive heart failure; *CHD*, congenital heart disease; *CVL*, central venous line; *K*, potassium; *Ca*, calcium; *AV*, atrioventricular; *PVC*, premature ventricular contractions; *RBBB*, right bundle branch block; *IVCD*, interventricular conduction delay; *WPW*, Wolff-Parkinson-White syndrome.

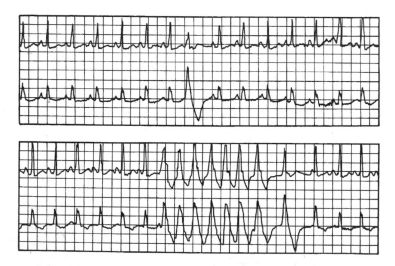

FIG. 55-12 Premature ventricular contractions and ventricular tachycardia. *Top panel:* A premature ventricular contraction: a wide, premature QRS not preceded by a P wave. A retrograde P wave is seen in the T wave of the PVC. The PVC is followed by a compensatory pause. *Bottom panel:* Ventricular tachycardia in the same patient. Note the similarity of the QRS complexes during VT with that of the PVC. *PVC*, premature ventricular contraction.

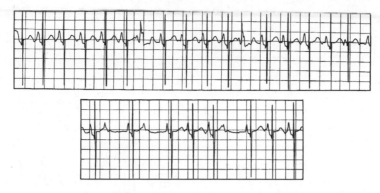

FIG. 55-13   Premature atrial contractions. *Top strip:* An early QRS complex preceded by an early P wave. As is often (but not always) the case, no compensatory pause follows the early beat. *Bottom strip:* The irregular rhythm caused by an early atrial contraction that does not conduct through to the ventricle, a "blocked" PAC. PAC, premature atrial contraction.

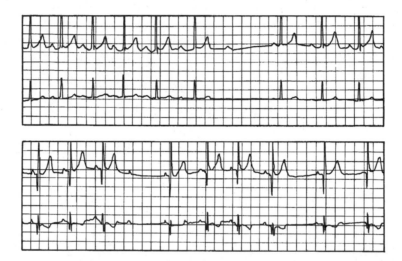

FIG. 55-14   Second-degree AV block. *Top panel:* Type I (Wenkebach) AV block. Note the progressive lengthening of the PR interval until a QRS is dropped. *Bottom panel:* Type II AV block. No change is seen in the PR interval preceding the dropped beat. AV, atrioventricular.

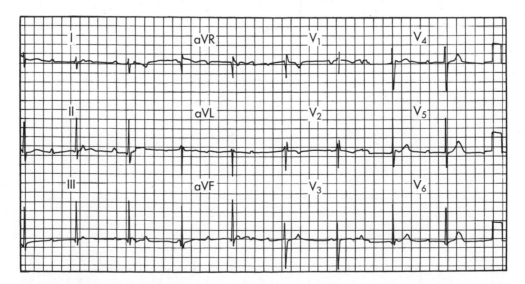

FIG. 55-15   Third-degree AV block. The P waves march through this strip at 90 beats/min; the junctional escape rate is 54 beats/min. Those P waves that should conduct (those outside the T wave, or more than 0.4 sec after the QRS) do not, as evidenced by the lack of change in the RR intervals.

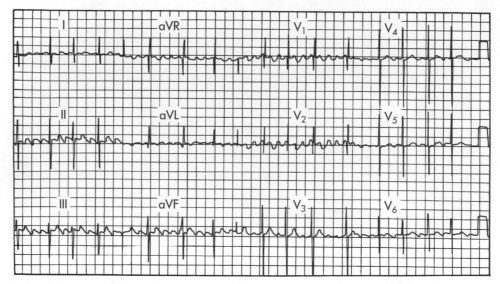

FIG. 55-16 Atrial flutter. Sawtooth flutter waves at a rate of approximately 300/min are seen especially well in II, III, V$_1$, and V$_2$. The flutter is conducted with varying (2:1 to 4:1) degrees of AV block. AV, atrioventricular.

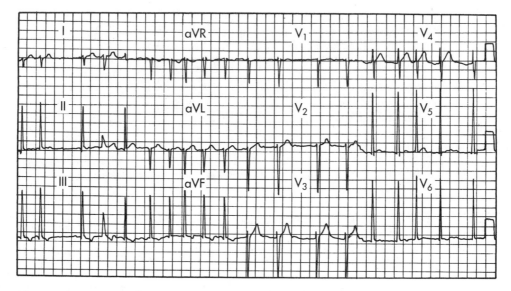

FIG. 55-17 Atrial fibrillation. The constantly varying RR intervals and the irregular baseline seen in this ECG are hallmarks of atrial fibrillation. ECG, electrocardiogram.

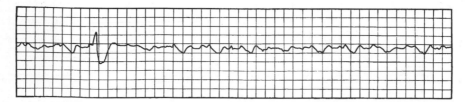

FIG. 55-18 Ventricular fibrillation. A single, very wide ventricular beat is followed by low-amplitude, rapid, irregular depolarizations characteristic of ventricular fibrillation.

2. Sinus slowing can occur.
3. The PR and QTc intervals may be prolonged.
4. Atrial fibrillation can occur but is most common in adults.

Medications. Many drugs affect the ECG and can be arrhythmogenic.*

Rhythm Interpretation. Table 55-2 may prove a useful guide for the diagnosis of common arrhythmias.

---

*For a review of the effects of cardiac medications, refer to Opie LH, Phil D, editors: *Drugs for the heart,* ed 4, Philadelphia, 1995, WB Saunders. For other medications, information on possible arrhythmogenesis and ECG effect is available from pharmacology texts, poison control centers, or manufacturer-supplied product information.

REFERENCES

1. Clochesy J, Cifani L, Howe K: Electrode site preparation techniques: a follow-up study, *Heart Lung* 20(1):27-30, 1991.
2. Davignon A, Rautaharju P, Boisselle E, et al: Normal ECG standards for infants and children, *Pediatr Cardiol* 1:123-152, 1979.
3. Ellison RC, Freedom RM, Keane JF, et, al: Indirect assessment of severity in pulmonary stenosis, *Circulation* 56:I15-20, 1977.
4. Garson A: *The electrocardiogram in infants and children: a systemic approach,* Philadelphia, 1983, Lea & Febiger.
5. Hoffman J: Primary T wave changes in children, *Praxis* 64:803-811, 1975.
6. Rogers M, Zakha KG, Nugent SK, et al: Electrocardiographic abnormalities in infants and children with neurological injury, *Crit Care Med* 8:213-214, 1980.
7. Sachder J, Puri D: Electrocardiographic alterations in diphtheria, *Indian J Pediatr* 34:429-431, 1967.
8. Wagner HR, Weidman WH, Ellison RC, et al: Indirect assessment of severity in aortic stenosis, *Circulation* 56:20-23, 1977.

56 Temporary Cardiac Pacing

Christopher C. Erickson

For many patients inadequate cardiac output is caused by either hypovolemia, abnormal vascular resistance, or poor contractility. Therapy to correct these problems aims at increasing the stroke volume. However cardiac output also demands a minimal heart rate for a given stroke volume. Patients who have significant bradycardia, such as sinus bradycardia or arrest, and advanced second- or third-degree atrioventricular (AV) block often need a higher heart rate to sustain core perfusion.

The two commonly used approaches for increasing the heart rate are temporary pacing and pharmacologic agents. The more effective of these is pacing. The focus of this chapter is on pacing, with brief remarks on pharmacologic agents.

Beta-adrenergic agonists such as isoproterenol (0.01 to 0.1 µg/kg/min) or vagal blockers such as atropine (0.02 to 0.04 µg/kg/min) can aid in elevating the heart rate, but their effects are often limited in patients with structural disease of the cardiac conduction tissues. In addition it is often difficult to achieve a higher heart rate in patients in whom a relative tachycardia may be appropriate (e.g., septic shock with fever, cardiomyopathy). Some patients require pacing despite high doses of beta-agonists.

The rhythm disturbance and hemodynamic status determine the best therapy. When the ventricular rate is low but the blood pressure and perfusion are reasonably good, no therapy is appropriate despite the rhythm. If it appears that

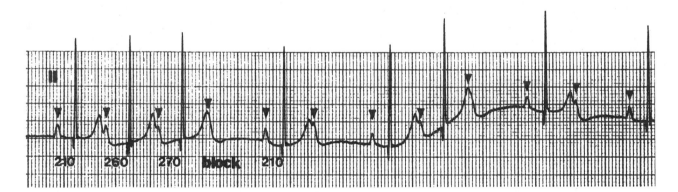

FIG. 56-1 Second-degree AV block. In this tracing note Wenckebach conduction where the P-R interval progressively lengthens. The arrowheads indicate P waves. The numbers below the tracing show the P-R intervals in milliseconds. Eventually a P wave cannot conduct to the ventricles (block). This arrhythmia may respond to beta-agonist agents to provide 1:1 conduction from atria to the ventricles. Paper speed, 25 mm/sec; AV, atrioventricular.

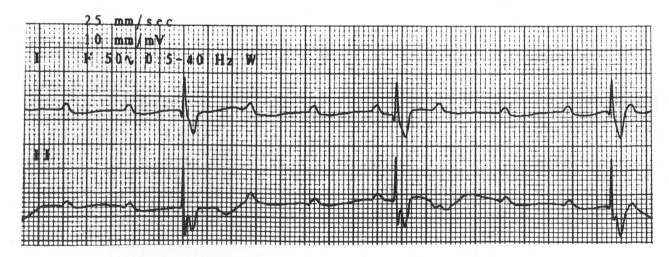

FIG. 56-2 Complete AV block. Note P waves with QRS complexes appearing regularly without any relationship to the P waves. Paper speed, 25 mm/sec.

second-degree (2-degree) AV block is present where some, but not all, P waves conduct to the ventricles (Fig. 56-1), then an isoproterenol infusion may work well to increase AV conduction. It may also work in cases where the sinus rate is inappropriately low for the patient's age, size, and clinical status. If advanced 2-degree or complete (3-degree) AV block is present (Fig. 56-2) or if severe sinus bradycardia or arrest is present, pharmacologic agents prove inadequate to increase the heart rate; initiate plans for temporary pacing immediately. Patients with sudden asystole or severe bradycardia with very few escape beats are candidates for temporary pacing.

Five methods of temporary pacing are possible. These include (1) transvenous intracardiac, (2) esophageal, (3) transcutaneous, (4) transthoracic, and (5) postoperative temporary pacing wires. The indications for each method vary as a result of the pacing needs and condition of the patient.

TRANSVENOUS INTRACARDIAC PACING
Indications

This method involves placement of a pacing catheter directly inside the right ventricle. It is the most reliable way to achieve capture (cardiac contraction after a pacing stimulus).[13,24] Use this method in patients with advanced forms of AV block or significant sinus bradycardia. Another indication for transvenous pacing is right-sided cardiac catheterization of patients with left bundle branch block or bifascicular block that includes right bundle branch.[9] This method of pacing is easier in those patients who already have access to a large vein (either femoral, internal jugular, or subclavian) via indwelling venous sheath. Pace patients who need emergency pacing, but without access to a large vein, by other means (transcutaneous or transthoracic) while obtaining access to a large vein.

Contraindications

Absolute. For patients with prosthetic mechanical tricuspid valves do not place temporary pacing wires into the right ventricle because damage to the valve or catheter entrapment may result.[13,24] Instead, and only in life-threatening situations, place a temporary pacing wire into the femoral or brachial artery and pass it retrograde across the aortic valve into the left ventricle, but only for a brief time (e.g., up to 4 hours) while arranging other modes of pacing. This approach requires fluoroscopy and some degree of skill and experience to place the catheter correctly. In addition placement of a catheter into the left side of the heart poses the risk of thrombus formation that may lead to embolic phenomenon to the brain or coronary arteries. Therefore employ systemic anticoagulation with heparin (100 U/kg up to 5000 U).

Hypothermia is an absolute contraindication despite the heart rate or blood pressure.[24] Pacing in hypothermic patients may result in ventricular fibrillation that is refractory to usual therapy.

Relative. Bleeding diatheses,[13,24] digitalis toxicity,[24] and sepsis[24] are relative contraindications; judge the decision to use transvenous pacing with these conditions according to the patient's clinical status. Patients who have been asystolic for a prolonged period are not likely to recover and therefore attempts at transvenous pacing are futile.[24]

Complications

Many complications associated with this procedure result from problems with venous access (see Chapter 31). Perforation of the right ventricle can result in pericardial effusion and cardiac tamponade. Pericardial pain may be the only manifestation of a perforation. Normal pacing from the right ventricle should produce a left bundle branch block pattern. A change to a right bundle branch block pattern may suggest a perforation of the right ventricular free wall or interventricular septum.[13]

Other complications include infection, poor sensing or capture of cardiac tissue, as well as atrial or ventricular arrhythmias. Incorrect placement of the catheter in a location other than the right ventricle (atrium, inferior vena cava, proximal coronary sinus) results in inability to pace the ventricles. Also a patent foramen ovale or congenital heart defects may allow inadvertent passage of the catheter into the left side of the heart or systemic circulation. This may permit systemic embolization of any thrombi that could adhere to the catheter, resulting in stroke, myocardial infarction, or other embolic phenomenon.

Equipment

Transvenous catheters have a variety of configurations of electrodes and shapes (Fig. 56-3). The catheters used for temporary pacing are bipolar. They are available with or without a balloon tip.[11,24] When placing catheters without fluoroscopy, the balloon facilitates placement of the catheter into the right ventricle.[13,21,24] Other catheter designs are for placement into the right atrial appendage or have an electrode arrangement with distal ventricular electrodes and proximal atrial electrodes to allow for dual-chambered pacing.[13,24] In emergencies concerns about dual-chambered pacing should not interfere with prompt, efficient placement of a lead into the ventricle. In patients whose condition is relatively stable dual-chambered pacing helps optimize hemodynamic status.[11]

Discussion of temporary pacing pulse generators follows later in this chapter.

Fluoroscopy greatly enhances the ease and likelihood of correct catheter placement. Use it either in a cardiac catheterization laboratory or by means of a portable C-arm unit in the Emergency Department or intensive care unit. Many pediatric cardiac catheterization laboratories have both anterior-posterior and lateral viewing, further enhancing ease of placement.

Techniques

Place transvenous pacing catheters from any major vein; however blind placement without fluoroscopy is difficult from the femoral veins. The right subclavian and right internal jugular veins are the preferred locations for placing the catheter. They allow placement of a permanent pacemaker from the left subclavian approach.

Make a slight curve several centimeters from the catheter tip to aid in passage into the right atrium and tricuspid valve. Advance the catheter into the vein through an indwelling transvenous sheath. Then if the catheter has a balloon, inflate it. Be careful to deflate the balloon when withdrawing the catheter from the ventricle to prevent injury to the tricuspid

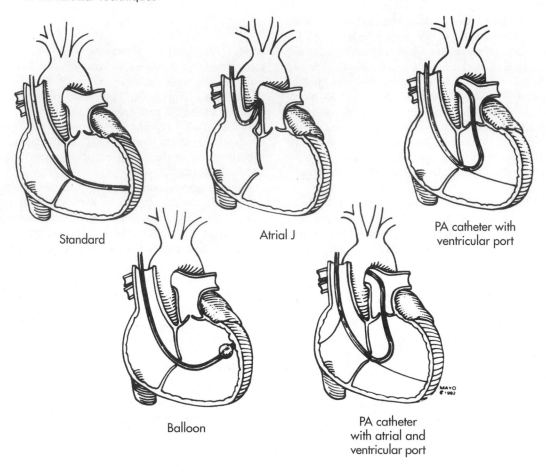

Standard

Atrial J

PA catheter with
ventricular port

Balloon

PA catheter
with atrial and
ventricular port

FIG. 56-3 A variety of pacing catheters are available. These diagrams demonstrate common varieties.

(Reprinted with permission from Furman S, Hayes DL, Holmes DR, editors: *A practice of cardiac pacing*, Mount Kisco, 1993, Futura.)

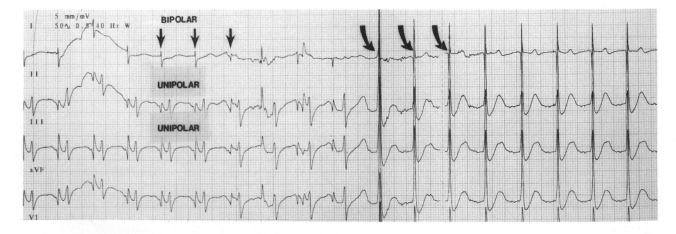

FIG. 56-4 Recording of electrograms during blind passage of a quadripolar pacing lead. The condition of the patient with intermittent bradycardia was too unstable for transfer to the catheterization laboratory to use fluoroscopy. Connect the distal two electrodes to the "right arm" and "left arm" leads on a standard electrocardiograph machine. This arrangement provides a bipolar electrogram in lead I and unipolar electrograms in leads II and III with hybridization of the electrograms in the remaining leads. The straight arrows indicate bipolar *atrial* electrograms where they align with atrial deflections in other leads. As the lead passes into the right ventricle, the sharp deflections, indicated by the curved arrows, become ventricular.

valve or chordal structures. Direct the catheter tip slightly to the left and anteriorly. If fluoroscopy is not available, connect one or both of the distal catheter connector pins (labeled as lead "D" or "1," and lead "2") to the "right arm" and "left arm" electrocardiogram leads, respectively. Also attach the "right leg" and "left leg" leads to the lower extremities, using only standard wet gel leads. Dried gel leads prevent the electrocardiogram machine from recognizing the pacing lead and indicating that leads are disconnected. When advancing the catheter, the electrocardiogram changes as the catheter passes from chamber to chamber.[13] Note large bipolar and unipolar atrial signals as the catheter moves through the right atrium (Fig. 56-4). This changes to large ventricular electrograms as the catheter enters the right ventricle. Observe the heart monitor for ventricular ectopy; once it appears, use small, twisting movements back and forth with the fingers and advance until encountering a *small* amount of resistance. Insert the distal electrode catheter pin (sometimes labeled "D" or "1") into the negative pin clamp on the pacemaker (Fig. 56-5). Place the proximal pin (sometimes labeled "2") into the positive pin clamp.

Begin pacing at high-output settings (10 mA) and test

thresholds. A discussion of threshold testing follows (see Temporary Pacemakers and Threshold Testing). Order a portable chest roentgenogram to verify the position of the catheter. The catheter tip should be toward the apex of the right ventricle (Fig. 56-6).

Once the position of the catheter is satisfactory after testing thresholds, secure the catheter and venous sheath to the skin with a clear adhesive dressing (Op-site, Tegaderm) (Fig. 56-7). It is important to secure the catheter to the skin *very well* so that movement of the catheter does not cause sudden loss of capture and hemodynamic consequences.

Remarks

If fluoroscopy is available, it is very beneficial in guiding catheters to the desired position. However, the urgency may

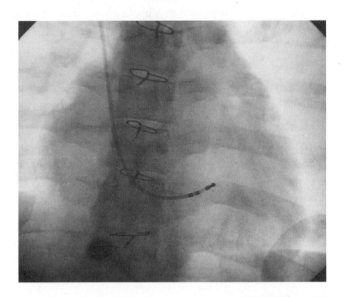

FIG. 56-6   Chest radiograph demonstrating the correct position of a temporary pacing catheter toward the apex of the right ventricle.

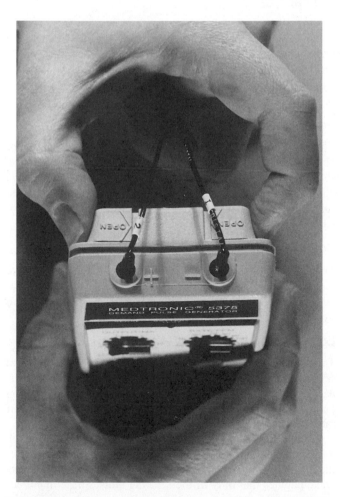

FIG. 56-5   Correct placement of the pacing catheter pins into the temporary pacemaker. The holes for pin insertion have spring-loaded push buttons to keep the pins in place. To insert the pins, squeeze these buttons and place the "D" or "1" pin into the negative hole. Place the pin marked "2" into the proximal hole.

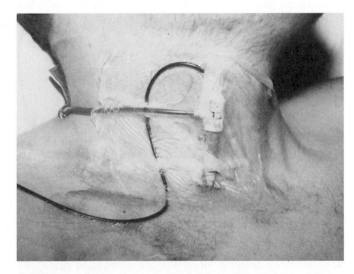

FIG. 56-7   Transvenous pacing lead in place through a venous sheath into the right internal jugular vein. The catheter tip is in the right ventricle. The pins on the other end of the catheter (not shown) attach to a temporary VVI pacemaker.

prohibit the time required to obtain and use fluoroscopy; do not delay the procedure to do so. Keep the patient on bed rest to minimize catheter movement.

Recheck pacemaker thresholds daily and set the power output at twice the threshold. If thresholds increase to unacceptable levels (i.e., less than half of the maximal pacing output), adjust the catheter, using fluoroscopic guidance to obtain acceptable thresholds.

ESOPHAGEAL PACING

Indications

Esophageal pacing is an easy way to achieve atrial capture because of ease of passage via the nose or mouth. Esophageal pacing is indicated in patients with sinus bradycardia or junctional escape rhythm *with intact AV conduction.* Esophageal pacing is also indicated as a backup pacing mechanism when patients undergo conversion of supraventricular arrhythmias (see Chapter 57).

Contraindications

Esophageal pacing is contraindicated in patients with atrioventricular conduction block. However it is possible to use esophageal atrial pacing in conjunction with temporary transvenous or epicardial ventricular pacing connected to a dual-chamber temporary pulse generator. It is not possible to pace patients who have had cardiac transplantation effectively via the esophagus since the new heart is sewn to the recipient's old atrial tissue that remains in front of the esophagus. There is no electrical conduction between old atrial tissue (recipient) and new atrial tissue (donor). Patients who have had recent nasal, facial, pharyngeal, or esophageal surgical procedures are at somewhat higher risk of perforation of a suture line with passage of an esophageal catheter.

Complications

Complications are rare for esophageal pacing. The most common associated problem is chest pain. However the pain is only present while pacing. As mentioned, perforation of nasal, facial, pharyngeal, or esophageal structures is possible in patients who have recently had surgical procedures in these areas.

Equipment

The pacing leads and stimulators are identical to those described in Chapter 57. For bradycardia pacing a stimulator that has programmable functions is unnecessary.

Techniques

Lead placement and electrical connections are the same as described in Chapter 57. Begin pacing power output at 9 to 10 ms and 10 mA. Gradually increase the current until achieving atrial capture. If the current is greater than 15 to 20 mA, consider the need for pain medication.

Remarks

Nasogastric or feeding tubes that are already in place can interfere with esophageal capture. Remove these tubes before placing an esophageal lead.

TRANSCUTANEOUS PACING

Consider transcutaneous cardiac pacing in children when emergency pacing is necessary.[4,16-18,24] The prognosis of patients who receive emergency transcutaneous pacing with severe bradycardia or asystole is poor. Rosenthal demonstrated that transcutaneous pacing achieved capture in only 11 of 21 patients with asystole.[19] None of these patients survived to discharge from the hospital and only 2 of 11 patients with severe bradycardia survived to discharge. In addition early application of transcutaneous pacing before the patient reached the hospital produced very few survivors.[6,7,18] Despite these dismal statistics, in controlled situations transcutaneous pacing has proved efficacious.[2,15,16] Therefore transcutaneous pacing is most useful when immediately applied, such as during an in-hospital arrest or bradycardic event. One of the advantages of this form of pacing is that the pacing patches do not interfere with chest compressions.[24] The main disadvantages include significant pain in patients who have maintained consciousness and less reliable capture in patients who are obese or who have increased thoracic capacity, pericardial or pleural effusions, or poor lead placement.[24]

Indications

Reserve this form of pacing for patients in very critical condition with severe bradycardia or asystole when unable to obtain large venous access. In addition attempt transcutaneous pacing when technical difficulties prevent correct placement of a transvenous catheter in patients with venous access.

Contraindications

The main contraindication to transcutaneous pacing is major chest trauma that precludes placement of the pacing patches. *Prolonged* asystole (>30 minutes) before pacing begins is a contraindication because of the low likelihood of a successful recovery even with initiation of effective cardiopulmonary resuscitation after the arrest.

Complications

Transcutaneous pacing can be painful to patients who have retained some level of consciousness.[1,16,24] This is particularly true with higher energy thresholds.[24] In addition local hyperemia under the patches may occur.[1]

Equipment

Transcutaneous pacing units and patches are available from several manufacturers (Zoll Medical, Physio-Control, Laerdal, Medac) that provide a pulse width of 20 or 40 ms and an output current of 0 to 200 mA depending on the model. Heart rate selection ranges from 30 to 180 beats/min.

Electrode size is important in that a larger electrode patch decreases the pain from muscle stimulation.[3] Several manufacturers produce pediatric-sized patches. Manufacturers make patches that only fit their pacing units. Some manufacturers provide a larger ground patch for the back than for the front. It is sometimes necessary to use standard electrocardiogram leads to monitor the patient's intrinsic rhythm.

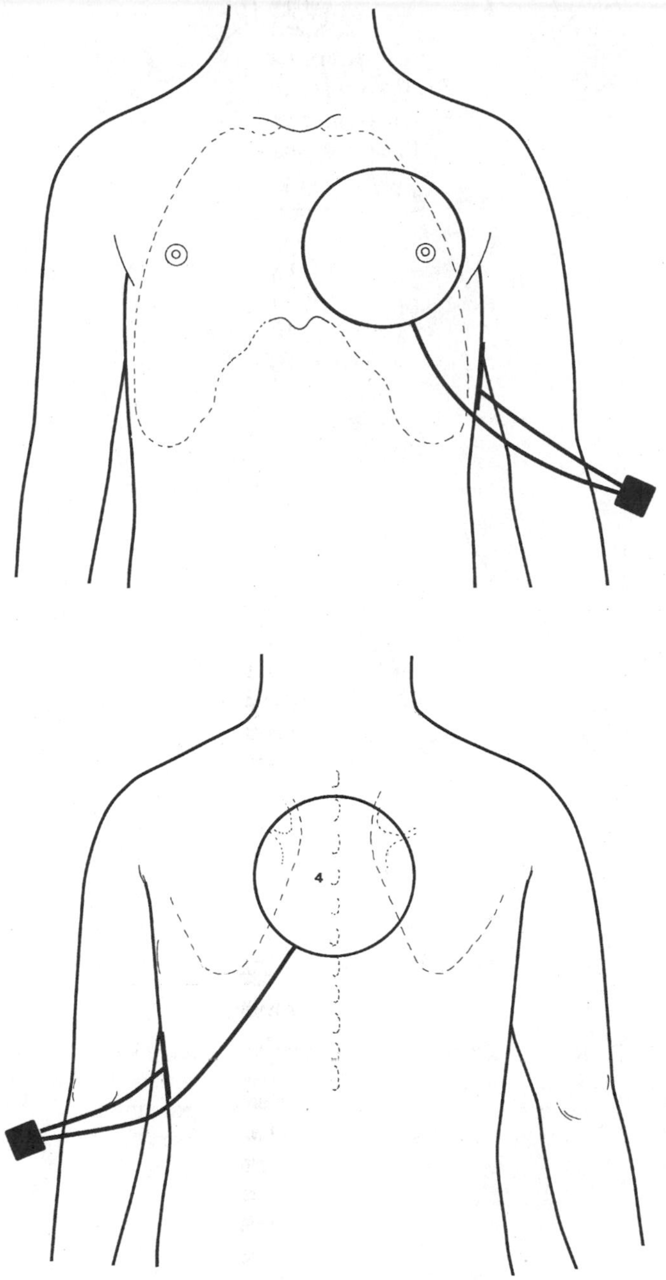

FIG. 56-8 Transvenous pacing patches in the optimal positions. **A,** Anteriorly place the patch in the electrocardiographic V₃ position. **B,** Posteriorly position the patch between the scapulae at the level of the fourth thoracic vertebral body. The two patches are joined by a plug that fits onto a cable from the pacing device.

Techniques

Select the appropriate size patch (pediatric vs. adult). Pediatric patients who weigh more than 15 kg can use the adult-sized patches.[4] If there is any doubt which size is appropriate, use the adult size because it lowers the impedance and current density despite a higher capture threshold.[4] Current density influences pain more than absolute output current.[4] Place one pacing patch on the left precordium in the V₃ electrocardiogram position.[19] Place the other patch pos-

teriorly in the region of the midscapula at the level of T₄ (Fig. 56-8). The wires from both patches are connected by a plug. Attach this plug to the cable from the pacing unit.

To begin pacing, select an output energy. For adult- or near-adult-size patients start with the maximum energy output, and then decrease it if ventricular capture occurs.[7,18,19,21] The mean threshold requirement in healthy adult volunteers is 65 to 81 mA.[3,8,12,14] In pediatric patients these values tend to be lower, but the threshold depends on the size of patch used.[4] Higher thresholds are likely to be present in patients with acidosis and with poor coronary circulation. Because of the difficulty in detecting capture,[19] confirm capture by either an arterial waveform tracing or a palpable pulse. If ventricular capture does not occur at maximal output, check to see that the patch placement is correct. A pericardial effusion may also interfere with capture.

Adjust the pacing rate according to age. Use normal to slightly higher than normal rates for age initially. Hemodynamic status may indicate the need for higher rates.

If transcutaneous pacing is successful, prepare for placement of a transvenous pacing catheter. Once this catheter is in place, discontinue transcutaneous pacing.

Remarks

Pain can be a limiting factor that determines success of transcutaneous pacing. If pain requires a reduction in the output current to a level below that required to capture the ventricle, then use medications to control the pain.

Acidosis may thwart ventricular capture; pursue correction of acidosis aggressively.

TRANSTHORACIC (TRANSMYOCARDIAL) PACING

Even beyond transcutaneous pacing reserve this form of pacing as the last resort to pace the ventricle. The procedure involves inserting a pacing catheter through the chest wall and into the right ventricle to achieve capture. If other pacing modalities have failed to provide an adequate heart rate or achieve ventricular capture, transthoracic pacing does not offer any greater ability to help the patient. White said that, despite mechanical capture in 33% of patients, there were no survivors.[23]

Indications

Only use transthoracic pacing in patients in desperate circumstances, and only after attempting other pacing modalities. One subset of patients who could potentially benefit from transmyocardial pacing are those with congenital heart disease who have undergone a Fontan-like operation. A Fontan procedure often isolates the right atrial chamber from the rest of the heart so that a transvenous pacing catheter does not pass into a ventricle from the venous system. Pacing using a catheter passed retrograde through the aortic valve is possible, but it is technically more difficult to place. This may be an indication for *emergency* transthoracic pacing.

Contraindications

Reserve this procedure for very rare circumstances that are extreme emergencies; therefore there are no absolute contraindications. However relative contraindications necessitate reevaluation of the possible benefit from this pacing mode in dire conditions. These include bleeding diatheses, septic shock, severe head or brain injury, and end-stage terminal diseases.

Complications

The potential for complications from transthoracic pacing is high as best demonstrated by Brown, who looked at injuries from transthoracic pacing attempts during autopsies in 20 patients.[5] They used six different approaches and all approaches demonstrated a significant incidence of trauma (15% to 100%) to structures in or around the heart besides the intended placement in the right ventricle. These injuries included perforations of the heart or nearby blood vessels, puncture of the lung or liver, and coronary artery laceration. In addition cardiac tamponade is a significant risk.

Equipment

Except for sterile preparation supplies the only equipment needed are a transthoracic pacing kit and a temporary pacemaker. The kit (Elecath, catalog number 11-KTM 1) includes a 6-inch, 18-gauge needle with stylet; a 34-cm bipolar pigtail pacing wire; and an electrical connector. Temporary pacing connector cables aid the connection from the pacing wire to the pacemaker.

A discussion of pacemakers and threshold testing follows later in this chapter.

Technique

Prepare the lower sternal area with sterile technique. Insert the introducer needle in the left xyphocostal angle at an angle of 30 degrees to the skin.[23] Aim the needle toward the left shoulder. After aspirating blood, advance the pacing wire through the needle into the right ventricle (Fig. 56-9). Slide the electrical connector onto the end of the pacing wire and fasten the plastic set screws. Attach the two plugs from the connector to the temporary pacemaker either directly or by using connector cables. Set the pacemaker at maximal output to see whether capture is present. If so withdraw the needle, leaving the pacing wire in place. Check the final position with a chest roentgenogram. Secure the pacing wire to the skin with a sterile transparent adhesive dressing. Keep the patient at bed rest.

TEMPORARY PACING WIRES AFTER CARDIAC SURGERY

Congenital heart defects requiring surgical repair pose a risk to the normal conduction system. In particular abnormalities such as ventricular septal defects, atrioventricular (AV) canal defects, and tetralogy of Fallot require placement of sutures close to the normal conduction system. With conduction system damage or destruction the resulting rhythm can range from sinus bradycardia to complete AV block with a very slow ventricular escape rhythm. These abnormalities can develop within the first 48 to 72 hours postoperatively. Edema in the region of the surgical repair often causes temporary dysfunction and AV block.

Postoperative arrhythmias are common in the pediatric

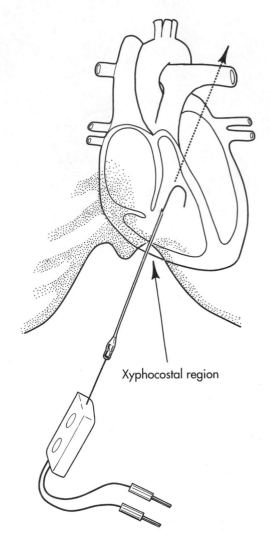

FIG. 56-9 Placement of a transthoracic pacing lead. Introduce the needle in the xyphocostal region pointed superiorly toward the left shoulder. Hold the needle securely and pass the pacing lead into the right ventricle. Remove the needle at this time. After capturing the ventricles secure the lead into place.

Xyphocostal region

population. Often it is difficult to make a precise diagnosis by surface electrocardiograms alone.

Temporary epicardial pacing wires placed during open heart surgical repair provide a means of increasing cardiac output in patients with bradycardic rhythms. Synchronous atrial and ventricular pacing provides a significant hemodynamic advantage[10,24] and affords precise atrial arrhythmia diagnoses.[22]

Indications

The surgeon should place atrial and ventricular epicardial wires in almost all pediatric patients having open heart surgery,[22] particularly those at higher risk for AV conduction problems or supraventricular arrhythmias such as junctional ectopic tachycardia. Although it is rarely necessary to use most wires, base the decision to use the temporary wires on the patient's hemodynamic status. Patients with arrhythmias also benefit because the wires are useful for both diagnosing and treating arrhythmias.

Contraindications

There are no absolute contraindications to temporary wires. Patients who seem to have fragile cardiac tissue, particularly in the atrium, may be at increased risk to lacerate the myocardium with wire removal, and therefore their placement may be contraindicated. Also patients with dense fibrous tissue from prior operations can experience difficulty in capturing the myocardium, but temporary wires may still be useful in diagnosis arrhythmias.

Complications

Problems caused by epicardial wires are rare.[22] Perhaps the most common is difficulty in removing the wires before discharge. Rarely complications such as perforations of the heart or fracture of the epicardial wire into a cardiac chamber can occur.[20] Anticoagulated patients require extra care when removing wires. Also epicardial wire stimulation thresholds tend to increase rapidly and may exceed the capacity of the temporary pacemakers to provide an adequate safety margin. If this should occur, consider placing a permanent pacemaker or transvenous pacing catheter.

Equipment

Wires for temporary epicardial pacing are available from several manufacturers (Medtronic, Ethicon). Temporary pacemakers are discussed later in this chapter.

Techniques

The surgeon places the wires at the conclusion of the heart operation, passing two atrial wires and one or two ventricular wires through the skin. If using only one ventricular wire, bury a second ground wire into the subcutaneous tissue. The wires exit the skin in standard locations so that one can know which wires are atrial and which are ventricular.[22] By convention the wires exiting the skin on the right side of the sternum are the atrial wires[22] (Fig. 56-10). The wires to the left of the sternum are the ventricular wires. When surgeons use a skin ground wire, they place it farthest to the left. Close inspection of the skin exit site or a chest radiograph can verify the location of wire attachment.

The wires have stainless steel terminal ends that easily fit into alligator clips or directly into the pacemaker. When pacing in a unipolar configuration, connect the wire attached to the myocardium to the negative terminal on the pacemaker. Attach the skin wire to the positive terminal. Begin pacing at high output settings (20 mA) and test thresholds. For a discussion of threshold testing, see Temporary Pacemakers and Threshold Testing. When it is unnecessary to use the wires immediately, wrap and tape them to the patient's abdomen.

Remarks

One can record atrial electrograms from the temporary wires. Use a standard electrocardiogram machine with liquid gel leads. After making a baseline recording, detach the right and left arm leads and connect the atrial wires to the leads to the machine. Record the atrial electrograms. Note sharp atrial

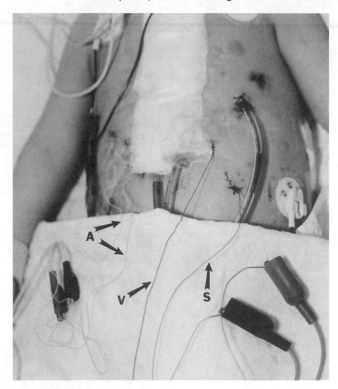

FIG. 56-10 Temporary epicardial wires in a postoperative cardiac patient. Note the position of the wires. The atrial wires (A) exit the skin on the patient's right side. A single ventricular wire (V) exits on the patient's left side. The wire farthest to the left (S) is a ground lead placed into the subcutaneous tissue. Attach both sets of wires to alligator clips and then attach to the temporary pacemaker.

electrograms among QRS complexes; use them to detect the underlying rhythm.

The surgeon should attach two atrial leads directly to the atrium (as opposed to one atrial and one skin ground) in order to provide dual-chamber pacing and accurate detection of bipolar atrial electrograms.

TEMPORARY PACEMAKERS AND THRESHOLD TESTING
Temporary pacemakers

A variety of temporary pacemakers that require nothing more than a 9-V battery for a power source are available. The simplest pacemaker is a single-chamber demand and inhibited form (AAI or VVI) (Fig. 56-11, *A*). For dual-chamber pacing one can use the DVI mode (paces both chambers, only senses the ventricle, inhibition occurs only with ventricular sensed events) (Fig. 56-11, *B*). Recently manufacturers released a new pacemaker that has full DDD function (paces and senses both chambers with appropriate inhibition on either channel) (Fig. 56-11, *C*). This allows sensing of the atrium; therefore the heart rate can reflect the hemodynamic status of the patient (e.g., increased rate with hypotension or hypovolemia). This also allows AV sequential pacing that optimizes cardiac stroke volume and output. One can use

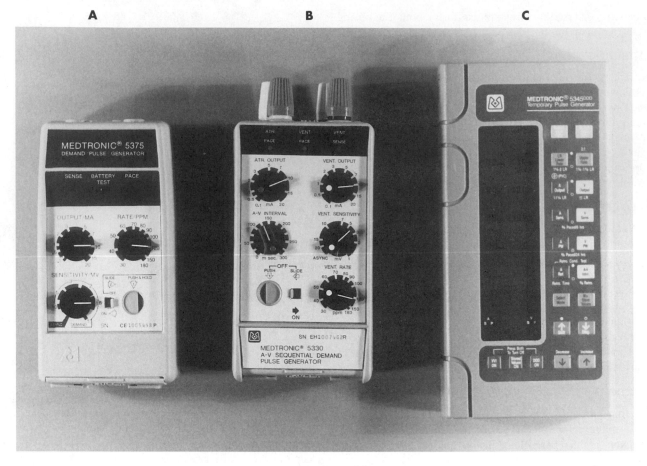

FIG. 56-11 Medtronic temporary pacemakers. **A,** Single-chamber pacemaker for use on atrial or ventricular leads or wires. This channel provides both pacing and sensing (AAI and VVI). **B,** Dual-chamber pacemaker programmed to the DVI mode with both atrial and ventricular leads or wires connected. This pacemaker paces the atrium and ventricle. It bases its timing on sensing from the ventricular channel; however the atrial channel cannot sense the atrium. With only ventricular leads or wires connected, the pacemaker works as a ventricular demand and inhibited pacemaker (VVI). By using the atrial leads or wires in the ventricular channel, it is possible to perform atrial demand and inhibited pacing (AAI). **C,** The dual-chamber pacemaker is programmable to a wide variety of modes. It can pace and sense from both the atrial and ventricular channels (DDD). This pacemaker has the added advantage of capacity to change the pulse width and refractory periods. In addition it can overdrive arrhythmias with high-rate atrial pacing.

these temporary pacemakers with transvenous, transthoracic, and epicardial pacing systems.

These pacemakers are not suitable for esophageal pacing. Esophageal pacing requires a much higher output to capture the atrium. Only a few stimulators that are available can provide enough output for this purpose (Medtronic, Bloom, Arzco). One can use these stimulators for the other pacing modalities mentioned, albeit with much lower settings.

Threshold testing

The pacing threshold is the minimal amount of energy, current, time, or amplitude required to cause the heart to contract with each pacing stimulus. In the single-chamber pacemaker and the DVI pacemaker the factory sets the pulse width and one cannot change it. It is also not possible to change the voltage amplitude; therefore only changes in the

current settings determine thresholds. On the DDD temporary pacemaker it is possible to control both pulse width and output current.

Procedure. Test temporary pacing systems at least daily, more often in patients who have poor underlying heart rates or evidence of elevated or rapidly increasing thresholds.

Before testing any pacing system, demonstrate the patient's underlying rhythm and use appropriate caution in patients with a very low underlying heart rate. *Do not* simply turn off the pacemaker. If suppression of the patient's underlying natural subsidiary pacemaker occurs, turning off the temporary pacemaker suddenly may result in prolonged asystole, giving the mistaken impression that the patient has no underlying rhythm. Instead program the pacemaker to the VVI mode at a rate similar to the current heart rate. To do this simply turn down the atrial current to zero on the DVI

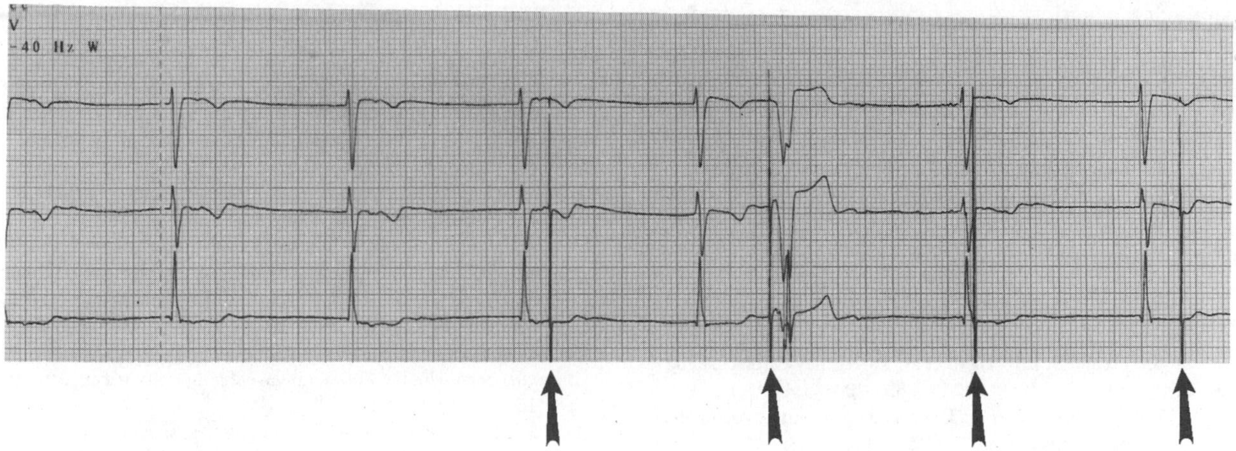

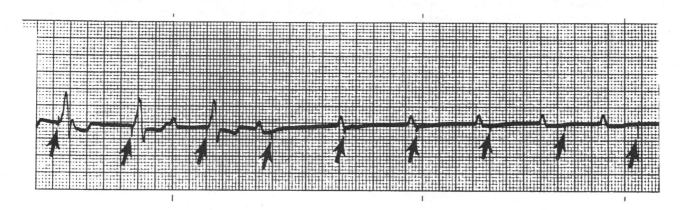

FIG. 56-12   Loss of sensing. Pacing artifacts (*arrows*) appear inappropriately after decreasing the sensitivity. There is no relationship between the pacing artifacts and the patient's intrinsic QRS complexes. To correct this problem, increase the sensitivity (decrease the number) on the pacemaker.

FIG. 56-13   Loss of capture. On the left side of this tracing, a QRS complex follows the first three pacing artifacts (*arrows*). On the right side of the tracing as the output energy decreases, QRS complexes do not follow the pacing spikes, indicating a loss of capture. Correct this problem by increasing the current or pulse width (increase the number).

pacemaker and reprogram the mode selection on the DDD pacemaker to VVI. When switching from DDD to VVI, select a lower rate limit that is similar to the patient's current atrial tracking rate to prevent a large heart rate drop. (In the DDD mode the lower rate limit may be 60 but the patient's intrinsic atrial rate may be 103. Because the DDD mode allows sensing of the atrium and triggering of the ventricle, the ventricular rate also is 103. Simply switching to VVI may result in a heart rate drop from 103 to 60. Instead switch to VVI at a rate of 100.) Slowly decrease the ventricular rate by 10 to 20 pulses/min every 10 to 15 seconds to allow the patient's autonomic system to adjust to the lower cardiac output. Check the patient to ensure that he or she is not becoming symptomatic and that perfusion has not significantly changed.

Once the patient's own QRS complexes appear, note the rhythm and decrease the sensitivity (make the number larger). When pacing spikes appear, the sensitivity threshold has been exceeded (Fig. 56-12). The sensing threshold is the lowest sensitivity (highest number) that still senses the ventricle. Set the sensitivity to twice threshold (half the number). If the patient's hemodynamic status is stable in the patient's underlying rhythm, test the atrial channel sensitivity in a similar manner by changing the DDD pacemaker to the AAI mode. The single-chamber and DVI pacemakers cannot sense atrial activity.

After testing sensitivity, increase the pacing rate to 20 to 30 pulses/min. Test the stimulation thresholds by slowly decreasing the output current until pacing spikes appear without corresponding QRS complexes (loss of capture) (Fig. 56-13). The lowest setting that still captures the ventricle is the threshold. Set the output at twice threshold.

Test atrial stimulation in a similar manner, but set the pacing rate higher than the *atrial* rate. Perform testing in the AAI, AOO, DOO, DDD, and DVI modes. Slowly turn down the atrial output until pacing spikes appear without corresponding P waves. Again the lowest setting that still captures the atrium is the threshold. Set the atrial output at twice threshold. Return the pacemaker to the desired mode and rate.

In summary a variety of temporary pacing methods are available in the intensive care setting. Transvenous pacing is the most reliable and safest, but performing it requires time and skill. Transcutaneous and transthoracic pacing are emergency and last-resort forms of pacing and carry a poor prognosis if not initiated within a few minutes of the bradycardic event. Temporary pacing wires are a reliable means for backup pacing in postoperative cardiac patients; they can also be used for diagnostic purposes.

REFERENCES

1. Altamura G, Toscano S, LoBianco, et al: Emergency cardiac pacing for severe bradycardia, Part II, *PACE* 13: 2038-2043, 1990.
2. Amar D, Gross JN, Burt M, et al: Transcutaneous cardiac pacing during thoracic surgery, *Anesthesiology* 79:715-723, 1993.
3. Bocka JJ: External transcutaneous pacemakers, *Ann Emerg Med* 18.1280-1286, 1989.
4. Beland MJ, Hesslein PS, Finlay CD, et al: Non-invasive transcutaneous cardiac pacing in children, *PACE* 10:1262-1270, 1987.
5. Brown CG, Gurley HT, Hutchins GM, et al: Injuries associated with percutaneous placement of transthoracic pacemakers, *Ann Emerg Med* 14:223-228, 1985.
6. Cummins RO, Graves JR, Larsen MP, et al: Out-of-hospital transcutaneous pacing by emergency medical technicians in patients with asystolic cardiac arrest, *N Engl J Med* 328:1377-1382, 1993.
7. Eitel DR, Guzzardi LJ, Stein SE, et al: Noninvasive transcutaneous cardiac pacing in prehospital cardiac arrest, *Ann Emerg Med* 16:531-534, 1987.
8. Falk RH, Zoll PM, Zoll RH: Safety and efficacy of noninvasive cardiac pacing, *N Engl J Med* 309:1166-1168, 1983.
9. Fitzpatrick A, Sutton R: A guide to temporary pacing, *Br Med J* 304:365-369, 1992.
10. Hartzler GO, Maloney JD, Curtis JJ, et al: Hemodynamic benefits of atrioventricular sequential pacing after cardiac pacing, *Am J Cardiol* 40:232-236, 1977.
11. Hayes DL, Holmes DR: Temporary cardiac pacing. In Furman S, Hayes DL, Holmes DR, editors: *A practice of cardiac pacing,* Mount Kisco, NY, 1993, Futura.
12. Heller MB, Kaplan RM, Peterson J, et al: Comparison of performance of five transcutaneous pacing devices, *Ann Emerg Med* 16:493, 1987.
13. Jafri SM, Kruse JA: Temporary transvenous cardiac pacing, *Crit Care Clin* 8:713-725, 1992.
14. Kaplan RM, Heller MB, Paris PM, et al: The effect of different combinations of external pacemakers and pads on pacing thresholds, capture rate, and patient tolerance, *Ann Emerg Med* 17:750, 1988.
15. Kelly JS, Royster RL, Angert KC, et al: Efficacy of noninvasive transcutaneous cardiac pacing in patients undergoing cardiac surgery, *Anesthesiology* 70:747-751, 1989.
16. Madsen JK, Meibom J, Videbak R, et al: Transcutaneous pacing: experience with the Zoll noninvasive temporary pacemaker, *Am Heart J* 116:7-10, 1988.
17. Noe R, Cockrell W, Moses HW, et al: Transcutaneous pacemaker use in a large hospital, *PACE* 9:101-104, 1986.
18. Quan L, Graves JR, Kinder DR, et al: Transcutaneous cardiac pacing in the treatment of out-of-hospital pediatric cardiac arrests, *Ann Emerg Med* 21:905-909, 1992.
19. Rosenthal E, Thomas N, Quinn E, et al: Transcutaneous pacing for cardiac emergencies, *PACE* 11:2160-2167, 1988.
20. Roth JV: Temporary transmyocardial pacing using epicardial pacing wires and pacing pulmonary artery catheters, *J Cardiothorac Vasc Anesth* 6:663-667, 1992.
21. Syverud SA, Dalsey WC, Hedges JR: Transcutaneous and transvenous cardiac pacing for early bradyasystolic cardiac arrest, *Ann Emerg Med* 15:121-124, 1986.
22. Waldo AL, MacLean WAH: *Diagnosis and treatment of cardiac arrhythmias following open heart surgery,* Mount Kisco, NY, 1980, Futura.
23. White JD, Brown CG: Immediate transthoracic pacing for cardiac asystole in an emergency department setting, *Am J Emerg Med* 3:125-128, 1985.
24. Wood M, Ellenbogen KA: Bradyarrhythmias, emergency pacing, and implantable defibrillation devices, *Crit Care Clin* 5:551-569, 1989.

57 Acute Treatment of Tachyarrhythmias

Christopher C. Erickson

Cardiac arrhythmias in children, particularly infants, can be asymptomatic or may lead to sudden death. The appearance of tachycardia or irregular rhythm on a patient's heart monitor in the Emergency Department (ED) or pediatric intensive care unit (PICU) necessitates prompt attention despite the absence of symptoms.

A variety of medications treat tachyarrhythmias either alone or in concert with techniques discussed later. This chapter discusses the indications, contraindications, potential complications, equipment, and techniques available to treat stable and unstable tachyarrhythmias as well as irregular rhythms. Section IX describes techniques and pharmacologic management of pediatric cardiac arrest rhythms.

VAGAL MANEUVERS

Supraventricular tachycardia (SVT) is the most common form of sustained symptomatic arrhythmia in infants and children.[2,21,38] It most frequently occurs as a reentry form involving an accessory pathway.[2,21,38] This provides a reciprocating circuit of depolarization between the atrium and ventricle, usually with the atrioventricular (AV) node providing a critical part of that circuit (Fig. 57-1). The term *reciprocating tachycardia* indicates this form of SVT. Since increased vagal tone can slow or even stop conduction through the AV node, techniques to increase vagal tone can easily and noninvasively terminate an episode of reciprocating tachycardia.* This is also true for AV nodal reentrant tachycardia that is seen in older children and adolescents. In patients whose condition is stable use these vagal maneuvers before more invasive techniques. In addition one can teach vagal maneuvers to parents and patients to help prevent prolonged episodes and ED visits.[39]

Vagal techniques include Valsalva's maneuver or abdominal pressure, rectal stimulation, carotid massage, gagging, administration of ipecac to induce vomiting, and facial immersion in cold water.[16,21,38] Facial immersion,[33] using a washcloth soaked in ice-cold water, or a bag filled with ice, is most effective in infants and small children.[6,16,21,38]

Indications

Vagal maneuvers are indicated in the following patients: children with stable, narrow QRS tachycardia (heart rate greater than expected with sinus tachycardia); patients with a tachyarrhythmia and a history of reciprocating tachycardia, even with a wide QRS complex; patients with a known bundle branch block in sinus rhythm that have tachycardia. Vagal maneuvers in general do not convert atrial flutter or fibrillation but may provide temporary slowing of the ventricular response to aid in the diagnosis of the arrhythmia;

they may also slow sinus tachycardia. Waxman described 9 of 15 ventricular tachycardia patients in whom vagal maneuvers produced conversion;[40] therefore although vagal maneuvers are not indicated as first-line therapy in known ventricular tachycardia, in the hemodynamically stable patient they may still have some role and are unlikely to pose risk.

Contraindications

The only absolute contraindication for these procedures is hemodynamically unstable tachycardia, when immediate direct current cardioversion is imperative.

Ocular pressure can cause an increase in vagal tone; however avoid using it because of the potential for eye injury.

Known tachycardias that result from automatic or ectopic mechanisms (atrial ectopic tachycardia, junctional ectopic tachycardia, and ventricular tachycardias displaying automatic behavior), as well as atrial flutter and fibrillation, do not respond to vagal maneuvers. However, the response to vagal stimulation may aid in diagnosing the arrhythmia.

Complications

Perform vagal maneuvers in almost any setting, particularly once the patient's history for reciprocating tachycardia is known.[6] However, there is a small risk of ventricular arrhythmias or severe bradycardia,[21] and therefore monitoring of a patient who is experiencing his or her first episode is advisable.

Use direct facial immersion, an iced washcloth, or an ice bag with infants cautiously to guard against aspiration during the maneuver.

Equipment

Except for a washcloth and iced water or an ice-filled bag, most vagal maneuvers require nothing more than patient cooperation. Manual manipulation for carotid massage, rectal massage, or abdominal pressure to create Valsalva's maneuver may be necessary in young children. The physician may require additional assistance to hold an infant to apply the facial immersion techniques. In rare instances syrup of ipecac may be necessary to induce vomiting and a strong vagal response.

Techniques

Ensure availability of oxygen and suction. Have intravenous (IV) equipment and perhaps IV needles available in case bradycardia develops. Hook the patient to an electrocardiography (ECG) machine and have a defibrillator and crash cart nearby. Monitor the patient with a running 3- or 6-lead electrocardiogram during the vagal maneuver, particularly for the patient's first episode of tachycardia.

Facial immersion techniques. There are several ways to apply a cold water stimulus to the face, including using a

---

*References 6, 16, 21, 32-34, 38, and 39.

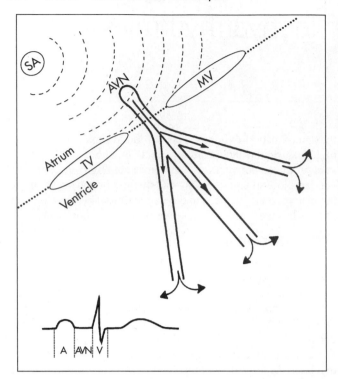

A

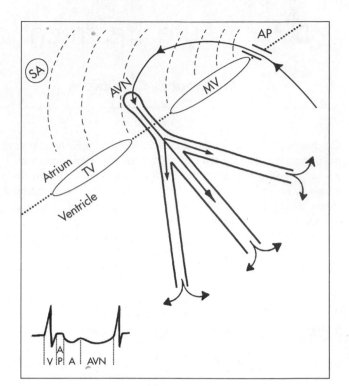

B

FIG. 57-1 Patterns of conduction. **A,** Sinus rhythm with conduction beginning in the sinus node, which causes sequential depolarization of the atrium, AV node, and His-Purkinje system, finally ending in the ventricles. **B,** Reentry tachycardia involving an accessory connection. Conduction from the atrium proceeds through the AV node, into the His-Purkinje system, and down to the ventricles. Conduction then continues as it returns retrograde to the atrium via an accessory connection. Finally it goes back to the AV node, beginning the sequence again in an endless loop or reciprocating manner. This is a reciprocating form of supraventricular tachycardia. **C,** AV nodal reentry tachycardia where the reentry circuit is entirely within the region of the AV node. For each time conduction completes the reentry circuit an impulse may fire to both the atria and ventricles simultaneously. A, Atrium; AP, accessory connection; AVN, AV node; MV, mitral valve; SN, sinus node; TV, tricuspid valve; V, ventricle.

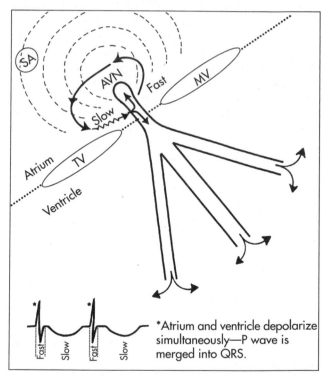

C

washcloth soaked in iced water or an iced-filled bag and physically immersing the child's face in iced water. Immersion of the child's face may work well in older children who can hold their breath; the risk of aspiration is greater in infants and toddlers.[6] Place a washcloth soaked in iced water or a bag filled with ice over the child's entire face until the tachycardia breaks, but for no more than 15 seconds[6] (Fig. 57-2). Cover both the mouth *and* nose. Straining of the infant against a closed airway can create Valsalva's maneuver simultaneously.

Valsalva's maneuver. Have the patient take in a deep breath and strain the abdominal muscles to increase intrathoracic pressure for 10 to 15 seconds. Releasing the strain and held breath increases systolic pressure, which, in turn, causes a vagal reflex that may stop the tachycardia[24,38,39] (Fig. 57-3). In younger, less cooperative children use abdominal pressure to create the same effect.[21]

Rectal massage. For infants insert a well-lubricated fifth digit into the rectum and massage the vault, while recording the rhythm strip. Enlist the assistance of a caretaker or medical provider to restrain the child gently.

Carotid massage. To perform carotid massage apply constant pressure on the area lateral to the thyroid cartilage just anterior to the sternocleidomastoid muscle for 5 to 10 seconds.[18,21] This technique works better in older children than in infants and toddlers.

Gagging. To elicit gagging, use a tongue depressor or culturette swab to touch or press lightly on the posterior oropharynx briefly.

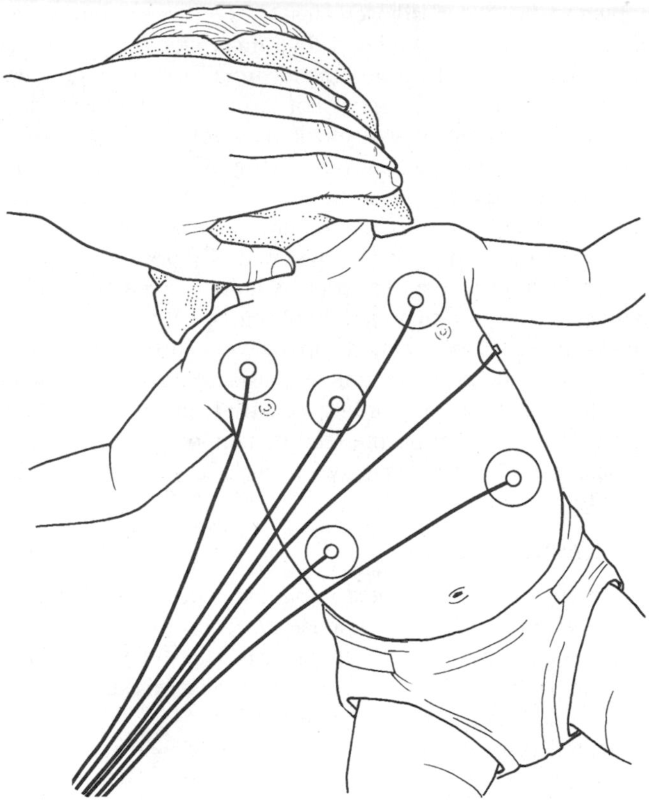

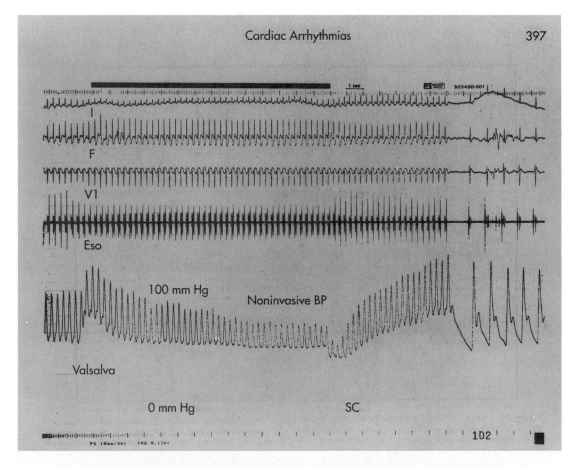

FIG. 57-2   Application of a washcloth soaked in ice water to the face of an infant to elicit a vagal response to stop tachycardia. When converting patients with an initial presentation of tachycardia, run a multichannel ECG rhythm strip while applying the washcloth. Cover the nose and mouth with the washcloth for no more than 15 seconds or until the tachycardia breaks. *ECG*, electrocardiogram.

Cardiac Arrhythmias 397

FIG. 57-3   Patient tracing of electrocardiogram, esophageal tracing, and plethysmography during Valsalva maneuver to stop supraventricular tachycardia. Note that tachycardia does not break until after a terminal rise in the blood pressure.

(From Walsh EP, Saul JP: *Nadas' pediatric cardiology,* Philadelphia, 1992, Hanley & Belfus.)

Remarks

Try vagal techniques three times before moving on to the next level of treatment, such as drug therapy, esophageal pacing, or direct current (DC) cardioversion. Older children may have already found that holding their breath can terminate most episodes; ask them to try these maneuvers before proceeding to more invasive methods.

ADENOSINE ADMINISTRATION
Introduction

Adenosine is one of the most important recent innovations to treat and diagnose arrhythmias. It has rapidly become the drug of choice for treating or diagnosing arrhythmias, particularly reciprocating tachycardia, because of its efficacy and safety. Adenosine has a more rapid onset of action than either digoxin or verapamil and is safe to give to infants, whereas verapamil has been associated with fatal outcomes.[16] In addition adenosine has an extremely short half-life as a result of its metabolism in blood.[9,23,27,30] This short half-life necessitates the use of a special procedure for administration.

One disadvantage of adenosine is that it often stimulates a reflex tachycardia after conversion. This tachycardia may produce another episode of AV nodal or reciprocating tachycardia.

Indications

Therapeutic. Adenosine is ideal for stopping reentry tachycardias that rely on the AV node for part of the reentry loop. Adenosine causes complete AV block that interrupts conduction and converts the patient's arrhythmia to normal sinus rhythm[9,23,25,27,30] (Fig. 57-4).

Diagnostic. Adenosine creates temporary AV block that can aid in diagnosis of other arrhythmias such as atrial flutter or fibrillation, atrial ectopic tachycardia, and junctional ectopic tachycardia. These may not terminate with adenosine. Increased or complete AV block may reveal classic flutter waves or atrial ectopic P waves[25] (Fig. 57-5). Atrial ectopic tachycardia may briefly stop, only to be followed by the characteristic "warm-up" as the tachycardia resumes.

Sinus tachycardia also slows with adenosine, then resumes. In cases where one suspects junctional ectopic tachycardia, but 1:1 ventriculoatrial (retrograde P wave) conduction is present, producing temporary AV dissociation with adenosine without disruption of the tachycardia helps confirm the diagnosis. Recording of atrial electrograms from either an esophageal pacing lead or temporary pacing wires in postoperative patients may be necessary to detect atrial activity.[25]

Contraindications

Adenosine is contraindicated in patients with unstable tachycardia when the time to prepare the dose may exceed the time to DC cardiovert the patient. It may also be contraindicated in patients with severe reactive airway disease because of possible bronchospastic properties.[9,11]

Several drug interactions have occurred with adenosine. Dipyridamole potentiates adenosine's effect,[9,27] whereas methylxanthines, such as theophylline and caffeine, antagonize it.[5] Because adenosine has vasodilating properties, use caution when administering it in the presence of vasodilating agents.[9,27] There are no contraindications to using adenosine in the presence of other antiarrhythmic agents including digoxin, verapamil, quinidine, flecainide, amiodarone, and disopyramide.[25,30,35]

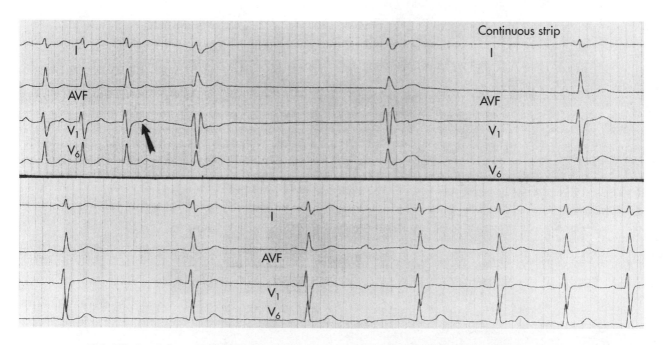

FIG. 57-4 Supraventricular tachycardia converted with adenosine. Note the termination of the tachycardia with a P wave indicating block in the AV node (*arrow*) followed by sinus arrest. The next two beats during sinus arrest are junctional escape beats. Paper speed is 25 mm/sec. AV, Atrioventricular.

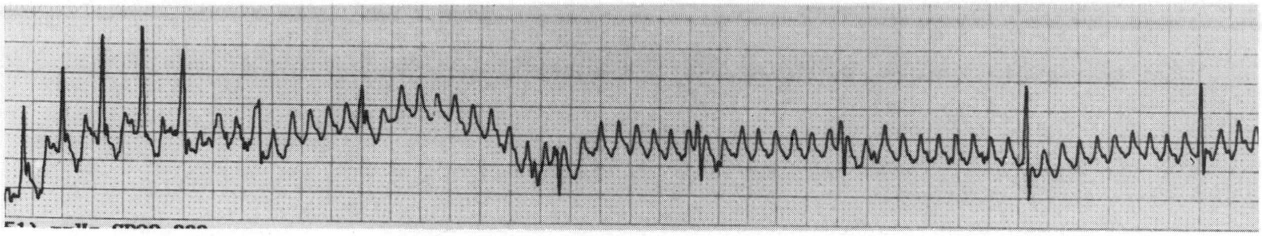

FIG. 57-5   Atrial flutter unmasked by adenosine. On the left-hand portion of the strip a narrow QRS tachycardia at 250 beats/min is visible but P waves are difficult to detect. With adenosine AV block reveals rapid atrial flutter waves at 500 beats/min but fails to terminate the arrhythmia. Paper speed is 25 mm/sec.

Complications

Several potential problems exist with adenosine administration. The greatest concern revolves around the possibility of inducing bronchospasm. The patients at greatest risk for potential problems are those with severe pulmonary disease, although some investigators have experienced no problems among this subset of patients.[5,11,25] Temporary vasodilation can occur as well.[9]

Equipment

The key to giving adenosine effectively is delivering the dose as a bolus quickly enough for it to reach the heart before being metabolized in the blood. To deliver the dose, use an intravenous line that is as proximal to the heart as possible. If possible, use a large-bore central venous line. For most patients in the ED, particularly infants, this may not be possible or practical. In school-age and older children an IV in the antecubital fossa is effective. In infants who have poor perfusion use *any* IV, although success may only occur with larger dosage.

Connect the IV directly to tubing with either a rubber diaphragm for medication administration or a stopcock close to the catheter (Fig. 57-6). Prepare a syringe of normal saline solution (5 ml for infants and toddlers, 10 ml for school-age and older children). Put the adenosine in a separate syringe.

Techniques

The proper initial dose of adenosine is 0.05 to 0.1 mg/kg up to a maximum single dose of 6 mg.[5,9,11,30,35] Increase subsequent doses to 0.15 to 0.2 mg/kg up to a maximum single dose of 12 mg and repeat as needed. It is available in a concentration of 3 mg/ml. Decrease the dose in patients receiving dipyridamole and increase it in those on methylxanthines.[5,9,27]

With the IV in place, insert the needles of both the adenosine syringe and the saline solution syringe through the rubber diaphragm of the IV connector (Fig. 57-6). Start a 3- or 6-lead rhythm strip. Clamp the tubing from the IV to the IV fluid bag to prevent retrograde injection of drug. Inject the adenosine with one hand, then immediately inject the saline solution with the other. Hold in the plunger on the adenosine syringe so that adenosine and saline solution do not reflux into the syringe.

Alternatively attach each syringe to a separate port on a stopcock or switch syringes on a single IV port. Although

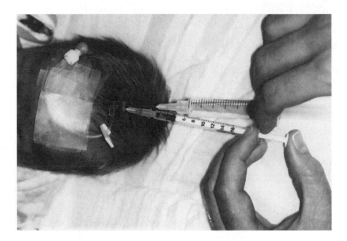

FIG. 57-6   Dual-syringe technique of adenosine administration through a heparin lock in an infant's scalp. Administer the adenosine (small syringe) first; follow with a rapid saline solution flush (large syringe).

these methods are effective, they are not as easy and any delay in switching stopcock directions or syringes raises concerns about partial metabolism of the adenosine dose before flushing of the bolus.

After delivering the dose a brief period of marked sinus arrest or completed AV block may follow. The adenosine effect only lasts for seconds and, in general, accelerated sinus or junctional escape rhythm, as well as premature atrial beats, follow. Occasionally reciprocating tachycardia may recur. Overholt reported a patient with severe sinus bradycardia after conversion that lasted 2 to 3 minutes and required temporary pacing.[25]

Remarks

Remove any air from both syringes to minimize the need for aspiration of blood back into the line.

The tachycardia and premature beats that frequently follow conversion of reciprocating tachycardia may precipitate other episodes of reciprocating tachycardia.[35] If this occurs after several doses of adenosine, use another drug, esophageal pacing, or elective DC cardioversion to terminate the tachycardia permanently.

ESOPHAGEAL RECORDING AND OVERDRIVE PACING

Introduction

Esophageal pacing has proved to be very effective for terminating supraventricular arrhythmias including reciprocating tachycardias and atrial flutter.* The proximity of the esophagus to the left atrium makes the technique of esophageal recording and pacing very easy (Fig. 57-7). The advantages of using an esophageal lead for treating arrhythmias include (1) confirmation of the diagnosis by observing atrial electrograms, (2) physiologic treatment of the arrhythmia without the side effects of medications, (3) ability to pace the heart if there is suppression of the sinus node and junction after termination of the tachycardia, and (4) ability to keep the lead taped in place when infants require repetitive conversion until drug levels are therapeutic.

Indications

Use esophageal pacing in the acute setting for the diagnosis and conversion of reciprocating tachycardias (SVT) and atrial flutter. It is also useful for backup pacing when one anticipates severe bradycardia after overdrive pacing or cardioversion of atrial arrhythmias.[22] Do not rely on esophageal pacing to pace bradycardia in patients who have advanced second- or third-degree AV block. However esophageal pacing with epicardial ventricular wires in postoperative cardiac patients can provide atrioventricular synchronous pacing if the necessary equipment is available.

Patients with postoperative junctional ectopic tachycardia caused by heart surgery may benefit from suppressing the tachycardia by pacing the atrium.[38] Atrial pacing with esophageal or epicardial atrial wires at a rate slightly faster than the junctional ectopic tachycardia can provide atrioventricular synchrony and improve cardiac output.

In addition cardiologists can use esophageal leads to induce reciprocating tachycardia for diagnosing the cause of palpitations and for drug testing.

Contraindications

Esophageal overdrive pacing is not effective in patients with known automatic tachycardias, such as atrial and junctional ectopic tachycardias or ventricular tachycardia.

There is no contraindication to using esophageal pacing with any medication, including digoxin.[22]

Esophageal pacing is contraindicated in patients who may have congenital anomalies of the esophagus (e.g., tracheoesophageal fistula).

Complications

Major problems with esophageal pacing are rare. When problems do occur, the most common is chest discomfort.[10,12,22,36] No major complications were reported, although Dick, et al.[12] described inhibition of ventricular pacing in a patient with a dual-chamber pacemaker who underwent esophageal pacing in an asynchronous mode for atrial flutter.

Occasionally attempts to treat atrial flutter may result in

---

*Reference 8, 10, 12, 13, 17, 34, 36, and 38.

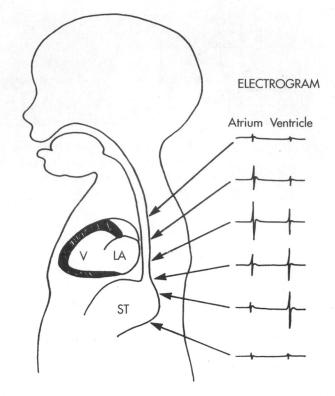

FIG. 57-7 Esophageal anatomy relative to the left atrium. The amplitude of the atrial and ventricular signals (electrograms) correlates with the depth of catheter insertion. *V*, Ventricle; *LA*, left atrium; *ST*, stomach.

(From Walsh EP, Saul JP; *Nadas' pediatric cardiology*, Philadelphia, 1992, Hanley & Belfus.)

conversion to atrial fibrillation. Dick, et al.[12] reported that three of eight patients with atrial flutter converted to atrial fibrillation briefly before spontaneously converting to sinus rhythm.[12] Three other patients converted to atrial fibrillation or a faster flutter and required direct current cardioversion. One patient converted to SVT. Gallagher reported induction of ventricular tachycardia after rapid atrial pacing in two of four patients with ventricular tachycardia.[14] Benson, Campbell, and Gallagher have reported patients in whom esophageal leads produced ventricular, rather than atrial, pacing.[3,10,14]

Equipment

Leads. The esophageal lead is bipolar (two electrodes); a soft, pliable material, such as silicone, encases it.

Many esophageal leads are actually endocardial pacing leads designed for permanent atrial pacing in the coronary sinus (Medtronic No. 6992, 6992A, 6902, 6904A, or 6901R). Because they are silicone and they have a tapered end with 29-mm (6992), 28-mm (6901R), 22-mm (6904A), or 15-mm (6992A and 6902) electrode spacing, they have provided excellent atrial electrograms with minimal discomfort in patients of all sizes (Fig. 57-8).

Other companies also make bipolar leads especially for esophageal pacing and recording (Arzco, Elecath). The Arzco 4 French esophageal lead (TAPCATH) has 13-mm electrode spacing and is ideal for infants because it is possible to tape it into place for patients who need repetitive

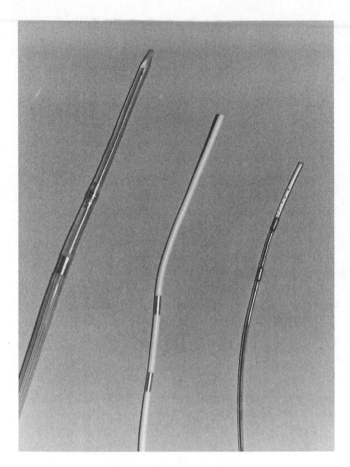

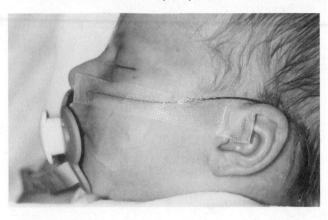

FIG. 57-9   Infant with an esophageal lead taped in place for easy overdrive pacing for recurrent reciprocating tachycardia. The catheter can stay in place for several days when beginning drug therapy. The lead is well tolerated by infants, and they can feed while it is in place.

FIG. 57-8   Esophageal bipolar recording and pacing catheters. On the left is a Medtronic coronary sinus lead (model No. 6992A) used for esophageal pacing in patients of all sizes. In the middle is a catheter made by Elecath. On the right is an esophageal pacing catheter (Arzco 4 French TAPCATH) that is ideal for infants, for whom leaving the catheter in place is desirable.

overdrive pacing of tachycardia while beginning drug therapy (Fig. 57-9). Arzco also makes a pill electrode (TAPSUL) with 13-mm spacing that is a suitable alternative in older patients who can swallow a pill.

Attach the lead to either an electrocardiogram or a pacing box with a standard temporary pacing connecting cable.

Recording Device. Record atrial electrograms either on a standard ECG machine (preferably the multichannel strip type) or a multichannel physiologic recorder. Record leads I, AVF, V_1, and V_6 simultaneously at a minimum.

Attach the standard ECG leads, using either standard gelled leads or ECG lead paste. Newer dried gel leads do not allow for proper recording from the esophageal lead because of differences in lead resistance that the recorder interprets as a detached lead.

Electronic Stimulator. Several companies make stimulators either suitable for or manufactured for esophageal pacing (Medtronic, Inc., Arzco Medical Electronics, and Bloom Associates) (Fig. 57-10). Esophageal pacing requires higher pulse widths and pulse currents to achieve capture of the left atrium.[4,12,14] Esophageal stimulators have a pulse width range up to 10 ms and an output current up to 20 mA. Use a programmable stimulator that can provide premature

stimuli, as well as constant and rapid atrial pacing. This feature allows reinduction of tachycardia for drug testing and for later study of the mechanism of the tachycardia.

Techniques

Placement of Lead. In conscious patients use sedation to place the lead. Infants do well with midazolam (Versed) 0.1 mg/kg intranasally into each of the nares (total dose = 0.2 mg/kg). Sedate older children with a combination of narcotic for pain and either a benzodiazepine or an antihistamine, such as promethazine or hydroxyzine, for sedation.

Placement of the lead to the correct depth aids in capture of the left atrium. Benson et al. demonstrated a correlation between patient height and minimal pacing capture threshold[4] (Fig. 57-11). Measure the lead depth from the distal electrode and place tape on the lead to mark the correct depth, as determined from Fig. 57-11. Coat the tip of the lead with viscous lidocaine and then insert it into one of the patient's nares. Advance the lead to the tape marker. Asking the patient to swallow several times aids placement of the lead. Then connect to the lead to the recorder. Determine the ideal depth, that is, that with the maximal atrial electrogram (electrical signal from atrium), by slowly advancing and withdrawing the lead. When the electrograms are optimal, tape the lead to the patient's face and make a recording of the electrogram and surface ECG (Fig. 57-12). Then connect the lead to the stimulator with a standard temporary pacing cable.

Overdrive Pacing. For pacing to be of value, atrial capture (atrial contraction response to the electric impulse) must occur. The minimum energy requirement for atrial capture is the threshold. This can be difficult to determine if the patient is already in tachycardia. For esophageal pacing use a pulse width of 10 ms. Start the output current at 8 mA and progressively increase until capture occurs. Adjust the output current for overdrive pacing slightly above the threshold value, keeping in mind that significant discomfort can occur at currents higher than 15 mA.[3,14]

Before pacing start the recorder. To perform conversion of reciprocating tachycardia, place single or double premature impulses into the tachycardia, timed from the sensed

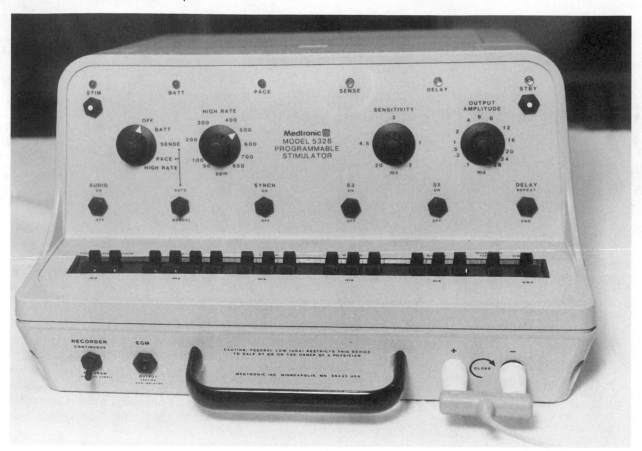

FIG. 57-10 Programmable stimulator used for esophageal overdrive pacing (Medtronic, Inc., model No. 5328). This stimulator can provide many extra stimuli with a long pulse width and wide range of output currents.

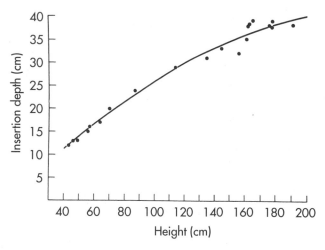

FIG. 57-11 Relationship of patient height to ideal insertion depth for an esophageal pacing catheter. Patients less than 60 cm had esophageal depths measured from the mouth to the distal electrode. Patients more than 60 cm had depths measured from the nares.

(From Benson DW et al: Transesophageal atrial pacing threshold; Role of interelectrode spacing, pulse width and catheter insertion depth, Am J Cardiol 53:63, 1984.)

atrial electrograms (Fig. 57-13). If this fails, use short bursts of atrial pacing for up to 10 seconds at 10 to 80 ms less than the tachycardia cycle length to terminate the tachycardia[12,17,36] (Fig. 57-14). Decrease the pacing cycle length by 10 ms or increase the length of the burst each time until the tachycardia breaks.

Atrial ectopic tachycardia does not terminate with overdrive pacing. Only very brief pauses in atrial activity occur, followed by rapid resumption of the tachycardia (Fig. 57-15).

Perform overdrive pacing for atrial flutter by using burst pacing. Each burst should begin 30 to 50 ms less than the flutter cycle length. The duration of each burst should be 1 to 10 seconds, beginning at 15 mA.[8,10,13] Decrease each successive burst by 10 ms and/or the duration of the burst.

Remarks

Detecting atrial capture can be difficult. The pacing artifact distorts the baseline, making P wave detection difficult. One way to detect atrial capture is to note conduction of the QRS complexes. More rapid atrial pacing should change either the ventricular rate or conduction to the ventricles.

For patients with reciprocating tachycardia who have had recurrent episodes of tachycardia after administration of adenosine or other medications tape the esophageal lead to the patient's face so that it is available for repeat esophageal pacing as needed. Once successful chronic therapy has begun, remove the lead.

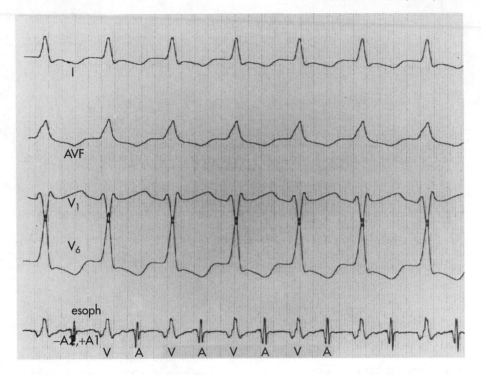

FIG. 57-12   Reciprocating tachycardia with leads I, AVF, V$_1$, V$_6$, and an esophageal electrogram. A, Atrial electrogram; *esoph,* esophageal lead; V, ventricular electrogram.

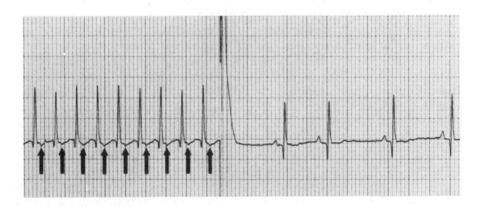

FIG. 57-13   Reciprocating tachycardia in lead III terminated with a single premature paced beat. Arrows show the retrograde P waves. Note that sinus recovery is not prolonged. Paper speed 25 mm/sec.

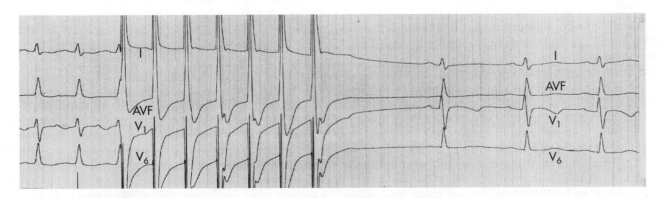

FIG. 57-14   Esophageal overdrive pacing of reciprocating tachycardia to sinus rhythm. Minimal sinus bradycardia is present. Scale: 4 cm = 1 second.

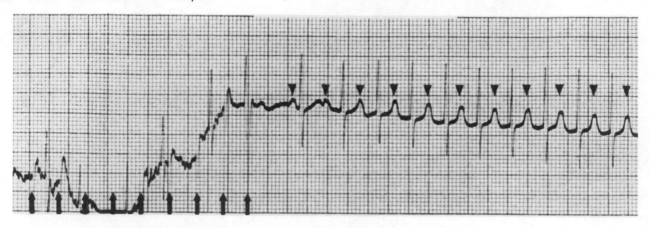

FIG. 57-15 Esophageal overdrive pacing in a patient with atrial ectopic tachycardia. Arrows indicate esophageal pacing spikes. Arrowheads demonstrate resumption of atrial ectopic tachycardia after momentary slowing in the tachycardia.

Atrial flutter often requires longer bursts to be successful. However, it is best to start with short bursts.

DIRECT CURRENT CARDIOVERSION AND DEFIBRILLATION
Introduction

The delivery of direct current for cardioversion of many tachyarrhythmias is one of the most effective and rapid forms of treatment.[21,22,41] According to the American Heart Association/American College of Cardiology/American College of Physicians Task Force on Elective Direct Current (DC) Cardioversion is the delivery of precisely timed electrical energy to the heart to convert an organized, but abnormal, rhythm to one that is more hemodynamically ideal. In contrast defibrillation is the delivery of a random high-energy shock to a heart that has ventricular fibrillation.[41,42]

Ventricular fibrillation is rarely the presenting rhythm of a pulseless and apneic child.[31,37,42] Even among patients with congenital heart disease it is uncommon, and it is even more rare in infants.[31,37] Losek showed that defibrillation for an asystolic rhythm produced a rhythm change in only 10 of 49 (20%); resuscitation was successful in only 3 of these 10, and none survived.[20]

Indications

Base the decision to use direct current to treat an arrhythmia on two factors: (1) the hemodynamic status of the patient and (2) the type of arrhythmia.

Hemodynamically unstable rhythm. It is not essential to know the precise rhythm diagnosis for patients in whom tachyarrhythmias are obviously causing significant hemodynamic compromise. Direct current cardioversion is first-line therapy in all patients with moderate to severely unstable tachyarrhythmias, including narrow QRS tachycardias.[42] This is particularly true when the nature of the tachyarrhythmia is unknown and the delay required to make an exact electrocardiographic diagnosis or to prepare medications may cost valuable time. On the other hand if the arrhythmia is hemodynamically stable, take time to analyze the arrhythmia for clues to guide therapy and to prepare appropriate antiarrhythmic medications.

Assess the stability of a patient's condition with an arrhythmia by evaluating the level of consciousness, systemic blood pressure, distal perfusion, and systemic oxygenation.[41] An infant with a wide QRS tachycardia who is alert and has a systolic blood pressure of 60 mm/Hg with mild diaphoresis may not require cardioversion as first-line therapy. However perform immediate cardioversion on an 8-year-old with a narrow QRS tachycardia who is syncopal and has a systolic blood pressure of 50 mm/Hg with poor capillary refill and cool extremities.

Type of arrhythmia. Many arrhythmias respond to cardioversion. These include supraventricular and ventricular tachycardias with reentry mechanisms such as those involving an accessory pathway (Wolff-Parkinson-White), AV nodal reentry tachycardia, atrial flutter, and ventricular tachycardia associated with myocardial damage (e.g., cardiomyopathy, repair of congenital heart disease).[21,22,33,41] Atrial flutter and fibrillation may respond to medical conversion, although it is not unusual for these arrhythmias to be refractory and require DC cardioversion.[7,15,28] Of course ventricular fibrillation requires immediate conversion with direct current.[20,42] Automatic or ectopic arrhythmias (atrial ectopic tachycardia, junctional ectopic tachycardia, and automatic ventricular tachycardia) are not treatable by cardioversion.

Contraindications

The contraindications for cardioversion are mostly relative, including conditions that are stable but that, if left unaltered, may eventually deteriorate.

Digoxin lowers the fibrillation threshold. Cardioversion of a patient on digoxin may rarely result in ventricular fibrillation. Therefore administer IV lidocaine, 1 mg/kg, before cardioversion.[21,28] Suspected or documented digoxin toxicity contraindicates elective cardioversion until serum levels fall into a therapeutic range or symptoms resolve.[22,41]

Another relative contraindication to cardioversion is chronic atrial fibrillation because clots may have formed on the atrial wall. Atrial thrombi may dislodge and embolize at the time of the first coordinated atrial beat after conversion.

Radford reported that 3 of 35 pediatric patients with atrial fibrillation had cerebral embolism.[29] Short-term systemic anticoagulation (3 weeks) is indicated before elective cardioversion.[28,41]

Complications

Although there are few lasting effects of DC cardioversion, serious complications can result. New and sometimes more serious arrhythmias may develop. In addition progressively higher delivered energy produces a greater incidence of myocardial damage.[26] This is also true for shocks that are close together in time.[26] Box 57-1 lists some of the complications of cardioversion. Moak provides an excellent review of the literature about problems following cardioversion that are beyond the scope of this chapter.[22]

Equipment

Perform direct current cardioversion or defibrillation with a standard defibrillator. Newer models may feature lower power outputs to accommodate lower energy requirements for atrial arrhythmias in children (Fig. 57-16). Several features available on defibrillators are particularly important for pediatric patients, including ability to select lower energy outputs, R wave synchronization, easy switching to pediatric or infant paddles, on-screen monitoring and paper recording, and portability. The ability to change from standard paddles to electrode patches is helpful during elective cardioversions.

BOX 57-1   COMPLICATIONS OF CARDIOVERSION

Tachyarrhythmias

Atrial fibrillation
Supraventricular tachycardia
Ventricular tachycardia
Ventricular fibrillation

Bradyarrhythmias

Sinus arrest or bradycardia
Atrioventricular block
Bundle branch block

Myocardial damage or necrosis

Depression of Ventricular function

Embolic phenomenon

Adapted From Moak JP: Electrical treatment of arrhythmias. In Garson A, Bricker JJ, In *The science and practice of pediatric cardiology*, Philadelphia, 1990, Lea & Febiger.

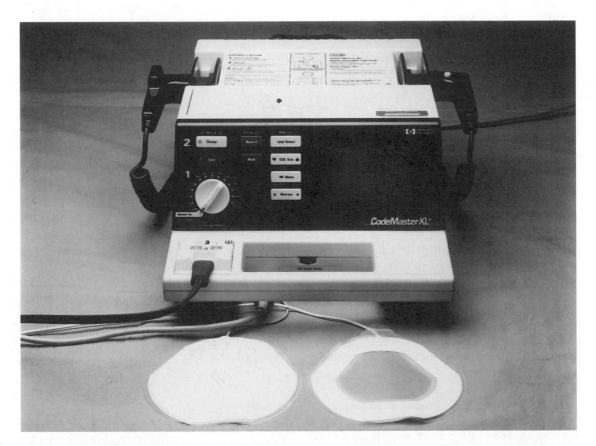

FIG. 57-16   Standard hospital defibrillator. Pediatric defibrillators should have a selection of low-energy outputs and synchronization available. Standard paddles mount on the sides of the defibrillator. In front are the defibrillator patches to apply before elective cardioversion and connect to the defibrillator unit.

During elective cardioversions run a simultaneous six-lead rhythm strip with leads I, II, III, AVF, V$_1$, and V$_6$, for more accurate assessment of the success of each energy application, particularly with atrial fibrillation and atrial flutter. With emergency arrhythmias a single-lead monitor screen is adequate.

Determine the size of electrode paddles by the size of the patient. Atkins demonstrated a much lower transthoracic impedance when using adult-size paddles and recommended their use when the size of the child's chest allowed for adequate contact, at about 10 kg or 1 year of age.[1]

Techniques

Emergency cardioversion or defibrillation. For patients who have life-threatening arrhythmias cardioversion should follow an efficient sequence of events *after* airway and ventilation are ensured.

First decide whether the arrhythmia is ventricular fibrillation or not. This should be easy to detect on any monitor and dictates whether synchronized cardioversion is indicated. *If the patient is in ventricular fibrillation, the defibrillator does not discharge while in the synchronized mode.* Treat all other arrhythmias with *synchronized* cardioversion to prevent the development of more malignant arrhythmias. In an occasional patient with ventricular tachycardia with an attempt at synchronization the defibrillator is unable to identify the QRS and thus does not fire. When synchronization is not possible, asynchronous cardioversion is permissible.

Second, select the energy level. For emergency arrhythmias begin with 1 J/kg. If this setting is not successful, double the setting for a repeat shock.

Next apply electrode jelly or paste to the paddle surfaces, rubbing each paddle with the other to spread it completely and evenly. Do not use alcohol pads. Saline-solution-soaked gauze may cause solution to drip from one paddle to the other and result in arcing current.

At this point apply the paddles directly to the skin. Place one paddle near the base of the heart and the other near the apex (see Fig. 57-17, *A*).

Charge the paddles by pressing the *charge* button on one of the paddles or on the defibrillator. Make sure that all personnel do not have direct contact with the patient or the bed. Then deliver the energy by pressing the button at the top of each paddle simultaneously.

Finally check the monitor for the rhythm that returns after energy delivery. Be ready for any rhythm from severe bradycardia to ventricular fibrillation. If the first charge was in the synchronized mode, be sure to switch to unsynchronized if ventricular fibrillation is the return rhythm.

Elective cardioversion. Performing elective cardioversions in the catheterization laboratory or PICU after the patient has ingested nothing for 6 hours is ideal. Have an IV

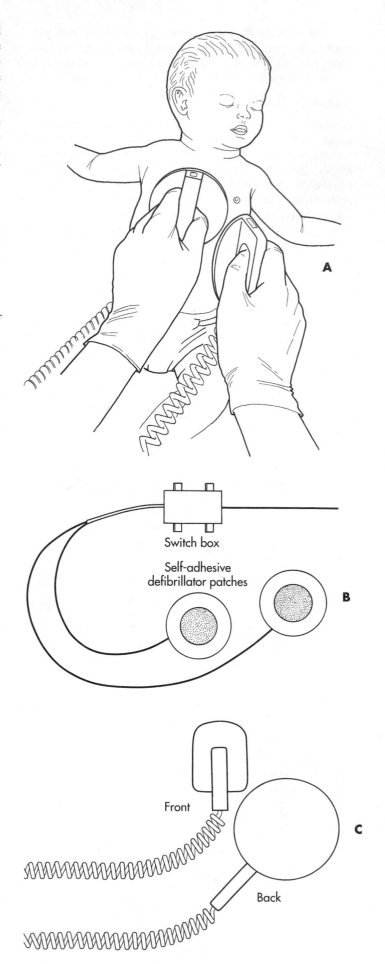

FIG. 57-17 Methods of delivering direct current. **A,** Standard defibrillator paddles applied to the sternum and the apex of the heart. **B,** Self-adhesive defibrillator patches with a switch box to deliver the charge. **C,** Defibrillator paddles including one designed for placement on the back with the other standard paddle over the left precordium.

in place and consider using general anesthesia administered by an anesthesiologist. This guarantees total anesthesia and amnesia with a physician dedicated to watching the patient's airway and breathing pattern. Use very short-acting anesthetic agents such as propofol or methohexital so that the patient can recover complete consciousness in 5 to 10 minutes. For patients in whom general anesthesia is unavailable or too risky use conscious sedation with the aid of an anesthesiologist, if available. Use ketamine 0.5 to 1 mg/kg IV or diazepam 0.1 mg/kg IV if no anesthesiologist is available.[22] Have a pediatric crash cart at hand.

Prepare to perform esophageal or intravascular pacing if the return rhythm may be significant bradycardia. Administer lidocaine 1 mg/kg IV if the patient is on digoxin. Attach a multichannel ECG recorder and run it continuously during energy delivery.

Select the method of delivering the energy. Traditional paddle placement is near the base and apex of the heart (Fig. 57-17, A). An alternative method is delivery of current in an anterior to posterior direction by placing a specialized back paddle (which requires electrode gel or paste) just inferior to the left scapula and a standard defibrillator paddle over the left precordium (Fig. 57-17, B). Alternatively one can place pregelled defibrillation electrode patches (Cardiotronics, Hewlett-Packard Company, R2 Medical Systems, Inc., Zoll Medical Corporation) in the same positions (Fig. 57-17, C). These pads are made in adult and pediatric sizes.

Select the desired energy dose. Moak suggests using an initial dose of 0.25 to 0.5 J/kg for atrial arrhythmias and an initial dose of 0.5 to 1.0 J/kg for ventricular tachycardia.[22] Double the doses if unsuccessful.

Make sure the defibrillator is in the synchronized mode. Always use synchronization for elective cardioversion. However if the return rhythm is ventricular fibrillation, turn off the synchronization to deliver the next charge.

Proceed from this point with the steps outlined for emergency cardioversion or defibrillation.

Remarks

Transthoracic impedance falls with firm contact and after the first shock.[19] This means that the heart receives more energy on subsequent shocks.

Consider the patient's acid-base status as well as any electrolyte abnormalities. Hypokalemia, hypoxia, and acidosis may reduce the likelihood of converting an arrhythmia.[19,42]

Spread electrode gel or paste over the entire paddle surfaces to prevent skin burns. However, do not spread gel or paste on the skin in the area that lies between the two paddles to prevent arcing of the electric current.[42] Skin burns may result even with proper application of electrode gel or paste. If they do, hydrocortisone cream may help promote healing and relieve irritation.

REFERENCES

1. Atkins DL, Sirna S, Kieso R, et al: Pediatric defibrillation: importance of paddle size in determining transthoracic impedance, *Pediatrics* 82:914-918, 1988.
2. Benson DW, Dunnigan A, Benditt DG: Follow-up evaluation of infant paroxysmal atrial tachycardia: transesophageal study, *Circulation* 75:542-549, 1987.
3. Benson DW Jr, Dunnigan A, Sterba R, et al: Atrial pacing from the esophagus in the diagnosis and management of tachycardia and palpitations, *J Pediatr* 102:40-46, 1983.
4. Benson DW Jr, Dunnigan A, Benditt DG, et al: Transesophageal atrial pacing threshold: Role of interelectrode spacing, pulse width and catheter insertion depth, *Am J Cardiol* 53:63-67, 1984.
5. Berul CI: Higher adenosine dosage required for supraventricular tachycardia in infants treated with theophylline, *Clin Pediatr* 32:167-168, 1993.
6. Bisset GS, Gaum W, Kaplan S: Theice bag: A new technique for interruption of supraventricular tachycardia, *J Pediatr* 97:593-595, 1980.
7. Bjerkelund C, Orning OM: An evaluation of DC shock treatment of atrial arrhythmias: immediate results and complications in 437 patients, with long-term results in the first 290 of these, *Acta Med Scand* 184:481-491, 1968.
8. Butto F, Dunnigan A, Overholt ED, et al: Transesophageal study of recurrent atrial tachycardia after atrial baffle procedures for complete transposition of the great vessels, *Am J Cardiol* 57:1356-1362, 1986.
9. Camm AJ, Garratt CJ: Adenosine and supraventricular tachycardia, *N Engl J Med* 325:1621-1629, 1991.
10. Campbell RM, Dick M, Jenkins JM, et al: Atrial overdrive pacing for conversion of atrial flutter in children, *Pediatrics* 75:730-736, 1985.
11. Clarke B, Till J, Rowland E, et al: Rapid and safe termination of supraventricular tachycardia in children by adenosine, *Lancet* 1:299-301, 1987.
12. Dick M, Scott WA, Serwer GS, et al: Acute termination of supraventricular tachyarrhythmias in children by transesophageal atrial pacing, *Am J Cardiol* 61:925-927, 1988.
13. Dunnigan A, Benson DW, Benditt DG: Atrial flutter in infancy: diagnosis, clinical features, and treatment, *Pediatrics* 75:725-729, 1985.
14. Gallagher JJ, Smith WM, Kerr CR, et al: Esophageal pacing: a diagnostic and therapeutic tool, *Circulation* 65:336-341, 1982.
15. Garson A Jr, Bink-Boelkens M, Hesslein PS, et al: Atrial flutter in the young: a collaborative study of 380 cases, *J Am Coll Cardiol* 6:871-878, 1985.
16. Garson A Jr: Medicolegal problems in the management of cardiac arrhythmias in children, *Pediatrics* 79:84-88, 1987.
17. Gikonyo BM, Dunnigan A, Benson DW: Cardiovascular collapse in infants: association with paroxysmal atrial tachycardia, *Pediatrics* 76:922-926, 1985.
18. Josephson ME: Sinus node function. In *Clinical cardiac electrophysiology*, Philadelphia, 1993, Lea & Febiger.
19. Kerber RE, Jensen SR, Gascho JA, et al: Determinants of defibrillation: prospective analysis of 183 patients, *Am J Cardiol* 52:739-745, 1983.
20. Losek JD, Hennes H, Glaeser PW, et al: Prehospital countershock treatment of pediatric asystole, *Am J Emerg Med* 7:571-575, 1989.
21. Ludomirsky A, Garson A Jr: Supraventricular tachycardia. In Garson A Jr, Bricker JT, McNamara DG, editors: *The science and practice of pediatric cardiology*, Philadelphia, 1990, Lea & Febiger.
22. Moak JP: Electrical treatment of arrhythmias. In Garson A Jr, Bricker JT, McNamara DG, editors: *The science and practice of pediatric cardiology*, Philadelphia, 1990, Lea & Febiger.
23. Moak JP: Pharmacology and eletophysiology of antiarrhythmic drugs. In Gillette PC, Garson A Jr, editors: *Pediatric arrhythmias: electrophysiology and pacing*, Philadelphia, 1990, WB Saunders.
24. O'Laughlin MP, McNamara DG: Syncope. In Garson A Jr, Bricker JT, McNamara DG, editors: *The science and practice of pediatric cardiology*, Philadelphia, 1990, Lea & Febiger.
25. Overholt ED, Rheuban KS, Gutgesell HP, et al: Usefulness of adenosine for arrhythmias in infants and children, *Am J Cardiol* 61:336-340, 1988.
26. Patton JN, Allen JD, Pantridge JF: The effects of shock energy, propranolol, and verapamil on cardiac damage caused by transthoracic countershock, *Circulation* 69:357-368, 1984.
27. Pelleg A: Adenosine in the heart: its emerging roles, *Hosp Pract* 28:71-99, 1993.
28. Porter CJ: Atrial flutter and atrial fibrillation. In Garson A Jr, Bricker JT, McNamara DG, editors: *The science and practice of pediatric cardiology*, Philadelphia, 1990, Lea & Febiger.

29. Radford DJ, Izukawa T: Atrial fibrillation in children, *Pediatrics* 59:250-256, 1977.

30. Reyes G, Stanton R, Galvis AG: Adenosine in the treatment of paroxysmal supraventricular tachycardia in children, *Ann Emerg Med* 21:1499-1501, 1992.

31. Schoenfeld PS, Baker MD: Management of cardiopulmonary and trauma resuscitation in the pediatric emergency department, *Pediatrics* 91:726-729, 1993.

32. Sperandeo V, Piero D, Palazzolo P, et al: Supraventricular tachycardia in infants: use of the diving reflex, *Am J Cardiol* 51:286-287, 1983.

33. Sreeram N, Wren C: Supraventricular tachycardia in infants: response to initial treatment, *Arch Dis Child* 65:127-129, 1990.

34. Sugrue DD, McLaran C, Hammill SC, et al: Refractory supraventricular tachycardia in the neonate: treatment with temporary antitachycardial pacing, *Mayo Clin Proc* 60:169-172, 1985.

35. Till J, Shinebourne EA, Rigby ML, et al: Efficacy and safety of adenosine in the treatment of supraventricular tachycardia in infants and children, *Br Heart J* 62:204-211, 1989.

36. Twidale N, Roberts-Thomson P, Tonkin AM: Transesophageal electrocardiography and atrial pacing in acute cardiac care: Diagnostic and therapeutic value, *Aust NZ J Med* 19:11-15, 1989.

37. Walsh CK, Krongrad E: Terminal cardiac electrical activity in pediatric patients, *Am J Cardiol* 51: 557-561, 1983.

38. Walsh EP, Saul JP: Cardiac arrhythmias. In Fyler DC, editor: *Nadas' pediatric cardiology,* Philadelphia, 1992, Hanley & Belfus.

39. Waxman MB, Wald RW, Sharma AD, et al: Vagal techniques for termination of paroxysmal supraventricular tachycardia, *Am J Cardiol* 46:655-664, 1980.

40. Waxman MB, Wald RW, Finley JP, et al: Valsalva termination of ventricular tachycardia, *Circulation* 62:843-851, 1980.

41. Yurchak PM, Williams SV, Achord JL, et al: Clinical competence in elective direct current (DC) cardioversion: a statement for physicians from the AHA/ACC/ACP task force on clinical privileges in cardiology, *Circulation* 88:342-345, 1993.

42. Zaritsky A: Cardiopulmonary resuscitation in children, *Clin Chest Med* 8:561-571, 1987.

PULMONARY TECHNIQUES

58 Respiratory Monitoring

Karl H. Karlson, Jr.

Hospitals generally monitor respiration by measurement of impedance across the chest wall. *Impedance* is a measure of those factors that oppose the flow of current through a conductor. In the human body resistance is the major component of impedance, although the capacitance created by cell membranes may contribute a small amount to the total thoracic impedance. Changes in the thoracic impedance are proportional to changes in thoracic volume.[2,4] The monitors process these measured changes in impedance electronically so that they produce the respiratory pattern on the monitor along with a digital display of the respiratory rate. Most respiratory monitors in the Emergency Department (ED) or pediatric intensive care unit (PICU) are modular parts of complete systems for cardiopulmonary monitoring.

Indications

The indications for respiratory monitoring include any illnesses in which information about the respiratory rate and pattern is necessary. Monitoring for central apnea or hypopnea (shallow respiration) as well as respiratory rate is possible with impedance monitors.

Contraindications

The only contraindication for such monitoring is any skin lesion that would preclude the placement of electrodes.

Equipment and Techniques

There are many brands of monitors on the market and most do not require calibration when connecting a patient for monitoring. Begin monitoring by placing the electrodes just inferior to the nipples on the chest wall (Fig. 58-1) after cleaning the skin to ensure good contact. Appropriate positioning of the electrodes is important to obtaining reliable data.[1] After connecting the leads to the monitor, select alarm parameters to match the child's clinical status.

Remarks

Although the concept of impedance across a body surface appears simple and evaluation has shown that detection systems are relatively reliable,[5] the actual measurement is complex. As a result both false alarms and missed events occur (see Table 58-1).[3] Cardiac oscillations can deform the thorax enough to be mistaken for breaths by the detection circuits of the monitor, and it is possible to miss true apnea. False alarms in the absence of apnea are most commonly associated with loose leads, positional changes, and shallow breathing (particularly in small infants) that is not detectable because of the limits of the sensitivity of the monitor.

Table 58-1 Causes of False and Missed Alarms

False alarms	Missed alarms
Loose leads	Obstructive apnea
Poor position	Cardiogenic oscillations
Shallow breaths	
Motion artifact	

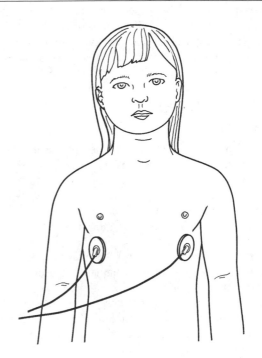

FIG. 58-1 Place electrodes just inferior to the nipples on the chest walls.

REFERENCES

1. Baird TM, Goydos JM, Neuman MR: Optimal electrode location for monitoring the ECG and breathing in neonates, *Pediatr Pulmonol* 12:247-250, 1992.
2. Baker LE, Geddes LA, Chaput CJ: Physiological factors underlying transthoracic impedance variations in respiration, *J Appl Physiol* 21:1491-1499, 1966.
3. Brouillette RT, Morrow AS, Weese-Mayer DE et al: Comparison of respiratory inductive plethysmography and thoracic impedance for apnea monitoring, *J Pediatr* 111:377-383, 1987.
4. Olson T, Victorin L: Transthoracic impedance, with special reference to newborn infants and the ratio air-to-fluid in the lungs, *Acta Pediatrica Scand* 207(suppl):1-57, 1970.
5. Wilson AJ, Franks CI, Freeston IL: Algorithms for the detection of breaths from respiratory waveform recordings of infants, *Med Biol Eng Comput* 20:286-292, 1982.

59 Flexible Fiberoptic Bronchoscopy

George B. Mallory, Jr. and Paul C. Stillwell

The flexible fiberoptic bronchoscope has become an essential tool for specialists who care for infants and children with respiratory disease.* Before 1981, access to the intrathoracic airways of most pediatric patients for inspection, therapeutic intervention, or diagnostic testing required the use of a rigid bronchoscope under general anesthesia in the operating room. This technology was generally the province of the surgical subspecialist. Compared to the rigid bronchoscope, the flexible fiberoptic bronchoscope has the advantage of permitting the examination of the entire airway without distorting airway anatomy and, because the patient is breathing spontaneously, in the presence of near-normal transmural pressures (Table 59-1).[29] Bronchoscopy in the pediatric population is most useful on an elective basis for diagnosis of a variety of chronic airway and lower respiratory disorders.[12,42] For the acutely ill child, access to the airway for diagnosis and therapy via the flexible fiberoptic bronchoscope is helpful in a number of clinical scenarios.[10]

Indications

The list of indications for flexible fiberoptic bronchoscopy in pediatric patients is long (Box 59-1). The two most common broad indications at present are suspected abnormalities of airway anatomy and severe pneumonia. Reviews of the standard indications exist in detail elsewhere.[10,12,38,42] Box 59-2 lists indications which are most likely to arise in the critically ill or injured child.

Airway anatomy. Inspection of airway anatomy is often indicated in patients with unexplained acute or progressive chronic respiratory failure.[28,34] Extrathoracic airway obstruction is an uncommon primary cause of respiratory failure in infants and children. The presence of pharyngeal obstruction during sleep causing obstructive sleep apnea is an important clinical entity and may contribute to respiratory failure in patients with neuromuscular disease [33] and chronic obstructive pulmonary disease. It may be the primary pathogenetic mechanism of disordered gas exchange in patients with craniofacial disorders[17] and in some children with massive tonsils and adenoids.[22] Flexible fiberoptic bronchoscopy can define upper airway anatomy and determine the site of obstruction in these clinical scenarios. It is especially useful in patients with neuromuscular disease in whom dynamic airway collapse at different levels of the pharyngeal airway often occurs.

In an awake patient obstruction at or near the glottis may be acute and severe, as in epiglottitis, laryngotracheobronchitis, or bacterial tracheitis.[7] Generally, physical examination and plain radiographs of the airway define the pathology and guide therapy; thus bronchoscopy is avoided. There are some occasions when precise definition of the supraglottic, glottic,

and subglottic anatomy is indicated in an acutely ill child. Experienced personnel can safely perform flexible fiberoptic endoscopy with clarification of anatomic lesions, even in ill infants and children. Use extreme caution when examining the child with acute upper airway obstruction because acute mucosal swelling or acute laryngospasm may be life-threatening. Usually surgeons who are prepared to do an emergency tracheostomy should examine these children in the operating room under general anesthesia.

Vocal cord dysfunction often masquerades as severe unresponsive asthma.[5] If unrecognized, this condition leads to recurrent Emergency Department (ED) visits, prolonged and/or repeated hospitalization, and pediatric intensive care unit (PICU) stays. Differentiation from true asthma is usually possible by localization of the adventitious sounds over the laryngeal area and characteristic pulmonary function tests.[3,5] Laryngoscopy at the time of airway obstruction demonstrates adduction of the true and/or false vocal cords during both inspiration and expiration, leaving only a tiny posterior glottic opening. If the endoscopic examination occurs between episodes of severe airway obstruction, the laryngeal function is normal; the bronchoscopist can induce the vocal cord adduction by adverse imagery and hyperventilation in many patients. Many children with vocal cord dysfunction also have asthma, which adds to the diagnostic confusion, although it is uncommon for both to be active at the same time.[3] Treat vocal cord dysfunction by voice training, behavior modification, and relaxation techniques. It is poorly responsive to pharmacologic manipulation.

At times, intubated infants and children manifest respiratory symptoms of tracheal obstruction during mechanical ventilation or preceding extubation. Flexible fiberoptic bronchoscopy has been highly effective in defining distal airway pathology in this situation.[6,10,24,31] The potential variations in airway pathology are even greater in the pediatric patient with a tracheostomy tube.[44] In a tracheotomized patient it is possible to advance the flexible fiberoptic bronchoscope either through the tube or via the nasal route, permitting inspection of the larynx, the subglottis, the stoma (where granulation tissue commonly grows), and distal tracheal structures (Fig. 59-1).[38,42] When using the transnasal route, the physician can inspect the entire airway while maintaining effective ventilation through the tracheostomy tube. It is usually possible to pass the scope adjacent to the tracheostomy tube into the distal airway. After examination with the tube in place, the scope should be withdrawn carefully to inspect the stoma site further. In this way, the bronchoscopist can define airway pathology that might interfere with ventilation with the tube in situ or that might hinder decannulation. If airway pathology within the mid and distal trachea is the primary indication for bronchoscopy, pass the appropriate-sized instrument through the tracheostomy tube (or stoma with the tube temporarily removed). The patient's

---

*References 10,14,15,38, and 45.

Table 59-1   Comparison of Flexible and Rigid Bronchoscopy

	Flexible	Rigid
Advantages	Less airway trauma	Best optics
	Conscious sedation	Ventilating via sidearm
	Spontaneous breathing	Instrumentation with laser or forceps
	Dynamic changes	
	Peripheral view	
	BAL	
	Portable	
Disadvantages	Breathe around scope	General anesthesia
	No/small suction channel	Splinting airway open
		Central view only
		Higher cost

BAL, Bronchoalveolar lavage.

BOX 59-1   **COMMON INDICATIONS FOR PEDIATRIC FLEXIBLE FIBEROPTIC BRONCHOSCOPY**

Stridor
Hoarse cry
Wheezing unresponsive to bronchodilator therapy
Persistent cough
Lobar or whole lung emphysema
Suspected congenital airway anomalies
Obstructive sleep apnea
Proven or suspected recurrent aspiration
Hemoptysis
Parenchymal masses
Persistent, severe, or recurrent pneumonia
Bronchiectasis
Atelectasis
Airway trauma

BOX 59-2   **INDICATIONS FOR BRONCHOSCOPY IN THE CRITICALLY ILL CHILD**

Extrathoracic

Acute stridor
Postextubation stridor
Neck trauma
Compressing neck mass

Obstructive apnea
Acute hoarseness
Difficult intubation

Intrathoracic

Wheezing
  Unexplained
  Unilateral
  Poorly responsive
Pneumonia
  Very severe
  Compromised host
  Nosocomial
  Not responding to antibiotics
Mediastinal mass
Hemoptysis
Vague history of foreign body aspiration
Atelectasis (unresponsive)
Localization of endotracheal tube
Airway obstruction despite intubation or tracheostomy

---

size and respiratory status and the preference of the operator determines the choice of approach.

Some intubated pediatric patients require precise delineation of the location of the endotracheal or tracheostomy tube tip in relation to the carina; a chest radiograph may not be appropriate because of clinical urgency or the setting, such as a draped patient in the operating room.[10] With the ultrathin scope, this application to the critically ill neonate is now possible.[9,27,35,39] It is possible to maintain ventilation with insertion of an endotracheal tube suction adaptor in line to admit the scope. If the endotracheal tube is out of position, reposition it under direct vision.

Bronchoscopy often proves to be a valuable tool for the small subset of infants and children who pose difficult challenges for endotracheal intubation with the usual technique of direct laryngoscopy.[27] The context may be an elective procedure in the operating room or it may be an acute respiratory emergency elsewhere. Infants and children in this category have a variety of structural factors that may make adequate visualization of the glottis difficult. Such factors include micrognathia with or without anteriorly placed glottis[11,30]; macroglossia due to Beckwith-Wiedemann syndrome or mucopolysaccharidosis[41]; short, congenitally or surgically fixed

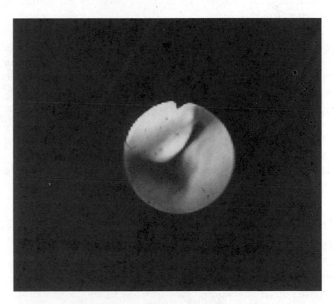

FIG. 59-1   Upper trachea with bronchoscope just above tracheostomy stoma. The tracheostomy tube is visible on the anterior wall (9 o'clock to 1 o'clock position).

cervical vertebrae preventing adequate neck extension; temporomandibular ankylosis[20]; unstable cervical vertebrae at risk of subluxation; and obscuring of the hypopharynx by trauma, edema, or acquired mass lesion.[2,36] In rare patients, such as a child with a massive mediastinal lymphoma, adequate ventilation may be difficult in the supine position because of gravitational forces compromising intrathoracic airway patency.

Another urgent indication for flexible fiberoptic bronchoscopy may be the presence of lobar or whole lung atelectasis refractory to standard ventilation, suctioning, and physiotherapy.[25] Infants and young children with severe or chronic pulmonary conditions are at highest risk for significant recalcitrant atelectasis. With the flexible fiberoptic bronchoscope, it is possible to inspect the airway, identify airway anomalies (if any), and visualize and aspirate mucus plugs. It maybe necessary to administer liquefying solutions, including normal saline, isotonic sodium bicarbonate, *N*-acetylcysteine, or DNase, through the suction channel to dislodge and remove plugs. At times results are dramatic, although efforts are not universally successful.

Pneumonia. Severe pneumonia is a cause of significant morbidity and mortality in the pediatric age group. Use of flexible fiberoptic bronchoscopy has increased for identifying a specific etiology.* Patients at greatest risk for opportunistic lung infection include children with human immunodeficiency virus infection, organ transplant patients (especially lung, heart-lung, and bone marrow recipients), patients with severe immunodeficiency syndromes, cancer patients on chemotherapy, and chronically intubated patients. Bronchoalveolar lavage (BAL) from a segment or subsegment of affected lung is the most common technique to obtain deep lower respiratory specimens in pediatric and adult patients. The suction channel of the Olympus BF3C10 is large enough to instill and collect BAL samples, but is too small for the currently available protected brush devices. BAL is usually satisfactory for diagnosing lower respiratory infections in pediatric patients.

Airway Foreign Body. Rigid bronchoscopy is the approach of choice in pediatric patients with foreign bodies in the airway. If the history is not convincing or if the aspiration event occurred in the remote past, the flexible fiberoptic bronchoscope may be the method for diagnosis (Fig. 59-2).[43] Upon discovering a foreign body in an infant or toddler, the bronchoscopist should consider terminating the procedure and arranging for removal by rigid bronchoscopy. Notify the appropriate surgeon promptly to execute definitive therapy. Rarely, in older children, it is possible to use a larger flexible fiberoptic bronchoscope with forceps removal of a foreign body.

Contraindications

The most important and common contraindication to flexible fiberoptic bronchoscopy is severe respiratory failure with clinical instability when the insertion of the bronchoscope, even through an endotracheal tube, is likely to worsen the patient's condition. This scenario is most common in infants with narrow-caliber endotracheal tubes. All contraindications to flexible fiberoptic bronchoscopy are relative; for each case, weigh the risk of the procedure against the risk of not obtaining the information available from the procedure.

Complications

In the stable child in a controlled setting, there are almost no serious complications of flexible fiberoptic bronchoscopy. The complications that do occur are usually minor and easy

*References 1,4,8,13,16,21,23, and 26.

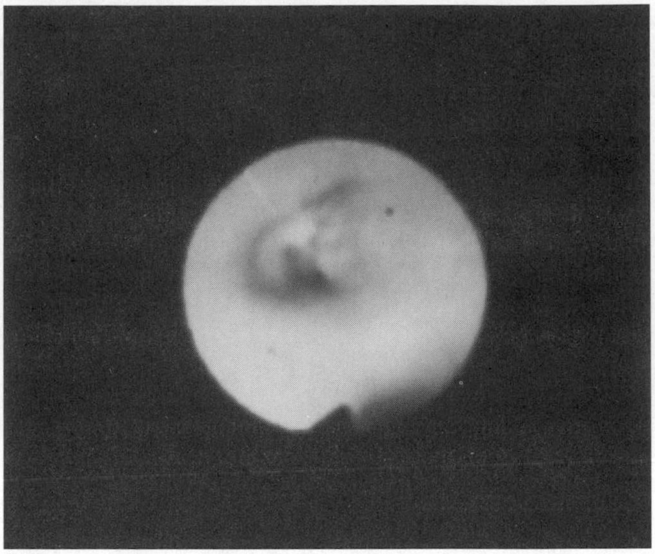

FIG. 59-2 Foreign body within the bronchus with surrounding granulation tissue.

BOX 59-3 RISKS AND COMPLICATIONS

Sedation

Allergic reaction
Hypoventilation
Inadequate for comfort
Idiosyncratic reaction

Trauma

Epistaxis
Airway edema
Perforation
Vocal cord avulsion
Pneumothorax

Mechanical

Laryngospasm
Hypoxemia
Atelectasis
Remote fever after bronchoalveolar lavage
Airway obstruction
Respiratory failure
Death

---

to handle (Box 59-3).[10,15,38,44] Recognition of potential complications in the more severely ill child should allow the bronchoscopist to prepare for them adequately and thus prevent or minimize them.

A significant proportion of the complications relate to sedative agents. Fortunately allergic reactions are rare, usually mild, and easily treated with antihistamines. Occasionally narcotics may produce a nonimmunologic release of histamine; the resulting local urticaria usually requires no therapy. More significant is hypoventilation, which is often avoidable by initially using small doses of short-acting drugs and repeating doses during the procedure as needed to provide adequate comfort. Hypoventilation is often transient. If associated with frank apnea or desaturation, manage it by assisted ventilation via anesthesia bag and face mask. Resume the procedure after spontaneous ventilation returns. It is rare that a child will require naloxone and/or flumazenil to reverse narcotic and benzodiazepine agents, respectively. A major advantage of using the combination of a narcotic and a benzodiazepine is that both are potentially reversible if hypoventilation occurs.

Equally problematic is inadequate sedation. Excessive coughing or struggling not only makes the procedure more difficult for the bronchoscopist, but increases the risk of airway trauma and damage to the equipment. The solution is carefully monitoring, titrating medication to effect, and promptly treating untoward side effects. Patients with a history of tolerance to benzodiazepines may benefit from the combination of ketamine and midazolam.

Minor epistaxis from the passage of the scope through the nasopharynx is common in small children. Bleeding usually stops spontaneously and does not generally interfere with the procedure. In patients who are at high risk for bleeding difficulties, obtain coagulation studies and a platelet count before the procedure. If necessary, correct laboratory abnormalities by exogenous agents to decrease the risk of bleeding. If the bronchoscopist is careful to keep the bronchoscope away from the airway walls, there should be minimal problems with edema. If the patient is uncooperative or coughs violently, airway trauma is common, but the usual residual injury is only mucosal petechiae. The bronchoscopist should not force the scope through areas of constriction and should never advance the bronchoscope without visualization of a clear path.

Adequate topical analgesia will usually avoid laryngospasm. Because the patients must breathe around the scope, transient partial large airway obstruction may cause hypoxemia, which is easy to treat with supplemental oxygen via oral or nasal route or through the suction port of the bronchoscope.[32] Limited focal atelectasis is common following bronchoscopy, especially with BAL, and usually resolves in a matter of hours. It rarely produces clinically significant deterioration, but patients are at risk, particularly if they have intrinsic pulmonary disease, for mild desaturation for 2 to 4 hours following bronchoscopy. Therefore, if a patient's oxygenation is marginal before the procedure, pay extra attention to his or her oxygenation during and following the procedure.

Approximately 50% of children will have a fever several hours following BAL. The fever generally requires no specific therapy and is self-limited. Anticipate such a fever to avoid an excessive evaluation.

Serious complications after pediatric flexible fiberoptic bronchoscopy are rare. Pneumothorax occurs almost exclusively in patients who undergo bronchoscopy while on positive-pressure ventilation with high inspiratory and expiratory pressures. In patients undergoing transbronchial biopsy, pneumothorax occurs in 1% to 2% of procedures. A small-caliber thoracostomy tube for 24 hours usually suffices to evacuate pleural air and permit healing. Respiratory failure caused by bronchoscopy, intravenous sedation, or BAL is rare. There is only one report of death following flexible fiberoptic bronchoscopy in a child.[40]

Equipment

The instruments available for flexible fiberoptic bronchoscopy in infants and children have evolved over the past 12 years. The most commonly used "pediatric" instrument over the past decade has been the Olympus BF3C4 or its newer models the BFC310 and BF3C20, all of which have a 3.5- to 3.7-mm outer diameter and a 1.2-mm suction channel. Another commonly used pediatric instrument is the Olympus BFN20 (or "ultrathin" scope) with a 2.2-mm outer diameter and no suction channel. Each instrument has wide angulation, permitting views of the apical segments of the upper lobes without difficulty. Many pediatric bronchoscopists also use the smallest adult-type instrument for procedures that require a larger suction channel. The Olympus PD10, PD20, and PD30 have an outer diameter of 4.9-mm and a 2.2-mm suction channel through which biopsy forceps can fit. Table 59-2 provides a comparison of currently available pediatric and small adult instruments.

Besides the bronchoscope itself, a suction outlet with tubing, a light source and a pulse oximeter are essential. In most situations, it is also advisable to monitor patients via continuous electrocardiography and frequent sphygmomanometry. Although not essential, photographic equipment, still or video, is ideal for documentation of findings (Fig. 59-3). A fully equipped resuscitation cart must be nearby. Keep oxygen and an anesthesia bag with an appropriate-size mask within easy reach during the procedure. The American Thoracic Society has recently adopted standards for pediatric flexible fiberoptic bronchoscopy.[15]

The patient's clinical state, the availability of equipment, and the judgment of the bronchoscopist determine the choice of setting for bronchoscopy. It is most common to perform the procedure in a designated procedure area. However, flexible fiberoptic bronchoscopy equipment is portable, and it is often preferable to perform the procedure at the bedside on the ward (usually only under special circumstances), in the ED or PICU, or in the operating room.

In addition to the bronchoscopist, there is need for at least two assistants, one responsible for the patient's clinical status (respiratory, cardiac, and anesthetic) and the other responsible for the equipment and related procedures (i.e., BAL and/or transbronchial biopsy). The personnel must be competent in patient monitoring, pediatric cardiopulmonary re-

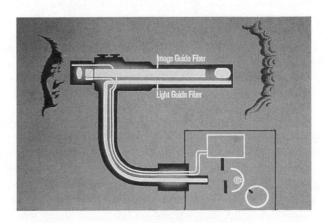

FIG. 59-3 Schematic view of bronchoscopic equipment.

Table 59-2 Bronchoscopic Equipment Used in Children

Manufacturer	Olympus	Olympus	Olympus	Pentax	Pentax
Model	BF3C10 BF3C20	BFP30 BFP20 BFP10	BFN20 BF	FB10X	FB15X
Outer diameter	3.5 mm	4.9 mm	2.2 mm	3.4 mm	4.8 mm
Diameter, second channel	1.2 mm	2.2 mm	—	1.2 mm	2.2 mm
Field of view	90°	100°	75°	95°	100°
Flexion	160°, 100°	180°, 100°	160°, 90°	180°, 130°	180°, 130°
Working length	550 mm	550 mm	550 mm	600 mm	600 mm
Smallest endotracheal tube	4.5	6	2.5 / 3	4.5	6
Age of use	Term infant and older	≥7 years*	Premature infant and older	Term infant and older	≥7 years*

* It is possible to bronchoscope younger patients safely with the larger instruments under special circumstances if a larger suction channel is necessary for instrumentation.

suscitation, administration of intravenous and topical medications, equipment care, and proper handling of specimens.[15]

Technique

Bronchoscopy. Carefully evaluate the patient's cardiopulmonary status before sedation and during the procedure itself. Review the child's history, physical state at the time of the bronchoscopy, relevant laboratory results (blood gas, Sao_2, spirometry) and radiographic findings. The bronchoscopist should define the specific goals of the procedure a priori. Communicate these goals to the parents, the patient (if age appropriate), and other members of the patient care team present.

A relaxed atmosphere is essential for preparing a child for flexible fiberoptic bronchoscopy. It is often desirable to allow parents in the procedure area, at least until the sedation of the patient is complete. The bronchoscopist should try to foster a quiet, pleasant environment for the procedure. Where possible, dim the lights. Developmentally adapted explanations are useful to minimize patient anxiety. A comfortable child in the company of trusted adults is easy to sedate with lower doses of medication than an anxious or stressed patient.

After baseline vital signs and oximetry, begin pharmacologic sedation (Table 59-3). Most patients will have intravenous lines in place. Do not use intramuscular sedation for bronchoscopy because of variable absorption, variable timing of sedation effect, and the difficulty titrating dose to effect with repeated injections.

In years past, bronchoscopists commonly used an intramuscular "lytic cocktail" of demerol, promethazine, and thorazine (DPT) for sedation. Most bronchoscopists have now abandoned this regimen, however, in favor of shorter-acting and more effective combinations of a narcotic and benzodiazepine given by the intravenous route.

The goal of sedation is to provide enough comfort for the bronchoscopy experience to be minimally uncomfortable while permitting adequate respiratory effort during scope insertion and manipulation within the airway. Many bronchoscopists consider agents such as benzodiazepines, which result in amnesia for the events, highly desirable. Intravenous sedation combined with topical anesthesia is successful in the vast majority of patients without undue side effects. Use

Table 59-3 Intravenous Sedating Agents for Flexible Fiberoptic Bronchoscopy

		Common initial dose
Narcotic	Fentanyl	1 µg /kg
	Meperidine	1 mg/kg
Narcotic antagonist	Naloxone	0.01 mg/kg (repeat if necessary)
Benzodiazepine	Midazolam	0.05 mg/kg
	Diazepam	0.1 mg/kg
Benzodiazepine antagonist	Flumazenil	0.02 mg (repeat if necessary)
Barbiturate	Methohexital	2-5 mg/kg
	Pentobarbital	1-3 mg/kg
Psychotropic	Ketamine	1-2 mg/kg

aerosolized lidocaine in a dose of 20 to 40 mg before sedation, then titrate intravenous midazolam and fentanyl to provide an adequate level of comfort to the patient (see also Chapter 12). The initial dose of midazolam is 0.05 to 0.1 mg/kg; slowly increase until clinical effect is adequate. The initial fentanyl dose is 1 µg/kg. Some bronchoscopists use meperidine in lieu of fentanyl, usually with an initial dose of 1 mg/kg. If further sedation is necessary, use additional doses of benzodiazepine and narcotic alternately.

Midazolam is an anxiolytic benzodiazepine with amnestic properties, whereas fentanyl is an analgesic with antitussive effects. Meperidine is similar to fentanyl, but has a longer pharmacologic half-life. A combination of midazolam and ketamine can be highly effective and appears to have a lower tendency to produce hypoventilation than midazolam and fentanyl. Table 59-3 lists other pharmacologic options.

After achieving initial sedation, further doses may be necessary, depending on the duration of the procedure. Most patients are awake within 1 hour of the end of the procedure if the bronchoscopist uses short-acting agents.

As a rule, place the patient in the supine position (Fig. 59-4). For the bronchoscopist's convenience, the procedure can be performed with the patient sitting or in the lateral decubitus position, if necessary. Just before insertion of the

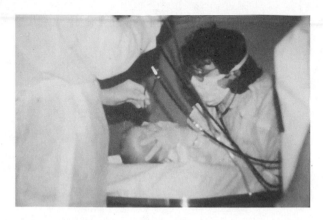

FIG. 59-4   Bronchoscopy in progress.

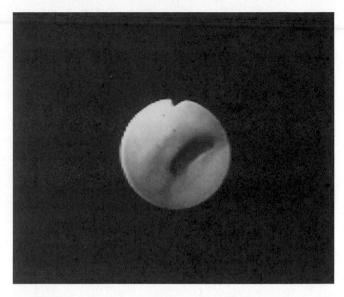

FIG. 59-5   View of the distal trachea in an infant with VATER association and tracheomalacia.

scope, apply lidocaine solution or jelly to the naris via a cotton tip applicator and gently and gradually pass it posteriorly to the adenoids. Establish patency of the nasal airway in this way before passing the bronchoscope. Some physicians also routinely use topical vasoconstrictors to maximize nasal patency and parenteral atropine (especially if using ketamine) to reduce airway secretions. Apply additional lidocaine to the larynx and tracheobronchial tree through the suction channel of the scope under direct vision, except in young infants in whom the ultrathin scope is necessary because of the absence of a suction channel. Since lidocaine is readily absorbable across mucous membranes, keep the cumulative dose of lidocaine below 7 mg/kg as a general guideline.

As the bronchoscope passes through the airway, observe the static and dynamic anatomy of the pharynx, larynx, and tracheobronchial tree. The greatest visual challenge in pediatric flexible fiberoptic bronchoscopy is often identifying pharyngeal and supraglottic landmarks because of the narrow dimensions and dynamic state of this part of the airway. Careful, controlled manipulation of the scope requires coordination and experience. After identifying the larynx, administer lidocaine solution through the suction channel directly onto the vocal cords to ensure adequate topical anesthesia of this critical portal to the intrathoracic airway. When patient sedation and laryngeal anesthesia are adequate, traverse the vocal cords with a quick, gentle thrust.

Apply suction at several different levels of the airway to attain a sense of the relative compliance of the airway. Severe narrowing of the trachea or bronchus during expiration or with applied suction may indicate clinically significant airway malacia (Figs. 59-5 and 59-6). Familiarity with normal degrees of collapsibility of the intrathoracic airways of infants and children will help to interpret the significance of dynamic airway behavior.

Note the presence of blood, mucus, and pus. Copious amounts of material within the airway may obscure visualization, and instillation of saline is often necessary to liquefy secretions to permit clearance via suctioning.

It is often clinically relevant to evaluate the frequency and intensity of the patient's cough and the patency of the large intrathoracic airways during coughing. Forceful diaphragmatic contractions result in the movement of the tracheobronchial tree in a caudal direction. Diaphragmatic paralysis

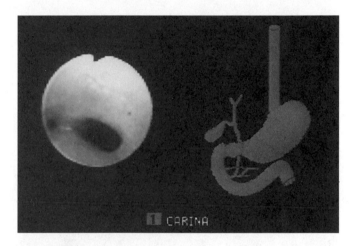

FIG. 59-6   Asymmetric carina with reduction in anterior-posterior diameter of the right mainstem bronchus in an infant with Down's syndrome and bronchomalacia.

will be manifest by rostral movement of the tracheobronchial tree toward the bronchoscopist.

Observe and photograph anatomic abnormalities. Avoid trauma to critical parts of the airway by keeping the scope in the central part of the airway and never forcing it through a severely stenotic large airway (Figs. 59-7 and 59-8).

It is possible to pass the flexible fiberoptic bronchoscope through an endotracheal tube, if present, or if the bronchoscopist believes that this approach is preferable. In intubated patients maximize oxygenation with the administration of supplemental oxygen (FIo_2 usually at least 0.40). The ultrathin scope passes through a 2.5-mm endotracheal tube, but concomitant ventilation is only possible through a 3-mm endotracheal tube. Similarly, the BF3C10 fits through a 4.5-mm endotracheal tube, but ventilation may be difficult via a 4.5-mm tube and may require a minimum of a 5-mm endotracheal tube, especially if underlying lung disease compromises gas exchange. The PD20 passes through a

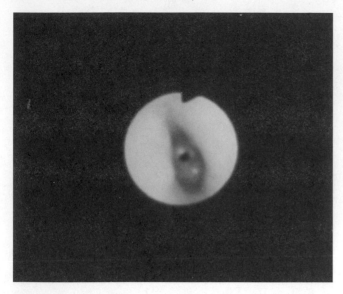

FIG. 59-7 View through the glottis demonstrating subglottic stenosis.

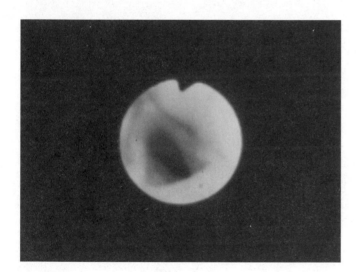

FIG. 59-8 View through the glottis demonstrating a subglottic hemangioma.

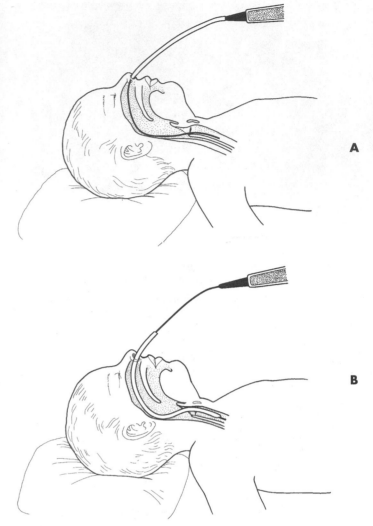

FIG. 59-9 Sequence for bronchoscopic endotracheal intubation. **A,** Thread the endotracheal tube over the bronchoscope and insert it into the airway. **B,** After advancing the scope through the larynx into the distal trachea, slide the endotracheal tube over the bronchoscope.

5.5-mm tube, but ventilation is possible with a 6-mm endotracheal tube. When using the smallest-sized endotracheal tube, optimal lubrication of the scope is mandatory as is careful monitoring of the patient's ventilatory status. When the fit is tight, manual ventilation of the patient via anesthesia bag with an FIo_2 of 0.6 or higher may be necessary, especially if the patient has significant underlying lung disease.

Bronchoscopic Intubation. Thread an appropriate-sized endotracheal tube over the bronchoscope before inserting the scope into the patient's airway. Pass the bronchoscope through the naris (or insert a plastic mouthpiece between the teeth) into the hypopharynx. After advancing the scope through the larynx into the distal trachea, slide the endotracheal tube over the bronchoscope. When tube position is satisfactory, withdraw the bronchoscope (Fig. 59-9 *A* and *B*).

Bronchoalveolar Lavage. Many studies have described techniques for performing BAL.* Although standardization of technique is still evolving, there is general agreement concerning the essentials. Pass the bronchoscope into the lower airway by the usual route and try to limit the amount of suctioning within the extrathoracic airway. Wedge the tip of the bronchoscope into the smallest airway in the appropriate region of the lung. Instill physiologic sterile nonbacteriostatic saline in aliquots, usually 10 to 25 ml, and aspirate or suction into a sterile container after each instillation. The total volume of fluid is variable but is no more than 10% of the estimated functional residual capacity, or 20 ml/kg. Two aliquots are often sufficient to obtain the necessary volume for several microbiologic and staining procedures. For a fully grown adolescent, aliquots may range from 50 to 150 ml. Promptly label and send them to the laboratory (Box 59-4).

---

*References 1,4,8,13,16,21,23, and 26.

Efficiency and expertise within the laboratory are critical to an accurate diagnosis.

Diagnose *Pneumocystis carinii* by silver stain or newer antigen detection methodologies. Seek viral pathogens by fluorescent antibody, shell vial assay for cytomegalovirus and traditional culture techniques. Culture fungi quantitatively; however, the interpretation of clinical significance is difficult, especially in intubated patients who grow *Candida* spp.[18] The identification of bacterial pathogens is problematic since the bronchoscope passes through the contaminated environ of the pharynx on its way to the lower airway. A method of quantitating bacterial cultures may be useful[19]; most patients with bacterial lower respiratory infections grow pathogens in a colony density $\geq 10^6$.[10,19,37] Lesser quantities signify upper airway contamination, colonization, or a partially treated infection. With these considerations in mind, BAL is helpful and generally accurate in the diagnosis of pneumonia in critically ill or immunocompromised children.

Foreign Body Removal. To remove a foreign body, secure the object via forceps and then withdraw the instrument and forceps from the lower airway together. This is only possible in older children using a large flexible bronchoscope. It is usually preferable to use rigid bronchoscopy for foreign body removal.

Remarks

The development of small pediatric instruments has made direct visualization of the pediatric airways a common part of the evaluation and treatment of many pediatric respiratory disorders. Each pediatric tertiary care center should develop a practice style of managing children with acute and chronic respiratory disease that best suits the individual strengths of the attending physicians. The frequency of flexible fiberoptic bronchoscopy procedures is likely to increase as indications continue to expand and more choices in equipment are available. A significant proportion of the examinations done in each institution will be in critically ill children, most commonly in the PICU, but occasionally in the ED or the operating room. There should be few complications from this procedure in experienced hands.

REFERENCES

1. Abadco DL, Amaro-Galvez R, Rao M, et al: Experience with flexible fiberoptic bronchoscopy with bronchoalveolar lavage as a diagnostic tool in children with AIDS, *Am J Dis Child* 146:1056-1059, 1992.
2. Baines DB, Goodrick MA, Beckenham EJ, et al: Fiberoptically guided endotracheal intubation in a child, *Anaesth Intensive Care* 17:354-356, 1989.
3. Barnes SD, Grob CS, Lachman BS, et al: Psychogenic upper airway obstruction presenting as refractory wheezing, *J Pediatr* 109:1067-1070, 1986.
4. Bye MR, Bernstein L, Shah K, et al: Diagnostic bronchoalveolar lavage in children with AIDS, *Pediatr Pulmonol* 3:425-428, 1987.
5. Christopher KL, Wood RP, Eckert RC, et al: Vocal cord dysfunction presenting as asthma, *N Engl J Med* 308:1566-1570, 1983.
6. Davis DA, Tucker JA, Russo P: Management of airway obstruction in patients with congenital heart defects, *Ann Otol Rhinol Laryngol* 102:163-166, 1993.
7. Davis HW, Gartner JC, Galvis AG, et al: Acute upper airway obstruction: croup and epiglottis, *Pediatr Clin North Am* 28:859-880, 1981.
8. de Blic J, McKelvie P, Le Bourgeois M, et al: Value of bronchoalveolar lavage in the management of severe acute pneumonia and interstitial pneumonitis in the immunocompromised child, *Thorax* 42:759-765, 1987.
9. Deres M, Kosack K, Waldschmidt J, et al: Airway anomalies in newborn infants: detection by tracheoscopy via endotracheal tube, *Biol Neonate* 58: 50-53, 1990.
10. Fan LL, Spark LM, Fix FJ: Flexible fiberoptic endoscopy for airway problems in a pediatric intensive care unit, *Chest* 93:556-560, 1988.
11. Finer NN, Muzyka D: Flexible endoscopic intubation of the neonate, *Pediatr Pulmonol* 12:48-51, 1992.
12. Fitzpatrick SB, Marsh B, Stokes D, et al: Indications for flexible fiberoptic bronchoscopy in pediatric patients, *Am J Dis Child* 137:595-597, 1983.
13. Frankel LR, Smith DW, Lewiston NJ: Bronchoalveolar lavage for diagnosis of pneumonia in the immunocompromised child, *Pediatrics* 81:785-788, 1988.
14. Godfrey S: Problems in practice: bronchoscopy in childhood, *Br J Dis Chest* 81:225-231, 1987.
15. Green CG, Eisenberg J, Leong A, et al: Flexible endoscopy of the pediatric airway, *Am Rev Respir Dis* 145:233-235, 1992.
16. Grigg J, Van den Borre C, Malfroot A, et al: Bilateral fiberoptic bronchoalveolar lavage in acute unilateral lobar pneumonia, *J Pediatr* 122:606-608, 1993.
17. Handler SD: Upper airway obstruction in craniofacial anomalies: diagnosis and management, *Birth Defects* 21:15-31, 1985.
18. Jones JM: Pneumonia due to *Candida, Aspergillus,* and mucorales species. In Shelhamer J, Pizzo PA, Parrillo JE, et al, editors: *Respiratory disease in the immunosuppressed host,* Philadelphia, 1991, JB Lippincott.
19. Kahn FW, Jones JM: Diagnosing bacterial respiratory infection by bronchoalveolar lavage, *J Infect Dis* 155:862-869, 1987.
20. Kleeman PP, Jantzen JAH, Bonfils P: The ultrathin bronchoscope in the management of the difficult paediatric airway, *Anaesthesiology* 34:606-608, 1987.
21. McCubbin MM, Trigg ME, Hendricker CM, et al: Bronchoscopy with bronchoalveolar lavage in the evaluation of pulmonary complications of bone narrow transplantation in children, *Pediatr Pulmonol* 12:43-47, 1992.
22. Menashe VD, Farrehi C, Miller M: Hypoventilation and cor pulmonale due to chronic upper airway obstruction, *J Pediatr* 67: 198-203, 1965.
23. Milburn HJ, Prentice HG, du Bois RM: Role of bronchoalveolar lavage

in the evaluation of interstitial pneumonitis in recipients of bone marrow transplants, *Thorax* 42:766-772, 1987.

24. Miller RW, Peak W, Kellman RK, et al: Tracheobronchial abnormalities in infants with bronchopulmonary dysplasia, *J Pediatr* 111:779-782, 1987.

25. Nussbaum E: Pediatric flexible bronchoscopy and its application in infantile atelectasis, *Clin Pediatr* 24:379-382, 1985.

26. Pattishall EN, Noyes BE, Orenstein DM: Use of bronchoalveolar lavage in immunocompromised children with pneumonia, *Pediatr Pulmonol* 5:1-5, 1988.

27. Rucker RW, Silva WJ, Worcester CC: Fiberoptic bronchoscopic nasotracheal intubation in children, *Chest* 76:56-58, 1979.

28. Ruggins NR, Milner AD: Site of upper airway obstruction in preterm infants with problematic apnea, *Arch Dis Child* 66:787-792, 1991.

29. Sackner MA. State of the art: bronchofiberoscopy, *Am Rev Respir Dis* 111: 62-88, 1975.

30. Scheller JG, Schulman SR: Fiberoptic bronchoscopic guidance for intubating a neonate with Pierre Robin syndrome, *J Clin Anesth* 3:45-47, 1991.

31. Schellhase DE, Graham LM, Fix EJ, et al: Diagnosis of tracheal injury in mechanically ventilated premature infants by flexible bronchoscopy, *Chest* 98:1219-1225, 1990.

32. Schnapf BM: Oxygen desaturation during fiberoptic bronchoscopy in pediatric patients, *Chest* 99:591-594, 1991.

33. Seid AB, Martin PJ, Pransky SM, et al. Surgical therapy of obstructive sleep apnea in children with severe mental deficiency, *Laryngoscope* 100:507-510, 1980.

34. Sher AE, Shprintzen RJ, Thorpy MJ: Endoscopic observations of obstructive sleep apnea in children with anomalous upper airways; predictive and therapeutic value, *Int J Pediatr Otorhinolaryngol* 11:135-146, 1986.

35. Shinwell ES, Higgins RD, Auten RL, et al: Fiberoptic bronchoscopy in the treatment of intubated neonates, *Am J Dis Child* 143:1064-1065, 1989.

36. Tassonyi E, Lehmann C, Gunning K, et al: Fiberoptically guided intubation in children with gangrenous stomatitis, *Anesthesiology* 73:348-349, 1990.

37. Thorpe JE, Baughman RP, Frame PT, et al: Bronchoalveolar lavage for diagnosing acute bacterial pneumonia, *J Infect Dis* 155:855-861, 1987.

38. Tutor JD, Kiernan MP, Beckerman RC: Pediatric bronchoscopy: improved tools, expanding uses, *J Respir Dis* 12:1016-1035, 1991.

39. Vigneswaran R, Whitfield JM: The use of a new ultra-thin fiberoptic bronchoscope to determine endotracheal tube position in the sick newborn infant, *Chest* 80:174-177, 1981.

40. Wagener JS: Fatality following fiberoptic bronchoscopy in a two-year-old child, *Pediatr Pulmonol* 3:197-199, 1987.

41. Wilder RT, Belani KG: Fiberoptic intubation complicated by pulmonary edema in a 12-year-old child with Hurler syndrome, *Anesthesiology* 72:205-207, 1990.

42. Wood RE: The diagnostic effectiveness of the flexible bronchoscope in children, *Pediatr Pulmonol* 1:188-192, 1985.

43. Wood RE, Gauderer MWL: Flexible fiberoptic bronchoscopy in the management of tracheobronchial foreign bodies in children: the value of a combined approach with open tube bronchoscopy, *J Pediatr Surg* 19:693-698, 1984.

44. Wood RE, Postma D: Endoscopy of the airway in infants and children, *J Pediatr* 112:1-6, 1988.

60 Bedside Pulmonary Function Tests and Pulmonary Mechanics

Tom B. Rice

During the past 35 years pulmonary function testing (PFT) has developed from the realm of physiologic research to become a widely used clinical tool. Technologic advances during the past decade have stemmed from the enhanced understanding of lung structure and function, and of the pathogenesis and therapy of lung disease. Advances in PFT appear to have been much more rapid and have had a greater impact on the care of adults than of children.[33]

This chapter discusses bedside PFT and pulmonary mechanics in the management of critically ill and injured pediatric patients. The focus is on two clinical situations: (1) preventing and/or identifying respiratory failure in the high-risk spontaneously breathing child and optimizing therapy and (2) monitoring therapy, optimizing ventilator management, preventing severe complications, and prognosticating outcome in the acutely ill child requiring assisted ventilation.

PULMONARY FUNCTION TESTING

PFT assesses functional status, facilitates diagnosis, and includes both complex and technique-dependent methods.[32]

Indications

Box 60-1 lists indications for performing PFT. The major clinical indications include assessing the type and magnitude of the physiologic abnormalities in patients with respiratory distress (especially those with known asthma or obstructive pulmonary disease). PFT is not usually diagnostic for specific disorders; however, it can define whether the functional impairment is consistent with the clinical findings. PFT in infants can also help monitor the progression of respiratory disorders. In many instances it provides more sensitive, objective information about lung function than the physical examination and chest radiograph. PFT can also assist in monitoring therapy of both acute and chronic pulmonary disorders, such as determining the effectiveness of bronchodilator therapy, or mechanical ventilation. It is also useful in the determination of impairment and in perioperative planning for both general anesthesia and postoperative mechanical ventilation needs.

Contraindications

To obtain reliable, valid, objective PFT the various ventilatory maneuvers required for spirometry and peak flow determination must be reproducible. Children younger than 5 or 6 years of age are usually unable to inspire to total lung capacity, exhale to residual volume, or produce maximal inspiratory effort on request. Because of this, reproducibility is difficult in younger children. In addition older children who refuse to cooperate, who have difficulty in following directions, or who, because of their medical condition, are unable to cooperate or sustain the effort necessary to complete the required maneuvers may not be able to produce valid and consistent results.[41,42]

PFT is also difficult to perform in the intubated patient. A contraindication for bedside pneumotachography in the intubated patient is the presence of an air leak around the endotracheal tube because it introduces inaccuracy into volume measurement. It is also difficult to measure functional residual capacity (FRC) in mechanically ventilated patients since high oxygen concentrations make gas dilution determinations inaccurate.

Complications

A technical complication of PFT is failure to obtain a high-quality study because of lack of cooperation, air leak, or other artifact.

Spirometry

Spirometry is the measurement of lung volume change. It is the simplest way to monitor lung function in the nonintubated patient. The technique can produce either a spirogram of expired or inspired gas volume plotted against time or a flow-volume curve, a display of volume versus simultaneous flow rate. Unfortunately in the intubated patient these effort-dependent maneuvers may be unreliable.

Equipment. The spirometer assesses expired volume directly, either by measuring physical volume displacement of water or by using a dry rolling seal spirometer. The spirometer is the gold standard for tidal volume measurements.

The American Thoracic Society and the American College of Chest Physicians have standardized requirements for instrumentation in the past decade.[5,6,20,21,43] Recent technological advances have produced small portable spirometers that meet these rigorous standards and produce the required documentation. See Box 60-2 for recommendations on equipment, personnel, procedures, and interpretation.*

Technique. Ideally perform spirometry with the child in a seated position. When possible in the stable patient use nose clips; however this may not always be possible in the sick child. Instruct the patient to take a deep breath (to total lung capacity), to hold the breath for 1 to 2 seconds, and then to perform a forced expiratory effort, a maximal expiration effort completely emptying the lungs to residual volume. In children, obtain three or more trials in order to elicit the child's best effort.[14]

SPIROGRAM. The volume-time spirogram is the simplest

---

*References 4-6, 20-22, 43, and 58.

BOX 60-1 INDICATIONS FOR PEDIATRIC PULMONARY FUNCTION TESTING

Detection of respiratory disease
Quantification of respiratory disease
Monitoring of respiratory disease progression
Monitoring of respiratory disease therapy
Determination of impairment/disability
Assessment of perioperative risk

BOX 60-2 RECOMMENDATIONS FOR SPIROMETRY EQUIPMENT AND TESTING

Equipment
- Responsive to small volumes/flows
- Meets minimums specified by American Thoracic Society (ATS)[4-6]
- Periodically calibrated as specified by ATS[20-21]
- Appropriate-sized mouthpieces for patient
- Hard Copy documentation of test results

Interpretations
- Best of three attempts at maximum effort flow volume curve used for evaluation[26]
- Uniform selection of starting point for forced vital capacity (FVC)
- All values corrected to barometric temperature pressure saturated (BTPS)[3, 43]

Personnel
- Experienced with children
- Technologist able to provide motivation to obtain maximal performance
- Technologist comments on patient cooperation[3, 22]

Facility/Procedures
- Comfortable testing area without distractions[26]
- Adequate time allowed for teaching/coaching

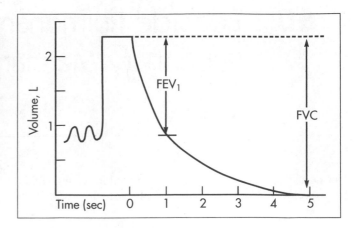

FIG. 60-1 Volume-time spirogram illustrating the forced vital capacity (FVC) and forced expiratory volume in 1 second (FEV_1).

---

script.[43] Consider values exceeding the 95% confidence limit (±2 standard deviations [SDs]) as abnormal. A change of more than 1 SD or more than 10% in serial testing indicates a clinically significant change in lung function.

Low FVC and normal FEV_1 are evidence of restrictive pulmonary disease. Patients with low FEV_1 and normal FVC values probably have obstructive airway disease. FEV_1 is a satisfactory index for predicting asthmatic patients' need for hospitalization. Asthmatic individuals who have an FEV_1 of less than 20% to 30% of the predicted value and who do not improve by more than 35% at the end of 1 hour of intense treatment require hospital admission.[17,50]

FLOW-VOLUME LOOP. The graphic display of volume versus instantaneous flow rate during forced exhalation and inspiration is a flow-volume loop (Fig. 60-2). Miller and Hyatt were the first to demonstrate the use of a maximum effort flow-volume curve (MEFVC) in the detection and evaluation of airway lesions.[36,37] The MEFVC is extremely useful for diagnosis of diseases of the airways in both adults and children.[8,27] The actual shape of the curve changes with obstructive disease of both small and large airways, as well as with restrictive pulmonary disease.[13] Evaluation of various patterns of the MEFVC can provide insight as to the causes of the flow limitations.[9,60]

A MEFVC requires a maximum respiratory effort and therefore subject cooperation.[28] To obtain MEFVC in infants and young children attempt simulated maximal effort techniques such as the crying vital capacity obtained with the use of a mask and pneumotachograph; however abnormal flow rates caused by vocal cord apposition often confound these techniques.[63]

In adults the pattern of significant airway obstruction during forced exhalation also occurs during tidal breathing.[57] When compared to the MEFVC the tidal breathing flow-volume curve (TBFVC) loop provides similar objective measurement of airway caliber and assists in evaluating therapeutic efforts.[31,40] It is possible to obtain tidal breathing flow-volume curves in sleeping infants or children.[37] Such TBFVCs display reproducible patterns of inspiratory and expiratory flow during tidal breathing.

TBFVC airway patterns are often identifiable in the ab-

---

form of spirometry obtained at the bedside. The two most useful and reproducible measurements obtained from the spirogram are the forced vital capacity (FVC) and the forced expiratory volume in 1 second (FEV_1).

From the spirogram record the volume of the FVC. FEV_1 is the maximum volume that the patient can exhale from a complete inspiration in 1 second. Thus it is a measurement of both volume and flow over the first second (Fig. 60-1). Record the largest value for the FVC and the FEV_1 even if the two values are not from the same curve.

Normal values vary with age (height), gender, and race and numerous tables lists reference values (Table 60-1).[42,43] For a more comprehensive listing refer to Quanjer's manu-

Table 60-1   Predicted Normal Values for Pediatric Pulmonary Function Studies

Study	Summary Regression Equation	% Standard Deviation
Peak expiratory flow rate (PEFR)	PEFR (L/min) $-$ 2425.5714 + 5.2428 $\times$ Ht. (cm)	13
Vital capacity (VC)	Boys: Log VC(ml) = -2.3554 + 2.6727 $\times$ log Ht. (cm) Girls: Log VC(ml) = -2.4756 + 2.7194 $\times$ log Ht. (cm)	13
Maximal voluntary ventilation (MVV)	MVV (L/min) = 299.507 + 1.276 $\times$ Ht. (cm)	21
Forced expiratory volume, second (FEV$_1$)	log FEV$_1$ (ml) = 2.6781 + 2.7986 $\times$ log Ht. (cm)	8.8
FEV$_1$/VC	%FEV$_1$/VC = 100 $\times$ FEV$_1$ (ml)/VC (ml)	

Adapted from Polgar G, Promadhat: *Pulmonary function testing in children: techniques and standards,* Philadelphia, 1971, WB Saunders.

sence of respiratory symptoms. TBFVC pattern characteristics are similar to those found in MEFVC of older children and adults who can cooperate. Therefore use the MEFVC in cooperative children above the age of 6 and the TBFVC in sleeping infants and children. Both maneuvers are simple screening procedures that can direct further diagnostic and therapeutic intervention.

Fig. 60-2 demonstrates the MEFVC loop in a normal child of 8 years of age and a TBFVC of a 1-year-old. Fig. 60-3 demonstrates some of the major reproducible patterns in adults, older children, and infants. Pattern 1 demonstrates a normal TBFVC. The normal TBFVC is round or oval and has a similar shape in adults, children, and infants.[2,29] Pattern 2 demonstrates a decelerating expiratory limb of the TBFVC (a concave expiratory curve), usually seen in children with obstructive or small airways disease. The most common

diagnosis associated with this pattern is bronchial asthma; however, in neonates a similar pattern occurs with bronchopulmonary dysplasia or bronchiolitis.[31,37] Note the improvement after administration of a bronchodilator. Pattern 3, with low, flat expiratory flow and minimal fluctuation, occurs in children and infants who have an intrathoracic airway obstruction. Pattern 4 represents a high flow to volume relationship. In this instance tidal volumes are much smaller than normal and the respiratory rate higher. Such findings usually occur with restrictive pulmonary diseases such as acute respiratory distress syndrome (ARDS) in children or neonates with severe respiratory distress syndrome (RDS) or cardiac failure.[39,61] Pattern 5 demonstrates limited inspiratory flow. This pattern occurs with extrathoracic obstruction of the upper airway such as laryngomalacia.[52] Pattern 6 shows flat inspiratory and expiratory curves or a "box"

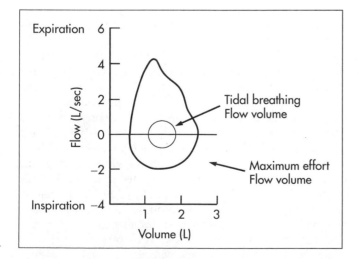

FIG. 60-2   Maximum expiratory flow-volume curve of a normal 8-year-old child and tidal breathing flow-volume loop of a 1-year-old child.

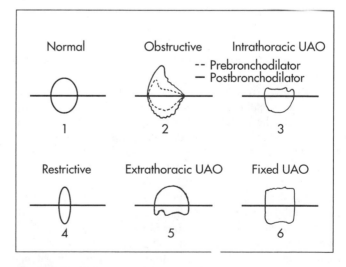

FIG. 60-3   Tidal breathing flow-volume curve patterns. *UAO,* Upper airway obstruction.

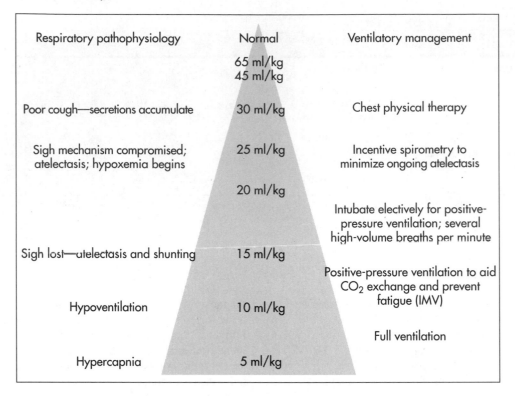

FIG. 60-4 In mechanical ventilatory failure the gradual decline in vital capacity determines the associated respiratory pathophysiologic condition and recommended ventilatory management.

(Adapted from Ropper AH: Management of Guillain-Barré syndrome. In Ropper AH, Kennedy SK, Zervas NT, editors: *Neurological and neurosurgical intensive care*, Baltimore, 1983, University Park Press.)

shape indicating a fixed lesion. Such a pattern occurs with subglottic hemangioma or tracheal web.[1]

Peak Flow Determination

The peak flow meter provides a simple alternative to spirometry for peak expiratory flow rate (PEFR) measurement at the bedside in spontaneously breathing patients. Simply defined, *PEFR* is the maximum flow attainable on forced expiration. The inexpensive instrumentation and relative accuracy contribute to its value.[11]

Equipment. New extra-small, portable peak flowmeters are now available to measure flows as low as 30 L/min with accuracy.

Technique. Spontaneously breathing children as young as 5 years are capable of cooperating with peak flow determination. Ask the child to remove any gum or food from the mouth. Move the pointer on the peak flowmeter to zero. Ask the child to stand, if possible, or at least sit up straight in bed. Hold the meter in a horizontal position with fingers away from the vent holes and numbers. Ask the child to breathe in slowly as deeply as possible with the mouth wide open. Place the mouthpiece on the tongue and the lips around the mouthpiece and have him or her blow hard and fast, a short, sharp blast. The meter records the fastest flow. Repeat for a total of at least three tries, allowing at least 10 seconds between attempts, and record the best (highest) flow.

Table 60-1 includes predicted values for peak flow. PEFR values of less than 16% of the predicted value and failure to improve by more than 16% within 15 to 20 minutes after administration of a bronchodilator usually indicate need for hospitalization.[7,17,50]

Bedside Pulmonary Function Tests

Although bedside PFT is commonly employed in the neonatal, pediatric, and adult intensive care units, few data establish its usefulness in the infant and the older child. In contrast considerable data demonstrate the utility of PFT in adults in predicting successful weaning and extubation of ventilator-dependent patients. VC greater than 10 ml/kg with a maximum negative inspiratory force (NIF) greater than −20 cm H_2O usually predicts successful extubation.[62] In infants or children who cannot cooperate, crying vital capacity greater than 15 ml/kg predicts a NIF greater than −45 cm H_2O and possibly successful extubation.[49] Although criteria such as these have gained acceptance in the literature for weaning from mechanical ventilation,[38,47,56,64] they are often of little value in the pediatric ventilator-dependent patient[10,18,55] (see also Chapter 29). On the other hand vital capacity and negative inspiratory force measurements are helpful in the evaluation and monitoring of respiratory muscle strength in patients with weakness secondary to neuromuscular disease. Elective intubation is appropriate for this group when the vital capacity falls below 20 ml/kg (Fig. 60-4).[45]

Equipment. In the intensive care unit a small hand-held respirometer provides bedside measurement of volumes and an anaeroid manometer provides measurement of negative inspiratory force.

Technique. To measure vital capacity (VC) ask the patient to inspire maximally then exhale slowly and completely through the respirometer. Maximal voluntary ventilation (MVV) is the total volume recorded after instructing the patient to breathe as deeply and rapidly as possible for 15 seconds. Record the total volume after 10, 12, and 15 seconds and extrapolate the volume over 1 minute to report a flow rate in liters per minute. The MVV maneuver exacerbates air trapping and exertion of the respiratory muscles; therefore significant obstructive lung disease reduces MVV. In lung disease the MVV_{12} and MVV_{15} often decrease in relation to the MVV_{10} as a result of respiratory muscle fatigue.[46] Normal values vary by as much as 30%, so interpret modest decreases with caution.[46] Healthy young adult males average 170 L/min.[46] Values are lower in healthy women and decrease with age in both sexes.[46]

To measure negative inspiratory force (NIF) first warn the patient to expect brief airway occlusion. Then occlude the airway or endotracheal tube at or near functional residual capacity (FRC) for 20 seconds with an attached pressure manometer. The maximum deflection associated with the patient's effort is the NIF. In cooperative patients measure the maximal inspiratory pressure (MIP) by performing airway occlusion at residual volume, rather than at FRC, then measuring the pressure generated by the first breath after release of the occlusion. Patients who are unstable hemodynamically may not tolerate the airway occlusion maneuver required for measurement of negative inspiratory force or maximal inspiratory pressure.

Sahn reported that NIF values greater than −30 cm H_2O are usually present in healthy adult patients.[47] Similarly Platzker reported normal NIF values for children as above −35 cm H_2O.[41] It is difficult to sustain normal spontaneous ventilation when values for NIF decline to less than −20 cm H_2O. Normal MIP values in children are greater than −96 ± 35 cm H_2O (boys) and greater than −90 ± 20 cm H_2O (girls).[44]

PULMONARY MECHANICS

Pulmonary mechanics are tools for clinicians to evaluate the effectiveness of mechanical ventilation. Systems providing online pulmonary mechanics from mechanical ventilators have developed rapidly over the past several years.

Equipment and Technique

Systems for pulmonary mechanics employ a differential pressure pneumotachometer to measure tidal volume. A transducer on both sides of a flow resistor measures changes in pressure ($\dot{V} = \Delta P/R$); the flow signal is integrated with time and is proportional to pressure. Options for pressure measurement include pleural pressure, transpulmonary pressure, and pressure across the entire respiratory system. This process requires calibration for gas concentration, humidity, and temperature. The accuracy of pneumotachography also depends on absence of an air leak, which is difficult to accomplish with uncuffed endotracheal tubes. Coupling this system with a high-speed computer allows rapid data manipulation, permitting breath-to-breath analysis. Such systems typically display waveforms of the airway pressure, flow, and tidal volume in real time, producing flow-volume loops and pressure-volume curves.[15,19,23-25,35]

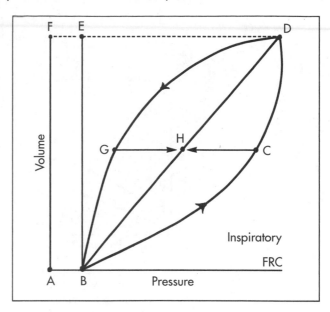

FIG. 60-5 Pressure-volume loop in a child with normal lungs. Area ABCDFA, total work of breathing; slope of BHD, lung compliance (C_{dyn},l); distance CH, inspiratory pressure; distance GH, expiratory pressure; distance GHC/delta flow (C–G), total lung resistance (R_L).

From the pressure-volume curves derive estimates of total static lung compliance (C_L) and respiratory system resistance (R_{rs}) and assess the degree of lung distention. Compliance (C_{rs}) reflects the elastic properties of the respiratory system and is the change in volume per unit change in pressure (milliliters per centimeter of water [ml/cm H_2O]). To measure static compliance press the inspiratory pause; hold and read the plateau pressure on the light-emitting diode (LED) display after equilibration (2 to 4 seconds). Calculate compliance using the formula

$$C = \Delta V/\Delta P$$

or (tidal volume − compressible volume)/(plateau pressure − positive end-expiratory pressure [PEEP]). Estimate compressible volume as 1 mL/cm H_2O pressure for permanent tubing and 3 mL/cm H_2O pressure for more compliant disposable tubing.[53]

Resistance of the respiratory system is a reflection of the friction encountered by gas flowing through the airways and by tissue moving against tissue. It is the change in pressure required for a unit change in flow (cm H_2O/L/sec). See Fig. 11-16.

Work of breathing integrates elastic and resistive properties and is the cumulative product of pressure and volume at any instant during a respiratory cycle; it determines the hysteresis of the dynamic pressure-volume curve. It is possible to calculate work of breathing by measuring the area of a pressure-volume loop (Fig. 60-5).[16]

Figs. 60-6 and 60-7 illustrate pressure-volume curve patterns representing common conditions in the pediatric intensive care unit (PICU). Prebronchodilator and postbronchodilator assessments of resistance are useful in evaluating the effectiveness of therapy in obstructive lung disease (Fig. 60-7).

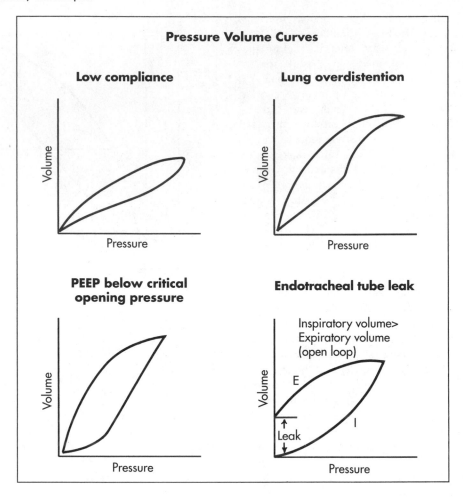

FIG. 60-6 Pressure-volume curves.

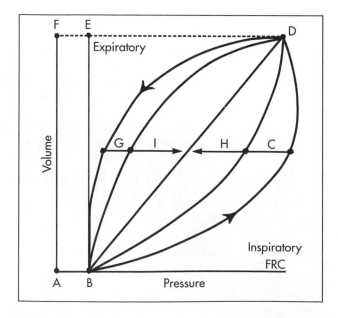

FIG. 60-7 Prebronchodilator pressure-volume curve (BCDGB) and postbronchodilator pressure-volume curve (BHDIB). Lung resistance (R_L) for the prebronchodilator curve = (GC/delta flow C–G) and for the postbronchodilator curve = (IH/delta flow H–I).

In order to provide optimal pulmonary gas exchange, match the ventilator settings to the mechanical properties of the respiratory system. This requires understanding the time course of air flow within a breath, a concept described by the time constant τ. If accurate measurements of compliance and resistance are available (requires an esophageal balloon to estimate pleural pressure), one may calculate the time constant (T) from compliance (C) and resistance (R) by using the formula

$$\tau = RC$$

Alternatively, one may compute T from the slope of the linear portion of the flow-volume curve[14] or from the slope of the volume-time waveform collected during passive exhalation to atmospheric pressure.[48] Remove the patient from the ventilator before making these measurements.

Patients experience auto-PEEP or intrinsic PEEP when the time required for passive exhalation exceeds the ventilator's set expiratory time (i.e., inadequate time constants). By convention the number of seconds required for lung volume to return passively to 95% of equilibrium after a tidal inflation is equal to three time constants (3T). Therefore mechanical ventilator rates (breaths per second) greater than

3T progressively increase FRC and diminish dynamic compliance by "stacking breaths," causing auto-PEEP. One strategy to prevent stacking breaths is to use a mechanical ventilator rate lower than 60÷3T breaths/min.[54] Unfortunately different time constants may exist for different lung units in many disease processes; this method provides only an estimate.

To assess auto-PEEP press the expiratory pause button during a regular ventilator cycle. The cycle stops at the end of expiration with inspiratory and expiratory valves closed. The airway pressure falls over 2 to 4 seconds until a plateau is reached. This plateau pressure corresponds to auto-PEEP. Auto-PEEP is high in some patients with obstructive lung disease (up to 22 cm H_2O) and in some with ARDS (up to 8 cm H_2O).[30]

Levy et al.[30] describe in detail a method to develop static pressure-volume curves using online information from the Siemens Servo 900C by measuring static pressure at different inflation volumes alternately using the expiratory hold and the inspiratory hold features. Refer to the original reference for more details on this technique. Although beyond the scope of this chapter a methods paper by Sly et al. describes the interrupter technique for measuring resistance and compliance on ventilated patients.[51]

Many modern pediatric ventilators provide a display of tidal volume, respiratory frequency, and inspiratory flow rate.[12,34,59] These systems usually detect apnea and hypopnea by measuring flow or a change in lung volume by using a pneumotach.

Minute ventilation ($\dot{V}e$) is the product of tidal volume and frequency; the alveolar ventilation, dead space ventilation, and central drive determine $\dot{V}e$. Newer ventilators often display this value. However in patients with decreased compliance ventilated with high peak inspiratory pressure the ventilator display may overestimate the volume received by the patient if using distensible ventilator circuits because of the compressible volume in the circuit. Estimate normal minute ventilation with the equation[65]

$$\log(\dot{V}e, ml/min) = 0.3035 + 1.6815 (\log height, cm)$$

REMARKS

There is a broad distribution of values on normal PFT data in pediatric patients around the mean for each test. Therefore each laboratory should develop its own normal values using its own equipment even though normal pediatric pulmonary function data are available for most tests performed on children above the age of 6 years.

REFERENCES

1. Abramson AL et al: The use of tidal breathing flow-volume loop in laryngotracheal disease of neonates and infants, *Laryngoscopy* 92:922, 1982.
2. Adler SM, Wohl MEB: Flow-volume relationship at low lung volumes in healthy term newborns, *Pediatrics* 61:636, 1978.
3. American Thoracic Society: Lung function testing: selection of reference values and interpretative strategies, *Am Rev Respir Dis* 144:1202-1218, 1991.
4. American Thoracic Society: Single-breath carbon monoxide diffusing capacity (transfer factor): recommendations for a standard technique, *Am Rev Respir Dis* 136:1299-1307, 1987.
5. American Thoracic Society: Snowbird workshop on standardization of spirometry, *Am Rev Respir Dis* 119:831-838, 1979.
6. American Thoracic Society: Standardization of spirometry, *Am Rev Respir Dis* 136:1285-1298, 1987.
7. Banner AS, Shah RS, Addington WW: Rapid prediction of need for hospitalization in acute asthma, *JAMA* 235:1337, 1976.
8. Bouhoys A: *Breathing,* New York, 1974, Grune & Stratton.
9. Carilli AD et al: The flow-volume loop in normal subjects and in diffuse lung disease, *Chest* 66:5, 1974.
10. Chiswick MI, Milner RDG: Crying vital capacity: measurement of neonatal lung function, *Arch Dis Child* 51:22, 1976.
11. Clark NM, Evans D, Mellins RB: Patient use of peak flow monitoring, *Am Rev Respir Dis* 145:722-725, 1992.
12. Cunningham DM: Intensive care monitoring of pulmonary mechanics for preterm infants undergoing mechanical ventilation, *J Perinatol* 9:56, 1989.
13. Davidson FF, Burke GW: Physiologic differentiation of upper and lower airway obstruction, *Ann Otol Rhinol Laryngol* 86:630-632, 1977.
14. Davis G, Coates AL: Pulmonary mechanics. In: Hilman BC, editor: *Pediatric respiratory diseases: diagnosis and treatment.* Philadelphia, 1993, WB Saunders.
15. England SJ: Current techniques for assessing pulmonary function in the newborn and infant: advantages and limitations, *Pediatr Pulmonol* 4:48, 1988.
16. Eyck Ten LG: The work of breathing in normal and diseased individuals, *Arkos* 1:4, 1989.
17. Fanta CH, Rossing THE, McFadden ER Jr: Emergency room treatment of asthma, *Am J Med* 72:416, 1982.
18. Fiastro J et al: Comparison of standard weaning parameters and the mechanical work of breathing in mechanically ventilated patients, *Chest* 94:232, 1988.
19. Fisher JB et al: Identifying lung overdistension during mechanical ventilation by using volume-pressure loops, *Pediatr Pulmonol* 5(1):4, 1988.
20. Gardner RM, Clausen JL, Cotton DJ et al: Computer guidelines for pulmonary laboratories, *Am Rev Respir Dis* 134:628-629, 1986.
21. Gardner RM, Clausen JL, Crapo RO et al: Quality assurance in pulmonary function laboratories, *Am Rev Respir Dis* 134:625-627, 1986.
22. Gardner RM, Clausen JL, Epler G et al: Pulmonary function laboratory personnel qualifications, *Am Rev Respir Dis* 134:623-624, 1986.
23. Gerhardt T, Bancalari E: Chestwall compliance in full term and premature infants, *Acta Paediatr Scand* 69:359, 1980.
24. Heaf DP et al: The accuracy of esophageal pressure measurement sin convalescent and sick intubated infants, *Pediatr Pulmonol* 2:5, 1986.
25. Heldt GP et al: Dynamic lung compliance, closure of the patent ductus arteriosus and surfactant therapy, *Pediatr Res* 23:510A, 1988 (abstract).
26. Hilman BC, Allen JL: Clinical applications of pulmonary function testing in children and adolescents. In Hilman BC, editors: *Pediatric respirtory disease diagnosis and treatment,* Philadelphia, 1993, WB Saunders.
27. Hyatt RE, Black LF: The flow volume curve, *Am Rev Respir Dis* 107:191-199, 1973.
28. Hyatt RE, Schilder DP, Fry DL: Relationship between maximum expiratory flow and degree of lung inflation, *J Appl Physiol* 13:331-336, 1958.
29. Karlberg P: Respiratory studies in newborn infants, *Acta Paediatr* 49:345-357, 1960.
30. Levy P, Similowski T, Corbeil C et al: A method for studying the status volume-pressure curves of the respiratory system during mechanical ventilation; *J Crit Care* 4:83-89, 1989.
31. Lonky SA, Tisi GM: Determining changes in airway caliber in asthma: the role of submaximal expiratory flow rates, *Chest* 77:741-748, 1980.
32. MacDonald KD, Wirtchafter DD: Applied pulmonary mechanics, *Neonatal Intens Care* 6:41, 1992.
33. Marini JJ: Monitoring during mechanical ventilation, *Clin Chest Med* 9:73, 1988.
34. Maunder RJ, Hudson LD: Respiratory monitoring in the intensive care unit. In Shoemaker WC, Abraham E, editors: *Diagnostic methods in critical care,* New York, 1987, Marcel Dekker.

35. McCann EM, Goldman SL, Brady JP: Pulmonary function in the sick newborn infant, *Pediatr Res* 4:313, 1987.

36. Miller RD, Hyatt RE: Obstructing lesions of the larynx and trachea: clinical and physiologic characteristics, *Mayo Clin Proc* 44:145-161, 1969.

37. Milner AD, Saunders RA, Hopkin IE: Tidal pressure volume and flow volume respiratory loop patterns in human neonates, *Clin Mol Med* 54:257-264, 1978.

38. Montgomery A et al: Prediction of successful weaning using airway occlusion pressure and hypercapnic challenge, *Chest* 91:496, 1987.

39. Morgan WJ et al: Partial expiratory flow-volume curves in infants and young children, *Pediatr Pulmonol* 5:232, 1988.

40. Morris MJ, Lane DJ: Tidal expiratory flow pattern in airflow obstruction, *Thorax* 36:135-142, 1981.

41. Platzker A, Keens T: Pulmonary function testing in pediatric patients. In: Wilson AF, editor: *Pulmonary function testing indications and interpretations,* Orlando, Fla, 1985, Grune & Stratton, pp 275-292.

42. Polgar G, Promadhat V: *Pulmonary function testing in children: techniques and standards,* Philadelphia, 1971, WB Saunders.

43. Quanjer PH, Stocks J, Polgar G et al: Compilation of reference values for lung function measurements in children, *Eur Respir J* 2(suppl 4):184S-261S, 1989.

44. Rochester DF, Arora NS: Respiratory muscle failure, *Med Clin North Am* 67:573-597, 1983.

45. Ropper AH: Management of Guillain-Barré syndrome. In Ropper AH, Kennedy SK, Zervas NT, editors: *Neurological and neurosurgical intensive care,* Baltimore, 1983, University Park Press.

46. Ruppel G: *Manual of pulmonary function testing,* St. Louis, 1982, Mosby.

47. Sahn S, Lakshminarayan S: Bedside criteria for discontinuation of mechanical ventilation, *Chest* 63:1002, 1973.

48. Shannon DC: Rational monitoring of respiratory function during mechanical ventilation of infants and children, *Intens Care Med* 15:S13-16, 1989.

49. Shimada Y et al: Crying vital capacity and maximal inspiratory pressure as clinical indicators of readiness for weaning of infants less than a year of age, *Anesthesiology* 51:456, 1979.

50. Silver RB, Ginsburg CM: Early prediction of the need for hospitalization in children with acute asthma, *Clin Pediatr* 23:81, 1984.

51. Sly PD, Bates JHT, Milic-Emili J: Measurement of respiratory mechanics using the Siemens Servo Ventilator 900C, *Pediatr Pulmonol* 3:400-405, 1987.

52. Smith GJ, Cooper DM: Laryngomalacia and inspiratory obstruction in later childhood, *Arch Dis Child* 56:345-349, 1981.

53. Spearman CB, Sheldon RL, Egan DF: *Egan's fundamentals of respiratory therapy,* ed 4, St. Louis, 1982, Mosby.

54. Strieter RM, Lynch JP: Complications in the ventilated patient, *Clin Chest Med* 9:127, 1988.

55. Sutherland JM, Ratchcliff JW: Crying vital capacity, *Am J Dis Child* 101:93, 1961.

56. Tahvanainen J, Salmenpera M: Extubation criteria after weaning from intermittent mandatory ventilation and continuous positive airway pressure, *Crit Care Med* 11:702, 1983.

57. Takishima T et al: Flow-volume curves during quiet breathing, maximum voluntary ventilation and forced vital capacities in patients with obstructive lung disease, *Scand J Respir Dis* 48:384-393, 1967.

58. Taussig LM: Standardization of lung function testing in children, *J Pediatr* 97:668, 1980.

59. Tobin MJ: Respiratory monitoring in the intensive care unit, *Am Rev Respir Dis* 138:1625, 1988.

60. Tophan JM, Empey DW: Practical assessment of obstruction in the larynx and trachea, *J Laryngol Otolaryngol* 88:1185-1193, 1974.

61. Wall MA, Misley MC, Dickerson D: Partial expiratory flow-volume curves in young children, *Am Rev Respir Dis* 129:557, 1984.

62. Weisman IM, Rinaldo JE, Rogers RM et al: Intermittent mandatory ventilation, *Am Rev Respir Dis* 127:641, 1983.

63. Wise PH et al: Flow volume loop in newborn infants, *Crit Care Med* 8:61-63, 1980.

64. Yang K, Tobin M: A prospective study of indexes predicting the outcome of trials of weaning from mechanical ventilation, *N Engl J Med* 324:1445-1450, 1991.

65. Zapletal A: Small airway function in children and adolescents, methods, reference values. In Hegzog H, editor: *Progress in respiratory research,* vol 22, Basel, Switzerland, 1987, Karger-Basel.

PART XII

GASTROENTEROLOGY TECHNIQUES

61 Rectal Examination

Nicholas Tsarouhas

Despite its importance, the rectal examination is one of most commonly omitted parts of the pediatric physical examination. Some believe that this examination involves only testing the stools for occult blood. However, the digital exploration and palpation of the rectal vault allows for proper evaluation of an important part of the gastrointestinal (GI) tract.

Though referred to as "the rectal examination," this examination also should include the "perianal" examination, which includes the detailed inspection of the perianal mucosa and skin. The careful examiner can gain important information. The abdominal examination is not complete without the evaluation of the most distal aspect of the gastrointestinal tract: the rectum and perianal area.

Indications

The rectal examination is a key part of the pediatric physical examination. It is essential in any patient with abdominal or GI complaints. One of the more common indications is rectal bleeding. One goal is to ascertain whether blood is actually present. Many foods and medicines may falsely make the stool appear bloody or black and tarry. Box 61-1 lists some of the more common culprits. Once the presence of blood is proven, the source of the bleeding must be determined. Stools with bright red blood (hematochezia) are classically described as coming from below the ligament of Treitz, whereas black, tarry stools (melena), usually originate from above the ligament.

The presence of gross blood on the examining finger may herald a severe, ischemic intestinal insult such as malrotation with volvulus.[4] Alternatively, it may point to an infectious colitis. Bloody mucus may be a clue to an intussusception, the classic "currant jelly stools." Blood-streaked stools most likely originate more distally, such as from a rectal polyp or anal fissure. Box 61-2 lists some of the more common causes of lower GI bleeding by age group.

Although the search for the exact location of the bleeding is important, do not forget to consider the hemodynamic consequences of rectal bleeding. Monitor the cardiovascular and neurologic status of these patients. Diminished or absent anal sphincter tone may be a harbinger of serious neurologic injury.

In cases of severe abdominal pain, the rectal examination is again vital. Rectal tenderness may occur with appendicitis. This is true not only in a retrocecal or pelvic appendicitis but also in the common presentation.[5] A boggy mass on palpation may indicate an appendiceal abscess. The examiner may palpate a similar mass with an intussusception.

Constipation is another indication that mandates a thorough rectal examination. The palpation of a large amount of hard stool in the rectal vault could point to several diagnoses. An acute presentation of constipation could be secondary to an anal fissure. Hard stools could cause a traumatic fissure

---

BOX 61-1 SUBSTANCES THAT MAY MIMIC RECTAL BLEEDING

Red stools	Black stools
Food coloring (Kool-Aid/Jell-O)	Licorice
Beets	Bismuth (Pepto-Bismol)
Tomatoes	Iron
Grapes	Charcoal
Antibiotics (ampicillin)	
Serratia marcescens (Red diaper syndrome)	

---

that could cause the child to withhold stools because of the pain involved with their passage. A viral illness, though commonly known to cause diarrhea, may also cause constipation. Finally, many drugs are known to cause constipation, including aluminum-containing antacids, anticholinergics, antidepressants, iron, lead, muscle relaxants, narcotics, and psychotropics.[2] In a chronic presentation, "functional" or "idiopathic" would be the most likely diagnosis. However, hypothyroidism, neuromuscular disease, and even pregnancy could present with constipation. The rectal examination is crucial in a patient suspected of having Hirschsprung's disease. In this disorder, the ampulla is devoid of feces despite a history of constipation.

Perianal inspection is indicated to evaluate rectal pain. A chief complaint of rectal pain could point to hemorrhoids. External hemorrhoids can be recognized as a tender, swollen, bluish mass at the anus that causes extreme pain with defecation and sitting. In contrast, internal hemorrhoids are not readily visible and often cannot be palpated.[1] The only clue on examination may be bright red blood on the examining digit.

Other important findings on the perianal inspection might include a pilonidal cyst or sinus. These congenital midline structures are usually found at the level of the coccyx or lower sacrum. These structures may herald an underlying spinal defect such as spina bifida occulta. Often the only clue is a subtle sacral dimple or a tuft of hair.

Examination of the perianal area is indicated if the child complains of rectal itching. Perianal pruritis, especially nocturnal, should raise the suspicion of a pinworm infestation. The child often excoriates the perianal area as a result of the intense itching. One way to confirm the diagnosis is to find the small white worms; another way is to press clear cellophane tape to the anus and then locate the eggs under the low-power setting of a microscope.

A perianal examination is especially important if there is a complaint of rectal pain with fever. A perianal abscess can be recognized as a tender, erythematous mass at the anal

---

BOX 61-2 CAUSES OF RECTAL BLEEDING

Neonate (Birth-1 mo)	Infant (1 mo-2 yr)	Preschool (2 yr-5 yr)	School-age (> 5 yr)
1. Swallowed maternal blood	1. Anal fissure	1. Infectious colitis	1. Infectious colitis
2. Nasopharyngeal or oropharyngeal trauma or manipulation	2. Allergic colitis	2. Polyps	2. Inflammatory bowel disease
3. Anal fissure	3. Infectious colitis	3. Meckel's diverticulum	3. Polyps
4. Allergic colitis	4. Intussusception	4. Intussusception	4. Epistaxis
5. Coagulopathy	5. Meckel's diverticulum	5. Hemolytic-uremic syndrome	5. Hemmorrhoids
6. Hemmorrhagic disease of the newborn	6. Hirschsprung's disease	6. Henoch-Schönlein purpura	6. Pseudomembranous enterocolitis
7. Malrotation with volvulus	7. Volvulus	7. Anal fissure	7. Hemolytic- uremic syndrome
8. Necrotizing enterocolitis	8. Esophagitis	8. Epistaxis	8. Peptic ulcer
9. Infectious colitis	9. Peptic ulcer	9. Inflammatory bowel disease	9. Esophagitis
10. Sepsis	10. Intestinal duplication	10. Pseudomembranous enterocolitis	10. Meckel's diverticulum
11. Hirschsprung's disease	11. Polyps	11. Peptic ulcer	11. Vascular malformation
12. Intestinal duplication	12. Inflammatory bowel disease	12. Esophagitis	
13. Meckel's diverticulum	13. Hemolytic-uremic syndrome	13. Lymphonodular hyperplasia	
14. Intussusception	14. Henoch-Schönlein purpura	14. Vascular malformation	
15. Gastritis	15. Vascular malformation		
16. Peptic ulcer	16. Pseudomembranous enterocolitis		
17. Vascular malformation	17. Lymphonodular hyperplasia		

---

margin. Skin tags are another common finding around the anus. Although usually not important, they may be a red flag for the diagnosis of Crohn's disease. Perianal warts support the diagnosis of a sexually transmitted infection. Perianal bruising or abrasions support a suspicion of child abuse.

Contraindications

There are few contraindications to a pediatric rectal examination. One relative contraindication involves the neutropenic patient. Many believe that there exists the possibility that even relatively minor trauma to the rectal mucosa may induce a transient but dangerous bacteremia. Another relative contraindication is the performance of a rectal examination on a patient with a recent history of anal surgery.

Complications

The most common complication of the rectal examination is discomfort. Warn the patients and the parents before the examination. Pain is another possible complication and often signals that the finger has entered too rapidly or that there is inadequate lubrication. Fortunately, most patients complain only of discomfort and not actual pain. Pain is often secondary to the underlying pathologic condition of the area. Mild traumatic bleeding may occasionally be noted.

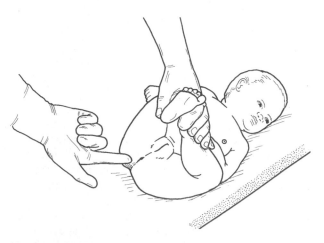

FIG. 61-1 Technique for the rectal examination of the infant.

Equipment

The equipment needed for the rectal examination is minimal. The materials generally required are gloves, a lubricant (Surgilube), and the blood-testing reagent and pads (Hemoccult or Hemotest).

Techniques

Rectal Examination. The most important first step in the rectal examination is to prepare the patient and parent by alerting them to the possibility of discomfort while stressing the importance of the examination. Next, position the patient. In the infant, the supine position is probably optimal. Hold the feet together and flex the knees and hips onto the abdomen. While the nondominant hand controls the legs, gently insert the gloved and lubricated index or fifth finger of the dominant hand into the anus (Fig. 61-1). The index finger is preferred for its greater tactile sensitivity.

Another method places the patient in the side-lying position. This position is better for slightly older pediatric patients. Place the patient onto the left side, with the buttocks close to the edge of the examination table and the knees and hips slightly flexed (Fig. 61-2).

There are other considerations for even older patients. With a female adolescent, for instance, perform the rectal examination at the conclusion of the pelvic examination and while the patient is still in the lithotomy position. If no pelvic examination is to be performed, use the left lateral decubitus position. The careful examiner often palpates the cervix through the anterior rectal wall.[1]

The older male adolescent should have his prostate examined. Insert the finger into the rectum as far as possible and ask the patient to bear down "as if having a bowel movement." Palpate the posterior surface of the prostate, anteriorly in the rectum. The median sulcus is normally flanked by two nontender, anodular, rubbery, lateral lobes. Tenderness to palpation might suggest prostatitis.

Disimpaction. The rectal examination may be extended to include digital disimpaction. Digital disimpaction involves

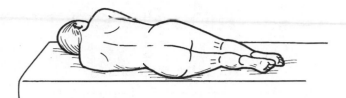

FIG. 61-2   Positioning for the rectal examination of an older child.

the manual breaking up and digital removal of hard or retained stool particles in the rectal vault. This procedure is often necessary in severe cases of constipation. However, digital disimpaction is not the ultimate solution. A complete regimen for constipation involves colonic evacuation with enemas, laxatives, and behavioral conditioning.[3]

References

1. Bates B, Hoekelman RA: *A guide to physical examination and history taking,* ed 5, Philadelphia, 1991, JB Lippincott.
2. Ludwig S: Constipation. In Fleisher G, Ludwig S, editors: *Textbook of pediatric emergency medicine,* ed 3, Baltimore, 1993, Williams & Wilkins.
3. Pettei MJ, Davidson M: Idiopathic Constipation. In Walker WA, Durie PR, Hamilton JR, et al, editors: *Pediatric gastrointestinal disease,* vol 2, Philadelphia, 1991, Decker.
4. Schnaufer L, Mahboubi S: Abdominal Emergencies. In Fleisher G, Ludwig S, editors: *Textbook of pediatric emergency medicine,* ed 3, Baltimore, 1993, Williams & Wilkins.
5. Silen W: Acute appendicitis. In Braunwald E, Isselbacher KJ, Petersdorf RG, et al, editors: *Harrison's Principles of internal medicine,* ed 11, New York, 1987, McGraw-Hill.

62 Tube Placement

Nicholas Tsarouhas

NASOGASTRIC/OROGASTRIC/TRANSPYLORIC TUBES

Nasogastric (NG) and orogastric (OG) tubes are important both diagnostically and therapeutically in many situations. The transpyloric tube is a special type of feeding tube that is designed to pass into the intestinal tract. All feeding tubes do not need to be transpyloric. In fact, most pediatric feeding tubes are placed into the stomach. Because of their similarities, the NG, OG, and transpyloric tubes are considered together in this section.

Indications

One of the most important *diagnostic* uses of the NG and OG tubes involves gastrointestinal (GI) bleeding. This type of tube is essential in evaluating a possible upper GI bleed. Aspiration of gastric contents through the tube gives a rapid indication of the presence or absence of bleeding. Bright red blood usually denotes an active or recent bleed, whereas dark brown "coffee grounds" indicate an older bleed. A large amount of blood is more worrisome than scant flecks of blood. NG- and OG-tube aspiration gives important information about the location, rate, extent, and age of the bleeding.

Ingestions are another scenario in which a gastric tube is useful diagnostically. Aspiration of recently ingested capsules or tablets allows both confirmation and possible identification of the ingestant. This is a case in which an OG tube is more useful. A *large-bore* gastric tube is preferred to increase the possibility of pill or pill-fragment withdrawal; the smaller nasal anatomy of the child may make passage of a large-bore NG tube difficult.

Instillation of contrast dyes through NG and OG tubes allow for diagnostic imaging studies of the GI tract. The radiographic appearance of an NG tube coiled up in the esophagus may be the initial clue to the diagnosis of esophageal atresia. Determination of gastric pH by NG- or OG-tube aspirate allows for evaluation of the efficacy of medications used to treat ulcers, gastritis, and esophagitis.

One of the most common *therapeutic* indications for the use of NG- or OG- tubes is the delivery of enteral nutrition. Delivery is usually accomplished through the use of NG feeding tubes. However, an alternative method involves placing a transpyloric tube. Hospitalized patients, especially the critically ill who have decreased gastric emptying time, may tolerate this route better. Transpyloric feedings may decrease the risk of aspiration. There is, however, considerable controversy regarding this issue.

There are many other therapeutic indications for use of NG or OG tubes. Aspiration of gastric contents within 1 hour of an ingestion may remove a significant amount of ingestant whether in pill *or* liquid form. In this case, the tube is already in the proper place to begin gastric decontamination with activated charcoal and, in selected cases, whole-bowel irri-gation. A convulsing infant with a known history of water intoxication or near-drowning can have a significant amount of water aspirated from the stomach. This procedure can lessen the hyponatremia.

Gastric lavage with saline is an important first step in the management of an active gastric bleed. Decompression of the stomach and proximal bowel is a key component in the management of patients with an ileus or obstruction. Pancreatitis and protracted vomiting are two additional indications for placement of NG or OG tubes.

Finally, evacuation of the stomach before endotracheal intubation is often used to lessen the risk of aspiration. Similarly, in a child hand-ventilated with a bag and mask, the stomach may need decompression to enhance diaphragmatic excursion.

Contraindications

There are several important contraindications to the passage of NG, OG, and transpyloric tubes. First, because aspiration is a common complication in a patient with an altered mental status, the placement of a tube is contraindicated in patients who do not have protective airway reflexes. Grave consequences include aspiration and respiratory failure.

With an esophageal stricture or recent history of alkali ingestion, there is risk of esophageal perforation if a tube is forced through the esophagus. In addition, tube passage may trigger gagging, which may stimulate profuse bleeding in an awake trauma patient with a penetrating cervical wound. Similarly, tube-induced gagging can injure the spinal cord in a child with an unstable cervical spine.

A contraindication unique to the NG and transpyloric tubes is passage through the nose of a patient with a facial fracture and suspected cribriform plate injury. Passage of the tube may result in a catastrophic intracranial intubation.

Complications

Complications with the use of NG, OG, and transpyloric tubes can be divided into three categories: insertion, placement, and use.

Insertion. Passage into the trachea is an occasional complication and can usually be recognized by the presence of gagging, coughing, a color change, or an inability to speak. When this event occurs, immediately withdraw the tube. Minimize this complication by having the patient swallow or drink during insertion.[8] Further complications include pneumothorax, bronchopleural fistula, pneumonia, empyema, and pulmonic instillation of enteral fluid. Fortunately, these complications are rare in pediatric patients.

The nasal or oropharyngeal mucosa may be abraded during tube passage, which may result in minor bleeding or epistaxis. Abrasion usually can be avoided if the well-lubricated tube is advanced gently and not forced. If resistance still occurs, try the other nostril or a smaller tube.

Occasionally the tube may come out of the mouth. If removal and reinsertion are unsuccessful, stiffen the tube with ice-water immersion. In a study of 121 endotracheally intubated adults, Ratzlaff, Heaslip, and Rothwell[11] found that Salem Sump tubes that were iced for 10 minutes required fewer insertion attempts than more flexible tubes.

Placement Check. When checking placement of a tube, do not assume that any fluid aspirated confirms gastric placement. Fluid can be aspirated from both the lungs and the pleural space. Another false-positive placement involves the auscultation of insufflated air in the stomach area. These "whooshing" or "gurgling" sounds may be transmitted from the thorax to the upper abdomen. On the other hand, do not be misled about a truly properly placed tube without fluid return. These false-negatives may occur if the wall of the NG or OG tube collapses during attempted fluid aspiration or if the side ports are above the fluid level.[10]

Use. Two placement concerns are also potential problems of use. Prevent tube-wall collapse by using a smaller syringe for aspiration or a lower suction pressure. Minor repositioning usually corrects problems with the side ports. Additionally, always check the tube for leaks and patency before use. If aspiration or saline flushes do not clear a block, try a solution of one part vinegar and two parts water.

A complication unique to the OG tube involves biting on the tube by the patient. Avoid this complication by using a bite block or oral airway. Occasional complications of a transpyloric tube are diarrhea and ileus. Minor discomfort is a complication of all tubes. Finally, enteral erosion and perforation are very rare complications that occur with tubes left in place for prolonged periods.

Equipment

The most important equipment for tube placement is the correct tube. The basic types of tubes include the Levin tube, the Salem Sump tube, and the Entriflex or Dobbhoff feeding tubes (Fig. 62-1). The Levin tube is a standard single-lumen, nonradiopaque tube. It is good for instillation, aspiration, and low intermittent suction. The Salem Sump tube is a double-lumen, radiopaque tube. The smaller second lumen permits continuous vent for airflow when constant suction is applied (Fig. 62-2). This tube rarely collapses or sucks in gastric mucosa.[3] Both tubes have multiple distal ports and measuring marks for placement. The feeding tubes are essentially the same as Levin tubes except that they come with a stylet and distal weight to optimize proper placement. Table 62-1 compares and contrasts these tubes.

When choosing sizes for pediatric NG or OG tubes, choose the largest-bore tube that is easily passable. Rough guidelines to follow are as follows: 8 French for an infant, 10-12 French for a small child, 14-16 French for an older child, and 18 French for an adolescent. Alternatively, use a tube size that is twice the estimated endotracheal tube size (i.e., *[Age (yrs) + 16] ÷ 2*).

Additional equipment for tube placement includes lubricant jelly, tape, a rubber band, a safety pin, catheter-tip syringes, saline, a basin, a stethoscope, a glass of water, and a flexible straw. Other useful items might include a pacifier, an ice bath, DuoDERM hydroactive dressing, Cetacaine anesthetic spray, 2% lidocaine gel, and oxymetazoline (Afrin) or phenylephrine (Neo-Synephrine) nasal spray. Meto-

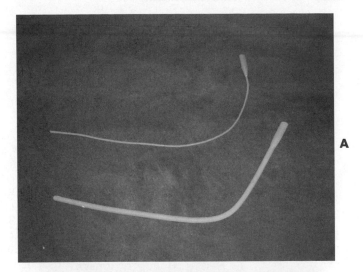

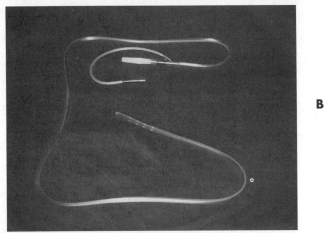

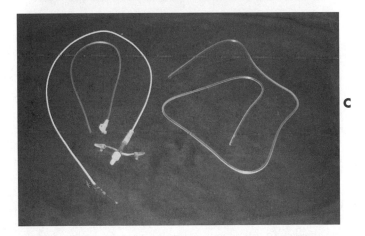

FIG. 62-1   **A,** Levin tubes. **B,** Salem Sump tube. **C,** Feeding tubes.

clopramide (Reglan), a prokinetic agent, may be useful for the passage of the transpyloric tube.

Techniques

Insertion of a Nasogastric Tube. When inserting an NG tube, first select the proper style tube, size, and route for passage. Make sure there are no leaks or blocks in the tube. Estimate the distance that the tube is to be passed. A useful method for estimating is to measure the distance from the tip of the nose to the earlobe to the upper abdomen (Fig. 62-3).

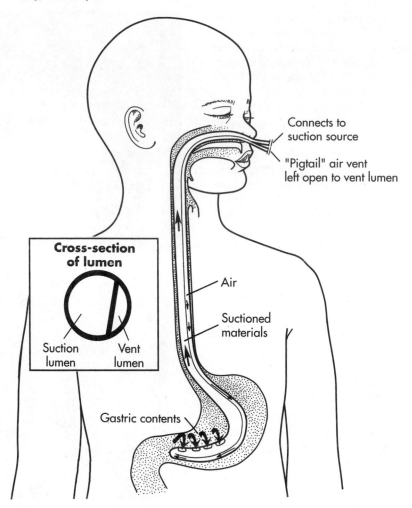

Cross-section
of lumen

Suction
lumen

Vent
lumen

Connects to
suction source

"Pigtail" air vent
left open to vent lumen

Air

Suctioned
materials

Gastric contents

FIG. 62-2 Salem Sump tube in place in a child. Note that air is sucked downward through the proximal "pigtail" of the smaller lumen as gastric contents enter the distal "eyes" and are aspirated upward through the larger lumen.

If possible, have the patient flex his or her neck. The use of a pacifier in an infant and sips of water through a flexible straw in an older child may facilitate passage. Lubricate the end of the tube and liberally insert it into the nostril. It is important to insert along the floor of the nose and to push gently posteriorly, *not* superiorly (Fig. 62-4).

If the child is in pain or if passage is difficult, try oxymetazoline or phenylephrine to vasoconstrict the nasal mucosa and 2% lidocaine gel topically to achieve nasal anesthesia. To minimize gagging, spray Cetacaine into the pharynx.[3] Once the tube is down, check placement (see Placement Check later in this section). When proper placement is ensured, tape the tube to the nose or affix it to the patient's face with DuoDERM hydroactive dressing, which adheres well yet can be peeled off easily (Fig. 62-5).

Insertion of an Orogastric Tube. The procedure for inserting an OG tube essentially is the same as that for an NG tube, except that it is passed through the oropharynx. The passage of an OG tube is usually more comfortable for the patient. However, the NG tube is more comfortable once it has been placed. Lubrication of an OG tube is not necessary.

Insertion of a Transpyloric Feeding Tube. The passage of a transpyloric feeding tube is similar to the passage of an NG

tube, with a few notable exceptions. A feeding tube has a stylet to facilitate passage. Before the tube is inserted, lubricate it by removing the stylet and injecting 10 ml of water through the tube, which activates a preapplied lubricant. Re-insert the stylet after lubrication.

Introduce and pass the lubricated, weighted end in the same manner as for an NG or OG tube. Advance the tube and roll the patient onto his or her right side. The stylet can now be withdrawn. Note that this technique is the same as for passing a gastric feeding tube except for the right-sided positioning.

In a study of 33 adults, Schulz et al.[12] proposed a new modification that adds stomach insufflation with 0.5 to 1 L of air just before the tube is advanced. This study reported an 88% immediate success rate and a 93% overall success rate. They also reported a 0% immediate success rate with the "old" method.[12] Additionally, intravenous (IV) metoclopramide may be useful in stimulating gastric peristalsis.[7]

Placement Check. Several methods can be used to check tube placement. One of the more common methods involves attaching a catheter-tip syringe to the NG or OG tube and aspirating stomach contents. If doubt exists, test the pH of the aspirate. The pH of gastric secretions is usually 1 to 3.5

Table 62-1   Comparison of Levin, Salem Sump, and Feeding
Tubes

Advantages	Disadvantages
Levin tubes	
Easy to pass	Single lumen cannot control amount of suction
Simple to use	
Good for instillation, aspiration, and low intermittent suction	May become occluded with (and cause damage to) gastric mucosa
	Nonradiopaque
Salem sump tubes	
Double lumen allows constant airflow for controlled suction	Venting "pigtail" is sometimes clamped (defeats purpose of the tube)
Minimizes occlusion with (and damage to) gastric mucosa	
Radiopaque	
Feeding tubes	
Thin, flexible, and soft; therefore more comfortable	Passage more difficult; usually requires a stylet
Distal weight to optimize proper placement	Collapses with aspiration
Radiopaque	Need x-ray study to check placement
	Clogs with thick feeds
	May dislodge with retching or forceful cough

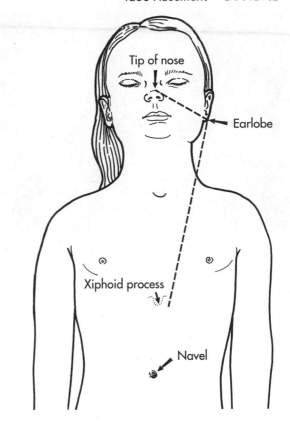

FIG. 62-3   Technique for measuring the distance to pass the NG tube.

(duodenal pH is 6.5, and jejunal pH is 7.5).[13] Another common method involves injecting air through the tube and listening with a stethoscope for "gurgling" or "whooshing." If doubt still exists, obtain an abdominal x-ray study. A properly placed transpyloric tube (in the duodenum or jejunum) should have its tip to the right of the midline on the x-ray study. Once in proper position, the tube need not be changed.

Nasogastric Tube Lavage in Upper GI Bleeding. A saline lavage at room temperature is the optimal solution for patients with upper GI bleeding. Approximate volumes are 50 ml for an infant and 100 to 200 ml for older children. Allow the saline 2 to 3 minutes to dwell and then aspirate by gentle suction. Lavage the stomach until clear. Note, however, that continuation offers little benefit if the lavage has not cleared after 10 minutes. Leave the tube in place for gravity drainage or low suction and consult a gastroenterologist and surgeon. Irrigate the tube every 15 to 30 minutes.

Remarks

Considerable controversy exists regarding the utility of transpyloric feeding tubes. In a two-part prospective study, Marian et al.[7] found a low incidence of spontaneous duodenal passage of transpyloric tubes in critically ill, ventilated adults. Furthermore, they found gastric feeding to be safe and effective. In a review of the literature, Lazarus, Murphy, and Culpepper[6] concluded that there was no difference in the

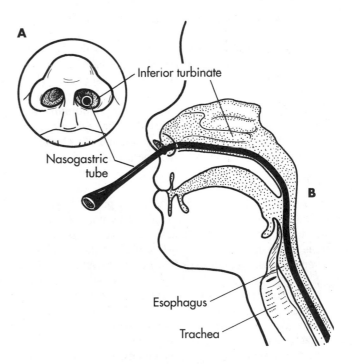

FIG. 62-4   **A,** Slide the NG tube along the floor of the nose. **B,** Sagittal view of NG tube in the nasopharynx.

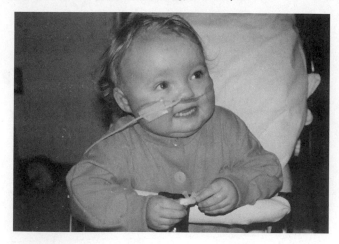

FIG. 62-5 NG tube affixed to child's face with DuoDERM hydroactive dressing.

rates of pulmonary aspiration between transpyloric and gastric feedings. Studies by Grahm, Zadrozny, and Harrington[4] and Strong et al[13] have drawn similar conclusions.

GASTROSTOMY TUBES

The use of gastrostomy tubes (G tubes) with pediatric patients is becoming increasingly common. It is therefore important for the emergency and critical care physician to be familiar with the various types of G tubes and apparatus, their complications, and how to manage them. Furthermore, the physician must have some insight into both the underlying pathologic condition that made the tube necessary and the underlying anatomy.

The surgeon usually inserts the G tube in the operating department with the use of a general anesthetic. Alternatively, the gastroenterologist may percutaneously insert the tube in the endoscopy suite with a local anesthetic. The incision or percutaneous insertion is made through the abdominal wall and into the stomach, midway along the greater curvature. The tube is secured with a purse-string suture, and the stomach is anchored to the peritoneum at the operative site.[14]

Indications

G tubes are most commonly placed in patients who are projected to be unable to take adequate nourishment by mouth for a long period. Esophageal atresia is a good example of an anatomic anomaly that might require a G tube. Children with this condition often need a G tube, not only until the surgeon reconnects the esophagus and stomach but also until the child "learns to eat." Chronic malabsorptive syndromes are another indication for a G tube. For example, an infant who has undergone bowel resection secondary to necrotizing enterocolitis has a continuous GI tract, but his or her short gut syndrome makes supplemental feeds mandatory.

Children who have undergone extensive craniofacial reconstruction to correct congenital anomalies may require G tubes. Similarly, patients with severe facial injuries secondary to trauma may require temporary G-tube placement.

Children with severe neurologic impairments often need G

tubes. Many simply have no urge to eat, whereas others have disorders of chewing or swallowing. Additionally, these children often suffer from severe gastroesophageal reflux. A G tube and Nissen fundoplication are often necessary to prevent aspiration. The special needs of these children require a great deal of nursing and parent time. The G tube simplifies care while also providing a convenient route for long-term enteral nutrition.

Complications

One of the most severe complications of a G tube is gastric outlet obstruction. The child usually experiences a sudden onset of emesis. Emergent management involves pulling back the G tube. Pull on the G tube until there is resistance and the tube is snug against the abdominal wall. Alternatively, it may be safer to pull out the tube completely. The tube may also cause emesis by blocking the esophagus.

Another complication is cellulitis around the stoma. The site is often tender, erythematous, and edematous. The patient may or may not have fever or other systemic symptoms. Therapy involves local care and antibiotics. The differential diagnosis of bacterial infection includes local irritant dermatitis, allergic hypersensitivity reaction, and fungal rash.

A local irritant dermatitis may develop as a result of a small amount of gastric leakage around the tube. Therapy again requires local care. Various protective barriers are also available. Occasionally the gastrostomy site widens, and the leak becomes more excessive. In rare cases of large leaks, the physician may need to discontinue the feeds until the hole narrows. Attempting to solve a leakage problem by replacing the leaky tube with a larger tube is rarely successful. Another complication of a larger stoma is that the tube is more likely to fall out.

Allergic hypersensitivity reactions may be caused by various brands of adhesives or cleaning solutions. Topical hydrocortisone and a brand change are usually palliative. A fungal rash may also develop. This infection, usually with *Candida albicans,* appears as fiery red plaques. An antifungal cream such as clotrimazole is curative. Finally, granulation tissue may develop around the stoma. Silver nitrate swabs usually handle this problem effectively.

Another complication of the G tube is a clog. Parents occasionally complain that the tube will not infuse. If aspiration and gentle flushes with saline or water and vinegar are not effective, try repositioning the tube. If these steps are not successful, the tube may need to be replaced. Do not try to pull out a new tube that has been in place for only a few weeks without surgical or gastroenterologic consultation because the tract may not yet have healed.

A tube that has fallen out is a more common complication. If a tube becomes dislodged in the first few weeks after the ostomy is created, replace it with a smaller Foley catheter. This technique may prevent pushing the newly fixed stomach away from the anterior abdominal wall. If doubt exists regarding the placement of the newly inserted tube, consider a dye study. Extravasation of dye indicates a problem that may require operative correction.

Replace an older tube that has fallen out as soon as possible. If this tube is not replaced immediately, the stoma may narrow and become impassable to that same tube. *Forcing* a tube into a small stoma may result in bleeding,

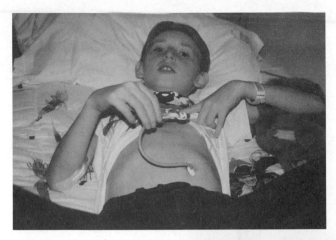

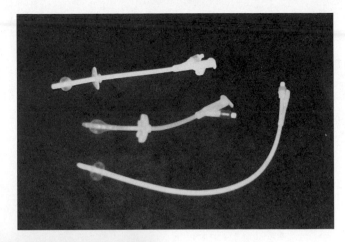

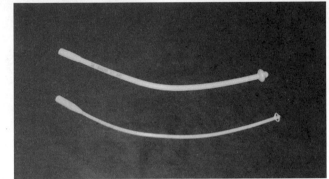

FIG. 62-6   **A,** G tube in a child with tube position guard at skin. **B,** G tubes with distal securing balloons. **C,** G tubes with distal securing mushrooms.

tract disruption, gastric perforation, and undue pain. Reinsert a smaller tube or Foley catheter to keep the tract patent until consultation can be obtained.

Equipment

Reinsertion of a G tube requires Luer-Lok syringes, a catheter-tip syringe, a clamp, a water-soluble lubricant (K-Y jelly), and saline. Additional G-tube equipment may include tube position guards (Fig. 62-6, *A*) and obturators.

There are many types of G tubes. The basic tube has one or two proximal ports for infusing liquids. Many G tubes have an additional proximal port to inflate a distal securing balloon (Fig. 62-6, *B*). Alternatively, the G tube may have a distal "mushroom" tip to secure the tube (Fig. 62-6, *C*). Tubes with this type of tip usually come with an obturator for insertion (Fig. 62-7). The distal end may have one or many ports for exit.

The Gastroport, or button G tube, deserves special note because it is different from the others (Fig. 62-8, *A*). This tube is nearly flush with the patient's abdomen (Fig. 62-8, *B*) and has a proximal button to close it when finished. This tube has a one-way valve at the proximal end that minimizes reflux and eliminates the need for clamping. Do not check residuals with this type of tube because doing so may damage the one-way valve.[14] Attach an adapter into the proximal end of the button to infuse the desired fluid. The distal end may or may not have a mushroom tip.

Techniques

Insertion of a Mushroom-Tip Gastrostomy Tube. Insertion of a mushroom-tip G tube requires an obturator. Insert the obturator through the G tube and into the mushroom to stretch and extend the tip. Hold the lubricated, obturator-fitted G tube perpendicular to the abdomen. Rest the distal hand on the abdomen while applying firm, steady pressure with the proximal hand.

The resistance abruptly decreases when the mushroom enters the stomach. Advance the mushroom a few more centimeters into the stomach so that the mushroom can open properly. Be careful not to continue pushing forcefully once the resistance decreases; doing so could injure the opposite wall of the stomach. Remove the obturator and gently pull on the tube until the resistance of the mushroom hitting the stomach is felt. Apply a tube guard, or bolster, to prevent forward progression of the tube toward the pylorus. If this device is not available, tape the tube in place (see Fig. 62-7).

Insertion of a Balloon-Tip Gastrostomy Tube. Insertion of a balloon-tip G tube is very similar to the insertion of a mushroom-tip G tube. First, check the balloon for leaks. Inject 5 ml of saline into the Y end of the tube using a 5-ml Luer-Lok syringe. The balloon should inflate and have no leaks. Withdraw the saline by aspirating through the same syringe.

After passing the lubricated balloon tip into the stomach, use saline again to reinflate the balloon. Remove the syringe

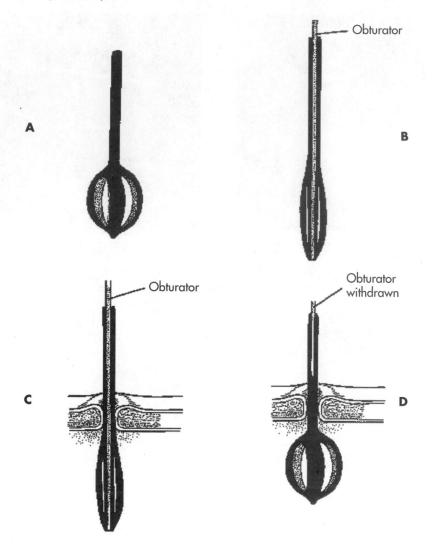

FIG. 62-7 **A,** Mushroom tip of G tube. **B,** Inserted obturator stretches mushroom. **C,** Obturator guides G tube through gastrostomy. **D,** Withdrawn obturator allows mushroom to reopen to secure G tube.

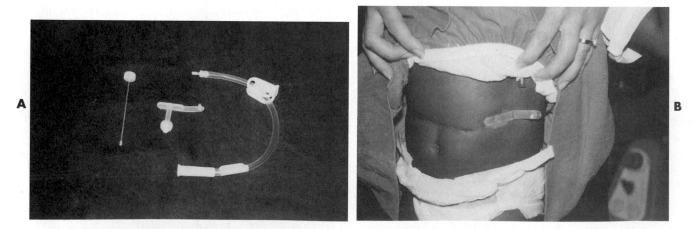

FIG. 62-8 Gastroport, or button, G tubes. **A,** Obturator, G tube, and adapter (*left to right*). **B,** G tube in child.

and pull gently on the tube until it meets resistance. The tube can now be secured and clamped.

SENGSTAKEN-BLAKEMORE TUBE

Upper GI bleeding constitutes 90% of all major GI bleeding.[1] Esophageal varices are the cause of one of the most severe types of bleeds. In 1950, Sengstaken and Blakemore introduced the concept of balloon tamponade for the control of bleeding esophageal varices. Though developed for the adult, the technique is similar in the child.[5]

The Sengstaken-Blakemore tube (Fig. 62-9) is a triple-lumen tube with a gastric and an esophageal balloon. Two of the lumens inflate the gastric and esophageal balloons, and the third lumen is used to aspirate gastric contents. Another type of tube, the Linton tube, has only a single-lumen gastric balloon. The Sengstaken-Blakemore tube is more effective than the Linton tube for esophageal bleeding, whereas the Linton tube with its bigger gastric balloon is more effective for gastric bleeding.[2] The Sengstaken-Blakemore tube is used more often and has a success rate of 50% to 80%.[1]

Indications

The initial management of upper GI bleeding includes airway protection, oxygen, access with large-bore catheters, aggressive volume resuscitation, crossmatching for blood component transfusions, and NG-tube lavage. If bleeding continues after 10 to 15 minutes of NG-tube lavage and the patient's vital signs are stable, the surgeon or gastroenterologist may consider flexible endoscopy. When emergent endoscopy confirms the diagnosis of bleeding varices, options include sclerotherapy, metoclopramide and a vasopressin infusion, and/or the Sengstaken-Blakemore tube. The Sengstaken-Blakemore tube is indicated in situations of massive life-threatening hemorrhage or continued bleeding despite IV vasopressin and blood transfusions.

Contraindications

Contraindications for the use of the Sengstaken-Blakemore tube include recent esophageal surgery and known esophageal stricture. The patient with a loss of pharyngeal reflexes should be intubated with a cuffed endotracheal tube before using the Sengstaken-Blakemore tube. However, with persistent hemorrhage even these contraindications become rela-

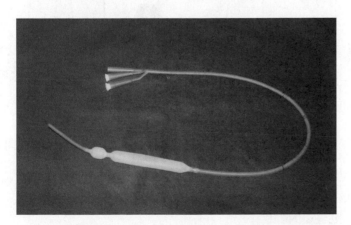

FIG. 62-9   Sengstaken-Blakemore tube.

tive.[12] In patients with massive hemorrhage that is unresponsive to lavage and blood component therapy, operative intervention is imperative and precludes gastric intubation.

Complications

One of the most severe complications of the Sengstaken-Blakemore tube is airway occlusion, which is usually caused by the migration of the esophageal balloon up and into the hypopharynx. This migration may result from excessive traction on the tube. Treatment involves emergent cutting of the tube just below the triple ports (to deflate the balloons) and immediate removal of the tube.

Another airway complication is aspiration, which is usually secondary to the accumulation of secretions in the esophagus. Avoid this complication by placing an NG tube in the esophagus for suction. Alternatively, consider definitive airway protection with a cuffed endotracheal tube.

Esophageal rupture is another very severe complication of the Sengstaken-Blakemore tube. Inflation of the gastric balloon in the esophagus is usually the cause. A more chronic complication is esophageal or gastric erosion secondary to excessive or prolonged pressure from the balloons. Such complications illustrate the importance of periodic (at least every 6 hours) deflation of the balloons.

If the bleeding persists despite tube placement, consider suboptimal balloon placement as well as erroneous diagnosis. Some less life-threatening complications include retrosternal chest discomfort, agitation, epistaxis, and hiccups.[2] The overall complication rate is 9% to 35%, with a mortality rate of 5% to 20%.[1]

Equipment

The equipment necessary for placement of a Sengstaken-Blakemore tube includes an NG tube, suction equipment (source, collection receptacle, tubing), catheter-tip syringes, saline, anesthetic spray (e.g., oxymetazoline HC1 0.05%), several rubber-tipped hemostats, scissors, tape, a mercury manometer, and lubricant. There is a special Sengstaken-Blakemore tube for children less than 13 years of age.

Techniques

Before inserting a Sengstaken-Blakemore tube, test the balloons. Inflate the balloons under water; inflate the esophageal balloon to 50 mm Hg (Fig. 62-10); the gastric balloon gets 250 ml of air.[2] If no leaks are detected, deflate the balloons. Next, check the patency of all lumens.

Premeasure the distance that the NG tube will be placed into the *esophagus*. Place the NG tube next to Sengstaken-Blakemore tube with tip of the NG tube just above the proximal portion of the esophageal balloon. Place tape around the proximal end of the NG tube as a marker.[2]

Empty the stomach before passing the Sengstaken-Blakemore tube; this step lessens the chance of aspiration. Applying a local vasoconstrictor (e.g., oxymetazoline HC1 0.05%) to the nasal mucosa is also helpful.[1]

Pass the lubricated tube into the nose (or the mouth in small pediatric patients). When the tube is completely in, inflate the gastric balloon with 50 to 100 ml of air and clamp the gastric balloon port. Pull the tube gently until the resistance of the stomach is met. Confirm the proper place-

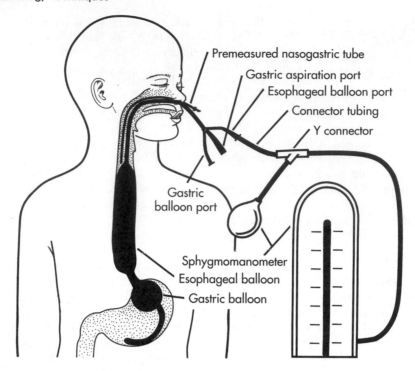

FIG. 62-10 Diagram of Sengstaken-Blakemore tube attached to manometer to inflate esophageal balloon to proper pressure.

ment of the gastric balloon with an immediate abdominal x-ray study.

The physician may now choose to add air into the gastric balloon—up to 150 ml in the pediatric balloon and 250 ml in the adult balloon. Pull the tube slightly until taut then tape it at the nose. The majority of bleeds stop with the inflation of the gastric balloon.[1]

After the gastric balloon is inflated and secured, pass the premeasured NG tube. This step controls the accumulation of saliva and blood that can lead to aspiration. If the esophageal bleeding continues, inflate *that* balloon too. As depicted in Fig. 62-10, attach the inflow tube of the Sengstaken-Blakemore tube to a sphygmomanometer; inflate the esophageal balloon to the minimum required to control the bleeding (up to a maximum of 40 mm Hg). Clamp the intake port of the esophageal balloon to prevent air leaks. Fig. 62-11 depicts a properly placed Sengstaken-Blakemore tube in a child.

Remarks

Do not spray the topical anesthetic in the pharynx because doing so may depress the gag reflex and possibly increase the likelihood of aspiration. Use only *air* to inflate the balloons; the use of liquids may make emergency deflation of the balloons more difficult.[2] For this reason, keep a pair of scissors at the bedside at all times.

It is also useful to keep the patient's head at a 30- to 45-degree angle, which helps keep the stomach empty and decreases nausea and aspiration. Remember to irrigate the gastric lumen to maintain its patency. Finally, check the esophageal pressure every 30 minutes to ensure that it is optimal.[1]

Most physicians usually keep the balloons inflated for approximately 24 hours. Deflate the esophageal balloon first;

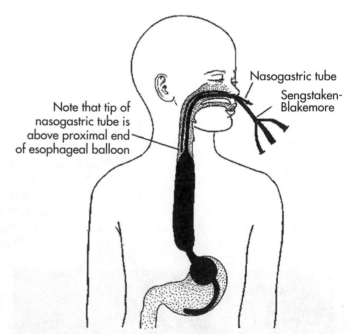

FIG. 62-11 View of Sengstaken-Blakemore tube properly inflated in a child.

deflate the gastric balloon 1 hour later. Monitor the complication of rebleeding by irrigating and aspirating through the gastric tube every ½ hour for the next 1 to 2 hours.[1] If there is no new blood, remove the tube.

REFERENCES

1. Boyle JT: Gastrointestinal Emergencies. In Fleisher G, Ludwig S, editors: *Textbook of pediatric emergency medicine,* ed 3, Baltimore, 1993, Williams & Wilkins.

2. Glauser J: Balloon tamponade of gastroesophageal varices. In Roberts JR, Hedges JR, editors: *Clinical procedures in emergency medicine,* ed 2, Philadelphia, 1991, WB Saunders.

3. Glauser J: Nasogastric Intubation. In Roberts JR, Hedges JR, editors: *Clinical procedures in emergency medicine,* ed 2, Philadelphia, 1991, Saunders.

4. Grahm TW, Zadrozny DB, Harrington T: The benefits of early jejunal hyperalimentation in the head-injured patient, *Neurosurgery* 25:729-735, 1989.

5. Kline JJ: Modification of the adult Blakemore tube for use in children with bleeding esophageal varices, *J Pediatr Gastroenterol Nutr* 5(1):153-154, 1986.

6. Lazarus BA, Murphy JB, Culpepper L: Aspiration associated with long-term gastric versus jejunal feeding: a critical analysis of the literature, *Arch Physical Med Rehabil* 71:46-53, 1990.

7. Marian M, Rappaport W, Cunningham D, et al: The failure of conventional methods to promote spontaneous transpyloric feeding tube passage and the safety of intragastric feeding in the critically ill ventilated patient, *Surgery* 176:475-479, 1993.

8. May M, Nellis KJ: Nasogastric intubation: avoiding complications, *Res Staff Phys* 30(7):60-62, 1984.

9. McCormick PA, Burroughs AK, McIntyre N: How to insert a Sengstaken-Blakemore tube, *Br J Hosp Med* 43:274-276, 1990.

10. Metheny N: Measures to test placement of nasogastric and nasointestinal feeding tubes: a review, *Nurs Res* 37(36):324-329, 1988.

11. Ratzlaff C, Heaslip JE, Rothwell ES: Factors affecting nasogastric tube insertion, *Crit Care Med* 12(1):52-53, 1984.

12. Schulz MA, Santanello SA, Monk J, et al: An improved method for transpyloric placement of nasoenteric feeding tubes, *Internat Surg* 78:79-82, 1993.

13. Strong RM, et al: Equal aspiration rates from postpylorus and intragastric-placed small-bore nasoenteric feeding tubes: a randomized, prospective study, *J Pediatr Enter Nutr* 16:59-63, 1992.

14. Volden C, Grinde J, Carl D: Taking the trauma out of nasogastric intubation, *Nurs 80* 10(9):64-67, September 1980.

63 Anoscopy

Evaline A. Alessandrini

Anoscopy is a valuable diagnostic tool in the evaluation of anorectal diseases in infancy and childhood. It can be performed using commercially available anoscopes, otoscopes, and glass test tubes, or by manual eversion of the anus. Adequate visualization of the anal canal can be accomplished by any of these simple procedures.

A review of anatomy will simplify the performance and interpretation of the procedure (Fig. 63-1). The mucosa of the anal canal consists of stratified squamous epithelium. Distally it ends at the anal verge, which is also known as the perianal region. Proximally, the anorectal line marks the junction of the anal canal with the rectal ampulla. Here the rectal mucosa forms the columns of Morgagni and the anal crypts that are involved in fissures, abscesses, and other proctocologic conditions. The anal sphincter mechanism surrounding the anal canal consists of an internal sphincter of involuntary smooth muscle and a striated voluntary muscle capable of strong contraction.

Indications

Indications for performing anoscopy with or without an anoscope include a variety of conditions[1,3] (Box 63-1). The most common indication is exploring the etiology of blood-streaked stools or blood in the diaper or on the toilet tissue.[1] Anoscopy may reveal an anal fissure in a child of any age or hemorrhoids in an adolescent. Rectal pain or pain with defecation may disclose anal fissures, perianal abscesses, or hemorrhoids. Pruritis of the anal region warrants anoscopy for the evaluation of pinworms or other causes of inflammation. The etiology of recurrent constipation, diarrhea, or nonspecific abdominal pain may be elucidated. The diagnosis and treatment of anal foreign bodies can be accomplished. Anoscopy also plays a role in the evaluation of sexual abuse as demonstrated by anal tears. Sexually transmitted diseases such as genital warts or gonorrhea can be cultured and diagnosed. Investigation of mucous stools can be pursued for inflammation or infection. In some cases, patients may complain of perianal discomfort or a mass, and anoscopy reveals a rectal prolapse or prolapsed polyp. Collection of samples for heme testing and stool culturing are easily obtainable during anoscopy.

BOX 63-1 **INDICATIONS FOR ANOSCOPY**

Blood-streaked stools	Pain with defecation
Blood in diaper or on toilet tissue	Pruritis of the anal region
	Anal foreign body
Mucous discharge from the anus	Presence of perianal mass or lesion
Rectal pain	

Contraindications

There are few absolute contraindications to anoscopy. However, do not not perform this procedure on a patient with an imperforate anus or on one with a history of repaired imperforate anus.[2] Perform a digital rectal examination before using an anoscope.[4] Obstruction, stenosis, or severe pain also preclude anoscopy with instrumentation.[6] In these cases, perform only a visual inspection. Other relative contraindications include neutropenia, acute peritonitis, rectal abscess, acute inflammatory bowel disease, and toxic megacolon.[10]

Complications

The most common complication encountered during anoscopy is irritation of the anal mucosa, especially bleeding from small tears or fissures. When using a glass test tube for anoscopy, ensure that the glass does not break while it is in the anal canal. A theoretical complication of anoscopy is bacteremia. Bacteremia has been described in 8% to 10% of all patients undergoing sigmoidoscopic evaluation[11] but has not been described in the pediatric population during anoscopy. Proceed cautiously with patients with neutropenia. The most severe complication includes perforation of the rectum if the anoscope is not correctly positioned or has been advanced too far.

Equipment

Gloves and a water-soluble lubricant are necessary for a digital rectal examination. Select a commercially available anoscope of the appropriate size for the child being examined. For an infant, use a 1-cm outer diameter anoscope with a length of 8 to 10 cm; for children, use a 1.5-cm outer diameter anoscope with a length of 12 to 25 cm.[9] An adult anoscope is adequate for most adolescents (Fig. 63-2). Anoscopes are available with a powered light source or as disposables for which an extrinsic light source is necessary.[8]

Adequate examination of the anal canal is also possible with a glass test tube and an external light source such as an otoscope light, a floor lamp, or a penlight. A special head can be fitted onto the handle of a traditional otoscope for anoscopy.[5] Other equipment needed at the bedside includes cotton balls or swabs for clearing the anal lumen and culture material as required for diagnostic purposes.

Techniques

After the appropriate equipment has been assembled, proper positioning of the child is crucial (Fig. 63-3). To examine infants, place them in the supine position with the legs flexed at the hips and slightly abducted by an assistant standing at the head.[9] To perform anoscopy in children, place them in either the left lateral decubitus position or in a prone knee-to-chest position. When using the left lateral decubitus position, keep the patient's left leg straight and the right leg

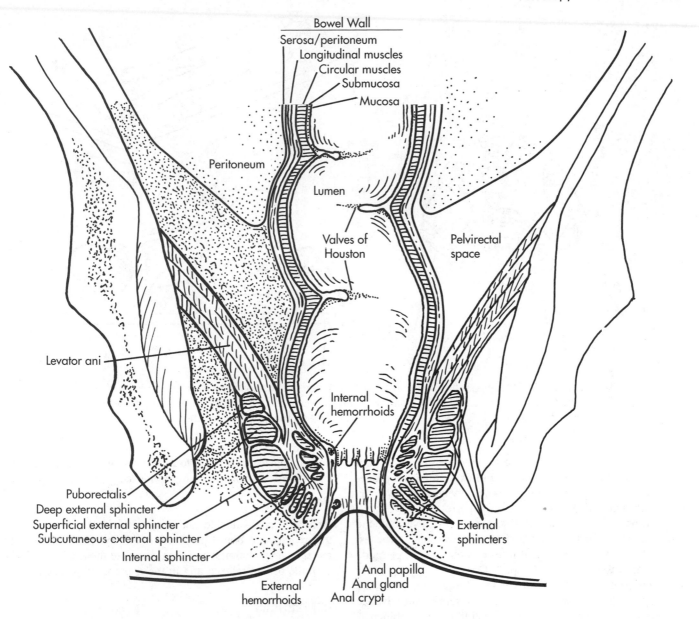

Bowel Wall
Serosa/peritoneum
Longitudinal muscles
Circular muscles
Submucosa
Mucosa

Peritoneum

Lumen

Valves of
Houston

Pelvirectal
space

Levator ani

Internal
hemorrhoids

Puborectalis
Deep external sphincter
Superficial external sphincter
Subcutaneous external sphincter
Internal sphincter

External
sphincters

External
hemorrhoids

Anal papilla
Anal gland
Anal crypt

FIG. 63-1   Coronal section of the anal canal and rectum.

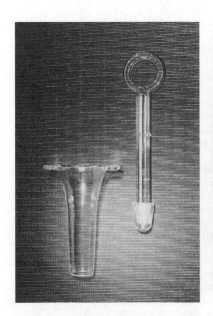
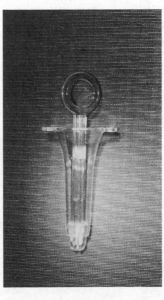

FIG. 63-2   Adult-sized disposable anoscope with obturator.

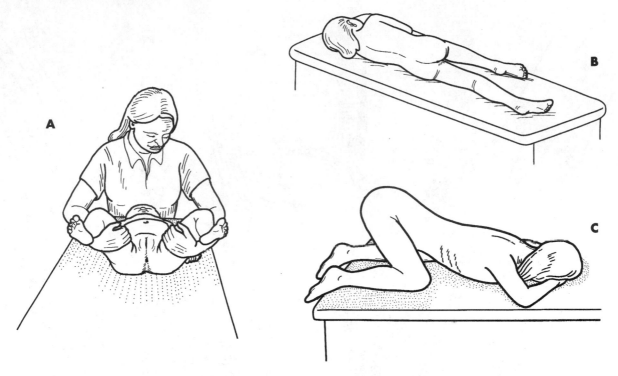

FIG. 63-3 Proper positioning for infants and children during anoscopy. **A,** Infant supine with hips flexed and abducted by assistant. **B,** Child in lateral decubitus position with upper knee drawn toward chest. **C,** Child in prone position resting on knees and upper chest.

flexed and drawn toward the chest. Alternatively, draw both legs toward the chest. Reassuring and explaining the procedure to the child and parent reduces anxiety and improves the ease with which the procedure can be performed.

Next, perform a digital rectal examination to determine the direction of the anal canal and to discover any stenoses, obstructions, or severely painful lesions that would preclude examination with the anoscope.[4] Once the appropriately sized anoscope has been chosen and lubricated, place the anoscope with the obturator at the anal verge, and advance with slow gentle pressure in the direction of the umbilicus.[8] Ask an older child to bear down to relax sphincter muscles and facilitate advancement of the anoscope.[7]

When the anoscope has been inserted to the desired length, remove the obturator. Do not advance the anoscope further or reinsert the obturator because doing so may cause a nipping of the anal mucosa.[6] Once the obturator has been removed, examine the anal canal and obtain cultures and specimens while slowly and steadily withdrawing the anoscope and rotating it in a 360-degree manner.

Many Emergency Departments and pediatric intensive care units are not equipped with an anoscope. In this case, perform this examination by manually spreading the buttocks of the child to evert the anal canal. Some physicians are able to visualize the more proximal anal canal by inserting a test tube and shining a light source into it. The walls of the anal canal can be seen easily through the clear test tube. Accomplish the anal canal examination by using a special head for an otoscope or a nasal speculum to spread the anal mucosa, and look for any pathologic conditions with an external light source. In the event that the anoscopy proves to be nondiagnostic, consider a referral to a pediatric gastroenterologist or surgeon for flexible proctosigmoidoscopy or colonoscopy.

Remarks

Anoscopy is a valuable and easy-to-perform diagnostic tool that requires no bowel preparation. Always perform a digital rectal examination first and then complete the anoscopy easily with the patient relaxed and in the appropriate position.

REFERENCES

1. Berry R, Perrault J: Gastrointestinal bleeding. In Walker WA, Durie PR, Hamilton JR, et al, editors: *Pediatric gastrointestinal disease*, vol 1, Philadelphia, 1991, BC Decker.
2. Bockus HL, editor: *Gastroenterology*, vol 2, Philadelphia, 1976, WB Saunders.
3. Brown CH, editor: *Diagnostic procedures in gastroenterology*, St. Louis, 1967, Mosby.
4. Christian RL: Anorectal disorders. In Branch WT, editor: *The office practice of medicine*, Philadelphia, 1982, WB Saunders.
5. Cucchiara S, Guandalini S, Staiano A, et al: Sigmoidoscopy, colonoscopy and radiology in the evaluation of children with rectal bleeding, *J Pediatr Gastroenterol Nutr* 2:667-671, 1983.
6. Ellis DJ, Beran PG: Proctoscopy and sigmoidoscopy, *Br Med J* 281:435-437, 1980.
7. Farmer KCR, Church JM: Open sesame: tips for traversing the anal canal, *Dis Colon Rectum* 35(11):1092-1093, 1992.
8. Glauser JM: Anoscopy and sigmoidoscopy. In Roberts JR, Hedges JR, *Clinical procedures in emergency medicine*, ed 2, Philadelphia, 1991, WB Saunders.
9. Hijmans JC: Proctoscopy of the infant, *Am J Dis Child* 105:113-115, 1963.
10. Otto P, Klause E: *Atlas of rectoscopy and colonoscopy*, Berlin, 1973, Springer-Verlag.
11. Simon RR, Brenner BE: Proctoscopy in the infant. In *Emergency procedures and techniques*, ed 2, Baltimore, 1987, Williams & Wilkins.

64 Reduction of Rectal Prolapse

Evaline A. Alessandrini

Rectal prolapse is a rare condition characterized by an abnormal protrusion of the rectum through the anus. Partial prolapse involves the mucosa and submucosa and is most common in children who are less than 3 years of age. Peak incidence occurs in the 1- to 2-year age group and may be a result of recently acquired erect posture and voluntary control over defecation.[5] Prolapse of the entire rectal wall is termed *procidentia* and occurs more often both in older children with underlying disease and in debilitated elderly adults.[1]

In most cases of childhood rectal prolapse, the cause is unknown. Diarrhea or straining with bowel movements is a common provoking factor. Children with weak rectal musculature—such as those with meningomyelocele, prune-belly syndrome, and exstrophy of the bladder—are predisposed to rectal prolapse.[2] Procidentia in an older child warrants an investigation for diseases associated with this condition, such as cystic fibrosis, rectal polyps, or illnesses associated with ascites or a sustained cough.

Patients with rectal prolapse present with a painless protrusion from the rectum that often resolves spontaneously. Stools may contain much mucus and small amounts of blood. On physical examination, mucosal prolapse appears as radial folds of mucosa protruding through the anus.[7] Full-thickness prolapse is characterized by circular folds in the prolapsed mucosa.[5] Rectal prolapse must be differentiated from hemorrhoids, a prolapsed rectal polyp, or an intussusception extruded via the anus.

Indications

Manual reduction of a rectal prolapse that has not reduced spontaneously is always indicated. Reduction is also necessary if the prolapse is prolonged or if passive congestion or bleeding has occurred. Unlike with adults, simple mucosal prolapse in the pediatric population does not require surgical evaluation unless it is recurrent or recalcitrant to routine management. Prolapse as a complication of anorectal surgery requires specialized surgical procedures for its correction.[3,6]

Contraindications

There are no absolute contraindications for the reduction of a rectal prolapse. If vascular compromise of the prolapsed segment is evident, perform reduction immediately. Admit these patients to the hospital because they are at risk for bowel perforation.

Complications

The rectal prolapse itself may be complicated by bleeding or ulceration. Rarely, the prolapsed bowel can become gangrenous if the prolapse is prolonged. Rupture of a vascularly compromised segment could occur during manual reduction but has not been reported in the pediatric literature.

Equipment

The only equipment required for reducing a rectal prolapse are gloves, a lubricant, and some gauze pads. A sedative that is appropriate for the age of the patient and the level of anxiety may be necessary (see Chapter 12).

Techniques

Place the adequately sedated patient in a prone position over the parent's lap or in the knee-chest position on the examination table. Use lubricated gloves to place 4 × 4 gauze pads at the 3 and 9 o'clock positions of the prolapse (Fig. 64-1). Gauze improves grip on the mucosa. Apply firm, gentle pressure to reduce the direction of the prolapse. Such pressure can be achieved by pressing on the prolapse with both thumbs while stabilizing the hands on the buttocks (see Fig. 64-1). Alternatively, the index and middle fingers may be used to compress the prolapse while an assistant holds the patient (Fig. 64-2). As much as 15 minutes of pressure is often required to complete the reduction. Perform a digital rectal examination to ensure that the reduction is complete.[5] Instruct the patient to lie on his or her side after the procedure. If the prolapse recurs immediately, tape the buttocks temporarily.

Surgery may be warranted if there is no response to conservative management. Surgery includes perirectal injection of sclerosing agents, with which many authors report an excellent success rate.[4,8] Major surgical procedures as performed on adults are rarely necessary in children.[4,8] Major surgical procedures as performed on adults are rarely necessary in children.[4]

Remarks

In the case of acute rectal prolapse in children, it is first necessary to ascertain the diagnosis by distinguishing it from hemorrhoids, a prolapsed polyp, or extruded intussusception. Hemorrhoids occur primarily in adolescents, are purple in color, and are contiguous with one wall of the anal mucosa so that a palpating finger cannot encircle the entire hemorrhoid. Prolapsed polyps often are palpable within the rectum as a small growth on a stalk. Again, they arise from a single wall of the rectum and not from the entire circumference. Intussusception is a diagnosis suspected on clinical grounds in a lethargic child who is vomiting. On physical examination the circular folds of the mucosa of the intussusception may appear as a full-thickness rectal prolapse. The extent of the prolapse and the clinical history and examination lead to the diagnosis of intussusception. After manual reduction, it is of utmost importance to address the primary problem. Because straining with stools is the most common inciting event for rectal prolapse, prescribe stool softeners and lubricants such as mineral oil. In addition, recommend a child toilet seat for toilet-trained children to reduce the spreading of the gluteal

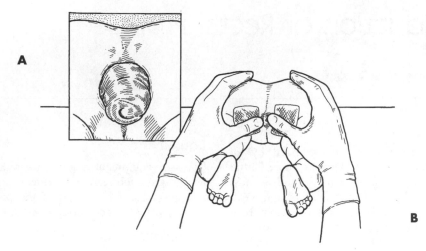

FIG. 64-1 Manually reducing a rectal prolapse. **A,** Illustration of prolapse before reduction. **B,** Thumb method for reduction.

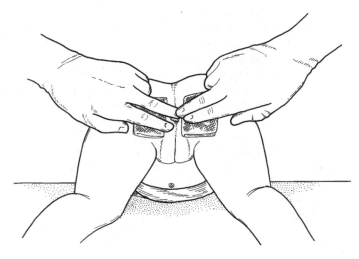

FIG. 64-2 Finger method for reduction (see text for explanation).

folds during defecation. Patients with recurrent prolapse require a work-up for cystic fibrosis and a barium enema to rule out rectal polyps or other lesions that may act as a lead point for the prolapse.

REFERENCES

1. Altemeier WA, Culbertson WR, Schowengerdt C, et al: Nineteen years' experience with one-state perineal repair of rectal prolapse, *Ann Surg* 173:993, 1971.
2. Armstrong AL, Bivins BA, Sachatello CR: Rectal prolapse: a brief review, *J Ky Med Assoc* 76:329, 1978.
3. Caouette-Laberge L, Yazbeck S, Laberge JM, et al: Multiple-flap anoplasty in the treatment of rectal prolapse after pull-through operations for imperforate anus, *J Pediatr Surg* 22:65-67, 1987.
4. Kay NRM, Zachary RB: The treatment of rectal prolapse in children with injections on 30% saline solutions, *J Pediatr Surg* 5:334, 1970.
5. Leape LL: Other disorders of the rectum and anus. In Welch KJ, Randolph JG, Ravitch, MM, et al, editors: *Pediatric surgery*, vol 2, ed 4, Chicago, 1986, Year Book Medical.
6. Nixon HH, Puri P: The results of treatment of anorectal anomalies: a thirteen to twenty year follow-up, *J Pediatr Surg* 12:27-37, 1977.
7. Schwartz SI, Lillenei RC, Shires GT, et al, editors: *Principles of surgery*, ed 3, New York, 1977, McGraw-Hill.
8. Wyllie GG: The injection treatment of rectal prolapse, *J Pediatr Surg* 14:62, 1979.

65 Enemas

Evaline A. Alessandrini

Occasionally a health-care provider may find it necessary to prescribe or administer an enema to an infant or child for a variety of bowel problems.

Indications

Enemas may be classified as therapeutic, diagnostic, or cleansing. Cleansing enemas are indicated for evacuation of the lower bowel before radiologic or surgical procedures. The most common diagnostic enema is the barium enema, which is used to diagnose conditions of the lower gastrointestinal tract. Therapeutic enemas are directed at the treatment of several disease states. Many different types of enemas are used to treat constipation and fecal impaction. Warm fluid enemas may be used as therapy for hypothermia in children. Barium or air enemas are used in the radiologic suite not only to diagnose but also to reduce intussusception in pediatric patients.

Further discussion of radiologic enemas and cleansing enemas for surgery is beyond the scope of this text. This chapter concentrates on the use of therapeutic enemas for constipation and fecal impaction in the pediatric population. In most instances, immediate evacuation of an enema is all that is required for the treatment of constipation. However, use a retention enema in children with severe fecal impaction or obstipation. Tape or squeeze together the buttocks of a younger child or ask the older child to contract the perineal muscles.

Contraindications

Do not administer enemas to patients with intestinal disorders that predispose them to perforation. Such diagnoses include inflammatory bowel disease, appendicitis, diverticulitis, or other illnesses characterized by peritonitis or vascular compromise. Immunosupression is another contraindication to enema therapy.[8]

Imperforate anus and toxic megacolon are cases in which enemas must be used discriminately. In these diseases, evacuation of the enema fluid is delayed or impeded and may result in metabolic abnormalities as the fluid is absorbed through the intestinal lumen.

Use enemas, particularly those of the phosphate variety, with great caution in children with renal disease because this therapy can promote hypocalcemia and hyperphosphatemia. Because phosphate binds with the aluminum and magnesium found in antacids, children taking these antacids should not receive phosphate enemas.

Complications

Many children experience mild abdominal pain and cramping or anal irritation and pruritis after receiving an enema. Children may develop a dependence on enemas to defecate if they are used repetitively. Hypothermia may complicate enema therapy, particularly in infants, if the fluid is not warmed to body temperature before administration. Transient bacteremia is a recognized but unusual complication of enema treatments.[8]

Perforation of the rectum may occur if the rectal catheter is not properly positioned during fluid instillation or if an enema is given to a patient who has an inflammatory intestinal contraindication.

Metabolic abnormalities resulting from enema therapy have been reported in the pediatric literature. These abnormalities most commonly include hyperphosphatemia and hypocalcemia from the administration of phosphate enemas.[3,4,7] Hypernatremia and dehydration have also been described as complications of sodium phosphate enemas.[1,3] Hyponatremia has been described with the use of tap-water enemas in infants.[2] Consequently, judicious use of enemas in children includes selection of the proper fluid, the appropriate volume, adequate and timely fluid evacuation, and the ability to monitor for complications, particularly metabolic derangements.

Equipment

Materials to be assembled before enema administration include nonsterile gloves, lubricant, a bed pan or diapers for the younger child, towels, and a waterproof pad for the bed. A commercially available enema kit may be used. CB Fleet Company, Inc. in Lynchburg, Virginia, makes several effective over-the-counter enema solutions. Other fluids administered as enemas include tap water, mineral oil, soapsuds, and even milk and molasses. The use of these substances has not been well-investigated in children; consequently, the correct doses and side effects of these enemas have not been definitively established.[8] Mineral oil is an effective enema for lubrication for hard fecal impactions and allows the stool to exit the rectal vault more easily. Controlled trials evaluating the advantages of different types of enema solutions in children have not been performed. Many recommendations are based on anectodal experience. Sodium phosphate enemas are most commonly and safely used in children. In the event that an enema kit is not available, enema fluids may be administered via a 10 or 12 French catheter[6] (Table 65-1). Warm the enema fluid to body temperature (37.7° C) to increase peristalsis; avoid heating to more than 40° C.[5] To prevent hypothermia, always warm enema fluids for infants less than 1 year of age.

Technique

After all equipment has been assembled and the procedure has been explained to the patient and parent, properly position the patient. Place the infant or young child in a supine position, place a bed pan under the buttocks and a pillow under the head and back because the patient will be

Table 65-1 Types of Commercially Available Enema Fluid

Fluid	Mechanism	Dosage	Dosage supplied
Sodium phosphate and biphosphate	Laxative, direct cleansing action	<2 yr—75 ml >2 yr—135 ml	135 ml 75 ml
Mineral oil	Lubricates stool in cases of fecal impaction	2-6 yr—75 ml > 6 yr—135ml	135 ml
Bisacodyl	Stimulates peristalsis through colonic mucosa	2-6 yr—15 ml >6 yr—30 ml	30 ml

Table 65-2 Enema Volume and Catheter Advancement by Age

	Fluid volume	Catheter advancement distance
Infant (5-10 kg)	100-250 ml	1 in
Preschool child (10-25 mg)	200-300 ml	2 in
School-age child (25-50 mg)	250-500 ml	3 in
Adolescent (>50 kg)	500-700 ml	3-4 in

unable to retain the fluid after administration. Rest the older child in the left lateral recumbent position with the knees drawn toward the chest.

Lubricate the rectal catheter. Commercially available enema kits are packaged with a prelubricated catheter. The distance of catheter insertion into the rectum and the volume of fluid to be administered varies with the age of the child and the type of fluid used (Table 65-2). After the catheter has been appropriately positioned, instill the fluid either by gravity by raising the bag no more than 18 inches above the rectum or by squeezing the plastic bottle from the commercially prepared enema. If a retention enema is required, hold together the buttocks of the infant or toddler for a short time to retain the fluid.[5] The older child may remain on his or her side after enema therapy and may evacuate the contents into the bed pan or toilet as preferred.

Remarks

Carefully choosing the type of enema fluid is critical to minimize the risk of metabolic derangements in children requiring enema therapy. For severe constipation or fecal impaction, enema administration may be repeated under a physician's direction for 3 or 4 consecutive days.

REFERENCES

1. Davis RF, Eichner JM, Bleyer A, et al: Hypocalcemia, hypophosphatemia, and dehydration following a single hypertonic phosphate enema, *J Pediatr* 90:484-485, 1977.
2. Fitzgerald JF: Constipation in children, *Pediatr Rev* 8:299-302, 1987.
3. Martin RR, Lischora GR, Braxton M, et al: Fatal poisoning from sodium phosphate enemas, *JAMA* 257:2190-2192, 1987.
4. McCabe M, Sibert JR, Routledge PA: Phosphate enemas in childhood: cause for concern, *Br Med J* 302:1074, 1991.
5. Skale N: Enemas. In *Manual of pediatric nursing procedures,* Philadelphia, 1992, JB Lippincott.
6. Smith MJ, Goodman JA, Rockwood NL: *Child and family: concepts of nursing practice,* ed 2, New York, 1991, McGraw-Hill.
7. Sotos JF, Cutler EA, Finkel MA, et al: Hypocalcemic coma following pediatric phosphate enemas, *Pediatrics* 60:305-307, 1977.
8. Sutphen JL: Gastrointestinal procedures. In Lohr JA, editor: *Pediatric outpatient procedures,* Philadelphia, 1991, JB Lippincott.

66 Parenteral Nutrition

Stephanie A. Storgion and Emily B. Hak

The critically ill or injured child has substrate requirements that exceed baseline metabolic needs. However, previously healthy individuals who sustain an acute injury or illness can tolerate the resultant catabolic state for several days without long-term sequelae. Those who have chronic illness or decreased protein and calorie reserves or those who are in the rapid phases of growth, such as occurs in early childhood and adolescence, are less capable of tolerating these losses and should be considered for early nutrition intervention. Several studies have demonstrated that malnourished adults who receive perioperative nutritional supplementation have an improved postoperative course over a similar group who receive no nutritional intervention.[10,39] Whenever possible, use the gastrointestinal tract for feeding; but critically ill patients often have metabolic factors or technical complications that preclude enteral feeding. In those patients who cannot or should not be enterally fed, parenteral nutrition is an effective alternative.

Indications

Critically ill or injured children who have medical or surgical problems that make enteral nutrition undesirable or not feasible require parenteral nutrition. These medical problems include ileus, necrotizing enterocolitis, pancreatitis, inflammatory bowel disease, and aspiration. Surgical problems necessitating parenteral nutrition include necrotizing enterocolitis, congenital bowel defects, burns to or grafting from specific areas of the body (to avoid stool contamination of wounds), abdominal trauma, and chylothorax. In most cases, patients who refuse oral feedings can be tube fed. However, in patients who have significant irritation or inflammation in the upper gastrointestinal tract, such as is seen in Stevens-Johnson syndrome, placement of a feeding tube may traumatize tissue.

Contraindications

There are few contraindications for parenteral nutrition.[49] Hypersensitivities to components of parenteral nutrition solutions have been reported and include parenteral vitamins or the diluent, preservatives, and fat emulsion. Individuals who have anaphylactic reactions to eggs should not receive fat emulsion because egg phospholipids are used as the emulsifier.

In those patients who require parenteral nutrition, begin enteral feedings, even a very low volume electrolyte or dextrose solution, as soon as possible. Many patients receive a combination of parenteral and enteral feedings throughout most of their stay in the intensive care unit.

Complications

Parenteral nutrition-related complications are technical, metabolic, and infectious. Technical complications include those that occur during catheter placement, dislodgment after placement, breakage, and occlusion. Repair broken permanent central venous catheters under aseptic conditions. Treat partial catheter occlusions according to the suspected type of occlusion, in an attempt to clear the catheter (Table 66-1).* Choose the product appropriate for the type of occlusion and instill a volume equivalent to the catheter volume; allow it to dwell for several hours. At the end of the dwell time, withdraw the volume and withdraw approximately 3 to 5 ml of blood to ensure removal of the occluding material. In some cases, use continuous infusion (see Table 66-1). Although heparin (1 to 2 units/ml of dextrose/amino acid solution) is effective in prolonging the time before infiltration of parenteral nutrition solutions infused peripherally,[1] there is a lack of evidence of a beneficial effect on clot formation in patients receiving solutions centrally. Monitor platelet concentrations in patients who are receiving even small amounts of heparin because of the potential development of heparin-induced thrombocytopenia.[34]

Metabolic toxicities associated with the administration of parenteral nutrition affect the neurologic, hepatic, renal, immunologic, and hematologic systems.[49] Use forethought to minimize iatrogenic electrolyte abnormalities. Cholestasis and osteoporosis are more commonly seen in premature infants who receive long-term parenteral nutrition.[37,40] Parenteral nutrition–associated cholestasis is a diagnosis of exclusion, with lack of enteral stimulation, sepsis, medications (e.g., furosemide), and underlying hepatic disease being important factors. In general, laboratory evidence of cholestasis related to parenteral nutrition is not seen until after at least 10 days of therapy. Early laboratory markers of cholestasis include 5′-nucleotidase, direct bilirubin, and γ-glutamyl transpeptidase, whereas increases in transaminases occur later. If cholestasis occurs, institute small-volume enteral feedings and cycle the patient off of parenteral nutrition for a few hours during the day. Phenobarbital is not effective in the treatment of cholestasis.[22]

Infectious complications are a significant problem. Initially treat suspected central-line infections with coverage for methicillin-resistant *Staphylococcus aureus* and gram-negative organisms, including *Pseudomonas* species. After the organism has been identified, base antibiotic therapy on organism sensitivity. Infuse antibiotics through the catheter port that is thought to be infected.[20] While the catheter is not being used, use antibiotic or antifungal dwell treatment to increase the exposure to the antimicrobial.[2,21,41] Fibrin deposition in and around the catheter begins soon after insertion and provides a place for organisms to reside. Failure to eradicate organisms in the fibrin results in reinfection; there-

---

*References 4,8,15,18,31,32,38,46,52, and 56.

379

Table 66-1   Treatment Methods for Central Venous Catheter Occlusions

Occlusion type	Drug	Dosage
Fibrin	Urokinase	200 U/kg/hr continuous infusion;[4] 5000 U/ml dwell[16,31]
	Streptokinase	5000 U/hr × 20 or 24 hr resolved thrombus in two adults[32,38]
	TPA	Loading dose of 2 mg in a 3 year old or 5 mg in adults followed by 0.5 mg/kg (dissolved in sterile water and diluted in NS) over 24 hours for 109-190 hours (151 hr in child) plus continuous infusion heparin in anticoagulant doses[52]
Calcium phosphate precipitate, medications soluble in acid (e.g., etoposide)	HCl	0.1 N HCl dwell[8,18,31,56]
Medications soluble in alkali (e.g., ticarcillin/clavulanic acid, oxacillin, heparin, phenytoin)	NaHCO₃	1 mEq/ml dwell[31]
Soap formation	EtOH−	70% ethanol in sterile-water dwell[31,46]

fore consider using fibrinolytic dwell therapy concomitantly with antibiotics. Consider the potential for the release of organisms or endotoxins from dissolved fibrin that are then flushed into the systemic circulation. This approach has not been evaluated in an organized study. In some cases, removal of the catheter is essential to the eradication of the infection. Dextrose/amino acid solutions are not good bacterial growth media because of solution hypertonicity; however, fungi grow well in these solutions. Both bacteria and fungi grow in fat emulsions.

At least 50% of the fatty acid content in fat emulsions is from linoleic acid, an ω-6 polyunsaturated fatty acid (PUFA) that is a precursor of prostaglandins and leukotrienes.[60] Because prostaglandins and leukotrienes are mediators of immune function, fat emulsion has the potential to promote infection. In addition, fatty acids have been shown to enhance immune function and are effectively used as a calorie source during infection. On the other hand, triglyceride tolerance may be decreased during sepsis. Therefore during infection, use modest doses of lipid and monitor triglyceride tolerance.

Equipment

Use percutaneous catheters that are either centrally or peripherally inserted, tunneled catheters, and implanted ports for central venous access.[43] Percutaneous catheters can have multiple lumens but are not intended to be used for extended periods of time. They tend to crack with age, which increases the risk for infection. Silastic catheters can be multilumen and, like implanted ports, are intended for long-term central venous access. Infuse parenteral nutrition using a volumetric infusion device.

Techniques

Substrate. The usual daily doses of macronutrients and micronutrients are listed in Table 66-2[14]; however, these doses may require modification during critical illness. In extremely catabolic patients, it is often impossible to provide sufficient substrate because of access limitations, fluid restriction, disease, medications, and organ dysfunction. How-

Table 66-2   Daily Nutritional Requirement

Nutrient	Adult	Pediatric
Macronutrients		
Protein	1.5-3 g/kg	1.5-3 g/kg
Glucose	25-30 kcal/kg	30-100 kcal/kg
Lipid	1-2 g/kg	1-4 g/kg
Micronutrients		
Sodium	60-150 mEq	2-6 mEq/kg
Potassium	80-200 mEq	2-5 mEq/kg
Chloride	40-100 mEq	2-3 mEq/kg
Acetate	10-40 mEq	
Phosphorous	10-60 mMol	1-2 mMol/kg
Calcium	4.8-19.2 mEq	0.5-2 mEq/kg
Magnesium	10-45 mEq	0.3-0.5 mEq/kg
Zinc	3-10 mg	100-300 µg/kg
Copper	1-1.5 mg	20-60 µg/kg
Chromium	10-15 µg	0.14-0.2 µg/kg
Manganese	150-800 µg	2-10 µg/kg
Selenium	40-120 µg	3 µg/kg
Vitamins		
MVI Pediatric for infusion	—	5 ml
MVI-12 Multivitamin infusion	10 ml (both vials)	—

From Cochran EB, Kamper CA, Phelps SJ, et al: Parenteral nutrition in the critically ill patient, *Clin Pharm* 8:783–799, 1989.

ever, estimate the usual daily macronutrient and micronutrient requirements as initial substrate goals and adjust these according to clinical response.

FLUIDS. The fluid volume available for parenteral nutrition is a common limitation to the ability to provide adequate nutrition to critically ill children. Components of parenteral nutrition are specific concentrations of amino acids, dextrose, electrolytes, minerals, trace elements, and vitamins (Table 66-3). Thus there are concentration limits for parenteral nutrition solutions that may result in suboptimal dosing of one or more components. Solution orders for a patient receiving maintenance fluids or 50% maintenance fluids are compared in Table 66-4. To compound the solution to be infused at 50 ml/kg (i.e., 50% maintenance), 151 ml of components would need to be removed. One solution involves decreasing the original protein content (20 g in 333 ml) to 10.9 g, which would require 182 ml of 6% amino acids. Alternatively, use a 10% amino acid product (200 ml of volume) and decrease the dextrose concentration to 22% to achieve the same goal.

Table 66-3 Concentrations of Selected Components of Parenteral Nutritional Solution

Solution	Concentration
Protein	6% (6 g/100 ml), 10% (10 g/100 ml)
Dextrose	50 g/100 ml ($D_{50}W$), 70 g/100 ml ($D_{70}W$)
Sodium chloride	2.5, 4 mEq/ml
Sodium acetate	2, 4 mEq/ml
Sodium phosphate	2 mEq Na/ml, 1.3 mMol P/ml 4 mEq Na/ml, 2.7 mMol P/ml
Potassium chloride	1.5, 2, 3 mEq/ml
Potassium acetate	2, 4 mEq/ml
Potassium phosphate	4.4 mEq K/ml, 3 mMol P/ml
Calcium gluconate	0.456 mEq (100 mg) /ml
Magnesium sulfate (50%)	4.1 mEq/ml
Selenium	40 µg/ml
L-cysteine hydrochloride	50 mg/ml

Na, Sodium; *K,* potassium; *P,* phosphorus.

In many cases, fluid-restricted patients can have their continuous infusion medications (e.g., dopamine, dobutamine, fentanyl, midazolam) concentrated and prepared in a compatible high-dextrose concentration diluent, thereby providing a significant amount of carbohydrate calories. Because carbohydrate calories are provided outside the parenteral nutrition solution, the volume that would otherwise be used for dextrose is available for amino acids. However, with concentrated parenteral nutrition solutions, small increases in rate can result in significant increases in doses of substrate. For example, a fluid-restricted patient who is receiving 50% maintenance fluids with normal daily doses of protein, calcium, and potassium will receive potentially harmful amounts of these substrates if the solution rate is increased to maintenance.

Conversely, manage patients who require large amounts of fluid by using a parenteral nutrition solution volume that provides fluids at a maintenance rate concomitantly with an electrolyte solution that is providing the additional fluid. Patients who require excess fluids often have rapidly changing fluid requirements, and this approach ensures the adequate provision of substrate in the face of changing fluid requirements.

PROTEIN. Failure to provide adequate calories results in the conversion of amino acids to glucose, an expensive calorie source. When appropriate amounts of calories are provided, a nonprotein calorie (carbohydrate- or lipid-to-nitrogen ratio of approximately 150:1) has been found to result in positive nitrogen balance.[47] Each gram of nitrogen is equal to 6.25 g amino acids. Use this ratio as a guide for protein and carbohydrate dosing.

Amino acid products are available as standard adult formulations and pediatric products that contain a greater concentration of essential amino acids and a variety of nonessential amino acids.[28,29] A higher-quality amino acid

Table 66-4 Sample Orders Showing the Volume of Each Component (in milliliters) Required to Compound a Solution for an 8-kg Child Who Has Received 100 ml/kg or 50 ml/kg

	100 ml/kg (800 ml)	50 ml/kg (400 ml)
Protein (2.5 g/kg) = 20 g		
Amino acid 6% g/100 ml	333	333
Dextrose (final concentration of 25%)		
$D_{70}W$ = 70 g/100 ml	286	143*
Sodium (2 mEq/kg = 16 mEq)		
chloride (16-12.8 = 3.2 mEq)	1.3	1.3
phosphate (1.2 mMol/kg = 12.8 mEq)	4.3	4.3
Potassium (2 mEq/kg)	10.7	10.7
Calcium gluconate (2 mEq/kg = 16 mEq)	35	35
Magnesium sulfate (0.3 mEq/kg = 2.4 mEq)	0.6	0.6
Vitamins	5	5
Trace elements (PTE-4, Fujisawa)	1.6	1.6
Selenium (3 µg/kg = 24 µg)	0.6	0.6
L-cysteine HCl (40 mg/g pediatric amino acid)	16	16
Total fluids required for compounding	694.1	551.1
Sterile water	105.9	−151.1*

*400 ml (available for parenteral nutrition solution) −551.1 ml (total volume of desired components) = 151.1 ml (negative free water).
If compounded as written, the final dextrose concentration would be 18% instead of 25%, and the final amino acid concentration would be 3.6% instead of 5%. Ultimately, the patient would receive 38% less substrate than ordered. Final concentrations of calcium and phosphorus should be considered.

may be used more efficiently, and positive nitrogen balance has been achieved in stable postsurgical neonates who received 2.2 g of a pediatric amino acid/kg/day and 60 to 70 kcal/kg/day.[12] Protein needs in critically ill children likely are increased, but this need is difficult to assess because of difficulties in performing nitrogen balance, the influence of hydration on visceral protein concentrations, and fluid shifts that affect weights. Therefore make these assessments but interpret them with an understanding of the limitations.

To determine needs in patients with ongoing protein losses, measure the protein concentration of peritoneal drains, chest tube outputs, and wound losses to determine the protein loss, and develop a plan to replace these losses. Accomplish this replacement therapy by increasing the amount of protein in the parenteral nutrition solution and replacing the fluid and electrolytes through a concomitant infusion. In hypoalbuminemia, add albumin to the parenteral nutrition solution and use a suitable fluid and electrolyte solution to replace volume losses. Alternatively, use an electrolyte and albumin replacement fluid to replace the fluid and protein losses without altering the parenteral nutrition solution.

Protein doses may need to be decreased for patients with acute renal failure or hepatic failure or for premature neonates. Lower protein doses in acute renal failure may help preserve glomeruli because infusion of amino acids increases glomerular filtration rate. In hepatic disease, products with low concentrations of aromatic amino acids may prevent or reverse the progression of hepatic encephalopathy, but data do not support their use in patients who are not in fulminant hepatic failure. In moderate hepatic disease, give patients conservative doses of a higher quality amino acid product and evaluate by assessing clinical response and serum ammonia and blood urea nitrogen (BUN). Premature infants may not be able to eliminate renally the acid load delivered through amino acid infusions. Start very low–birth weight infants with pediatric amino acid products and use lower doses of amino acids (0.5 to 1 g/kg/day) initially. Advance by 0.5 to 1 g/kg/day as tolerated. Adjust electrolyte anions to minimize problems with acidosis.

CARBOHYDRATE. Glucose provides 3.4 kcal/g and is the carbohydrate source used in most parenteral nutrition solutions. Most parenteral nutrition dextrose concentrations range from 20% to 40%. In small infants, use initial doses of 5 to 10 g/kg/day (3.5 to 7 mg/kg/min) and gradually increase to approximately 25 g/kg/day (17 mg/kg/min) as tolerated. As children grow, the glucose oxidation rate gradually decreases and in adults is approximately 5 to 8 g/kg/day. Base incremental dose increases on g/kg increases and not on solution dextrose concentration. Doses that exceed the glucose oxidation rate result in fat accumulation and not the accretion of lean body mass. Additionally, glucose is metabolized to water and CO_2 which, in the face of excessive carbohydrate doses, can contribute to CO_2 retention. During the acute phase of critical illness and glucocorticoid therapy, many patients experience intolerance to even modest doses of glucose, which can be managed with insulin. Evaluate patients who have had stable blood glucose concentrations and suddenly develop hyperglycemia or hypoglycemia with no change in glucose dose for sepsis. Alternatively, a compounding error in dextrose concentration or a dramatic change in infusion rate may be responsible for unexplained changes in blood glucose. Determine temporal relationships between changing solutions or rates to rule out these factors as the cause of glucose intolerance.

Use insulin to manage significant hyperglycemia. An initial dose for very low–birth weight infants is 0.05 units/kg/hr, whereas older infants and children need 0.1 units/kg/hr. Insulin drips are compatible with dextrose amino acid solutions and can be concomitantly infused. When insulin is used, initially monitor blood glucose at frequent intervals (every 1 to 2 hours) and titrate the insulin dose accordingly. Hyperglycemia may resolve quickly; thus continued blood glucose monitoring is important. Insulin drives potassium and phosphate intracellularly; therefore monitor potassium and phosphate status and adjust the doses of these electrolytes accordingly. If a patient stabilizes on a specific dose of insulin, add this amount to the parenteral nutrition solution. Alternatively, add a conservative insulin dose (i.e., 1 unit/4 g dextrose) to the parenteral nutrition solution and titrate the dose as needed. The addition of insulin directly to the solution ensures its discontinuation when the solution is stopped. With concomitant infusion, titrate the insulin dose immediately in response to blood glucose concentration.[6,54] Failure to discontinue the insulin infusion when the dextrose solution is discontinued can result in significant hypoglycemia.

ELECTROLYTES. Electrolytes are eliminated renally, and factors that affect renal function result in altered needs.[33] Intense diuretic therapy to manage fluid overload increases urinary electrolyte elimination.[59] Correct resultant electrolyte deficiencies either by bolus administration or by increasing the amount in the parenteral nutrition solution.

Sodium. Provide sodium as the chloride, phosphate, or acetate salt. The amount of sodium and the salt form depends on the condition of the patient. When evaluating appropriateness of dosing, consider all sources of sodium intake. Hidden sources may include intravenous line flushes, medications, and arterial lines. A careful evaluation of total body stores, fluid balance, and underlying disease is important in determining the cause and subsequent management of hypernatremia or hyponatremia.

Potassium. Provide potassium as the chloride, phosphate, or acetate salt. The potassium concentration that can be infused centrally is based on need; however, the rate of administration should not exceed 0.5 to 1 mEq/kg/hr from all sources. Avoid transiently high potassium concentrations by increasing the amount of potassium delivered continuously to minimize the frequency of intermittent potassium infusions. Intracellular potassium is exchanged for H+ in acidosis, which results in an increase in serum potassium concentration; opposite occurs in alkalosis. Thus consider acid-base status and potential therapeutic interventions that may affect serum potassium concentration.

Limit peripheral infusions of potassium to 40 to 60 mEq/L because more concentrated solutions are very irritating to veins. Do not infiltrate solutions containing large amounts of potassium because doing so can result in serious sequelae, including tissue sloughing and necrosis.

Chloride, Acetate Phosphorus. Add sodium and potassium as chloride, acetate, or phosphorus depending on patient need. Those who receive large doses of diuretic, particularly loop diuretics, may require relatively large amounts of chloride. Sodium and chloride are lost with nasogastric suction, and both water and electrolytes may need to be replaced. Acetate is efficiently converted to bicarbonate and can help correct acidosis. Do not use bicarbonate because of the potential formation of calcium carbonate. Sodium phosphate contains 0.75 mMol of PO_4 /mEq of sodium, whereas potassium phosphate contains 0.67 mMol of PO_4 /mEq of potassium. Do not exceed a phosphorus delivery rate of 0.05 mMol/kg/hr because of the potential for complexation with calcium and resultant precipitation of calcium phosphate in soft tissue or vasculature.

Calcium. Calcium accretion rates determined in the developing fetus are up to 7.5 mEq/kg/day—a calcium dose that cannot be provided through enteral or parenteral nutrition.[35] More important than providing an absolute dose of calcium is the provision of the appropriate ratio of calcium and phosphorous, which for infants has been described as a molar ratio of 1:1 or 1.3:1 or as a weight ratio of 1.3:1 to 1.7:1.[37]

Calcium and phosphorus solubility is enhanced by lower solution pH and lower temperatures. In general, amino acid products are acidic, but the pH varies widely. Both an increased amino acid concentration and an increased dextrose concentration decrease solution pH and enhance calcium and phosphorous solubility. Solubility curves for various amino acid products have been published and provide guidelines for the amounts of calcium and phosphorus that are soluble.[19] To enhance solubility, adjust solution pH by using hydrochloric acid, glacial acetic acid, or L-cysteine HCl.[55] Heat lamps, ultraviolet lights, or warming beds raise the temperature of solution and may cause precipitation within the infusion line; in some cases, solutions warmed by body temperature have precipitate in the catheter itself.[51]

Gluconate is the preferred calcium salt because it dissociates less readily than the chloride salt and is less likely to form a precipitate with phosphorus. Because calcium is a divalent cation, it alters the electrical charge around lipid particles, which increases the potential for lipid coalescence and formation of a soap that can clog the catheter. Solutions with relatively high calcium concentrations should not have lipids directly added to them. Instead, infuse lipids concomitantly either through a Y-site injection port proximal to the patient or through a separate intravenous line.

As with potassium, calcium is irritating to the tissue and can result in significant tissue damage should concentrated solutions infiltrate.

Vitamins/Trace Elements. In otherwise healthy children, provide vitamin and trace element reserves that are adequate to meet their immediate needs.[24] Premature neonates have limited nutrient stores. Promptly address their needs for vitamin and trace elements. Decrease vitamin doses in patients with renal insufficiency.

Because zinc is important in wound healing and tissue repair, provide it early in the course of parenteral nutrition. The renal elimination of zinc is increased following long bone fractures and burns and with the infusion of histidine or cysteine, which is an amino acid added to solutions compounded with pediatric amino acid products.[3,11,61] Copper and manganese undergo biliary elimination; decrease the doses of these trace elements in patients with significant cholestasis. Supplement post–liver transplant patients who

have a biliary drain because there will be no enterohepatic recirculation of copper and manganese. Selenium and chromium are renally eliminated, and doses may need to be adjusted in patients with renal insufficiency that persists.

Iron dextran is compatible with parenteral nutrition solutions, which makes this treatment reasonable for those with iron deficiency anemia who cannot take iron enterally. The response to parenteral iron is delayed and not likely to be of immediate benefit; therefore its use in critically ill children is limited. In addition, gram-negative organisms metabolize iron, which places infected patients at risk for deleterious effects.[30] Anaphylaxis has been reported with the infusion of iron dextran.

Fat Emulsion. Intravenous fat emulsion provides a concentrated source of calories (2 calories/ml in 20%) and can be an important source of calories in a fluid-restricted patient. Use doses up to 3 g/kg/day in preterm neonates and 4 g/kg/day in infants (see Table 12-8).[15] Give older children and adolescents up to 2 g/kg/day. Concomitant infusion of fat emulsion with dextrose amino acid solution that peripherally increases the time before infiltration occurs, which is important in patients with limited venous access.[48]

In critical illness, lipid clearance can be decreased; therefore monitor serum triglycerides to assess tolerance.[44] Patients who are not being given enough calories to meet their needs may mobilize endogenous fat stores to meet calorie needs and therefore may have hypertriglyceridemia. Check the plasma or serum for turbidity to obtain a subjective assessment of exogenous chylomicron concentration in the plasma. Continue fat emulsion for those who have increased serum triglycerides but have clear plasma, and even consider a dose increase. Follow triglyceride concentrations closely; increases of 5% to 10% are likely not of concern. Most often, triglyceride concentrations decrease when calorie needs, either as fat emulsion or carbohydrate, are being met.

Neonates with indirect hyperbilirubinemia may be at risk for kernicterus as a result of fatty-acid displacement of bilirubin from binding sites on albumin; however, they are also at risk for essential fatty-acid deficiency.[45] Neonates with physiologic jaundice who have albumin concentrations within the age-related normal range can probably be given modest lipid doses (0.5 to 1 g/kg/day as a continuous infusion) without ill effects. Intravenous fat is delivered directly into the circulation and bypasses lymphatic transport; therefore chylothorax is not a contraindication to fat infusions.

Fat emulsions of 20% are the most concentrated source of parenteral calories, providing 2 kcal/ml. With 10% fat emulsions, the ratio of phospholipid to triglyceride is greater, resulting in an increase in lipoprotein X–type particles that sequester cholesterol and may compete with triglycerides for clearance.[25] Therefore use the 20% products.

ASSESSMENT. Assess baseline nutritional status by anthropometric and biochemical indexes.[26,27,42,57] Weights and other anthropometric measurements often cannot be obtained because of patient instability; when they are obtained, they may be difficult to interpret because of the large fluid fluxes. Concentrations of visceral proteins may not be helpful in determining baseline nutritional status in the acutely ill patient because plasma proteins may leak into the tissues or be avidly consumed during critical illness. In addition, visceral proteins (albumin, transthyretin or prealbumin, retinol-binding protein) are affected by hydration status and may not accurately reflect the adequacy of nutrition intake.[17,23] The shorter half-life visceral proteins, prealbumin and retinol-binding protein, may be better predictors of protein repletion.

Perform nitrogen balance, but remember that the percentage of urea nitrogen in the urine varies widely in critical illness.[7,36] Total urinary nitrogen measurements are the preferred method; however, the equipment to perform this analysis is not available in most hospital clinical laboratories. The resting energy expenditure in adults can be estimated by using indirect calorimetry, but small lung volumes and the use of uncuffed endotracheal tubes make this technology currently unreliable in critically ill children.[50] Assessment of the baseline nutritional stages and of the response to the nutrition supplement in the pediatric intensive care unit is difficult, with clinical impression being one of the most important assessment tools.[5]

Remarks

Carbohydrates. Many drugs that are commonly used in the intensive care setting are compatible with 25% dextrose. Continuous infusion of medications in 25% dextrose provides calories, which allows the remaining fluids to be used primarily for protein, fat, and micronutrient administration.

Fat emulsion. Infuse both the 10% and 20% fat emulsions peripherally or centrally to provide calories, even in those patients with the most restricted fluid regimens. The 20% products are preferred.

Concentrated Formulas. Patients receiving formulations with concentrated amounts of protein or electrolytes (particularly potassium and calcium) should not have infusion rates adjusted without considering the impact on nutrient doses. Liberalize fluids using a separate dextrose electrolyte solution that is Y-ed into the parenteral nutrition solution fluids.

Albumin. Add albumin to dextrose amino acid solutions; however, solutions containing more than 25 g albumin/L may be difficult to infuse through a 0.22 micron filter. Additionally, when added to a concentrated dextrose solution, the half-life of albumin is decreased, in part, as a result of glycosylation of the albumin.[53] Using albumin in asymptomatic patients with hypoalbuminemia is controversial. However, patients with a serum albumin concentration of <2 g/dl may deserve replacement.[9,58] In patients without ongoing losses, 1 g/kg should increase the serum concentration by 0.3 g/dl.[13]

Medication Compatibility. Medications with an increased pH are likely to be incompatible with parenteral nutrition solutions that are typically acidic. Alterations in pH can cause precipitation of the drug or of calcium phosphate. Give most medications concomitantly through a Y-site injection port and do not add directly to the parenteral nutrition solution. Phenytoin, amphotericin, and bicarbonate are incompatible with solutions, and ampicillin is relatively incompatible.

REFERENCES

1. Alpan G, Eyal F, Springer C, et al: Heparinization of alimentation solutions administered through peripheral veins in premature infants: a controlled study, *Pediatrics* 74:375-378, 1984.
2. Arnow PM: *Malassezia furfur* catheter infection cured with antibiotic lock therapy, *Am J Med* 90:128-130, 1991.
3. Askari A, Long CL, Blakemore WS: Net metabolic changes in zinc, copper, nitrogen and protein balance in skeletal trauma patients, *Metabolism* 31:1185-1193, 1982.
4. Bagnall HA, Gomperts E, Atkinson JB: Continuous infusion of low-dose urokinase in the treatment of central venous catheter thrombosis in infants and children, *Pediatrics* 83:963-966, 1989.
5. Baker JP, Detsky AS, Wesson DE, et al: Nutritional assessment: a comparison of clinical judgment and objective measurements, *N Engl J Med* 306:969-972, 1982.
6. Binder ND, Raschko PK, Benda GI, et al: Insulin infusion with parenteral nutrition in extremely low–birth weight infants with hyperglycemia, *J Pediatr* 1114:273-280, 1989.
7. Boehm KA, Helms RA, Storm MC: Assessing the validity of adjusted urinary urea nitrogen as an estimate of total urinary nitrogen in three pediatric populations, *JPEN J Parenter Enteral Nutr* 18:172-176, 1994.
8. Breaux CW, Duke D, Georgeson KE, Mestre JR: Calcium phosphate crystal occlusion of central venous catheters used for total parenteral nutrition in infants and children: prevention and treatment, *J Pediatr Surg* 22:829-832, 1987.
9. Brown RO, Bradley JE, Bekemeyer WB, et al: Effect of albumin supplementation during parenteral nutrition on hospital morbidity, *Crit Care Med* 16:1177-1182, 1988.
10. Campos ACL, Meguid MM: A critical appraisal of the usefulness of perioperative nutritional support, *Am J Clin Nutr* 55:117-130, 1992.
11. Carr G, Wilkinson AW: Zinc and copper urinary excretions in children with burns and scalds, *Clin Chim Acta* 61:199-204, 1975.
12. Chessman K, Johnson M, Fernandes E, et al: Changing parenteral substrate requirements in neonates receiving pediatric amino acid formulations, *JPEN J Parenter Enteral Nutr* 12:105 (abstract), 1988.
13. Cochran EB, Hogue SL: Prediction of serum albumin concentration after albumin supplementation in pediatric patients receiving parenteral nutrition, *Clin Pharm* 10:704-706, 1991.
14. Cochran EB, Kamper CA, Phelps SJ, et al: Parenteral nutrition in the critically ill patient, *Clin Pharm* 8:783-799, 1989.
15. Committee on Nutrition, American Academy of Pediatrics: Use of intravenous fat emulsion in pediatric patients, *Pediatrics* 68:738-743, 1981.
16. Curnow A, Idowu J, Behrens E, et al: Urokinase therapy for Silastic catheter–induced intravascular thrombi in infants and children, *Arch Surg* 120:1237-1240, 1985.
17. Doweiko JP, Nompelggi DJ: The role of albumin in human pathophysiology, Part III. Albumin and disease states, *JPEN J Parenter Enteral Nutr* 15:476-483, 1991.
18. Duffy LG, Kerzner B, Gebus V, et al: Treatment of central venous catheter occlusion with hydrochloric acid, *J Pediatr* 114:1002-1004, 1989.
19. Fitzgerald K, MacKay M: Calcium and phosphate solubility in neonatal parenteral nutrient solutions containing TrophAmine, *Am J Hosp Pharm* 43:88-93, 1986.
20. Flynn PM, Shenep JL, Stokes DC, et al: In-situ management of confirmed central venous catheter–related bacteremia, *Pediatr Infect Dis J* 6:729-734, 1987.
21. Gaillard JL, Merlino R, Pajot N, et al: Conventional and nonconventional modes of vancomycin administration to decontaminate the internal surface of catheters colonized with coagulase-negative staphylococci, *JPEN J Parenter Enteral Nutr* 14:593-597, 1990.
22. Gleghorn EE, Merritt RJ, Subramanian N, et al: Phenobarbital does not prevent total parenteral nutrition–associated cholestasis in noninfected neonates, *JPEN J Parenter Enteral Nutr* 10:282-283, 1986.
23. Grant JP: Nutritional assessment in clinical practice, *Nutr Clin Pract* 1:3-11, 1986.
24. Greene H, Hambridge K, Schanler R, et al: Guidelines for the use of vitamins, trace elements, calcium, magnesium and phosphorous in infants and children receiving total parenteral nutrition: report of the Subcommittee on Pediatric Parenteral Nutrient Requirements from the Committee on Clinical Practice Issues of the American Society for Clinical Nutrition, *Am J Clin Nutr* 48:1324-1342, 1988.
25. Haumont D, Deckelbaum RJ, Richelle M, et al: Plasma lipid and plasma lipoprotein concentrations in low–birth weight infants given parenteral

nutrition with twenty or ten percent lipid emulsion, *J Pediatr* 115:787-793, 1989.

26. Helms RA, Miller JL, Burckart GGJ, et al: Clinical outcome as assessed by anthropometric parameters, albumin and cellular immune function in high-risk infants receiving total parenteral nutrition, *J Pediatr Surg* 18:564-569, 1983.

27. Helms RA, Dickerson RN, Ebbert ML, et al: Retinol-binding protein and prealbumin: useful measures of protein repletion in critically ill, malnourished infants, *J Pediatr Gastroenterol Nutr* 5:586-592, 1986.

28. Helms RA, Christensen ML, Mauer EC, et al: Comparison of a pediatric versus standard amino acid formulation in preterm neonates requiring parenteral nutrition, *J Pediatr* 110:466-470, 1987.

29. Heird WC, Dell RB, Helms RA, et al: Amino acid mixture designed to maintain normal plasma amino acid patterns in infants and children requiring parenteral nutrition, *Pediatrics* 80:401-408, 1987.

30. Hershko C, Peto TEA, Weatherall DJ: Iron and infection, *Br Med J* 296:660-664, 1988.

31. Holcombe BJ, Forloines-Lynn S, Garmhausen LW: Restoring patency of long-term central venous access devices, *J Intraven Nurs* 15:36-41, 1992.

32. Jacobs MB, Yeager M: Thrombotic and infectious complications of Hickman-Broviac catheters, *Arch Intern Med* 144:1594-1599, 1984.

33. Khilanani P: Electrolyte abnormalities in critically ill children, *Crit Care Med* 20:241-250, 1992.

34. King DJ, Kelton JG: Heparin-associated thrombocytopenia, *Ann Intern Med* 100:535-540, 1984.

35. Knight P, Buchanan S, Clatworthy H: Calcium and phosphate requirements of preterm infants who require prolonged hyperalimentation, *JAMA* 243:1244-1246, 1980.

36. Konstantinides FN, Konstantinides NN, Li JC, et al: Urinary urea nitrogen: too intensive for calculating nitrogen balance studies in surgical clinical nutrition, *JPEN J Parenter Enteral Nutr* 15:189-193, 1991.

37. Koo WWK: Parenteral nutrition–related bone disease, *JPEN J Parenter Enteral Nutr* 16:386-394, 1992.

38. Kramer FL, Goodman J, Allen S: Thrombolytic therapy in catheter-related subclavian venous thrombosis, *J Can Assoc Radiol* 38:106-108, 1987.

39. Meguid MM, Campos AC, Hammond WG: Nutritional support in surgical practice: Part 1, *Am J Surg* 159:345-358, 1990.

40. Merritt RJ: Cholestasis associated with total parenteral nutrition, *J Pediatr Gastroenterol Nutr* 5:9-22, 1987.

41. Messing B, Peitra-Cohen S, Debure A, et al: Antibiotic-lock technique: a new approach to optimal therapy for catheter-related sepsis in home parenteral nutrition patients, *JPEN J Parenter Enteral Nutr* 12:185-189, 1988.

42. Moskowitz SR, Pereira G, Spitzer A, et al: Prealbumin as a biochemical marker of nutritional adequacy in premature infants, *J Pediatr* 102:749-753, 1983.

43. Orr ME, Ryder MA: Vascular access devices: perspectives on designs, complications, and management, *Nutr Clin Pract* 8:145-152, 1993.

44. Park W, Paust H, Brosicke H, et al: Impaired fat utilization in parenterally fed low–birth weight infants suffering from sepsis, *JPEN J Parenter Enteral Nutr* 10:627-630, 1986.

45. Paulsrud JR, Pensler, L, Witten CF, et al: Essential fatty acid deficiency in infants induced by fat-free intravenous feedings, *Am J Clin Nutr* 25:897-904, 1972.

46. Pennington CR, Pithie AD: Ethanol lock in the management of catheter occlusion, *JPEN J Parenter Enteral Nutr* 11:507-508, 1987.

47. Peters C, Fischer JE: Studies on calorie-to-nitrogen ratio for total parenteral nutrition, *Surg Gynecol Obstet* 151:1-8, 1980.

48. Phelps SJ, Cochran EB: Effect of the continuous administration of fat emulsion on the infiltration of intravenous lines in infants receiving peripheral parenteral nutrition solutions, *JPEN J Parenter Enteral Nutr* 13:628-632, 1989.

49. Phelps SJ, Brown RO, Helms RA, et al: Toxicities of parenteral nutrition in the critically ill patient, *Crit Care Clin* 7:725-753, 1991.

50. Rasanen J: Continuous breathing circuit flow and tracheal tube cuff leak: sources of error during pediatric indirect calorimetry, *Crit Care Med* 20:1335-1340, 1992.

51. Robinson LA, Wright BT: Central venous catheter occlusion caused by body heat–mediated calcium phosphate precipitation, *Am J Hosp Pharm* 39:120-121, 1982.

52. Rodenhuis S, van't Hek LGFM, Vlasveld LT, et al: Central venous catheter–associated thrombosis of major veins: thrombolytic treatment with recombinant tissue plasminogen activator, *Thorax* 48:558-559, 1993.

53. Rothschild MA, Oratz M, Schreiber SS: Serum albumin, *Hepatology* 8:385-401, 1988.

54. Sajbel TA, Dutro MP, Radway PR: Use of separate insulin infusions with total parenteral nutrition, *JPEN J Parenter Enteral Nutr* 11:97-99, 1987.

55. Schmidt GL, Baumgartner TF, Fischischweiger W, et al: Cost containment using cysteine HCl acidification to increase calcium/phosphate solubility in hyperalimentation solutions, *JPEN J Parenter Enteral Nutr* 10:203-207, 1986.

56. Shulman RJ, Reed T, Pitre D, et al: Use of hydrochloric acid to clear obstructed central venous catheters, *JPEN J Parenter Enteral Nutr* 12:509-510, 1988.

57. Thomas MR, Massoudi M, Byrne J, et al: Evaluation of transthyretin as a monitor of protein-energy intake in preterm and sick neonatal infants, *JPEN J Parenter Enteral Nutr* 12:162-166, 1988.

58. Velanovich V: Crystalloid versus colloid fluid resuscitation: a meta-analysis of mortality, *Surgery* 105:65-71, 1989.

59. Vileisis R: Furosemide effect on mineral status of parenterally nourished premature neonates with chronic lung disease, *Pediatrics* 85:316-322, 1990.

60. Wan JM, Teo TC, Babayan VK, et al: Invited comment: lipids and the development of immune dysfunction and infection, *JPEN J Parenter Enteral Nutr* 12:43S-48S, 1988.

61. Zlotkin SH: Nutrient interactions with total parenteral nutrition: effects of histidine and cysteine intake on urinary zinc excretion, *J Pediatr* 114:859-864, 1989.

PART XIII

RENAL TECHNIQUES

67 Acute Hemodialysis

Phillip L. Berry

Although hemodialysis techniques have been in use in adult critical care units since the 1960s,[23] pediatric units did not use the technique widely until the 1970s[22] and, even then, on a limited basis because the dialysis hardware, artificial kidneys, and tubing were produced predominately to meet the needs of adults. In the early 1980s,[27] just as pediatric nephrologists were perfecting their improvisations with available equipment and developing smaller devices with the manufacturers, innovations in the area of chronic peritoneal dialysis[19] brought about a sweeping change in emphasis. The advent of new catheters, a wide variety of new dialysis solutions, and automated peritoneal cycling machines heightened the enthusiasm of pediatric nephrologists for peritoneal dialysis, used for many years in the acute setting, leading to the preferential use of this technique over hemodialysis.[4] Nonetheless, peritoneal dialysis is not always appropriate in the treatment of acute renal failure and other disorders encountered in the pediatric intensive care unit (PICU); thus hemodialysis and hemofiltration (see Chapter 67 and 69) remain useful and essential to the care of very ill children.

General Principles of Hemodialysis

Hemodialysis replaces, albeit inadequately, three normal kidney functions: solute removal or clearance, water removal or ultrafiltration, and correction of acidosis. Solute removal depends mainly on passive diffusion of substances across the semipermeable membrane of the "artificial kidney" or hemodialyzer.[14] The major driving force for diffusion is the solute concentration gradient across the membrane. The net movement of solute decreases as the solute concentration in the blood and dialysate compartments of the dialyzer approach equilibrium. Furthermore, movement of solutes is bidirectional, allowing substances in the dialysate to enter the blood if the concentration gradient so mandates. To maximize diffusion, adjust blood flow and dialysate flow independently to achieve clearance rates that are within the capacity of the dialyzer (Table 67-1) yet safe for the patient (see Complications). Although blood flow varies greatly according to patient size and type of access, most systems function efficiently using a dialysate flow rate of 500 ml/minute. Fig. 67-1 illustrates the relationship between clearance and blood flood, a curve that is flow rate dependent, plateauing at a rate of about 300 ml/minute in the case of urea. The molecular weight and protein binding characteristics of other solutes principally determine their membrane permeability.

Dialysis removes water, called ultrafiltration, by applying hydrostatic pressure across the membrane.[15] The amount of fluid removed over time by any dialyzer depends on its permeability to water and its surface area. This characteristic, the ultrafiltration co-efficient, kUf, is different for each dialyzer (see Table 67-1). The kUf determines the milliliters of water removed each hour per millimeter of mercury pressure across the dialyzer membrane. Positive pressure in the blood path (venous resistance) and/or negative pressure within the dialyzer (vacuum) determine the amount of transmembrane pressure. Modern dialysis delivery systems measure and adjust pressures internally so that they apply just the right amount of transmembrane pressure to the dialyzer to effect the desired rate of fluid removal, a parameter selected by simply adjusting a dial. High ultrafiltration rates will cause some increase in clearance, especially of higher-molecular-weight substances (middle molecules) that convective mass transfer drags across the membrane.[16]

The backflux of solute from dialysate to blood allows the correction of acidosis as a result of the transfer of bicarbonate into the blood. The same concept applies for correcting other electrolyte disturbances such as hypokalemia or hyponatremia.[30] "Tailor" the dialysate to correct such disturbances through internal concentration adjustments or by actually adding the solute of interest to the dialysate.

Indications

Use hemodialysis to aid patients with oliguria or acute renal failure after attempts to correct the underlying disorder have failed and before a life-threatening crisis occurs. A delay in the implementation of dialysis until the "bitter end" will almost always result in futile therapy. Although individual indications for dialysis are relative, most nephrologists consider them to be rather straightforward signals for dialytic intervention. Box 67-1 lists the most common indications for dialysis in the PICU.

Acute oliguria and ongoing requirements for intravenous infusions lead to fluid overload, which may produce simple peripheral edema or pulmonary congestion and hypertension. The definition of oliguria is urine output less than 240 ml/m^2/day. After establishing that the urine output will not respond to conservative corrective maneuvers or to diuretics, perform dialysis. On occasion, simple ultrafiltration (i.e., fluid removal without use of dialysate) may suffice; however, in most instances involving a critically ill child with acute renal failure, the dialysis component of the procedure is necessary to remove uremic toxins and restore electrolyte balance.

Hyperkalemia is the most dangerous of the electrolyte disturbances amenable to dialytic intervention.[1] The blood level of potassium that mandates dialysis is the level that causes cardiac conduction disturbances or dysrhythmias in an individual patient. Conservative therapy with glucose, insulin, calcium, bicarbonate, and ion exchange resins is seldom sufficient to control hyperkalemia; and their use should prompt immediate dialysis. Treat blood levels of potassium above 7.5 mEq/L, even without serious electrocardiogram abnormalities, with dialysis, especially if accompanied by other electrolyte disturbances, increased catabolism, cell

Table 67-1 Hemodialyzers Commonly Used in Pediatrics

Company	Model	Material	Type	Sterilization	Surface area (M²)	Priming 100	Vol 200	TMP 300	kUf ml/ mm Hg/hr	50	Urea CL at QB (ml/min) 100	150	200	300
Gambro	Mini-minor	CU	Plate	ETO	0.23	20	?	?	0.5	25	51		61	
	1L	CU	Plate	ETO	0.23	32	38	40	1.0	36	50	56		
	1N	CU	Plate	ETO	0.40	43	56	63	1.5	46	76	64		
	3L	CU	Plate	ETO	0.80	76	87	91	3.8		94		150	185
	3N	CU	Plate	ETO	0.80	77	90	95	4.3		95		156	185
	5N	CU	Plate	ETO	1.10	106	123	134	5.5		96		170	215
Baxter	CA-50	CA	HF	ETO	0.50	38	38	38	1.8	55	90	105	128	
	CA-70	CA	HF	ETO	0.70	55	55	55	2.5		97		153	
	CA-90	CA	HF	ETO	0.90	64	64	64	3.2		99		169	
	CA-110	CA	HF	ETO	1.10	80	80	80	5.3		100		176	
	CA-170	CA	HF	ETO	1.70	110	110	110	7.6		100		194	
	HT-80	HP	HF	ETO	0.80	50	50	50	3.2		98		160	189
	HT-100	HP	HF	ETO	1.00	69	69	69	4.6		99		170	207
Cobe	100-HG	HP	HF	GAMMA	0.22	18	18	18	2.0	50	82	102		179
	200-HG	HP	HF	GAMMA	0.60	34	34	34	3.5		120		150	206
	300-HG	HP	HF	GAMMA	0.80	44	44	44	4.5		125		167	
Fresenius	F-40	PS	HF	ETO	0.65		45		20.0				165	
	F-50	PS	HF	ETO	0.90		63		30.0				176	

kUf, Ultrefiltration co-efficient; *TMP*, transmembrane pressure; *CU*, cuprophan; *CA*, cellulose acetate; *HP*, hemophan; *PS*, polysulfone; *HF*, hollow fiber; *ETO*, ethylene oxide; *GAMMA*, gammaray; *Cl*, clearance; *Qb*, blood flow.

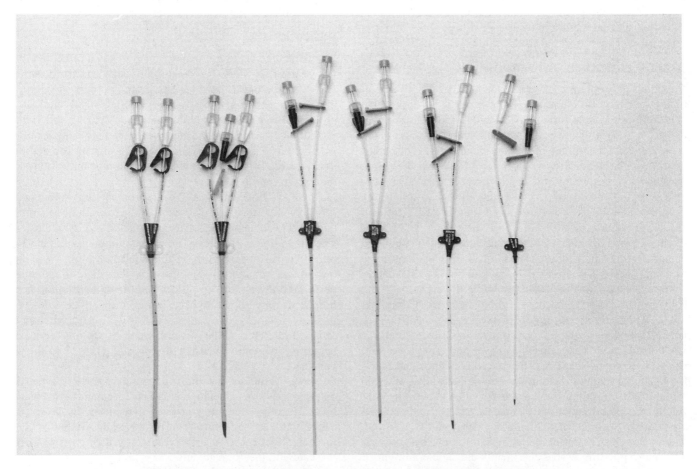

FIG. 67-1 Catheters suitable for pediatric hemodialysis (Arrow International, Reading, PA). *Left to right*: AK22122 (12F, 16-cm, 12-gauge, 12-gauge); AK22123 (12F, 16-cm, 12-gauge, 12-gauge, 16-gauge); AK25802 (8F, 20-cm, 14-gauge, 14-gauge); AK22802 (8 Fr, 16-cm, 14-gauge, 14-gauge); AK12802 (8F, 16 cm, 14-gauge, 14-gauge). Not pictured, CS 14502 (5F, 13-cm, 18-gauge, 20-gauge).

BOX 67-1   INDICATIONS FOR DIALYSIS IN THE IN-
TENSIVE CARE UNIT

Fluid retention
  Pulmonary edema
  Severe peripheral edema
  Hypertension
Electrolyte disturbances
  Hyperkalemia
  Hyponatremia
  Hypocalcemia
  Hyperphosphatemia
Metabolic acidosis
Metabolic alkalosis
Uremia
  Bleeding
  Central nervous system abnormalities
  Pericarditis
  Vomiting
Nutrition
Other
  Hypercalcemia
  Hyperuricemia
  Hypothermia
  Drug intoxication*

*See also Chapter 103.

A blood urea nitrogen (BUN) level greater than 100 mg/dl usually mandates dialysis, especially if it is rising rapidly. Although uremic symptoms are not usually apparent at that level, they may become more obvious as the BUN approaches 150 mg/dl, a level at which dialysis is almost always indicated. The underlying disease may often cause clinical conditions identical to those associated with a high BUN, such as bleeding in patients with liver failure or pericarditis following open-heart surgery. Spend little time sorting out these fine distinctions until after dialysis has eliminated the uremic factors. Likewise, many factors other than uremia cause central nervous system depression. Nonetheless, dialysis usually improves the mental status of severely ill uremic patients. Other nonspecific symptoms such as nausea, vomiting, and anorexia may improve markedly after only a few dialysis treatments. If alleviation of the uremia does not abrogate the symptoms thought to be related to the uremic syndrome, begin a search for other causes of these symptoms, or implement other therapy aimed at individual symptoms. Uremic symptoms may also improve with the initiation of nutritional support sufficient to prevent a catabolic state.[21] In many instances this is possible by administration of parenteral alimentation fluids in volumes tolerated only with concomitant use of ultrafiltration with dialysis. Consider the use of dialysis to ensure the ability to deliver adequate nutrition to be a sole and sufficient criterion for dialysis.[13] Other indications listed in Box 67-1 uncommonly mandate dialysis in pediatric medicine, although, when conservative management of these disorders is unsuccessful, dialysis provides efficient correction.

Contraindications

Although no absolute contraindications to hemodialysis exist, certain conditions may render the process hopelessly difficult or futile. Even so, some state laws guarantee dialysis to anyone who desires it, regardless of the severity of his illness. When a patient is too young or otherwise unable to state his wishes and the family is unavailable or indecisive, the institutional ethics committee may guide such decisions.

Complications

The most common complications of hemodialysis are hypotension, cramps, nausea and vomiting, headache, chest pain, back pain, itching, and fever and chills; but the possible complications are far more numerous (Box 67-2). Very often the blood pressure falls during acute hemodialysis.[11] A variety of factors produce this hypotension, including plasma water loss via ultrafiltration, osmotic shifts of fluid from the intravascular to the extravascular space with acute lowering of the blood urea level, autonomic unresponsiveness, and left ventricular dysfunction in certain patients. Use of acetate-containing dialysate, which causes vasodilation and myocardial depression, or low-sodium dialysate, which causes water to shift out of the intravascular compartment, may aggravate hypotension.[29]

Hypotension may occur secondary to the lack of vasoconstriction in the setting of ultrafiltration-induced blood volume depletion. Acetate-containing dialysate may produce an inadequate vasoconstrictive response, and warm dialysate causes core warming and a resultant venous and arteriolar dilation.[25] Cooler dialysate, 34° to 36° C, may prevent hypotension, but

---

lysis, infection, gastrointestinal bleeding, trauma, or rhabdomyolysis.

Other electrolyte disturbances are usually not as life-threatening as hyperkalemia; nonetheless in the setting of acute renal failure, they are almost impossible to correct without dialysis.[30] Hyponatremia caused by water overload in oliguric patients responds well to hemodialysis. Hypocalcemia usually improves promptly, mainly in response to the resolution of hyperphosphatemia, which occurs rapidly with hemodialysis.

Metabolic acidosis requires dialytic intervention when further administration of sodium bicarbonate would likely produce hypernatremia, intolerable volume overload, or hypercarbia. Patients with metabolic acidosis resulting from drugs (e.g., aspirin) or other exogenous acid ingestions benefit from hemodialysis rather than peritoneal dialysis because of the efficiency of drug removal and the highly efficient transport of base into the patient. Also treat patients with severe lactic acidosis from enzyme deficiencies or from hepatocellular dysfunction preferentially with hemodialysis solutions containing bicarbonate or acetate buffers instead of lactate, the standard peritoneal dialysate buffer. Since acetate is a known vasodilator and causes dialysis-related morbidities (such as dialysis-related hypoxemia), its use in the acute setting has diminished with the widespread availability of bicarbonate delivery systems.[6]

Metabolic alkalosis may accompany acute renal failure in postoperative patients receiving nasogastric suction. Under these conditions the standard dialysate solutions does not allow correction of the alkalemia. Consider using low acetate-high chloride or low-bicarbonate dialysate preparations in such instances.[3,26]

BOX 67-2 COMPLICATIONS OF HEMODIALYSIS

Hypotension
  Hypovolemia
  Lack of vasoconstriction
  Cardiac dysfunction
  Other
    Cardiac tamponade
    Myocardial infarction
    Hemorrhage
    Sepsis
    Arrhythmia
    Dialyzer reaction
    Hemolysis
    Air embolism
Cramps
Nausea and vomiting
Headache
Chest pain
Itching
Fever and chills
Neurologic
  Disequilibrium syndrome
  Intracranial bleeding
  Seizures
Infectious
  Vascular access
  Transfusion related
  Contaminated equipment
Metabolic
  Acidosis and alkalosis
  Hypokalemia
Hematologic
  Anemia
  Leukopenia
  Complement activation
Pulmonary
  Hypoxemia

---

it causes discomfort and chills. Food ingestion during dialysis causes splanchnic vasodilation and hypotension; thus the patient must not eat during a treatment.[5] If hypotension is severe enough to cause tissue ischemia, adenosine release from the ischemic area can amplify the hypotension.[31] Adenosine, a vasodilator itself, also blocks norepinephrine release. This mechanism may be most important in the severely anemic patient; thus correct the hematocrit to at least 30% in the acute setting.[10] Last, prevent inadequate vasoconstriction by the avoidance of antihypertensive medications and other vasodilators on the day of dialysis. Treat hypotension by placing the patient in the Trendelenburg position, reducing the ultrafiltration rate, and giving isotonic saline.

A discussion of the vast array of cardiac factors that may predispose to hypotension during hemodialysis is beyond the scope of this text.[28] If hemodynamic instability is a portentous concern, avoid hemodialysis and use more gentle renal replacement therapies such as hemofiltration or peritoneal dialysis.

The second most common complication of hemodialysis is muscle cramping, presumably related to a reduction in limb perfusion.[7] Predisposing factors include hypotension, dehydration (dialyzing below the "dry weight"), and low-sodium dialysate. Immediately treat the combination of hypotension and cramps by discontinuing ultrafiltration and volume expansion with isotonic saline. Cramps alone may respond to hypertonic saline, 50% glucose, or mannitol. With modern hemodialysis machines, program dialysate sodium to start the treatment with a relatively high concentration of 150 to 155 mEq/L, and gradually reduce it to 135 to 140 mEq/L during the treatment.[10] Removing a greater proportion of the excess fluid in the early phase of the treatment or removing fluid by simple ultrafiltration before using the dialysis mode may also reduce cramping.

Nausea and vomiting occur in about 10% of dialysis treatments, usually related to hypotension or to the disequilibrium syndrome described in the following paragraph. Lower blood flow rate, avoidance of hypotension, and measures similar to those used to prevent cramping may prevent vomiting. Headache, the cause of which is unknown, responds to the same interventions. Chest pain and back pain rarely occur in children undergoing dialysis. Treat such occurrences, thought to be the result of complement activation induced by some dialyzer membranes, with antihistamines and nasal oxygen and use an alternative dialyzer.

Two less common but serious complications deserve further comment. The disequilibrium syndrome, which can occur during or after dialysis, results from the osmotically induced shift of water from the plasma into brain cells following the rapid removal of solutes from the blood.[17] Minor symptoms include headache, lethargy, twitching, and nausea and vomiting; but these may progress to the major complications of disorientation, obtundation, seizures, and coma.[2] In the acute setting, prevent disequilibrium by prescribing a modest reduction of urea nitrogen (30%) and by using low blood flow rates to maintain the urea clearance rate less than 3 ml/kg/minute. Treat mild disequilibrium with blood flow reduction or discontinuation of dialysis. More severe symptoms mandate cessation of dialysis. Consider administration of 1 g/kg of mannitol intravenously. Provide supportive treatment and search for other causes of central nervous system deterioration.

The last noteworthy complication is hypoxemia, which occurs routinely during dialysis but is of no consequence unless the patient has significant cardiac or pulmonary disease.[8] Dialysis may cause a reduction in Po_2 of 5 to 30 mm Hg by causing hypoventilation and possibly by producing an intrapulmonary diffusion block mediated by lung sequestration of leukocytes. Avoid acetate-buffered and high bicarbonate dialysate, which produce alkalosis-associated hypoventilation. Nasal oxygen administration is sufficient therapy for most patients.

Equipment

Vascular Access. Successful acute hemodialysis depends on the establishment of excellent vascular access.[9] Dialyze the newborn through the umbilical vein using a 5 to 8.5 Fr umbilical catheter and a single-needle system or via a combination of umbilical arterial and venous catheters using a standard system. Although the traditional approach to

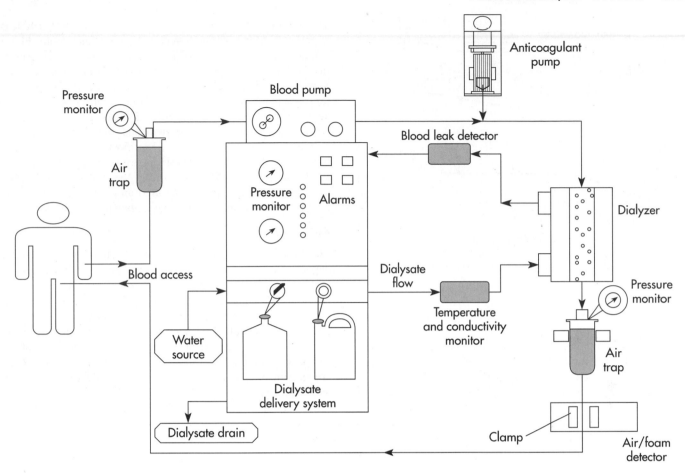

FIG. 67-2   Basic components of a single-patient hemodialysis system.

vascular access in the older infant or child is insertion of two single-lumen femoral venous catheters, the availability of a wide variety of dual and multilumen catheters (Fig. 67-2) provides safe and effective access for children of all sizes. Place these catheters in the femoral, jugular, or subclavian veins by the Seldinger technique. If anticipating a prolonged need for hemodialysis, insert a cuffed silicone catheter (Hickman or Pediatric Quinton Permcath) in larger children through the jugular or subclavian vein into the right atrium.[20] The cuff allows these catheters to "seal in," providing some protection against infection and dislodgment. Complications of catheter placement include laceration of the vein, pneumothorax, hemothorax, pneumomediastinum, vascular occlusion, thrombosis, and infection.

Extracorporeal Circuit.   The extracorporeal blood circuit should not exceed 10% of the patient's total blood volume; thus only a few of the many available lines, dialyzers, and machines are appropriate for use with babies and small children. Table 67-2 lists hemodialysis machines that accommodate pediatric and neonatal blood lines. Table 67-1 lists common pediatric hemodialyzers. Add the priming volume of the artificial kidney to the arterial and venous blood line volume to determine the extracorporeal circuit volume. If this total exceeds 10% of the patient's blood volume, prime the circuit with blood. Note that the priming volume of parallel plate dialyzers increases with increasing transmembrane pressure, which can lead to extracorporeal volume expansion during use. The best dialyzers for most situations

Table 67-2   Dialysis Systems for Infants and Children

Company/ machine	Neonatal line volume (arterial+venous [ml])	Pediatric line volume (arterial+venous [ml])
Cobe/Centry 3	40	80
Fesenius/2008H	20	62
Baxter/SPS 550	20	62
Gambro/AK 10	32	70

are low-flux hollow fiber filters that are nondistensible and require relatively less heparinization than plate dialyzers.[9]

The dialysis machine reduced to its essence delivers blood and dialysate to the artificial kidney. Fig. 67-3 shows a typical hemodialysis circuit. Components of the machine include a blood pump, a dialysate delivery system, and some safety devices. The blood pump controls blood flow and thus clearance. The typical dialysate delivery system draws up concentrated dialysate and bicarbonate from jugs, dilutes it with purified water in a 34:1 proportion, and pumps it through the artificial kidney and down the drain.

Several safety features guard against the possible catastrophic consequences of a system failure. Continuous monitoring of the electrical conductivity of the diluted dialysate ensures the maintenance of proper ionic concentrations and prevents the occurrence of dialysate-free water, which can cause massive hemolysis. Temperature controls keep the

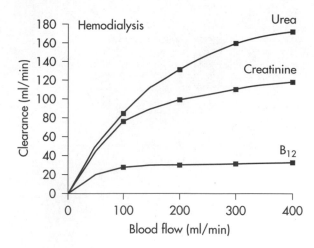

FIG. 67-3 Idealized clearance curves for a standard hemodia lyzer.

dialysate from overheating and hemolyzing the blood. An air detector turns off the blood pump if air enters the blood line, and a blood detector alarms if any blood enters the dialysate circuit. Pressure sensors prevent dialyzer rupture by stopping blood flow when the intra-dialyzer pressures exceed safe limits. Machines with ultrafiltration control continuously monitor fluid removal and display the net volume removed. To carefully control the ultrafiltration rate, use only dialysis systems with volumetric ultrafiltration regulation. Older equipment may cause obligatory fluid losses that are uncontrollable and difficult to measure. In such an environment, use portable bed scales.

Techniques

Individual patient needs, including consideration of patient size, hemodynamic stability, and tolerance of anticoagulation, guide dialysis techniques. Children weighing less than 8 kg require an extracorporeal circuit primed with whole blood or 5% albumin in isotonic saline. The use of blood as a priming solution may predispose to dialyzer clotting and hyperkalemia; therefore, if the patient is stable and has an adequate hematocrit, 5% albumin in saline is usually sufficient. Carefully control ultrafiltration and clearance and replace excess fluid removal during the procedure. When the target weight at the end of the treatment is 95% of the starting weight and the ultrafiltration rate is less than 0.2 ml/kg/min, patients usually tolerate the procedure well. Accomplish the removal of wastes slowly, especially if the BUN is greater than 100 mg/dl; set the blood flow rate so as not to exceed 5 ml/kg/min. By using the solute clearance curve (see Fig. 67-1) packaged with each type of dialyzer, the blood flow rate that will produce the desired clearance can be determined. In the acute setting, strive for urea clearance less than 3 ml/kg/min to avoid disequilibrium.[18] To prevent hypotension and disequilibrium when greater fluid and waste removal is desirable or accidentally occurs, give intravenous mannitol at 1 g/kg by continuous infusion throughout the treatment.[24]

Achieve anticoagulation by systemic heparinization, using 20 to 50 U/kg of heparin as a loading dose, followed by continuous infusion of 10 to 25 U/kg:Slhour. Patients who

are at high risk for bleeding may do well with much less heparin.[12] Monitor anticoagulation via the whole blood activated clotting time (ACT), which is easy to perform at the bedside using the Hemochron Automated Coagulation System (International Technidyne, Edison, NJ). The normal range of the ACT is 90 to 140 seconds. During hemodialysis keep the ACT between 1.25 and 1.5 times the normal range.

The frequency and duration of hemodialysis treatments vary according to patient needs, but most children require no more than three to four sessions per week. As the uremic syndrome comes under control after the first few treatments, dialysis efficiency can be increased and therefore fewer, but longer and more intensive, treatments can be delivered.

Remarks

The decision to use hemodialysis rather than peritoneal dialysis depends on several factors, including local availability, patient preference, clinical condition of the patient, and diagnosis. Hemodialysis is definitely preferable in two situations: for rapid solute removal or when it is not possible to perform peritoneal dialysis (see Chapter 68). Hemodialysis is difficult to use in patients with severe vascular disease, active bleeding, and severe cardiovascular instability. Although infants and small children are historically poor candidates for hemodialysis, it is now technically possible to perform the procedure on almost any small patient by using carefully selected catheters, lines, and dialyzers made for pediatric use.

REFERENCES

1. Allon M: Treatment and prevention of hyperkalemia in end-stage renal disease, *Kidney Int* 43(6):1197-1209, 1993.
2. Arieff A, et al: Brain water and electrolyte metabolism in uremia: effects of slow and rapid hemodialysis, *Kidney Int* 4:177-187, 1973.
3. Ayus J, Olivero J, Adrogue H: Alkalemia associated with renal failure: correction by hemodialysis with low-bicarbonate dialysate, *Ann Intern Med* 140(4):513-515, 1980.
4. Baum M, et al: Continuous ambulatory peritoneal dialysis in children: comparison with hemodialysis, *N Engl J Med* 307:1537-1542, 1982.
5. Brandt JL, et al: The effect of oral protein and glucose feeding on splanchnic blood flow and oxygen utilization in normal and cirrhotic subjects, *J Clin Invest* 34:1017-1025, 1955.
6. Buyer DR, et al: Regional blood flow redistribution due to acetate, *J Am Soc Nephrol* 4:91-97, 1993.
7. Canzanello VJ, Burkart JM: Hemodialysis associated with muscle cramps, *Semin Dial* 5:299-304, 1992.
8. Chen TS, et al: Hemodynamic changes during hemodialysis: relationship to arterial Po_2, *Proc Clin Dial Transplant Forum* 9:66-71, 1979.
9. Donkerwolke R, Bunchman T: Hemodialysis in infants and small children, *Pediatr Nephrol* 8:103-106, 1994.
10. Daugirdas JT, et al: A double blind evaluation of sodium gradient hemodialysis, *Am J Nephrol* 5:163-168, 1985.
11. Daugirdas JT: Preventing and managing hypertension, *Semin Dial* 7:276-283, 1994.
12. Geary D, et al: Low dose and heparin free hemodialysis in children, *Pediatr Nephrol* 5:220-224, 1991.
13. Goldstein D, Strom J: Intradialytic parenteral nutrition: evolution and current concepts, *J Renal Nutr* 1(1):9-22, 1991.
14. Gotch FA, Keen Marcia: Dialyzers and delivery systems. In Cogan MG, Garovoy M, editors: *Introduction to dialysis*, New York, 1985, Churchill Livingstone.
15. Henderson LW: Biophysics of ultrafiltration and hemfiltration. In Drukker W, Parsons F, Mahero J, editors: Replacement of renal function by dialysis, Boston, 1983, Martinus Nijhoff.
16. Hootkins R, Bourgeois B: The effect of ultrafiltration on dialyance: mathematical theory and experimental verification, *ASAIO Trans* 37:M375-M377, 1991.

17. Kennedy AC, et al: The pathogenesis and prevention of cerebral dysfunction during dialysis, *Lancet* 1:790-792, 1964.

18. Kiellstrand CM: Hemodialysis for children. In Friedman E, editor: *Strategy in renal failure*, New York, 1978, John Wiley & Sons.

19. Kohaut EC: Continuous ambulatory peritoneal dialysis: a preliminary experience, *Am J Dis Child* 132:270-271, 1981.

20. Mahan J, Mauer M, Nevins T: The Hickman catheter: a new hemodialysis access device for infants and small children, *Kidney Int* 24:694-697, 1983.

21. Moore L, Acchiardo S: Aggressive nutritional supplementation in chronic hemodialysis patients, *CRN Q* 11(3):13-14, 1987.

22. Potter D, et al: Treatment of chronic uremia in childhood, II, *Hemodial Pediatr* 46:647-689, 1970.

23. Quinton W, Dillard D, Scribner B: Cannulation of the blood vessels for prolonged hemodialysis, *Trans Am Soc Artif Intern Organs* 6:68-73, 1960.

24. Rosa AA, et al: The importance of osmolality fall and ultrafiltration rate in hemodialysis side effects: influence of intravenous mannitol, *Nephron* 27:134-141, 1981.

25. Sherman RA, et al: Effect of variation in dialysate temperature on blood pressure during hemodialysis, *Am J Kidney Dis* 4:66 68, 1984.

26. Swartz RD, et al: Correction of postoperative metabolic alkalosis and renal failure by hemodialysis, *Ann Intern Med* 86(1):52-55, 1977.

27. Trachtman H, Hackney P, Tejani A: Pediatric hemodialysis; A decade's (1974-84) perspective, *Kidney Int* 30:515-522, 1986.

28. Travis M, Henrich W: Factors which affect cardiac performance curing hemodialysis, *Semin Dial* 2:241-245, 1989.

29. Van Stone J, Bauer J, Carey J: The effect of dialysate sodium concentration on body fluid compartment volume, plasma renin activity, and plasma aldosterone concentration in chronic hemodialysis patient, *Am J Kidney Dis* 2:58-64, 1982.

30. Ward R, et al: Hemodialysate composition and intradialytic metabolic, acid-base, and potassium changes, *Kidney Int* 32:129-135, 1987.

31. Wooliscroft JO, Fox IH: Increased body purine levels during hypotensive events: evidence for ATP degration, *Am J Med* 81:472-478, 1986.

Phillip L. Berry

Use of the peritoneal cavity for treatment of critically ill children has existed for at least three quarters of a century. The first report of successful treatment of dehydration with intraperitoneal saline occurred in 1918.[7] Reports of the use of the peritoneum to treat children with renal failure first appeared in 1948 and 1949.[8,35] Because of advances in the production of synthetic tubing and catheters and the widespread availability of commercially prepared dialysis solutions, peritoneal dialysis soon became the most commonly used dialytic method for the treatment of acute renal failure in children.[18] In the 1970s the application of peritoneal dialysis for end-stage renal disease led to technical improvements in peritoneal dialysis machines and disposable equipment, which brought peritoneal dialysis into the forefront as the treatment of choice for children with both acute and chronic renal disease.[9,11,26,33] Despite the recent report indicating that hemofiltration techniques are supplanting other dialysis modalities, peritoneal dialysis remains the first choice for treatment of acute renal failure in 37% of pediatric medical centers.[6]

General Principles of Peritoneal Dialysis

Like hemodialysis, peritoneal dialysis replaces only three normal kidney functions: solute removal or clearance, water removal or ultrafiltration, and correction of acidosis.[20] This type of dialysis takes place between the capillaries in the interstitium of the peritoneal membrane and the infused dialysis solution across the peritoneal membrane.[25] Because children have approximately twice the peritoneal membrane surface area per unit body weight as adults, the technique has been very successfully applied in pediatric medicine.[17] The peritoneal membrane acts as an imperfect semipermeable membrane, allowing small molecules and water to pass through faster than larger molecules.

Solutes diffuse across the membrane by diffusion and convection. Diffusion through peritoneal membrane pores and intercellular clefts is a spontaneous process whereby particles in liquid reach a uniform concentration by random movement throughout the solvent. The net diffusion rate of a substance between the blood and peritoneal cavity depends on the solute concentration difference, the pressure difference across the membrane, the membrane surface area, and the media temperature. Convective transport refers to the transfer of molecules moving in the same direction as part of total fluid movement. Convective transport occurs during dialysis in concert with ultrafiltration, or the net movement of water caused by a water concentration difference that is induced by the instillation of hyperosmotic dialysate into the peritoneal cavity. As seen in Fig. 68-1, these events occur at maximal rate with initial instillation of the dialysate; i.e., at the beginning of the "exchange."[25] At this time the glucose concentration in the peritoneal cavity is maximal, effecting

maximal net transcapillary ultrafiltration. Glucose concentration decreases exponentially as absorption of glucose into the bloodstream and dilution with ultrafiltrate dissipate the glucose gradient. The transfer of solute from blood to the peritoneal cavity is also maximal early in the exchange and decreases as the solute approaches equilibrium across the peritoneal membrane. When corrected for body surface area, membrane kinetics in children are strikingly similar to those of adults.[37] Studies verify that significant differences in peritoneal membrane performance exist from patient to patient when tested under optimal conditions. During rapidly changing clinical circumstances the efficiency of the membrane is much less predictable; thus clinicians often determine dialysis parameters empirically.

Indications

The indications for peritoneal dialysis are the same as those listed for hemodialysis in Box 67-1. The urgency to correct one of these abnormalities guides the selection of the dialytic modality. Peritoneal dialysis is approximately one-sixth to one-eighth as efficient as hemodialysis in terms of small solute clearance and approximately one-fourth as efficient regarding fluid removal when applied intermittently.[39] However, patients in the intensive care unit (ICU) usually undergo peritoneal dialysis on a continuous basis 24 hours per day; therefore the overall effect on plasma solute and water removal approximates that of hemodialysis applied intermittently.[28] Base the choice between hemodialysis and peritoneal dialysis on personal preference and individual clinical circumstances (mainly contraindications) that could sway the decision toward one modality or the other.

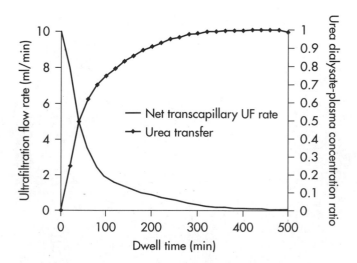

FIG. 68-1 Urea transfer (—♦—) and ultrafiltration (—) vs. dwell-time curves, illustrating the highest activity in the first hour of the peritoneal dwell cycle.

BOX 68-1   COMPLICATIONS OF ACUTE PERITONEAL DIALYSIS

Catheter-related

Bowel perforation
Bladder perforation
Vessel perforation
Preperitoneal installation
Catheter migration
Fibrin encasement
Omental encasement
Luminal obstruction
Subcutaneous leakage
Exit-site leakage
Cuff erosion

Infectious

Exit-site infection
Tunnel infection
Peritonitis

Dialysis-related

Hypervolemia/hypovolemia
Hypernatremia/hyponatremia
Hyperkalemia/hypokalemia
Acidosis/alkalosis
Hyperglycemia
Hypoproteinemia
Hypertriglyceridemia

Other

Abdominal wall hernia
Inguinal hernia
Pleural leak
Abdominal pain
    Inflow, dwell, outflow
Pneumoperitoneum
Peritoneal eosinophilia
Peritoneal sclerosis

Contraindications

Widely accepted contraindications to acute peritoneal dialysis are related to a lack of integrity of the peritoneal membrane or cavity. Do not treat babies who have diaphragmatic hernia, omphalocele, and gastroschisis with peritoneal dialysis. Abdominal surgery with residual drains or fistulae and surgery that creates a thoracoabdominal connection usually prevents successful peritoneal dialysis. Patients with recent gastrointestinal and urinary tract surgery and even extraperitoneal renal transplantation are candidates for peritoneal dialysis,[1] but hemofiltration or hemodialysis may offer advantages in certain situations. Patients who have undergone extensive or multiple abdominal procedures or who have had peritonitis may have widespread adhesions that can prevent dialysate flow and contact with the peritoneal membrane. Patients with cardiac failure or shock of any cause

may perfuse the peritoneal membrane so poorly that peritoneal dialysis becomes extremely inefficient; opt for hemofiltration in these conditions. Finally, the presence of a ventriculoperitoneal shunt represents a relative contraindication to peritoneal dialysis.[2]

Complications

Box 68-1 lists complications of peritoneal dialysis, most of which are manageable without discontinuing the procedure. Complications related to insertion of the peritoneal dialysis catheter stem from the type of catheter placed and the method of placement. The percutaneous placement of an acute catheter carries the highest risk of serious complications. Grossly bloody effluent, a fall in the hematocrit, or shock signal the occurrence of an intraabdominal blood vessel laceration.[10] This most serious of complications necessitates an emergency laparotomy. Unexplained polyuria and glycosuria may signal the accidental puncture of the urinary bladder. Feces or gas in the peritoneal effluent or the abrupt onset of watery diarrhea that has a high glucose concentration is indicative of bowel perforation.[31] These three complications usually prevent further treatment with peritoneal dialysis, at least for several days.

A less serious problem related to acute percutaneous catheter insertion is preperitoneal installation, or the insertion of a catheter into the abdominal wall instead of into the peritoneal cavity, which causes pain and local swelling during dialysate influx. The problem is easy to diagnose and readily correctable by replacing the catheter. Once the catheter is in place, a number of problems may befall it. Catheters can migrate out of the pelvic gutter into other abdominal locations that prevent the easy influx and drainage of dialysate. For instance, a catheter located over the dome of the liver does not function properly. Inadequate drainage may also occur when omentum or fibrin encases the catheter. In addition, fibrin may enter the catheter and produce an intraluminal clot that is difficult to dislodge, even with vigorous dialysate infusion. Nonetheless, forceful infusion of saline followed by withdrawal of dialysate may occasionally dislodge this material and open the catheter. Even a well-placed and functioning catheter may present problems. Subcutaneous leakage of dialysate into the abdominal wall tissues surrounding the insertion site or leakage of fluid through the exit site to the outside are relatively common problems with acute catheters that do not have one or more cuffs. Even cuffed catheters may leak and require surgical intervention. Cuffs may also migrate and erode through the skin or out of the exit site. Remove an eroding superficial cuff as soon as inflammation appears around it.

Peritonitis is the most frequent serious complication of acute peritoneal dialysis.[24] Approximately one fifth of the cases of peritonitis occur in temporal association with exit site or tunnel infections.[19] *Staphylococcus aureus* causes exit site infections.[29] When infected, the catheter exit site appears red and crusty with or without purulent exudate. Local care with antibacterial solutions such as 3% saline, dilute hydrogen peroxide, or povidone iodine may be curative. If such agents fail, administer a 10-day course of oral antistaphylococcal antibiotics or intravenous (IV) vancomycin. Chronic catheters traverse from the exit site through a subcutaneous tunnel before dropping into the peritoneal cavity. Exit site infections may extend down the tunnel, causing pain, swelling, nodularity, and redness over the subcutaneous portion of the catheter. Tunnel infections are very difficult to treat and, in many cases, result in catheter removal. Both exit site and tunnel infections predispose a patient to peritonitis, but peritonitis may also occur alone.[29] The pathogenesis of peritonitis in chronic dialysis patients is controversial; improper aseptic technique that allows bacteria to gain access to the peritoneal cavity through the catheter lumen probably causes most episodes.

Diagnostic criteria for peritonitis include the following: (1) symptoms and signs of peritoneal inflammation, (2) cloudy peritoneal fluid with an elevated peritoneal fluid cell count ($>100/\mu l$, $>50\%$ neutrophils), (3) demonstration of bacteria in the peritoneal effluent Gram stain or culture.[24] Patients may experience abdominal pain, nausea, vomiting, or diarrhea, but cloudy peritoneal effluent is the usual hallmark and may occur without the classic signs of peritonitis. Carefully analyze the peritoneal fluid, because other causes of cloudy fluid such as fibrin, chyle, or mild bleeding may lead to an erroneous diagnosis. A careful physical examination that reveals abdominal pain in concert with cloudy fluid almost always accurately diagnoses peritonitis. Although bacteria cause 80% to 90% of all cases of peritonitis, between 5% and 20% of the cases are culture negative. *Staphylococcus epidermidis* and *S. aureus* account for as many as 60% of the cases, with gram-negative organisms accounting for approximately 20%. Miscellaneous organisms such as fungi cause the remainder of the cases.

The treatment of peritonitis is standardized only in patients undergoing chronic maintenance peritoneal dialysis.[24] The application of these treatment protocols in the pediatric intensive care unit is highly questionable, but some principles are useful. Administer antimicrobials, including vancomycin and another antibiotic such as a third-generation cephalosporin or an aminoglycoside for gram-negative coverage, intraperitoneally and on the initial day of treatment. Add antimicrobials to the dialysate in a concentration equal to typical plasma concentration targets for those medications. Signs and symptoms of peritonitis should subside within 5 days after the initiation of therapy; continue antibiotic therapy for between 10 and 14 days. It is possible to cure most cases of peritonitis without catheter removal; however, some gram-negative infections, such as *Pseudomonas* infections, may be resistant to therapy.[23] Fungal peritonitis generally mandates catheter removal.[15]

Complications related to the dialysis itself are similar to those experienced by patients undergoing hemodialysis.[2] Hypovolemia is a common problem, particularly in smaller patients who may become inadvertently volume depleted, especially with continuous treatment. Hypervolemia may also occur when the obligatory IV fluids exceed the ultrafiltration capacity of the dialysis prescription. This complication is extremely common in the critically ill child who is receiving multiple IV infusions delivered by separate IV systems in addition to intermittent infusions of blood and albumin. This same scenario may produce hypernatremia, especially when high concentrations of dialysate glucose are used to effect rapid ultrafiltration. Dialysate containing very high concentrations of glucose may also cause hyperglycemia, which depresses serum sodium by 1.3 mEq/L for every increase of 100 mg/dl in the serum glucose concentration. Manage severe hyperglycemia by using parenteral insulin or, in some cases, by adding insulin to the dialysate.

Hypoproteinemia may occur as a result of substantial protein diffusion from the blood into the dialysate. During a routine daily dialysis treatment, patients lose an average of 0.2 g of protein/kg virgule of body weight.[5] For that reason, patients may need extra protein supplementation in addition to the usual amounts recommended for critically ill children, which in practical terms usually amounts to a daily protein intake of approximately 2 to 3 g/kg.[32]

A number of other annoying but usually benign complications may occur in patients undergoing peritoneal dialysis. Abdominal wall hernias develop in approximately 10% of all patients undergoing chronic peritoneal dialysis, but the incidence is much less in supine patients cared for in critical care units. On the other hand, inguinal hernias are more common, even in patients who are bedridden. Children often develop scrotal or labial edema and, in some patients, severe penile edema. Overt inguinal hernias or occult dialysate leaks from catheter tracks may cause this edema.[16] Obtain a diagnosis by physical examination, by a computed tomography scan with contrast, or by peritoneal scintigraphy. Inguinal hernias cause most of these complications. If the fluid collection is severe, it may interfere with peritoneal dialysis; perform herniorrhaphy before resuming dialysis.

Although uncommon, leakage into the pleural cavity also prevents continuation of peritoneal dialysis.[14] Most of these leaks occur through defects on the right side of the diaphragm and lead to pleural effusions that may become large. Such complications are relatively common after cardiothoracic surgery but may occur spontaneously, presumably as a result of congenital defects in the diaphragm. Diagnose diaphragmatic leaks by thoracentesis to yield fluid, the composition of which is similar to peritoneal dialysate. Scanning demonstrates that technetium-tagged microaggregated albumin injected into the peritoneal space enters the chest in such circumstances.[34] Some patients may continue supine peritoneal dialysis if the communication is small. However, if the diaphragmatic leak is sufficient to cause recurrent high volume hydrothoraces, repair the defect in the diaphragm before continuing peritoneal dialysis. Attempt pleurodesis in patients who are unable to transfer to some other form of dialytic therapy.

Abdominal pain may be an indication of peritonitis, but also consider other causes. Low pH of the peritoneal dialysis solution or the position of the catheter tip may produce pain during inflow. Overdistention of the peritoneal cavity produces pain during dwell; reduce overdistention by decreasing the dialysate dwell volume. Excessive drain time, which allows the peritoneal catheter to pull against abdominal structures after evacuation of the dialysate volume, usually causes pain during outflow. Shortening the drain time usually relieves this complication. Pneumoperitoneum caused by air entering the abdomen during the dialysate inflow is a common finding that may cause pain or may be an incidental radiologic finding. Do not immediately assume that air under the diaphragm indicates a perforated viscus.

The final complications of note are peritoneal fluid eosinophilia[22] and peritoneal sclerosis.[13] The eosinophil count may become elevated in peritoneal effluent, usually soon after peritoneal catheter insertion. The cause of this elevated count remains unknown but may be the effect of plasticizers leached from the peritoneal dialysis solution containers and tubing. Instillation of antibiotics for treatment of peritonitis may cause some later cases of peritoneal eosinophilia. Fungal or parasitic infections of the peritoneum occasionally produce eosinophilia. Peritoneal sclerosis is an unusual but serious complication characterized by the formation of thick fibrous tissue that covers the abdominal and pelvic viscera. The effectiveness of peritoneal dialysis decreases, and intestinal obstruction may occur. The cause of peritoneal sclerosis remains unknown, but it is more common in patients with recurrent episodes of peritonitis. No satisfactory treatment for this condition exists.

Equipment

Catheters. Successful application of peritoneal dialysis depends in large part on the function and longevity of the peritoneal dialysis catheter. There are two general categories of catheters: acute or chronic. Insert acute catheters over a stylet or flexible wire at the bedside.[38] Most of these catheters are straight or slightly curved with numerous side holes at the distal end. Because it is possible to place acute catheters at the bedside, dialysis may commence without delay or surgical consultation. However, acute catheters do not have felt cuffs to protect against bacterial migration; therefore the incidence of peritonitis increases with their use, and leakage is more common. If dialysis extends for a prolonged period, use chronic peritoneal catheters, even in the acute setting. Chronic dialysis catheters usually are made of flexible Silastic tubing with numerous perforations at one end, a connector at the other, and one or two Dacron felt cuffs in the middle.[36] These catheters require surgical placement through the rectus muscle, usually below the umbilicus. The surgeon drops the perforated end of the catheter into the peritoneal cavity through a small incision, directs it toward the pelvic gutter, and secures the Dacron cuff within the rectus muscle according to described methods.[3,4] This procedure forms an almost water-tight seal instantly, and dialysis may begin shortly after surgery.

During healing, fibroblasts grow into the Dacron cuff, which anchors the catheter firmly in place, provides a barrier to bacterial migration, and prevents dialysate leakage. Draw the catheter through a subcutaneous tunnel to an exit site several inches from the secured cuff. Insert a titanium connector into the external catheter segment. Although controversy exists regarding the virtue of straight catheters vs. curled catheters, single-cuffed catheters vs. double-cuffed catheters, and exotic modifications of these two standard types, no catheter design has emerged as undeniably best.[12] A number of pediatric centers have verified success with adult- and pediatric-sized curled Tenckhoff catheters.[30] Although the details of placement and usage vary from center to center, this catheter works well in children of all sizes. It is easy to place and, because of its curled design, seldom becomes entrapped by omentum or migrates to a dysfunctional position.[21]

Dialysate. After inserting the peritoneal dialysis catheter, begin dialysate infusion at a volume of 10 to 20 ml/kg/exchange.[2] The choice of dialysate in the initial hours of the treatment depends on the treatment goals. Four standard

Table 68-1   Composition of Peritoneal Dialysis Solution

Substance	Concentration
Sodium	132 mEq/L
Magnesium	1.5 mEq/L
Chloride	102 mEq/L
Calcium	3.5, 2.5 mEq/L
Lactate	35 mEq/L
Dextrose	1.5, 2.5, 3.5, 4.25 g/dl
Osmolarity	346, 396, 447, 485 mOsm/L
pH	5.5

Table 68-2   Peritoneal Dialysis Solution Containing Bicarbonate

Solution	Amount (ml)
NaCl (0.45%)	896
NaCl (2.5 mEq/ml)	12
NaHCO$_3$ (1 mEq/ml)	40
MgSO$_4$ (10%)	1.8
D$_{50}$W	50
Total	**999.8**

Total Solute Concentration in mEq/L

Sodium	139
Chloride	99
Magnesium	1.5
Sulfate	1.5
Bicarbonate	40
Dextrose	2.5 g/L
Osmolality	423 mOsm/kg

Modified from Nash MA, Russo JC: Neonatal lactic acidosis and renal failure: the role of peritoneal dialysis, *J Pediatr* 91:101-105, 1977.

solutions are available and differ only in their dextrose concentration. The commercially available solutions contain 1.5%, 2.5%, 3.5%, or 4.25% dextrose. Any of these solutions may be helpful, but in most critically ill children, a starting solution containing 2.5% dextrose is usually sufficient to effect a safe rate of fluid removal while avoiding hyperglycemia. Table 68-1 lists the composition of a typical peritoneal dialysis solution.

Although lactate is the standard buffer in peritoneal dialysis solutions, some patients are unable to tolerate lactate, which is readily absorbed across the peritoneal membrane. These patients have an ongoing metabolic acidosis that partly results from accumulation of endogenous lactic acid; additional lactate absorbed from the dialysate may worsen this condition. Ask the hospital pharmacy to formulate a bicarbonate-containing dialysate as needed to treat these patients.[27] Table 68-2 provides a recipe for this type of peritoneal dialysis solution. Bicarbonate-containing dialysate solutions contain no calcium; give calcium intravenously to avoid hypocalcemia during the procedure. Dialysate is commercially available in clear plastic bags that are underfilled, which makes it easy to place additives into the bags using aseptic technique. Commonly used additives are potassium chloride, heparin, and antibiotics.

Automated Cyclers. Because of the development of auto-

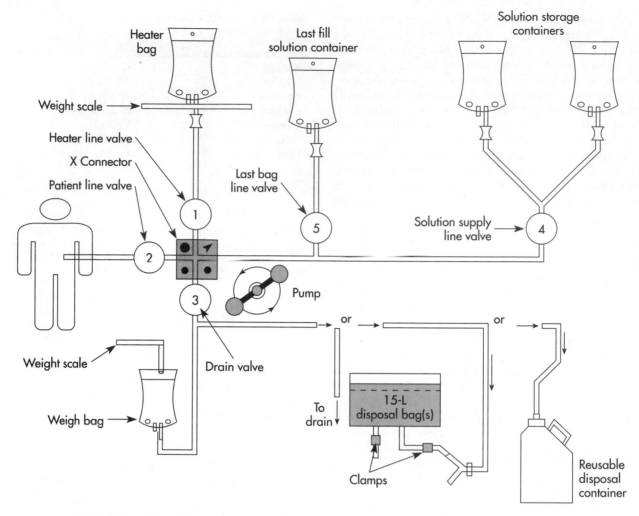

FIG 68-2   Schematic representation of the automated peritoneal dialysis cycler (Baxter, Deerfield, Ill). The circuit controls dialysate flow at five points. The patient fills and drains by gravity. The pump fills the heater bag and empties the weigh bag.

mated cycling peritoneal dialysis machines that can deliver an intraperitoneal volume as low as 50 ml, over the past 10 years the technique of peritoneal dialysis has evolved from a manual procedure to a fully automated procedure. Thus the use of manual systems is rare except with the smallest of patients. The system that pediatricians have used most extensively is the Pac X-tra (Baxter, Deerfield, Ill). Fig. 68-2 shows a schematic representation of this machine. Such a cycler minimizes nursing time; dialysis personnel can set up the machine, and ICU nurses can monitor it. It is possible to hang a series of dialysate bags on the machine for 24 hours or longer. This ability provides adequate dialysate volume for lengthy treatments. At the beginning of the treatment, the dialysis staff adjusts the fill volume of dialysate and timers that regulate inflow, dwell time, and drainage time. It is easy to train ICU personnel to troubleshoot the machine and monitor the alarms.

Techniques

Consult a surgeon or nephrologist to perform Tenckhoff catheter placement in the operating room. After surgical placement of the Tenckhoff catheter, perform rapid exchanges of saline or dialysate in volumes of 10 to 20 ml/kg body weight to test for leakage. A leaking catheter renders peritoneal dialysis a lost cause; resecure it. Use a functional catheter immediately, but treat it gently for the first several days. During this "break-in" period, cycle small-dialysate dwell volumes continuously.

Modify the dialysis prescription to meet the needs of each patient. The dialysis prescription contains the following components: (1) session length, (2) exchange volume, (3) inflow time, (4) dwell time, (5) outflow time, (6) dialysate concentration (% dextrose), and (7) additives.

Session Length.   Customarily determine sessions or treatment periods for no longer than 1 day at a time. Depending on the treatment goals, continue the session for as many hours or days as necessary. It is common to accomplish some goals, such as resolution of hyperkalemia, well before other goals, such as resolution of anasarca; thus it is often necessary to make intradialytic adjustments of other treatment parameters (e.g., the dialysate concentration) while maintaining long treatment times.

Exchange Volume.   The amount of intraperitoneal fluid tolerated by most children is between 35 and 45 ml/kg body weight.[2] Approach this volume over a time period of approximately 1 week by starting at a volume of 10 to 20 ml/kg and increasing by increments of 5 to 10 ml/kg every other day. Immediately reduce dwell volumes that result in pain, respiratory embarrassment, or leakage to a volume that relieves the problem.

Inflow Time. Inflow of dialysate occurs by gravity. Automated peritoneal dialysis cyclers do not pump fluid into or out of the patient. The amount of time allowed for inflow depends on the exchange volume, the difference between the level of the patient and the level of the dialysate bags, and catheter patency. Minimize this time, usually no longer than 10 minutes.

Dwell Time. Dwell time is the period between the end of the inflow time and the start of the outflow time. It is the time during which dialysis occurs. Although peritoneal clearance of solutes and fluid removal occur throughout dwell times of up to 4 hours, the most efficient transport of wastes and water occurs during the first 30 minutes of the dwell (see Fig. 68-1). For that reason, dwell time is usually set between 30 minutes and 1 hour.

Outflow Time. Outflow occurs by gravity; dwell volume, differential patient and drain bag levels, and catheter function determine outflow. Patient position is sometimes also very important. Under optimal circumstances, complete drainage within 10 minutes. The dialysis nurse assesses outflow time during the initial cycles, sets the time empirically on the basis of the system's function, and reassesses frequently to ensure that fluid retention does not occur. Automated cyclers will alarm if fluid retention greater than 15% of the dwell volume occurs. Slow drainage or low drainage may be the earliest signs of catheter obstruction or peritonitis.

Dialysate Concentration. The main difference among the types of commercially available dialysis solutions is their dextrose concentrations and resultant osmolarities (see Table 68-1). Solutions of higher osmolarity effect a greater ultrafiltration rate; they cause water to move from the blood into the peritoneum in greater volume over a shorter time period. The choice of fluid is dictated by the amount of fluid removal desired and the urgency of such removal combined with the patient's ability to withstand hemodynamic changes. Most children will have a sufficient ultrafiltration, which simulates normal urine output, when treated with 2.5% dextrose-containing dialysate. Higher concentrations are necessary for patients with large parenteral fluid requirements or for those who have inefficient peritoneal membranes secondary to peritonitis or other peritoneal damage.

Additives. The addition of electrolytes and medications to the dialysate (using meticulously sterile technique) is a common procedure in the acute setting. Potassium chloride is the most common addition to the usual components because the dietary intake of potassium in critically ill children is either absent or very small. It is common to restrict parenteral infusion of potassium in patients receiving dialysis, even when they are receiving adequate parenteral nutrition. To prevent dangerous negative balance, add potassium chloride to all of the dialysate bags at an appropriate concentration, usually between 2 and 4 mEq/L.

Another common additive is sodium heparin. In concentrations of 500 to 1000 units/L of dialysate, heparin prevents fibrin accumulation in the Tenckhoff catheter. It is particularly useful for newly inserted catheters, during episodes of peritonitis, or when intraabdominal bleeding occurs for any reason.

Place antibiotics into the dialysate to treat peritonitis or to maintain blood levels of the antibiotics used to treat infection in other areas. Add antibiotics to the dialysate in concentrations that match the desired plasma concentration.

Remarks

The zealous use of peritoneal dialysis to treat children with end-stage renal disease has resulted in technical refinements that have greatly increased its utility in the critical care of children. The procedure has the distinct advantage of simplicity over the dialysis modalities that depend on an extracorporeal blood circuit. The patient needs no systemic anticoagulation, and it is safe to use peritoneal dialysis in patients with bleeding diathesis. Because it is less likely to cause hypotension or osmotic dysequilibrium, peritoneal dialysis is safer for hemodynamically unstable patients. Likewise it is safer for infants and small children in whom hemodialysis is more difficult to perform. The automated cycler has reduced the time commitment for the dialysis nursing staff and for the ICU nurses. Cyclers have eliminated the need for frequent violation of a sterile system, thus reducing the certainty of peritonitis (as was seen in previous years) to only a possibility. Although sluggish and inefficient, peritoneal dialysis is gentle and persistent—desirable qualities in the hectic atmosphere of the ICU.

REFERENCES

1. Alexander SR: Pediatric CAPD update—1983, *Perit Dial Bull (Suppl)* 3:515-522, 1983.
2. Alexander SR: Peritoneal dialysis in children. In Nolph KD, editor: *Peritoneal dialysis,* Dordrecht, The Netherlands, 1989, Kluwer Academic.
3. Alexander SR, Tank ES, Corneil AT: Five years' experience with CAPD/CCPD catheters in infants and children. In Fine RN, Sarer K, Mehls O, editors: *CAPD in children,* New York, 1985, Springer-Verlag.
4. Alexander SR, et al: Clinical parameters in continuous ambulatory peritoneal dialysis for infants and children. In Moncrief JW, Popovich RP, editors: *CAPD update,* New York, 1981, Masson.
5. Balfe JW, et al: The use of CAPD in the treatment of children with end-stage renal disease, *Perit Dial Bull* 1:35-38, 1981.
6. Belsha CW, Kohaut EC, Warady BA: Dialytic management of childhood acute renal failure: a survey of North American pediatric nephrologists, *Pediatr Nephrol* 9:362-363, 1995.
7. Blackfan KD, Maxcy KF: The intraperitoneal injection of saline solution, *Am J Dis Child* 15:19-28, 1918.
8. Bloxsum A, Powell N: The treatment of acute temporary dysfunction of the kidneys by peritoneal irrigation, *Pediatrics* 1:52-57, 1948.
9. Chan JCM: Peritoneal dialysis for renal failure in childhood, *Clin Pediatr* 17:349-354, 1978.
10. Chesney RW, et al: Acute renal failure: an important complication of cardiac surgery in infants, *J Pediatr* 87:381-388, 1975.
11. Day RE, White RHR: Peritoneal dialysis in children: review of 8 years' experience, *Arch Dis Child* 52:56-61, 1977.
12. Diaz-Buxo JA, Geissenter WT: Single cuff versus double cuff Tenckhoff catheter, *Perit Dial Bull* 4:S100, 1984.
13. Dobbie JW: Pathogenesis of peritoneal sclerosing syndromes (sclerosing peritonitis) in peritoneal dialysis, *Perit Dial Int* 12:14-27, 1992.
14. Edwards SR, Unger AM: Acute hydrothorax—a new complication of periteonal dialysis, *JAMA* 199:853-855, 1967.
15. Eisenberg EG, Leviton I, Soeiro R: Fungal peritonitis in patients receiving peritoneal dialysis: experience with 11 patients and review of the literature, *Rev Infect Dis* 8:309-321, 1986.

16. Engeset J, Youngson G: Ambulatory peritoneal dialysis and hernial complications, *Surg Clin North Am* 64:385-392, 1984.

17. Esparanca MJ, Collins DL: Peritoneal dialysis efficiency in relation to body weight, *J Pediatr Surg* 1:162-169, 1966.

18. Etteldorf UN, et al: Intermittent peritoneal dialysis in the management of acute renal failure in children, *J Pediatr* 60:327-339, 1962.

19. Gokal R, et al: Peritoneal catheters and exit site practices: toward optimum peritoneal access, *Perit Dial Int* 13:29-39, 1993.

20. Gruskin AB, Balvarte HJ, Dabbagh S: Hemodialysis and peritoneal dialysis. In Edelmann C, editor: *Pediatric kidney disease,* Boston, 1992, Little, Brown.

21. Hickman RO, Watkins S: Peritoneal dialysis access: an introduction, *Dial Transplant* 17:10-12, 1988.

22. Humayun HM, et al: Peritoneal fluid eosinophilia in patients undergoing maintenance peritoneal dialysis, *Arch Intern Med* 141:1172-1173, 1981.

23. Juergensen PH, et al: Pseudomonas peritonitis associated with continuous ambulatory peritoneal dialysis: a six-year study, *Am J Kidney Dis* 11:413-417, 1988.

24. Keane WF, et al: Peritoneal dialysis–related peritonitis treatment recommendations: 1993, *Perit Dial Int* 13:14-28, 1993.

25. Khana R, Nolph KD, Oreopoulos D: *The essentials of peritoneal dialysis,* Dordrecht, The Netherlands, 1993, Kluwer Academic.

26. Kohaut EC: Continuous ambulatory peritoneal dialysis: a preliminary pediatric experience, *Am J Dis Child* 135:270-271, 1981.

27. Nash MA, Russo JC: Neonatal lactic acidosis and renal failure: the role of peritoneal dialysis, *J Pediatr* 91:101-105, 1977.

28. Nolph KD, et al: Determinants of low clearances of small solutes during peritoneal dialysis, *Kidney Int* 13:117-123, 1978.

29. Piraino B: A review of *Staphlococcus aureus:* exit-site and tunnel infections in peritoneal dialysis patients, *Am J Kidney Dis* 16:89-95, 1990.

30. Rottembourg J, et al: Straight or curled Tenckhoff peritoneal catheter for CAPD, *Perit Dial Bull* 1:151-153, 1981.

31. Rubin J, et al: Peritonitis and bowel perforation in peritoneal dialysis, *Ann Intern Med* 81:402-403, 1974.

32. Salusky IB: Nutritional recommendations for children treated with CAPD/CCPD. In Fine RN, editor: *Chronic ambulatory peritoneal and chronic cycling peritoneal dialysis in children,* Boston, 1987, Martinus Nijhoff.

33. Salusky, et al: Continuous ambulatory peritoneal dialysis in children, *Pediatr Clin North Am* 29:1005-1012, 1982.

34. Spadaro JJ, Thakur V, Nolph K: Technitium-99 m-labelled macroaggregated albumin in demonstration of transdiaphragmatic leakage of dialysate in peritoneal dialysis, *Am J Nephrol* 2:36-38, 1982.

35. Swan H, Gordon HH: Peritoneal lavage in the treatment of anuria in children, *Pediatrics* 4:586-595, 1949.

36. Tenckhoff H, Schechter: A bacteriologically safe peritoneal access device, *Trans Am Soc Intern Organs* 14:181-187, 1968.

37. Warady BA: The peritoneal equilibration test (PET) in pediatrics, *Contemp Dial Nephrol,* pp 21-23, March 1994.

38. Weston RE, Roberts M: Clinical use of stylet catheter for peritoneal dialysis, *Arch Intern Med* 115:659-662, 1965.

39. Zawanda ET: Indications for dialysis. In Dougirdas JT, Ing TS, editors: *Handbook of dialysis,* Boston, 1994, Little, Brown.

69 Continuous Extracorporeal Hemofiltration

Curtis B. Pickert and Mark J. Heulitt

Critically ill infants and children may require large volumes of fluid for hemodynamic and nutritional support. However, some patients with primary or secondary renal insufficiency are unable to excrete urine of the quality and quantity necessary to maintain fluid and electrolyte homeostasis. Eventually they may develop one or more complications of this imbalance, including fluid overload, uremia, or hyperkalemia.

If there are no contraindications or limitations, temporary support with peritoneal dialysis or hemodialysis is an option until the primary disease process improves or until the child receives a transplanted kidney. However, there remains a subgroup of critically ill patients in whom peritoneal dialysis or hemodialysis is not feasible because of problems such as hemodynamic instability, intraperitoneal processes, or difficulty in securing dialysis access. In the past there was very little to offer these children, and in spite of having a curable primary disease they would succumb to massive fluid overload or to the metabolic complications of renal insufficiency. Over the past decade, continuous extracorporeal hemofiltration (CEH) has evolved as a modality for the regulation of fluid and electrolytes and the removal of metabolic toxins in pediatric patients with renal insufficiency.* Using either an arteriovenous or pump-assisted venovenous extracorporeal circuit with an in-line hemofilter, it is possible to continuously remove large volumes of an ultrafiltrate of plasma from even the most critically ill and hemodynamically unstable patients.[3,9,14-15,27]

The basic principle of CEH is remarkably simple. It uses a plastic "hemofilter" that is composed of an outer collecting chamber that surrounds a bundle of parallel hollow fibers permeable to water and small solutes but impermeable to larger circulating elements such as albumin and blood cells. The hemofilter is in-line in an extracorporeal arteriovenous or venovenous circuit (Fig. 69-1). The hydraulic pressure generated by the arterial pulse (arteriovenous) or pump (pump-assisted venovenous) pushes the blood through the fibers within the hemofilter. By the process of convection, plasma water and small solutes pass through micropores in the walls of the hollow fibers and into the outer collecting chamber of the filter, where they form the ultrafiltrate (Fig. 69-2). A chamber exit port is the outlet for fluid removal. A pump placed on the ultrafiltrate removal line can regulate the quantity of ultrafiltrate removed per unit of time. The remaining blood exiting the hemofilter returns to the patient via the venous return catheter or lumen.

The hemofilter is available in various sizes depending on the size of the patient and the rate of ultrafiltration required (Table 69-1; Figs. 69-3 and 69-4). Within individual hemofilters the fiber pore size also varies, generally allowing

*References 1, 2, 13, 16, 17, 21, 26-30, 37-40, 47, and 49-52.

Table 69-1 Hemofilter Specifications*

	Diafilter 30	Diafilter 20	Minifilter Plus	Minifilter
Typical ultrafiltration rate (ml/min)	12-100	7-50	1-8	0.5-1.5
Membrane area	0.7 m²	0.4 m²	800 cm²	150 cm²
Filter blood volume (ml)	58	38	15	6
Circuit blood volume (ml)†	105	85	35	35

Courtesy Amicon, Inc., Beverly, MA.
*Approximate values. Ultrafiltration rates depend on rate of blood flow.
†Includes tubing for pump-assisted CEH.

solutes with a mass less than 5000 Da to pass freely while inhibiting the passage of circulating elements with a mass greater than 50,000 Da (Table 69-2). Erythrocytes (7.5 μm), platelets (2 to 4 μm), granulocytes (12 to 15 μm), and lymphocytes (6 to 18 μm) will not pass through an intact fiber. The micropores, which have a diameter on the order of 2 nm, restrict the passage of circulating cells or substances with a diameter greater than 1 μm (Fig. 69-5). The filters are highly biocompatible, with no complement activation and no intrinsic platelet, leukocyte, or red blood cell destruction.

Inherent to the effectiveness of CEH is the need for sustainable, large bore vascular access.[22,36] Access for arteriovenous hemofiltration in pediatric patients can be in the axillary,[30] radial,[13,30,51] brachial,[30,51] femoral,[30,51] umbilical,[21,30] and pedal[28] arteries and in the umbilical, brachial, internal jugular, subclavian, and femoral veins.[28,51] It is also possible to obtain venovenous access in these large veins, and the use of a double-lumen, low-resistance hemodialysis or hemofiltration catheter allows for the use of a single site for both outlet and inlet ports (Fig. 69-6). There are no reports of recirculation with this method. Specific hemofiltration catheters are available; it is also permissible to use introducer sheaths for hemofiltration. It is imperative that the catheters be as large as is safe and feasible to reduce the resistance to flow in both ports.

The circuit requires anticoagulation and effective blood flow to prevent clotting of the filter. Plasma proteins, blood cells, and fibrinous matter can accumulate within the lumen of the fibers, increasing viscosity and obstructing flow. Frequent replacement of the hemofilter and circuit secondary to clotting in the fibers leads to blood loss, thrombocytopenia, and inefficient hemofiltration as a result of fiber obstruction and lost filtration time during circuit changes. Most clinicians use heparin for anticoagulation, but the use of citrate is also permissible.[34] Follow the activated clotting time (ACT) at the bedside to monitor the effectiveness of heparinization. Maximizing the lifespan of individual circuits

403

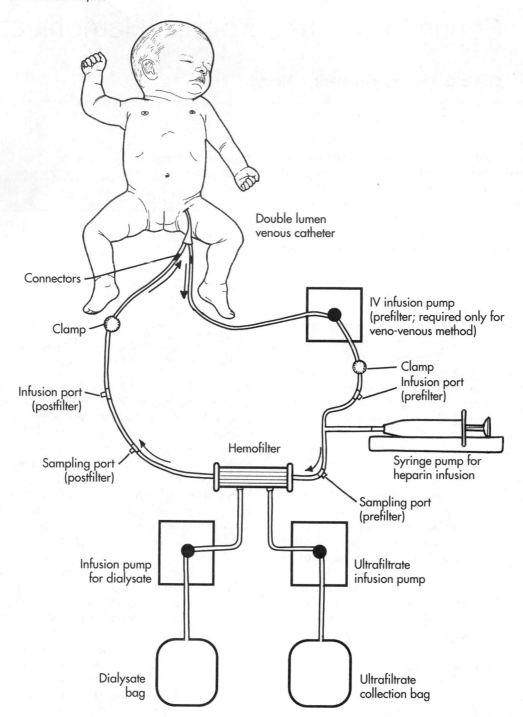

FIG. 69-1 Illustration of extracorporeal circuit used for venovenous, pump-assisted hemodia-filtration. Prefilter pump not necessary for arteriovenous method.

and filters requires good flow through the circuit. A strong arterial pulse or pump assistance facilitates flow and increases the longevity of the circuit. Administration of prefilter fluid (e.g., normal saline) may augment filter flow and reduce viscosity within the lumen of the fiber. To minimize anticoagulation of the patient, use regional heparinization with a post-filter protamine infusion.[24]

The CEH sieving coefficient, expressed mathematically as the ratio of ultrafiltrate concentration of a solute to plasma concentration of the same solute, describes the degree to which CEH removes a solute. This relationship dictates the replacement-fluid solute concentration necessary to maintain homeostasis. For small solutes such as sodium, potassium, or glucose, the sieving coefficient is approximately equal to 1.0 because these solutes pass through the fiber micropores by means of convection in a concentration essentially equivalent to that of plasma (Table 69-3). On the other hand, the sieving coefficient may be greater or less than 1.0, varying from a value of 0.008 for albumin, where CEH filters very little, to 1.124 for bicarbonate, where the ultrafiltrate concentration exceeds that of plasma.[25] The Gibbs-Donnan effect of negatively charged proteins at the membrane facilitates the pas-

Table 69-2 Approximate Molecular Weights of Circulating Humoral Factors

Substance	Molecular weight
Interleukin 1	15,000
Interleukin 2	30,000-35,000
Interleukin 3	40,000
Interleukin 4	20,000
Interferon alpha	25,000
Interferon gamma	20,000-25,000
T-suppressor factor	70,000
Migration inhibitory factor	15,000-70,000
Macrophage chemotactic factor	35,000-55,000
Lymphotoxin	10,000-200,000
Lymphocyte-stimulating factor	85,000
Proliferation inhibitory factor	70,000
Macrophage colony-stimulating factor	70,000
Macrophage growth factor	70,000
Migration inhibitory factor	70,000
Neutrophil chemotactic factor	750,000
Tumor necrosis factor (cachectin)*	40,000-45,000
Complement factors	25,000-400,000
Erythropoietin	38,000
Ferritin	440,000
Coagulation factors	
XIII	320,000
XII	80,000
XI	160,000
X	59,000
IX	57,000
VIII	330,000
VII	48,000
V	330,000
Prothrombin	72,000
Thrombin	34,000
Fibrinogen	340,000
Protein C	62,000
Protein S	69,000
Plasminogen	90,000
IgG	150,000
IgA (monomeric)	160,000
IgA (secretory)	400,000
IgM	900,000
IgD	180,000
IgE	190,000

*Dissociates into four subunits of molecular weight 17,000.

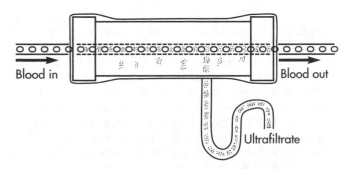

FIG. 69-2 Illustration of passage of blood through hemofilter with formation of ultrafiltrate by process of convection.

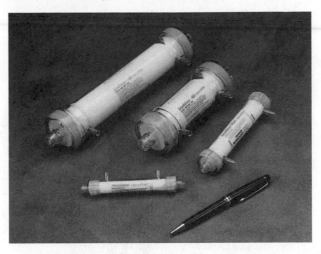

FIG. 69-3 Various sizes of hemofilters.

(Courtesy Amicon, Inc., Beverly, MA.)

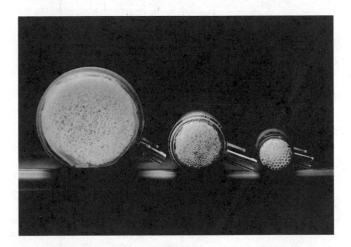

FIG. 69-4 Cross-sectional photo of hemofilter demonstrating fiber arrangement.

(Courtesy Amicon, Inc., Beverly, MA.)

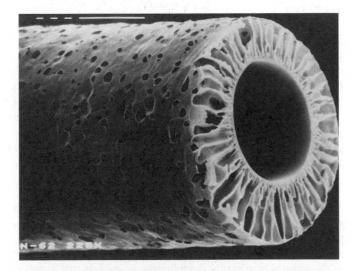

FIG. 69-5 Electron micrograph of single fiber (×225). Pore diameter approximately 60 angstrom.

(Courtesy Amicon, Inc., Beverly, MA.)

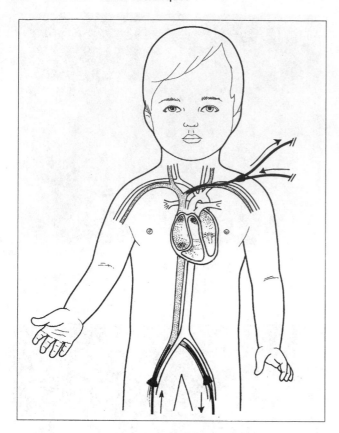

FIG. 69-6 Illustration of a single-lumen catheter placed in iliac veins (double site, arteriovenous or venovenous) vs. double-lumen catheter in left subclavian vein (single site, venovenous) for hemofiltration.

Table 69-3 Sieving Coefficients of Drugs and Solutes in CEH

	Sieving coefficient	Reference
Drug		
Amikacin	0.95	18
Amphotericin B	0.10	18
Ampicillin	0.80	18
Cefoperazone	0.10	18
Cefotaxime	0.62	18
Cefoxitin	0.30	18
Ceftriaxone	0.10	18
Cephapirin	0.55	18
Clindamycin	0.40	18
Digoxin	0.80	18
Erythromycin	0.30	18
Gentamicin	0.95	18
Imipenem	0.80	18
Metronidazole	0.80	18
Mezlocillin	0.68	18
N-acetyl procainamide	0.90	18
Nafcillin	0.20	18
Oxacillin	0.05	18
Penicillin	0.50	18
Phenobarbital	0.60	18
Phenytoin	0.10	18
Procainamide	0.86	18
Streptomycin	0.65	18
Theophylline	0.47	18
Tobramycin	0.95	18
Vancomycin	0.90	18
Solute		
Albumin	0.008	24
Bicarbonate	1.124	24
Bilirubin (direct)	0.030	24
Bilirubin (total)	0.030	24
Blood urea nitrogen	1.048	24
Calcium	0.637	24
Chloride	1.046	24
Creatinine	1.020	24
Creatinine phosphokinase	0.676	24
Glucose	0.043	24
Magnesium	0.879	24
Phosphorus	1.044	24
Potassium	0.985	24
Sodium	0.993	24
Uric acid	1.016	24

sage of anions and retards the passage of some cations across the membrane.[2,12,18] Because of this influence, calcium has an intermediate sieving coefficient (0.637). Sieving coefficients also are available for a number of pharmacologic agents; modify doses accordingly (Table 69-3).[5,12,18] Amino acids, glucose, lipids, vitamins, and minerals also have various sieving coefficients; thus individualize parenteral nutrition in the patient on CEH.[26,31]

It is possible to infuse dialysate fluid into and circulate it countercurrently through the outer chamber of the hemofilter, which creates an increased gradient for the removal of potassium, urea nitrogen, and other metabolic toxins from the blood. The term for this process is *hemodiafiltration*.[5,6,9,13] The infusion of dialysate fluid thus increases the amount of total fluid to remove from the outer chamber of the hemofilter and recover in the ultrafiltrate. The flow capabilities of the pump on the ultrafiltrate line may limit the rate of dialysate flow and ultrafiltration.

Indications

CEH is indicated in the critically ill patient who requires renal replacement therapy but in whom hemodialysis or peritoneal dialysis is not possible. These patients include infants or children without adequate vascular access for hemodialysis or patients in whom the hemodynamic status is too unstable to allow the procedure. Patients meeting this criteria typically are those with septic shock and postoperative cardiac surgical patients who develop secondary renal insufficiency.[37] Patients with intraperitoneal processes such as peritonitis, recent abdominal surgery, or extensive bowel adhesions from past surgery may not be candidates for peritoneal dialysis but do tolerate CEH well. Occasionally, severe lung disease restricts the use or effectiveness of peritoneal dialysis because of the limitations on filling volumes and the effect on ventilation; such patients may benefit from CEH. There is extensive experience with CEH in postoperative patients with acute renal failure.[32,33,44] Although CEH removes potassium and urea from the blood, it is generally a much slower process than either peritoneal dialysis or hemodialysis; consider CEH only when the other modalities are contraindicated.

CEH may also benefit patients with endotoxemia or septic

shock. In addition to providing renal replacement therapy, CEH may influence the course of the disease. Patients with this type of disease process may improve clinically while on CEH, principally because of the removal of circulating humoral mediators through the hemofilter.[6,7,19,43,46] More research must define the precise mechanism of benefit and whether the effect is significant enough to warrant reevaluation of the indications for CEH in this population. CEH also improves pulmonary gas exchange in patients with multiple organ-system failure CEH[3,16]; CEH may be a useful adjunct in the care of patients with concurrent hepatic and renal failure.[1,15] There are also reports of the successful treatment of life-threatening inherited metabolic defects in young infants with CEH. This method also has effectively controlled hyperammonemia.[41,42,45]

CEH may be the preferred method of renal replacement for patients with increased intracranial pressure.[14] Hemodialysis causes an increase in intracranial pressure with a concomitant decrease in mean arterial pressure, which results in a reduction in cerebral perfusion pressure. On the other hand, because CEH has no effect on either intracranial pressure or arterial pressure, it preserves cerebral perfusion pressure.

Other conditions in which CEH is beneficial include intoxication with iron[4] or lithium,[8] myoglobinuric renal failure after trauma,[10,11,48] tumor lysis syndrome,[20] and hypernatremia.[35]

Contraindications

An acute or recent intracranial or other systemic hemorrhagic event is a relative contraindication to the use of CEH because of the need for heparinization of the circuit, which typically results in some degree of heparinization in the patient. To minimize this occurrence, infuse protamine postfilter[24]; however, the risk of extending the hemorrhage remains significant. On the other hand, a coagulopathy is not an absolute contraindication and may actually prevent clotting in the hemofilter. Hypotension and cardiovascular instability are not contraindications and, in fact, may improve after beginning CEH.[15] Because of the relatively slow and continuous removal of ultrafiltrate, patients with such conditions typically tolerate the procedure very well.

Complications

Potential complications associated with CEH include bleeding, anemia, thrombocytopenia, thrombosis, metabolic acidosis, hyponatremia, hypovolemia, infection, and catheter-related problems. The need for long-term anticoagulation for days or weeks augments the risk of bleeding, which already has been increased because of the use of heparin. Anemia may occur because of bleeding. Each circuit replacement causes a significant loss of both red blood cells and platelets. Thrombosis may occur at line-insertion sites, with the potential for thromboembolic sequelae in both arterial and venous beds depending on the placement of the catheter. Because of the Gibbs-Donnan effect, there is an obligatory loss of bicarbonate in the ultrafiltrate.[2,18] Bicarbonate levels in the ultrafiltrate exceed that of plasma, resulting in a metabolic acidosis in many patients undergoing CEH. The acidosis is responsive to bicarbonate administration. Because the ultrafiltrate sodium concentration will be equal to the plasma concentration (sieving coefficient = 1), hyponatremia occurs

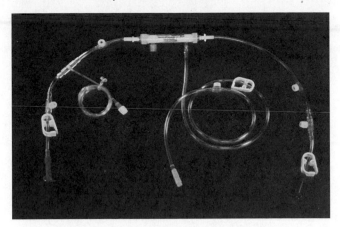

FIG. 69-7   *Example of extracorporeal circuit.*
(Courtesy Amicon, Inc., Beverly, MA.)

unless the fluids being administered to the patient are high in sodium.

Hypovolemia may occur if continuous and meticulous attention is not given to the input and output. Pump disfunction or inadvertently high pump rates on the ultrafiltrate collection line can lead to sudden, massive plasma-water loss. It is crucial to monitor not only the set pump rate but also the actual ultrafiltrate volume at frequent intervals to confirm that the desired volume is removed. Infection is an inherent risk in any procedure involving an extracorporeal system and relatively long-term vascular access. Circuit replacement typically occurs every 12 to 48 hours and increases the potential for introducing infection; perform this task using aseptic technique. Hypothermia may occur if exposure to ambient temperature cools the blood in the circuit.

Equipment

Commercially prepared CEH circuits are available that include the tubing for attachment to standard indwelling catheters, various sizes of filters (see Table 69-1), and access ports for prefilter and postfilter fluid and medication administration (see Fig. 69-1; 69-7). Maintain these circuits in a sterile environment and ensure that multiple sets in various sizes are readily available for circuit replacement.

A patient undergoing CEH may require the use of a flow-regulating pump for augmentation of prefilter blood flow (venovenous CEH), administration of countercurrent dialysate to the outer chamber of the hemofilter, or for regulation of the volume of hourly ultrafiltrate production. Specific hemofiltration pumps are available, but it is acceptable to use standard intravenous pumps.[23] Effective CEH requires high flow rates for augmentation of hydraulic pressure, and pumps typically must be capable of providing rates from between 500 and 2000 ml/hr, depending on the indication and size of the patient. If countercurrent dialysate is put through the outer chamber to enhance removal of urea or potassium, use similar pump-assisted high flow rates. Connect standard tubing from the outer chamber of the hemofilter to a fluid collection bag or bottle and, if desired, place a pump in-line to regulate the rate of ultrafiltration. Thus a circuit may require the simultaneous use of three pumps. Arteriovenous hemofiltration does not require pump assistance, but if the knowledge of precise ultrafiltrate volumes is desirable, place a pump on the ultrafiltrate collection line. If arterial blood flow is inadequate to maintain appropriate filter efficiency and longevity, augment it with pump assistance. Monitor blood pressure continuously if necessary.

A bedside device for determining ACT facilitates close monitoring of the degree of anticoagulation and is an important adjunct to the safe provision of CEH.

Techniques

After identifying the CEH patient, identify the type of hemofiltration. This identification primarily depends on the indication for the procedure and on the availability of arterial and venous access. Options available to the physician include arteriovenous or venovenous access, with or without the use of countercurrent dialysate.

The next priority is secure, sustainable vascular access. In infants, a 4 or 5 French introducer sheath provides large-bore access in the internal jugular, subclavian, or femoral veins, as well as the femoral artery. Intravenous catheters in the radial, dorsalis pedis, and posterior tibial arteries are options for the arterial limb in successful arteriovenous hemofiltration. In addition, 5 or 7 French double-lumen hemodialysis or hemofiltration catheters provide low-resistance access while requiring cannulation of a single vein. In older children and adolescents, use catheters of appropriately larger sizes. To minimize resistance and facilitate blood flow, use the largest catheter possible that will not compromise the vessel. Adolescents can undergo effective CEH with 5 to 7 French single-lumen or 9 to 13 French double-lumen catheters.

During placement of the vascular catheters, prepare the circuit and hemofilter. Base the choice of hemofilter and circuit primarily on the size of the patient and the volume of blood that will fill the circuit. Prime the circuit with heparinized, type-specific blood (one unit of heparin per ml of blood) or saline. As a general rule, the volume of the circuit should not exceed 10% of the patient's blood volume (see Table 69-1). If the volume of the circuit exceeds 5% of blood volume, use heparinized blood to prime the circuit.

Infuse heparin prefilter at a rate of 10 to 20 units kg/hr. Determine the ACT at the bedside hourly to ensure adequate heparinization, with the objective of maintaining the ACT in the range of approximately 160 to 240 seconds. Anticoagulation of the circuit also depends on good filter flow and in spite of high heparin doses will not be adequate in the presence of poor flow. If indicated, infuse protamine postfilter to reduce the degree of anticoagulation in the patient.

Begin hemofiltration after securing vascular access and priming the circuit and hemofilter. Using aseptic technique, connect the outflow limb of the extracorporeal circuit to the arterial or venous outflow catheter in the patient. Carefully avoid the introduction of air within the tubing. Keep the tubing clamped during this period to prevent premature flow through the system. Connect the venous return limb to the venous return catheter in the patient. Unclamp the circuit and simultaneously initiate any pump assistance to the prefilter limb. Blood will begin to flow through the circuit, and ultrafiltration will commence almost immediately. Gradually increase the pump that is augmenting flow through the catheter to the maximum flow that access will allow, typically between 500 and 1000 ml/hr. Specific bubble-trap

circuits for pediatric patients have not yet been developed; engineer this circuit individually, if desired. Avoid introducing air during circuit attachment to minimize the risk of air embolism.

Begin pump regulation of the ultrafiltration rate. Initially set the desired rate of plasma-water removal, knowing that this rate may require modification if the actual amount of ultrafiltrate is less than the desired amount. If flow is inadequate or the hemofilter begins to clot, the efficiency of ultrafiltration decreases. This decreased efficiency warrants increasing the ultrafiltration pump flow to attain the desired amount of output. When ultrafiltration decreases markedly, it is time to replace the hemofilter. A dark brown or black discoloration often appears at the dependent portion of the hemofilter as it is clotting off and signals the need for filter replacement. The hemofilter typically lasts between 12 and 48 hours before requiring replacement. The need to change filters more often than every 12 hours results in blood loss and significant inefficiency of filtration.

If indicated, infuse countercurrent dialysate into the outer chamber of the hemofilter countercurrent to the flow of blood. Use flow rates of 200 to 1000 ml/hr (depending on the hemofilter) to maximize the removal of substances such as potassium, urea nitrogen, and ammonia. Increase the ultrafiltrate pump flow by this amount to ensure removal of the dialysate from the outer chamber and to prevent it from passing into the fibers and circulating to the patient.

The administration of prefilter fluid at relatively high flow rates augments filter flow and increases longevity of the hemofilter. Infuse a physiologic fluid such as normal saline prefilter at a rate recoverable in the ultrafiltrate. In a given patient the total ultrafiltrate removed per hour may be the sum of the desired net ultrafiltrate (plasma water), the dialysate, and the prefilter fluid. The flow capabilities of the pump on the ultrafiltrate line may therefore limit rates for dialysate and prefilter fluid administration, as well as the rate of ultrafiltration.

Meet the patient's fluid requirements with any appropriate replacement fluid, including balanced salt solutions, total parenteral nutrition, or enteral feedings. Specific replacement solutions used in the past offer no advantage over fluids tailored to the patient's individual laboratory results.

Reduce the ultrafiltration rate gradually when there is evidence of improving hemodynamic status or renal function. When it appears that the patient is no longer dependent on ultrafiltration, remove the circuit, or reduce the net ultrafiltration rate to zero while maintaining flow through the circuit. In many cases, CEH provides a bridge to more permanent or long-term methods of dialysis. Discontinue CEH as the patient transitions to either peritoneal dialysis or hemodialysis.

Remarks

CEH may appear to appear to cause a "steal" phenomenon from the kidneys. For example, in one case a patient was treated with extracorporeal membrane oxygenation with ultrafiltration for 2 weeks followed by CEH alone for approximately 1 week. The patient remained oliguric throughout this time. When problems with the arterial access site necessitated the abrupt cessation of arteriovenous hemofiltration, the patient's intrinsic renal function returned within hours and required no further renal replacement therapy. CEH may have an effect on renal blood flow, "stealing" from the kidneys.

Calculate sieving coefficients easily by measuring the ultrafiltrate concentration of the solute or drug in question and dividing that into the serum concentration. Address the homeostasis of electrolytes and drug levels specifically in this manner.

Arteriovenous hemofiltration may be inferior to pump-assisted venovenous hemofiltration. The venovenous route allows avoidance of arterial access, use of a single venous site with a double-lumen catheter, and more predictable catheter flow. Some literature suggests that venovenous hemofiltration is the superior method of applying the modality.[9,44]

REFERENCES

1. Alarabi AA, et al: Artificial renal and liver support in a severe hepatorenal syndrome of childhood, *Acta Pediatr* 81(1):75-78, 1992.
2. Alexander SR: Continuous arteriovenous hemofiltration. In Levin DL, Morris FC, editors: *Essentials of pediatric intensive care,* St Louis, 1990, Quality Medical.
3. Bagshaw ON, Anaes FR, Hutchinson A: Continuous arteriovenous hemofiltration and respiratory function in multiple organ system failure, *Intensive Care Med* 18(6):334-338, 1992.
4. Banner W, Vernon D: Continuous arteriovenous hemofiltration in experimental iron intoxication, *Crit Care Med* 17(11):1187-1190, 1989.
5. Bellomo R, McGrath B, Boyce N: In vivo catecholamine extraction during continuous hemodiafiltration in inotrope-dependent patients, *ASAIO Trans* 37(3):324-325, 1991.
6. Bellomo R, Tipping P, Boyce N: Tumor necrosis factor clearances during venovenous hemodiafiltration in the critically ill, *ASAIO Trans* 37(3):322-323, 1991.
7. Bellomo R, Tipping P, Boyce N: Continuous venovenous hemofiltration with dialysis removes cytokines from the circulation of septic patients, *Crit Care Med* 21(4):522-526, 1993.
8. Bellomo R, et al: Treatment of life-threatening lithium toxicity with continuous arteriovenous hemofiltration, *Crit Care Med* 19(6):836-837, 1991.
9. Bellomo R, et al: A prospective comparative study of continuous arteriovenous hemodiafiltration and continuous venovenous hemodiafiltration in critically ill patients, *Am J Kidney Dis* 21(4):400-404, 1993.
10. Berns JS, Cohen RM, Rudnick MR: Myoglobinuric acute renal failure frequently develops in patients with traumatic rhabdomyolysis, *Am J Nephrol* 950:1-2, 1990.
11. Better OS, Stein JH: Early management of shock and prophylaxis of acute renal failure in traumatic rhabdomyolysis, *N Engl J Med* 322(12):825-829, 1990.
12. Bickley SK: Drug dosing during continuous arteriovenous hemofiltration, *Clin Pharm* 7:198-206, 1988.
13. Bishof NA, et al: Continuous hemodiafiltration in children, *Pediatrics* 85(5):819-823, 1990.
14. Davenport A, Will EJ, Davison AM: Early changes in intracranial pressure during haemofiltration treatment in patients with grade 4 hepatic encephalopathy and acute oliguric renal failure, *Nephrol Dial Transplant* 5:192-198, 1990.
15. Davenport A, Will EJ, Davidson AM: Improved cardiovascular stability during continuous modes of renal replacement therapy in critically ill patients with acute hepatic and renal failure, *Crit Care Med* 21(3):328-338, 1993.
16. DiCarlo JV, et al: Continuous arteriovenous hemofiltration/dialysis improves pulmonary gas exchange in children with multiple organ system failure, *Crit Care Med* 18(8):822-826, 1990.
17. Ellis EN, et al: Pump-assisted hemofiltration in infants with acute renal failure, *Pediatr Nephrol* 7:434-437, 1993.
18. Golper TA: Drug removal during continuous renal replacement therapies, *Dial Trans* 22(4):185-188, 1993.
19. Gomez A, et al: Hemofiltration reverses left ventricular dysfunction during sepsis in dogs, *Anesthesiology* 773(4):671-685, 1990.
20. Heney D, et al: Continuous arteriovenous haemofiltration in the treatment of tumor lysis syndrome, *Pediatr Nephrol* 4(3):245-247, 1990.
21. Jenkins RD, et al: Continuous renal replacement in infants and toddlers. In Sieberth HG, Mann H, Stummvoll HK, editors: Continuous hemofiltration, *Contrib Nephrol* 93:245-249, 1991.
22. Jenkins R, et al: Effects of access catheter dimensions on bloodflow in continuous arteriovenous hemofiltration. In Sieberth HG, Mann H, Stummvoll HK, editors: Continuous hemofiltration, *Contrib Nephrol* 93:171-174, 1991.
23. Jenkins R, et al: Accuracy of intravenous infusion pumps in continuous renal replacement therapies, *ASAIO Trans* 38(4):808-810, 1992.
24. Kaplan AA, Petrillo R: Regional heparinization for continuous arteriovenous hemofiltration (CAVH), *ASAIO Trans* 10(3):312-315, 1987.
25. Kaplan AA, Longnecker RE, Folkert VW: Continuous arteriovenous hemofiltration: a report of six-months' experience 100:358-367, 1984.
26. Kuttnig M, et al: Nitrogen and amino acid balance during total parenteral nutrition and continuous arteriovenous hemofiltration in critically ill anuric children, *Child Nephrol Urol* 11(2):74-78, 1991.
27. Leone MR, et al: Early experience with continuous arteriovenous hemofiltration in critically ill pediatric patients, *Crit Care Med* 14:1058-1063, 1986.
28. Lieberman KV: Continuous arteriovenous hemofiltration in children, *Pediatr Nephrol* 1:330-338, 1987.
29. Lieberman KV, Nardi L, Bosch JP: Treatment of acute renal failure in an infant using continuous arteriovenous hemofiltration, *J Pediatr* 106:646-649, 1985.
30. Lopez-Herce J, et al: Continuous arteriovenous hemofiltration in children, *Intensive Care Med* 15:224-227, 1989.
31. Maksym CJ: Parenteral nutrition considerations during continuous artiovenous hemofiltration and continuous arteriovenous hemofiltration-dialysis, *The Michigan Drug Letter* 6(12), 1-5, 1987.
32. Mault JR, et al: Continuous arteriovenous filtration: an effective treatment for surgical acute renal failure, *Surgery* 101(4):478-484, 1987.
33. Mault JR, et al: Continuous hemofiltration: a reference guide for SCUF, CAVH, and CAVHD, 1989, University of Michigan.
34. Mehta RL, et al: Regional citrate anticoagulation for continuous arteriovenous hemodialysis in critically ill patients, *Kidney Int* 38(5):976-981, 1990.
35. Moss GD, et al: Correction of hypernatraemia with continuous arteriovenous haemofiltration, *Arch Dis Child* 65(6):628-630, 1990.
36. Olbricht CH, et al: The influence of vascular access on the efficiency of CAVH. In Sieberth HG, Mann H, editors: Continuous hemofiltration, *Contrib Nephrol* 93:14-24, 1984.
37. Paret G, et al: Continuous arteriovenous hemofiltration after cardiac operations in infants and children, *J Thorac Cardiovasc Surg* 104(5):1225-1230, 1992.
38. Pearson D, et al: Pump-assisted hemofiltration (PAHF) in infants (abstract). Paper presented at the Southern Society for Pediatric Research, New Orleans, January 21-23, 1993.
39. Ronco C, et al: Treatment of acute renal failure in newborns by continuous arteriovenous hemofiltration, *Kidney Int* 29:908-915, 1986.
40. Schroder CH, Severijnen RS, Potting CM: Continuous arteriovenous hemofiltration (CAVH) in a premature newborn as treatment of overhydration and hyperkalemia due to sepsis, *European J Pediatr Surg* 2(6):368-369, 1992.
41. Sperl W, et al: Continuous arteriovenous haemofiltration in hyperammonaemia of newborn babies (letter), *Lancet* 336(8724):1192-1193, 1990.
42. Sperl W, et al: Continuous arteriovenous haemofiltration in a neonate with hyperammonaemic coma due to citrullinaemia, *J Inherit Metab Dis* 15(1):158-159, 1992.
43. Stein B, et al: Influence of continuous hemofiltration on hemodynamics and pulmonary function in porcine endotoxic shock, *Contrib Nephrol* 93:105-109, 1991.
44. Storck M, et al: Comparison of pump-driven and spontaneous continuous haemofiltration in postoperative acute renal failure, *Lancet* 337:452-455, 1991.
45. Thompson GN, et al: Continuous venovenous hemofiltration in the management of acute decompensation in inborn errors of metabolism, *J Pediatr* 118:879-884, 1991.

46. van Bommel EFH, Grootendorst AF, van Leengoed LAMG: Influence of high-volume hemofiltration on hemodynamics in porcine endotoxic shock (abstract). Tenth Annual Meeting of the International Society of Blood Purification, Oct 7-9, 1992, Louisville.

47. Werner HA, Herbertson MJ, Seear MD: Operating characteristics of pediatric continuous arteriovenous hemofiltration in an animal model, *Pediatr Nephrol* 7(2):189-193, 1993.

48. Winterberg B, et al: Hemofiltration in myoglobinuric acute renal failure, *Int J Artif Organs* 13(2):113-116, 1990.

49. Yorgin PD, Krensky AM, Tune BM: Continuous venovenous hemofiltration, *Pediatr Nephrol* 4:640-642, 1990.

50. Zobel G, Ring E, Zobel V: Continuous arteriovenous renal replacement systems for critically ill children, *Pediatr Nephrol* 3:140-143, 1989.

51. Zobel G, et al: Vascular access for continuous arteriovenous hemofiltration in infants and young children, *Artif Organs* 12(1):16-19, 1988.

52. Zobel G, et al: Continuous arteriovenous hemofiltration versus venovenous hemofiltration in critically ill pediatric patients, *Contrib Nephrol* 93:257-260, 1991.

Part XIV

GENITOURINARY/ GYNECOLOGIC TECHNIQUES

70 Transurethral Bladder Catheterization

Louis M. Bell

Transurethral bladder catheterization, whether for placement of an indwelling Foley catheter or as an intermittent procedure for obtaining a urine specimen, is an ancient technique that is performed in most cases without difficulty. Bladder catheterization can often establish a diagnosis of urinary tract infection in febrile infants and young children. Bladder catheterization is less traumatic and invasive than suprapubic bladder aspiration (see Chapter 71) and also is less likely to result in contamination of the urine specimen than a specimen collected via a urine bag.

Although the technique of transurethral bladder catheterization is most difficult in girls, with experience, knowledge of anatomy, and the proper equipment, physicians and nurses can perform this procedure with a minimal amount of discomfort.

Indications

Indications for bladder catheterization fall into two categories. Use an indwelling (Foley) catheter in children with acute urinary retention and an inability to void or for patients in whom measurement of urine output is vital. Critically ill or injured children, such as those with multiple traumatic injury or those with a shock syndrome, require careful measurement of urine output during the resuscitation phase of their illness. For indwelling use, select balloon-tipped catheters that are size 8 to 14 French. Use a straight indwelling catheter (feeding tube) in most newborn infants. Occasionally, consider using an 8 French Foley catheter in a full-term female infant. Consider using a balloon-tipped Foley catheter as the child grows beyond 6 months of age.

Intermittent bladder catheterization is indicated for the collection of a urine specimen for diagnostic purposes to rule out a urinary tract infection. Intermittent bladder decompression in patients with neurogenic bladders or for urologic study of urinary tract anatomy is also an indication for this procedure.

Contraindications

Before urethral catheterization, carefully evaluate any child with a pelvic injury or a blunt abdominal injury (Box 70-1). Do not attempt bladder catheterization in children who have blood at the urethral meatus, prostatic displacement on rectal examination (boys), an identifiable perineal hematoma, or an obvious pelvic fracture.

Urethral Injuries. Injuries to the male urethra occur in association with pelvic fractures, straddle injuries, and instrumentation. Blood at the urethral meatus is most commonly associated with injuries to the anterior urethral segments. Blind placement of a urethral catheter may convert a partial urethral tear into a complete transsection of the urethra. Diagnose urethral injuries by performing a retrograde urethrogram. Whereas anterior urethral injuries are often benign and may exist as isolated injuries, posterior urethral injuries

usually occur with severe multiple trauma and are usually associated with pelvic fractures in particular. Mortality rates in patients who have sustained a pelvic fracture may be as high as 30%.[1]

Trauma to the female urethra is rare except following surgical procedures or instrumentation. Injuries at the bladder or vesicle urethral junction are more common in females, particularly after blunt abdominal trauma in motor vehicle accidents. Urethral or bladder injuries often occur concurrently with vaginal injury.[1]

Bladder Injuries. Bladder injuries associated with pelvic fractures involve penetration of the bladder by a bony fragment in 80% of the cases. During childhood the bladder is found in a high abdominal location, which makes the organ more susceptible to injury than in adults, in which the bladder is found lower in the pelvis. In more than 90% of patients with rupture of the bladder, gross hematuria is the single most important symptom.[1] In patients with hematuria and a suspected pelvic or lower abdominal injury, obtain a plain radiograph to exclude pelvic fracture. If there is no pelvic fracture and no other sign of a bladder or urethral tear, such as blood at the meatus or abnormal position of the prostate on rectal examination, proceed with urethral catheterization and perform a retrograde cystogram. With a CT scan or intravenous pyelogram, evaluate the urinary tract of those who are stable following trauma and have microscopic hematuria exceeding 20 red blood cells per high-power field (RBC/HPF) in a spun specimen.[1]

Complications

Complications of bladder or urethral catheterization are rare in the pediatric population, primarily because these patients are generally healthy. The main complication of bladder catheterization occurs in those patients with indwelling catheters. Remarkably, 40% of all hospital-acquired infections in adults occur as urinary tract infections associated with indwelling bladder catheters or following other types of urologic instrumentation.[7] Risk factors for urinary tract infection in adults are female gender, older age, and degree of underlying illness. As is the case with adult patients, children in an intensive care unit setting are at an increased risk for nosocomial urinary tract infections. At The Children's Hospital of Philadelphia, 9% of nosocomial infections in the intensive care units are urinary tract infections (unpublished information, L. Bell) (Box 70-2).

The risk of infection increases with longer duration of catheter placement. In adults, a single catheterization of the urethra is associated with approximately a 1% to 8% risk of subsequent bacteruria.[7] Fecal bacteria colonize the distal centimeter of the urethra in both catheterized and noncatheterized individuals. During the process of urethral catheterization, some organisms from the distal urethra contaminate the bladder. However, in the vast majority of cases, these bacteria wash away without causing infection or symptoms in the patient. In general, remove indwelling catheters as soon as possible during the course of the hospital stay.

Although hematuria can occur during routine catheterization, it is rare (<1%).[4] In critically ill or injured infants, use feeding tubes transurethrally as indwelling catheters. In neonates, placement of the smaller caliber feeding tube may be less traumatic and as effective as a balloon-tipped catheter. Although rarely reported, there are at least seven case reports of catheter knotting within the bladder.[2] None of these patients had abnormal genitourinary anatomy. The use of a feeding catheter and the insertion of an excessive length of catheter into the bladder are major reasons for this type of complication. Knowledge of urethral length for age (Table 70-1) reduces the risk of catheter knotting in the bladder.

Equipment

Arrange the equipment for bladder catheterization before the procedure order. Order a "bladder catheterization tray," which includes the following equipment (except for the type and size of catheter needed): examination gloves, a sterile drape, povidone-iodine solution, absorbent cotton balls, for-

---

Table 70-1 Approximate Urethral Length in Children*

	Boy (cm)	Girl (cm)
Newborn	6 ± 2	1.5–2
2 years	8 ± 2	1.5–3
5 years	10 ± 2	1.5–3 ± 2
10 years	12 ± 2	1.5–3 ± 2
12 years	16–20 ± 2	4–6 ± 2

*To prevent inserting an excessive length of catheter into the bladder, which can (rarely) result in knotting, use these guidelines for urethral length in situations of intermittent catheterization of the bladder or if using feeding tubes as indwelling catheters for infants.

Table 70-2 Recommended Catheter Size for Children*

	Boy (French)	Girl (French)	Type
Newborn	3	3 or 5	Straight
1-2 years	5	5 or 8	Straight/balloon
3-5 years	8	8	Balloon-tipped
6-10 years	8 or 10	8 or 10	Balloon
12 years	10 or 12	12	Balloon
13 years and older	12	12 or 14	Balloon

*An indwelling double-lumen catheter with an inflatable balloon comes in sizes 8 to 14 French. For infants, especially newborn or premature infants, use a straight indwelling catheter and a feeding tube in sizes of 3, 5, 8, or 10 French.

---

ceps, lubricating jelly, a 10-ml prefilled inflation syringe, a sterile specimen container, and labels (Fig. 70-1). Choose the proper catheter size and type according to the age and gender of the patient. The older the child, the larger the catheter size. Females, in general, can accommodate larger catheters than males because the female urethra is shorter and straighter. The larger the catheter diameter, the more quickly the urine drains from the bladder. Table 70-2 provides a guideline for choosing catheter size. After urethral catheterization in uncircumcised boys, remember to pull the foreskin forward (or distally) to prevent paraphimosis.

Techniques

Bladder catheterization is easier with knowledge of both male and female anatomy. (Figs. 70-2 and 70-3). Arrange the catheter tray equipment. Open a sterile drape and place it near the genital area. Using sterile technique, open the catheter, drop it onto the sterile drape, and place lubricant onto the sterile drape. Prepare povidone-iodine wipes and a sterile basin for use on the drape. Begin the procedure by having an assistant or another health-care worker provide gentle but adequate restraint (see Fig. 70-1). If the patient is old enough, let him or her participate in this process. Take time to gain his or her confidence and allow him or her to understand the procedure.[3] At this point, don sterile gloves. In the female patient, separate the labia majora with the thumb and index finger. Swab the urethral meatus (see Fig. 70-3, *A*) from front to back three times with separate povidone-iodine swabs.

In the male patient, retract the foreskin with the thumb and index finger of the left hand if necessary to reveal the meatus

---

BOX 70-2 **COMPLICATIONS OF URETHRAL CATHETERIZATION**

Urethral or bladder trauma
Vaginal catheterization
Urinary tract infection
Paraphimosis
Hematuria
Intravesicle knot (rare)

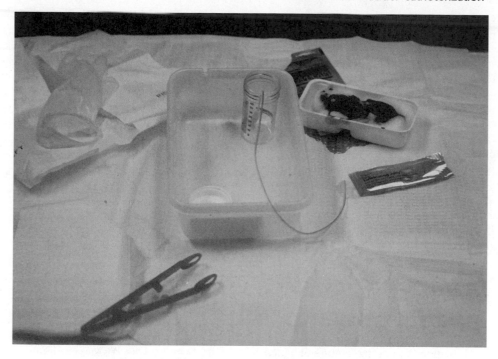

FIG. 70-1   Equipment for bladder catheterization.

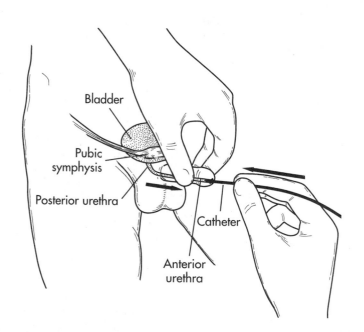

FIG. 70-2   Transurethral bladder catheterization; position and placement in the male.

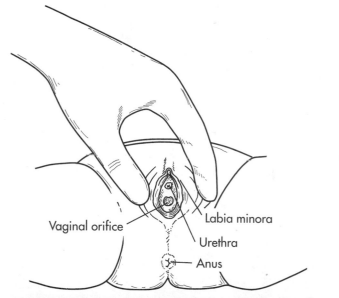

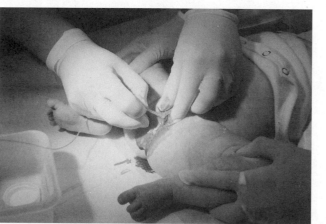

and glans; gently extend the penile or anterior urethra (see Fig. 70-2). Clean this area three times with povidone-iodine. While maintaining this position, lubricate the catheter tip with a water-soluble lubricant with the right hand. Place the distal end of the catheter into a sterile basin or sterile specimen container in which to collect the urine. Using the guidelines regarding urethral length, insert the catheter into the meatus of the urethra (see Table 70-1; Fig 70-3, *B*). Do not force the catheter if resistance is met. In older children, discard the first milliliter of urine to avoid contaminating the urine specimen with bacteria that colonizes in the distal urethra.[8]

FIG. 70-3   **A** and **B** Transurethral bladder catheterization; position in the female.

For straight intermittent bladder catheterization, remove the catheter after urine flow ceases. If an indwelling Foley catheter has been inserted into the urethra, Luer-Lok the prefilled syringe into the connection and inflate the balloon with the sterile water indicated on the bulb. Once the balloon has been inflated, pull on the catheter until resistance is met. To connect the indwelling catheter to a closed system, wipe the distal end of the catheter with povidone-iodine and insert it into the drainage tubing attached to the urine drainage bag. Keep the urine drainage bag in a position lower than that of the bladder. Tape the indwelling catheter or tubing to the inner thigh, leaving enough slack to allow for full movement of the leg without dislodging the catheter. For non–balloon-tipped (feeding-tube) catheters, use the same procedure except for taping. In the female neonate, tape the tube to the proximal inner thigh and adjacent to the labia majora. In the male neonate, tapc the tube with a ½-inch piece of tape that is placed along the shaft of the penis and extends to wrap around the tube. Take care not to tape the circumference of the glans penis or shaft.

Remarks

Suspect a urinary tract infection if the urine culture obtained by bladder catheterization reveals >1000 colony-forming units/ml of a single organism.[6] However, in children with urinary tract symptoms or fever, isolation of a single organism that has <1000 colony-forming units should still raise suspicion of an infection; repeat bladder catheterization in 24 to 48 hours. Start presumptive therapy in symptomatic children after the culture. In febrile neonates, consider the urinalysis abnormal if there are more than 10 white blood cells per high-power field and few bacteria or if bright-field microscopy on a spun specimen detects none. Urine specimens collected from an adhesive bag placed around the urethra are not used for bacteriologic cultures. However, urine cultures for viral (e.g., cytomegalovirus) or other chemical analyses may be obtained with this noninvasive technique.

REFERENCES

1. Garcia CT, Peters CA: Genitourinary trauma. In Fleisher GR, Ludwig S, Henretig FM, et al, editors: *Textbook of pediatric emergency medicine,* ed 3, Baltimore, 1993, Williams & Wilkins.
2. Kanengiser S, Juster F, Kogan S, et al: Knotting of a bladder catheter, *Pediatr Emerg Care* 5:37-39, 1989.
3. Lohr JA, Howards SS, Rein MF: Urogenital procedures. In Lohr JA, editor: *Pediatric outpatient procedures,* Philadelphia, 1991, JB Lippincott.
4. Pollack CV, Pollack ES, Andrew ME: Suprapubic bladder aspiration versus urethral catheterization in ill infants: success, efficiency and complication rates, *Ann Emerg Med* 23:225-230, 1994.
5. Ruddy RM: Section VIII, Procedures. In Fleisher GR, Ludwig S, Henretig FM, et al, editors: *Textbook of pediatric emergency medicine,* ed 3, Baltimore, 1993, Williams & Wilkins.
6. Shaw KN, Hexter D, McGowan KL, et al: Clinical evaluation of a rapid screening test for urinary tract infections in children, *J Pediatr* 118:733-736, 1991.
7. Stamm WE: Nosocomial urinary tract infections. In Bennett JV, Brachman PS, editors: *Hospital infections,* ed 3, Boston, 1992, Little, Brown.
8. Zbaraschuk I, Berger RE: Emergency urologic procedures. In Roberts JR, Hedges JR, editors: *Clinical procedures in emergency medicine,* Philadelphia, 1995, WB Saunders.

71 Suprapubic Bladder Aspiration

Louis M. Bell

Suprapubic bladder aspiration is used primarily for diagnosing urinary tract infections or for evaluating sepsis in the neonate or child up to 2 years of age. Suprapubic bladder aspiration is quick, simple to perform and, performed properly, has a very low complication rate. Its main advantage is that it bypasses the distal urethra, in which fecal bacteria normally colonize, thereby minimizing the risk of contamination. Over the years, numerous studies have shown that suprapubic aspiration is superior to other methods of collecting urine specimens for the diagnosis of urinary tract infection and has a urine contamination rate of approximately 4%. The rates of obtaining urine successfully using this technique range from 25% to 100%. Recently, efforts to improve aspiration success rates have focused on using portable ultrasound to determine if the bladder is full.[1]

Indications

The primary indication for suprapubic bladder aspiration is for diagnosising urinary tract infection in children less than 2 years of age. The procedure is rarely performed in older toilet-trained and cooperative children because it is usually possible to obtain an uncontaminated urine specimen by other means.

Contraindications

Contraindications to suprapubic bladder aspiration include evidence of an existing coagulopathy or thrombocytopenia (Box 71-1). Relative contraindications to this procedure include significant abdominal distention of unknown etiology, recent abdominal surgery, and suspicion of intestinal obstruction.[2]

Complications

Complications associated with suprapubic bladder aspiration include microscopic hematuria, which is usually less than 10 red blood cells per high-power field (Box 71-2). Fecal

---

> BOX 71-2 **COMPLICATIONS OF SUPRAPUBIC BLADDER CATHETERIZATION**
>
> Hematuria (microscopic hematuria is very common)
> Intestinal perforation (usually benign)
> Infection of the abdominal wall
> "Dry tap" (failure to obtain urine)

material aspirated into the syringe indicates a rare complication of intestinal perforation. Although anxiety provoking, this complication is usually benign; simply observe the patient for any signs or symptoms of peritonitis. An additional complication of this procedure may be infection of the abdominal wall and cellulitis surrounding the puncture site. There are no reports of significant hemorrhage associated with this procedure.

Equipment

Prepare equipment, including gloves, a 3- to 5-ml syringe to obtain the urine specimen, a 1- to 1½-inch 25-gauge needle for preterm infants and a 1½- to 2½-inch 22-gauge needle for other children, povidone-iodine pads to sterilize the skin, one sterile gauze pad, one adhesive strip, a sterile specimen container, and a label.

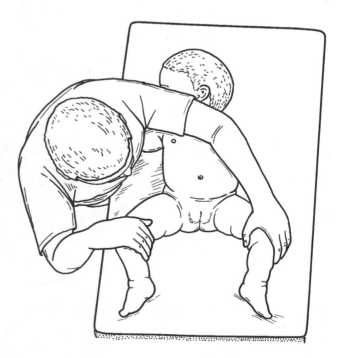

FIG. 71-1 Position used to restrain infant or child for suprapubic bladder aspiration.

> BOX 71-1 **INDICATIONS AND CONTRAINDICATIONS FOR SUPRAPUBIC BLADDER ASPIRATION**
>
> **Indications**
>
> Obtaining urine for diagnostic tests (usually a bacterial culture)
>
> **Contraindications**
>
> Coagulopathy
> Thrombocytopenia
> Abdominal distention
> Recent abdominal surgery
> Recent voiding (within the last ½ to 1 hour)

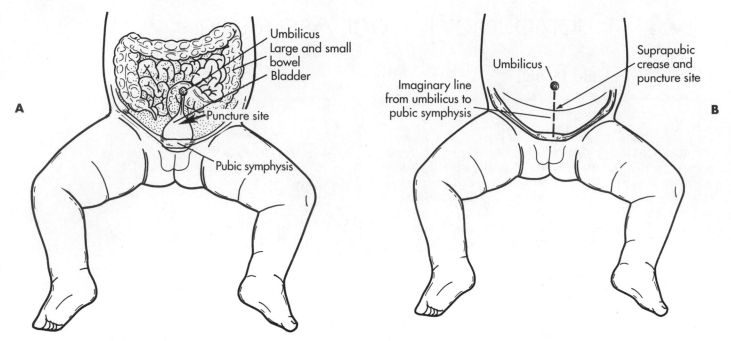

FIG. 71-2 A, Puncture site and external anatomy (frontal view) for suprapubic bladder aspiration. **B,** Puncture site and internal anatomy for suprapubic bladder aspiration.

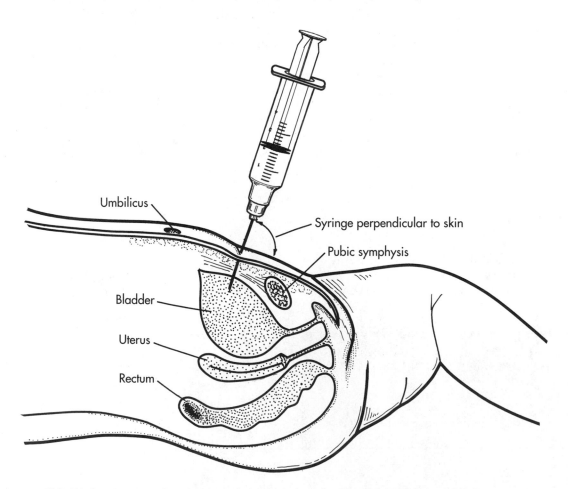

FIG. 71-3 Puncture site and anatomy (sagittal view) for suprapubic bladder aspiration.

Techniques

In general, ask parents to leave the room during this procedure. Position the patient in a frog-leg position and request that an assistant restrain him or her. Position the assistant to the side to hold the child's legs. Have the assistant's arm lightly restrain the upper body (Fig. 71-1). Draw an imaginary line from the umbilicus to the superior portion of the pubic symphysis. Perpendicular to this imaginary line, halfway or three fourths of the distance to the umbilicus, is a suprapubic crease (Fig. 71-2, A). Make the puncture in this area (Fig. 71-2, B). Remember that the bladder in an infant and young child is an abdominal and not a pelvic organ; this knowledge will aid in obtaining a successful urine specimen. In the male child, apply gentle compression to the penile shaft before cleansing the skin with the povidone-iodine swabs. This step will prevent the infant from voiding during the procedure. After identifying the suprapubic crease (see Fig. 71-1), insert the needle perpendicular to the skin and maintain gentle back pressure on the syringe until urine flows freely (Fig. 71-3). Stop the procedure if unsuccessful after a maximum of three passes.[3]

Remarks

Suprapubic bladder aspiration sometimes fails to yield urine. As many as 70% of all attempts fail, with "dry tap" being the only result. Despite this failure rate, this technique is the standard for comparison to other techniques.

Success rates have recently improved by using portable ultrasound to assist with urine collection. Using portable ultrasound in 1991, Gochman, Karasic, and Heller,[2] were successful in obtaining urine in 79% of their attempts at suprapubic aspiration (n = 19) vs. success in only 52% (n = 31) in the nonultrasound group. They attempted suprapubic aspiration only in those children who had a full bladder on ultrasound. All children were less than 2 years of age, and 82% were less than 2 months of age. In another investigation in neonates, 100% of the infants whose ultrasound revealed a full bladder had successful suprapubic aspiration vs. only 36% of neonates who had no ultrasound.

The major disadvantage of suprapubic bladder aspiration is a practical issue of time efficiency, especially in a busy urban emergency department with a high patient volume. The nursing staff can perform transurethral bladder catheterization with a high success rate, whereas physicians traditionally perform suprapubic aspirations. In most cases it is more time efficient for physicians to order the transurethral catheterization than to take the time to perform the suprapubic aspiration and have a significant chance of failure (or to wait an hour after urination before attempting suprapubic aspiration). In a recent prospective, randomized study, Pollack, Pollack, and Andrew[4] compared suprapubic bladder aspiration to urethral catheterization and noted no immediate complications. No child had evidence of postprocedure hematuria. However, the increased efficiency in specimen collection must be balanced against an increase in urine contamination rates. In one study of neonates undergoing a sepsis work-up at The Children's Hospital of Philadelphia, the urine contamination rate was 8.4% for transurethral catheterization vs. reported rates of 4% for suprapubic aspiration.[5] Urine specimens collected from an adhesive bag placed around the urethra are not used for bacteriologic cultures. However, urine cultures for viral (e.g., cytomegalovirus) or other chemical analyses may be obtained using this noninvasive technique.

REFERENCES

1. Baker MD, Bell LM, Avner JR: Outpatient management without antibiotics of fever in selected infants, *N Engl J Med* 329:1437-1441, 1993.
2. Gochman RF, Karasic RB, Heller MB: Use of portable ultrasound to assist urine collection by suprappubic aspiration, *Ann Emerg Med* 20:631-635, 1991.
3. Lohr JA, Howards SS, Rein MF: Urogenital procedures. In Lohr JA, editor: *Pediatric outpatient procedures*, Philadelphia, 1991, JB Lippincott.
4. Pollack CV, Pollack ES, Andrew MF: Suprapubic bladder aspiration versus urethral catheterization in ill infants: success, efficiency and complication rates, *Ann Emerg Med* 23:225-230, 1994.
5. Ruddy RM: Section VII, Procedures. In Fleisher GR, Ludwig S, et al, editors: *Textbook of pediatric emergency medicine*, ed 3, Baltimore, 1993, Williams & Wilkins.

72 Doppler Ultrasound Evaluation of the Scrotum

Joel A. Fein

The child who comes to the Emergency Department complaining of scrotal pain or swelling requires immediate attention. The differential diagnosis includes testicular torsion (torsion of the spermatic cord), torsion of the appendix testis, epididymitis, traumatic injuries such as rupture or hematoma, and incarcerated hernia. The ramifications of misdiagnosis can be severe. In the case of testicular torsion, early manual detorsion and subsequent operative fixation dramatically increase the chances of testicular salvage. Although a detailed history and physical examination are the most useful tools in the assessment of the acute scrotum, Doppler ultrasound of the testicle is an adjunct in the diagnoses of testicular torsion and epididymitis. In patients with testicular torsion, Doppler ultrasound has the most accuracy within the first 8 hours after onset of pain. However, the technique has limited sensitivity and specificity even in the most skilled hands. The physician evaluating the child with scrotal pain must be familiar not only with the technique of Doppler ultrasound but also with the interpretation of the results.

The normal scrotum contains two descended testes, each of which has a soft, curved epididymis positioned posterolateral to the testicle. Each spermatic cord contains the vessels and nerves that supply the testis, muscle fibers, and the vas deferens, which carries sperm from the testis and epididymis to the ejaculatory duct. The tunica vaginalis testis is a membrane that surrounds the testis on three sides and allows for fixation of the testis posteriorly in the scrotum.

Testicular torsion results when the spermatic cord twists on its own axis and is associated with a congenital malformation known as the "Bellclapper" deformity. In patients with this deformity, the tunica vaginalis testis completely envelops the testicle and prevents proper posterior fixation within the scrotum. Torsion occurs mainly in adolescents. Two-thirds of all patients with testicular torsion are between the ages of 12 and 18 years of age. The diagnosis is rare in patients under 6 years of age or older than 35 years of age. The patient usually complains of sudden, severe, unilateral scrotal pain. However, abdominal pain may be the only presenting complaint, especially in younger children. Nausea and vomiting are common. Physical examination may reveal a tender, high-riding, transversely located testicle within a edematous scrotal sac. The evaluation of the cremasteric reflex is a crucial part of the physical examination. A brisk retraction of the dartos muscle ipsilateral to the inner thigh stroke is extremely unlikely in testicular torsion.

Epididymitis is an inflammatory process and is often secondary to infection by sexually transmitted organisms. Like testicular torsion, this entity is most commonly diagnosed in adolescent boys. However, unlike torsion, the scrotal pain and swelling of epididymitis often occurs more insidiously than in testicular torsion. Physical examination may reveal a penile discharge and tenderness of the area just posterior to the testicle. The pain is occasionally bilateral and may extend to the testicle as an epididymo-orchitis. Only 30% of the urinalyses in patients with epididymitis reveal greater than five white blood cells per high-power field (WBC/HPF). In contrast to testicular torsion, nausea and vomiting are not commonly associated with epididymitis.

Indications/Contraindications

Use Doppler ultrasound to evaluate blood flow to the testicle. Apply the technique to patients who present with scrotal pain and/or swelling and in whom the history and physical examination indicate that blood flow to the testicle might be altered. The technique is especially helpful in evaluating the restoration of testicular blood flow after a manual detorsion procedure. There are no absolute contraindications to this technique, but do not delay urologic consultation or definitive management of testicular torsion because of Doppler ultrasound.

Complications

The potential complications of the Doppler ultrasound technique are related to the regional anesthetic and detorsion techniques that are described in the following paragraphs. After needle insertion, a localized hemorrhage can occur inside the spermatic cord, which could further compromise the arterial supply to the testis. Likewise, conversion of a partial torsion into a complete torsion may occur if the detorsion procedure is performed in the wrong direction.

Equipment

All commercially available Doppler flowmeters contain two components: a transducer probe for transmission and reception of ultrasound waves and an amplifier device such as a speaker, stethoscope, or headphone set (Fig. 72-1). An acoustic gel specifically designed to increase skin contact should be applied before the procedure.

Techniques

Cord Block. Before manipulating a painful scrotum, administer a regional anesthetic to the spermatic cord and testicle. To perform this procedure, isolate and stabilize the spermatic cord and inject 1% lidocaine directly into the cord. Inject between 2 and 10 ml of lidocaine depending on the patient's size. The patient should feel immediate relief of pain in the ipsilateral testicle. Some physicians argue that the use of a regional anesthetic obviates the physician's ability to assess the patient's relief of pain in response to manual

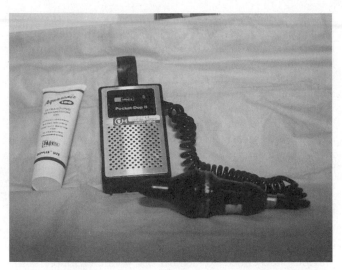

FIG. 72-1 Equipment for Doppler ultrasound.

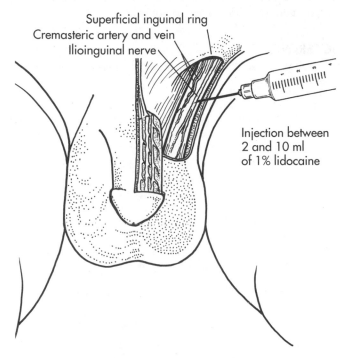

Superficial inguinal ring
Cremasteric artery and vein
Ilioinguinal nerve

Injection between
2 and 10 ml
of 1% lidocaine

FIG. 72-2 Technique for regional spermatic-cord block.

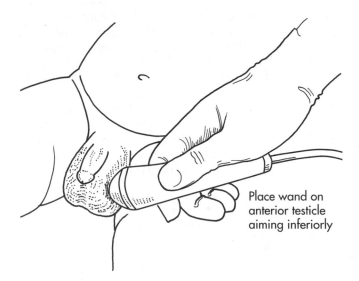

Place wand on
anterior testicle
aiming inferiorly

FIG. 72-3 Application of Doppler wand to testicle.

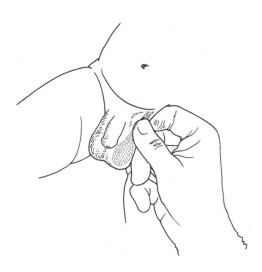

FIG. 72-4 The funicular compression test.

detorsion. A compromise would be to administer conscious
sedation instead of a regional cord block (see Chapter 12)
(Fig. 72-2).

To begin the Doppler study, hold the testicle with two
fingers on the medial and lateral sides and place the Doppler
wand in the center of the testicle, aiming inferiorly (Box
72-1). Adjust the probe to achieve maximum clarity of sound
(Fig. 72-3). If possible, examine the unaffected side first to
allow for evaluation of the technique and comparison with
the affected side.[2] If a sound is localized, perform the
funicular compression test to confirm that the sound is
originating from the testicular artery and not from the
surrounding tissues (Fig. 72-4). Compress the spermatic cord
while the probe is on the testicle and listen for a decrease in

flow associated with occlusion of the testicular artery. The sound should return when the cord is released.

Manual Detorsion. If the clinical picture suggests testicular torsion, use the Doppler flowmeter to assess the success of the manual detorsion procedure. To detorse the testicle, turn it about its axis to "untwist" the vessels in the spermatic cord. In torsion, the testicle usually twists medially, toward the center of the body. Therefore in the initial maneuver rotate the testicle 180 degrees laterally, toward the ipsilateral thigh.[4] Relief of pain and swelling and restoration of flow as assessed by Doppler ultrasound indicates a successful detorsion. If there is an increase in pain, perform the detorsion maneuver in the opposite direction.

Interpretation of Results. The absence of testicular blood flow as demonstrated by Doppler ultrasound supports the clinical diagnosis of testicular torsion. In addition, the initial absence of testicular blood flow and the subsequent restoration of that flow after manual detorsion can be demonstrated using this technique. If the detorsion is successful, the patient should also experience relief of symptoms.

Patients with epididymitis commonly have increased testicular blood flow, but such a finding on Doppler ultrasound examination does not eliminate the possibility of a late-presenting testicular torsion with reactive inflammation.[1]

Limitations of Procedure. A flow study that wrongly suggests the presence of testicular blood flow (false-positive) is the most dangerous misinterpretation of this technique. This misinterpretation can occur for one of four reasons. First, the probe can be directed superiorly instead of inferiorly, thus reflecting flow in the proximal spermatic cord but not in the distal arteries. Second, inflammation occurring 6 to 8 hours after the onset of torsion can transmit proximal flow

signals through the tissues. Third, if the technique is improper or if the testicle is small, flow from the examiner's finger can occasionally be detected, especially through a liquefying testicle. Finally, partial torsion can create a flow signal that is present but diminished. A diminished flow signal may also occur early in the course of torsion, when venous flow is obstructed but arterial flow is not.

Flow studies that suggest an absence of flow when there truly is flow present (false-negative) can occur if there is inadvertent compression of the cord during the procedure. A hydrocele that obliterates the transmission of flow from the artery to the transducer can also create false results.

Remarks

In a patient with suspected testicular torsion, do not delay urologic consultation to perform any of the procedures previously described. Remember that portable Doppler ultrasound studies of the scrotum have a low sensitivity and specificity and are used for ancillary data only. Although color Doppler ultrasound has greater sensitivity and specificity, this technique is not commonly performed by Emergency Department or critical care personnel.[3]

REFERENCES

1. Erden MI, Ozbeck SS, Sytac SK, et al: Color Doppler imaging in acute scrotal disorders, *Urol Int* 50:39-42, 1993.
2. Levy BJ: The diagnosis of torsion of the testicle using the Doppler ultrasonic stethoscope, *J Urol* 113:63-65, 1975.
3. Perri AJ, Slachta GA, Feldman AE, et al: The Doppler stethoscope and the diagnosis of the acute scrotum, *J Urol* 116:598-600, 1976.
4. Vordermark JS: The acute scrotum: management with the use of ancillary diagnostic techniques, *AUA Update Series* 3:2-8, 1984.

73 Reduction of an Incarcerated Inguinal Hernia

Louis M. Bell

The indirect inguinal hernia is the most common congenital anomaly found in children.[1] It is much more common in male children and has a strong familial incidence. The prevalence of inguinal hernia is less in term infants (3.5% to 5%) than in infants born prematurely (9% to 11%).[2] Incarcerated hernias are most commonly diagnosed in the first year of life and occur in females (39% vs. 22%) involving the ovary rather than the intestine.[1,2] Furthermore, major complications such as testicular or ovarian infarction, peritonitis, and prolonged hospitalization (resulting from infection) occur in 11% of those with incarcerated indirect inguinal hernias vs. only 0.6% of those without incarceration at the time of repair.[2] Therefore knowledge of the technique of reduction of the incarcerated inguinal hernia is very important. Ability to successfully reduce an incarcerated inguinal hernia eliminates the need for emergency surgery and the inherent surgical risks and complications.

Indications and Contraindications

In the absence of contraindications, always attempt to reduce an incarcerated inguinal hernia to prevent strangulation of the incarcerated bowel, ovaries, or other organs. Attempt reduction to allow for resolution of the edema, which is associated with the incarceration, and also to prevent the emergency surgery for an unreducable segment of bowel or ovary.

The contraindications to attempting reduction include obvious signs of peritonitis or free air in the abdomen.

Complications

The complications of this procedure are primarily discomfort for the child during the reduction. Lessen the discomfort with careful preparation and sedation, which is discussed under Technique. In addition, recognize when the reduction is only partially successful. Although the person performing the procedure may have reduced a significant part of the incarcerated bowel, unless reduction is complete, the child may be predisposed to bowl strangulation. Finally, although more rare, with aggressive attempts at reduction, testicular or ovarian rupture have been reported.

Equipment

No special equipment is needed for reduction of incarcerated inguinal hernia.

Technique

Knowledge of the anatomy of the inguinal area (Figs. 73-1 and 73-2) assists in proper positioning of the hands for reduction. Preparation before the actual reduction is most important. Put the child in a supine, mild Trendelenburg

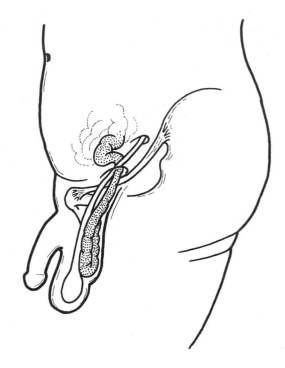

FIG.73-1   Indirect inguinal hernia: anatomical relationships.

position. Although it helps to have the child as calm as possible, this is often difficult because there is often pain associated with the incarceration and occasionally some vomiting. The child and parents may be anxious and upset. Attempt reduction initially without sedation by placing the left hand over the area of the external inguinal ring. Exert mild inferior pressure with the left hand. Use the right hand to gather the mass of bowel or other organs in a funneled approach and gently squeeze the mass, applying pressure to achieve reduction of the mass into the abdominal cavity (Fig. 73-2).

If reduction does not occur with this initial attempt, then sedate the patient with 0.1 mg/kg of morphine sulfate IV (and a benzodiazapine in some cases) and allow him or her to relax and fall asleep, if possible. Maintain the patient in the Trendelenburg position, dim the lights, and allow the patient to relax. After 30 minutes, check the patient to see if the mass has reduced spontaneously. If the mass is still present, repeat the procedure. If reduction is still unsuccessful after 10 minutes of effort with an adequately sedated patient, consult a surgeon.[3,4]

Remarks

If the child's incarcerated hernia is successfully reduced, consider prompt elective repair. In one study of 14 children with successfully reduced incarcerated indirect inguinal her-

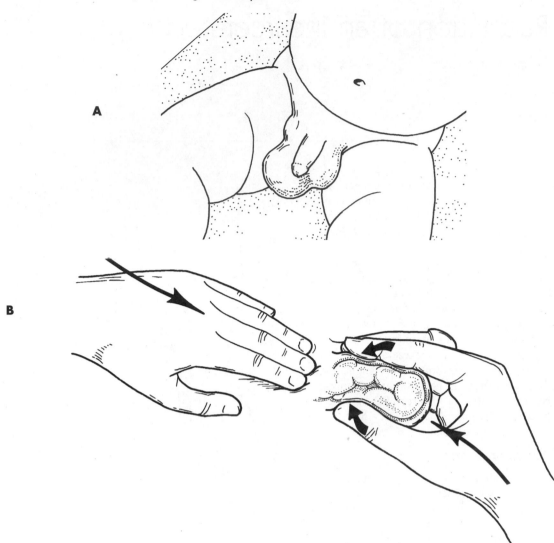

FIG.73-2 **A,** Indirect inguinal hernia positioning and techniques for reduction; **B,** manual decompression of the inguinal hernia.

nias, six (43%) presented *again* with an incarceration and required emergency reduction. Repair at 48 hours after the initial incarceration event would have prevented five of the six recurrences. In addition, for children younger than 10 years, semi-elective repair of indirect inguinal hernias undertaken within 7 days of diagnosis prevented greater than 86% of emergent surgery.[5]

Finally, if the physician is unsure of a complete reduction of the incarcerated abdominal contents, ultrasound examination may be helpful. In one study in Israel of 58 children under 2 years of age, the accuracy of diagnosis of groin swelling was 93% with ultrasonography.[6]

REFERENCES

1. Erez I, et al: Prompt diagnosis of "acute groin" conditions in infants, *Eur J Radiol* 15:185-189, 1992.
2. Glauser JM: Abdominal hernia reduction. In Roberts JR, Hedges JR, editors: *Clinical procedures in emergency medicine*, Philadelphia, 1985, WB Saunders, pp 777-783.
3. Moss RL, Hatch EI: Inguinal hernia repair in early infancy, *Am J Surg* 161:596-599, 1991.
4. Ruddy RM: Section VII procedures in Fleisher GR, Ludwig S, et al, editors: *Textbook of pediatric emergency medicine*, ed 3. Baltimore, 1993, Williams & Wilkens, pp 1640-1641.
5. Schnaufer L, Manhoubi S: Abdominal emergencies. In Fleisher GR, Ludwig S, et al, editors: *Textbook of pediatric emergency medicine,* ed 3. Baltimore, 1993, Williams & Wilkens, pp 1307-1335.
6. Stephens BJ, et al: Optimal timing of elective indirect inguinal hernia repair in healthy children: clinical considerations for improved outcome, *World J Surg* 15:952-957, 1992.

74 Penile Zipper Injuries

George A. Woodward

There is probably no other injury that strikes more fear into the heart of a young boy or man than a penile injury. With encouragement from the medical community to forego circumcision, more boys have foreskin entrapments in zippers. This most often happens in a boy between the ages of 3 and 6 years, who has better things to do than ensure complete replacement of his penis into his pants after urinating. Many children with this injury are not wearing underpants. Anxiety and fear, along with pain, will be evident in both the child and his or her caretaker. Before arrival in the Emergency Department (ED), there may have been several attempts at home to free the entrapped skin by attempting to unzip the zipper; the results of such efforts are often increased laceration, maceration, edema, pain, and entrapment and a distinct reluctance of the young boy to allow further medical intervention.

Before attempting removal, examine the zipper components and clarify its assembly and disassembly options. The zipper consists of teeth, which are interlocking, and a sliding component consisting of an anterior and a posterior plate connected by a median bar (diamond) (Fig. 74-1, A). A short review on the anatomy of a zipper is presented by Saraf and Rabinowitz.[4]

Indications

Free the entrapped foreskin as soon as possible.

Contraindications

There are no contraindications to freeing the penile foreskin.

Complications

Movement of the penis during attempted removal can result in severe pain. Further trauma to the skin of the penis can occur during removal. Infection is a rare sequela.

Equipment

Obtain a wire cutter if cutting the median bar is planned. Mineral oil is necessary for saturation of the skin and zipper. Use a 27- to 29-gauge needle, a 5-ml syringe, and 1% lidocaine without epinephrine for local anesthesia.

Technique

Although it is occasionally possible to unzip a zipper with entrapped skin, in most patients other techniques are easier and less traumatic. The technique of unzipping often results in increased pain. One simple way to remove skin that is stuck in the teeth of a zipper or underneath the slide is to cut the median bar (diamond) with a pair of wire or bone cutters (Fig. 74-1, B).[1,3,5] This allows the zipper to simply fall apart, releasing the entrapped skin. This can often be done without local or regional anesthesia, but consider restraint or conscious sedation (see Part III), depending on the child and

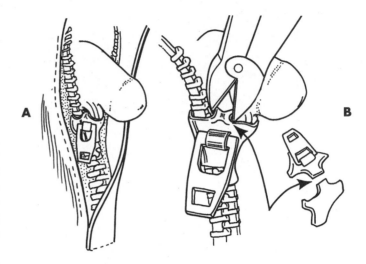

FIG. 74-1 **A** and **B,** Zipper view with entrapped skin (prepuce, redundant skin).

previous removal attempts. If local anesthesia is needed, inject local 1% xylocaine into the entrapped skin or perform a penile block (see Chapter 16).

Mineral oil may allow for a nontraumatic solution to this sticky situation.[2] Place mineral oil on the entrapped skin for approximately 10 minutes to allow for simple removal without the need for skin or zipper dissection. This technique proved useful in the reported cases when a wire cutter was not available and the zipper was of an unusual anatomy that did not allow the usual approach to removal. It is advantageous because it is relatively painless, the child is not frightened by needles or wire cutters, and mineral oil is readily available in most EDs. The authors[2] also describe three other techniques for removal. These include pushing the fastener away from the penis in the direction opposite the original entrapment, unfastening the teeth of the zipper one at a time from alternating sides, and cutting transversely through the cloth that holds the teeth in line, allowing the zipper to be removed from both sides.

Care of the lacerated or edematous penile tissue after removal depends on the severity of the injury. Treat most cases conservatively with warm soaks. Ensure that tetanus immunization is current. If the laceration is severe, incise the injured tissue. A circumcision may be needed. Consult with a urologist before performing tissue removal. Antibiotics are usually not necessary.

Remarks

Increased pain results whenever the zipper attached to the foreskin is moved. Thus the pants should be carefully supported at all times to avoid sudden movement of the attached zipper. Cutting the pants away (often done at home) may reduce the weight attached to the zipper and the chance of inadvertent movement.

REFERENCES

1. Gausche M, Seidel J: Releasing penile foreskin trapped in a zipper, *Pediatr Rev* 14:140, 1993.
2. Kanegaye JT, Schonfeld N: Penile zipper entrapment: a simple and less threatening approach using mineral oil, *Pediatr Emerg Care* 9:90-91, 1993.
3. Nolan JF, Stillwell TJ, Sands JP Jr: Acute management of the zipper-entrapped penis, *J Emerg Med* 8:305-307, 1990.
4. Saraf P, Rabinowitz R: Zipper injury of the foreskin, *Am J Dis Child* 136:557-558, 1982.
5. Snyder III HM: Urologic emergencies. In Fleisher GR, Ludwig S, editors: *Textbook of pediatric emergency medicine,* ed 3, Baltimore, 1993, Williams & Wilkins, p 1390.

Kathy N. Shaw

Although inspection of the external genitalia of the prepubertal child is ideally part of any routine physical examination, many physicians are unable to identify normal anatomy and are both inexperienced and uncomfortable with the examination.[8] In the emergency setting, examination of the child's genitalia is essential for diagnosis and treatment of suspected sexual abuse, vaginal bleeding in a girl, or abdominal pain in a boy. Figs. 75-1 and 75-2 review the normal anatomy of the external genitalia in prepubertal girls and boys.

There are many physiologic differences in prepubertal children compared to adolescents or adults. The labia majora do not completely cover the vulva in the prepubertal girl. The vaginal mucosa appears thin and red compared to the moist, dull pink, estrogenized mucosa of the pubertal child. The perihymenal tissue and hymen have a lacelike vascular pattern, also because of lack of estrogen.[2,5] In newborn boys, 4% have true undescended testes. Most of these descend by 1 year of age when the incidence decreases to less than 1%. However, an active cremasteric reflex often draws the testis up out of its normal position, giving the appearance of an undescended testis unless "milked" down[10] (Fig. 75-3). Physiologic phimosis is normal in infants and preschool boys. The foreskin of the penis is not fully retractable in 96% of newborns, 50% of 1-year-olds, and 10% to 20% of 3-year-olds.[3] Thus never force back the foreskin during an examination.

Indications

Indications for genital examination include symptoms or signs that point to the genitalia as a possible etiology for a problem. Common symptoms necessitating a genital examination include genital discharge or rash, vaginal bleeding, genital pain or swelling, inguinal or abdominal mass, lower abdominal pain, urinary or rectal symptoms, known or suspected vaginal foreign body, and suspected sexual molestation.[7]

Contraindications

Never physically restrain the child or force him or her to have a genital examination. If the child cannot or will not willingly participate, defer the examination to another time and setting or, if emergent, perform under general anesthesia.

Complications

There are few physical complications to the prepubertal genital examination. In girls do not perform routine speculum examination in the Emergency Department. Pain, inflammation, and secondary adhesions may occur in uncircumcised boys with forcible retraction of the foreskin. The primary complication to avoid in both sexes is psychologic stress to the child from forcible examination or examination without his or her consent and participation.

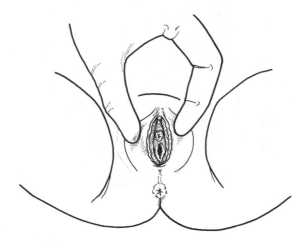

FIG. 75-1   External genitalia of the prepubertal girl.

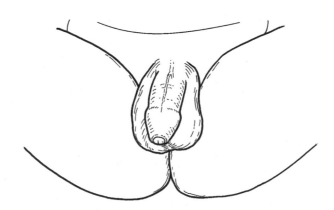

FIG. 75-2   External genitalia of the prepubertal boy—uncircumcised.

Equipment

Necessary equipment includes good lighting, an otoscope without a speculum or a hand-held magnifying lens, and gloves.

Techniques

Preparation for the Examination. Preparing the child is the most important part of the examination process and the most time consuming. Most children are hesitant and scared about being examined. Attempt to establish rapport, respect their privacy, let them maintain some control over the situation, and explain in detail each step before proceeding. A confident, relaxed, unhurried approach is most reassuring to the child. Use terminology for body parts with which the child is familiar. Let the child inspect any equipment, choose

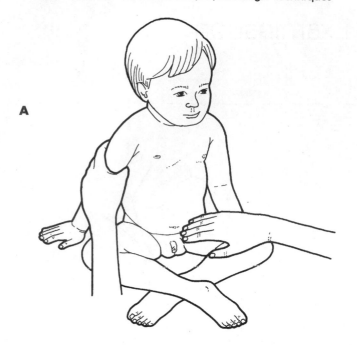

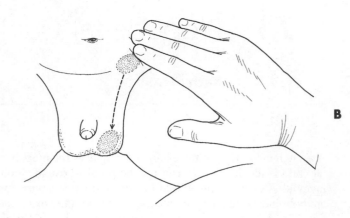

FIG. 75-3 **A** and **B,** Gentle milking of the retractile testis into the scrotum.

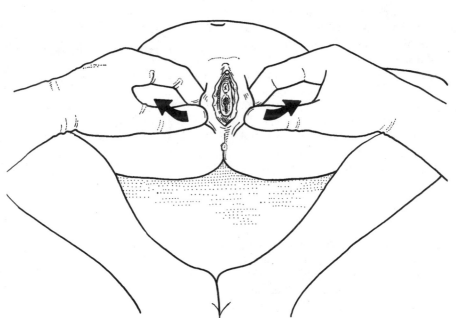

FIG. 75-4 Supine or "frog leg" position with traction for visualization of the prepubertal girl's genitalia.

who should be present during the examination, and ask questions. Make it clear to the child that, if he or she says "stop," the procedure will halt.[2,6]

Examination of the Prepubertal Female Genitalia. Positioning is essential to obtaining a clear view of the genitals and anus. The supine traction method (Fig. 75-4) and knee-chest positions are best for opening the vaginal introitus and exposing the edges of the hymen to allow visualization of at least a portion of the vaginal canal.[9] Most young children prefer examination on their mother's lap in the "frog-leg" position. Lay the child on her back with the hips fully abducted and the bottoms of the feet touching one another.

To visualize the anterior two thirds of the vaginal canal, apply gentle traction by grasping the lower portion of the labia majora between the thumb and index fingers and pull outward and slightly upward (see Fig. 75-4). Older girls are better able to cooperate for the knee-chest position. Ask the child to get up on her knees like she is going to crawl. Have her rest her head on her folded arms, facing her parent with her chest resting on the table in a sway-backed posture. Then place the examiner's thumb along the leading edge of the gluteus maximus at the level of the introitus and lift[9] (Fig. 75-5).

Carefully inspect the genitalia, especially the general

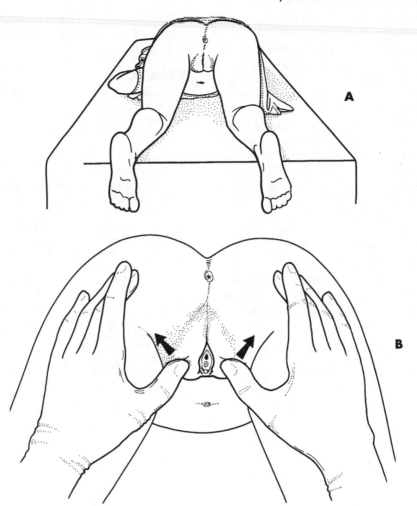

FIG. 75-5 **A** and **B,** Knee-chest position with gentle traction for visualization of the prepubertal girl's genitalia.

condition of the tissues, sexual maturation, presence of discharge, skin lesions, and normal anatomy (see Fig. 75-1). Often inexperienced examiners pay too much attention to irregularities in the hymen and the size of the hymenal orifice.[4] There is much variability in the typical hymenal appearance and orifice shape. The fundamental hymenal orifice shapes include annular or circumferential, posterior rim or crescentic, and fimbriated or redundant (Fig. 75-6). These, in turn, may have clefts, bumps, notches, tags, thickening, thinning, and elastic character.[1,2,4,5] The position of the child, degree of traction placed on the external genitalia, age, and degree of relaxation of the child can influence hymenal measurements. The presence and location of scarring or notching, especially from the 4 to 8 o'clock positions, may be more indicative of past trauma.[1]

Examination of the Prepubertal Male Genitalia.[10] Examination of the male genitalia should include the urethral meatus, the penis, and the scrotal contents (see Fig. 75-2). Although the young, uncircumcised baby often has physiologic phimosis, gentle, partial retraction usually allows visualization of the external urethral meatus at the tip of the glans penis. The urethra should be a cleft or slit at the tip of

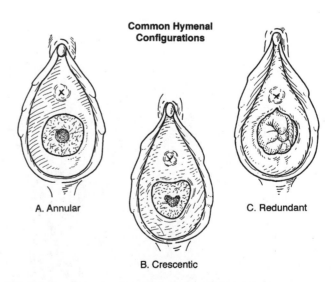

Common Hymenal Configurations

A. Annular

B. Crescentic

C. Redundant

FIG. 75-6 Common hymenal configurations or types.

the penis. The urethral opening may be abnormally located on the ventral surface of the penis (hypospadius) or rarely on the dorsal surface of the penis (epispadius). In obese boys the large mound of superficial fat may partially conceal the penis, making it appear small in size. Gentle retraction on this mound demonstrates a normal-length penis. Finally, evaluate the scrotal contents thoroughly. To palpate both testes, proceed downward from the external inguinal ring to the scrotum to counteract the active cremasteric reflex in infants. Older children may assume a squatting position or crossed-leg seated position to aid in "milking" the retractile testis down into the scrotum. (see Fig. 75-3). Inguinal hernias occur more frequently in premature infants and may appear only with crying or straining. Palpate them as inguinal or scrotal bulges that are usually reducible. Hydroceles are common in the newborn but usually subside spontaneously during the first few weeks of life. Hydroceles are collections of fluid within the tunica or processus vaginalis palpable as scrotal and sometimes inguinal masses. Often attached to the testes, they are nonreducible, nontender, and larger at night, and they can be transilluminated.

Remarks

The secret to a successful genital examination in the prepubertal child is time and patience. Engage the child as a willing participant. The examination itself usually takes less than 2 minutes if the child is cooperative.

REFERENCES

1. Berenson AB, Heger AH, Hayes JM, et al: Appearance of the hymen in prepubertal girls, *Pediatrics* 89:387-394, 1992.
2. Emans SJ, Goldstein DP, editors: Office evaluation of the child and adolescent. In *Pediatric adolescent gynecology*, ed 3, Boston, 1990, Little, Brown.
3. Gairdner D: The fate of the foreskin: a study of circumcision, *Br Med J* 2:1433-1437, 1949.
4. Gardner JJ: Descriptive study of genital variation in healthy, nonabused premenarchal girls, *J Pediatr* 120:251-260, 1992.
5. Giardino, et al: *A practical guide to the evaluation of sexual abuse in the prepubertal child,* Newbury Park, Calif, 1992, Sage Publications.
6. Horowitz DA: Physical examination of sexually abused children and adolescents, *Pediatr Rev* 9:25-29, 1987.
7. Huffman JW, Dewhurst CJ, Capraro VJ, editors: Examination of the premenarchal child. In *The gynecology of childhood and adolescence*, Philadelphia, 1981, WB Saunders.
8. Ladson S, Johnson CF, Doty RE: Do physicians recognize sexual abuse? *Am J Dis Child* 141:411-415, 1987.
9. McCann J, et al: Comparison of genital examination techniques in prepubertal girls, *Pediatrics* 85:182-187, 1990.
10. Walker RD: Presentation of urogenital disorders in children. In Kelalils PP, King LR, Belman AB, editors: *Clinical pediatric urology*, ed 2, Philadelphia, 1985, WB Saunders.

76 Pelvic Examination—Adolescent

Nanette C. Kunkel

An adolescent faces many fears when she undergoes a pelvic examination in the Emergency Department (ED). The fear of discovery of the unknown, of disease or pregnancy, and of loss of virginity all may increase her anxiety. Careful explanations and a calm approach may decrease this uneasiness. Despite physician and patient reluctance, the information gained from this examination is likely to influence patient care and may even be life saving.

Indications

The pelvic examination provides useful information in adolescent patients with abdominal pain, particularly when appendicitis and pelvic inflammatory disease are included in the differential diagnosis. When a vaginal discharge is present or a sexually transmitted disease is suspected, a speculum examination is required, since cultures from the endocervix for *Chlamydia trachomatis* and *Neisseria gonorrhoeae* are more reliable than vaginal cultures in the postpubertal female. Other indications for performing a pelvic examination in the ED include vaginal bleeding, suspected sexual assault, suspected pelvic mass or foreign body, and ectopic pregnancy or other suspected pregnancy-related complication. A pelvic examination is not necessary for a routine suspected pregnancy in the ED.

Contraindications

Suspected placenta previa is the only relative contraindication to performing the pelvic examination. An obviously pregnant adolescent (> 20 weeks) who comes to the ED with painless vaginal bleeding or a history of painless spotting may have an abnormal implantation of the placenta over or very near the cervical os. In this case, uncontrolled bleeding can sometimes be precipitated by a pelvic examination, necessitating premature delivery.[5] With such bleeding, perform a speculum examination carefully, but defer the digital examination of the cervix to an obstetrician in the delivery room.

Complications

Except for precipitating hemorrhage with a placenta previa, complications of the pelvic examination are usually equipment related. The cervix, vaginal wall, or external genitalia can be pinched by the speculum if it is closed too early or withdrawn improperly. If the light source emits heat, avoid burning the patient's thighs. In addition, some vaginal spotting may result from endocervical culture collection, particularly when a cytobrush is used for the chlamydia culture. Forewarn the patient that this may occur. Finally, teenagers sometimes worry that after a pelvic examination they will no longer be considered a "virgin." A careful explanation can help reassure them.

Equipment

The equipment needed for a pelvic examination is listed in Box 76-1. Have a variety of specula available. The pediatric speculum ($5/8 \times 3$ –inch) is usually too short and excessively wide and thus is rarely useful.[3,6] The Huffman speculum ($1/2 \times 4\frac{1}{4}''$ is useful for most adolescents, while the Pedersen speculum ($7/8 \times 4\frac{1}{2}$–inch) is better for sexually experienced adolescents. A diagram or model may be helpful when explaining the procedure to the patient and also for educating her about normal or abnormal findings.

Techniques

Explain the procedure thoroughly, and allow the patient to voice her fears or ask questions before beginning the pelvic examination. Ask her to void first, since an empty bladder makes palpation easier and more comfortable. A chaperone should be present for the examination in all cases and should be a female if possible. Sometimes conscious sedation is necessary (Section III). Patients usually prefer to be draped so that the examiner can view only the genitalia. Use a handheld mirror to help the patient view the examination or place the patient in a semi-sitting position as an alternative to the standard lithotomy position. Maintain privacy by doing the procedure in a closed room without interruptions.

External Genitalia. Visualize the external genitalia first,

BOX 76-1   EQUIPMENT NEEDED FOR A PELVIC EXAMINATION

Examining table with stirrups
Light source (height adjustable)
Drapes
Chair
Lubricant (water-soluble)
Warm water source
Disposable gloves
Specula (variety of sizes)
Absorbent swabs for clearing secretions
Cotton swabs for cultures and preparations
Hemoccult card
Saline
Culture media
Clear tube for wet prep, potassium hydroxide swab, slides for wet mounts
Papanicolaou smear supplies
Mirror (hand)
Diagrams of female anatomy, model

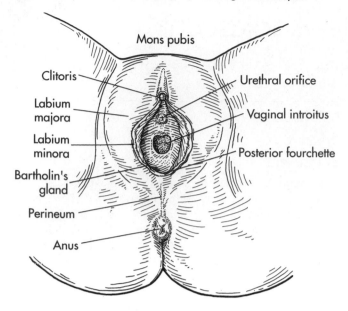

FIG. 76-1 Female external genitalia.

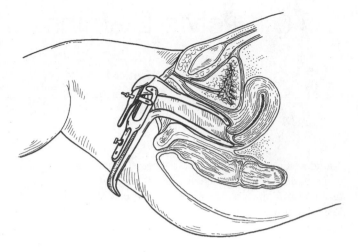

FIG. 76-2 Speculum examination.

and note any abnormalities or the presence of discharge or bleeding (Fig. 76-1). Inguinal adenopathy may be present with an infectious process. Skene's glands are located inside the urethra and are difficult to palpate. Bartholin's glands are located outside the hymen at 5 and 7 o'clock and can be palpated by placing one finger inside the hymenal ring. Both gland types can enlarge and produce a purulent discharge when infected.[3]

Apply gentle downward traction on the lower aspect of the labia minora to provide better visualization of the vaginal introitus. While inspecting this area, avoid casual comments about "normalcy" that can be misconstrued by the patient. Avoid direct manipulation of the clitoris since it may be uncomfortable.

Speculum Examination. Explain the procedure verbally and touch the thigh and external labia with the speculum before insertion to avoid surprises for the patient. Warm the speculum (not hot) and lubricate with plain water before insertion. Do not use other lubricants if cultures or a Papanicolaou (Pap) smear will be collected. Spread the labia; avoid pulling on any pubic hair. It is less traumatic to place the warmed speculum against the inner thigh before touching the perineum. The genitalia are very sensitive, and touching the thigh first allows the patient to anticipate the sensation of the speculum on the perineum. Ask the patient to perform a Valsalva maneuver to relax the muscles of the pelvic diaphragm and ease insertion of the speculum.[2] In a virginal or anxious teen, use a slow one-finger examination of the vagina to demonstrate the vaginal size and location of the cervix and help the pelvic muscles relax.[3] Then partially withdraw the finger and insert the speculum in a closed position, obliquely and posteriorly with a downward direction, gliding over the internal finger; then rotate it horizontally into place (Fig. 76-2). Open the speculum to allow visualization of the cervix. If the cervix is not visualized, close the speculum and readjust it. Avoid applying pressure upward on the anterior blade because it compresses the urethra and can be painful. Inspect the cervix for abnormali-

ties, discharge, or bleeding. Normal squamous epithelium is dull and pink. However, adolescents may have an ectropion, which is the presence of endocervical columnar epithelium on the exocervix. It is red and rough and is normal in adolescents. The junction between the two types of cells is called the squamocolumnar junction.

Collect vaginal secretions for microscopic evaluation or potassium hydroxide smear by placing a cotton swab in the pool of secretions found at the end of the speculum. Place the swab in a clean, dry tube with a few drops of saline added. Obtain cultures for *N. gonorrhoeae* by placing a sterile cotton swab in the endocervix and rotating it for about 30 seconds. Then streak the swab on a warmed Thayer-Martin culture medium. These cultures require a high CO_2 environment and need either rapid transport to the laboratory or a CO_2 capsule that is crushed in an airtight container. Other transport media exist for *N. gonorrhoeae* culture when laboratory facilities are not immediately available.[3] A Pap smear can also be obtained at this time. Rotate an Ayer spatula with pressure 360 degrees around the cervix and spread the collected material thinly on the slide, using both sides of the spatula.[3] The specimen is not adequate if the squamocolumnar junction is not sampled, and in an adolescent this may involve scraping laterally toward the vaginal wall.

Obtain an endocervical specimen by inserting a cytobrush or moistened cotton applicator into the os and twirling it. Roll this material onto a glass slide. Fix both slides immediately.[3] Obtain chlamydia cultures last since the objective is to obtain a good sample of endocervical lining cells with minimal contamination by vaginal secretions. First, wipe the face of the endocervix by using a large absorbent cotton swab. Specimens collected with the cytobrush yield an improved rate of isolation.[1] Swabs can be used but must be Dacron; avoid wooden shafts because the wood is often treated with chemicals that are toxic to cell cultures.[4] Rotate the swab or brush within the endocervical canal to obtain a good sample of columnar cells. Break the swab or brush so it remains in the liquid transport media. Place specimens in a refrigerator as soon as possible or transport directly to the laboratory. Chlamydia rapid testing may be cost-effective, depending on the prevalence rate of chlamydia infection in

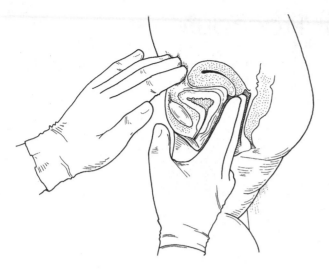

FIG. 76-3   Bimanual examination.

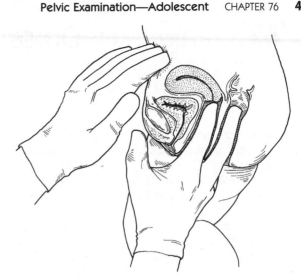

FIG. 76-4   Rectovaginal examination.

the population being tested; however, cultures are preferred particularly when documenting infection from sexual abuse.[8] Obtain specimens in the same manner. Instructions for preparing the slide are given in the kit. After culture collection, withdraw the speculum in a partially opened position while observing the vaginal wall for abnormalities.

Bimanual Examination. Perform the bimanual examination with either the right or left hand, although some examiners choose to switch hands during the procedure. With gloves on, lubricate the first two fingers of the examining hand with a water-soluble lubricating jelly, and place them in the vagina. When examining sexually inexperienced teens, occasionally only one finger may be comfortably introduced. Palpate the cervix and uterus internally, with help from the abdominal hand pressing anteriorly above the pubic bone (Fig. 76-3). Then move the vaginal fingers into the right lateral fornix as far as possible. Use the abdominal hand to produce pressure on the right lower abdomen, and use the fingers of the vaginal hand to sweep to the side for evaluation of the adnexal structures. The ovaries pass between the fingers of both hands as they are moving downward and toward the symphysis pubis. Some discomfort is always present on palpation of the ovaries; warn the patient beforehand. Repeat the examination on the opposite side. The adnexa are often not palpated if the patient is anxious or obese. Also evaluate the lateral walls and bony structure of the pelvis during the bimanual examination.

Rectovaginal Examination. Defer the rectovaginal examination if the rest of the examination is sufficient.[7] Change gloves before proceeding to heme test any stool, although with any vaginal bleeding, the results may still be uninterpretable. Lubricate the first two fingers of the examining hand, and place the middle finger in the rectum and the index finger simultaneously in the vagina (Fig. 76-4). Place the vaginal finger against the cervix and, with pressure from the abdominal hand, bring the uterus down so that its posterior

surface can be palpated with the rectal finger. Test the stool specimen if indicated for occult bleeding.

When finished, have the patient dress and then carefully review your findings with her.

Remarks

Disposable plastic specula can be difficult to open and close comfortably and may require practice before their first use. They also tend to make a sharp clicking noise when locking in the open position, and this can frighten the patient. Inform her of this possibility to prevent any sudden moves.

Controversy occasionally arises concerning the privacy and confidentiality of any findings. Individual physicians must understand state regulations and hospital policies. Carefully explain the importance of the diagnosis to the adolescent. Problems may arise when parents receive phone calls or bills concerning procedures and testing of which they had no previous knowledge.

REFERENCES

1. Bell TA: *Chlamydia trachomatis* infections in adolescents, *Med Clin North Am* 74(5):1229, 1990.
2. Carson SA: Gynecologic examination of the adolescent. In Koehler Carpenter SE, Roch JA, editors: *Pediatric and adolescent gynecology,* New York, 1992, Raven Press, pp 67-76.
3. Emans SJ, Goldstein DP: Pediatric and adolescent gynecology, Boston, 1990, Little, Brown, pp 17-45.
4. Martin DH: Chlamydial infections, *Med Clin North Am* 74(6):1378, 1990.
5. Pritchard JA, MacDonald PC, Gant NF: *Williams obstetrics,* ed 17, Norwalk, Conn, 1985, Appleton-Century-Crofts, p 409.
6. Rimza ME: An illustrated guide to adolescent gynecology, *Pediatr Clin North Am* 36(3):652, 1989.
7. Stewart DC, Neinstein LS: Gynecological examination of the adolescent female. In Neinstein LS: *Adolescent health care: a practical guide,* ed, Baltimore, 1991, Urban and Schwarzenberg, pp 641-647.
8. Vandeven AM, Emans SJ: Vulvovaginitis in the child and adolescent, *Pediatr Rev* 14(4):144, 1993.

77 Phimosis: Dorsal Slit Procedure

Kathy N. Shaw

Phimosis, the inability to retract the foreskin to expose the glans, is normal in infancy and common in childhood. Fully retractable foreskin is present in only 4% of newborns, 20% of boys at 6 months of age, and 50% at 1 year. By 3 years of age, the foreskin is retractable in 80% to 90% of uncircumcised boys.[2]

Physiologic phimosis or secondary nonretractility occurs in approximately 3% to 16% of uncircumcised boys[1,3] and may result from forcible and premature retraction in early childhood. This appears as a white "scarring" or thickened distal ring of foreskin at the tip of the prepuce that is not retractable.[5] If true or physiologic phimosis exists, the prepuce balloons with voiding.[4] Elective circumcision or surgical correction are the treatments of choice.

Indications and Contraindications

Do not perform dorsal slit of the phimotic foreskin for physiologic phimosis; perform this procedure in secondary phimosis only to allow urethral catheterization in an emergency situation. This is rarely necessary in children; ordinarily urologists should perform or direct dorsal slit procedures.

Complications

A dorsal slit procedure causes a "beagle-ear" deformity, often postponing elective circumcision. Other complications from this procedure include hemorrhage, infection, injury to the meatus and glans penis, secondary meatal stenosis, and avascular necrosis.

Equipment

Obtain necessary equipment, including sterile preparation solution, sterile drapes, and sterile gloves. Also prepare 1% lidocaine without epinephrine, a 5-ml syringe, a 27-gauge needle, one straight Crile clamp, one straight scissors, one needle holder, and 4-0 chromic catgut suture.

Techniques[6]

Clean the penis and drape with sterile towels. Using sterile technique, infiltrate the dorsal midline of the foreskin proximally to distally with 1% lidocaine without epinephrine along the course of the proposed slit. Test the foreskin, especially the inner surface, for anesthesia before starting the procedure. Consider a penile block (see Chapter 16) if anesthesia is inadequate (Fig. 77-1).

Carefully advance one jaw of a straight hemostat or Crile forceps under the foreskin but not into the glans or urethra. The foreskin should "tent up" at the coronal sulcus if the tip of the forceps is not in the urethra or under the glans. Once correctly placed, close the instrument. Remove the forceps after a few minutes and cut the serrated, crushed skin lengthwise with scissors. Close the edges of the incision with chromic suture. Now retract the foreskin to perform the emergency catheterization.

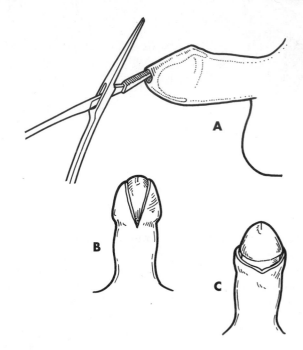

FIG. 77-1 Dorsal slit procedure. **A,** Placement of forceps with foreskin "tented" up; **B,** dorsal slit in phimotic foreskin; **C,** cut edges of foreskin brought back around glans penis and sutured around cut edges.

Remarks

Most cases of phimosis in children are physiologic and require no therapy. In fact, freeing these "adhesions" is unnecessary and unfounded physiologically or medically. Don't mistake normal penile adhesions in preschool boys with physiologic or secondary phimosis.[4] Even when true phimosis does exist, perform a dorsal slit procedure only in the rare case when emergency urethral catheterization is necessary.

REFERENCES

1. Fergusson DB, Hons BA, Lawton JM, et al: Neonatal circumcision and penile problems: an 8-year longitudinal study, *Pediatrics* 81:537-541, 1988.
2. Gairdner D: The fate of the foreskin: a study of circumcision, *Br Med J* 2:1433-1437, 1949.
3. Herzog LW, Alvarez SR: The frequency of foreskin problems in uncircumcised children, *Am J Dis Child* 140:254-256, 1986.
4. Kaplan GW: Circumcision—an overview. In Gluck L, editor: *Current problems in pediatrics,* Chicago, 1977, Year Book Medical Publishers, pp 1-33.
5. Rickwood AM, Hemglatha V, Batcup G, et al: Phimosis in boys, *Br J Urol* 52:147-150, 1980.
6. Zbaraschuk, Berger RE, Hedges JR: Emergency urologic procedures. In Roberts JR, Hedges JR, editors: *Clinical procedures in emergency medicine,* ed 2, edition, Philadelphia, 1991, WB Saunders.

78 Reduction of Paraphimosis

Kathy N. Shaw

Paraphimosis occurs with retraction of a mildly phimotic foreskin behind the glans. Venous congestion and edema result, which make it very difficult to reduce the foreskin back to a normal position. Since "physiologic" phimosis is common in most babies and many uncircumcised young boys, do not perform forceful retraction of the foreskin beyond the glans since it may result in symptomatic phimosis or paraphimosis.[2]

Indications

Reduce all cases of paraphimosis to prevent further edema and pain. If untreated, ischemia and gangrene can result. Attempt manual reduction first; if this fails, a slit through the preputial ring may be necessary. In cases in which surgical reduction is necessary, circumcision often follows after the swelling resolves.[2]

Contraindications

Consult the urologist for all cases of paraphimosis in children. If there will be a significant delay in the urologist's arrival, attempt manual reduction. If this is not successful, the urologist should perform or direct surgical reduction.

Complications

Ischemia of the glans can occur with excessive compression during manual reduction of the paraphimosis.[3] Complications from surgical reduction include infection; contusion or laceration to the penile shaft, glans, or urethra; and a tethered or hidden penis with incision too proximally of the skin on the penile shaft.

Equipment

Obtain equipment for *manual reduction of paraphimosis,* including lubricant jelly (1% lidocaine preferred), surgical glove or plastic bag, and crushed ice.

For *operative reduction of paraphimosis,* prepare sterile preparation solution, a sterile drape, and sterile gloves. Also needed are 1% lidocaine without epinephrine, a 5-ml syringe, a 27-gauge needle, a No. 15 surgical blade with handle, a needle holder, and 4-0 chromic suture.

Techniques

Manual Reduction of Paraphimosis. Coat the glans penis and the undersurface of the edematous foreskin with 1% lidocaine jelly to both lubricate and anesthetize the area. Surround the swollen foreskin and shaft of the penis by a crushed ice water compress made with a surgical glove or plastic bag. Using the "iced-glove" method,[1] insert the glans into the thumb of the glove, which is held invaginated into the ice water pouch of the body of the glove (Fig. 78-1). Apply steady manual compression to squeeze the edema from in front of the stricture to the shaft of the penis behind it.[4] Then reduce the paraphimosis by stabilizing the foreskin

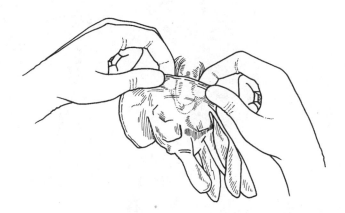

FIG. 78-1 Ice-glove method of decompression of edematous paraphimotic foreskin.

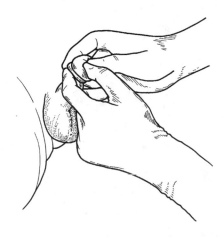

FIG. 78-2 Manual reduction of paraphimosis. Gentle traction of the foreskin with the second and third fingers and simultaneous counterpressure on the glans with the tips of the thumbs.

between the third and index fingers of both hands and using gentle traction while applying constant counter-pressure with the tips of the thumbs on the glans—as in turning a sock inside out[2,3] (Fig. 78-2).

Surgical Reduction of Paraphimosis.[2,4,5] Although surgical division of the foreskin is possible with sedation and local anesthesia, it is optimal for a urologist to perform the procedure in the operating room suite. Clean the shaft of the penis with sterile preparation solution and drape. Inject the dorsal area of the constricted ring and foreskin proximal and distal to it with 1% lidocaine without epinephrine at the 12-o'clock position. Make a longitudinal slit with the blade through the skin, the edematous subcutaneous layer, and the constricting ring, being careful not to injure the penile shaft below the dartos facia or the glans. Do not extend the

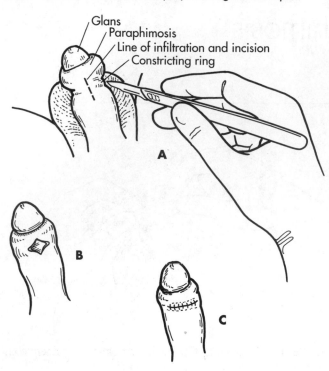

Glans
Paraphimosis
Line of infiltration and incision
Constricting ring

FIG. 78-3 Surgical reduction of paraphimosis. **A,** Vertical line on dorsum of penis for infiltration of local anesthesia and incision; **B,** diamond-shaped defect resulting from incision; **C,** closed transversely.

incision much beyond the constricting band in either direction. With complete incision of the constricting band, the retracted foreskin edges forms a diamond-shaped defect. Close the incision transversely, using chromic cat gut (Fig. 78-3).

Remarks

This procedure can be quite uncomfortable or painful. The age of the child and his ability to cooperate will aid in the decision to use local anesthesia with or without sedation versus general anesthesia. Consult a urologist in the beginning.

REFERENCES

1. Houghton GR: The 'ice-glove' method of treatment of paraphimosis, *Br J Surg,* 11:876-877, 1973.
2. Klauber GT, Sant GR: Disorders of the male external genitalia. In Kelalils PP, King LR, Belman AB, editors: *Clinical pediatric urology,* ed 2, Philadelphia, 1985, WB Saunders.
3. Neuwirth H, Frasier B, Cochran ST: Genitourinary imaging and procedures by the emergency physician, *Emerg Med Clin North Am* 7:1-28, 1989.
4. Schenck GR: The treatment of paraphimosis, *Am J Surg* 8:329, 1930.
5. Zbaraschuk I, Berger RE, Hedges JR: Emergency urologic procedures. In Roberts JR, Hedges JR, editors: *Clinical procedures in emergency medicine,* ed 2, Philadelphia, 1991, WB Saunders, pp 867-889.

79 Prepubertal Vaginal Bleeding

Kathy N. Shaw

Vaginal bleeding is abnormal after the first week of life and before menarche. Box 79-1 lists the many causes of reported prepubertal vaginal bleeding. As maternal hormones wane after birth, some babies slough estrogen-stimulated endometrial tissue, with resultant light vaginal bleeding. Vaginal bleeding in the prepubertal child is rarely caused by major trauma and may not actually be from the vagina itself. The urethra (urinary tract infection, urethral prolapse) or vulva (genital warts, inflammation, lichen sclerosis) may be the source of the bleeding. The most common causes of true vaginal bleeding during childhood are foreign body, infection, and minor trauma. One study of girls under 13 years of age found that 18% who presented with vaginal bleeding with or without discharge and 50% who presented with vaginal bleeding alone had a vaginal foreign body. [5] Other rare causes include tumors, transient isosexual precocity, cyclic vaginal bleeding without signs of pubertal development, and exogenous estrogen. [1-4]

Indications/Contraindications

With its heterogeneous and potentially serious or life-threatening causes, vaginal bleeding in the prepubertal child always warrants careful investigation by the emergency physician. Do not rely on the severity of the child's symptoms for reassurance. Vaginal lacerations do not always cause severe pain or bleeding. Conversely, the child may act quite distressed secondary to pinworms or vulvovaginitis. In many cases, simple examination of the external genitalia indicates the etiology. When a source of the bleeding is not easily discernible using the previously mentioned examination techniques, perform an internal examination under general anesthesia. Never restrain a child or force her to submit to a genital examination.

Complications

There are no physical complications from the procedure. Problems include an uncooperative child or failure to detect the source of bleeding. Both of these situations necessitate an examination under general anesthesia.

Equipment

Equipment needed for investigation of vaginal bleeding includes 2% lidocaine jelly, warm sterile saline, a rubber feeding tube or Foley catheter, a 30-ml syringe, and a basin. Also needed are gloves, sterile dressing sponges, culturettes and/or sterile swabs, an otoscope without the speculum or magnifying lens, and a good light source.

Techniques

Follow the procedure for the examination of the genitalia of the prepubertal child (see Chapter 75). Perform the initial examination in the supine frog-leg position with gentle traction to expose the anterior two thirds of the vaginal canal. In the older child use the knee-chest position to give a better view of the vaginal canal. Trauma to the vulva, urethral prolapse, and vulvovaginitis is usually evident on inspection. If a hymenal tear is present, suspect a penetrating injury. If an abrasion or cut is present, apply 2% lidocaine topically to minimize pain during further examination and irrigation. [1]

If no source of bleeding is obvious or if suspicion of vaginal injury exists, hold a basin underneath the perineum, and use a 30-ml syringe with a urinary catheter or rubber feeding tube attached with warm sterile saline to irrigate the vulva and vagina gently to identify the source of bleeding (Fig. 79-1). Gentle pressure with saline-soaked gauze or probing with saline-moistened curettes may help identify the source of bleeding. If no source is identifiable, check the urine for blood and inspect the rectum. If unable to perform a good examination or identify the source of bleeding, proceed to an examination under general anesthesia. [1,4]

BOX 79-1 **ETIOLOGIES OF REPORTED "VAGINAL BLEEDING" IN THE PREPUBERTAL CHILD**

More common

Neonatal hormone withdrawal
Foreign body
Vulvovaginitis: (with or without excoriation)
   Pinworms
   Group A β-streptococci
   Shigella
Urethral mucosa prolapse (peak age: 5-8 years)
Trauma—vulvar or vaginal
Urinary tract infection
Rectal bleeding

Rare

Genital warts
Tumors
Exogenous estrogen
Lichen sclerosis
Cyclic vaginal bleeding without signs of pubertal development

---

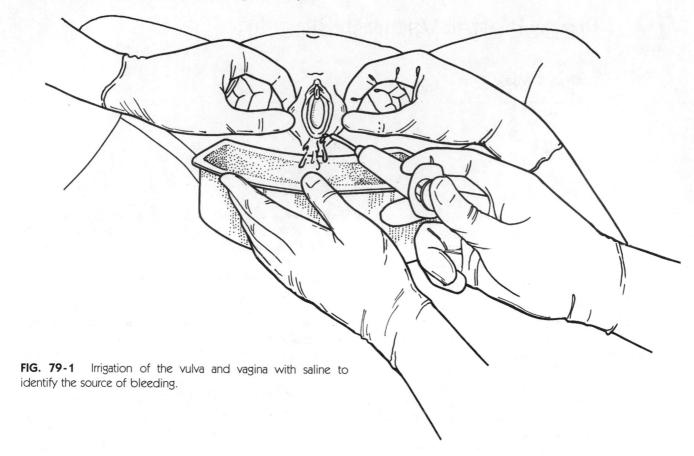

FIG. 79-1 Irrigation of the vulva and vagina with saline to identify the source of bleeding.

Remarks

As with any genital examination of the prepubertal child, use patience and take ample time for preparation. If vaginal trauma is in the differential, identify the source of bleeding since significant injury may be almost asymptomatic. Exclude sexual abuse in children with vaginal foreign bodies.

REFERENCES

1. Emans SJ, Goldstein DP, editors: Vulvovaginal problems in the prepubertal child, In *Pediatric adolescent gynecology,* ed 3, Boston, 1990, Little, Brown.

2. Heller ME, Savage MO, Dewhurst J: Vaginal bleeding in childhood: a review of 51 patients, *Obstetrics Gynaecology* 85:721-725, 1978.

3. Huffman JW, Dewhurst CJ, Capraro VJ, editors: Abnormal genital bleeding in childhood and adolescence. In *The gynecology of childhood and adolescence,* Philadelphia, 1981, WB Saunders.

4. Paradise JE: Vaginal bleeding. In Fleisher GR, Ludwig S, editors: *Textbook of pediatric emergency medicine,* ed 3, Baltimore, 1993, Williams & Wilkins, pp 494-501.

5. Paradise JE, Willis ED: Probability of vaginal foreign body in girls with genital complaints, *Am J Dis Child* 139:472-476, 1985.

80 Priapism: Aspiration of the Corpus Cavernosum

Kathy N. Shaw

Priapism, a persistent and often painful erection, is uncommon in children. Priapism may be classified as primary (idiopathic) or secondary to an underlying disease. Although there are many reported causes of priapism (Box 80-1), the overwhelming majority of cases of childhood priapism occur in boys with sickle-cell disease. Priapism occurs in 6% to 12% of patients with sickle-cell disease[2,9] and is secondary to the sludging of sickled cells, which impedes venous outflow from the corpora cavernosa. The sludging leads to local hypoxemia and acidosis, which in turn promotes further sickling of red blood cells. Attacks occur mainly at night and may be short (<3 hours) and self-limited or prolonged and require therapy.[2]

The goal of therapy for priapism is to allow detumescence of the penis by improving venous drainage of the corpora cavernosa, which is accomplished by treating the primary disease process (e.g., sickle-cell disease, leukemia) or by aspirating blood from the corpora. When the penis is in the flaccid state, the helicine arterioles and cavernous muscles contract secondary to α-adrenergic activity. This contraction limits blood flow to the corpora cavernosa, and the emissary veins relax.[3] Recently, local α-adrenergic agents have been used to reduce arterial blood flow.[4,7] In adults, systemic β-agonist therapy may improve venous outflow.[8] However, these agents are unproven for the treatment of childhood priapism. In addition, α-adrenergic agents should be used only in nonischemic priapism under the direction of a urologist.[6,7]

Look for an underlying etiology for priapism in children and treat the primary disease. In sickle-cell disease treatment involves hydration and hypertransfusion or exchange pheresis to increase the hemoglobin to 10 to 12 g/dl and to decrease the percentage of sickled cells to less than 30%. Concomitant supportive measures include analgesics and local application of ice packs. Most young patients with sickle-cell disease and priapism respond to conservative management and rarely develop impotence.[1,5,9] If priapism does not resolve in 48 to 72 hours, the urologist commonly performs surgical decompression with a shunting procedure.[2,9]

Indications

Earlier aggressive intervention and treatment is now recommended for some children or adolescents to prevent ischemia with its resultant thrombosis, fibrosis, and impotence.[6,7] The first and only therapy performed in the Emergency Department is simple needle aspiration and saline irrigation of the corpora, with or without α-adrenergic agents.

Obtain a urologic consultation immediately for the child with priapism. The Emergency Department physician should perform corporal aspiration and irrigation only if the urologist agrees that it is necessary but is unavailable to perform it.[7]

Contraindications

Medical treatment of sickle-cell disease is the first priority of the emergency physician for a child with sickle-cell disease and priapism.[2,9] Perform needle aspiration under the direction of a urologist.[6,7]

Patients with ischemic priapism as determined by blood gas analysis (pH <7.25; Po_2<30 mm Hg, Pco_2>60 mm Hg) or those in whom priapism has persisted for more than 36 to 48 hours are unlikely to respond to intracorporeal irrigation. The use of α-adrenergic agents may worsen or potentiate underlying tissue ischemia. In these cases, the urologist may elect to perform a surgical shunt procedure.[4,6,7]

Complications

Impotence is a complication of priapism itself and its duration before therapy; it is not secondary to either surgical or conservative medical treatment. The fact that only the more severe or prolonged cases receive surgical intervention may bias reports of greater potency after conservative (nonoperative) therapies. Early institution of treatment (<48

BOX 80–1 CAUSES OF PRIAPISM IN CHILDREN

Common

Sickle-cell disease

Less common

Leukemia
Medications
   Marijuana
   "Psychedelic" street drugs
   Antipsychotics
   Antihypertensives

Rare

Idiopathic
Blunt perineal trauma
Spinal cord injury
Fabry's disease
Nephrotic syndrome
Vasculitis
Coagulopathy
Congenital syphilis

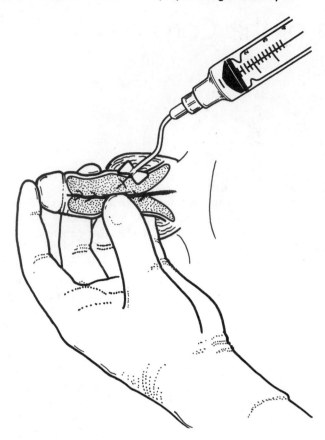

FIG. 80-1 Aspiration of the corpus cavernosum for priapism.

hours after onset of priapism) increases the likelihood that potency will be retained.[2,5,7]

The most common complication after aspiration of the corpora cavernosa for priapism is recurrence. Hematoma of the shaft and infections such as abscesses or cellulitis uncommonly occur. Other rare complications include necrosis, urethral fistulas, sloughing of penile skin, and megalophallus.[1,2,5] Hypertension and arrhythmias may occur with the use of α-adrenergic agents.[7]

Equipment

Equipment necessary for aspiration includes sterile drapes, sterile gloves, povidone-iodine or another preparation solution, and gauze sponges. Also needed are lidocaine 1% without epinephrine, a 3-ml syringe with a 25-gauge needle for lidocaine, 19 to 23-gauge butterfly needles for aspiration, two 30-ml syringes, a sterile basin, and a heparinized blood gas syringe.

In addition, normal saline is needed for irrigation and dilution of α-adrenergic agents as follows: 0.2 mg phenylephrine diluted to 10 ml,[6] 0.01 mg norepinephrine (10 ml of a 1 μg/ml solution),[4] and 2 to 3 ml of 1:100,000 epinephrine.[7]

Techniques

Using sterile technique, prepare and drape the penis and hold the shaft with the left hand. Stand on the right side of the bed. Position the thumb anteriorly to identify the dorsal neurovascular bundle, and place the index finger posteriorly over the urethra. Palpate the lateral aspect of one of the corpora

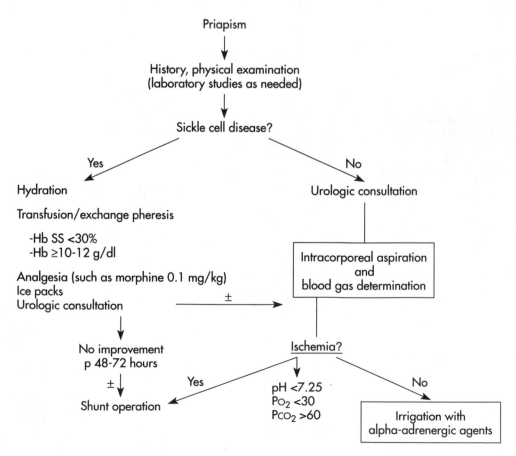

FIG. 80-2 Management of priapism.

cavernosa, and inject the skin with 1% lidocaine without epinephrine at a site at which there are no engorged veins. Because there are numerous anastamoses between the two corpora cavernosa, bilateral aspiration should not be necessary. Use a 23-gauge butterfly needle to puncture the corpus cavernosum, and aspirate blood while squeezing or "milking" the penis until bright red blood returns (Fig. 80-1). Aspirate approximately 100 to 500 ml.[6] Urinary retention is uncommon and catheterization is rarely necessary.[5]

A blood gas analysis on the initial blood can determine if ischemia exists (Fig. 80-2). Repeatedly perform gentle irrigation with 10 ml of normal saline solution. In patients with nonischemic priapism whose tumescence persists, a urologist should be consulted before an α-adrenergic agent such as phenylephrine or nonepinephrine is injected to maintain persistent detumescence.[6,7]

After removing the needle, apply digital compression for a few minutes to avoid hematoma formation. Do not use prolonged compression or surgical dressings because of the risk of penile skin necrosis. Fig. 80-2 reviews the management of priapism.

Many other therapies and maneuvers tried acutely in the past have been discounted on the basis of the proposed pathophysiology. These therapies include enemas, prostatic massage, estrogens, systemic heparin, hypotensive drugs, and spinal or epidural anesthesia.

Remarks

There is no universally accepted management for priapism. However, conservative management is indicated for priapism resulting from sickle-cell disease, which accounts for the majority of the cases in children.

REFERENCES

1. Bertram RA, Webster GD, Carson CC: Priapism: etiology, treatment, and results in a series of 35 presentations, *Urol* 26:229-232, 1985.
2. Hamre MR, Harmon EP, Kirkpatrick DV, et al: Priapism as a complication of sickle cell disease, *J Urol* 145:1-5, 1991.
3. Hauri D, Spycher M, Bruhlmann W: Erection and priapism: a new physiopathological concept, *Urol* 38:138-145, 1983.
4. Lue TF, Hellstrom WJC, McAninch JW, et al: Priapism: a refined approach to diagnosis and treatment, *J Urol* 136:104-108, 1986.
5. Macaluso JN, Sullivan JW: Priapism: review of 34 cases, *Urol* 26: 233-236, 1985.
6. Neuwirth H, Frasier B, Cochran ST: Genitourinary imaging and procedures by the emergency physician, *Emerg Med Clin North Am* 7:1-28, 1989.
7. O'Brien WM, O'Connor KP, Lynch JH: Priapism: current concepts, *Ann Emerg Med* 18:980-983, 1989.
8. Shantha TR, Finnerty DP, Rodriguez AP: Treatment of persistent penile erection and priapism using terbutaline, *J Urol* 141:1427, 1989.
9. Tarry WF, Duckett JW, Snyder HM: Urological complications of sickle cell disease in a pediatric population, *J Urol* 138:592-594, 1987.

PART X V

NEUROLOGY AND NEUROSURGERY TECHNIQUES

81 Management of Life-Threatening Intracranial Fluid Collections

Frederick A. Boop and Bruce J. Andersen

Shunt evaluation, a subdural tap, and burr holes are three commonly performed pediatric neurosurgical procedures that the emergency physician or pediatric intensivist can perform when a neurosurgeon is not available and when a child is not stable enough for transport (i.e., in the process of herniation). The nonneurosurgeon should not perform these procedures unless the treating physician has communicated with a neurosurgeon by telephone and been instructed by the neurosurgeon to act. These procedures carry a significant risk of causing brain damage or introducing infection into the brain if performed improperly; if possible, it is best to defer them until appropriately trained personnel are available.

In the normal adult, the intracranial pressure (ICP) is less than 150 mm of cerebrospinal fluid (CSF). In the newborn, ICP is generally less than 10 mm CSF, and in young children it is usually less than 50 mm CSF.[10] The ICP varies with intraabdominal pressure and may transiently rise as high as 70 mm CSF in a child who is crying or resisting the physician. For brain perfusion to occur, the perfusion pressure of the systemic blood must exceed the intracranial pressure, as illustrated by the following derivation:

$$CPP = MAP - ICP$$

in which CPP is the cerebral perfusion pressure and MAP is the mean arterial pressure.[17] When acutely elevated ICP compromises cerebral perfusion, the ischemic brainstem signals the body to increase perfusion by raising the systemic blood pressure. This action, which produces a decrease in heart rate and a widening of the pulse pressure, is termed the Cushing phenomenon. Concomitantly, the clinician will recognize a progression of neurologic dysfunction, which is initially an alteration in the level of consciousness. Therefore, the patient's level of consciousness is the most sensitive indicator of cerebral perfusion.

In the infant, macrocephaly may herald *slowly* expanding mass lesions, such as chronic subdural collections, hydrocephalus, or a neoplasm. The cranial sutures may be separated and the infant's eyes may be crossed (bilateral sixth–cranial nerve palsies) or down-driven in the orbit, which is termed *sunsetting*.[26] Because the cranial sutures are not fused in the infant or young child, an *acute* mass such as an epidural or acute subdural hematoma may present as a bulging fontanelle and irritability or as obtundation. In older individuals the cranial sutures have fused, and the intracranial volume is fixed. Therefore a space-occupying lesion produces the typical symptoms of raised ICP such as a headache or nausea and vomiting that often occurs out of sleep or on awakening in the morning.

Normally the cranium harbors extra space to allow for minor fluctuations in brain, blood, or CSF volume without an alteration in the ICP. This "compliance" allows a small intracranial mass to be present with few symptoms; however, as the mass enlarges, the intracranial compliance declines. Thereafter, small perturbations in intracranial volume will precipitate significant rises in ICP, as demonstrated by the intracranial pressure/volume curve (Fig. 81-1). This diagram explains why a person with an expanding epidural hematoma may be conscious and assist others immediately following an automobile crash, yet may be comatose and in the process of herniation on arrival at the Emergency Department (ED) a short time later.[2,27]

An understanding of perfusion pressure and the pressure-volume relationship forms the basis for the emergent treatment of raised ICP. When a patient is in a coma from blunt abdominal or chest trauma and is *hypotensive,* the coma may be secondary to inadequate cerebral perfusion. The first treatment is to replete the intravascular volume, which raises the systemic blood pressure and in turn may immediately improve neurologic function. However, if the obtundation accompanies an elevated systemic blood pressure and bradycardia, initiate treatment for presumed intracranial hypertension, recognizing that it is necessary to restore the cerebral perfusion pressure within 3 to 5 minutes to prevent irreversible ischemic damage.

The most rapid means of lowering ICP is by intubation and hyperventilation. Intubation of the comatose patient is preferable for airway protection, but hyperventilation alone begins to reduce intracranial volume within 30 seconds by eliciting a compensatory cerebral vasoconstriction in re-

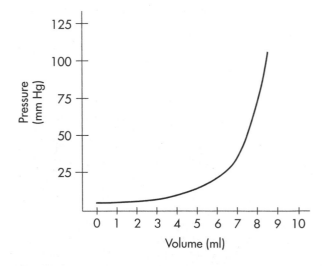

FIG. 81-1 This graph of the relationship between intracranial pressure and volume forms the basis for the emergent treatment of raised ICP. Note that small reductions in intracranial volume, such as that which hyperventilation or mannitol afford, allow significant reductions in ICP.

sponse to hypocarbia and a rising blood pH. This reduction in intracranial circulating blood volume may be only a few milliliters, but given the pressure-volume relationship, this reduction is often sufficient to restore cerebral perfusion.

The second order of treatment uses an osmotic diuretic. Give mannitol intravenously at a dose of 0.5 to 1 g/kg in combination with a diuretic such as furosemide. These agents reduce the intracranial volume and therefore ICP by raising the serum osmolality and drawing free water from the brain tissue by establishing an osmotic gradient. Mannitol requires 10 to 20 minutes to act, which is why hyperventilation is the best initial treatment. Once in effect, mannitol acts for 3 to 4 hours, which should allow the treating physician sufficient time to arrange transport or surgical assistance.[13] Do not give mannitol and furosemide to a patient who is hemodynamically unstable because the brisk diuresis that ensues will potentiate hemodynamic instability and may lead to cardiovascular collapse and further brain ischemia. When giving mannitol, place a Foley catheter to avoid overdistention of the bladder.

EVALUATION OF THE CEREBROSPINAL FLUID SHUNT

The normal adult produces approximately 0.5 L of CSF per day. The normal central nervous system may contain up to 140 ml of CSF in the subarachnoid space at any given time. Thus the turnover rate for CSF is 3 to 4 times per day.[1] When an acute imbalance between production and absorption occurs, the ICP begins to rise, and the patient rapidly becomes symptomatic.

Cerebrospinal-fluid shunts are made of flexible plastic (usually Silastic) and have three common components (Fig. 81-2). First is a ventricular catheter, which the neurosurgeon passes through a burr hole and through a relatively silent area of the brain to access the cerebral ventricle. The ventricular catheter connects to a pressure- or flow-regulating one-way valve that generally contains a reservoir or tapping chamber and distal tubing. The distal tubing is most often placed into the peritoneal cavity (ventriculoperitoneal [VP] shunt)[18] to allow drainage and absorption of CSF, but it can also be placed into the right atrium (ventriculoatrial [VA] shunt),[9] pleural cavity (ventriculopleural [V-pleural] shunt), or other body cavity.[25]

Although shunting is an effective treatment for hydrocephalus, it is not ideal. The placement of a shunt requires the presence of a foreign body under the skin, and there is an attendant risk of infection. Shunt infection rates vary widely but in general they should be no more than 8%.[8,15] The likelihood of infection increases in neonates who receive a shunt.[3] Shunt infections are rarely apparent during the hospitalization in which surgical placement occurred. The most common time for the child to come to the hospital with a shunt infection is 4 to 6 weeks following surgery. Eighty percent of all shunt infections occur within 6 months of shunt surgery, whether for the primary placement or for a revision.[23]

Infection may present with symptoms of malfunction or, more commonly, with irritability, malaise, nuchal rigidity, or abdominal pain.[9] Children with a shunt infection are not always febrile. By far the most common organism to infect a shunt is *Staphylococcus epidermidis,* an organism of low virulence; therefore the standard clinical signs of infection,

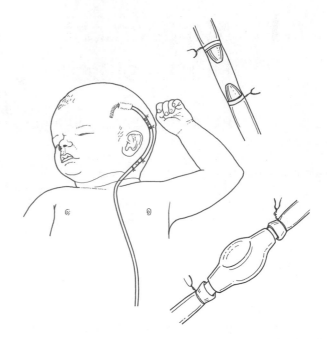

FIG. 81-2 The components of a ventriculoperitoneal shunt in situ. *Insets:* The configuration of two commonly used shunt valves, which are palpable through the skin before tapping.

such as sepsis, may be absent. The classic tachycardia, hepatosplenomegaly, and nephritis described with VA shunt infections is uncommon today because VA shunts have fallen into disfavor. When a shunt infection is possible, tap the shunt and analyze the CSF. The presence of polymorphonuclear leukocytes, hypoglycorrhachia (low CSF glucose), or a positive Gram stain indicates an infection; initiate antibiotic therapy appropriate for the Gram stain until cultures and sensitivities return that dictate otherwise.

Lifetime analysis of shunt function suggests that a malfunction occurs in more than 80% of shunts within 12 years following placement.[24] By far the most common cause of shunt malfunction is proximal obstruction of the ventricular catheter by choroid plexus. Distal obstruction is common in older children as they grow to the point that the extra tubing within the peritoneum pulls out of the cavity and interferes with drainage. Finally, Silastic tubing becomes brittle with age. Mobile segments, such as the tubing in the neck, are prone to fracture, causing the shunt to malfunction. Either insufficient tubing or a disconnection are easy to detect by radiographic imaging of the shunt.[1]

Indications

The indications for tapping a shunt are either diagnostic or therapeutic.[22] A therapeutic shunt tap is indicated in the individual who comes to the ED in extremis from a shunt malfunction. In such a case, the withdrawal of fluid may rapidly restore cerebral perfusion and sustain the patient until a neurosurgeon can repair the shunt.

Diagnostic shunt taps are indicated to determine the presence of either obstruction or infection. Although simple to perform, a shunt tap is a delicate procedure because the introduction of infection into an otherwise sterile system has major consequences. In a spina bifida population, McLone et al. have shown a significant reduction in intelligence in children who have had a shunt infection in comparison to those children who have never had a shunt infection.[19]

Contraindications

Before tapping a shunt, be certain that the child does not have a coagulopathy.[11] In the child who has hemophilia or leukemia or in the child who received a shunt for a malignant tumor and is undergoing either chemotherapy or craniospinal irradiation, document a normal prothrombin time, partial thromboplastin time, and platelet count. If questions regarding platelet function arise, a bleeding time may need to be documented. If the patient's condition permits, correct the coagulopathy before performing the tap.

Finally, in a child with sepsis from an obvious source such as pneumonia or a urinary tract infection, do not perform a shunt tap unless there is strong clinical suspicion. In the child with a shunt for documented communicating hydrocephalus, a lumbar puncture may yield useful information without risking the introduction of infection into the shunt; however, in a small percentage of shunt infections the lumbar CSF may not reflect the infection. In the face of ongoing sepsis, the risk of contaminating a shunt by tapping increases; therefore tapping the shunt is not a routine part of the evaluation for sepsis.

Equipment

The essential items for a shunt tap include a sterile 25-gauge butterfly needle, sterile gloves, sterile collection tubes, sterile gauze, and povidone-iodine solution. For convenience, all of the essential items except the sterile gloves and butterfly needle are included within a disposable pediatric lumbar puncture set.

The plastic dome of the shunt-tapping chamber is made of plastic that reseals itself as long as the needle punctures are no larger than 25 gauge. Larger-bore needles may damage the dome. Do not use lidocaine because it may increase the pain of the procedure. There are two advantages to using a butterfly needle. After needle insertion into the dome, it is possible to collect CSF through the tubing so that the needle does not change position relative to the skin if the child moves. Second, the tubing can be held upright and, by measuring the fluid column within, used as a manometer by which to gauge ICP.

Technique

Shunts come in a variety of shapes and sizes, but it is usually possible to palpate the reservoir under the skin not far from the burr hole. The flushing valve should be easy to depress and should refill within seconds of release. Do not shave the patient's hair to tap the shunt. In fact, several studies have indicated that shaving the hair just before surgery may actually increase the incidence of infection.[29]

Meticulously prepare the skin with alcohol and povidone-iodine solution. Once the preparation is complete, puncture the reservoir, observing meticulous sterile technique (Fig. 81-3). Fluid should flow slowly but spontaneously, and aspiration of the reservoir should not be necessary. If aspiration is necessary, do so only gently.

Once CSF flow begins, connect the Silastic catheter to the needle and hold it vertically to allow measurement of the fluid column, which should have a pulsatile meniscus. Because the shunt valve is at the ventricular level, the patient's

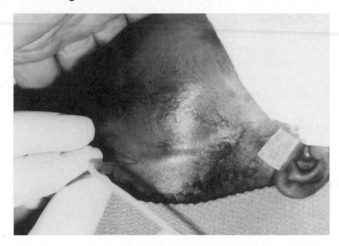

FIG. 81-3   Child undergoing a shunt tap. The hair has been shaved in this case to illustrate the shunt valve visible under the skin.

position is irrelevant. The height of the fluid column should correlate with the ICP. To verify the reliability of the measurement, have the cooperative patient perform Valsalva's maneuver; with the younger child, perform bilateral jugular compression (Queckenstedt's test) and watch for a rise in the meniscus. Two to three ml of fluid should be adequate for a Gram stain, culture and sensitivity, cell count with differential, and glucose and protein measurements. After collecting an adequate sample of fluid, withdraw the needle and maintain pressure with a sterile gauze until all bleeding has stopped.

Complications

If performed properly, the complication rate for a shunt tap is very low. Should no fluid be obtainable with the needle in the proper location, consider a proximal shunt obstruction. Not aspirating forcefully obviates the risk of creating an intraventricular hemorrhage. The major risk of the procedure is introducing infection into the sterile shunt system. If meticulous and proper sterile technique is observed, such a complication should occur in less than 0.5% of cases.[14]

Remarks

It is not uncommon for the child with a shunt malfunction to present with a low-grade fever in addition to irritability and vomiting.[7] If a shunt tap rules out infection, the child's fever may be secondary to malfunction rather than infection.

The interpretation of results following a shunt tap may not always be straightforward. *S. epidermidis* and *Staphylococcus aureus* are by far the most common organisms to infect a shunt. If a Gram stain demonstrates gram-positive cocci, a skin contaminant is not likely. On the other hand, the presence of coagulase-negative staphylococci on one 5-day subculture in the absence of associated CSF abnormalities *is* likely to represent a contaminant.

CSF flow is not a reliable means of determining shunt malfunction. The majority of shunt malfunctions result from proximal obstruction of the ventricular catheter by choroid plexus. A partial but high-grade obstruction may yield CSF at a slow rate, thereby giving false-negative results. The feel of the shunt during pumping is also notoriously unreliable.[21] A reliable mother's opinion or a computerized tomography scan of the ventricles is much more useful under such circumstances and does not risk infecting the shunt. At present, surgical exploration remains the gold standard for determining shunt patency.

EVACUATION OF SUBDURAL COLLECTIONS

Chronic collections of fluid in the subdural space are most common in children less than 2 years of age.[2] At this age, the cranial sutures are not fused and will separate under chronic pressure, allowing the typical presentation of macrocephaly, often with few associated symptoms. These subdural collections are most often a result of one of two causes. They follow trauma, with the fluid being typical of a chronic subdural hematoma,[6,20] or they occur as a postmeningitic effusion. If this effusion remains infected, it is a subdural empyema.

Indications

Subdural fluid accumulations require tapping for two reasons. First, for the child with progressive macrocephaly and neurologic compromise, the tap is therapeutic. Withdrawing fluid relieves the intracranial hypertension and helps resolve the subdural collection. Second, although postinfectious effusions often resolve spontaneously, a tap may be necessary to differentiate between a sterile effusion and empyema. A sterile effusion has normal or mildly xanthochromic fluid with a lymphocytosis, whereas empyema appears cloudy, contains polymorphonuclear leukocytes, and often has a positive Gram stain.

In the child who comes to the hospital with the question of nonaccidental trauma, on rare occasions a subdural fluid collection may require sampling for medicolegal reasons.

Contraindications

The contraindications for evacuating subdural collections are basically the same as for tapping a shunt. Additionally, in a child with a thin subdural collection (less than 0.5 cm), weigh the risk of inadvertent laceration of the cortex relative to the benefit of sampling the fluid. It is unlikely that such a minimal collection can cause neurologic deterioration in a child with open sutures; consider a primary brain insult instead.

Finally, as with other invasive procedures, the presence of a coagulopathy is a relative contraindication to subdural collection.

Complications

The complication rate from tapping a subdural collection of fluid is minimal.[22] Even if a bridging vein is punctured, it should stop bleeding before a significant accumulation forms if a small-bore needle has been used. If sterile technique is used and the patient is not bacteremic, there is little risk of introducing infection.

Minimize the risk of lacerating the brain by having an assistant hold the infant securely and by holding the needle immobile relative to the child's skull while withdrawing fluid from the tubing. In addition, infiltrate the scalp and periosteum with a small amount of lidocaine with epinephrine before the procedure.

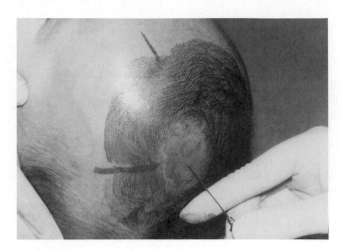

FIG. 81-4 Infant in the supine position undergoing percutaneous drainage of a chronic subdural hematoma. The lines mark the sagittal and coronal sutures, through which the needle passes just lateral to the anterior fontanelle. Direct the needle toward the ipsilateral lateral canthus.

Equipment

The setup contained in a disposable pediatric lumbar puncture kit is ideal. The kit contains sterile needles, lidocaine, sponges, gauze, and a basin for povidone-iodine solution. The only additional items necessary are sterile gloves. Use a 20- to 22-gauge needle with a needle stylet. An advantage to the teflon intravenous catheter set is that the rigid stylet can be withdrawn after placement, leaving in place only the soft plastic outer sleeve to minimize the risk of brain injury.

Technique

Begin the procedure with proper restraint and positioning of the infant (Fig. 81-4). Although preprocedural sedation is optional, it is best to avoid it in the child in whom postprocedural neurologic assessment is desirable. If sedation or analgesia is necessary, use short-acting, reversible agents such as midazolam and fentanyl.

Wrap the infant in a sheet or place him or her on a papoose board with an assistant holding the head in the supine position. Prepare the scalp over the anterior fontanelle and coronal sutures with alcohol and povidone-iodine. Do not shave the hair unless it is of sufficient thickness to obscure landmarks. Do not place towels over the infant's face. Infiltrate the skin just behind the coronal suture with a small amount of lidocaine and insert the needle 0.5 cm behind the coronal suture. Direct the needle 45 degrees laterally relative to the midline. After reaching the coronal suture, pass the needle through the suture at an oblique angle. The dura is a tough membrane and will give as the needle passes through it, similar to the sensation felt when performing a lumbar puncture. Remove the stylet and collect fluid (Fig. 81-5). When spontaneous flow ceases, withdraw the needle and apply pressure to the scalp with a sterile gauze until the bleeding stops.

Remarks

Allow for the spontaneous egress of subdural fluid. Avoid aspiration with a syringe, if possible, because using one may

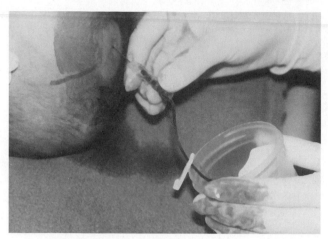

FIG. 81-5 Spontaneous drainage of a chronic subdural hematoma. Connect a 20-gauge teflon intravenous catheter to sterile extension tubing, which allows the fluid to be collected into a sterile container for analysis.

injure the cortex or bridging veins. If fluid flow is sluggish, mild manual pressure on the anterior fontanelle may raise the ICP sufficiently to improve flow. Gentle abdominal compression by the assistant may also hasten the flow. On rare occasions, fluid may continue to leak from the puncture site following needle withdrawal. A long subcutaneous needle tract helps prevent such a complication. Should it occur, painting the puncture site with nonflexible collodion may prevent leakage. If not, oversew the puncture site with a fine suture (e.g., 6-0 Prolene).

BURR HOLES

Even when inhouse neurosurgical services are available, the benefit of draining acute subdural or epidural hematomas in the ED or pediatric intensive care unit (PICU) is unclear.[5,14,16,28] Most studies agree that the patient who has a Glasgow Coma Scale score of 3 or who presents with ipsilateral pupillary dilation and contralateral hemiparesis has a poor prognosis for functional survival despite all efforts.[4,12,23] In light of these data, the nonneurosurgeon must consider realistic indications for performing this procedure under such conditions. Neuronal ischemic time is less than 5 minutes; even in the hands of an accomplished neurosurgeon, it takes longer than 5 minutes to set up equipment and to create burr holes. Therefore begin therapy with hyperventilation, mannitol, and furosemide. This procedure allows for a less hasty, more organized creation of the burr holes, which minimizes technical errors that cause brain injury.

Indications

The only indication for emergent burr holes is a rapidly expanding subdural or epidural hematoma that is unresponsive to hyperventilation, mannitol, and furosemide in a neurologically deteriorating patient. A traumatic hematoma may be intraparenchymal, epidural, or subdural. The clinical presentations of these hematomas are similar and include obtundation, localizing neurologic signs such as ipsilateral pupillary dilation and contralateral hemiparesis, and signs of local head trauma (e.g., scalp damage, swelling). The clinical presentation of an epidural hematoma often is one of a head injury and an initial lucid interval followed by progressive deterioration in the level of consciousness.[28]

Contraindications

The only absolute contraindication to burr-hole drainage is a coagulopathy, which may exist either premorbidly or may be the consequence of a severe brain injury. Make this judgment on the basis of oozing from puncture sites and other clinical signs suggestive of a coagulation disorder, because laboratory confirmation is usually not possible in the brief time frame. Relative contraindications to burr holes include the inability to treat the potential complications of burr-hole drainage associated with brain laceration or hemorrhage (i.e., the absence of a surgeon or person skilled in surgical hemostasis).

Complications

The worst possible complication of burr-hole drainage is that of plunging into the brain with the drill, which can either contuse or lacerate the underlying tissue. Uncontrollable bleeding may also occur either from the superficial temporal artery in the scalp or from the intracranial space if the procedure damages the middle meningeal artery or cortical surface vessels.

Equipment

Required equipment for burr-hole drainage includes a basic set of scalpels, hemostats, self-retaining retractors, tissue forceps, needle holders, and suture material. Suction, electrocautery, and a headlight are useful, and antibiotic irrigation solution for use before closure is advisable. Additional specialized equipment includes a Hudson brace and bit set, bone wax, a small straight curette (0 or 00 size) and a Penfield #3 dissector.

Technique

Stabilize the patient's head in the lateral position. Stabilization may require placement of a small roll under one shoulder. Rule out fractures or dislocations of the cervical spine before rotating the neck. If it is not possible to assess the cervical spine adequately, place the burr hole with the head in a neutral position. Ideally, place an emergency burr hole as a prelude to a formal craniotomy; therefore plan the incision to coincide with the subsequent craniotomy incision (Fig. 81-6, *A*).

Orient the scalp opening for the burr hole vertically just anterior to the ear and extending superiorly from the zygomatic arch 3 to 5 cm (Fig. 81-6, *B*). Infiltration of the scalp with 1% lidocaine containing epinephrine before draping decreases scalp bleeding. The incision should penetrate the entire scalp and underlying temporalis muscle. Use a small periosteal elevator or the back of a scalpel handle to dissect the temporalis musculature away from the underlying temporal bone, and insert a self-retaining retractor. The incision and exposure need only be large enough to insert the bit and allow visualization.

The bit used for the creation of burr holes is similar to a standard fluted twist drill that has been modified slightly; this modification decreases the likelihood of plunging into the

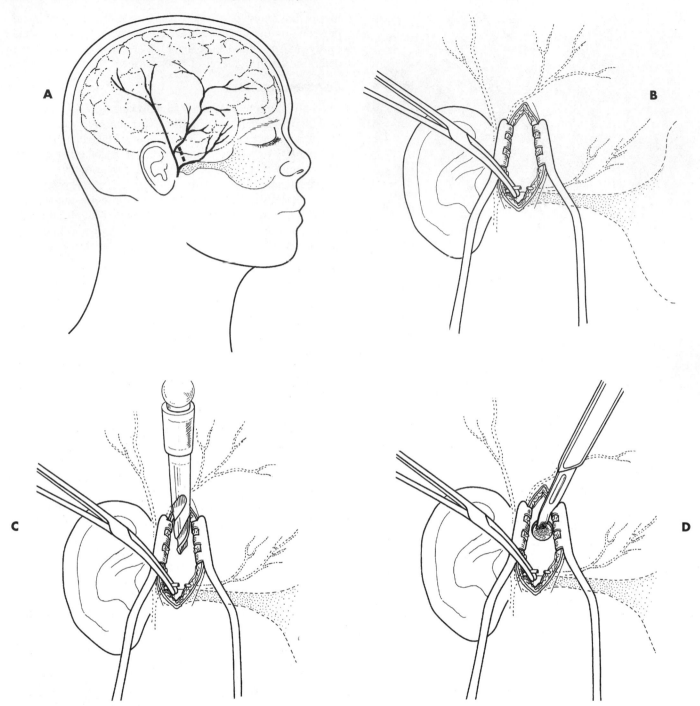

FIG. 81-6   Creation of burr holes. **A,** Turn the patient's head into the lateral position only after evaluating the cervical spine. The heavy dashed line represents the skin incision. Avoid the superficial temporal artery, which lies just beneath the skin with a palpable pulse. **B,** The skin incision is made through the scalp, through the temporalis muscle, and down to the bone. If there is bleeding from the superficial temporal artery, control it with a hemostat. **C,** Use a Hudson brace and fluted bit to create a burr hole. Take care not to plunge into the brain as the drill passes through the inner table of the bone. An epidural hematoma will evacuate once the inner table is open. **D,** After waxing the bleeding bone edges, coagulate and incise the dura, allowing the acute subdural hematoma to drain.

brain by tapering the distal third of the bit to create a slight "shoulder." This shoulder allows the tip of the bit to penetrate the inner table while preventing the rest of the bit from plunging. Monitor actual penetration either visually or tactilely, keeping in mind that the skull has an inner and outer table of hard cortical bone with a diploic space of cancellous bone. These layers are indistinct in younger persons, and frequent inspection is necessary as the bit penetrates the last of the inner table. In some individuals, the temporal squama can be very thin. Once the dura is visible, use a small, straight curette to remove the remaining thin shell of bone overlying the dura. Control bleeding from within the bone itself by applying bone wax to the fresh bone edges. If any epidural hematoma is present, it should evacuate spontaneously (Fig. 81-6, *C*).

If a bipolar electrocautery unit is available, coagulate the exposed dura to help control dural bleeding. If a unipolar (Bovie) electrocautery unit is available, place a hemostat, forceps, or scalpel blade in contact with the dura and make contact with the metal instrument to coagulate the dura. After coagulating the dura, incise it sharply in a cruciate pattern. The subdural hematoma should drain (Fig. 81-6, *D*). Facilitate this by placing a Penfield #3 dissector on the surface of the brain and gently depressing the cortex 2 to 4 mm below the dura and circumferentially around the burr hole. This procedure allows expression of more subdural blood by preventing the brain from obstructing the burr hole.

Remarks

Injecting epinephrine-containing solutions into the incision line reduces scalp bleeding if there is time for the vasoconstrictive actions of epinephrine to take effect. Laceration of a branch of the superficial temporal artery is common in the process of making the initial incision. Rather than spending time trying to ligate this artery, clamp it with a hemostat and continue with the procedure.

A middle cranial fossa epidural hematoma often underlies a skull fracture. When using a brace and bit near a fracture line, be aware that the inner table of bone may be comminuted. In such cases, the inner table of bone gives way with penetration of the outer table of bone, which causes the drill to plunge unexpectedly.

Do not allow minor distractions such as absolute scalp hemostasis, perfect placement of retractors, or other inconsequential "style points" slow the ultimate goal of evacuating the epidural or subdural hematoma.

REFERENCES

1. Aldrich EF, Harmann P: Disconnection as a cause of ventriculoperitoneal shunt malfunction in multicomponent shunt systems, *Pediatr Neurosurg* 16(6):287-291, 1991.
2. Alexander E, Jr: Chronic subdural hematoma in children. In Apuzzo MLJ, editor: *Brain surgery: complication avoidance and management*, vol 2, London, 1993, Churchill Livingstone.
3. Ammirati M, Anthony JR: Cerebrospinal fluid shunt infection in children: a study on the relationship between the etiology of hydrocephalus, age at the time of shunt placement and infection rate, *Childs Nerv Syst* 3:106-109, 1987.
4. Andrews BT, Ross AM, Pitts, LH: Surgical exploration before computed tomography scanning in children with traumatic tentorial herniation, *Surg Neurol* 32:434-438, 1989.
5. Andrews BT, Pitts LH: Functional recovery after traumatic transtentorial herniation, *Neurosurgery* 30(3):462, 1992.
6. Aoki N: Chronic subdural hematoma in infancy: clinical analysis of 30 cases in the CT era, *J Neurosurg* 73(2):201-205, 1990.
7. Ashkenazi E, Umansky F, Constantini S, et al: Fever as the initial sign of malfunction in noninfected ventriculoperitoneal shunts, *Acta Neurochir (Wein)* 114(3-4):131-134, 1992.
8. Camarata PJ, Haines SJ: Ventriculoatrial shunting. In Wilkins RH, Rengachary SS, editors: *Neurosurgical operative atlas,* Baltimore, 1991, Williams & Wilkins.
9. Choux M, Lorenzo G, Lang D, et al: Shunt implantation: reducing the incidence of shunt infection, *J Neurosurg* 77:875-880, 1992.
10. Cutler RPW: The cerebrospinal fluid. In Swash M, Kennard C, editors: *The scientific basis of clinical neurology,* London, 1985, Churchill Livingstone.
11. de Tezano Pinto M, Fernandez J, Perez Bianco PR, et al: Update of 156 episodes of central nervous system bleeding in hemophiliacs, *Haemostasis* 22(5):259-267, 1992.
12. Ersahin, Y, Mutleur S, Guzelbag E: Extradural hematoma: analysis of 146 cases, *Childs Nerv Syst* 9:96-99, 1993.
13. Hartwell RC, Sutton LN: Mannitol, intracranial pressure, and vasogenic edema, *Neurosurgery* 32(3):444-450, 1992.
14. Johnson DL, Duma C, Sivit C: The role of immediate operative intervention in severely head-injured children with a Glasgow Coma Scale score of 3, *Neurosurgery* 30(3):320-324, 1992.
15. Konty U, Hofling B, Gutjahr P, et al: CSF shunt infections in children, *Infection* 21(2):89-92, 1993.
16. Mahoney BD, Rockswold GL, Ruiz E, et al: Emergency twist drill trepanation, *Neurosurgery* 8:551-554, 1981.
17. Intracranial pressure concepts. In Marshall SB, Marshall LF, Vos HR, et al, editors: *Neuroscience critical care: pathophysiology and patient management,* Philadelphia, 1990, WB Saunders.
18. McCullough DC: Ventriculoperitoneal shunting. In Wilkins RH, Rengachary SS, editors: *Neurosurgical operative atlas,* vol 2, Baltimore, 1991, Williams & Wilkins.
19. McLone DG, Czyzewski D, Raimondi AJ, et al: Central nervous system infections as a limiting factor in the intelligence of children with myelomeningocele, *Pediatrics* 70(3):338-342, 1982.
20. Parent AD: Pediatric chronic subdural hematoma: a retrospective comparative analysis, *Pediatr Neurosurg* 18:266-271, 1992.
21. Piatt JH, Jr: Physical examination of patients with cerebrospinal fluid shunts: is there useful information in pumping the shunt? *Pediatrics* 89(3):470-473, 1992.
22. Rekatc HL: Shunt revision: complications and their prevention, *Pediatr Neurosurg* 17:155-162, 1991-1992.
23. Renier D, Lacombe J, Pierre-Kahn A, et al: Factors causing acute shunt infection: computer analysis of 1174 operations, *J Neurosurg* 61:1072-1078, 1984.
24. Sainte-Rose C, Piatt JH, Renier D, et al: Mechanical complications in shunts, *Pediatr Neurosurg* 17(1):2-9, 1991-1992.
25. Shurtleff DB, Stuntz JT, Hayden PW: Experience with 1201 cerebrospinal fluid shunt procedures, *Pediatr Neurosci* 12:49-57, 1985-1986.
26. Tzekov C, Cherninkova S, Gudeva T: Neuroophthalmological symptoms in children treated for internal hydrocephalus, *Pediatr Neurosurg* 17(6):317-320, 1991-1992.
27. Vilalta J, Rubio E, Castano CH, et al: Severe craniocerebral injuries with a lucid interval, *Neurologia* 8(2):49-52, 1993.
28. Wilberger JE, Jr, Harris M, Diamond DL: Acute subdural hematoma: morbidity, mortality, and operative timing, *J Neurosurg* 74(2):212-218, 1991.
29. Winston KR: Hair and neurosurgery, *Neurosurgery* 31(2):320-329, 1992.

82 Intracranial Pressure Monitoring

Mark W. Uhl

Elevation of intracranial pressure (ICP) is a common problem for many patients in the Emergency Department (ED) and pediatric intensive care unit (PICU). Causes of increased ICP may be primary, such as in head trauma, central nervous system (CNS) infections, CNS tumors, perinatal intracranial hemorrhage, acute hydrocephalus, ventriculoperitoneal shunt malfunction and obstruction; or secondary, as with metabolic, toxic, or hypoxemic-ischemic encephalopathies. Along with decreased cerebral blood flow, increased ICP remains one of the major factors in morbidity and mortality following CNS injury.[1,12,14,28] Increased ICP that results in CNS ischemia may occur hours to days after the initial insult and is a component of secondary brain injury.[3,9,23] The goal of ICP monitoring is to detect significant increases in ICP and to intervene appropriately to prevent secondary CNS injury as a result of compromised cerebral perfusion or herniation. ICP measurement, recording, and control are thus key elements in the management of patients in the PICU with serious neurologic injuries.

The skull should be considered as a closed space that contains three minimally compressible components: neuronal and supportive tissue (brain parenchyma), which accounts for approximately 80% of the intracranial volume, and blood and cerebrospinal fluid (CSF), each of which account for approximately 10% of the intracranial space. The addition of intracranial volume from a hematoma, a tumor, parenchymal edema, or an obstruction of CSF drainage causes an increase in ICP unless there is a compensatory decrease in volume from one of the other components. Usually this compensation occurs by shifting CSF to the spinal canal (assuming no obstruction to flow) or by cerebral vasoconstriction that reduces intracranial blood volume. After these compensatory mechanisms have been exhausted, further increases in intracranial volume cause a dramatic increase in ICP.[1,15]

Physical examination may not confirm the presence of elevated ICP. The classic triad of systemic arterial hypertension, bradycardia, and irregular respiratory effort (Cushing's triad) is a *variable* finding in children and occurs after ICP has reached life-threatening levels. Earlier signs suggesting the possibility of increased ICP include an impaired or deteriorating level of consciousness, abnormal posturing in response to stimulation, unilateral or bilateral pupil dilation, and papilledema. In infants, there may be bulging fontanelles and widened cranial sutures.[29] Unfortunately, such findings are not always present or may occur late in the development of significant intracranial hypertension. For these reasons and to allow early recognition and intervention, use ICP monitoring with seriously injured children for whom other forms of monitoring are not available or appropriate.

Indications

Indications for ICP monitoring include the following: (1) traumatic coma (Glasgow Coma Scale score ≤ 7), (2) a known intracranial pathologic condition in a setting in which it is not possible to monitor the neurologic examination adequately (e.g., general anesthesia in the operating room or sedative, analgesic, or muscle relaxant use in the PICU), (3) intracranial tumor with significant mass effect and altered level of consciousness, and (4) following evacuation of a mass lesion (especially traumatic hematoma). ICP monitoring may also guide management of metabolic encephalopathies (e.g., Reye's syndrome or diabetic ketoacidosis), hepatic encephalopathy, meningitis, and encephalitis.[15,29] ICP monitoring is rarely useful in severe hypoxemic-ischemic injury (e.g., near-drowning or other forms of asphyxiation) because the cerebral edema ("cytotoxic" edema) and increased ICP that results after these injuries reflects the inevitable progression of the initial anoxic insult. Unfortunately, patient outcome rarely improves by monitoring and aggressively treating elevated ICP in this setting.[4,29] ICP measurements may have some prognostic value after severe hypoxemic-ischemic injury; however, prognostic data are often available using less invasive methods such as evoked potentials.[10,11,30]

Contraindications

Specific contraindications to ventricular catheter placement include coagulopathy (prothrombin time >16 seconds or a platelet count <40,000/ml) or an inability to insert the catheter into the ventricle because of cerebral swelling or mass effect, which results in slitlike or effaced ventricles.[18]

A relative contraindication is hypoxemia-ischemia, for which knowledge or manipulation of the ICP does not alter outcome. The relative advantages and disadvantages of the different types of monitoring devices are discussed in the following paragraphs.

Complications

Risks associated with the ventricular catheter technique include infection and hemorrhage. Bacterial contamination from the scalp incision and/or craniotomy may result in ventriculitis or meningitis.[2,16] The risk of infection can be reduced significantly by tunneling the catheter in a subcutaneous position, similar to the technique used for surgically placed indwelling central venous catheters.[8] Some authors recommend replacing the ventricular catheter after 5 days; however, frequent monitoring of CSF profiles and Gram stains may obviate the need for an arbitrary schedule of catheter replacement. Hemorrhage, primarily from injury to cortical vessels during placement of the monitoring device, occurs in less than 2% of the cases.[20] Ventriculostomy causes injury to neurons along the catheter tract, but placement rarely causes any neurologic deficit.

Equipment

The two major types of ICP monitors are fluid-coupled devices with remote pressure transducers and fiberoptic or electronically coupled direct-pressure sensors (transducer-tipped catheters). Zero fluid-coupled devices at the level of the ventricular system, and they must remain in that position relative to the patient. Zero the direct pressure sensors at the time of insertion; their position relative to the patient does not affect the reading. Another distinction among monitors is the intracranial site used to monitor ICP.

Ventricular Catheter. The ventricular catheter (ventriculostomy) is the gold standard of ICP monitoring. It is a relatively simple device (a hollow, fluid-filled catheter) that the neurosurgeon inserts into the lateral ventricle to enable measurement of CSF pressure (ICP) at the transducer. Advantages of a ventriculostomy include the ability to drain CSF to reduce ICP, the ability to assess intracranial compliance by volume-pressure determinations, and easy ventricular access for the delivery of drugs such as antibiotics.[1,13,14,24]

Subdural and Subarachnoid Screws or Bolts. There are many variations in design for the subdural or subarachnoid bolt.[17,18,27] Placement of a bolt requires less technical precision than a ventriculostomy and because there is no penetration of the brain parenchyma, the risk of infection, hemorrhage, or traumatic edema is reduced.[27] Significant disadvantages include the inability to drain CSF to treat elevated ICP, the frequency of occlusion of subarachnoid devices, and the tendency to underestimate the true ICP. Underestimation of ICP is most common (and most worrisome) when ICP is significantly elevated.[17] Another drawback is the inability to use the subarachnoid devices in infants because their thin skulls do not allow sufficient stabilization of the monitoring device.

Fiberoptic Transducers. Fiberoptic transducers are pressure transducers that use fiberoptic technology to sense changes in light as reflected by a pressure-sensitive diaphragm in the catheter tip. A major advantage of these transducers is the flexibility of placing these catheters in any of several intracranial locations, including epidural, subdural, subarachnoid, ventricular, and intraparenchymal sites. The catheter does not require recalibration or rezeroing after initial calibration and insertion. The closed system also poses less risk of infection.[6,26] The major disadvantage is the inability to withdraw CSF, but one company has addressed this problem by combining the fiberoptic pressure transducer with a hollow ventricular catheter (Camino Laboratories Models 110-4H and 110-4HM, San Diego, Calif.).

Technique

Only a qualified neurosurgeon using standard surgical procedure should perform a ventriculostomy. The specific technique may vary. See Box 82-1 for equipment and supplies. When possible, place the catheter in the nondominant hemisphere (usually the right hemisphere). Place the patient in the supine position and immobilize the head. Shave the head and prepare it using sterile technique, and infiltrate the skin using 1% lidocaine with epinephrine. Make two transverse scalp incisions (Fig. 82-1). Make one incision anterior to the coronal suture (located in the coronal plane at

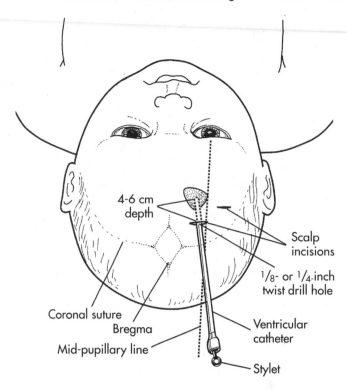

FIG. 82-1   Positioning of patient for placement of ventricular catheter (see text).

the auditory meatus) and in line with the ipsilateral pupil (2 to 4 cm from midline). Make the twist-drill craniotomy at this site. Puncture the dura carefully with a needle. If using a stabilizing bolt (Camino system),* use care not to strip the threads (skull thickness is 2 to 3 mm in neonates, 3 to 5 mm in children, and 5 to 10 mm in adults). Insert the ventricular catheter with stylet through the bolt and into the ventricle by directing the tip toward the medial canthus of the ipsilateral eye. Orient it in the coronal plane at the external auditory meatus or as indicated by the location of the lateral ventricle on a computed tomography (CT) scan (Fig. 82-2). After entering the ventricle and obtaining CSF, remove the stylet and cap the catheter (Fig. 82-3). Slide the compression cap and secure the bolt.* If not using a stabilizing bolt system, use a stylet or ventricular needle to cannulate the lateral ventricle with the ventriculostomy catheter. With the stylet in the catheter, insert it into the ventricle. Tunnel the proximal end of the ventricular catheter below the dermis (above the galea) from the incision to a separate incision at least 2.5 cm away (Fig. 82-4). Suture the incisions and use an additional stitch to secure the catheter to the scalp.[8,25] Connect the catheter to the appropriate pressure tubing, stopcock, fluid-collecting system (external ventricular drain), and transducer. Zero the system as appropriate for the device (zero the fiberoptic devices *before* insertion). Confirm proper placement by noting a nondampened waveform (Fig. 82-5) with appropriate cardiac and respiratory cycle variations.[1]

---

*Ventricular Bolt Pressure Monitoring Kit Model 110-4H or 110-4HM (micro); Camino Laboratories, 5955 Pacific Center Blvd, San Diego, CA 92121.

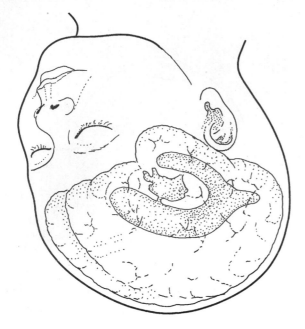

FIG. 82-2 Orientation of the lateral ventricle.

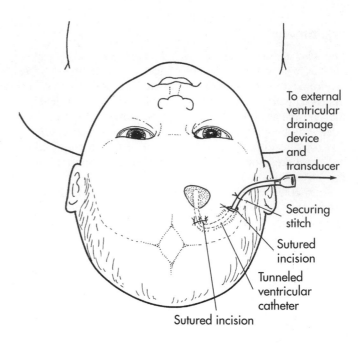

FIG. 82-4 Tunneled catheter ready for attachment to pressure tranducer.

To external ventricular drainage device and transducer

Securing stitch

Sutured incision

Tunneled ventricular catheter

Sutured incision

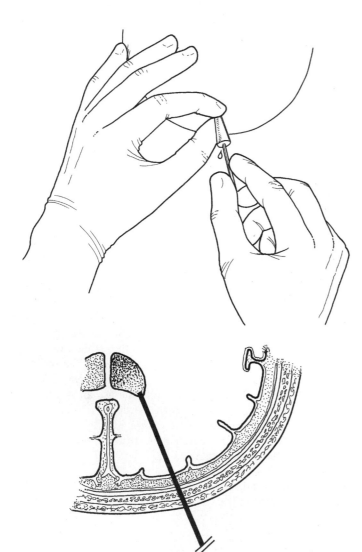

FIG. 82-3 Catheter tip in proper position in lateral ventricle with return of CSF.

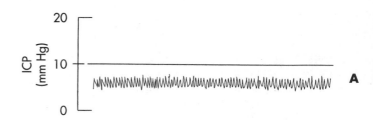

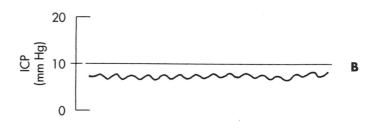

Cardiac cycle variation

Respiratory cycle variation

0 mm Hg

C

FIG. 82-5 Normal pulsatile ICP waveform with cardiac and respiratory variations. **A,** High chart recorder speed illustrates cardiac cycle variations. **B,** Slower speed shows respiratory cycle variations. **C,** ICP waveform during one respiratory cycle.

(Modified from Marmarou A, Tabaddor K: Intracranial pressure: physiology and pathophysiology. In Cooper PR, editor: *Head injury,* Baltimore, 1982, Williams & Wilkins.)

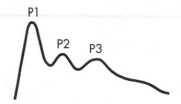

FIG. 82-6   Normal ICP wave with three components: the percussion wave (P_1), the tidal wave (P_2), and the dicrotic wave (P_3).

(Modified from Cardoso ER, Rowan JO, Galbraith S: Analysis of the cerebrospinal fluid pulse wave in intracranial pressure, *J Neurosurg* 59:817-821, 1983.)

Interpretation

The ICP waveform itself has several distinct components.[5] The main wave (P_1 or percussion wave) represents transmitted arterial pulsation from the intracranial arteries and choroid plexus (Fig. 82-6). The second component (P_2 or tidal wave) reflects intracranial compliance. It becomes more prominent as the brain becomes stiff (Fig. 82-7); it diminishes with hyperventilation or other maneuvers that reduce cerebral blood volume.[21] The third component (P_3 or dicrotic wave), represents venous pulsations and changes with variation in intrathoracic pressure. Normal ICP is less than 10 mm Hg.

Pathologic waveforms include the plateau wave (Fig. 82-8), which is a significant and sustained elevation in ICP above an elevated baseline. Plateau waves occur in the setting of decreased intracranial compliance and elevated ICP. They occur following decrements in systemic blood pressure and cerebral perfusion pressure (CPP) (CPP = mean arterial blood pressure − ICP). Plateau waves occur as a result of increased cerebral blood volume (intact autoregulation causing vasodilation), and they resolve when CPP increases above threshold (usually 70 to 80 mm Hg in adults). Plateau waves may last 5 to 20 minutes and are an ominous prognostic sign.[7,21]

Remarks

The foremost goal of patient management on the basis of ICP monitoring is to prevent secondary injury to the brain. The focus of routine intensive-care monitoring is on avoiding hypotension, hypoxemia, hypercarbia, and increased cerebral metabolism (fever, seizures, pain, and agitation). Avoid cerebral ischemic injury by maintaining an adequate cerebral perfusion pressure. Recent evidence suggests that efforts to raise CPP to at least 70 to 80 mm Hg may have beneficial results on outcome after traumatic brain injury.[22] A step-by-step algorithm may be appropriate if sustained ICP above 15 mm Hg continues to be a problem. The initial intervention is sedation with narcotics plus neuromuscular blockade to allow mechanical control of ventilation. The desired Pco_2 is 35 ± 2 mm Hg. Prolonged hyperventilation to low Pco_2 values may be detrimental.[19] If the ICP remains elevated, drain CSF to reduce the ICP to 10 mm Hg. If drainage fails to control ICP, give mannitol (0.25 to 1.0 g/kg). Administer repeated doses of mannitol until the serum osmolarity reaches 320 mOsm/L. The goal of fluid management and osmotic therapy is hypertonic euvolemia.

For intractable intracranial hypertension or signs of acute herniation, a repeat CT scan is mandatory to rule out a surgical mass lesion. If no surgical mass exists, hyperventilation to a Pco_2 of 30 mm Hg is an appropriate next intervention. If hyperventilation fails to control ICP, consider undertaking cerebral metabolic suppression with etomidate or barbiturates (phenobarbital or pentobarbital). Mild hypo-

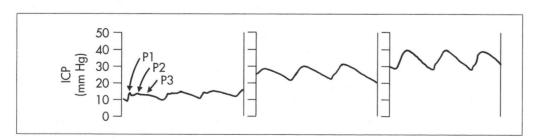

FIG. 82-7   Change in shape of the ICP waveform with reduced brain compliance. Note elevation of the P_2 and P_3 components as the ICP increases.

(Modified from Cardoso ER, Rowan JO, Galbraith S: Analysis of the cerebrospinal fluid pulse wave in intracranial pressure, *J Neurosurg* 59:817-821, 1983.)

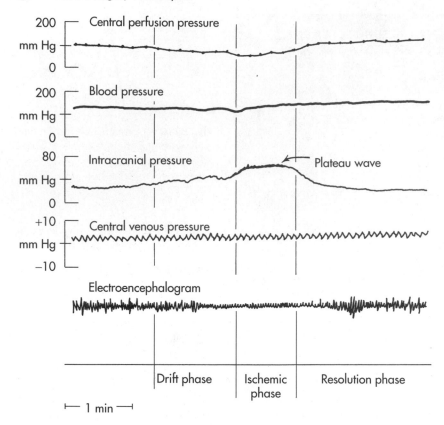

FIG. 82-8 Pathologic ICP plateau wave and its relationship to changes in blood pressure, central venous pressure, and cerebral perfusion pressure.

(Modified from Rosner MJ, Becker DP: Origin and evolution of plateau waves: experimental observations and a theoretical model, *J Neurosurg* 60:312-324, 1984.)

thermia to a core temperature of 90° F to 92° F also suppresses CNS metabolism. Experimental drug therapies under investigation include superoxide anion and free-radical scavengers, 21-aminosteroids, gangliosides, high-dose corticosteroids, and excitatory neurotransmitter receptor–blocking agents.

REFERENCES

1. Allen R: Intracranial pressure: a review of clinical problems, measurement techniques and monitoring methods, *J Med Eng Technol* 10:299-320, 1986.
2. Aucoin PJ, Kotilainen HR, Gantz NM, et al: Intracranial pressure monitors: epidemiologic study of risk factors and infections, *Am J Med* 80:369-376, 1986.
3. Becker DP, Miller JD, Ward JD, et al: The outcome from severe head injury with early diagnosis and intensive management, *J Neurosurg* 47:491-502, 1977.
4. Bohn DJ, Biggar WD, Smith CR, et al: Influence of hypothermia, barbiturate therapy, and intracranial pressure monitoring on morbidity and mortality after near-drowning, *Crit Care Med* 14:529-534, 1986.
5. Cardoso ER, Rowan JO, Galbraith S: Analysis of the cerebrospinal fluid pulse wave in intracranial pressure, *J Neurosurg* 59:817-821, 1983.
6. Crutchfield JS, Narayan RK, Robertson CS, et al: Evaluation of a fiberoptic intracranial pressure monitor, *J Neurosurg* 72:482-487, 1990.
7. Dean JM, Moss SD: Intracranial hypertension. In Fuhrman BP, Zimmerman JJ, editors: *Pediatric critical care*, St Louis, 1992, Mosby.
8. Friedman WA, Vries JK: Percutaneous tunnel ventriculostomy: summary of 100 procedures, *J Neurosurg* 53:662-665, 1980.
9. Fruin AH, Taylon C: Intracranial monitoring in patients with head trauma, *Surg Annu* 23:225-237, 1991.
10. Goitein KJ, Amit Y, Fainmesser P, Sohmer H: Diagnostic and prognostic value of auditory nerve brainstem evoked responses in comatose children, *Crit Care Med* 11:91-94, 1983.
11. Goodwin SR, Friedman WA, Bellefleur M: Is it time to use evoked potentials to predict outcome in comatose children and adults? *Crit Care Med* 19:518-524, 1991.
12. Langfitt TW, Gennarelli TA: Can the outcome from head injury be improved? *J Neurosurg* 56:19-25, 1982.
13. Leggate JR, Minns RA: Intracranial pressure monitoring: current methods. In Minns RA, editor: *Clinics in developmental medicine: problems of intracranial pressure in childhood*, Oxford, 1991, McKeith Press.
14. Lehman LB: Intracranial pressure monitoring and treatment: a contemporary view, *Ann Emerg Med* 19:295-303, 1990.
15. Marshall WK: Intracranial pressure. In Lake CL, editor: *Clinical monitoring*, Philadelphia, 1990, WB Saunders.
16. Mayhall CG, Archer NH, Lamb VA, et al: Ventriculostomy-related infections, *N Engl J Med* 310:553-559, 1984.
17. Mendelow AD, Rowan JO, Murray L, et al: A clinical comparison of subdural screw pressure measurements with ventricular pressure, *J Neurosurg* 58:45-50, 1983.
18. Mollman HD, Rockswold GL, Ford SE: A clinical comparison of subarachnoid catheters to ventriculostomy and subarachnoid bolts: a prospective study, *J Neurosurg* 68:737-741, 1988.
19. Muizelaar JP, Marmarou A, Ward JD, et al: Adverse effects of prolonged

hyperventilation in patients with severe head injury: a randomized clinical trial, *J Neurosurg* 75:731-739, 1991.

20. Narayan RK, Kishore PR, Becker DP, et al: Intracranial pressure: to monitor or not to monitor? *J Neurosurg* 56:650-659, 1982.

21. Rosner MJ, Becker DP: Origin and evolution of plateau waves: experimental observations and a theoretical model, *J Neurosurg* 60:312-324, 1984.

22. Rosner MJ, Coley IB: Cerebral perfusion pressure, intracranial pressure, and head elevation, *J Neurosurg* 65:636-641, 1986.

23. Saul TG, Ducker TB: Effect of intracranial pressure monitoring and aggressive treatment on mortality in severe head injury, *J Neurosurg* 56:498-503, 1982.

24. Shapiro K, Marmarou A, Shulman K: Characterization of clinical CSF dynamics and neural axis compliance using the pressure-volume index. I. The normal pressure-volume index, *Ann Neurol* 7:508-514, 1980.

25. Shillito J: *An atlas of pediatric neurosurgical operations,* Philadelphia, 1982, WB Saunders.

26. Sundbärg G, Nordström C, Messeter K, et al: A comparison of intraparenchymatous and intraventricular pressure recording in clinical practice, *J Neurosurg* 67:841-845, 1987.

27. Vries JK, Becker DP, Young HF: A subarachnoid screw for monitoring intracranial pressure: technical note, *J Neurosurg* 39:416-419, 1973.

28. Woster PS, LeBlanc KL: Management of elevated intracranial pressure, *Clin Pharm* 9:762-772, 1990.

29. Yatsiv I: Central nervous system evaluation and monitoring. In Holbrook PR, editor: *Textbook of pediatric critical care,* Philadelphia, 1993, WB Saunders.

30. Zentner J, Rohde V: The prognostic value of somatosensory and motor evoked potentials in comatose patients, *Neurosurgery* 31:429-434, 1992.

83 Doppler Evaluation of Cerebral Circulation

Joanna J. Seibert

High-resolution ultrasonography (US) that uses the anterior fontanelle as a window exquisitely depicts the intracranial contents of the newborn. The fine detail of high-resolution US and the portability of this bedside technique has made neurosonography the major imaging modality of the critically ill newborn. Continuous-wave and pulsed-duplex Doppler monitoring of cerebral circulation in the neonate through the anterior fontanelle are accepted methods of evaluating for brain death, asphyxia, cerebral edema, patent ductus arteriosus (PDA), hydrocephalus, arteriovenous malformations, and extracorporeal membrane oxygenation (ECMO) stability.[2,8,11,16]

Ultrasonographers most often study the anterior cerebral, internal carotid, and middle cerebral arteries through the anterior fontanelle. Velocity, waveform analysis, and indexes such as the Pourcelot resistive index (RI) are the most-used measurements in Doppler evaluation. The RI measurement is easily obtained and is calculated by subtracting the diastolic flow from the systolic flow and dividing by the systolic flow. The RI eliminates errors in velocity readings when the ultrasonographer is unable to perform angle correction in these small intracerebral vessels. With a 2-MHz transducer, these same measurements are possible after fontanelle closure and through the thin temporal bone in older children. Ultrasonographers typically study the anterior and middle cerebral vessels with this transtemporal approach.

The RI in the neonate ranges from 65 to 85.[11] The normal RI in older children and adults ranges from 50 to 60. Before closure of the fontanelle, the normal RI is between 60 and 70.[12] However, the RI is more valuable for observing trends and changes over time rather than for obtaining specific values. Table 83-1 summarizes changes in RI and systolic velocity with various intracranial abnormalities.

Indications

There are six conditions in which intracranial Doppler evaluation is most useful in the critically ill infant and child: (1) hydrocephalus, (2) subdural effusions, (3) asphyxia, (4) brain death, (5) cerebral edema and its treatment, and (6) arteriovenous malformations.[8-12]

Contraindications and Complications

There are neither contraindications to nor complications of Doppler evaluation of cerebral circulation.

Equipment

Perform the evaluation of cerebral circulation with duplex color Doppler equipment so that it is easy to visualize the insonated vessels. Use a 2-MHz transducer for the transtemporal approach or a 5- or 7-MHz transducer through the anterior fontanelle in infants.

Techniques

Through the anterior fontanelle, identify the anterior cerebral and internal carotid vessels. Find the anterior cerebral artery in the sagittal view as its branches sweep over the corpus callosum. Locate the intracranial internal carotid artery in the coronal view on either side of the sella turcica. With the transtemporal approach, identify the middle and anterior cerebral arteries at their bifurcation, where there is flow in the middle cerebral toward the transducer and flow in the anterior cerebral away from the transducer. Calculate the RI after determining the maximum and minimum velocity in each vessel.

Interpretation

Hydrocephalus and Subdural Effusions. The RI is most helpful in following the infant with hydrocephalus and/or subdural effusions.[11] With increasing pressure, the RI is elevated in both conditions. This elevation may relate to increased external compression of the cerebral vessels by dilated ventricles and/or edematous or compressed tissue that produces a decrease in diastolic flow. After the ventricles have been drained and pressure has been relieved, the RI returns to normal as diastolic flow increases.[11]

Asphyxia. A decrease in the RI of intracranial vessels is a useful measure of the presence of significant perinatal asphyxia within 24 to 48 hours after the asphyctic insult.[15] This decrease theoretically occurs because of vasodilation and asphyxia to the brain with an increase in the diastolic flow. This low RI also is a predictor of significant neurologic injury with probable severe neurodevelopmental handicaps.[15]

A low RI also occurs in older children with significant asphyxia *early* in their disease. This low RI can be a sign of significant injury before the patient's computed tomography (CT) scan shows signs of cerebral edema (Fig. 83-1). As cerebral edema increases, the diastolic flow decreases and the RI becomes elevated.

Brain Death. McMenamin and Volpe[5] described a characteristic sequence of deterioration of flow-velocity waveform in the anterior cerebral arteries in neonatal brain death. First there is a loss of forward diastolic flow followed by reversal of diastolic flow, which is followed by a decrease in systolic flow and, finally, no detectable flow in the anterior cerebral artery. With this loss of forward diastolic flow, the RI increases, becoming >100 as the diastolic flow reverses. As is evident in Table 83-1, many factors can increase the RI to above 100 in the neonate; increased intracranial pressure with or without hydrocephalus and PDA are the most common factors. A markedly elevated RI (100 to 200) in a full-term infant with no evidence of hydrocephalus or PDA is strongly suggestive of brain death.[2] The neonate who is clinically brain dead occasionally has normal or decreased RI

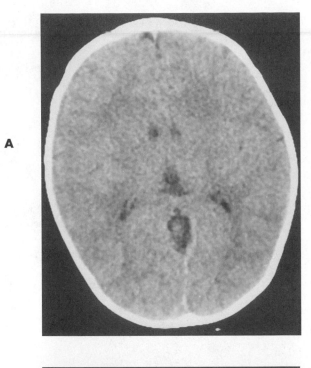

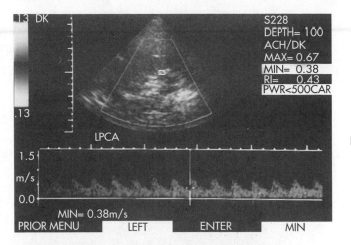

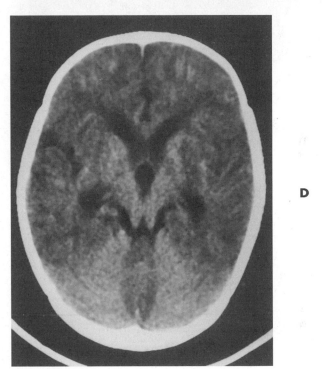

FIG. 83-1   **A,** A 1-year-old infant after respiratory arrest with a normal CT scan, but **B,** an abnormal Doppler evaluation with a low RI of 43 (50 to 60 normal for age). **C,** A CT scan 2 days later shows cerebral edema. **D,** A CT scan 1 month later shows marked atrophy.

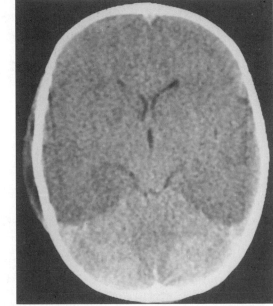

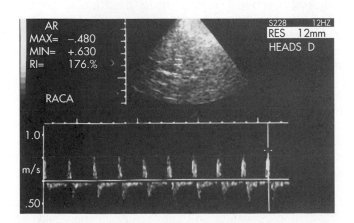

FIG. 83-2   A 3-year-old with acute encephalopathy, clinically brain dead with an RI of 176 with reversal of diastolic flow.

as well as intracranial perfusion as shown by nuclear medicine scan.[2] After fontanelle closure, an RI >100 in the middle or anterior cerebral arteries in a child with no evidence of hydrocephalus is a reliable predictor of brain death (Figs. 83-2 and 83-3).[7,14]

Cerebral Edema. Just as there is a direct relationship between an increased RI with a decrease in diastolic flow in patients with increased intracranial pressure with hydrocephalus,[12] there is an increase in RI with a loss of forward diastolic flow in patients with increased intracranial pressure secondary to cerebral edema from a variety of other causes.[3] An elevated RI is a measure of the presence of cerebral edema and varies with the course of the cerebral edema.

The RI is inversely related to P_{CO_2}. Increasing P_{CO_2} causes

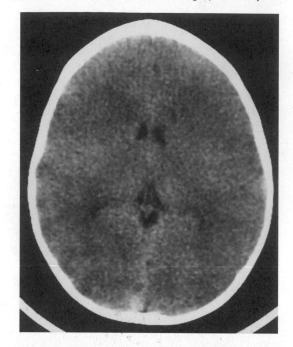

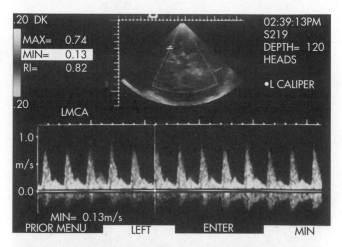

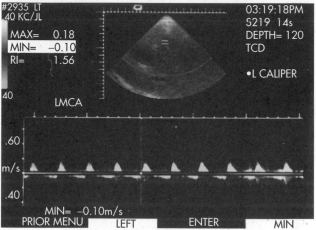

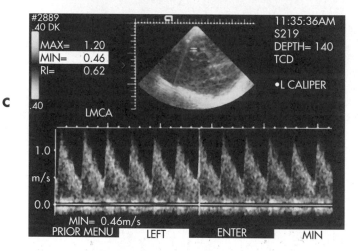

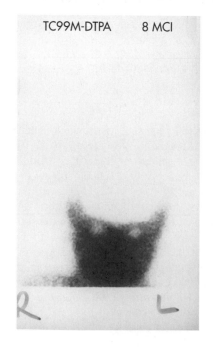

FIG. 83-3 A 1½-year-old with near-drowning. **A,** A CT scan shows cerebral edema. **B,** A Doppler evaluation shows an elevated RI of 82 from the left middle cerebral artery. **C,** A Doppler evaluation 2 days later shows that the RI has decreased to 62 with treatment. **D,** A Doppler evaluation 4 days later shows brain death with decreased velocity and reversal of diastolic flow with an RI of 156. **E,** A brain scan done at this time also shows brain death with no cerebral perfusion.

vasodilation with an increase in diastolic flow and a decrease in the RI. When the P_{CO_2} drops, there is vasoconstriction with a decrease in diastolic flow and an elevation of the RI. CO_2 reactivity is measurable using the RI. The cerebral blood flow should rise 4% for each mm Hg rise in CO_2.[1,3,4,8] The absence of change in the RI as the patient's hyperventilation increases is an absent CO_2 reactivity test and is a sign of severe brain injury.[6]

It is also possible to use RIs to monitor hyperventilation therapy in cerebral edema associated with head trauma.[10] As hyperventilation decreases the P_{CO_2}, the RI increases with the concomitant vasoconstriction of cerebral vessels. Increasing cerebral edema also increases the RI. Therefore it is necessary to correlate this measurement closely with other clinical and laboratory findings. For example, a patient who is on hyperventilation treatment and whose RI increases in the face of no change in intracranial pressure may benefit from decreased hyperventilation. The hyperventilation may be producing too much vasoconstriction.

Vascular Abnormalities. Intracranial Doppler evaluation is

TABLE 83-1 Cerebral Doppler Changes

	RI	Systolic velocity
Intracranial abnormalities		
Intracranial bleed	Increased	(Beat-to-beat variation, risk factor for intraventricular hemorrhage)
Periventricular leukomalacia	Increased	
Asphyxia	Decreased, acutely	
Brain edema	Increased	
Hydrocephalus	Increased, reverses after drainage	
Subdural hematoma	Increased	
Brain death	Increased	Decreased, reverse diastolic
ECMO	Decreased	
Vascular malformation stenoses	Decreased	Increased, turbulence
Extracranial abnormalities		
PCO$_2$	Inverse relationship	
Heart rate	Inverse relationship	
Shock		Decreased systolic diastolic
PDA	Increased	
Pneumothorax	Increased	
Cardiac ischemia	Increased	
Gastrointestinal bleed	Increased	
Polycythemia, hyperviscosity	Increased	Decreased
Drugs		
Indomethacin	Increased	Decreased
Maternal cocaine		Increased
Exogenous surfactant		Increased

very sensitive for the bedside detection of vascular malformations in the distressed neonate. It is possible to image the vascular malformation with color on the ultrasound; the vessels will show increased diastolic flow and turbulence. In addition, intracranial Doppler evaluation can detect a stroke in the neonate and older child.[13]

Intracranial Doppler evaluation is a useful tool for determining the cerebral vasculature status of the acutely ill child. Because it is a bedside technique, it is one of the most valuable imaging procedures available.

Remarks

For best results, perform Doppler evaluation for asphyxia as early as possible following admission. Before interpreting the results, look at all of the factors that can change the RI.

REFERENCES

1. Bode H, editor: *Pediatric applications of transcranial Doppler sonography,* New York, 1988, Springer-Verlag.
2. Glasier CM, Seibert JJ, Chadduck WM, et al: Brain death in infants: evaluation with Doppler US, *Radiology* 172:377-380, 1989.
3. Klingelhofer J, Conrad B, Benecke R, et al: Evaluation of intracranial pressure from transcranial Doppler studies in cerebral disease, *J Neurol* 235:159-162, 1988.
4. Lindegaard KF, Aaslid R, Nornes H: Cerebral arteriovenous malformations. In Aaslid R, editor: *Transcranial Doppler sonography,* New York, 1986, Springer-Verlag.
5. McMenamin JB, Volpe JJ: Doppler ultrasonography in the determination of brain death, *Ann Neurol* 14:302-307, 1983.
6. Newell DW, Seiler RW, Aaslid R: Head injury and cerebral circulatory arrest. In Newell DW, Aaslid R, editors: *Transcranial Doppler,* New York, 1992, Raven Press.
7. Petty GW, Mohr JP, Pedley TA, et al: The role of transcranial Doppler in confirming brain death: sensitivity, specificity, and suggestions for performance and interpretation, *Neurology* 40:300-303, 1990.
8. Raju TNK: Cerebral Doppler studies in the fetus and newborn infant, *J Pediatr* 119(2):165-174, 1991.
9. Raju TNK: Cranial Doppler applications in neonatal critical care, *Crit Care Med* 8(1):93-111, 1992.
10. Saliba EM, Laugier J: Doppler assessment of the cerebral circulation in pediatric intensive care, *Progress Pediatr Crit Care* 8(1):79-92, 1992.
11. Seibert JJ, McCowan TC, Chadduck WM, et al: Duplex-pulsed Doppler US versus intracranial pressure in the neonate: clinical and experimental studies, *Radiology* 171:155-159, 1989.
12. Seibert JJ, Glasier CM, Leithiger RE Jr, et al: Transcranial Doppler using standard duplex equipment in children, *Ultrasound Q* 8(3):167-196, 1990.
13. Seibert JJ, Miller SF, Kirby RS, et al: Cerebrovascular disease in symptomatic and asymptomatic patients with sickle cell anemia: screening with duplex transcranial Doppler US—correlation with MR imaging and MR angiography, *Radiology* 189:457-466, 1993.
14. Shiogai T, Sato E, Tokitsu M, et al: Transcranial Doppler monitoring in severe brain damage: relationships between intracranial haemodynamics, brain dysfunction and outcome, *Neurol Res* 12:205-213, 1990.
15. Stark JE, Seibert JJ: Cerebral artery Doppler ultrasonography for prediction of outcome after perinatal asphyxia, *J Ultrasound Med,* 13:595-600, 1994.
16. Taylor GA: Current concepts in neonatal cranial Doppler sonography, *Ultrasound Q* 9(4):223-244, 1992.

84 Jugular Bulb Catheterization for Measurement of Cerebral Oxygenation

Timothy C. Frewen and Narenda C. Singh

The integrated functions of cellular components depend on the continuous supply of substrate. The combined functions of the respiratory and circulatory systems provide these substrates through the microvascular circulation and the functional integrity of the cellular components. Therefore the measurement of substrate (oxygen, glucose, lactate) delivered and extracted provides valuable information about the functional integrity of this complex system. For example, the adequacy of tissue oxygen delivery and use can be inferred from systemic venous oxygen saturation (Sv_{O_2}).

The principle of measurement of tissue oxygen delivery and extraction is also useful to assess cerebral function through measurement of jugular bulb venous oxygen saturation (Sj_{O_2}) and oxygen content. Such monitoring is only recently available although many therapeutic interventions such as hyperventilation, hypothermia, diuretic therapy, and barbiturates used to treat brain edema significantly influence oxygen delivery and extraction. Recent data suggest that brain injury alters cerebral venous oxygen content in children and that normal or elevated cross-brain oxygen extraction values are associated with functional neurologic recovery.[6] In addition, recent literature suggests that bedside cannulation of the jugular venous bulb is feasible and safe.[6,8] Consequently, there is renewed interest in routine monitoring of cerebral venous oxygen saturation and content.

Indications

The indications for monitoring jugular venous indexes are expanding with increasing knowledge regarding the usefulness of the information obtained and the limited complications associated with the procedure.[20,21,22] With this technique, clinicians are able to continuously or intermittently monitor cerebral venous oxygen saturation and content, which rapidly reflects changes in oxygen delivery and use. Other useful information reflecting cerebral function includes cross-brain use of glucose and lactate.[33] If the clinician is also able to measure cerebral blood flow (CBF), he or she can calculate cross-brain oxygen extraction ratios to drive the cerebral metabolic rate of oxygen (CMR_{O_2}) and ratios of CBF/CMR_{O_2} to determine the coupling of flow and function, which may aid in prognostication.[1,39]

In addition, determination of cerebral arteriovenous oxygen difference has been used to estimate cerebral blood flow[34,36] and to therefore detect cerebral hypoperfusion. Transcranial Doppler evaluation along with Sj_{O_2} monitoring is useful in identifying patients with decreased cerebral perfusion pressure and therefore may be useful in patients without ICP monitoring.[3,4,5] The measurement of these variables in a variety of clinical situations has aided in detecting cerebral hypoxemia, assessing the efficacy of various therapeutic interventions, and determining prognosis.

Investigators have extensively studied cerebral oxygen delivery and CBF in patients with head injuries to detect impending global cerebral ischemia,* to monitor the effects of increasing ICP on the ratio of CBF to cerebral metabolic rate (CBF/CMR),[9,36] and to monitor the effects of therapeutic interventions.[2,13,16,29,30]

The measurement of cross-brain oxygen extraction and CMR_{O_2} is also useful in prognostication in pediatric near-drowning[6] and in other forms of hypoxemic ischemic injury.[1,18,21] It has facilitated the study of cerebral metabolism during hypothermic cardiopulmonary bypass in children[40] and adults.[32]

To a limited extent, the measurement of cross-brain oxygen extraction has been helpful in infectious and toxic encephalopathies, intracranial hemorrhage, and poisoning.[21,23] In a single patient, the lack of cross-brain oxygen extraction facilitated the diagnosis of brain death.[23]

Contraindications

Cannulation of the jugular venous bulb (JVB) is relatively safe. Previously, intracranial hypertension was a relative contraindication for JVB catheterization.[15,26,37] However, Goeting et al.[21] have demonstrated that this procedure is safe in patients with increased ICP. Other contraindications to JVB cannulation include local infection, local neck trauma, or any impairment to cerebral venous drainage. Bleeding diathesis is not a contraindication;[13] patients with coagulopathy have undergone JVB catheterization without significant local hematoma formation.[21]

Complications

In the hands of skilled personnel, few complications arise from JVB cannulation. Inadvertent puncture of the carotid artery is a possible occurrence.[20,21] Both venous and arterial hematomas occasionally occur; prevent or limit them by applying immediate local pressure.[21] There are reports of malpositioning of the catheter in the facial vein and transverse venous sinus[41] along with catheter looping.[20,21] Reposition the catheter if such a situation is detected radiographically. As with any other form of vascular access, catheter sepsis is a known complication and requires removal of the infected catheter.[20] Venous thrombosis is a theoretical complication, but autopsy studies in a small number of children have not demonstrated the presence of thrombosis.[20] The lack of thrombosis formation may be attributed to continuous infusion of heparinized saline through the catheter.[20,21] Theoretical complications are phrenic and recurrent laryngeal nerve damage and Horner's syndrome as a result of injury to other structures in the neck.

---

*References 3-5, 9, 18, 20, 27, 29, 35.

462

Equipment

See Box 84-1.

Techniques

The first description of clinical venipuncture of the jugular bulb occurred in 1927,[28] and this technique was essential to Kety and Schmidt's technique of nitrous oxide cerebral blood flow measurement.[25] In 1972, Persson, Settergren, and Dahlquist[31] described a technique for measurement involving direct puncturing of the anterior internal jugular vein to cannulate the jugular bulb in children. More recent techniques have involved direct puncture of the jugular bulb inferior to the mastoid process and retrograde insertion of a catheter into the jugular venous bulb through the internal jugular vein.

Two techniques involve retrograde insertion for pediatric patients. One technique involves placing the head down in a horizontal supine position and rotating the head, which digitally displaces the common carotid artery; the second technique provides for retrograde cannulation by maintaining the head in a slightly elevated position with the head slightly extended but otherwise neutral, with the concurrent application of skin traction over the clavicle.

Make the clinical decision to cannulate either the left or right internal jugular bulb on the basis of the nature and location of the brain injury. The right jugular bulb is best for right-sided, diffuse or multifocal bihemisphere disease because it is usually larger with higher flow.[17,41] Left-sided catheterization is best in left-sided focal disease, open-neck trauma, and right-sided ventriculoperitoneal shunts.

Horizontal Supine Head-turn Technique. To insert the cannula into the jugular bulb using the horizontal supine head-turn technique, place a surgical towel behind the child's shoulders to extend the neck with the head turned to the opposite side. Following the appropriate sterile procedure, palpate the carotid artery at the midpoint of an imaginary line that connects the suprasternal notch and the tip of the mastoid process; displace this artery medially. Depending on the clinical condition, infiltrate a local anesthetic 1 cm lateral to the midpoint of this line (Fig. 84-1). Use a 21-gauge thin-walled, short-bevelled needle to enter the skin 1 cm

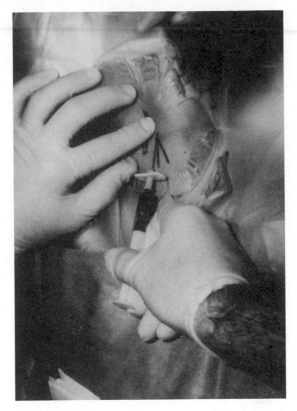

FIG. 84-1   Horizontal supine head-turn technique. The needle enters at a midpoint between the suprasternal notch and the mastoid process lateral to the carotid artery at a 30- to 45-degree angle directed toward the foramen magnum.

lateral to the midpoint of the line previously described. Use a 21-gauge needle to pierce the skin at a 30- to 45-degree angle from the horizontal plane and direct it cephalad toward the foramen magnum. While applying gentle suction pressure to the syringe, enter the internal jugular vein and, with the return of venous blood, disconnect the syringe and insert a 0.45-mm guide wire through the needle in a retrograde direction. Insert the wire until it meets resistance at the superior bulb, making sure that the external length of the wire exceeds that of the catheter when placed into the vein. Remove the needle, hold the guide wire in the vein, and insert an appropriate-length polyethylene catheter until it meets resistance at the superior bulb of the vein. Remove the guide wire and connect the catheter to a three-way stopcock. Infuse a heparinized solution (1 U/ml) of normal saline or dextrose water through a pump at 1 ml/hr to maintain catheter patency. Suture the catheter to the skin to avoid malpositioning of the catheter tip.

Head-up Position. The head-up position technique is preferable for patients with a suspected or confirmed cervical spine injury. Position the patient with his or her head slightly extended but otherwise neutral, often with a rolled towel between the neck and upper back. Prepare the skin in a similar manner to that previously described and identify the puncture site slightly lateral to the carotid impulse at the level of the inferior border of the thyroid cartilage. For small infants, this site may be slightly lower. Apply skin traction by pulling the skin downward over the clavicle with the hand

BOX 84-1   **EQUIPMENT REQUIRED FOR CANNULATION OF THE JUGULAR BULB**

Antiseptic solution
Sterile drapes
21-gauge needle
3-ml syringe
Local anesthetic (2%)
Guide wire (0.45 mm)
Polyethylene catheter
(2.5-8 cm)
Heparinized saline
(1 U/ml)
Suture
Sterile dressing

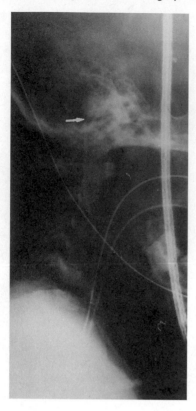

FIG. 84-2   The lateral skull x-ray study demonstrates the correct position of the catheter at the base of the skull.

stabilizing the syringe to enter the internal jugular vein successfully. This technique does not require palpation or displacement of the carotid artery.

If inadvertent carotid artery puncture occurs, withdraw the needle, apply pressure for 5 minutes, and then attempt percutaneous catheterization of the jugular bulb a second time on the same side; if unsuccessful, attempt catheterization on the other side. Standard cut-down techniques have also been used. After JVB cannulation, a lateral skull x-ray examination is necessary to confirm catheter placement at the base of the skull (Fig. 84-2).

Remarks

Catheterization of the jugular bulb is an essential first step to understanding cerebral oxygen delivery and use. *Oxygen content* of venous and arterial blood requires the measurement of venous and arterial saturation, hemoglobin, (Hgb) and PaO_2, as illustrated by the following equation:

$$O_2 \text{ content} = 1.36 \text{ ml/g} \times \text{Hgb} \times O_2 \text{ saturation} + (0.003 \times Pao_2).$$

Calculate the *cross-brain oxygen content difference* ($AVDO_2$) by subtracting the oxygen content of the jugular venous blood from the systemic arterial oxygen content. The normal arteriojugular difference in oxygen content in children is 4 to 8 vol%.[24] Calculate the *cerebral extraction of oxygen* (CEO_2) by obtaining the difference between the systemic arterial and jugular venous oxyhemoglobin saturation levels, since hemoglobin and hemoglobin-carrying capacity are similar in arterial and venous blood. The normal cerebral extraction of oxygen is 31.6%.[14] If capabilities are available to measure cerebral blood flow (CBF), one may calculate the cerebral metabolic rate for oxygen ($CMRO_2$)

(ml/min/100g) as $CMRO_2 = AVDO_2 \times CBF$. The normal range for $CMRO_2$ is 4.3 to 6.2 ml/min/100 g; however, values vary with both age and mental status. In certain clinical situations, a new variable, termed *cerebral consumption of oxygen* (CCO_2), may be more reflective of cerebral oxygen consumption than cerebral oxygen extraction.[11] Calculate the CCO_2 (ml/min/100 g) as $CCO_2 = CEO_2 \times CBF$. The normal range for CCO_2 is 4.6 to 5.3 ml/min/100 g. Continuous monitoring of jugular bulb oxyhemoglobin saturation using fiberoptic catheter oximetry may also permit early detection of oligemic cerebral hypoxemia as indicated by abnormally low jugular oxygen saturation in the presence of normal arterial oxygen saturation.[7-10,14,19,38] Jugular bulb oximetry may also be useful because it allows early identification of impaired cerebral oxygenation, even in the presence of normal cerebral perfusion pressure.

REFERENCES

1. Beckstead JE, Tweed WA, Lee J, et al: Cerebral blood flow and metabolism in man following cardiac arrest, *Stroke* 9:569-573, 1978.
2. Bricold AP, Glick D: Barbiturate effects on acute experimental intracranial hypertension, *J Neurosurg* 55:397-406, 1981.
3. Chan K-H, Dearden MN, Miller JD: The significance of posttraumatic increase in cerebral blood flow velocity: a transcranial Doppler ultrasound study, *Neurosurgery* 30:697-700, 1992.
4. Chan K-H, Miller JD, Dearden NM, et al: The effect of changes in cerebral perfusion pressure upon middle cerebral artery blood flow velocity and jugular bulb venous oxygen saturation after severe brain injury, *J Neurosurg* 77:55-61, 1992.
5. Chan K-H, Dearden NM, Miller JD, et al: Multimodality monitoring as a guide to treatment of intracranial hypertension after severe brain injury, *Neurosurgery* 32:547-553, 1993.
6. Connors R, Frewen TC, Kissoon N, et al: Relationship of cross-brain oxygen content difference, cerebral blood flow and metabolic rate to neurologic outcome after near-drowning, *J Pediatr* 121:839-844, 1992.
7. Cruz J: Continuous versus serial global cerebral hemometabolic monitoring: applications in acute brain trauma, *Acta Neurochir (Wien)* 42 (suppl) :35-30, 1988.
8. Cruz J: Combined continuous monitoring of systemic and cerebral oxygenations in acute brain injury: preliminary observations, *Crit Care Med* 21:1225-1232, 1993.
9. Cruz J, Miner ME: Modulating cerebral oxygen delivery and extraction in acute traumatic coma. In Miner ME, Wagner KA, editors: *Neurotrauma,* vol 1, Boston, 1986, Butterworth.
10. Cruz J, Gennarelli TA, Alves WM: Continuous monitoring of cerebral oxygenation in acute brain injury: multivariate assessment of severe intracranial "plateau" wave (case report), *J Trauma* 32:401-403, 1992.
11. Cruz J, Gennarelli TA, Alves WM: Continuous monitoring of cerebral hemodynamic reserve in acute brain injury: relationship to changes in brain swelling, *J Trauma* 32:629-635, 1992.
12. Cruz J, Jaggi JL, Hoffstad OJ: Cerebral blood flow and oxygen consumption in acute brain injury with acute anemia: an alternative for the cerebral metabolic rate of oxygen consumption? *Crit Care Med* 21:1218-1224, 1993.
13. Cruz J, Miner ME, Allen SJ, et al: Continuous monitoring of cerebral oxygenation in acute brain injury: injection of mannitol during hyperventilation, *J Neurosurg* 73:725-730, 1990.
14. Cruz J, Miner ME, Allen SJ, et al: Continuous monitoring of cerebral oxygenation in acute brain injury: assessment of cerebral hemodynamic reserve, *Neurosurgery* 29:743-749, 1991.
15. Dean JM, Rogers MC, Traystman RJ: Pathophysiology and clinical management of the intracranial vault. In Rogers MC, editor: *Textbook of pediatric intensive care,* Baltimore, 1987, Williams & Wilkins.
16. Dearden NM, Miller JD: Paired comparison of hypotonic and osmotic therapy in the reduction of intracranial pressure after severe head injury. In Hoff JT, Betz AL, editors: *Intracranial pressure VIII,* New York, 1989. Springer-Verlag.

17. Edwards EA: Anatomic variations of the cranial venous sinuses, *Arch Neurol Psychiatry* 26:801, 1931.

18. Frewen TC, Sumabat WO, Del Maestro RF: Cerebral blood flow, metabolic rate and cross-brain oxygen consumption in brain injury, *J Pediatr* 107:510-513, 1985.

19. Garlick R, Bihari D: The use of intermittent and continuous recordings of jugular venous bulb oxygen saturation in the unconscious patient, *Scand J Clin Lab Invest* 47 (suppl 188):47-52, 1987.

20. Gayle MO, Frewen TC, Armstrong RF, et al: Jugular venous bulb catheterization in infants and children, *Crit Care Med* 17:385-388, 1989.

21. Goetting MG, Preston G: Jugular bulb catheterization: experience with 123 patients, *Crit Care Med* 18(11)1220-1223, 1990.

22. Goetting MG, Preston G: Jugular bulb catheterization does not increase intracranial pressure, *Intensive Care Med* 17:195-198, 1991.

23. Hantson PH, Mahieu P: Usefulness of cerebral venous monitoring through jugular bulb catheterization for the diagnosis of brain death (correspondence), *Intensive Care Med* 18:59, 1992.

24. Kennedy C, Sokoloff L: An adaptation of the nitrous oxide method to the study of the cerebral circulation in children: normal values for cerebral blood flow and cerebral metabolic rate in children, *J Clin Invest* 36:1130-1137, 1957.

25. Kety S, Schmidt CF: Determination of cerebral blood flow in man by use of nitrous oxide in low concentration, *Am J Physiol* 143:53-56, 1945.

26. McGee WT, Mallory DL: Cannulation of the internal and external jugular veins, *Problems Crit Care* 2:214-217, 1988.

27. Muizelaar JP, Ward JD, Marmarou A, et al: Cerebral blood flow and metabolism in severely head-injured children, Part 2: autoregulation, *J Neurosurg* 71:72-76, 1989.

28. Myerson A, Halloran RD, Hirsch HL: Technique of obtaining blood from the internal jugular vein and internal carotid artery, *Arch Neurol Psychiatry* 17:807, 1927.

29. Nordstrom CH, Messeter K, Sundbarg G, et al: Cerebral blood flow, vasoreactivity and oxygen consumption during barbiturate therapy in severe traumatic brain lesions, *J Neurosurg* 68:424-431, 1988.

30. Obrist WD, Langfitt, TW, Jaggi JL, et al: Cerebral blood flow and metabolism in comatose patients with acute head injury: relationship to intracranial hypertension, *J Neurosurg* 61:241-253, 1984.

31. Persson B, Settergren G, Dahlquist G: Cerebral arteriovenous differences of acetoacetate and d-β-hydroxybutyrate in children, *Acta Pediatr* 61:273, 1972.

32. Prough, DS, Rogers, AT, Stump DA, et al: Cerebral blood flow decreases with time whereas cerebral oxygen consumption remains stable during hypothermic cardiopulmonary bypass in humans, *Anesth Analg* 72:161-168, 1991.

33. Rivers EP, Paradis NA, Martin GB, et al: Cerebral lactate uptake during cardiopulmonary resuscitation in humans, *J Cereb Blood Flow Metab* 11:479-484, 1991.

34. Robertson CS, Narayan RK, Gokaslan ZL, et al: Cerebral arteriovenous difference as an estimate of cerebral blood flow in comatose patients, *J Neurosurg* 61:241-253, 1984.

35. Robertson CS, Grossman RG, Goodman JC, et al: Predictive value of cerebral anaerobic metabolism and cerebral infarction after head injury, *J Neurosurg* 67:361-368, 1987.

36. Robertson, CS, Narayan RK, Gokaslan ZL, et al: Cerebral arteriovenous oxygen difference as an estimate of cerebral blood flow in comatose patients, *J Neurosurg* 70:222-230, 1989.

37. Rubenstein JS, Hageman JR: Monitoring of critically ill infants and children, *Crit Care Clin* 4:621-639, 1988.

38. Sheinberg M, Kantar MJ, Robertson CS, et al: Continuous monitoring of jugular venous oxygen saturation in head-injured patients, *J Neurosurg* 76:212-217, 1992.

39. Singh NC, Kochanek PM, Schiding JK, et al: Uncoupled cerebral blood flow and metabolism after severe global ischemia in rats, *J Cereb Blood Flow Metab* 12:802-808, 1992.

40. van der Linden J, Priddy R, Ekroth R, et al: Cerebral perfusion and metabolism during profound hypothermia in children, *J Thorac Cardiovasc Surg* 102:103-114.

41. Woodhall B: Variations of the cranial venous sinuses in the region of the torcular Herophili, *Arch Surg* 33:297, 1936.

85 Determination of Brain Death

Kristan Outwater

Over the past few decades, technologic advances in resuscitation and intensive care have made it necessary to expand the conventional view of death. The ability to temporarily support the cardiopulmonary system of patients with severe brain injury has presented an added requirement for the assessment of brain function.[2] There are two primary reasons for establishing criteria for brain death: (1) continuing support of patients who are dead provides no benefit to the patient and places a great physical, emotional, and financial burden on families, hospitals, and staff; (2) uniform standards and guidelines are imperative to help resolve controversy surrounding organ harvest for transplantation.

Many states now have legally recognized brain-death statutes. Most states do not establish medical criteria for determining brain death but authorize hospital boards to do so on the basis of accepted medical practice. In 1968, the Ad Hoc Committee of Harvard Medical School published guidelines that, although not redefining death, used brain-based rather than cardiopulmonary-based criteria for declaring death.[2,11] Subsequently, similar guidelines have been prospectively validated; once a patient meets certain medical and laboratory criteria and it is possible to definitively ascertain an irreversible loss of all brain function, the physician should consider the patient dead even if maintenance of cardiopulmonary function is temporarily possible.[1,36]

Three sets of suggested guidelines for the determination of brain death in children were published in 1987.[3,6,45] Clinical criteria used to document cessation of brain function are similar to those established in adults (Box 85-1).[13] The three sets of guidelines agree that the previously mentioned criteria are independent of the age of the patient (excluding children less than 7 days of age). However, differences of opinion continue regarding the determination of irreversibility of findings and the need for confirmatory testing.

The determination of irreversibility implies a period of observation of neurologic status. Patients admitted following cardiac resuscitation from hypoxemic ischemic injury (e.g., near-drowning, sudden infant death syndrome, severe respiratory failure leading to cardiopulmonary arrest) with initial absence of brain stem function may gradually achieve return of function over a period of hours. A hasty judgment of "poor prognosis" is not a determination of death. An observation period of 6 to 48 hours is appropriate and varies depending on the cause of coma,[3] the availability of confirmatory laboratory tests,[6] and the age of the patient.[45] Unfortunately, no studies to date have prospectively validated optimal observation periods in children.

The need for confirmatory testing is also controversial. The electroencephalogram (EEG) documents the presence or absence of cerebral activity but does not add information about brain stem function.[5,36a] Cerebral flow studies document whether the amount of blood flow to the brain is compatible with life. Lack of cerebral blood flow can confirm brain death in adults and children, but newborns may have a flow too low to detect and still have a return of brain stem function.[15,24,39]

Indications

Perform rigorous application of brain-death testing when a comatose patient loses cortical and brain stem function. Although a physician can withdraw life support from a patient who has been deemed terminally or hopelessly ill without having to document a loss of all brain functions, at least two factors warrant the consideration of actually establishing brain death. First, it is necessary to declare death to harvest organs for transplantation; families may find some measure of comfort in agreeing to donate organs. Second, families often find the decision-making process surrounding the withdrawal or the withholding of life support to be traumatic and burdensome. Determining brain death allows the intensivist to relieve the family of any burden of decision making by discontinuing life support soon after declaration of death without asking families to make a choice about whether to continue support.

Equipment

The equipment required for the determination of brain death is minimal because in most cases only knowledge of the cause of the coma, a lack of any mitigating circumstances, and a careful physical examination are necessary. To confirm brain death, it is ideal to consult a second examiner, preferably a pediatric neurologist or neurosurgeon.

Confirmatory testing such as EEG, evoked potentials, and cerebral flow studies may be necessary if the clinical examination is not adequate (e.g., if the patient has hypothermia, if sedative drug levels are too high, or if hypotension or bradycardia require prematurely halting the apnea test) or if a rapid determination of death becomes important. The EEG is a portable noninvasive procedure performed at the bedside and is quite specific for the diagnosis of brain death. When properly performed, an EEG that documents electrical silence helps confirm a lack of cerebral activity (but not brain stem function); irreversible absence of brain stem function clinically confirms brain death.[6,9,31]

The EEG may show electrocerebral silence even when the patient is still alive.[5,36a] Obtain a cerebral blood flow study rather than an EEG if it is not possible to test adequately any aspect of brain stem function. Conversely, electrical activity may remain even after death has occurred.[5,18] Use another confirmatory test if electrical activity remains but the history and clinical examination are consistent with brain death. Obtaining a technically adequate EEG in the electrically charged atmosphere of the intensive care unit may be

BOX 85-1   **DETERMINATION OF BRAIN DEATH**

History

Establish cause of coma sufficient to result in severe brain injury

Absence of confounding factors

Hypothermia (temperature $< 32°$ C), hypotension, sedation, neuromuscular blockade, surgically correctable conditions, toxic-metabolic derangements, paralysis

Absent cerebral function

Flaccid tone
No spontaneous movements, no response to verbal or painful stimulation

Absent brainstem function

Fixed, unresponsive, midposition, or fully dialated pupils
No eye movements; spontaneous, oculocephalic, or oculovestibular testing
No corneal, oropharyngeal, gag, cough, or respiratory reflexes

Apnea test

No response to $PaCO_2 > 55$ mm Hg

Age

Clinical examination applicable to all ages < 7 days: insufficient data; guidelines may be applied at the discretion of the attending physician and neurologist

Observation period

At least 6 hours; longer time depending on cause of coma, age, and use of confirmatory testing at the discretion of the attending physician, neurologist, and hospital policy

Confirmatory testing

Not obligatory unless unable to adequately perform any part of the clinical examination (e.g., presence of sedative drugs) or unless there is a need to make a rapid determination of brain death

---

difficult. In addition, performing and interpreting an EEG requires an experienced technician and electroencephalographer; such services are not always available on a 24-hour basis. Newborns may have transient electrocerebral silence for a variety of reasons, which renders the EEG an inadequate diagnostic tool for brain death in this age group.[7,10,50]

Evoked potential (EP) testing may provide additional evidence of the lack of brain stem function.[26,28,43,53] Several studies have documented the usefulness of brain stem auditory evoked potentials (BAEPs) in combination with somatosensory evoked potentials (SEPs) in corroborating the diagnosis of brain death.[26,43] EPs are a composite series of extremely small potentials; unlike with EEG tracings, sedative drugs do not suppress them. Flat responses are present in brain-dead patients but may also represent an interruption anywhere along the specific anatomic pathway being tested. However, recognize the shortcomings of EP testing; do not use EPs in isolation.[22,28,53]

The absence of blood flow to the brain is absolute evidence of brain death. Conventional cerebral angiography is the gold standard for documenting lack of blood flow to the brain. Although it is extremely accurate, it is also complex and costly. It is not portable, and the contrast material is potentially damaging to patients who are not brain dead.[19]

Some hospitals use radionuclide cerebral flow studies with isotope tracers in place of four-vessel angiography because a nuclear medicine scan can be performed at the bedside, is noninvasive, and is less costly. Establish a diagnosis of brain death if there is no carotid circulation above the base of the skull and no intracranial arterial circulation.[15,16,19,24] A small percentage (16%) of patients demonstrate venous filling, which is thought to reflect an arterial flow too low to detect followed by detectable venous pooling.[42] Radionuclide flow studies may be problematic in infants because there have been reports of persistent flow in babies who were clinically brain dead and undetectable flow in babies who later survived.[7,42] When diethylene triamine pentaacetic acid (DTPA) labelled with technetium 99m is the isotope tracer, radionuclide cerebral angiography does not evaluate blood flow to the entire brain because it does not determine blood flow to the midbrain, medulla, and cerebellum. Both white and gray matter take up technetium 99m–labelled hexamethyl propyleneamine oxine (HMPAO); it can mark the presence or absence of subtentorial flow.[25] Although HMPAO is costlier and technically more difficult to use, it may provide more information.[23,25,39]

Although magnetic resonance angiography has been proposed as another alternative to four-vessel angiography because it is less invasive than conventional angiography,[4] it is not portable and requires a prolonged period in which

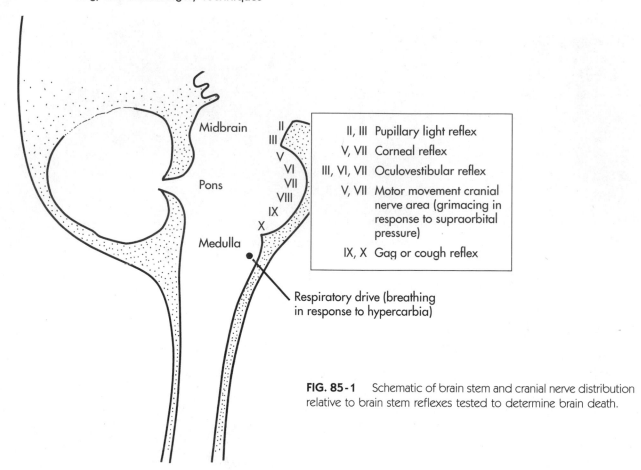

FIG. 85-1 Schematic of brain stem and cranial nerve distribution relative to brain stem reflexes tested to determine brain death.

intensive monitoring may not be optimal. The role of HM-PAO radionuclide scans and magnetic resonance angiography in detecting brain death in newborns is not known.

Techniques

Clinical Examination. Establish a diagnosis of brain death when the clinical evaluation discloses cerebral unreceptivity and unresponsivity and absent brain stem reflexes (see Box 85-1). This diagnosis requires a determination of irreversibility: an established cause of coma sufficient to account for loss of brain function; no possibility of recovery, exclusion of other drug and metabolic disorders, and the passage of a sufficient amount of time without a return in function. A rigid application of the clinical examination is imperative; it is necessary to have knowledge of when the clinical examination cannot be definitive (e.g., as a result of drugs or preexisting disease), as well as other means to make the diagnosis.

Confirmation of cerebral unreceptivity and unresponsivity requires that the patient exhibit no spontaneous movement and not respond to verbal, auditory, cutaneous, or painful stimuli. In addition, the pulse rate will not change in response to these stimuli. The presence of seizures or decorticate or decerebrate posturing is evidence that death has not occurred.

Key brain stem functions for testing include pupillary light, corneal, oculocephalic, oculovestibular, oropharyngeal, and respiratory reflexes (Fig. 85-1). Use a bright light to test the pupils; in brain death they are fixed, either dilated or in midposition. Oval pupils suggest residual midbrain function. Do not perform the test for oculocephalic reflexes (Fig. 85-2)

in patients at risk for cervical spine injury. Fig. 85-3 illustrates testing for the oculovestibular reflex. Test oropharyngeal reflexes by passing a suction catheter through the endotracheal tube to the carina; pass the same catheter through the mouth and into the posterior pharynx. Note a lack of responsiveness.

The apnea test (allowing carbon dioxide to accumulate in the blood stream to stimulate respiration) may be the most important test for lack of brain stem function and is the only way to test respiratory center (medulla) function.[8,30,34,41] Perform the apnea test (Fig. 85-4) over a time period estimated to allow the arterial Pa_{CO_2} to rise above 55 mm Hg and the pH to fall below 7.35 (usually approximately 5 minutes).[34] If it is necessary to terminate the apnea test prematurely because of hypoxemia, repeat the test after preoxygenation with 100% oxygen and the placement of a catheter through the endotracheal tube to administer oxygen during the period of apnea. An inability to formally test for apnea renders the entire clinical examination inadequate and necessitates ancillary testing to document brain death.

Spinal reflexes may be present in patients who are brain dead; these reflexes are often mistaken for spontaneous movements of the extremities or for respiratory effort.[48,49] In addition, spinal reflexes or a humoral response may mediate a hemodynamic response to surgical stimulation despite brain death.[51]

Confirmatory Testing. If confirmatory testing is necessary, a cerebral blood flow study is most often appropriate. With the radiologist who will perform the test and interpret the results, discuss the choice of isotope tracer for use in the

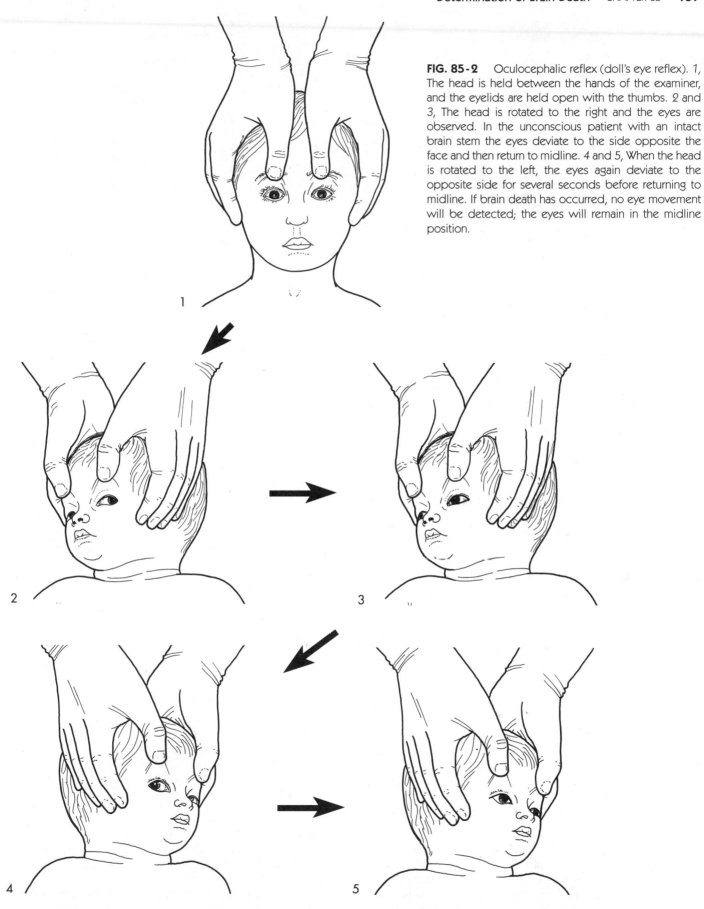

FIG. 85-2   Oculocephalic reflex (doll's eye reflex). *1,* The head is held between the hands of the examiner, and the eyelids are held open with the thumbs. *2* and *3,* The head is rotated to the right and the eyes are observed. In the unconscious patient with an intact brain stem the eyes deviate to the side opposite the face and then return to midline. *4* and *5,* When the head is rotated to the left, the eyes again deviate to the opposite side for several seconds before returning to midline. If brain death has occurred, no eye movement will be detected; the eyes will remain in the midline position.

**Unconscious
(Brain stem intact)**

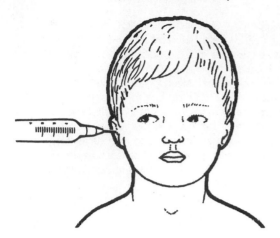

Brain death

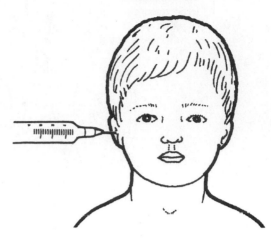

Eyes deviate to side of stimulation,
then slowly return to midposition.

No movement.

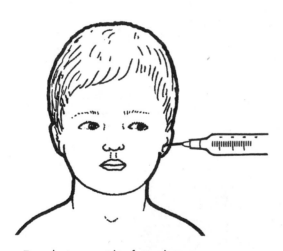

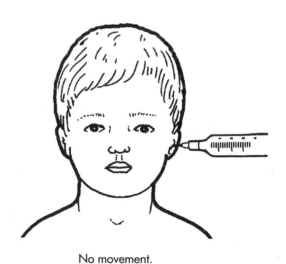

Eyes deviate to side of stimulation,
then slowly return to midposition.

No movement.

FIG. 85-3 To evaluate the oculovestibular reflex (cold caloric test), elevate the patient's head 30 degrees and ensure that the external auditory canal is clear and that the tympanic membrane is intact. Then fill a 10-ml syringe and attach the syringe to a short catheter. Place the catheter in the external ear canal and flush the ice water into the canal slowly over 1 minute. In the unconscious, brain stem–intact patient, the eyes deviate toward the side of irrigation before slowly returning to midline. No nystagmus is present in the unconscious patient. If the patient is brain dead, no eye movement will occur. Test the other side after a 5-min waiting period to allow the oculovestibular system to reequilibrate.

radionuclide scan or the use of four-vessel angiography or magnetic resonance angiography.

Approaching the Family. A thorough understanding of the concept and diagnosis of brain death is important to present the facts and finality of the situation to the family. The period of observation becomes important not only to document irreversibility but also to allow the family time to understand, to begin grieving, and to assemble additional family or

friends for support during a difficult time. Do not neglect to address the emotional impact on the hospital staff.[55]

Once the patient fulfills the criteria for brain death, the team in the pediatric intensive care unit can orchestrate the final minutes or hours to meet the needs of the family. To ensure understanding by the parents, review the concept of brain death with the family, even if the team discussed details at a previous meeting. As much as possible, use the term

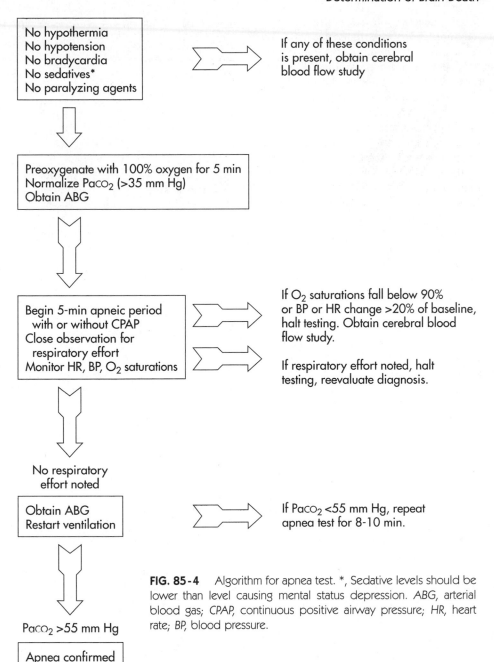

No hypothermia
No hypotension
No bradycardia
No sedatives*
No paralyzing agents

If any of these conditions
is present, obtain cerebral
blood flow study

Preoxygenate with 100% oxygen for 5 min
Normalize $PaCO_2$ (>35 mm Hg)
Obtain ABG

Begin 5-min apneic period
with or without CPAP
Close observation for
respiratory effort
Monitor HR, BP, O_2 saturations

If O_2 saturations fall below 90%
or BP or HR change >20% of baseline,
halt testing. Obtain cerebral blood
flow study.

If respiratory effort noted, halt
testing, reevaluate diagnosis.

No respiratory
effort noted

Obtain ABG
Restart ventilation

If $PaCO_2$ <55 mm Hg, repeat
apnea test for 8-10 min.

$PaCO_2$ >55 mm Hg

Apnea confirmed

FIG. 85-4 *Algorithm for apnea test.* *, *Sedative levels should be lower than level causing mental status depression.* *ABG*, *arterial blood gas;* *CPAP*, *continuous positive airway pressure;* *HR*, *heart rate;* *BP*, *blood pressure.*

death rather than *brain death.* Delay the withdrawal of cardiopulmonary support or the transfer to the operating room to allow additional family members or the chaplain to arrive or to allow the family to spend time at the bedside. The physician chooses the time of death somewhat arbitrarily; it often coincides with the time of completion of the brain death evaluation.[27] If the death was accidental or intentional, call the medical examiner and inform the family that an autopsy is necessary. Otherwise discuss autopsy with the family and obtain informed consent. The family should understand that the pathologists cannot perform an autopsy on harvested organs.

Organ-Donor Maintenance. Despite efforts to support the cadaver, brain death invariably results in hemodynamic collapse.[29] Asystole occurs, probably as a result of loss of vasomotor tone, hypothermia, and metabolic derangements from pituitary death and hormone depletion.[21,32,51] There are

also reports of myocardial high-energy phosphate and glycogen-storage depletion with brain death.[52] Aggressive therapy can forestall hemodynamic collapse and preserve organs for transplantation.[54] Fluid restriction, hyperosmolar therapy, hyperventilation, and steroids are necessary in some patients to control intracranial pressure and may contribute to the problems seen in cadaver organ donors. Care of the cadaver organs may actually be easier once management of intracranial hypertension is no longer necessary.

Hemodynamic stability is necessary to preserve all organs. In addition to achieving an optimal blood pressure, maintain adequate perfusion (good pulses, skin perfusion, urine output). Crystalloid or colloid infusions and inotropic support may be necessary. In adults, dopamine is the preferred agent[12,47]; however, no studies are available to guide the choice of inotropic drugs in the pediatric patient. Either dopamine or dobutamine is effective in many patients;

epinephrine is occasionally necessary to correct bradycardia or increase blood pressure. Be aware that inotropic and pressor agents may exacerbate dysrhythmias. Avoid excessive fluid administration because of the possibility of pulmonary insufficiency and water accumulation in the lung.[12,29]

Anticipate metabolic and hormonal abnormalities in the cadaver organ donor.[13,14,21,35] Hypothermia, diabetes insipidus, hypokalemia, and hyperglycemia are present in more than half of all pediatric donors.[21] These derangements worsen hemodynamic instability through fluid depletion and increased risk of arrhythmias. Treatment of diabetes insipidus includes replacement of urine losses with 5% dextrose in water; however, in many cases this large quantity of fluid replacement worsens hyperglycemia and complicates nursing management. A constant infusion of aqueous vasopressin (begin with 0.01 U/kg/hour, then titrate to achieve a urine output of 2 ml/kg/hr) allows for antidiuretic hormone effect without vasopressor effects and avoids the unevenness of fluid management with intermittent doses of vasopressin or desmopressin (DDAVP). Hyperglycemia may require a constant infusion of insulin.

Decreased thyroid hormone levels may occur in patients who are brain dead and may contribute to hemodynamic instability.[33] Studies of the efficacy of thyroid hormone administration in maintaining hemodynamic stability of cadaver organ donors have shown conflicting results,[17,20,32,38] and hormone replacement therapy is still experimental.

Remarks

Despite general societal and medical acceptance of the concept of brain death, controversy surrounds both the concept and the essential medical criteria for such a diagnosis.[44,46,56] In the United States, the diagnosis of brain death requires the demonstration of irreversible cessation of all functions of the entire brain, including the brain stem.[40] However, patients who are brain dead may have EEG activity, may have hypothalamic endocrine activity, may retain a hemodynamic response to external stimuli, and may have spinal reflexes.[46] How much cellular function can remain below the threshold for detection with present technology? Is that patient's brain dead or dying?[27,46] It is imperative to have a healthy respect for what current criteria can and cannot ascertain and to continue exploration of the concept of death and criteria for death determination.

Although there are several published sets of guidelines for determining brain death in children, no studies have validated any of them, especially in newborns. The minimum observation period necessary in children should be the subject of research. Confirmatory tests such as conventional contrast angiography, HMPAO radionuclide scans, or magnetic resonance angiography also must be studied as potentially sensitive indicators of cerebral blood flow in children.

The determination of death by brain-based criteria is reliable only with strict application of these criteria. Discrepancies between the clinical examination and cerebral blood flow studies suggest that something has been overlooked (Table 85-1).[36,37]

Once it is clear that medical therapy is futile, the primary concern is to help family members cope with the tragedy they are facing. To prevent increased stress for family members, the intensivist and nursing staff should deal sensitively and efficiently with the issues surrounding organ

Table 85-1 Pitfalls in the Diagnosis of Brain Death

Findings	Possible Courses
Fixed pupils	Anticholinergic drugs
	Neuromuscular blockers
	Preexisting disease
No oculovestibular reflexes	Ototoxic agents
	Vestibular suppressants
	Preexisting disease
No respiration	Posthyperventilaiton apnea
	Neuromuscular blockers
No motor activity	Neuromuscular blockers
	"Locked-in" state
	Sedative drugs
Isoelectric EEG	Sedative drugs
	Anoxia
	Hypothermia
	Encephalitis
	Trauma

From Plum F, Posner J: *Diagnosis of stupor and coma,* ed 3, London, 1980, FA Davis.

harvest, the urgent need for the bed now occupied by a heart-beating cadaver, and the needs of other critically ill patients.

A follow-up letter to the family in 2 or 3 weeks offering a meeting with the medical and nursing staff to reaffirm their experience, to answer any questions, and to review the autopsy findings may be appropriate.

REFERENCES

1. A Collaborative Study: An appraisal of the criteria of cerebral death, *JAMA* 237(10):982-986, 1977.
2. Ad Hoc Committee: A definition of irreversible coma, *JAMA* 205(6):85-88, 1968.
3. Ad Hoc Committee: Determination of brain death, *J Pediatr* 110(1):15-19, 1987.
4. Aichner F, et al: Magnetic resonance: a noninvasive approach to metabolism, circulation, and morphology in human brain death, *Ann Neurol* 32:507-511, 1992.
5. Ashwal S, Schneider S: Failure of electroencephalography to diagnose brain death in comatose children, *Ann Neurol* 6:512-517, 1979.
6. Ashwal S, Schneider S: Brain death in children, Part II, *Pediatr Neurol* 3(2):69-77, 1986.
7. Ashwal S, Schneider S: Brain death in the newborn, *Pediatrics* 84(3):429-437, 1989.
8. Benzel E, et al: Apnea testing for the determination of brain death: a modified protocol, *J Neuro Surg* 76:1029-1031, 1992.
9. Buchner H, Schuchardt V: Reliability of electroencephalogram in the diagnosis of brain death, *Eur Neurol* 30:138-141, 1990.
10. Coulter D: Neurologic uncertainty in newborn intensive care, *N Engl J Med* 316(14):840-842, 1987.
11. Dagi T: Death-defining acts. In Kaufman H, editor: *Pediatric brain death and organ/tissue retrieval,* ed 1, New York, 1989, Plenum.
12. Darby J, et al: Approach to management of the heartbeating brain-dead organ, *JAMA* 26(15):2222-2228, 1989.
13. Fackler J, et al: Age-specific characteristics of brain death, *Am J Dis Child* 142:999-1003, 1988.
14. Fiser D, et al: Diabetes insipidus in children with brain death, *Crit Care Med* 15(6):551-553, 1987.
15. Galaske R, et al: A new non-invasive method in determination of brain death in children, *Eur J Nucl Med* 14:446-452, 1988.
16. Goodman J, et al: Validity of radionuclide cerebral angiography for diagnosing brain death in infants. In Kaufman H, editor: *Pediatric brain death and organ/tissue retrieval,* New York, 1989, Plenum.

17. Gramm H: Acute endocrine failure after brain death, *Transplantation* 54(5):851-857, 1992.
18. Grigg M, et al: Electroencephalographic activity after brain death, *Arch Neurol* 44:948-954, 1987.
19. Heck L: Static and dynamic brain imaging. In Gottschalk A, Hoffer P, Potchen E, editors: *Diagnostic nuclear medicine,* Baltimore, 1988, Williams & Wilkins.
20. Keogh A: Pituitary function in brain stem–dead organ donors: a prospective survey, *Transplant Proc* 10(5):729-730, 1988.
21. Kissoon N, et al: Pediatric organ donor maintenance: pathophysiologic derangements and nursing requirements, *Pediatrics* 84:688-693, 1989.
22. Lang C: New criteria for brain death, *J Neurol Neurosurg Psychiatry* 54(11):1030-1031, 1991.
23. Larar G, Nagel J: Technetium-99-HMPAO cerebral perfusion scintigraphy: considerations for timely brain death declaration, *J Nucl Med* 33:2209-2213, 1992.
24. Laurin N, et al: Cerebral perfusion imaging with technetium-99m HMPAO in brain death and severe central nervous system injury, *J Nucl Med* 30:1627-1635, 1989.
25. Lutrin C: Radionuclide evaluation of brain death, *J West Med* 157(1):61-62, 1992.
26. Lutschg J, et al: Brain stem auditory evoked potentials and early somatosensory evoked potentials in neurointensively treated comatose children, *Am J Dis Child* 137:421-426, 1983.
27. Lynn J: Brain death: historical perspectives and current concerns. In Kaufman H, editor: *Pediatric brain death and organ/tissue retrieval,* New York, 1989, Plenum.
28. Machado C, et al: Brain stem auditory evoked potentials and brain death, *Electroencephalogr Clin Neurophysiol* 80:392-398, 1991.
29. Mackersie R, et al: Organ procurement in patients with fatal head injuries: the fate of the potential donor, *Ann Surg* 213:143-150, Feb 1991.
30. Marks S, Zisfein J: Apneic oxygen in apnea tests for brain death, *Arch Neurol* 47:1066-1068, 1990.
31. Moshe S: Usefulness of EEG in the evaluation of brain death in children, *Electroencephalogr Clin Neurophysiol* 73:272-275, 1989.
32. Novitzky D: Triiodothyronine replacement, the euthyroid sick syndrome, and organ transplantation, *Transplant Proc* 23(5):2460-2462, 1991.
33. Novitzky D, et al: Endocrine changes and metabolic response, *Transplant Proc* 10(5):33-38, 1988.
34. Outwater K, Rockoff M: Apnea testing to confirm brain death in children, *Crit Care Med* 12(4):357-358, 1984.
35. Outwater K, Rockoff M: Diabetes insipidus accompanying brain death in children, *Neurology* 34(9):1243-1246, 1984.
36. Pallis C: ABCs of brain-stem death: reappraising death, *Br Med J* 285:1409-1412, 1982.
36a. Pallis C: ABCs of brain-stem death: the argument about the EEG, *Br Med J* 286:284-287, 1983.
37. Plum F, Posner J: *Diagnosis of stupor and coma,* ed 3, London, 1980, FA Davis.
38. Randell T, Hockerstedt K: Triiodothyronine treatment in brain-dead multi-organ donors: a controlled study, *Transplantation* 54(4):736-738, 1992.
39. Reid R, et al: Clinical use of technetium-99m HMPAO for determination of brain death, *J Nucl Med* 30:1621-1626, 1989.
40. Report of the medical consultants on the diagnosis of death to the President's Commission: Guidelines for the determination of death, *JAMA* 246(10):2184-2186, 1981.
41. Ropper A, et al: Apnea testing in the diagnosis of brain death, *J Neuro Surg* 55:942-946, 1981.
42. Schwartz J, et al: Detection of blood flow to the brain by radionuclide cerebral imaging. In Kaufman H, editor: *Pediatric brain death and organ/tissue retrieval,* New York, 1989, Plenum.
43. Setzer N, et al: Evoked potential determinations in children with brain death, *Anesthesiology* 59(3):130, 1983.
44. Shewmon A: Commentary on guidelines for the determination of brain death in children, *Ann Neurol* 24(6):789-791, 1988.
45. Task force for the determination of brain death in children: Guidelines for determination of brain death in children, *Pediatrics* 80:298-299, 1987.
46. Truog R, Fackler J: Rethinking brain death, *Crit Care Med* 20(13):1705-1713, 1992.
47. Turcotte J: Conventional management of the brain-dead potential multi-organ donor, *Transplant Proc* 10(5):5-8, 1988.
48. Turmel A: Spinal man after declaration of brain death, *Neurosurgery* 28(2):298-301, 1991.
49. Urasaki E, et al: Preserved spinal dorsal horn potentials in a brain-dead patient with Lazarus' sign, *Neurosurgery* 76:710-713, 1992.
50. Volpe, JJ: Brain-death determination in newborns, *Pediatrics* 10(2):239-297, 1987.
51. Wetzel R, et al: Hemodynamic responses in brain-dead organ-donor patients, *Anesth Analg* 64:125-128, 1985.
52. Wicomb W, et al: The effects of brain death and 24-hour storage by hypothermic perfusion on donor heart function in the pig, *J Thorac Cardiovasc Surg* 91:896-909, 1986.
53. Ying Z, et al: Motor and somatosensory evoked potentials in coma: analysis and relation to clinical status and outcome, *J Neurol Neurosurg Psychiatry* 55:470-474, 1992.
54. Yoshioka T: Prolonged hemodynamic maintenance by the combined administration of vasopressin and epinephrine in brain death: a clinical study, *Neurosurgery* 18(5):565-567, 1986.
55. Younger S, et al: Psychosocial and ethical implications of organ retrieval, *N Engl J Med* 13(5):321-323, 1985.
56. Younger S, et al: "Brain death" and organ retrieval: a cross-sectional survey of knowledge and concepts among health professionals, *JAMA* 261(15):2205-2210, 1989.

OPHTHALMOLOGY TECHNIQUES

86 Basic Ophthalmic Examination

Alfred D. Sacchetti and Russell H. Harris

Children with eye-related injuries or illnesses are common visitors to all Emergency Departments (EDs). Techniques for managing these patients are relatively few in number and are easily mastered. This chapter reviews ED pediatric ophthalmic procedures. Patient cooperation is essential to any adequate eye examination. Administer sedatives and/or analgesics to children who are too anxious or distressed to permit a complete evaluation.

ANATOMY

Fig. 86-1 represents the basic gross anatomy of the eye. Although slit-lamp examination readily evaluates the anterior chamber, iris, and lens, most actual ED procedures involve only the lids, conjunctiva, and cornea. The lids are composed of three layers: the skin, tarsal plate, and conjunctival surface. This sandwich-type construction is evident at the lid margin, where the tarsal plate can be seen as a gray line just beneath the eye lashes. The conjunctiva originates on the inner surface of the lid and forms a thin membrane that covers all exposed areas of the eye except the cornea. A deep cul-de-sac is formed at the reflection of the upper conjunctiva, creating a potential space for foreign bodies to lodge. Blood vessels for the anterior eye lie in the space between the conjunctiva and sclera but are generally not visible unless some form of inflammatory process exists.

The cornea is composed of an epithelial-covered gelatin-like protein matrix. To maintain clarity the cornea has no blood vessels and receives oxygen and nutritional support through diffusion. Behind the cornea but in front of the iris lies the anterior chamber. Suspended posterior to the iris is the lens.

BASIC EYE EXAMINATION
Indications and Contraindications

Any patient with an eye-related complaint requires at least a basic eye examination. In cases of penetrating trauma or potential globe rupture, avoid portions of the examination that involve applying pressure to the eye, lids, or surrounding area. Portions of the examination that may increase intraocular pressure (IOP) include lid eversion, forced abduction of lids, and contact tonometry. Forgo the examination altogether in cases involving penetrating injuries with protruding foreign bodies still in place. Stabilize the foreign body in place, patch the unaffected eye closed, and immediately obtain a consultation.

Complications

Increasing IOP may worsen existing eye injuries and may occur with aggressive manipulation of an injured eye. If care is taken and if those portions of the examination that increase IOP are omitted, there are few if any complications.

Equipment

The equipment necessary for a basic eye examination include the following: a hand-held penlight, an ophthalmoscope, fluorescein, a cobalt blue light source, cotton-tipped applicators, topical anesthetics, a Snellen chart, lid retractors, and pH paper. Advanced visual acuity equipment is optional and is discussed later in this chapter.

Technique

Begin the basic eye examination with an inspection for obvious injuries, conjunctival injection, and pupillary shape. Simple inspection may be accomplished with the child held on a parent's lap. Difficulty with examination of the eye itself may be encountered if the child refuses to open the eye or if there is pronounced swelling of the lids. Patience and creative cajoling are generally successful in overcoming most voluntary resistance to eye inspection. Forced spreading of the lids is almost universally unsuccessful and with penetrating injuries may even be dangerous. In infants, forced abduction of the lids often produces inadvertent eversion of the upper lid and an unfavorable response from the child's parent. If a child persists in refusing to permit an eye examination, use a mild sedative or anxiolytic combination to encourage cooperation.

If a corneal injury is suspected, place one or two drops of a topical anesthetic such as tetracaine or proparacaine into the eye before the examination to relieve involuntary blepharospasm. Such immediate pain relief not only permits a more complete examination but also creates a favorable image for the medical team with the child. In some institutions the placement of topical anesthetics into the eye is part of the triage protocol. Such policies permit the patient and family to wait more comfortably until seen by the physician and also facilitate initial examination. The effects of topical anesthetics last less than 15 to 20 minutes.

Grossly swollen eyes may make examination difficult or even impossible. Encourage the patient to open the eye voluntarily to permit inspection. If the lids can be separated even a few millimeters, a full view of the eye may be afforded by having the patient rotate the eye across the exposed lid margins. If the eye cannot be voluntarily opened, expose the eye by applying gentle traction to the lids. Generally the examiner's fingers can be used to retract the lids, but in infants and small children cotton-tipped applicators may serve better. Whenever this maneuver is attempted, exert pressure parallel to the eye and only along the axis of the lid—never down onto the globe itself. Applying direct pressure to the eye may produce disastrous results if a penetrating injury exists or if the globe has been ruptured. Fig. 86-2 demonstrates lid retraction through external trac-

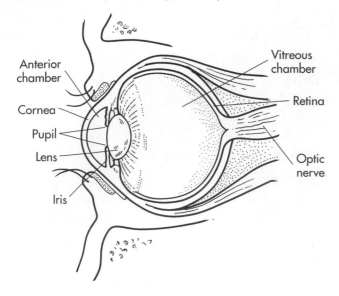

FIG. 86-1 Anatomy of the eye.

Anterior chamber
Cornea
Pupil
Lens
Iris
Vitreous chamber
Retina
Optic nerve

Table 86-1 Visual Function Battery

Test	Normal Reaction
Reaction to high-intensity light	Squinting, avoidance
Fixation	Orients towards penlight or familiar object
Following (horizontal and vertical)	Gaze tracks large object
Fix and follow red rod	Gaze tracks red rod in horizontal and vertical
Optokinetic nystagmus	Nystagmus produced by moving tape with 5-cm vertical stripes in front of child (see section of optokinetic nystagmus)
Grab large object	Successfully grabs large bottle or toy when presented
Grab large red object	Successfully grabs large red object
Obstacle course	Ability to avoid objects such as chairs when walking or crawling

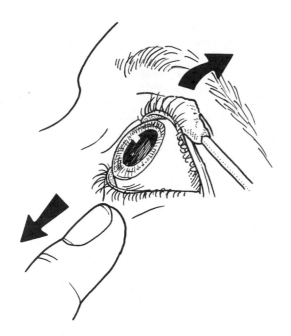

FIG. 86-2 Retraction of the upper and lower lids.

tion. If the lids cannot be separated in this manner, anesthetize the cornea and conjunctiva with a topical agent and use a lid retractor.

Specific retractors (Desmarres) are available, but if necessary a serviceable substitute can be fashioned from a paper clip. Applying the blunt, rounded edges gently to the lids rarely causes corneal injury.[2] Fig. 86-3 demonstrates the use of retractors to provide enough exposure to permit a screening examination of the cornea and anterior eye. When the retractors are placed, position them carefully over the scleral portion of the globe and slide them along the conjunctival surface of the lid to the center point of the lid.

An excellent complete screening examination is the Visual Function Battery (VFB), which evaluates all key aspects of a child's vision.[7] Table 86-1 contains the basic VFB. With this test even agitated children may receive a good assessment of their visual competence. A parent or less threatening companion may be substituted to test as many of the functions as possible and if properly coached may usually perform the entire battery.

The red-light portion of the examination screens for the function of cone vs. rod cells of the retina. This section of the VFB may be omitted for acute episodic examinations such as those following minor trauma or chemical exposures.

The obstacle course in the VFB requires independent locomotion capabilities in the child and may be omitted in very young infants. The obstacle course itself need not be elaborate and simply requires the child to navigate around another person or a chair to return to a parent.

The VFB may be quantitated if the progress of a child must be followed over time. To quantitate the VFB, perform three trials of each function and calculate a visual function quotient (VFQ). Determine the VFQ by dividing the total number of successfully completed tasks by the total number of tasks tested. The VFQ correlates with visual acuity as measured on a Snellen chart and has been used in place of formal visual acuity testing. After the initial examination, perform a more detailed and focused examination on specific portions of the eye as indicated.

Lid Eversion. Part of the ophthalmic examination includes upper lid eversion to exclude the possible presence of foreign bodies. These objects are most commonly found just behind the margin of the lid and are easily seen and removed following eversion.[2]

Applying a topical anesthetic before lid eversion makes the procedure much more comfortable and facilitates patient cooperation. To evert the upper lid, grasp the lashes and pull the lid away from the eye. Place a cotton-tipped applicator on the external surface of the lid and gently press inferiorly. This procedure flips the tarsal plate in the upper lid and successfully everts the lid (Fig. 86-4). The procedure may be easier if the child looks down during the eversion. In older and

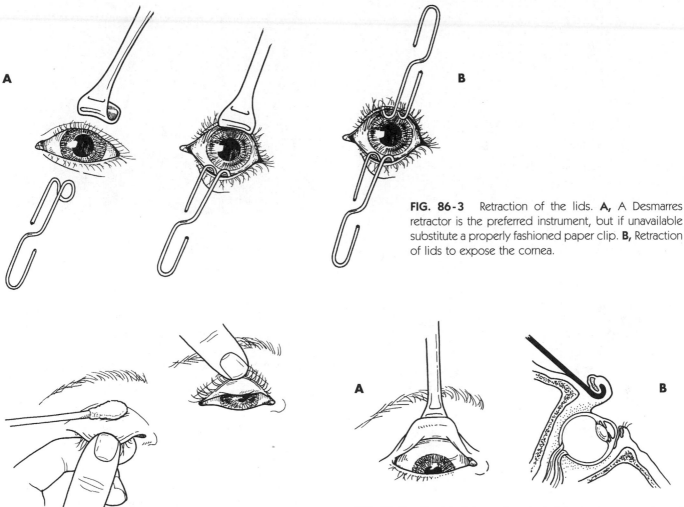

FIG. 86-3 Retraction of the lids. **A,** A Desmarres retractor is the preferred instrument, but if unavailable substitute a properly fashioned paper clip. **B,** Retraction of lids to expose the cornea.

FIG. 86-4 Lid eversion.

FIG. 86-5 Double lid eversion. **A,** A lid retractor or preshaped paper clip is used to first single-evert the lid. **B,** The retractor is angled back against the upper eyebrow to expose the fornix of the conjunctiva.

cooperative patients, simply looking up replaces the everted lid. In younger children replace the lid with a quick downward stroke on the lashes.

If a foreign body is suspected but not seen with simple lid eversion, perform double eversion of the lid. To perform this technique, insert a lid everter onto the outer portion of the lid and evert the lid in the normal fashion. Tilt the retractor back to completely expose the deep recesses of the upper-lid cul-de-sac (Fig. 86-5). If a lid everter is not available, use a paper clip that has been fashioned to resemble a lid everter.

Visual Acuity. Visual acuity is generally regarded as a patient's ability to see but is actually composed of four distinct subgroups (Box 86-1).[5] Detection acuity can be used to determine the presence or absence of vision in a particular patient. A child's ability to recognize that an object has been introduced into his or her visual field constitutes a test of detection acuity. Resolution acuity is commonly assessed when visual acuity is measured and is the ability of a patient to discriminate the internal features of an identified object or figure. Resolution acuity tests measure the patient's ability to distinguish features within a figure relative to the overall size

of the figure. The identification of letters on an eye chart is an example of resolution acuity testing.

Visual acuity testing requires not only an intact visual organ (the eye) but also a functioning neuroprocessing apparatus (the neuroophthalmic pathways and visual cortex). Children with neurologic deficits often require special compensating techniques and equipment to determine their visual acuity.

Snellen Chart. In the alert and cooperative verbal patient use a standard Snellen chart to determine visual acuity (Fig. 86-6, *A*). Ask literate patients to read letters of the alphabet while standing a fixed distance from the eye chart. In grading vision from a Snellen chart, define the patient's visual acuity as the smallest line in which the patient correctly identifies 50% of the letters.

Test nonliterate patients with a Snellen chart, but instead of having them read letters, ask them to indicate in which direction a letter E is facing. Alternate illiterate charts require the identification of simple black-and-white figures or drawings of hands pointing in different directions. Fig. 86-6, *B* demonstrates a typical pediatric nonliterate eye chart.

BOX 86-1 TYPES OF VISUAL ACUITY

Detection acuity

Ability to detect the presence or absence of an isolated object

Resolution acuity

Ability to discriminate distinct features of a visible object

Recognition acuity

Ability to recognize known features of an object from features of another object

Hyperacuity

Ability to localize features within a visible object

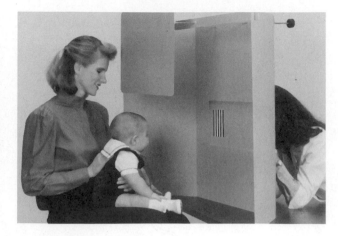

FIG. 86-7 Child sitting on mother's lap while undergoing preferred looking test with Teller cards.

(Courtesy Vistech Consultants, Inc., Dayton, OH)

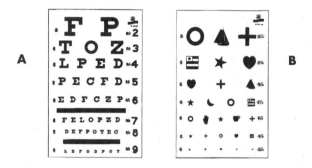

FIG. 86-6 Snellen visual acuity charts. **A,** Standard literate patient chart. **B,** Pediatric nonliterate figure chart.

(Courtesy Vistech Consultants, Inc., Dayton, OH.)

Optical Gratings. Individual figures need not be used to test resolution acuity. Their use is more a matter of convenience in verbal children. In nonverbal children use patterns of alternating black-and-white lines or sinusoid waves to test resolution acuity.* These patterns are termed *optical gratings* and are repetitive, predictable, and mathematically precise luminance variations. As the frequency of the pattern increases, it becomes progressively more difficult to resolve the patterns. The point at which the child can no longer distinguish the pattern is the child's visual acuity. Correlations of optical grating visual acuity with visual acuity measurements obtained from a Snellen chart exist but are imprecise. Regard these correlations as estimates only. Three tests use optical gratings for visual acuity testing: optokinetic nystagmus, preferential looking tests, and visual evoked potentials.

OPTOKINETIC NYSTAGMUS. Optokinetic nystagmus (OKN) is the response of a normal eye to the motion of a visual pattern across its visual field.[9,13] The eye tracks the pattern from a midposition to an extreme lateral gaze. As the pattern passes from view, the eye returns to the midposition to repeat the procedure. The eye must distinguish the pattern to elicit this reflex. In OKN testing an optical grating is used for the

pattern. Determine visual acuity by varying the frequency of the grating and observing the child's response. Because the child must be able to distinguish the pattern for OKN to occur, the grating frequency at which the nystagmus extinguishes is the child's visual acuity.

To perform this test, spin a wheel with a square-wave or striped pattern in front of the child to produce the nystagmus. Although resolution is required to distinguish the optical grating, OKN is generally regarded as a detection acuity test and not a resolution test.

PREFERENTIAL LOOKING TESTS. During preferential looking tests (PLTs), optical grating figures are presented to children to establish a gaze preference.* The test is based on the notion that a child preferentially looks at a distinct figure as opposed to a simple gray background. Black-and-white luminance variations appear gray at the threshold of a patient's resolution. By presenting the child with a choice of optically grated figures or a gray background, the examiner can determine whether the child preferentially looks at the figure or demonstrates no looking preference. Observing the child's reaction to variations in the grating frequencies allows the examiner to determine a point at which the child no longer demonstrates a looking preference. This grating frequency represents the child's visual acuity.[6]

Perform PLTs with the child sitting on a parent's lap while optical gratings are presented. The gratings are contained on one end of a card that has a gray background. The examiner or an assistant who is blinded regarding the position or frequency of the grating records the child's response and any looking preference. Fig. 86-7 demonstrates a child undergoing a PLT with a set of Teller cards, which are named after the physician who first described this phenomenon.[16] Multiple modifications of this technique have been described, including a screening examination in which gloves imprinted with optical gratings are substituted for the Teller cards.[12]

VISUAL EVOKED POTENTIALS. Visual evoked potentials (VEPs) monitor a child's ability to distinguish optical grat-

---

*References 5, 10, 11, 13, 16, and 17.

*Refences 6, 10, 11, 13, 16, and 17.

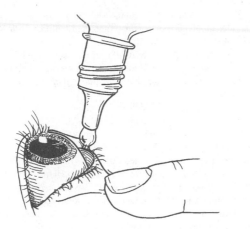

FIG. 86-8 Administration of ophthalmic medication.

ings through the use of electroencephalographic (EEG) monitoring.[5,16] As with PLTs, children are presented with optically grated images to determine resolution acuity. The measured event in VEP testing is not a motor response as with OKN or PLT but is the brain activity over the visual areas of the occipital cortex and brain stem. Although the most sophisticated of the visual acuity tests, VEPs are expensive and require specialized equipment and technical expertise. Their optimal value is for children who are unable to cooperate for PLTs or for whom more intensive investigation is required after screening tests have identified a problem.

Test visual acuity in each eye separately and with both eyes. When testing monocular vision, occlude the nontested eye with an opaque card while allowing it to remain open. Having the patient actively close one eye forces the patient to squint, which may distort the vision of the open eye.

Medication Administration. The proper technique for the placement of ophthalmic medications is to extend the lower lid and place the medication into the lower conjunctival reflection (Fig. 86-8). This approach works equally well for both drops and ointments. Holding pressure on the skin overlying the lacrimal duct or having the patient forcefully close the eye increases the conjunctival duration of the medication.[18] Dropping medications directly onto the cornea is painful and may frighten children for subsequent examinations. Use single-unit dose preparations of all ophthalmic drugs to prevent cross-contamination between patients.[1]

Determination of pH. The pH of the conjunctival sac should be determined if a chemical exposure to the eyes has occurred.[4] To perform this test expose the conjunctiva of the lower lid by providing gentle traction on the skin just under the lower lid. Touch the tip of a piece of pH paper to the conjunctiva and allow it to remain in place until well moistened, which usually requires 2 to 4 seconds. Remove the strip and compare its color to the reference color chart provided with the pH paper. If pH paper is not available, substitute the pH indicator on a urine dipstick.[2] Normal conjunctival pH is approximately 7.4.[4] Prior placement of ophthalmic solutions may alter the pH; if there is any question repeat the test after the eye has equilibrated for 20 minutes. Determination of pH takes only a few seconds and is important, particularly in alkali burns. However, rapid irrigation of such injuries is even more important; do not delay irrigation to perform pH measurements.[3,14]

Fluorescein Examination. Fluorescein examination is indicated in most patients with eye-related complaints. Perform the examination with sodium fluorescein, an orange dye that fluoresces under the proper pH conditions when exposed to a blue light source. The corneal subepithelial membrane (Bowman's membrane) has an alkaline pH compared with the normal epithelial pH of 7.4. Fluorescein taken up in this area fluoresces a bright green under a cobalt blue light. This phenomenon can be used to identify areas of the cornea that are missing the epithelial covering and serves as the basis for fluorescein testing for corneal abrasions. Other causes of epithelial defects, such as keratitis, burns, and lacerations, also fluoresce with this test.[8,15]

If pH determination is indicated, determine it before fluorescein staining because the orange color of the fluorescein may invalidate the colormetric comparisons used in pH determination. Soft contact lenses readily absorb the fluorescein dye; warn the patient and caregiver not to replace the child's contact lenses for at least 1 hour after the fluorescein dye has been instilled.

Fluorescein placement is performed in a manner similar to that of conjunctival pH testing. The only difference in fluorescein testing is that the strip of fluorescein-impregnated paper is moistened first with a drop of nonpharmacologic ophthalmic solution before placement in the conjunctival sac. The use of multidose premixed fluorescein solutions should be discouraged because of the risks of bacterial growth in the solution and cross-contamination between patients. Once the fluorescein has been placed into the conjunctival sac, instruct the patient to blink 2 to 3 times to spread the chemical across the cornea. Use a cobalt blue light to illuminate the cornea and identify any lesions. If too much fluorescein is placed into the conjunctiva, the entire surface of the eye occasionally picks up the stain and a diffuse haze appears over the cornea. If this reaction occurs, flush the eye with a small amount of a neutral solution and reexamine the eye.

Fluorescein staining may also be used to help identify lacrimal duct lacerations. Because the duct in the lower lid drains into the nose, any fluorescein in the conjunctiva traverses the duct and empties into the nasal cavity. If the lacrimal system is intact and functioning, fluorescein should appear in the nasal mucus within 20 minutes of conjunctival instillation. The best way to check for the fluorescein is to have the patient blow his or her nose and examine the tissue for the orange dye.

Remarks

Eye examinations are best performed in a specific eye room in the ED. If such a room is not possible or if the examination is to be performed in the intensive care unit, the necessary eye equipment should be assembled onto an eye tray or cart.

REFERENCES

1. Aylward GW, Wilson RS: Contamination of dropper bottles with tear fluid in an ophthalmic outpatient clinic, *Br Med J* 294:1587, 1987.
2. Barr DH, Samples JR, Hedges JR: Ophthalmologic procedures. In Roberts J, Hedges JR, editors: *Clinical procedures in emergency medicine,* Philadelphia, 1991, WB Saunders.

3. Burns FR, Paterson CA: Prompt irrigation of chemical eye injuries may avert severe damage, *Occup Health Saf* 58:33-36, 1989.

4. Campochiparo PA, Fogle JA, Spyker DA: Chemical and drug injury to the eye. In Haddad LM, Winchester JF, editors: *Poisoning and drug overdose,* ed 2, Philadelphia, 1990, WB Saunders.

5. Chandra A: Natural history of the development of visual acuity in infants, *Eye* 5:20-26, 1991.

6. Courage ML, Adams RJ: Visua acuity assessment from birth to three years using the acuity card procedure: cross-sectional and longitudinal samples, *Optom Vis Sci* 67:713-718, 1990.

7. Droste PJ, Archer SM, Helveston EM: Measurement of low vision in children and infants, *Ophthalmology* 98:1513-1518, 1991.

8. Glaser J: Neuro-ophthalmic examination: general consideration and special techniques. In Duane TD, Jafler ED editors: *Clinical ophthalmology,* vol 2, New York, 1987, Harper & Row.

9. Hopkisson G, Arnold P, Billingham B, et al: Visual assessment of infants: vernier targets for the Catford drum, *Br J Ophthalmol* 75:280-283, 1991.

10. Jackson GR, Jesup NS, Kavanaugh BL, et al: Measuring visual acuity in children using preferential looking and sine wave cards, *Optom Vis Sci* 67:590-594, 1990.

11. Katsumi O, Kronheim JK, Mehta MC, et al: Measuring vision with temporally modulated stripes in infants and children with ROP, *Invest Ophthalmol Vis Sci* 34:496-502, 1993.

12. Kronheim JK, Katsumi O, Matsui Y, et al: Visual hand display (VHD) as an introductory procedure for measuring vision in infants and young children with visual impairment, *J Pediatr Ophthal Strabismus* 29:305-311, 1992.

13. Lamkin JC: Can this baby see? Estimation of visual acuity in the preverbal child, *Int Ophthalmol Clin* 32:1-23, 1992.

14. Poe CA: Eye-irrigating lens more effective if applied seconds after accident, *Occup Health Saf* 59:43-47, 1990.

15. Sexton R: Herpes simplex keratitis. In Wilson LA, editor: *External diseases of the eye,* Hangerstown, Md, 1979, Harper & Row.

16. Teller DY, Morse R, Borton R, et al: Visual acuity for vertical and diagonal grating in human infants, *Vision Res* 14:1433-1439, 1974.

17. Vital-Durand F: Acuity care procedures and the linearity of grating resolution development during the first year of human infants, *Behav Brain Res* 49:99-106, 1992.

18. Zimmerman TJ, Kooner KS, Kandarakis AS, et al: Improving the therapeutic index of topically applied ocular drugs, *Arch Ophthalmol* 102:551-553, 1984.

87 Slit-Lamp Examination

Alfred D. Sacchetti and Russell H. Harris

Slit-lamp examination (SLE) permits a magnified stereoscopic view of the eye from the lashes to the lens.[4] The slit lamp itself consists of a binocular microscope mounted horizontally in a frame specifically designed to accommodate the patient's head. An adjustable light source is contained on a separate mount in the frame (Fig. 87-1). The viewing lens and light source can be positioned in all planes and may be rotated around the patient's eyes to permit both direct and oblique views. Various filters for the light source are available, but generally only the blue filter is commonly used when performing fluorescein staining.

Indications and Contraindications

SLE is indicated for any patient requiring a detailed examination of the eye. The only contraindications to this examination are patients who are too unstable to submit to the examination or those who are unable to cooperate with the procedure.

Equipment

In addition to the slit lamp, other equipment necessary for performing an SLE includes cotton-tipped applicators, topical anesthetic, and fluorescein.

Technique

Before the patient is placed in the slit lamp, the lens can be adjusted to the clinician's preference. The eyepieces are set in the same manner as a conventional binocular microscope. A finger placed at the expected position of the patient's eye can be used as a focus point for adjusting the individual eyepieces.

To perform a slit-lamp examination, a patient must be able to sit upright while holding the head stable. Younger children may sit on a parent's lap for the examination. Fig. 87-2 shows a patient and clinician properly positioned at a slit lamp. It is very important to have the patient not only rest his or her jaw in the chin slot but also to rest his or her forehead against the upper strap. This position maintains the patient in a vertical plane 90 degrees to the lens, which keeps both the upper and lower portions of the eye in simultaneous focus. Darken the room for SLE evaluation both for patient comfort and to facilitate portions of the examination.

Set the light source for the slit lamp to a narrow vertical rectangle or slit with the lowest possible brightness. Many clinicians use the bridge of the nose directly between the eyes as a focus source to set the light's intensity and shape. Using this area also allows the clinician to gauge a good starting distance for the slit-lamp examination. Knowing this distance is useful because, as with a microscope, minimal depth movements dramatically change the focus of an object. It is more comfortable for the patient if the gross depth positioning is adjusted while the light source is on the nose rather than shining in an irritated eye. In performing the examination itself, some clinicians place the light source in direct alignment with the viewing lens; however, for patient comfort offset the light source to 45 degrees to avoid direct illumination of the retina. Once the light source and depth are set, the ophthalmic examination can begin.

The slit lamp can be moved through the use of a joystick located at the base of the scope. The joystick provides very fine control over the viewing field and is used to adjust the depth of focus and the lateral motion of the lens.

The exact order in which an SLE is performed is a matter of personal preference and convenience. As with other portions of the physical examination, the development of an organized approach results in a more consistent examination with less possibility of omitting any component.

Logistically it is easiest to begin the examination with superficial structures and progress to deep structures. Beginning at one end of the eye, scan the lid margin of one of the lids; scan the opposite lid in the reverse direction. If a foreign body is suspected, evert the upper lid and use the slit lamp to examine underneath the lid. Because of the curve of the eye, the slit lamp must be moved in an arc as it scans across the eye and not just in a straight lateral direction. Following examination of the lid, examine the cornea, conjunctiva, and sclera. Again perform the examination with as narrow and tall a light slit as possible and with the same arclike scanning motion. Inspect isolated objects from different angles or magnifications.

Inspect the iris, pupil, and lens with the light set in this same manner. Pay particular attention to the lower portion of the anterior chamber and look for collections of blood (hyphema), which may pool in this area.

Visualize the anterior chamber proper by narrowing the light beam to a very small square and angling it across the cornea into the pupil (Fig. 87-3).[1,4] Occasionally to produce this effect the light source must be positioned at an angle that is greater than 45-degrees to the viewing lenses. Use the joystick to adjust the view so that the eye is viewed directly while the light is projected tangentially through the cornea, anterior chamber, and pupil and onto the lens. When adjustments are made properly, the eye will remain dark with the exception of the narrow beam of light. If the anterior chamber is quiet, the only light that is seen is that which is illuminating the anterior portion of the cornea and striking the lens. When iritis is present, the debris in the anterior chamber produces what is termed a *cell-and-flare reaction,* which resembles a sunbeam passing through a dusty room. The degree of cell and flare is roughly proportional to the severity of the patient's iritis.

Following the plain-light examination, return the light source to the slit configuration and repeat the cornea examination with the blue filter and fluorescein stain. With the slit lamp, microscopic lesions that cannot be visualized with the naked eye may be seen. Because deep abrasions may permit

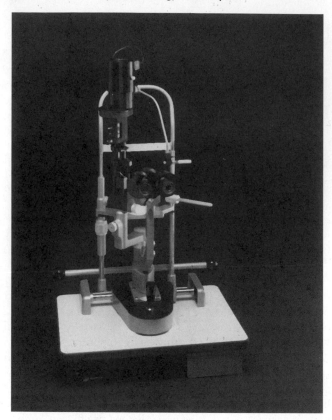

FIG. 87-1 Basic ophthalmic slit lamp.

(Courtesy Marco Ophthalmic, Inc., Jacksonville, Fla.)

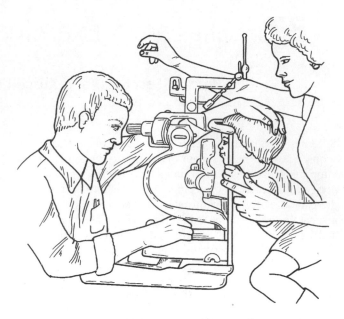

FIG. 87-2 Child properly positioned in slit lamp. Note that forehead rests completely against headrest to maintain proper alignment.

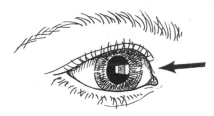

FIG. 87-3 Examination of the anterior chamber. Direct the small and narrow slit-lamp beam tangentially through the anterior chamber from the cornea to the lens. Set up the slit lamp to view the anterior chamber perpendicular to the direction of the beam of light.

the fluorescein dye to leak into the anterior chamber, the presence of dye in this area does not necessarily indicate a corneal laceration.

One observation that can be made during an SLE and that *does* indicate penetration of the anterior chamber is demonstration of the Seidel effect. With this effect, a steady stream of clear fluid can be seen washing out the fluorescein dye from a corneal defect, which indicates a communication between the anterior chamber and the surface of the cornea.[2,3]

Remarks

The more often an SLE is performed, the more comfortable the procedure becomes and the faster it can be performed. An experienced clinician can usually perform the entire examination in approximately 5 minutes.

REFERENCES

1. Barr DH, Samples JR, Hedges JR: Ophthalmologic procedures. In Roberts J, Hedges JR, editor: *Clinical procedures in emergency medicine,* Philadelphia, 1991, WB Saunders.
2. Cain W, Sinckey RM: Detection of anterior chamber leakage with Seidel's test, *Arch Ophthalmol,* (99):201-203, 1981.
3. Friedberg MA, Rapuano CJ: *Wills Eye Hospital office and emergency room diagnosis and treatment of eye diseases,* Philadelphia, 1990, JB Lippincott.
4. Tate GW, Safir A: The slit lamp: history, principles and practice. In Duane TD, editor: *Clinical ophthalmology,* vol 1, New York, Harper & Row, 1981.

88 Tonometry

Alfred D. Sacchetti and Russell H. Harris

Tonometry is the measurement of the intraocular pressure (IOP) of the eye. IOP is determined by deforming the cornea through the application of a metered force. When the force deforming the specific part of the eye is equal to the IOP, an equilibrium is reached; this equilibrium point corresponds to the IOP. The method used to deform the cornea and the device used to measure the equilibrium point differentiate the various detection techniques. Normal pediatric IOPs are noted in Table 88-1.[9]

Indications and Contraindications

Tonometry is indicated for any child in whom a derangement of IOP is suspected. Do not perform emergent measurement of IOP in any child with a penetrating ocular injury, a potential global rupture, or a possible detached retina.

Equipment

A number of different devices are available for the performance of tonometry (Table 88-2).

Schiötz Tonometer. The Schiötz tonometer allows direct mechanical measurement of the global pressure. This device uses a floating weighted plunger inside a fixed footplate to deform the cornea and deflect an indicator needle across a calibrated scale. A conversion factor based on the weight used calculates the IOP from the scale.

To perform Schiötz tonometry, thoroughly anesthesize the eye and place the patient in the supine position. Do not place the patient in even a slight Trendelenberg position because doing so may artificially raise the IOP. Ask the patient to focus with the opposite eye on a point on the ceiling directly above the stretcher. Retract the lids of the tested eye but do not exert any pressure on the globe through the lids; direct any pressure onto the bony rim surrounding the eye. Lower the footplate of the tonometer onto the cornea until the upper portion of the device is floating freely. Fig. 88-1 demonstrates a Schiötz tonometer in place on a cornea. Measure the opposite eye for a comparison, especially if there is any question that the readings on the affected eye are spurious.

The advantages of Schiötz tonometry are that it is relatively inexpensive and easily learned. The major disadvantage is that it requires significant patient cooperation.

Applanation Tonometer. The Goldmann applanation tonometer uses a refractive lens to indent a specifically sized area of the cornea (3 mm). Pressure equilibration is detected using the change in light of the cornea contacting the lens surface. To perform applanation tonometry, anesthesize the eye and stain it with fluorescein. Using a tonometer-equipped slit lamp with the blue filter in place, touch the applanation lens to the cornea. To view the tonometer, look through only the slit-lamp lens that is on the same side as the eye being tested. Fig. 88-2 demonstrates Goldmann tonometry. Two half-circles will appear in the lens when the eye is touched (Fig. 88-3). Adjust the tonometer until the inner edges of the

Table 88-1 Normal IOPs for Children by Age

Age (years)	Mean (mm Hg)	Standard deviation
Birth	9.59	2.30
0 - 1	10.61	3.10
1 - 2	12.03	3.19
2 - 3	12.58	3.19
3 - 4	13.73	2.05
4 - 5	13.56	2.00
5 - 6	14.41	1.99
6 - 7	14.15	2.32
7 - 8	13.95	2.49
8 - 9	14.32	1.73
9 - 10	13.96	2.67
10 - 11	14.59	2.51
11 - 12	13.97	2.42
12 - 13	14.89	1.89
13 - 14	13.94	1.78
14 - 15	14.09	2.47
15 - 16	15.18	2.43

Modified from Pensiero S, DaPozzo S, Perissutti P, et al: Normal intraocular pressure in children, *J Pediatr Ophthalmol Strabismus* 29:79-84, 1992.

two circles just touch.[2] When correctly set, the circles fluctuate with the patient's pulse pressure. Read the IOP from the tonometer.

The advantage of Goldmann applanation tonometry is its precision. This device is the gold standard against which other tonometers are measured. Nevertheless, there are a number of disadvantages to this device, including the need for a slit lamp, the necessity for a cooperative sitting patient, and a significant learning curve before the procedure can be mastered.

Tono-Pen Tonometer. The Tono-Pen is a small handheld contact tonometer.[3,6] As with the Schiötz tonometer, there is a central plunger and surrounding footplate. With this instrument, the central plunger is connected to an electronic strain gauge that calculates the equilibrium point from a waveform generated when the footplate touches the cornea.[1] To activate the Tono-Pen, the device need only be touched to the cornea until a click is heard, which signifies that the pen has registered a pressure. Perform multiple trials and average these trials to determine the IOP.

The major advantage of the Tono-Pen is its speed and simplicity. Because the cornea need only be touched, it may be used in uncooperative patients and children. The footplate is smaller than that of either a Goldmann applanation tonometer or Schiötz tonometer, which makes it better suited for irregular corneas or small children.

Cross-contamination is not a problem with a Tono-Pen because the tip is covered with a latex shield that is discarded

Table 88-2 Comparison of Different Tonometry Devices

	Device			
	Schiötz	Goldmann	Tono-Pen	Pulsair
Accuracy	Good	Excellent	Good	Good
Training	Minimal	Extensive	Minimal	Minimal
Difficulty	Simple	Complex	Simple	Simple
Cost	Low	Moderate	High	High
Position	Supine	Seated	Any	Any
Cross-contamination potential	Yes	Yes	No	No
Pediatric use	Difficult	Difficult	Simple	Simple
Portability	Yes	No	Yes	No

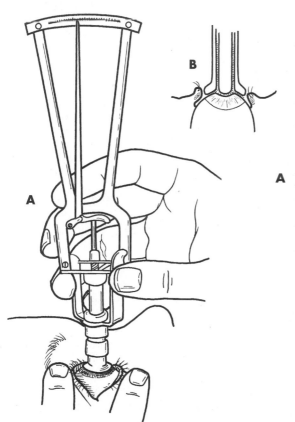

FIG. 88-1 **A,** Schiötz tonometer in place on eye. **B,** Close-up of footplate deforming cornea.

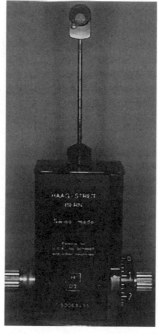

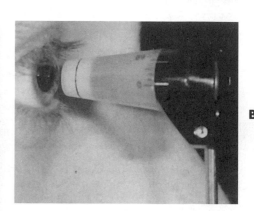

FIG. 88-2 Goldmann applanation tonometer. **A,** Applanation tonometer. **B,** Goldmann tonometer touching anterior cornea.

(From Ragge NK, Easty DL: *Immediate eye care,* St Louis, 1990, Mosby.)

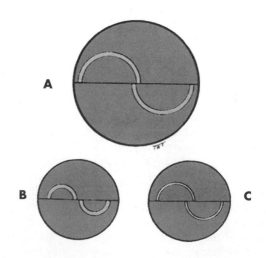

FIG. 88-3 Slit-lamp view of applanation tonometer in place. **A,** Proper alignment. **B,** Underapplanation or too much fluorescein. **C,** Overapplanation or too little fluorescein.

(From Ragge NK, Easty DL: *Immediate eye care,* St Louis, 1990, Mosby.)

after each patient. The disadvantages of this device include cost and accuracy. The device tends to differ slightly from the Goldmann standard in the normal range but in one study was 91% sensitive and 95% specific with IOPs in excess of 21 mm Hg.

Noncontact Tonometer. With the use of noncontact tonometers, IOP can be measured without touching the cornea.[4] These devices direct a graded impulse of air at the cornea.[7,10] A series of photodetectors measure the corneal flattening and correlate it with the pressure at the point at which the flattening occurred.[1] The Keeler Pulsair device is a handheld instrument through which the clinician visualizes the eye to be tested. When the instrument is properly positioned, an air stream is automatically triggered and the pressure is monitored.[1,5,8]

The major advantages of a noncontact tonometer are its portability and lack of direct patient contact with the instrument. Because the cornea is not touched, there is no need for pretreatment with topical anesthetics. In addition, the risk of cross-contamination with other patients is greatly decreased. The automated nature of the device makes it relatively easy to use, and it has been used with good success in children.[4] Disadvantages of the Keeler Pulsair device are similar to those of the Tono-Pen. The device correlates well with Goldmann applanation tonometers and in one study demonstrated a 93% sensitivity and 94% specificity in detecting IOPs in excess of 21 mm Hg.[1]

Remarks

The selection of a tonometry technique often depends more on the available equipment than on personal preference.

REFERENCES

1. Armstrong TA: Evaluation of the Tono-Pen and the Pulsair tonometers, *Am J Ophthalmol* 109:716-720, 1990.
2. Barr DH, Samples JR, Hedges JR: Ophthalmologic procedures. In Roberts J, Hedges JR, editors: *Clinical procedures in emergency medicine*, Philadelphia, 1991, WB Saunders.
3. Boothe WA, Lee DA, Panek WC, et al: The Tono-Pen: a manometric and clinical study, *Arch Ophthalmol* 106:1214-1217, 1988.
4. Buscemi M, Capoferri C, Garavaglia A, et al: Noncontact tonometry in children, *Optom Vis Sci* 68:461-464, 1991.
5. Fisher JH, Watson PG, Spaeth G: A new handheld air impulse tonometer, *Eye* 2:238-242, 1988.
6. Hessemer V, Rossler R, Jacobi KW: Tono-Pen: a new tonometer, *Int Ophthalmol* 13:51-56, 1989.
7. Kretz G, Demailly P: X-PERT NCT advanced logic tonometer evaluation, *Int Ophthalmol* 16:287-290, 1992.
8. Pearce CD, Kohl P, Yolton RL: Clinical evaluation of the Keeler PULSAIR tonometer, *J Am Optom Assoc* 63:106-110, 1992.
9. Pensiero S, DaPozzo S, Perissutti P, et al: Normal intraocular pressure in children, *J Pediatr Ophthalmol Strabismus* 29:79-84, 1992.
10. Vernon SA: Noncontact tonometry in the postoperative eye, *Br J Ophthalmol* 73:247-249, 1989.

89 Irrigation

Alfred D. Sacchetti and Russell H. Harris

Irrigation of the eye is a cleansing technique that uses the continuous flow of liquid across the external eye in an attempt to remove particulate material or to dilute a corrosive chemical.

Indications and Contraindications

Irrigation of the eye is indicated for any chemical or body-fluid exposure to the eye. The use of a continuous fluid stream can also be used to flush out small bits of nonembedded foreign material. There are no true contraindications to emergent eye irrigation. The more serious the chemical injury to the eye, the more important the irrigation.

Equipment

The equipment needed for irrigation of the eye is as follows: irrigation solution, intravenous tubing, intravenous catheter, Morgan lens (recommended).

Techniques

Unlike with wound irrigations in which high pressure is used, a steady, gravity-fed stream of saline is used with irrigation of the eye to flush the conjunctiva and cornea. Intravenous (IV) fluid dripped through standard IV tubing held a few millimeters above an anesthetized eye is the traditional method of irrigation.[1]

Retract the lids intermittently to expose redundant areas of the conjunctiva while moving the tip of the tubing to different positions over the eye. In general, 1 L of irrigation solution is considered the optimum amount for most chemical exposures. In small children and infants, proportionately less irrigant may be required. The one major exception to this standard volume of irrigation involves alkali burns. Because of the penetrating nature of these agents, prolonged irrigation—sometimes in excess of 24 hours—is required to treat this type of injury.

Intravenous normal saline solution (NSS) is the fluid most commonly used for eye irrigations. NSS itself can be irritating, and neutralizing the solution with sodium bicarbonate to a pH of 7.4 has been shown to relieve some of this discomfort.[3] Preanesthetizing the eye before irrigation can eliminate this problem. A commercial irrigation solution BSS Plus (Alcon) has been shown to be less irritating than either

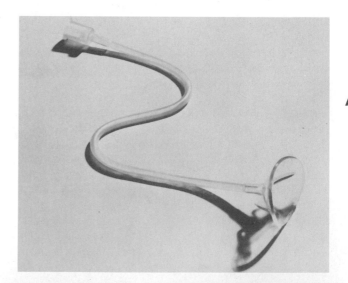

A

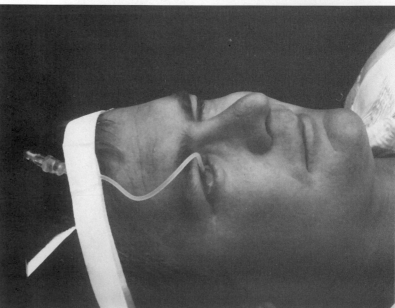

B

FIG. 89-1 Continuous irrigation contact lens. **A,** Morgan lens. **B,** Morgan lens in place.

(Courtesy Mor-Tan, Inc., Missoula, MT.)

NSS or NSS plus bicarbonate, but it is considerably more expensive.[3] The best use of these types of solutions may be for brief, small-volume irrigations such as those used to flush out a specific conjunctival foreign body.

When treating chemical exposures to the eye, the irrigation solution itself may be less important than the timing of the irrigation. The immediate application of tap or distilled water to an affected eye has been shown to be very effective in minimizing chemical corneal damage.[2,4]

A continuous irrigating contact lens may help irrigate a patient's eye. These devices are designed to permit unattended and prolonged irrigation of the cornea and conjunctiva.[4] The Morgan lens is a commercially available irrigation lens that provides a fast and efficient way to irrigate the eye in cases of thermal and chemical burns (Fig. 89-1). For more information, call Mor-Tan, Inc. at (800) 423-8659. Place the lens on an anesthetized eye and hold it in position with the upper and lower lids. Attach a standard IV tubing apparatus to the lens and irrigate the eye.

Another continuous irrigation system can be fabricated from the small tubing attached to a pediatric butterfly needle.[5] Cut the needle apparatus from the tubing and seal the end with a suture or cautery. Create multiple small holes in the tubing with the butterfly needle. Fashion the tubing into a loop and hold it in this position with a piece of silk suture. After administering a topical anesthetic, place the loop onto the conjunctiva and hold it in place with the lids. Attach standard IV tubing and irrigation solution to the loop of tubing and perform the irrigation. This system may be useful in infants who are too small for the commercial irrigation lenses. One other advantage of this system is that it permits repeated slit-lamp examination with the irrigation loop in place.

If both eyes require irrigation, fashion a continuous system from a standard nasal oxygen cannula. Place the oxygen prongs across the bridge of the nose so that a single prong rests on either side. Introduce IV solution through the oxygen tubing and allow it to flush across the patient's eyes.

Remarks

The use of topical anesthetics greatly facilitates irrigation of an eye and should be used liberally in conjunction with this procedure.

REFERENCES

1. Barr DH, Samples JR, Hedges JR: Ophthalmologic procedures. In Roberts J, Hedges JR, editors: *Clinical procedures in emergency medicine,* Philadelphia, 1991, WB Saunders.
2. Burns FR, Paterson CA: Prompt irrigation of chemical eye injuries may avert severe damage, *Occup Health Saf* 58:33-36, 1989.
3. Herr RD, White GL, Bernhisel K, et al: Clinical comparison of ocular irrigation fluids following chemical injury, *Am J Emerg Med* 9:228-231, 1991.
4. Poe CA: Eye-irrigating lens more effective if applied seconds after accident, *Occup Health Saf* 59:43-47, 1990.
5. Yamabayashi S, Furuya T, Gohd T, et al: Newly designed continuous corneal irrigation system for chemical burns, *Ophthalmologica* 201:174-179, 1990.

90 Eye Patching

Alfred D. Sacchetti and Russell H. Harris

Eye patching is a commonly performed ophthalmic procedure. The passive lid closure afforded by the patch relieves blepharospasm and provides a dark, moist environment to promote healing. When performed correctly, eye patching can increase a patient's comfort and provide a protective covering for the eye.

Indications and Contraindications

The primary indication of eye patching in the acute setting is to provide symptomatic relief from traumatic iritis and corneal abrasions. Patching is contraindicated in infectious conditions and penetrating injuries, where it may actually worsen the existing condition.[1]

Eye shields are indicated in instances of penetrating injuries or global rupture. In these situations, the shields are generally temporizing measures used to prevent further damage and are placed across the bony structures surrounding the eye without exerting pressure on the eye itself. If a commercial shield is unavailable, fashion a serviceable substitute from a small drinking cup.

Equipment

The only equipment required to perform an eye patching is an eye patch (or clean, dry gauze) and tape.

Technique

Commercial eye patches are generally too thin when used alone and are best used by combining two patches, with one folded in half and applied directly over the lid and the other layered on top of the first. Hold the patches in place with multiple rows of tape that originate from the ipsilateral corner of the mouth and cross over the patch to end on the forehead. Ideally the tape should form a fan-shaped pattern from the mouth across the patch (Fig. 90-1). In small children and infants, a single eye patch folded in half provides ample bulk to effectively patch the eye. To facilitate patching, remove skin oils with an alcohol swab.

Recheck pressure patches in 24 hours. Short-term patching for 1 to 2 days should be all that is ever indicated in the Emergency Department setting and is safe in almost all children. Patching for longer periods may adversely affect stereoscopic vision in infants; therefore avoid doing so without ophthalmic consultation.

Remarks

Eye patching has generally been routine in patients with corneal abrasions. More recently, many clinicians have begun leaving small abrasions unpatched and simply dilating the eyes and instructing the patients to use dark glasses. This approach seems appropriate for small abrasions but is probably inadequate for larger corneal injuries.

REFERENCE

1. Friedberg MA, Rapuano CJ: *Wills eye hospital office and emergency room diagnosis and treatment of eye diseases,* Philadelphia, 1990, JB Lippincott.

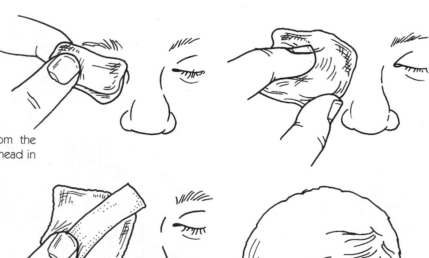

FIG. 90-1 Pressure patch. Tape the patch from the corner of the mouth and across the eye to the forehead in a fan-shaped pattern.

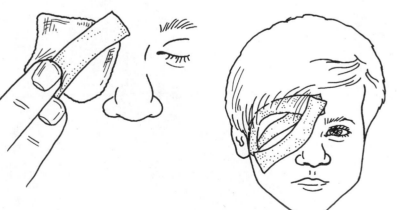

PART XVII

PERINATOLOGY TECHNIQUES

91 Newborn Delivery

Jacalyn S. Maller

In rare instances, neonate delivery occurs in the pediatric Emergency Department (ED). The typical patient is an adolescent who has had no prenatal care and who comes to the ED with lower abdominal pain and fetal crowning at the vaginal introitus. The United States has one of the highest adolescent pregnancy rates among all developed countries, with a disturbing increase in pregnancy in those under 15 years of age.[3]

The tendency of the adolescent to deny the possibility of pregnancy despite amenorrhea, weight gain, and fetal movements may result in a pregnancy going "unnoticed" until the onset of severe labor pains, particularly in a teenager who is obese. These pregnancies are high risk because of the lack of prenatal care and the tendency of adolescents to deliver low–birth weight or premature neonates. Poor nutrition, substance abuse, and the high prevalence of genital infections compound the likelihood of neonatal complications.[3]

Indications

If time allows, transport the woman in labor to a labor and delivery suite, where there are optimal conditions for aseptic technique, appropriate monitoring equipment, and experienced obstetric and neonatal personnel.[5] If delivery is imminent, do not transport the patient to an obstetric suite; the emergency physician must instead perform a vaginal delivery.

Determine the onset, timing, progression, and location of the contractions. Also determine the date of the last menstrual period to help assess the age of the fetus. Differentiate "true" labor from "false" labor or Braxton Hicks contractions by observing a progressive shortening of intervals and increasing intensity of contractions with pain localized to the back and abdomen.[1] Ultimately, the major differentiation between true and false labor is that only the former causes cervical changes and eventual expulsion of the fetus.

The multiparous patient progresses more rapidly than the primiparous patient through the various stages of labor. The first stage of labor lasts from the onset of contractions to full cervical dilation (10 cm) and can range from 5 hours in the multiparous patient to at least 8 to 12 hours in the primiparous patient. The second stage of labor begins with full cervical dilation and descent of the fetus and ends with the birth of the neonate. The woman develops the urge to defecate because of the pressure of the fetus against the rectum. Uterine contractions occur less than 2 minutes apart, with little resting between contractions. The second stage can also be highly variable in length and range from 20 minutes or less in the multiparous patient to at least 1 hour in a primiparous patient.[1] Transport of the patient is not an option at this stage, but the emergency physician may call for obstetric support, if available.

Determine whether the membranes have ruptured and whether there has been any bloody discharge or active bleeding. Bloody discharge, or "bloody show," consists of blood-tinged mucus that is extruded from the cervical canal once cervical dilation and effacement has begun. Distinguish this type of bleeding from third-trimester vaginal bleeding, which may indicate placenta previa or abruptio placentae, both of which are life threatening. Do *not* perform a vaginal examination if there is a history of active bleeding.[1]

The occurrence of ruptured membranes may be difficult to assess if fluid leakage has been slow. Various tests, such as using nitrazine paper to test the pH of vaginal fluid (alkaline if rupture has occurred, but false-positive when bleeding occurs) or checking for "ferning" on a microscope slide containing dried vaginal fluid, may be helpful but too often are unreliable or not immediately possible. The importance of ruptured membranes is twofold. If the presenting part is not fixed in the pelvis, the likelihood of umbilical cord prolapse increases. Prolonged rupture of membranes (>24 hours) may increase the risk of intrauterine infection and a compromised neonate once delivery occurs.[1] If ruptured membranes are suspected, perform a sterile speculum examination to minimize bacterial contamination.

In the most common ED scenario, delivery of the neonate is imminent. The physician rarely needs to perform a speculum examination or assess for cervical effacement, dilation, fetal station, or presenting part. Instead, perform an external vaginal examination to demonstrate the presenting part, which is the occiput in >95% of term deliveries.[2] With a stethoscope or Doppler ultrasonography, auscultate the fetal heart rate simultaneously with the maternal heart rate and immediately following a contraction, when signs of fetal distress are most evident. Normal fetal heart rate ranges from 120 to 160 beats/min. Suspect fetal distress if the heart rate falls below 120 beats/min following a contraction or if the resting fetal heart rate is abnormal.

Contraindications

In the cardiovascularly stable patient who is not actively contracting and before the second stage of labor, consider transferring the patient to a facility with obstetric services. Factors influencing this decision include the parity of the patient, the extent of cervical dilation (preferably <6 cm), the frequency of contractions, and the proximity of obstetric facilities. Once the second stage has begun, delivery may occur very rapidly, especially in the multiparous patient. The emergency physician may call in an obstetrician or may solicit a phone consultation if an obstetrician is not available. Prepare for possible neonatal resuscitation if the neonate is premature or if any risk factors, such as prolonged rupture of membranes, meconium-stained amniotic fluid, maternal fever, or evidence of fetal distress, are present.

Do not encourage vaginal delivery if there is a prolapsed

umbilical cord, suspected cephalopelvic disproportion, breech presentation, or fetal distress. Under these circumstances, arrange for a cesarean section.

Complications

Fetal Distress. Suspect fetal distress when there is an abnormal resting heart rate (<120 or >160 beats/min) or a decrease in fetal heart rate to less than 120 beats/min following a contraction. Manage the patient with oxygen and intravenous fluids and turn the patient to the left lateral decubitus position to maximize uterine blood flow and relieve possible umbilical cord compression. Ultimately the treatment for fetal distress is delivery of the neonate, often by cesarean section.

Prolapsed Umbilical Cord. Rupture of the amniotic membranes may result in umbilical cord prolapse through the cervix with compromised circulation to the fetus. Signs of a prolapsed umbilical cord may include a sudden drop in fetal heart rate. Confirm the diagnosis by palpating the cord in the vagina. To minimize fetal hypoxemia, deliver the neonate immediately (most often by cesarean section if the cervix is not completely dilated). Until delivery occurs, the physician can place his or her hand into the patient's vagina and elevate the presenting part to relieve cord compression. Attempt other therapy, including those maneuvers described previously for treatment of fetal distress.[4]

Postpartum Hemorrhage. Postpartum hemorrhage may result from external bleeding as a result of vaginal, cervical, or perineal lacerations or from internal bleeding caused by uterine atony or a retained placenta or placental fragments. Treat the external bleeding with direct pressure and repair of the lacerations (by an obstetrician and with the patient under general anesthesia) in the cervix or upper vagina. Treat internal bleeding with intravenous crystalloid and blood products, if necessary. Because of the relative hypervolemic state of pregnancy, blood loss may exceed 1.5 L before any clinical changes in vital signs occur. If palpation reveals a boggy uterus (a sign of uterine atony), improve uterine contractions by massaging the uterine fundus with one hand on the abdomen and massaging the uterus through the vaginal wall with the knuckles of the second hand. Give oxytocin to induce uterine contractions and decrease bleeding in conjuction with massage. If bleeding persists despite these measures, use methylergonovine (0.2 mg intramuscularly) to stimulate contractions, except in patients with hypertension.[2]

Breech Presentation. Breech presentation is more common with prematurity and congenital anomalies and results in higher incidences of umbilical cord prolapse, fetal distress, and increased morbidity and mortality. In most cases, a cesarean extraction minimizes some of the morbidity associated with breech deliveries. When faced with a vaginal breech delivery, allow the neonate to deliver spontaneously, preferably at least to the umbilicus, without any manipulation. Techniques of breech extraction—which are indicated when fetal distress develops, vaginal delivery is imminent, and no obstetrician is available—are beyond the scope of this chapter but are found in several obstetric texts and should be reviewed.[1]

Uterine Inversion. Although rare, uterine inversion may cause life-threatening hemorrhage. The most common asso-

---

> **BOX 91-1 EMERGENCY DEPARTMENT STERILE NEONATE DELIVERY PACK**
>
> Absorbent towels
> Obstetric gown
> Sterile drapes
> Sanitary pads
> Placenta basin
> Bulb syringe
> Baby blanket
> Hemostats (to clamp umbilical cord)
> Surgical scissors
> Umbilical tape
> Gauze sponges (4 × 4)
> Sterile gloves

> **BOX 91-2 NEONATAL RESUSCITATION EQUIPMENT**
>
> Overhead warmer
> Suction equipment
>   Bulb syringe
>   Wall suction
>   Suction catheters (5, 8, 10 French)
>   Meconium aspirator
> Bag and mask
> Oral airways
> Laryngoscope (Miller 0, 1)
> Endotracheal tubes (uncuffed, 2.5-4.0 mm)
> Stylet
> Medications
>   Epinephrine (1:10,000)
>   Naloxone (1 mg/ml)
>   Normal saline
>   Sodium bicarbonate (diluted 1:1 to 0.5 mEq/ml)
>   Dextrose 10%

---

ciated factor is traction on the umbilical cord and fundal pressure during the third stage of labor. The patient develops severe bleeding, abdominal pain, and shock in 50% of these cases. Promptly recognize this condition, give intravenous fluids and transfusion, and reposition the uterus to improve clinical outcome.[2]

Equipment

Box 91-1 lists the equipment needed for an emergency vaginal delivery. Many EDs have a sterile "obstetric pack" that contains these materials as well as a heated Isolette and equipment for neonatal resuscitation (Box 91-2).[6]

Techniques

Delivery is imminent when the perineal membranes are bulging or when the fetal head appears at the vaginal introitus. Place the patient in the dorsal lithotomy position with her legs separated and knees and hips flexed. Although vaginal delivery is never a completely sterile procedure, use sterile technique, including handwashing, sterile gloving,

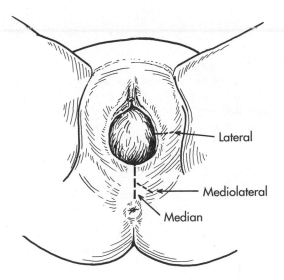

FIG. 91-1 Preferred sites for median and mediolateral episiotomy.

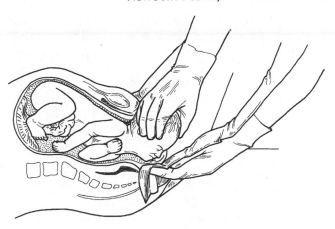

FIG. 91-2 Modified Ritgen maneuver.

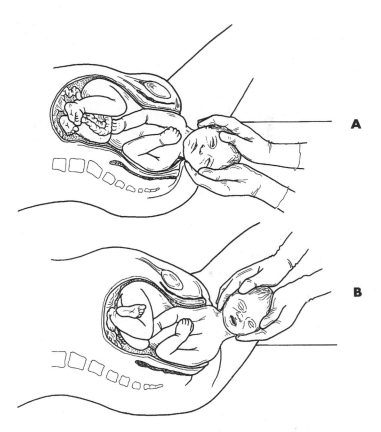

FIG. 91-3 **A** and **B,** Delivery of the fetal shoulders.

gowning, and perineal cleansing with povidone-iodine (Betadine) and draping if time allows.

With each contraction, the vaginal opening and vulva progressively dilate until they encircle the biparietal diameter of the fetal head (crowning). Although some clinicians question the utility of an episiotomy, it theoretically shortens the second stage of labor and minimizes damage to the fetal head and maternal perineum by substituting a straight surgical incision for the irregular, jagged laceration that often results from the stretching and thinning of the perineum to accommodate the fetal head. The timing of the episiotomy is critical because excessive maternal bleeding occurs when performed too early. If done too late, damage to the maternal tissues may already have occurred. Perform an episiotomy when 3 to 4 cm of the fetal head is visible.[1] The median episiotomy is preferable to the mediolateral incision because it is easier to repair, heals better, and results in less pain, blood loss, and dyspareunia. The major advantage of a mediolateral incision is the lower likelihood of damage to the anal sphincter (Fig. 91-1).[1] It is often possible to avoid episiotomy in multiparous patients. Contraindications include certain patients with inflammatory bowel disease, severe perineal scarring, and coagulation disorders.[5]

Anesthetize the perineum with 1% or 2% lidocaine. Make an incision with surgical scissors through the midline of the perineum and toward the anal sphincter.[2] Perform episiotomy repair following delivery of the placenta.

As the fetal head appears, ask the patient not to push but instead to breathe through the nose or pant. The physician's palm should be placed against the fetal occiput to provide countertraction and control the delivery. Exert upward pressure against the fetal chin through the perineum, the so-called modified Ritgen maneuver (Fig. 91-2), with the second hand covered with a sterile towel to protect the fetus from fecal excretions. After delivering the head, wipe the neonate's face and mouth and use a bulb syringe to suction the nose and mouth to avoid aspiration of amniotic or other secretions with the first breath.

Examine the neck for an encircling nuchal cord. If it is present and adequately loose, slip it over the neck. If the cord is too tight, place two clamps approximately 2 inches apart and cut the cord between the clamps.

Before delivery of the shoulders, the fetus will rotate into the anterior posterior plane of the pelvis. If this rotation is not occurring spontaneously, deliver the anterior shoulder by placing both hands on either side of the head and exerting gentle downward traction. Deliver the posterior shoulder similarly except with upward traction as necessary (Fig. 91-3).

The remainder of the body usually delivers easily. If not, exert moderate traction on the head in the longitudinal axis of the fetus to complete the delivery and to prevent any neck or brachial plexus injuries. The neonate is very slippery; hold it carefully with the head lower than the body to facilitate drainage of secretions. Suction the airway once again as needed.

Double-clamp the umbilical cord and cut it with sterile scissors approximately 30 to 60 seconds after delivery. Place umbilical tape around the cord approximately 1 cm from the navel. Dry the spontaneously breathing neonate in a warm blanket and give the neonate to the mother. Refer to Chapter 92 for a discussion of care of the distressed neonate.

Delivery of the placenta (the third stage) occurs spontaneously within 20 to 30 minutes. Signs of impending delivery are a firmer, contracting uterus, a sudden gush of blood, and lengthening of the umbilical cord.[1] In most cases, the mother's intraabdominal pressure is adequate to expel the placenta. If not, apply gentle pressure to the body of the uterus with the hand on the abdomen to elevate the uterus and aid in placental delivery. Avoid excessive traction on the umbilical cord because such traction may cause uterine inversion.

After cutting the placenta, massage the uterus to maintain a contracted state and minimize postpartum bleeding. Give oxytocin intramuscularly or intravenously by slow infusion (20 units added to 1 L of normal saline run at 10 ml/min until the bleeding slows).[1] Examine the vulva, vagina, cervix, and anal sphincter for lacerations. Take a sample of cord blood from the placenta for syphilis and Coombs' testing, and examine the placenta for any gross abnormalities.

Remarks

Most emergency full-term vaginal deliveries occur spontaneously. The role of the emergency physician is to assist in a controlled delivery, to provide encouragement and support for the patient in active labor, and to prepare to resuscitate the neonate if the need arises.

REFERENCES

1. Cunningham FG, MacDonald PC, Gant NG: Conduct of normal labor and delivery. In *Williams obstetrics,* ed 18, Norwalk, Conn, 1989, Appleton & Lange.
2. Doan-Wiggins L: Emergency childbirth. In Roberts JR, Hedges JR, editors: *Clinical procedures in emergency medicine,* ed 2, Philadelphia, 1991, WB Saunders.
3. Emans SJH, Goldstein DP: *Pediatric and adolescent gynecology,* ed 3, Boston, 1990, Little, Brown.
4. Gianopoulos JG: Emergency complications of labor and delivery, *Emerg Clin North Am* 12:201, 1994.
5. Higgins SD: Emergency delivery: prehospital care, emergency department delivery, perimortem salvage, *Emerg Med Clin North Am* 5:529, 1987.
6. Khan NS, Luten RC: Neonatal resuscitation, *Emerg Med Clin North Am* 2:239, 1994.

92 Neonatal Resuscitation

Constance McAneney

The birth and resuscitation of a neonate in the Emergency Department (ED) is an uncommon event. Fortunately, the majority of neonates do not need intervention beyond drying, warming, tactile stimulation, and suctioning.[2] For those neonates who require more resuscitation, the ideal setting is a delivery room or an intensive care nursery, but such placement may not be possible. Unfortunately, many patients who deliver in the ED are from high-risk groups, (i.e., teenage mothers, those without prenatal care, those who use drugs, and those with abnormal etiologies for labor (such as trauma or placental abruption). Therefore a delivery in an ED can be a combination of a high-risk delivery and a less-than-ideal setting.

One of the keys to a successful neonatal resuscitation is advance preparation of staff and equipment. Many times there is little immediate preparation time with the patient at the doorstep and fetal crowning. Therefore the most important preparation involves keeping the staff educated in neonatal resuscitation and designating an area with appropriate neonatal equipment ready. Organize the neonatal resuscitation equipment so that it is easy to use, and check it regularly. Include resuscitation charts with medication doses and equipment sizes for different weights (Table 92-1). Teach the staff where the equipment is and how to use it.

Timely neonatal assessment and treatment requires an understanding of the basic physiologic events that take place at birth. With the first breaths (thought to be stimulated by a combination of hypoxemia, acidosis, interruption of umbilical circulation, and thermal changes) the lungs expand, the Pao_2 increases, the pH increases, the Pco_2 decreases, and pulmonary vascular resistance falls.[2,4] Right-to-left shunting decreases at the foramen ovale and the ductus arteriosus. The ductus arteriosus and the foramen ovale remain open for a variable time. Hypoxemia can lead to an increase in pulmonary vascular resistance, which causes a closed ductus to reopen and increases the right-to-left shunting. Within the first minute of life, spontaneous respiration begins in the neonate, with the normal rate being 30 to 40 times/minute. The normal heart rate begins at 100 to 200 beats per minute (bpm) and stabilizes at 120 to 140 bpm. Although the cold environment of birth may help stimulate respiration, hypothermia increases oxygen consumption and prolongs acidosis.[1,4,6]

Asphyxia in the neonate initially causes an increase in the depth and frequency of respirations for approximately 3 minutes (primary hyperpnea), which is followed by hypoventilation that lasts approximately 1 minute (primary apnea). The neonate begins to gasp rhythmically eight to ten times per minute and then ceases to breathe (secondary apnea).[4,6,7] Aggressive ventilatory and circulatory resuscitation must take place for the neonate to survive. The primary and secondary apnea (the asphyxial event) may have occurred in utero, and immediate intervention is therefore imperative.

Table 92-1 Neonatal Resuscitation Equipment Sizes

Weight (g)	Endotracheal tube size (mm)	Suction catheter (French)	Laryngoscope blade
≤ 1000	2.5	5	0
2000	3.0	6	0
3000	3.0-3.5	6-8	0-1
4000	3.5	8	1

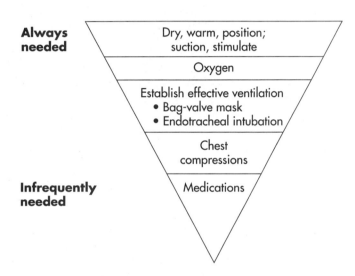

FIG. 92-1 Order of increasingly aggressive interventions in neonatal resuscitation.

(From Chameides L, Hazinski MF, editors: American Academy of Pediatrics and the American Heart Association: *Textbook of pediatric advanced life support*, Dallas, 1994, The American Heart Association.)

Indications

All neonates need some degree of intervention; most do not need full resuscitation. The inverted pyramid taught in Pediatric Advanced Life Support (American Heart Association) gives a pictorial representation of the frequency and sequence of increasingly aggressive interventions (Fig. 92-1).

Contraindications

The criteria to not resuscitate a neonate at birth are the same criteria for not initiating CPR in anyone: injury incompatible with life, dependent lividity, rigor mortis, and decomposition. In addition, there is a special consideration with the resuscitation of a neonate: gestational age. There is controversy surrounding the point at which a neonate is too immature to be viable. It is best to develop the protocol prospectively with consulting neonatologists at the primary institution or referral institution.

BOX 92-1 **NEONATAL RESUSCITATION EQUIPMENT**

Suction equipment with manometer
Suction catheters (5 - 10 French)
Bulb syringe
Meconium aspirator
Oxygen
Face masks (sizes 00, 0, 1, 2)
Self-inflating bag with oxygen reservoir (500 ml) or anesthesia bag with manometer
Laryngoscope, extra battery and bulb, straight blades (No. 0,1)
Endotracheal tubes (2.5, 3.0, 3.5, 4.0) and stylet
Feeding tube (5, 8 French)
Chest tubes (8, 10 French)
Three-way stopcocks
Umbilical catheters (3.5, 5.0 French)
Umbilical catheter tray
Towels
Hemostats and cord clamp
Syringes (10, 20 ml)
Medications
  Epinephrine 1:10,000
  Sodium bicarbonate
  Dextrose 10%, 25%
  Naloxone
  Volume expanders
  Normal saline flush
Resuscitation chart or length-based resuscitation tape

Table 92-2 Apgar Score

Sign	Score		
	0	1	2
Heart rate	Absent	Below 100	Over 100
Respiratory effort	Absent	Slow, irregular	Crying, rhythmic
Muscle tone	Flaccid	Some flexion	Good flexion, active
Reflex irritability	None	Grimace	Cry
Color	Blue or pale	Pink with blue extremities	Completely pink

Equipment

To perform neonatal resuscitation, a radiant warmer is essential, as well as monitors (cardiorespiratory and pulse oximeter) (Box 92-1).

Techniques

Basic Interventions. Open the neonatal equipment, check it for proper functioning, draw up medications that may be needed, and turn on the radiant warmer to warm the bed and blanket on which the neonate will be placed. Obtain a brief obstetric history.

At delivery, place the neonate head down and clamp the cord. Place the neonate under the warmer in the supine position with the neck extended and the head to the side. Place a towel under the shoulders and suction the mouth and then the nose. Use a bulb syringe if there is inadequate time to set up wall suction. With wall suction, do not allow pressure to exceed −100 mm Hg.[2] Have one person suction while another assesses heart rate by listening to the chest or feeling the pulsations of the umbilical cord. Remember also that deep suctioning of the oropharynx may cause bradycardia and apnea through vagal stimulation. Do not suction for more than 5 seconds at a time, and allow time between suctioning. Begin drying the neonate to help decrease heat loss and to provide stimulation. Provide additional stimulation by slapping the soles of the feet or rubbing the back. More vigorous stimulation is not warranted. If these methods

fail to stimulate respiration, use positive-pressure ventilation. Accomplish these steps, as well as an overall assessment, within the first minute of life.

A good guide to assessing the neonate is the Apgar score (Table 92-2).[3] Assess the neonate at 1 minute and 5 minutes of life. If resuscitation has been prolonged, give a 10-minute Apgar. This scoring system teaches the personnel attending to the neonate to observe more than one sign at a time and serves as a guide to the need for resuscitation. Do not delay resuscitation if the neonate displays inadequate respirations or an inadequate heart rate.

Assisted Ventilation. Respiratory rate should increase with brief stimulation. If it is not adequate, initiate positive-pressure ventilation. Evaluate heart rate by listening to the chest with a stethoscope, palpating the pulse from the umbilical cord, or palpating the femoral pulse. If the heart rate is greater than 100 bpm and the neonate is breathing spontaneously, continue the assessment. If the heart rate is below 100 bpm, initiate positive-pressure ventilation. Assess the neonate's color and give blow by oxygen to the neonate with cyanosis if the heart rate is greater than 100 bpm with spontaneous respirations. Acrocyanosis (blue hands and feet) is common at the beginning of life and is not an indication for oxygen therapy.

Be especially vigilant with the neonate who requires positive-pressure ventilation. The indications for this therapy are a heart rate less than 100 bpm, apnea, or cyanosis despite oxygen.[2,4,6,7] Use a mask that has a tight seal with the face, a bag that is no larger than 500 ml, and a manometer in line to avoid overinflation and iatrogenic pneumothoraces. The neonate generally requires inspiratory pressures of 30 to 40 cm H_2O, but it is important to watch the chest move and listen to breath sounds. Place an orogastric tube to avoid gastric distention if the neonate requires positive-pressure ventilation for more than 3 minutes. Provide the assisted ventilatory rate of 40 to 60 breaths per minute.

If after initiating positive-pressure ventilation the heart rate is above 100 bpm with spontaneous respiratory efforts, stop ventilatory support. Observe the neonate for rate and character of respirations. If he or she develops apnea, bradycardia, or cyanosis, restart positive-pressure ventilation.

Begin chest compressions if the neonate's heart rate is below 80 and falling despite positive-pressure ventilation. Provide smooth compressions at a rate of 120 times per minute with pauses for positive-pressure ventilation with 100% oxygen. Use a 3:1 ratio of compressions to ventila-

line under sterile conditions in the intensive care nursery and check placement with an x-ray study. Remember that the endotracheal tube is another route for the administration of epinephrine and naloxone (see Chapter 39).[2,5] Do not give sodium bicarbonate by this route.

Postresuscitation Management. Once successful resuscitation has taken place, continually reassess the neonate. Take care to prevent complications and anticipate problems (e.g., pneumothorax, hypothermia, hypovolemia, endotracheal tube dislodgment or plugging). Correct hypovolemia (with aliquots of 10 ml/kg of volume expander), hypoglycemia (with 4 ml/kg of D10), and metabolic acidosis (with 2 mEq/kg of half-strength sodium bicarbonate). Monitor blood gases and vital signs. Prepare for transport to the intensive care nursery or a tertiary care center.

Take special care for neonates who have suspected meconium aspiration; controversy surrounds the best approach. Thin, watery, meconium-stained amniotic fluid with an asymptomatic neonate usually does not require endotracheal intubation, but suction the mouth and nose at the perineum. However, if particulate meconium is present in the amniotic fluid, suction the neonate as the head is delivered, before the first breath. After delivery, visualize the neonate's glottis with a laryngoscope and intubate if meconium is present. Connect the meconium aspirator to suction on one end and to the endotracheal tube on the other (Fig. 92-2). Withdraw the endotracheal tube while applying suction. Reintubate and repeat if necessary. Failure to clear the airway requires endotracheal intubation for pulmonary toilet and tracheal suctioning.

Remarks

Remember that all neonates have some amount of respiratory acidosis at birth, but the asphyxiated neonate has more profound hypoxemia and acidosis and requires quick recognition and resuscitation. Hypothermia aggravates acidosis by causing an increase in oxygen consumption and eventually apnea. Resuscitation of the neonate requires ventilatory and circulatory support as well as correction of metabolic derangements.

If a neonate remains apneic and/or bradycardic, recheck the position of the airway. It is very easy to either hyperextend or flex the neck because of the large occiput. Recheck hand position over the mask. Do not let fingers touch the soft tissue of the neck because it is extremely easy to occlude the airway.

The neonate who has a sudden decompensation can be an enigma. Always check the airway first and make sure tube placement is correct. Listen for breath sounds. After a vigorous resuscitation, an ill neonate may develop a pneumothorax. If this condition seems to be occurring, perform needle aspiration of the chest and withdraw air. A chest tube may be needed.

Neonatalogists no longer recommend DeLee suction devices. Direct mouth suctioning of the endotracheal tube is contraindicated.

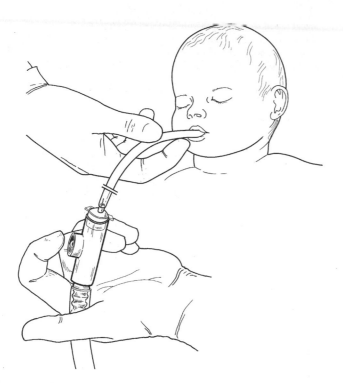

FIG. 92-2 Attaching a meconium aspirator to a wall suction tube and an endotracheal tube.

tions, which results in 90 compressions and 30 breaths per minute (see Chapter 52). Prepare to perform endotracheal intubation.

Intubation is indicated for those neonates in whom positive-pressure ventilation is ineffective or prolonged and for those who require continued suctioning (i.e., thick meconium aspiration).[2,4,6,7] Check all equipment before attempting intubation. Generally, do not use drugs for intubation of the neonate. Remember to consult a chart or length-based resuscitation tape (Chapter 51) for proper equipment sizes. Check placement of the endotracheal tube by listening to breath sounds; obtain a chest x-ray examination.

Delivery of Resuscitation Drugs. The neonate may remain bradycardic (heart rate less than 80 bpm) despite intubation and adequate ventilation with 100% oxygen. In this case, continue chest compressions and administer medications and fluids in an effort to correct acidosis and shock. The most accessible vascular route for the administration of medications is the umbilical vein. Loosely tie the cord with umbilical tape and cut it with a scalpel approximately 2 cm above the abdominal wall. Wash the cord with povidone-iodine (Betadine). The cord has three vessels: two thick-walled arteries and one larger, thin-walled vein. Attach the 5.0 French umbilical catheter (or feeding tube if an umbilical catheter is unavailable) to the three-way stopcock, flush it with normal saline, and slowly insert it into the vein. Because this line is placed in an emergency for resuscitation fluids and drugs, advance it just beyond the skin of the abdomen. There should be a good blood return. If the catheter is advanced too far (i.e., into the liver), necrosis can occur from the medication infusion. At this point infuse epinephrine, volume expanders, bicarbonate, and/or naloxone as needed. Remove this line after the resuscitation. Place a more secure

REFERENCES

1. Adamsons K, Gandy G, James LS: The influence of thermal factors upon oxygen consumption of the newborn infant, *J Pediatr* 66:495, 1965.

2. Chameides L, Hazinski MF, editors: American Academy of Pediatrics and the American Heart Association: *Textbook of pediatric advanced life support,* Dallas 1990, The American Heart Association.

3. Apgar V: A proposal for a new method of evaluation of the newborn infant, *Anesth Analg* 32:260, 1953.

4. Fisher DE, Paton JB: Resuscitation of the newborn infant. In Klaus MH, Fanaroff AA, editors: *Care of the high-risk neonate,* ed 3, Philadelphia, 1986, WB Saunders.

5. Greenberg M, Roberts J, Baskin S: Use of endotracheally administered epinephrine in the pediatric patient, *Am J Dis Child* 135:767, 1981.

6. James LS: Emergencies in the delivery room. In Fanaroff AA, Martin RJ, editors: *Neonatal-perinatal medicine: diseases of the fetus and infant,* St Louis, 1987, Mosby.

7. Schafermeyer RW: Neonatal resuscitation. In Fleisher GR, Ludwig S, editors: *Textbook of pediatric emergency medicine,* Baltimore, 1993, Williams & Wilkins.

93 Temperature Control and Monitoring

Constance McAneney

Thermoregulation is an important factor in the care of the neonate. Neonates, especially premature neonates, have difficulty with temperature control because they have a large ratio of surface area to weight, poor insulation (less subcutaneous fat tissue), and small mass.[3] They also do not possess the behaviors necessary to conserve heat, such as changing posture (flexing the extremities) and adjusting clothing. The goal is to maintain the neonate in a neutral thermal environment, which is defined as the range of thermal environment that permits normal core temperature in a neonate whose oxygen consumption and metabolic rate are minimal.[2] This neutral thermal range is narrow for naked neonates and falls slightly with advancing age.[1] The temperatures are higher than what is considered comfortable for adults and are different for various weights, gestational ages, and neonate conditions.[1]

A neonate exchanges heat by conduction, convection, evaporation, and radiation. Radiation accounts for the major proportion of heat loss in naked neonates in an incubator.[1] Heat loss from the head is clinically significant; a layered hat can decrease heat loss (see Chapter 3).[4] Insensible water loss is an important consideration with any neonate under a radiant warmer.

The most common method of maintaining a neutral thermal environment while resuscitating a neonate is to dry the neonate and place him or her under a radiant warmer. Monitor temperature by rectal or axillary probe. The most common continuous method of monitoring neonatal temperature under a radiant warmer is via skin thermistors (with servocontrol).

Servocontrolled equipment (whether incubators or radiant warmers) regulate temperature with a skin sensor taped to the abdomen of the neonate. If the neonate's temperature drops, the heating source increases heat output. Conversely, if the neonate's temperature increases, the heat output decreases.

Indications

Use radiant warmers as part of the resuscitation of any neonate. Frequent monitoring of temperature provides essential information to aid in the success of the resuscitation. Continuous monitoring with the skin probe (with servocontrol) is both the easiest and least invasive approach. It provides the advantage of decreasing the incidence of wide temperature fluctuations that may cause episodes of apnea.

Contraindications

There are no contraindications to providing a neutral thermal environment to a neonate during resuscitation via a radiant warmer.

Complications

Servocontrol devices can cause overheating if the probe detaches, or they may hide signs of temperature instability in a septic neonate. Such devices may subject a neonate with a fever to cold stress. Temperature regulation and monitoring by servocontrol devices requires orientation of the nursing and physician staff and the added expense of the equipment.

Equipment

The equipment necessary for providing a neutral thermal environment includes a radiant warmer, thermometer, and skin thermistor.

Techniques

Start the radiant warmer ahead of time to warm the surface on which the neonate is placed. Place the neonate under the warmer. Dry the skin and place the skin probe on the exposed surface of the abdomen. Because the radiant warmer heats the skin probe, cover it with a foam plastic pad and aluminum foil. Set the radiant warmer on servocontrol and set the temperature. The ideal skin temperature is 36° C for a 2-week-old, full-term neonate; 36.5° C for a small newborn; and 36.8° C for a very low–birth weight premature neonate.[3] When time permits, obtain the neonate's rectal or axillary (premature neonate) temperature to get a baseline. Periodically check the temperature with a thermometer to ensure a well-functioning and servocontrolled radiant warmer.

Remarks

Remember that the servocontrolled radiant warmer can not compensate for insensible water loss. Placing a plastic covering over the intubated neonate can decrease the water loss.[5] Make careful fluid adjustments on the basis of insensible water loss.

The thermistor probe must be on a skin surface on the trunk of the body that is exposed to the air. If the neonate is lying on the probe, the temperature gives a falsely high reading, and the heat source decreases its output.

REFERENCES

1. Hey EN: The care of babies in incubators. In Gairdner D, Hull D, editors: *Recent advances in paediatrics,* London, 1971, Churchill Livingstone.
2. Hey EN: Thermal neutrality, *Br Med Bull* 31:69, 1975.
3. Hey EN: Thermoregulation. In Avery GB, Fletcher MA, MacDonald MG, editors: *Neonatology: pathophysiology and management of the newborn,* ed 4, Philadelphia, 1994, WB Saunders.
4. Stothers JK: Head insulation and heat loss in the newborn, *Arch Dis Child* 56:530, 1981.
5. Yeh TF, Anema P, Lilien LD, et al: Reduction of insensible water loss in premature infants under the radiant warmer, *J Pediatr* 94:651, 1979.

94 Transillumination

Constance McAneney

Throughout the United States, intensive care nurseries use transillumination with variable frequency. Richard Bright[10] first described the technique in 1831; sites for transillumination have included the skull,[2,8] the abdomen,[6] the chest to detect pneumothoraces,[3] and the extremities for venipuncture and arterial puncture.[4,7,9] The technique is easy; descriptions of the techniques for transillumination of the hand and wrist for line placement are described in the following paragraphs.

Indications

Transillumination is indicated as a tool to aid in the placement of intravenous catheters and arterial lines and in venipuncture and arterial puncture for blood sampling.

Contraindications

There are no contraindications for using a transilluminator as long as the light has been commercially manufactured for this purpose. It is important not to use just any light source for transillumination because doing so may cause iatrogenic burns.

Complications

Complications from the use of the transilluminator itself are basically a result of burns to the skin when the light is held at the surface of the skin for a prolonged period.[5] The disadvantages to transilluminator use are that it is still difficult to visualize the vessels in an obese neonate and that it may take two people to immobilize the extremity and hold the light against the skin.

Equipment

In addition to a transilluminator, other supplies necessary for transillumination include those needed for vessel cannulation or puncture.

Technique

Gather all the supplies needed for the vessel puncture. Turn on the transilluminator and dim the room lights. Place the transilluminator probe tip against the extremity and opposite the arterial site (i.e., radial, dorsalis pedis, posterior tibial) (Fig. 94-1). Before radial artery puncture, perform the Allen's test to ensure collateral circulation.[1] The artery will appear to be pulsating and linear. Prepare the skin for puncture and enter it with a 25-gauge butterfly needle at a 30-degree angle (see Chapter 33). Vessels may appear more superficial under direct observation with the transilluminator. Draw blood in the usual manner. Remove the needle and compress the area until the bleeding has stopped.

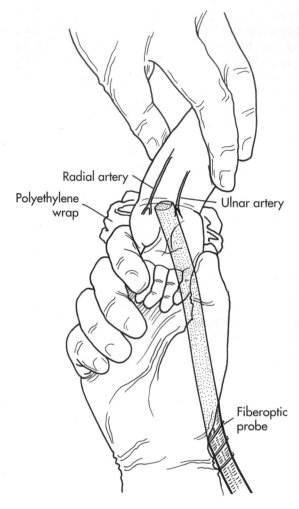

Radial artery

Polyethylene wrap

Ulnar artery

Fiberoptic probe

FIG. 94-1 Position of hand and wrist for radial artery puncture using the transilluminator.

REFERENCES

1. Allen EV: Thromboangiitis obliterans: methods of diagnosis of chronic occlusive arterial lesions distal to the wrist with illustrative cases, *Am J Med Sci* 78:237-244, 1929.

2. Dodge PR, Porter P: Demonstration of intracranial pathology by transillumination, *Arch Neurol* 5:30, 1961.
3. Kuhns LR, Bednarek FJ, Wyman ML, et al: Diagnosis of pneumothorax or pneumomediastinum in the neonate by transillumination, *Pediatrics* 56:355, 1975.
4. Kuhns LR, Martin AJ, Gildersleeve S, et al: Intense transillumination for infant venipuncture, *Radiology* 116:734, 1975.
5. McArtor RD, Saunders BS: Iatrogenic second-degree burn caused by transilluminator, *Pediatrics* 63:422, 1979.
6. Mofenson HC, Grensher J: Transillumination of the abdomen in infants, *Am J Dis Child* 115:428, 1968.
7. Pearse RG: Percutaneous catheterization of the radial artery in newborn babies using transillumination, *Arch Dis Child* 53:549-554, 1978.
8. Shurtleff DB: Transillumination of skull in infants and children, *Am J Dis Child* 107:14, 1964.
9. Wall PM, Kuhns LR: Percutaneous arterial sampling using transillumination, *Pediatrics* 59:1032, 1977.
10. Wyman ML: Uses of transillumination in the newborn nursery, *Perinatol Neonatol* 1:25, 1978.

95 Umbilical Vessel Catheterization

Constance McAneney

Neonatologists commonly use umbilical vessel catheterization in critically ill neonates for emergent vascular access during resuscitation, central venous access, blood sampling, blood pressure monitoring, and acid-base monitoring.[2,15] The umbilical vessels are extremely accessible, especially in very low–birth weight neonates, but catheterization can have some serious complications. Carefully consider the risks and benefits for each neonate before beginning the procedure.[3,9,14]

Indications

The major indications for umbilical line placement are vascular access for resuscitation, exchange transfusion, short-term central venous access, continuous blood pressure monitoring, and frequent blood gas sampling.[15]

Contraindications

Umbilical vessel catheterization is contraindicated in a neonate who is only mildly to moderately ill and in whom placement of a peripheral line to give parenteral fluids is possible.

Complications

Many of the complications resulting from umbilical vessel catheterization are serious and unavoidable. The presence of the catheter itself may promote clot formation.[6,12,16] A thrombus can form with the release of microemboli. If the tip of the venous catheter lies in a branch of the portal vein, liver necrosis can ensue following infusions of medications or parenteral nutrition.[2] If the tip of the arterial catheter is left near the origin of the renal arteries, thrombosis of the kidneys can occur.[6] Spontaneous perforation of the vessel wall and perforation of the colon have also occurred.[5] Neonates have also hemorrhaged secondary to inadvertent removal of the catheter or loose connections.[10] Infections can complicate umbilical vessel catheterizations.[8] Neonatal hypertension may relate to catheter placement.[1,13]

Equipment

A sterile gown, gloves, and mask must be worn when performing the line placement. Other equipment needed for umbilical vessel catheterization is listed in Box 95-1.

Techniques

Umbilical Vein Catheterization. Prepare all equipment before beginning the catheterization. Flush the umbilical catheter with saline and attach the stopcock. Place the neonate in the supine position and under a radiant warmer with the extremities restrained. Place a cardiorespiratory monitor and pulse oximeter in easy visibility with audible alarms on.

Wash the umbilical cord and abdomen from the xyphoid to the symphysis pubis with povidone- iodine (Betadine). Apply

---

> **BOX 95-1 EQUIPMENT FOR UMBILICAL VESSEL CATHETERIZATION**
>
> Umbilical tape and 3.0 silk suture with a needle
> Povidone-iodine (Betadine) solution
> Sterile gauze pads
> Gown, gloves, mask
> Sterile drapes
> Scalpel
> Umbilical catheters (3.5 and/or 5.0 French)
> Saline, heparinized saline for umbilical arterial line
> Three-way stopcocks
> Hemostats, smooth-curved iris forceps, iris scissors, needle holder
> Syringes

---

drapes. Loosely tie umbilical tape or insert a 3.0 silk purse-string suture at the base of the umbilical cord; cut it 1 to 2 cm from the skin at the base (Fig. 95-1). Visualize the vessels; there should be two thick-walled arteries and one thin-walled vein (see Fig. 95-1). Remove any clot from the vein. Hold the umbilical cord with a hemostat and gently insert the flushed 5.0 French umbilical catheter into the vein while applying gentle pressure (Fig. 95-2). There may be slight resistance at the abdominal wall. Apply gentle traction on the umbilical cord with steady but gentle pressure on the catheter. The catheter may meet a second resistance at the portal system. Withdraw the catheter slightly, rotate it, and then reinsert. If unsuccessful in getting past this point, do not force the catheter. Continue to withdraw, rotate, and reinsert it. When the catheter advances beyond the portal system (7 to 12 cm), withdraw fluid from the catheter, look for blood return, and suture the catheter in place. Tape the catheter to the abdominal wall to better secure it (Fig. 95-3). Obtain an x-ray study to check placement. Do not infuse medications or fluids until after confirming placement. If the catheter is in too far (it should be just beyond the ductus venosus in the inferior vena cava), withdraw the proper amount. However, if it is not in far enough, withdraw the catheter completely and start the process from the beginning to ensure aseptic technique. Do not infuse anything into the liver.

Umbilical Artery Catheterization. For an umbilical artery catheterization, prepare all equipment as for an umbilical vein catheterization. Flush the umbilical catheter with heparinized saline (1 U/ml heparin). Attach the stopcock to the catheter. Position the neonate in the supine position with the extremities restrained. Place a cardiorespiratory monitor and pulse oximeter in easy visibility with audible alarms on.

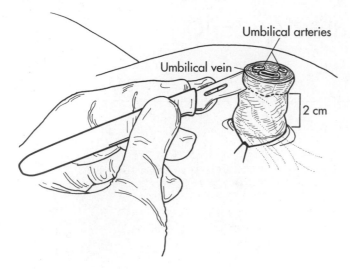

FIG. 95-1 Cutting the umbilical cord for line placement.

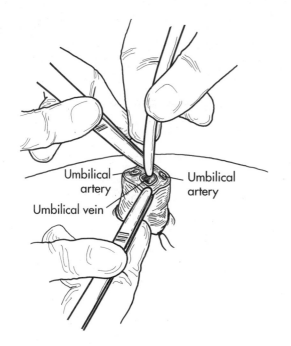

FIG. 95-2 Insertion of umbilical catheter.

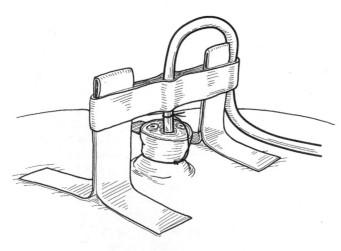

FIG. 95-3 Taping the catheter to the abdominal wall.

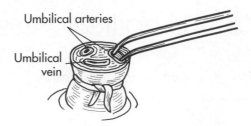

FIG. 95-4 Dilating the lumen of the artery.

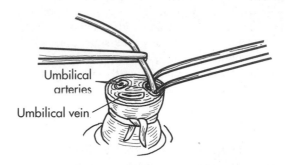

FIG. 95-5 Placement of arterial catheter.

Measure the neonate from the umbilicus to the shoulder. Mark the catheter at a point equal to 60% of this distance,[4] which is the length of the catheter to insert. Wash the umbilical cord and abdomen with povidine-iodine solution. Apply drapes. Loosely tie umbilical tape or insert a silk purse-string suture at the base of the umbilical cord; cut it 1 to 2 cm from the abdomen (see Fig. 95-1). Visualize the vessels. There should be two thick-walled arteries and one thin-walled vein (see Fig. 95-1). Attach two hemostats on either side of the umbilical cord and evert the clamps. With the smooth-curved iris forceps, slowly dilate the lumen of the artery. Do this procedure multiple times, gently advancing the forceps each time to approximately 1 cm (Fig. 95- 4).

Pick up the catheter flushed with heparinized saline, place it between the iris forceps in the artery, and advance it using constant gentle pressure (Fig. 95-5). There will be resistance below the abdominal wall and where the artery turns toward the iliac artery. There should be a good blood return when the catheter enters the iliac artery (Fig. 95-6).

Advance the catheter to the premeasured mark and secure it by tightening the purse-string suture. Tie square knots from the purse-string suture around the umbilical cord to the catheter. If using umbilical tape initially, place a suture in the umbilical cord and tie square knots from this suture to the catheter. Tape the catheter to the abdominal wall (see Fig. 95-3). Obtain an abdominal x-ray examination to verify placement.

Remarks

There is controversy over whether to use "high" or "low" umbilical artery lines.[7,11] With "low" lines, the tip of the catheter should be below L3. With "high" lines, the tip of the catheter should be at T7 to T8. If blanching or cyanosis of the lower extremity occurs, remove the catheter immediately and use the other artery.

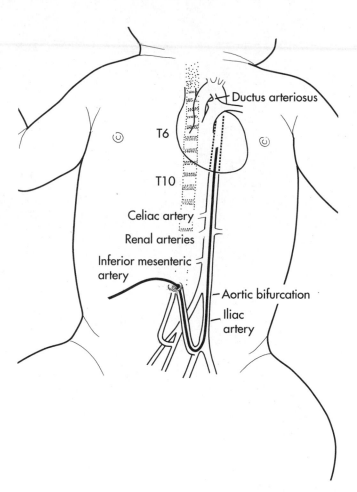

FIG. 95-6   Catheter in iliac artery.

REFERENCES

1. Bauer SB, Feldman SM, Gillis SS, et al: Neonatal hypertension: a complication of umbilical artery catheterization, *N Engl J Med* 293:1032, 1975.
2. Cochran WD, Heather TD, Smith CA: Advantages and complications of umbilical artery catheterization in the newborn, *Pediatrics* 42:769-777, 1968.
3. Dorand RD, Cook LN, Andrews BF: Umbilical catheterization: the low incidence of complications in a series of 200 newborn infants, *Clin Pediatr* 16:569, 1977.
4. Dunn P: Localization of umbilical catheter by postmortem measurement, *Arch Dis Child* 41:69, 1966.
5. Friedman A, Abellera R, Lidsky I, et al: Perforation of the colon after exchange transfusion in the newborn, *N Engl J Med* 282:796, 1970.
6. Goetzman BW, Stadalnik RC, Bogren HG, et al: Thrombolic complications of umbilical artery catheters: a clinical and radiographic study, *Pediatrics* 56:374, 1975.
7. Harris MS, Little GA: Umbilical artery catheters: high, low, or no, *Perinatal Med* 6:15, 1978.
8. Krauss AN, Albert RF, Kannan MM: Contamination of umbilical catheters in the newborn infant, *J Pediatr* 77:965, 1970.
9. Lemons JA, Honeyfield PR: Umbilical artery catheterization, *Perinatal Care* 2:17, 1978.
10. Miller D, Kirkpatrick BV, Kodroff M, et al: Pelvic exsanguination following umbilical artery catheterization in neonates, *J Pediatr Surg* 14:264, 1974.
11. Modrohisky S, Levine R, Blumhagen J, et al: Low positioning of umbilical artery catheters increases associated complications in newborn infants, *N Engl J Med* 299:561, 1978.
12. Neal WA, Reynolds JW, Jarvis CW, et al: Umbilical artery catheterization: demonstration of arterial thrombosis by aortography, *Pediatrics* 50:6, 1972.
13. Plumer LB, Kaplan GW, Mendoza SA: Hypertension in infants: a complication of umbilical arterial catheterization, *J Pediatr* 89:802, 1976.
14. Tooley WH, Myerberg DZ: Should we put catheters in the umbilical artery? *Pediatrics* 62:853, 1978.
15. Weaver RL, Ahlgren EW: Umbilical artery catheterization in neonates, *Am J Dis Child* 122:499, 1971.
16. Wigger HJ, Bransilver BR, Blanc WA: Thrombosis due to catheterization in infants and children, *J Pediatr* 76:1-11, 1970.

PART XVIII

INFECTIOUS DISEASE TECHNIQUES

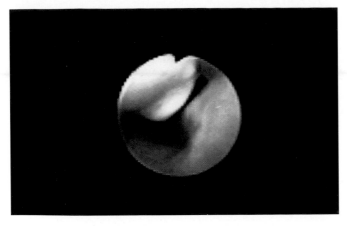

Plate 1 Upper trachea with bronchoscope just above tracheostomy stoma. The tracheostomy tube is visible on the anterior wall (9 o'clock to 1 o'clock position).

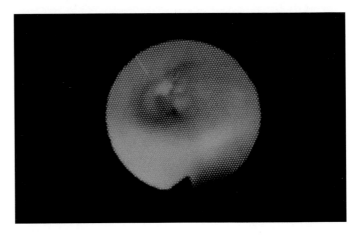

Plate 2 Foreign body within the bronchus with surrounding granulation tissue.

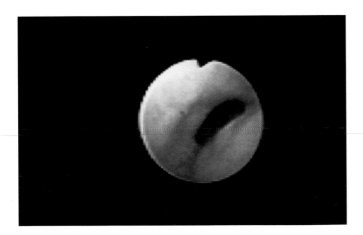

Plate 3 View of the distal trachea in an infant with VATER association and tracheomalacia.

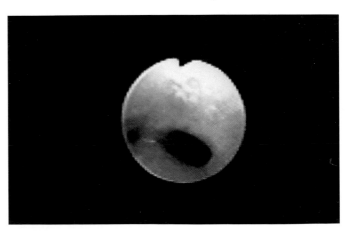

Plate 4 Asymmetric carina with reduction in anterior-posterior diameter of the right mainstem bronchus in an infant with Down syndrome and bronchomalacia.

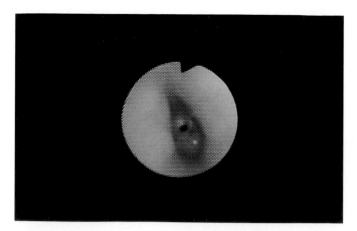

Plate 5   View through the glottis demonstrating subglottic stenosis.

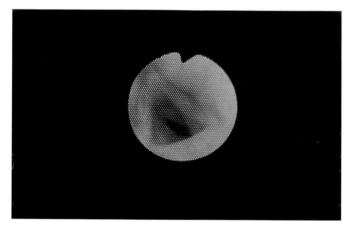

Plate 6   View through the glottis demonstrating a subglottic hemangioma.

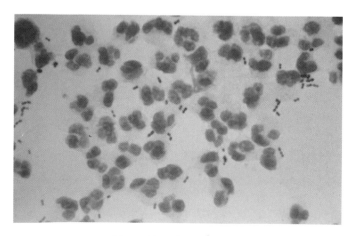
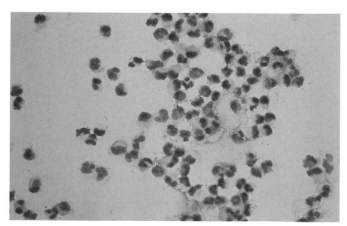

Plates 7 and 8   Gram stains of cerebral spinal fluid specimens. **Left,** Gram-positive lancet-shaped diplococci, *Streptococcus pneumoniae.* **Right,** Gram-negative coccobacilli, *Haemophilus influenzae.* (Courtesy R. Wheeler.)

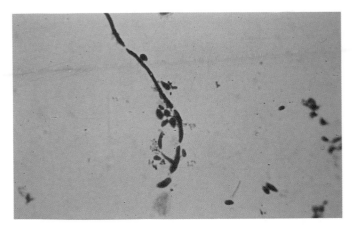

Plate 9 Typical appearance of the pseudohyphae of *Candida* spp.

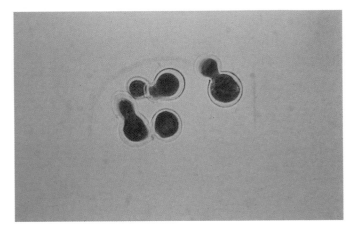

Plate 10 Broad-based budding yeast of *Blastomyces dermatitidis.*

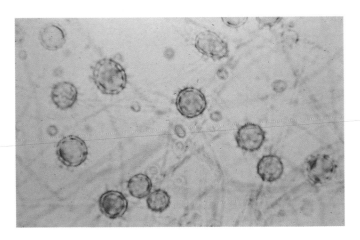

Plate 11 Yeast forms of *Histoplasma capsulatum.*

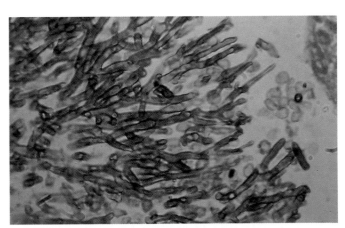

Plate 12 Septated branching hyphae of *Aspergillus* spp.

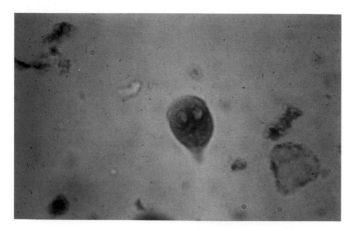

Plate 13 Trophozoite form of *Giardia lamblia.*

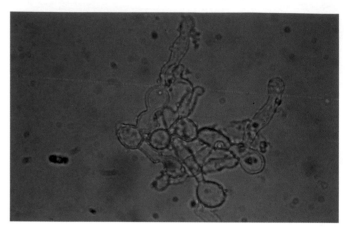

Plate 14 KOH preparation of a sputum, which demonstrates thick-walled, broad-based budding yeast, *Blastomyces dermatitidis.*

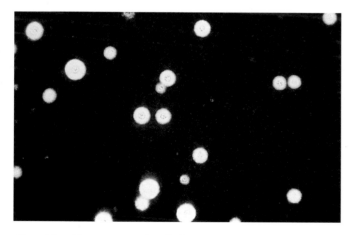

Plate 15 Clear surrounding halo caused by the large capsule of *Cryptococcus* with the India ink stain.

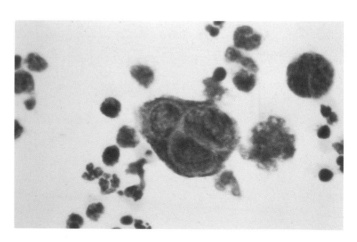

Plate 16 Tzanck prep using the Wright staining technique and demonstrating multinucleated giant cells and infection with the herpes simplex virus.

J. Thomas Cross and Gordon E. Schutze

Infectious diseases are everyday occurrences in pediatric emergency and critical care. The majority of these processes are self-limited viral infections or localized bacterial infections that respond to empiric antimicrobial therapy. In the normal host, a limited number of predictable pathogens cause most bacterial infections (e.g., otitis media, sinusitis, pneumonia, cellulitis, impetigo), which permits empiric outpatient therapy. However, a child or infant occasionally acquires a pathogen that results in invasive disease and systemic illness. In these instances, the clinician needs to optimize antimicrobial therapy using culture identification and sensitivities.

With the increasing incidence of acquired immunodeficiency syndrome (AIDS), advances in organ transplant techniques, the increasing population of patients on chronic corticosteroid therapy, and more aggressive chemotherapeutic protocols, there are more immunocompromised children than ever. These patients have alterations in at least one of their bodies' natural defense mechanisms (e.g., defects in phagocytic defenses, T-cell dysfunction, or humoral immune dysfunction), which predisposes them to infectious complications. Therefore the clinician must evaluate any potential source of infection in the immunocompromised patient to obtain a microbiologic identification and allow for early, pathogen-directed therapy. Techniques for the acquisition of clinical specimens and specimen handling, rapid diagnostic tests, and common diagnostic procedures vary with each institution.

BLOOD CULTURES

Blood cultures can be one of the most useful diagnostic tools available to the clinician.[11,14] In many cases, blood cultures give the only clue to the etiology of a patient's illness. If performed properly, it is a moderately sensitive but highly specific diagnostic procedure.

Indications

The indications for obtaining a blood culture are numerous and vary with the clinical setting. The usual situations in the pediatric intensive care unit (PICU) include a sudden change in temperature or pulse rate; the occurrence of chills, lethargy, or hypotension; fever with a heart murmur; and clinical evidence of sepsis. In the Emergency Department (ED), indications are fewer, including patients with possible occult bacteremia, clinical sepsis, or any serious bacterial infections (e.g., pneumonia, meningitis, urinary infections, pyarthrosis, or superficial infections with fever or leukocytosis). Children between the ages of 3 and 36 months who have a fever of 39° C or greater and a white blood cell count higher than 15,000/mm³ should also have a blood culture.[1]

Contraindications

There are no contraindications.

Complications

The most common complications of blood cultures are those associated with any phlebotomy, including bleeding at the site, development of such conditions as bruising and hematomas, and needlestick injuries associated with poor needle disposal. However, the most important "complication" relates to the recovery of a common skin organism in the blood culture. In some instances it is difficult to assess if the organism is really a pathogen or a contaminant, and the patient may receive unnecessary antibiotics or procedures. Repeated blood cultures in sets as well as clinical correlation are very important.

Equipment

The equipment required to obtain a blood culture includes a tourniquet, a 2% tincture of iodine, 70% alcohol, gloves, 2 × 2 sterile gauze, a needle or minicatheter (21, 23, or 25 gauge, depending on the size of the patient), and a Band-aid. Adults and older children also require two 100-ml vacuum culture bottles or two 50-ml vacuum bottles and an isolator tube (or if available, BactecPlus 30-ml bottles containing antimicrobial resins).[10] For infants and small children, the required equipment includes two 50-ml or two 100-ml vacuum culture bottles or a pediatric isolator and a 50- or 100-ml vacuum culture bottle.

Techniques

Use proper aseptic technique when obtaining a blood culture. Box 96-1 suggests guidelines for obtaining blood cultures and discusses the technique for obtaining peripheral venous blood cultures. However, a culture can also be obtained from arterial blood or blood sampled from an indwelling catheter after carefully prepping the needle insertion site. A positive culture from an indwelling catheter may reflect catheter colonization rather than bacteremia if a concurrent peripheral blood culture is sterile. Quantitative cultures may facilitate interpretation. Colony counts that are five to ten times higher on cultures obtained from central venous catheters compared to concurrent cultures of peripheral blood are consistent with catheter-related infections.[7,13]

Remarks

Do not change needles between the time of performing the venipuncture and depositing blood into the culture bottles; doing so serves only as a chance for contamination and increases the risk of needlestick injuries. A common means of contamination involves touching the venipuncture area with nonsterile gloves. Inform the laboratory if the presence of a slow-growing organism is likely so that the cultures can be held longer than the standard 1-week time period. For example, *Brucella* species often require as long as 4 weeks, and fungi and mycobacteria may not grow for 4 to 6 weeks. If fungemia is likely, use fungal isolators with standard blood

BOX 96-1 **TECHNIQUE FOR OBTAINING BLOOD CULTURES**

Use only sterile equipment and strict aseptic technique.

Apply a tourniquet and locate a fixed vein.

Prepare the skin by applying a 2% tincture of iodine, beginning with the site of proposed puncture and then cleansing in widening circles. Remove the iodine with 70% alcohol and allow to dry.

Do not touch the skin after this cleaning except with sterile gloves

Perform venipuncture and withdraw 20 ml of blood for adults and older children and 2 to 6 ml for infants; however, some systems require amounts as small as 0.2 ml.

Do not change needles.[5,9,12]

Immediately add the blood to the vacuum bottles, with 10 ml per bottle for adults and one half of the total amount for infants and children; allow the vacuum to draw the blood. For the pediatric isolator, add 0.5 to 1.5 ml and put any remaining blood into standard vacuum bottles. (Note: The optimum volume of blood varies with the type of culture bottles used. For best results, consult manufacturers' recommendations.)

Discard the needles and syringe (do not recap) into the appropriate receptacles for disposal.

Take specimens to the laboratory promptly or place them in an incubator at 37° C.

culture bottles. For the diagnosis of endocarditis, perform three sets of blood cultures. The first two blood cultures yield the etiologic agent in approximately 90% of the cases.[15] In 80% of patients, the bacteremia of endocarditis continues with less than 100 colony-forming units (CFU) per ml of blood.[2]

THROAT SWABS

Most sore throats result from viral infection, but 10% to 20% are bacterial infections. Group A β-hemolytic streptococcus, diphtheria, gonorrhea, and fusospirochetal (Vincent's) organisms may all appear as pharyngitis. In addition, fungal infections such as with *Candida* organisms can appear as exudative pharyngitis. Common viral etiologies of severe pharyngitis include the Epstein-Barr virus, enterovirus, adenovirus, and herpes simplex virus.

Indications

Prepare a throat culture for patients who complain of a sore throat or who have physical examination findings consistent with pharyngitis or tonsillitis, such as exudates, erythema, or pustules.

Contraindications

Do not swab the throat of a patient who has suspected epiglottitis or who has an unstable airway until the airway is secure.

Complications

Pain, bleeding, gagging, and vomiting are the most commonly encountered complications of obtaining a throat swab. In a patient with epiglottitis, acute respiratory compromise is possible with gagging.

Equipment

Most hospitals have available a system similar to the Marion Scientific Culturette specimen transport system, with one head for rapid streptococcal testing and another head for culture. In addition, assemble a tongue blade and light source.

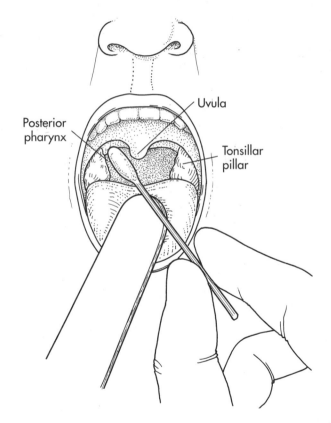

FIG. 96-1 Technique for obtaining a throat culture.

Techniques

Have the patient open his or her mouth. Usually, it is helpful to have the patient elevate the soft and hard palates by phonating the word "Ah" or a similar word. Direct the swab toward any pustular material or, if none is visible, sample each tonsillar area (Fig. 96-1). Place the culture tip into culture material immediately or, if not possible, place it in a Stuart or Amies transport medium. If the swab is dry, it is still acceptable to prepare a culture for up to 2 hours. Notify the laboratory of specific suspected pathogens, particularly if the organism does not grow on routine culture media (e.g., gonorrhea).[8,11]

RESPIRATORY SYNCYTIAL VIRUS ENZYME-LINKED IMMUNOSORBENT ASSAY AND CULTURE

Respiratory syncytial virus (RSV) is the most important respiratory virus that affects infants and young children.[8] Infections most commonly occur during the winter and early spring. Outbreaks in communities are associated with infant mortality estimated to be near 2%, and morbidity is quite high. For patients in high-risk groups (e.g., congenital heart disease, bronchopulmonary dysplasia, cystic fibrosis, or certain premature infants), the mortality rate may be much higher and the use of ribavirin may be indicated. Hospitals may experience outbreaks, which can cause havoc during epidemics.

Indications

Patients with upper respiratory–type infections that occur during the winter or spring are likely to have RSV infection depending on the occurrence of the virus in the community. Most mildly ill patients do not require specific therapy for this infection; therefore testing for this virus in usually not indicated. However, test symptomatic infants and young children (<2 years of age) who are severely ill or who are at high risk for developing severe lower respiratory tract disease with RSV, particularly those patients who might benefit from specific therapy (ribavirin).

Contraindications

There are no contraindications.

Complications

Trauma may result from inserting the swab into an unrestrained child. Sneezing can also occur, and the person performing the procedure may become infected.

Equipment

If using the catheter collection method, equipment for swabbing includes a protective gown and gloves, an 8-cm 10-French catheter for nasopharyngeal suctioning, and suction apparatus. If using the swab technique, use sterile swabs and viral transport media or, if not available, sterile saline in a test tube. Obtain a cup of ice to transport the specimen to the laboratory. An RSV Enzyme-Linked Immunosorbent Assay (ELISA) antigen kit is also necessary for rapid diagnostic testing.

Techniques

Place and restrain the child on his or her back. For catheter suctioning, insert the thin tubing through one of the nostrils and into the posterior pharynx. Withdraw the tubing while simultaneously applying suction, and aspirate the nasopharyngeal contents into a sterile container. Inoculate the contents onto a swab and into transport media and, if available, onto an RSV ELISA antigen-testing kit.

For the swab technique, insert the swab as shown in Fig. 96-2. Gently advance the swab into the nose and to the posterior pharynx until there is resistance. Inoculate the swab

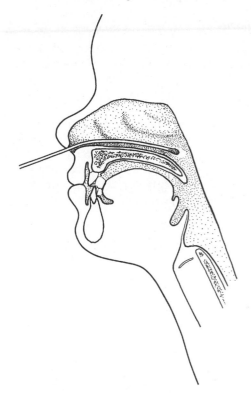

FIG. 96-2   Nasal swab collection.

into transport media and, if available, onto the RSV ELISA antigen-testing kit. For both techniques, transport the media on ice to the laboratory.

Remarks

The sensitivity of the ELISA antigen-detection system varies according to the kit used and the quantity and quality of specimen aspirated (50% to 80%). If available, perform an RSV culture at the same time to increase the sensitivity of the test.

RECTAL SWAB

The rectal swab is important for detecting bacterial organisms and viruses that produce gastroenteritis, proctitis and, occasionally, systemic disease.

Indications

Stool cultures are not indicated for all cases of acute diarrhea because most episodes are mild and self-limited. However, stool cultures are indicated in cases of moderate-to-severe disease, in protracted courses of diarrhea, when there is blood or mucus in the stool, or to determine if patients are shedding specific organisms (e.g., *Salmonella* carriers).

Contraindications

Patients with neutropenia or recent rectal surgery should not have rectal manipulation.

Complications

Besides local discomfort, there should not be complications as a result of a rectal swab. With forceful insertion, there is a risk of perforation, but this occurrence is exceedingly rare.

Equipment

The equipment necessary to perform a rectal swab includes a routine culture swab, gloves and, if desired, viral culture media.

Techniques

To perform a rectal swab, spread the buttocks and insert the swab gently into the rectal vault past the anal sphincter (approximately 3 to 5 cm in adults and 1 cm in infants and children). Rotate the swab several times and withdraw it. Plate the swab immediately or place it in a transport medium (either for bacterial or viral isolates).[6]

Remarks

With a rectal swab, it is not possible to examine specimens by direct microscopic analysis. The small amount of material collected may be inadequate to identify carriers who may be shedding small numbers of organisms at infrequent intervals. Notify the laboratory of the suspected organisms because certain bacteria require unique media or temperatures for incubation and proper identification. For example, *Campylobacter* organisms require a selective culture media referred to as a ''selective campy blood agar,'' and the best medium with which to detect *Yersinia* organisms is cefsulodin irgasan novobiocin (CIN) agar.

CONJUNCTIVAL AND LID CULTURES AND SCRAPINGS

Along with lid cultures and, occasionally, corneal cultures, conjunctival cultures can be a useful diagnostic aid for patients with conjunctival disease.

Indications

Conjunctival and lid cultures and scrapings are mandatory in patients with neonatal conjunctivitis, hyperacute conjunctivitis, membranous conjunctivitis, corneal ulcers, postoperative infections, Parinaud's oculoglandular syndrome, orbital cellulitis, and periocular abscesses, as well as preoperatively with any patient with one eye and an ocular prosthesis.[3,4]

Contraindications

Do not perform conjunctival and lid cultures in patients with herpes dendritic keratitis and other such infections before examination by an ophthalmologist.

Complications

Pain, local bleeding, and irritation are the most common problems encountered with eye cultures and scrapings.

Equipment

The equipment needed for eye cultures includes sterile cotton-tipped or calcium alginate applicators, thioglycollate broth, sterile spatulas, proparacaine hydrochloride drops for topical anesthesia, glass slides, and fixative solution or methyl alcohol. Routine culture media include blood, chocolate, colistin-nalidixic and MacConkey agars. If gonococcal infection is possible, include a Thayer-Martin agar as well. Place cultures for chlamydia into a chlamydia transport medium.

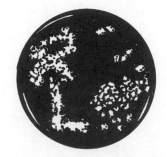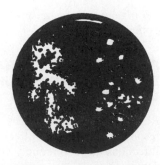

FIG. 96-3 Typical streak plate for lid and conjunctival cultures.

Techniques

Conjunctival Cultures. Obtain conjunctival cultures before lid margin cultures to reduce the false-positive rate resulting from the mechanical action of lid cultures. Use horizontal streaks on the culture plate for the conjunctival specimens and R- and L-shaped streaks to represent the lid specimens. Divide each plate into four quadrants and place each of the specimens into one of the quadrants (Fig. 96-3).

Use a sterile cotton-tipped or calcium alginate applicator moistened in thioglycollate broth to obtain this culture. Have the patient look up, and wipe the swab across the lower conjunctival cul-de-sac of the right eye from the temporal to the nasal margin. With a horizontal streak, inoculate the right upper quadrant of the agar plate. Place the tip of the applicator into thioglycollate broth and twirl it. Break off the tip and discard the upper portion of the applicator. Repeat the same procedure for the left eye, and place a horizontal streak in the right lower quadrant of the agar plate.

Lid Cultures. To obtain the lid cultures, swab another moistened applicator along the lower lash margin from the temporal to the nasal margin of the right eye. Inoculate the lid sample on the left upper quadrant of the agar plate using an R-shaped streak. Perform the same procedure for the left lid and inoculate it in the lower left quadrant of the agar plate with an L-shaped streak. Place both applicators into thioglycollate broth.

Conjunctival Scrapings. Use a sterile spatula to obtain conjunctival specimens for cytologic examination. Take samples from the upper tarsus area. To scrape the upper tarsal conjunctiva, instill one or two drops of proparacaine hydrochloride into the eye. Have the patient look down and evert the upper lid to expose the upper conjunctiva. Gently but firmly scrape the exposed conjunctiva, but do not precipitate bleeding. Spread the sample onto the center of a glass slide, making sure to turn over the spatula. Fix the slide immediately or allow it to air dry and then fix it in methyl alcohol. To scrape the lower conjunctiva, instill the anesthetic and have the patient look up. Pull down the lid and scrape across the epithelial surface. Apply the scrapings to the slide and fix it. An adequate sample should contain 500 to 1000 cells.

Remarks

When performing the conjunctival scraping, stay at least 2 to 3 mm away from the lid margins to avoid scraping the area of naturally occurring keratinized epithelial cells. Perform conjunctival cultures before lid cultures to prevent contamination of the conjunctival area with lid material.

REFERENCES

1. Baraff LS, Bass JW, Fleisher GR, et al: Practice guidelines for the management of infants and children 0 to 36 months of age with fever without source, *Pediatrics* 92:1-12, 1993.
2. Beeson PB, Brannon ES, Warren JV: Observations on the sites of removal of bacteria from the blood of patients with bacterial endocarditis, *J Exp Med* 84:9-23, 1945.
3. Brinser JH, Burd EM: Principles of diagnostic ocular microbiology. In Tabbara KF, Hyndiuk RA, editors: *Infections of the eye,* Boston, 1986, Little, Brown.
4. Brinser JH, Weiss A: Laboratory diagnosis in ocular disease. In Tasman W, Jaeger E, editors: *Duane's clinical ophthalmology,* Philadelphia, 1992, JB Lippincott.
5. Chapnick EK, Schaffer BC, Gradon JD, et al: Technique for drawing blood cultures: is changing needles truly necessary? *South Med J* 84:1197-1198, 1991.
6. Dalton HP, Nottebart HC: *Interpretive medical microbiology,* New York, 1986, Churchill Livingstone.
7. Flynn PM, Shenep JL, Stokes DC, et al: In situ management of confirmed central venous catheter-related bacteremia, *Pediatr Infect Dis J* 6:729-734, 1987.
8. Henry JB, editor: *Clinical diagnosis and management,* ed 18, Philadelphia, 1991, WB Saunders.
9. Isaacman DJ, Karasic RB: Lack of effect of changing needles on contamination of blood cultures, *Pediatr Inf Dis J* 9:274, 1990.
10. Isenberg HD, Washington JA, Doern G, et al: Specimen collecting and assembly. In Balows A, editor: *Manual of clinical microbiology,* Washington, DC, 1991, American Society of Microbiology.
11. Jawetz E, Melnick JL, Adelberg EA: *Medical microbiology,* ed 19, Norwalk, Conn, 1991, Appleton & Lange.
12. Krumholz HM, Cummings S, York M: Blood culture phlebotomy: switching needles does not prevent contamination, *Ann Intern Med* 113:290-292, 1990.
13. Raucher HS, Hyatt AC, Barzilai A, et al: Quantitative blood cultures in the evaluation of septicemia in children with Broviac catheters, *J Pediatr* 104:29-37, 1984.
14. Washington JA: Medical bacteriology. In Henry JB, editor: *Clinical diagnosis and management by laboratory methods,* ed 18, Philadelphia, 1991, WB Saunders.
15. Werner AS, Cobbs CG, Kaye D, et al: Studies on the bacteremia of bacterial endocarditis, *JAMA* 202:199, 1967.

Steven L. Hickerson and Richard F. Jacobs

GRAM STAIN

The Gram stain is probably one of the most useful screening tools available to the clinician. It can provide rapid, early information for more pathogen-directed antimicrobial therapy. The Gram stain is a differential, direct stain used to separate bacteria into gram-positive and gram-negative categories on the basis of the properties of their cell walls (Fig. 97-1). Because of the thick cell wall of gram-positive bacteria, crystal violet (the primary stain) remains after decolorization and appears deep blue or purple. Gram-negative organisms are unable to retain the primary stain following decolorization and instead stain with the safranin counterstain and appear red.

Indications

Gram stains are performed on a broad array of clinical specimens, including sterile body sites or fluids (cerebrospi-

nal fluid, peritoneal or pleural fluids, and tissue biopsy specimens) or nonsterile specimens (sputum, tracheal aspirates, abscess fluid, spun or unspun voided urine, or eye, nasopharyngeal, or rectal specimens).

Equipment

The reagents necessary for a Gram stain include crystal violet (2 g 90% crystal violet dye in 20 ml ethyl alcohol, 0.8 g ammonia oxalate, and 100 ml distilled water), Gram iodine solution (1 g iodine crystals with 2 g potassium iodide in 100 ml distilled water), decolorizer (50 ml acetone with 50 ml of 95% ethyl alcohol), and safranin (2.5 g of 99% safranin O dye in 100 ml of 95% ethyl alcohol that is added to 100 ml of distilled water).[9]

Techniques

To prepare a Gram stain, smear the specimen evenly over a clean glass microscope slide. Allow the specimen to air dry and fix it onto the slide by passing it over a Bunsen burner flame three to four times. An alternate method involves fixing the smear by flooding the slide with methanol or ethyl alcohol and allowing it to stand for a few minutes. Once the smear has cooled, place the slide on a staining rack and flood

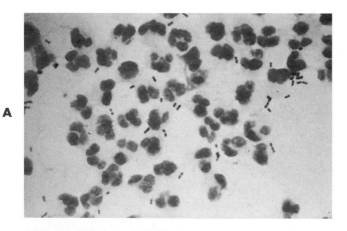

A

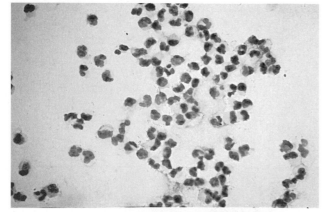

B

FIG. 97-1 Gram stains of cerebral spinal fluid specimens. **A,** Gram-positive lancet-shaped diplococci, *Streptococcus pneumoniae.* **B,** Gram-negative coccobacilli, *Haemophilus influenzae.* (Courtesy R. Wheeler.)

Table 97-1 Gram Stain Interpretation

Staining characteristics	Morphology	Suspected pathogens
Gram-positive	Lancet-shaped diplococci	*Streptococcus pneumoniae*
	Cocci in chains	Streptococci
	Large cocci in tetrads or clusters	Staphylococci
	Rods	*Bacillus* spp.
		Clostridium spp.
		Listeria monocytogenes
	Branching filaments	*Nocardia* spp.
		Actinomyces spp.
Gram-negative	Diplococci	*Neisseria* spp.
	Coccobacilli	*Haemophilus* spp.
	Rods	Enterobacteriaceae
		Enterobacter spp.
		Escherichia spp.
		Klebsiella spp.
		Proteus spp.
		Salmonella spp.
		Serratia spp.
		Shigella spp.
		Yersinia spp.
		Pseudomanas spp.
	Curved rods	*Vibrio* spp.

it with crystal violet. After exposing the smear to the crystal violet primary stain for 1 minute, rinse it thoroughly with water. Flood the smear with Gram iodine solution and allow it to stand for 1 minute; again rinse the smear with water. Hold the slide at a 45-degree angle and rinse it with a few drops of acetone-alcohol decolorizer until no more crystal violet can be removed. The usual duration of decolorization is 10 seconds or less. Thoroughly rinse the slide with water and place it on the staining rack. Cover the smear with safranin and allow it to stand for 1 minute; rinse it with water and blot it dry. Examine the slide under the low-power objective and then under oil immersion. Table 97-1 discusses the interpretation of Gram stain results.[7,9]

WET PREPARATION OR SALINE MOUNT

Indications

The wet preparation allows for direct examination of unstained clinical specimens and permits visualization of unaltered cells and microorganisms. This technique also detects motile microorganisms. Wet prep examination is primarily useful in the evaluation of vaginal or urethral infections; perform a wet prep on all patients with suspected vaginitis, vaginosis, or pelvic inflammatory disease because coinfection with sexually transmitted diseases can occur. This method is also useful for examining sputum specimens or stool samples for parasites.

Equipment

The equipment necessary for a wet prep includes a cotton-tipped applicator, sterile saline, a clean glass slide, and a coverslip.

Techniques

When obtaining a sample for a wet prep, use a cotton-tipped applicator to collect a sample of the discharge or to swab the secretions in the vaginal vault. Place the swab into a tube containing 2 ml of sterile saline. Place a drop of this suspension in the center of a clean glass slide and cover it with a glass coverslip. Examine the prep under low- and high-power objectives; close the iris of the microscope slightly to reduce the light source. *Trichomonas vaginalis* appears as pear-shaped, flagellated protozoa that are motile and slightly larger than white blood cells (WBCs). The presence of clue cells (epithelial cells that have numerous bacteria clinging to their surface) is indicative of infection with *Gardnerella vaginitis*. Budding yeast or hyphal elements may be visualized with this technique, but usually requires the digestion of epithelial cells with potassium hydroxide for visualization of fungal elements. To examine sputum, mix a small amount of the sputum with 1 to 2 drops of saline on a microscope slide and cover it with a coverslip. Examine the preparation under the high-power objective to investigate a presumptive diagnosis of a pulmonary mycosis. *Candida* spp. appear as budding yeast with pseudohyphae (Fig. 97-2), whereas *Blastomyces dermatitidis* appears as a broad-based budding yeast form (Fig. 97-3). *Histoplasma capsulatum* is typically a tiny yeast form (Fig. 97-4) but is rarely visible with direct examination; the presence of septated, branching hyphae is suggestive of *Aspergillus* spp. (Fig. 97-5).

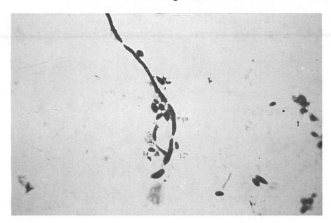

FIG. 97-2   Typical appearance of the pseudohyphae of *Candida* spp.

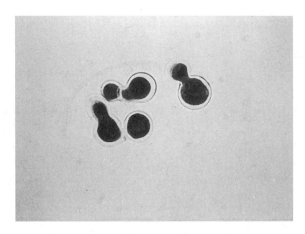

FIG. 97-3   Broad-based budding yeast of *Blastomyces dermatitidis*.

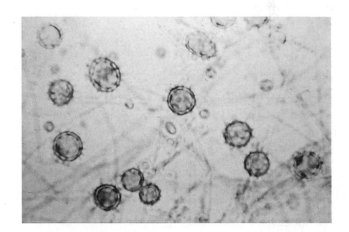

FIG. 97-4   Yeast forms of *Histoplasma capsulatum*.

To examine a stool specimen, emulsify a small amount of fecal material in 1 to 2 drops of saline on a clean glass slide.[9] Place a coverslip on this mixture and examine it under low- and high-power objectives. Protozoan cysts appear refractile using this technique, and motile trophozoites can be observed (Fig. 97-6). Because of poor delineation of the internal

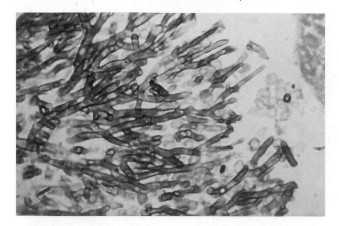

FIG. 97-5 Septated branching hyphae of *Aspergillus* spp.

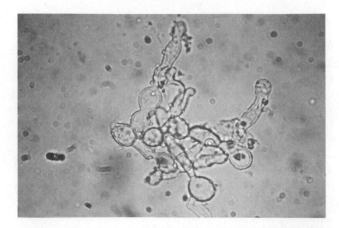

FIG. 97-7 KOH preparation of a sputum, which demonstrates thick-walled, broad-based budding yeast, *Blastomyces dermatitidis.*

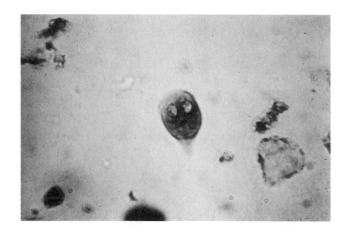

FIG. 97-6 Trophozoite form of *Giardia lamblia.*

structures, it is impossible to establish a definitive identification of parasites by this procedure; an iodine stain is usually required.

POTASSIUM HYDROXIDE WET PREPARATION
Indications

The potassium hydroxide (KOH) wet preparation technique is useful for the direct examination of clinical specimens, which allows for visualization of fungal elements. KOH digests cellular components of the specimen more rapidly than fungal elements and therefore clears the specimen of epithelial cells, inflammatory cells, and debris (Fig. 97-7). This procedure is often difficult to interpret because of persistent cellular debris. A negative KOH wet preparation does not exclude fungal disease.

Equipment

The equipment necessary to prepare a KOH prep includes a clean glass slide and coverslip, a Bunsen burner, and either 10% KOH solution or 10% KOH–dimethyl sulfoxide solution.

Techniques

Place the specimen (e.g., skin scrapings, hair, nails, pus, tissue, or sputum) onto a clean glass microscope slide. Place

1 to 2 drops of 10% KOH solution or 10% KOH–dimethyl sulfoxide solution onto the specimen. Cover the specimen with a glass coverslip and, if using KOH solution, gently heat the preparation by passing it over a Bunsen burner flame two or three times. Avoid boiling the preparation. If using the KOH–dimethyl sulfoxide solution, do not heat the preparation. View the specimen under a low-power objective and confirm the identification using the high-power objective. Thick specimens may take longer for adequate digestion by KOH.[1,5]

INDIA INK PREPARATION
Indications

The India ink preparation is a negative stain used to identify encapsulated yeast (e.g., *Cryptococcus neoformans)* in clinical specimens. Its primary use is to examine cerebrospinal fluid (CSF) in patients at risk for cryptococcal meningitis, such as organ transplant recipients, patients with lymphoreticular malignancies, patients on chronic corticosteroid therapy, and patients with acquired immunodeficiency syndrome (AIDS). However, the sputum specimens of patients suspected of having pulmonary cryptococcal disease can also be examined using the India ink technique. In CSF specimens, the India ink prep has a sensitivity of approximately 50%.[3] In many centers the cryptococcal latex agglutination test has supplanted the India ink preparation because it has a sensitivity of more than 90% in CSF.[6,8] However, the India ink prep remains a good and quick test for the presumptive diagnosis of cryptococcal meningitis, especially in centers in which the latex agglutination test is not readily available and in patient populations that have a high occurrence of *Cryptococcus* spp. (e.g., AIDS).

Equipment

The equipment necessary to perform an India ink prep includes a clean glass slide and coverslip and a drop of India ink.

Techniques

Add 1 drop of centrifuged specimen to the center of a clean microscope slide. Place a drop of India ink onto the specimen

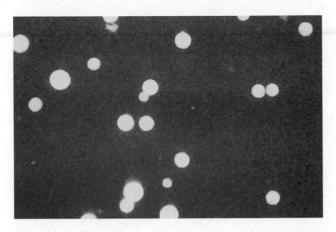

FIG. 97-8   Clear surrounding halo caused by the large capsule of *Cryptococcus* with the India ink stain.

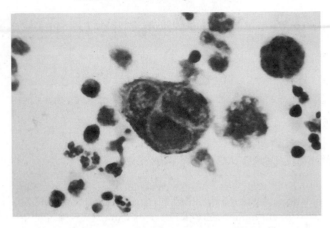

FIG. 97-9   Tzanck prep using the Wright staining technique and demonstrating multinucleated giant cells and infection with the herpes simplex virus.

and mix well. Place a coverslip over the preparation and view it under the high-power objective; scan the entire smear because few organisms may be present. The *Cryptococcus* spp. appears as a bright encapsulated yeast, usually 5 to 8μ with a clear surrounding halo caused by the large capsule on the black background (Fig. 97-8).[1,9]

TZANCK SMEAR

Indications

The Tzanck preparation was originally described in 1947 and is a rapid method for the identification of viral infectious etiologies (herpesvirus or Varicellavirus) of vesiculobullous diseases.[10] In many cases the diagnosis is evident on clinical grounds; however, early in the course of the illness the diagnosis may remain unclear and, if therapeutic intervention is under consideration, the Tzanck preparation may provide an expeditious diagnosis. Although different stains may be used for the technique, the end result remains the same—the identification of multinucleated giant cells (Fig. 97-9). The Tzanck preparation has a sensitivity of approximately 50%, and therefore many tertiary care centers have replaced it with direct fluorescence antibody (DFA) testing, which has higher sensitivity and specificity for herpes simplex virus types 1 and 2 and Varicella zoster. Nevertheless, the Tzanck prep remains a quick, uncomplicated technique for the identification of herpes viral infections when DFA testing is not available.

Equipment

The equipment necessary for a Tzanck preparation includes 70% alcohol, an 18-gauge needle, a cotton-tipped applicator or a No. 10 or 15 scalpel blade, and a clean glass microscope slide and coverslip. The options for the different stains of this procedure include the Giemsa stain,[4,11] Paragon Multiple Stain (PMS),[2] Wright stain, and methylene blue stain.

Techniques

Identify an intact vesicle or bulla and, using sterile technique, prepare the area with 70% alcohol. Using an 18-gauge needle, unroof the vesicle to expose the base. Using either a cotton-tipped applicator or No. 10 or 15 scalpel blade, firmly scrape the base of the vesicle. Smear this material onto a clean microscope slide and allow it to air dry. Cover the smear with the selected stain for 15 seconds and thoroughly rinse it with water. Allow it to air dry and view the slide directly, mount it using a mounting medium, or apply immersion oil and a coverslip. Under a high-power objective, examine the stained smear for multinucleated giant cells and intranuclear inclusions, which are pathognomonic for either herpes simplex or varicella zoster infections (Fig. 97-9). The Tzanck preparation cannot distinguish between herpes and varicella infections.

REFERENCES

1. Al-Doory Y: *Laboratory medical mycology,* Philadelphia, 1980, Lea & Febiger, pp. 81-82.
2. Barr RJ, Herten J, Graham HJ: Rapid method for Tzanck preparations, *JAMA* 237:1119-1120, 1977.
3. Bindschadler DD, Bennett JE: Serology of human cryptococcosis, *Ann Intern Med* 1968, pp 45-52.
4. Blank H, Burgoon CF, Baldridge GD, et al: Cytologic smears in diagnosis of herpes simplex, herpes zoster, and varicella, *JAMA* 146:1410-1412, 1951.
5. Campbell MC, Stewart JL: *The medical mycology handbook,* New York, 1980, John Wiley & Sons, pp. 163-164.
6. Gordon MA, Vedder DK: Serologic tests in diagnosis and prognosis of cryptococcosis, *JAMA* 197:961-967, 1966.
7. Hendrickson DA, Krenz MM: Reagents and stains. In Balows A, Hausler WJ Jr, Hermann KL, et al, editors: *Manual of clinical microbiology,* ed 5, Washington, DC, 1991, American Society for Microbiology, p. 1306.
8. Kaufman L, Blumer S: Latex-cryptococcal antigen test, *Am J Clin Pathol* 59:285-286, 1973.
9. Koneman EW, Allen SD, Dowell VR Jr, et al: *Color atlas and textbook of diagnostic microbiology,* ed 4, Philadelphia, 1992, JB Lippincott.
10. Tzanck A: *Le cytodiagnostic immediat en dermatologie, Bull Soc Fr Dermatol Syphiligr* 7:68, 1947.
11. Wheeland RG, Burgdorf WH, Hoshaw RA: A quick Tzanck smear, *J Am Acad Dermatol* 8:258-259, 1983.

Steven L. Hickerson and Gordon E. Schutze

BEDSIDE COLD AGGLUTININS TEST

The bedside cold agglutinins test is a useful screening diagnostic test when evaluating a patient with a community-acquired pneumonia or atypical pneumonia. The association of cold agglutinins with atypical pneumonia dates to the 1940s.[13] However, it was not until the 1960s that a definite association linked the atypical pneumonia syndrome with cold agglutinins and the Eaton agent, *Mycoplasma pneumoniae*.[3,12] Cold agglutinins are IgM antibodies that are directed to the I antigen of erythrocytes.[11,17]

Indications

The bedside cold agglutinins test may be useful in the diagnosis of *Mycoplasma* disease. A positive bedside cold agglutinins test corresponds to a cold agglutinin titer of at least 1:32 and is present in 50% to 75% of patients infected with *M. pneumoniae*.[2,5]

Contraindications

There are no contraindications to a bedside cold agglutinins test.

Equipment

The equipment required for a bedside cold agglutinins test includes a lancet, an alcohol preparation pad, a blue-top sodium citrate tube, and a cup of ice.

Techniques

To perform the bedside cold agglutinins test, obtain 0.2 ml or 4 to 5 drops of blood via a lancet fingerstick or venipuncture. Place the blood in a blue-top tube containing 0.2 ml of sodium citrate. Place the tube in the cup of ice water for approximately 10 minutes. Hold the tube at a 90-degree angle by the blue cap to avoid warming; rotate the tube to allow the contents to come in contact with the chilled tube. A positive test is represented by coarse follicular agglutination and results from an excess of cold antibody. Fine agglutination or no agglutination represents a negative test. Confirm the result by rewarming the tube in a hand and observing for the disappearance of agglutination.[9,10]

Remarks

The bedside cold agglutinins test is only a supportive test in the diagnosis of infection with *M. pneumoniae*. Although cold agglutinins in the setting of pneumonia most commonly occur in patients with *M. pneumoniae* infection, they are not specific for *Mycoplasma* disease. Cold agglutinins can also occur in other conditions, such as viral pneumonia, Epstein-Barr virus infection, adenoviral infection, mumps, measles, influenza, scarlet fever, malaria, atypical hemolytic anemia, Raynaud's disease, and paroxysmal nocturnal hemoglobin-uria. Cold agglutinins are not present in all patients with *Mycoplasma* disease and typically do not appear until the second week of illness; therefore a negative test does not exclude *M. pneumoniae* as the etiologic agent. Confirm the results by immunofluorescence or an enzyme-linked immunosorbent assay (ELISA) demonstration of antibody titers.

ANTIGEN TESTING

Antigen detection tests have become quite popular. These tests help to identify the potential infective agent in severely ill children. Common methods for performing bacterial antigen studies include counterimmunoelectrophoresis or latex agglutination. Viral and parasitic antigen tests involve a myriad of procedures, including immunofluorescence, enzyme immunoassay, and electron microscopy. The availability of each test varies with the institution.

Indications

Perform bacterial antigen testing on patients who come to the hospital with sepsis or meningitis and who received oral or parenteral antimicrobial agents before hospitalization. This form of testing may also be useful for symptomatic neonates born to mothers who were receiving antimicrobial agents at the time of delivery. The patient's history and physical examination guide other types of antigen testing. Table 98-1 outlines the common organisms identifiable through antigen testing.

Contraindications

There are no contraindications to antigen testing, but use these tests in a thoughtful manner. For instance, there is no reason to perform antigen testing if a child comes to the hospital with meningitis and if gram-positive diplococci are present on the Gram stain. Culture results will become available within 24 hours, and identifying the *Streptococcus pneumoniae* antigen 24 hours before the culture reveals the organism will certainly not change the initial antibiotic therapy for the child.

Techniques

Table 98-1 lists suggested sources of specimens for antigen testing. Transport all specimens to the laboratory in a timely manner. Refrigerate all specimens that are being kept overnight. For the best results, perform antigen testing on fresh specimens. Obtain urine for antigen testing by catheterization or suprapubic aspiration. Specimens obtained through bag collection have more false-positive results as a result of stool or skin contamination. To detect viruses in vesicular lesions, it is important to scrape the bottom of the lesion during sample collection.

Table 98-1   Antigen Detection by Organism

Organism	Suggested source of specimen*	Advantages	Limitations
Haemophilus influenzae, type B (Hib)	U, CSF, JF	Urine sensitivity is 91% to 100%[1]	Number of cases of invasive Hib disease has greatly declined; false-positives result from Hib immunizations[7,15]
Streptococcus pneumoniae	U, CSF	CSF sensitivity is 67% to 100%[1]	Urine sensitivity is 0 to 50%[1]
Neisseria meningitidis	CSF		Urine should not be used because of 0% sensitivity;[1] CSF results are only slightly better (0% to 50%); false-positives result from *E. coli*
Group B streptococci	U, CSF		False-positives with urine testing because of perineal and rectal colonization[16]
Escherichia coli	U, CSF		Not widely available
Cryptococcus neoformans	CSF, ST	Rapid diagnosis of disease in patient with HIV	CSF results are less sensitive than serum for meningitis[4]
Neisseria gonorrhoeae	UES	Better sensitivity than cervical Gram stain in female patients[18]	Equivalent to Gram stain in male patients
Group A Streptococci	T	Highly specific	Wide variation of sensitivity; negative results require a throat culture
Mycobacterium tuberculosis	CSF	More sensitive than direct staining of CSF[6]	Overall poor sensitivity limits usefulness
Chlamydia trachomatis	C, NP	Highly sensitive for respiratory specimens	Lack of specificity for use in evaluation of sexual abuse[14]
Herpes simplex virus	OGL	More specific than Tzanck smear	Limited data on other sources
Cytomegalovirus	BL	More sensitive than shell vial cultures[8]	Labor intensive; patient cannot have neutropenia
Varicellavirus	VF	More specific than Tzanck smear	
Respiratory syncytial virus	NP		Sensitivities vary by technique for sample acquisition
Influenza A	NP	Quick results	Varying results depending on the kit used
Rotavirus organisms	ST	Extremely sensitive and simple to perform	Seasonal variation of disease
Adenovirus *40/41*	ST	Highly sensitive and specific	Not widely available
Hepatitis B surface antigen	BL	Most important and commonly used marker	Detectable for only 12 weeks
Human immunodeficiency virus P-24 antigen	BL	Can be used to measure disease activity	Not useful in infants <6 months of age

*U, Urine; *CSF,* cerebral spinal fluid; *JF,* joint fluid; *UES,* urethral epithelial secretions; *T,* throat secretions; *NP,* nasopharyngeal secretions; *OGL,* oral genital lesions; *VF,* vesicular fluid; *ST,* stool; *BL,* blood; *C,* conjunctiva.

Remarks

Antigen detection is only as rapid as the individual performing the test. Communicating with laboratory personnel about suspected pathogens before submitting the sample may facilitate an answer. False-positives are associated with these tests because colonization or other site infection renders the test positive. Conversely, false-negatives occur in systemic infections and vary with the body fluid tested. For example, centrifuged urine, appears to have the highest sensitivity for *Haemophilus influenzae* bacterial antigens.

REFERENCES

1. Ballard TI, Roe MH, Wheeler RC, et al: Comparison of three latex agglutination kits and counterimmunoelectrophoresis for detection of bacterial antigens in a pediatric population, *Pediatr Infect Dis J* 6:630-634, 1987.
2. Chanock RM: Mycoplasma infections of man, *N Engl J Med* 273:1257-1264, 1965.
3. Chanock RM, Dienes L, Eaton MD, et al: *Mycoplasma pneumoniae:* proposed nomenclature for atypical pneumonia organism (Eaton agent), *Science* 140:662, 1963.
4. Chuck SL, Sande MAL: Infections with *Cryptococcus neoformans* in the acquired immunodeficiency syndrome, *N Engl J Med* 321:794-799, 1989.
5. Cordero L, Caudrado R, Hall CB, et al: Primary atypical pneumonia: an epidemic caused by *Mycoplasma pneumoniae, J Pediatr* 71:1, 1967.
6. Daniel TM: New approaches to the rapid diagnosis of tuberculous meningitis, *J Infect Dis* 155:599-602, 1987.
7. Darville T, Jacobs RF, Lucas RA, et al: Detection of *Haemophilus influenzae* type B antigen in cerebrospinal fluid after immunization, *Pediatr Infect Dis* 11:243, 1992.
8. Erice A, Holm MA, Gill PC, et al: Cytomegalovirus (CMV) antigenemia assay is more sensitive than shell vial cultures for rapid detection of CMV in polymorphonuclear blood leukocytes, *J Clin Microbiol* 30:2822-2825, 1992.
9. Garrow DH: A rapid test for the presence of increased cold agglutinins, *Br Med J* 2:206-208, 1958.
10. Griffin JP: Rapid screening for cold agglutinins in pneumonia, *Ann Intern Med* 70:701-705, 1969.

11. Janney FA, Lee LT, Howe C: Cold hemagglutinin cross-reactivity with *Mycoplasma pneumoniae, Infect Immun* 22:29-33, 1978.

12. Liu C, Eaton MD, Heyl JT: Studies on primary atypical pneumonia. Part II. Observations concerning the development and immunological characteristic of antibody in patients, *J Exp Med* 109:545, 1959.

13. Peterson OL, Ham TH, Finland M: Cold agglutinins (autohemagglutinins) in primary atypical pneumonias, *Science* 97:167, 1943.

14. Porder K, Sanchez N, Roblin PM, et al: Lack of specificity of chlamydiazyme for detection of vaginal chlamydial infection in prepubertal girls, *Pediatr Infect Dis* 8:358-360, 1989.

15. Rothstein EP, Madore DV, Girone JAC, et al: Comparison of antigenuria after immunization with three *Haemophilus influenzae* type B conjugate vaccines, *Pediatr Infect Dis* 10:311-314, 1991.

16. Sanchez PJ, Siegel JD, Cushion NB, et al: Significance of a positive urine group B streptococcal latex agglutination test in neonates, *J Pediatr* 116:601-606, 1990.

17. Smith CB, McGinniss MH, Schmidt PJ: Changes in erythrocyte I agglutinogen and anti-I agglutinins during *Mycoplasma pneumoniae* infection in man, *J Immunol* 99:333-339, 1967.

18. Stamm WE, Cole B, Fennell C, et al: Antigen detection for the diagnosis of gonorrhea, *J Clin Microbiol* 19:399-403, 1984.

99 Diagnostic Procedures

Steven L. Hickerson, J. Thomas Cross, Gordon E. Schutze, and Richard F. Jacobs

OTOSCOPY

Otoscopy, with an adequate medical history and a thorough physical examination, is usually sufficient to establish a clinical diagnosis of middle ear disease. Signs and symptoms associated with diseases of the ear and temporal bone include otalgia, otorrhea, hearing loss, swelling, vertigo, nystagmus, tinnitus, and facial paralysis.[6] It is best to diagnose ear disease by using pneumatic otoscopy, but a thorough physical examination may identify conditions that predispose the child to ear disease. For example the craniofacial anomalies of trisomy 21 are associated with an increased risk of ear disease.

Examine the ear itself, using a systematic approach. Signs of infection in the external auditory meatus, auricle, and so on can be quite helpful in discerning information about infection in the interior structures. For example postauricular disease may indicate infection in the periosteum or related structures.

Indications

Perform otoscopy on all patients with ear signs or symptoms and on all children with fever, leukocytosis, or head trauma.

Contraindications

Inability to restrain the child adequately can result in injury, so defer the examination.

Complications

Bleeding or trauma to the external auditory meatus and perforation of the tympanic membrane may result if the child moves suddenly. Excessive positive or negative pressure can be painful or produce rupture of the tympanic membrane. Pain may occur in the auditory canal with movement of the speculum across inflamed external auditory canal tissue as a result of acute otitis externa or chronical draining.

Equipment

Siegle and Bruening pneumatic otoscopes are similar, each consisting of an airtight chamber into which various specula fit according to the child's canal size. Today most standard otoscopes have the capability of assessing movement of the tympanic membrane by insufflation. A convex lens covers the proximal end. The side of the chamber contains a knob over which rubber tubing with a bulb attaches distally for insufflation. Specula of various sizes are necessary. A cerumen curette or dental irrigator may be necessary.

Techniques

Remove all cerumen obstructing the external auditory canal to allow adequate visualization of the canal and the tympanic membrane. To remove cerumen use a cerumen spoon or curette through a speculum under direct vision or employ gentle warm water irrigation if the tympanic membranes are intact.

To visualize the tympanic membranes use a speculum with the largest lumen that comfortably fits[1] in the child's external auditory meatus.[4] Restrain the child adequately.[7] Position the otoscope with the hand holding the otoscope while resting against the parietal area of the skull (Fig. 99-1).[49] Use the other hand to apply posterosuperior traction on the pinna in older children, or simple posterior traction in infants, to straighten the curve in the external canal. When the speculum is in the canal and there is good visualization of the tympanic membrane, squeeze and passively deflate the bulb and observe the tympanic membrane for movement. Inspection of the tympanic membrane includes evaluation of its color, degree of translucency, and mobility. The position and movement of the tympanic membrane are very important and allow determination of the presence of fluid in the middle ear (Fig. 99-2). The appearance of the tympanic membrane may be helpful. Normally there is a ground-glass appearance. A blue-yellow color indicates effusion; a red membrane, in the absence of other pathologic findings, may be normal because the blood vessels of the tympanic membrane may become engorged from crying or fever alone. Landmarks are visible in the normal ear (Fig. 99-3).

Remarks

The tympanic membrane of the neonate lies in a more horizontal plane than in the older child; thus the eardrum may appear to be smaller and retracted. Additionally the neonate's ear canal frequently contains vernix caseosa; however, it is easy to remove. The canals of the neonate are

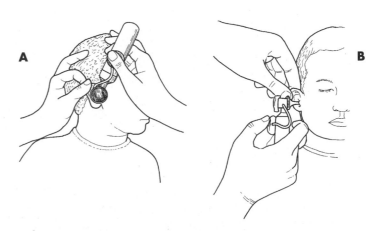

FIG. 99-1 Methods of positioning otoscope. **A,** Using both hands for restraint. **B,** Technique for cooperative child.

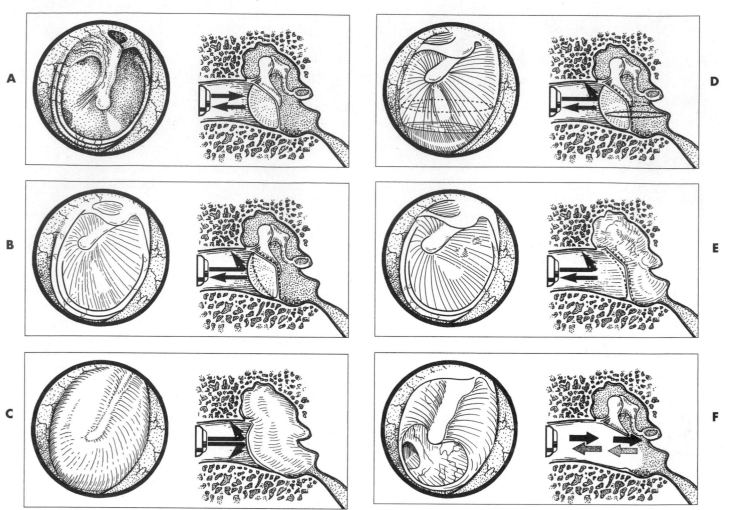

FIG. 99-2   **A** to **F,** Common conditions of the middle ear as assessed with the otoscope. **A,** Normal. **B,** Negative middle ear pressure. **C,** Acute otitis media. **D,** Fluid level. **E,** Otitis media with effusion. **F,** Perforation of the tympanic membrane.

(From Bluestone CD, Klein JO: *Otitis media in infants and children,* Philadelphia, 1988, WB Saunders.)

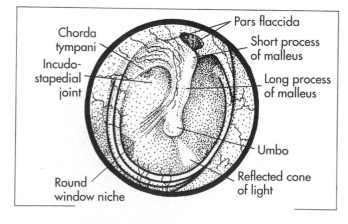

FIG. 99-3   Landmarks of the middle ear.

usually very pliable and collapse and expand with pneumatic otoscopy, thus making it more difficult to move the tympanic membrane.[15] To overcome this problem, carefully insert the speculum farther into the canal.

Otoscopy is extremely subjective and there are frequent interobserver differences.[46] Tympanocentesis for diagnostic fluid studies may be helpful in some patients.

TYMPANOCENTESIS

Tympanocentesis is a lost art for many recently trained clinicians. However the widespread use of broad-spectrum antibiotics, the acquired immunodeficiency syndrome (AIDS) epidemic, and the development of resistant bacteria have increased the need for tympanocentesis, particularly in patients with unresponsive middle ear effusions.

Indications

This procedure is useful in determining the infectious cause of many middle ear effusions.[8,9,55] The indications for the procedure vary; in general consider it for any seriously ill patient with concomitant otitis media. Perform it on patients with otitis media who have toxic signs or symptoms or suppurative complications, including mastoiditis with periostitis, meningitis, extradural abscess, subdural empyema, focal encephalitis, brain abscess, lateral sinus thrombosis, or otitic hydrocephalus.[10] Other indications include otitis media in the newborn, the very young infant (<3 months of age), or the immunocompromised child in whom presence of unusual organisms is possible. Finally consider tympanocentesis in patients who experience facial paralysis as an isolated complication of otitis media.[11]

Contraindications

The most important aspect of this procedure is the ability to immobilize the child properly; if this is not possible, then do not attempt the procedure. Inability to visualize the landmarks of the tympanic membrane and associated structures adequately is an absolute contraindication for this procedure, as damage to the middle ear structures is quite likely without adequate visualization.[50]

Complications

The most common complications of the procedure (usually associated with concomitant myringotomy) are persistent perforation and development of an atrophic scar.[50] Persistent otorrhea may follow the procedure and consequently an eczematoid external otitis may develop. Neurologic complications are rare but do occur. Severing the chorda tympani produces impairment of the sense of taste on the corresponding side of the tongue. Note that the nerve is occasionally visible at the posterior-inferior border of Shrapnell's membrane. Transient facial paralysis may also occur as the facial nerve lies immediately above the oval window. There are rare reports of fatal hemorrhage with laceration of the internal carotid artery that extends as far as the middle of the promontory of the tympanic membrane. In infants the bulb of the jugular vein may lie beneath the mucous membrane of the floor of the tympanic membrane without intervening bone. With excessive penetration fracture of the crura of the stapes may occur, as may dislocation of the incudostapedial joint.

Equipment

Equipment required includes material for body restraint; sterile gauze; a short-bevel 21- or 22-gauge, 8 to 10-cm spinal needle; or an Alden-Senturia trap (Storz Instrument Co., St. Louis, MO) with a needle attached.[9,50] Also needed are antiseptic solution, 70% alcohol; extension tubing from an infusion set; 10-ml syringe; otoscope with operative head; 20% cocaine solution (or other local anesthetic); and culture swab or Calgiswab (Falton, Oxnard, CA) moistened with trypticase soy broth.

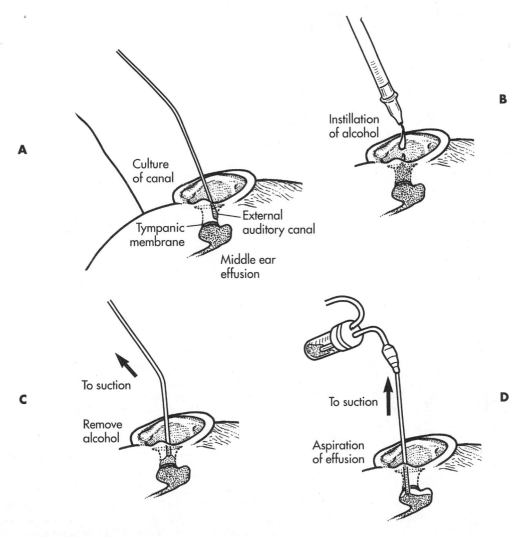

FIG. 99-4   A to **D,** Technique for tympanocentesis.

(From Bluestone CD, Klein JO: *Pediatric otolaryngology,* ed 2, Philadelphia, 1990, WB Saunders.)

BOX 99-1 TECHNIQUE OF TYMPANOCENTESIS

1. Clear the canal of cerumen, then insert the largest speculum that fits the external canal and visualizes the tympanic membrane.
2. Remove the otoscope. Obtain a culture specimen of the external ear canal before instillation of alcohol solution.
3. Instill the alcohol into the ear and then drain it with sterile gauze and a wick. Allow the alcohol to dry completely.
4. Bend the needle at half its length to an angle between 30 and 45 degrees with a complementary angle bent into the needle 2 to 3 cm proximal to the first bend (see Fig. 99-4).
5. Attach the extension tubing and syringe to the needle and have an assistant hold them.
6. Instill local anesthetic solution into the ear canal and leave it for at least 10 minutes to allow for adequate anesthesia.
7. Remove the local anesthetic with another gauze and wick.
8. Reinsert the otoscope and visualize the tympanic membrane.
9. Immobilize the patient securely.
10. Advance the bent needle slowly into the external auditory canal through the otoscope head in the direction of the inferior-posterior quadrant.
11. Advance the needle to the tympanic membrane; as the needle passes through the membrane direct the assistant to aspirate with the syringe; then, quickly withdraw the needle.
12. Cleanse the external auditory canal of any drainage or blood.
13. The quantity of material aspirated from the middle ear is usually quite small and remains in the needle or the extension tubing. Gently flush the tubing and needle with a few drops of sterile nonbacteriostatic saline solution onto the culture medium.

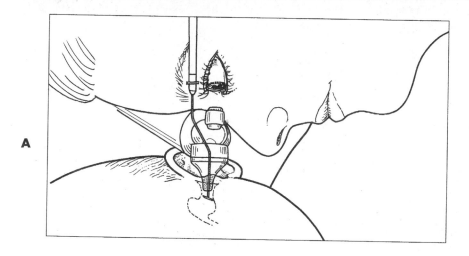

A

FIG. 99-5 **A** and **B,** Approach to tympanocentesis.

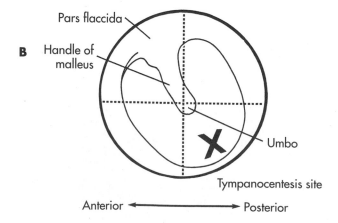

B

Pars flaccida

Handle of malleus

Umbo

Tympanocentesis site

Anterior ⟷ Posterior

Techniques

Fig. 99-4 illustrates the technique and Box 99-1 outlines the steps in performing tympanocentesis.[9,50] Fig. 99-5 depicts proper orientation of the needle. Restraining the child is of utmost importance.

Remarks

Before performing tympanocentesi, culture of the external ear canal can help to differentiate between contaminants from the external ear canal and pathogens from the middle ear.[1] Proper visualization is extremely important; problems encountered include cerumen and debris in the external canal, inadequate speculum size, wrong angle of insertion of the speculum, and a dim light source from the otoscope. Insufficient angulation of the tympanocentesis needle may also preclude adequate visualization.

It is important to immobilize the ear completely; if it is not possible to achieve proper restraint with local anesthesia and immobilization, consider the use of general anesthesia. Allow the alcohol to dry before performing the procedure, as puncture through a film of alcohol is more painful than incision of a dry membrane.

SOFT TISSUE ASPIRATION

Cellulitis and soft tissue infections are common disorders in children and are common Emergency Department (ED) problems. Although needle aspiration of soft tissue infections for Gram stain and culture is a useful diagnostic tool, the true efficacy of this procedure is unproved in normal children. Goetz first described needle aspiration of soft tissue infections in children with *Haemophilus influenzae* type b cellulitis,[37] and Uman and Kunin described the technique in adults with cellulitis and subcutaneous abscesses.[85] Recovery of pathogens occurred in a limited number of patients. Studies evaluating needle aspiration of areas of cellulitis in children have demonstrated recovery rates that range from 40% to 60%.[32,33,48] However two prospective studies in adults have demonstrated a lower recovery rate, with potential pathogens isolated in only 10% of patients.[47,61] Studies performed in patients with immunosuppression or underlying diseases that predispose to cellulitis produced greater yield of the offending pathogens via aspiration.[76]

Though there are numerous potential pathogens in cellulitis and soft tissue infections, in normal hosts with uncomplicated infection, a limited number of bacteria are the cause.[31] *Staphylococcus aureus* and *Streptococcus pyogenes* (group A) are the usual causative pathogens in uncomplicated cutaneous cellulitis involving the extremities and trunk, excluding facial cellulitis in children, for which *Hemophilus influenzae* type B frequently is the causative agent. Institute initial antimicrobial therapy with antistaphylococcal and antistreptococcal therapy alone, except in the case of facial cellulitis. Since the majority of patients respond to empiric therapy, routine cultures are not usually necessary. In the case of cutaneous abscesses the pathogens typically reflect the microflora of the anatomic region where the abscess developed. In normal host, the only therapy required for cutaneous abscesses are adequate incision and drainage. The addition of antibiotics typically does not affect the healing rate in this population and thus routine cultures are not indicated.

Indications

There are particular instances in which aspiration and culture of a region of cellulitis or an abscess are indicated. Consider aspiration and culture for patients who do not respond to the initial therapy, who experience recurrent cellulitis or abscesses, who have systemic toxicity, and who are immunocompromised.[59]

Equipment

The necessary equipment includes povidone-iodine solution, 70% alcohol, 4 × 4s, 1% lidocaine, 22-gauge needle, and 3-ml syringe for local anesthesia. Use an 18-gauge needle for the initial puncture and an 18- or 20-gauge needle for aspiration, a 5-ml syringe, and nonbacteriostatic, sterile saline solution.

Techniques

Previous literature suggested needle aspiration of areas of cellulitis at the leading edge of erythema; however a recent study demonstrated increased recovery of a causative agent with aspiration from the point of maximal inflammation.[47,48] Thus select the site to aspirate at the region of maximal inflammation, whether it be the leading edge of erythema, the

center of the cellulitis, or an area of apparent suppuration.[47,61,83] Thoroughly cleanse the area with povidone-iodine solution, then swab the site of puncture with 70% alcohol. Use of local anesthesia with 1% lidocaine is optional; however this typically produces more discomfort than the subsequent aspiration. To prevent occlusion of the aspiration needle use a separate 18-gauge needle for the initial puncture through the skin.[83] Advance the collection needle through this site to the appropriate depth, avoiding vital structures. To aspirate an area of facial cellulitis use a 22-gauge needle instead.[37] Apply gentle negative pressure while withdrawing the needle. If unsuccessful in obtaining fluid, inject 0.1 to 0.2 ml of nonbacteriostatic sterile saline solution and aspirate immediately. However the saline solution may extrude any material aspirated into the needle and, typically, increases the pain associated with the procedure.[83]

Send fluid obtained from aspiration for Gram stain and aerobic cultures; however for perirectal cellulitis or abscesses also perform anaerobic cultures. If there is no fluid, streak the needle on a blood agar plate. In the immunocompromised patient or patient with an atypical process, perform fungal and acid-fast bacteria (AFB) stains and, if enough specimen is available, cultures.

Remarks

Reserve needle aspiration of soft tissue infections for patients who are predisposed to atypical pathogens or in whom the infection cannot be localized; in these individuals the yield of isolation of a clinically relevant pathogen is increased and may directly affect antimicrobial therapy.

THORACENTESIS
Indications

Pleural fluid accumulation has varied causes, both infectious and noninfectious. Aspiration of effusions frequently helps to determine whether they are exudative or transudative as a clue to their cause (Table 99-1 outlines values for both exudates and transudates). As a general rule sample new effusions for diagnosis. Patients with large amounts of pleural fluid resulting in respiratory compromise or discomfort may require "therapeutic" thoracentesis. In addition, perform the procedure for emergency diagnosis and treatment of suspected tension pneumothorax or evacuation of simple stable pneumothorax. The procedure is also necessary for instillation of specific chemotherapeutic agents to the pleura.

Contraindications

There are no absolute contraindications to diagnostic thoracentesis (removing relatively small amounts of fluid, between

Table 99-1 Characteristics of Exudative Effusions

Test	Value	Fluid/serum ratio
Protein	>3 g/dl	>0.5
Lactate dehydrogenase (LDH)	>200 units/L	>0.6
White blood cell count	>1000 cells/mm^3	—
pH	<7.20	—

30 and 50 ml); there are, however, several relative contraindications,[16] including bleeding disorders and anticoagulation, which can result in hemothorax. Ordinarily however, careful thoracentesis in a child with a coagulopathy does not cause serious hemothorax. Locating effusions of very small volume can be a problem. Sonography or fluoroscopy may be necessary to localize the collection accurately. In addition patients with contralateral lung compromise are at great risk if a pneumothorax should occur on the "good" side. Mechanical ventilation is also a relative contraindication as thoracentesis may produce a tension pneumothorax under positive-pressure conditions. Patients with an ipsilateral ruptured diaphragm are at great risk as well.

Do not insert the needle through an area of infection, as it may "seed" the pleura with the infecting skin agent (particularly with *Herpes* and *Staphylococcus* species). Managing pleural adhesions is difficult because the risk of piercing the closely adherent visceral pleura and lung is high. The main factor to consider is whether the risk of the procedure is greater than the benefit if it is successful.

Complications

Pneumothorax is the most common serious side effect of this procedure and occurs in 25% to 40% of patients. In recent years the use of ultrasound guided thoracentesis has reduced this proportion to as low as 5%.[41] Syncope occurs on occasion as a result of the pleuropulmonary reflex. Air embolus has also occurred.[63] With removal of more than 1000 to 1500 ml at one time in an older child or adult pulmonary edema can develop. Unilateral pulmonary edema may occur but is rare.[84] Fatal hemorrhage can result from insertion of the needle into the lung, heart, liver, or great vessels; significant bleeding can also result from laceration of smaller vessels, including intercostals. Infection from contaminated instruments or poor sterile technique occurs in 2% of cases.[7] It is not possible to obtain fluid in up to 12% of patients.[20]

Equipment

Today most hospitals have kits prepared for thoracentesis. However if a commercially available product is not available, it is easy to perform the procedure using standard equipment. Necessary equipment includes antiseptic solutions (70% alcohol and povidone-iodine); sterile gloves; four sterile towels; ampule of 1% lidocaine; 5-ml and 10-ml syringes; 26- and 22-gauge needles; gauze sponges; and an 18-gauge short-bevel needle, 7.5 cm long. Other equipment required includes a three-way stopcock; rubber tube, 45 cm long, with adapter to fit the female port of the stopcock; hemostat; sterile test tubes, one plain (red top) and one with anticoagulant (purple top); and a No. 11 scalpel blade.[14,51,70]

Techniques

Position the patient in a sitting position on a treatment table with arms resting on a bedside table or supported by an assistant.[14,50] Hold an infant against an assistant's chest in the "burping" position for a posterior or posterolateral approach. The point for aspiration depends on the location of the pleural fluid. Choose the most inferior site so that gravity helps drain the fluid. Physical examination and roentgenogram usually determine the site. However, many physicians employ ultrasound-guided studies for loculated fluid. The usual site is the base of the thorax in the posterior axillary line. Clean the site in a circular motion, spreading outward with povidone-iodine, then remove the cleanser with 70% alcohol.

Don sterile gloves and place sterile towels above and below the puncture site so that is possible to visualize it well. Fill a 5-ml syringe with 1% lidocaine and place a 26-gauge needle on the syringe. Place an anesthetic wheal over the rib below the interspace for planned needle insertion (Fig. 99-6). Infiltrate the skin and underlying tissues through the wheal down to the rib periosteum and pleura, aspirating before each injection. If the patient is a larger child or adult, a longer 22-gauge needle may be necessary to complete anesthesia. It can be helpful to determine with the smaller needle the depth at which it is possible to obtain the pleural fluid. Attach the 18-gauge needle to the male port of the three-way stopcock. Attach the plastic tubing to one of the female ports and attach a 10-ml syringe to the hub.

Hold the needle with only as much length exposed as is

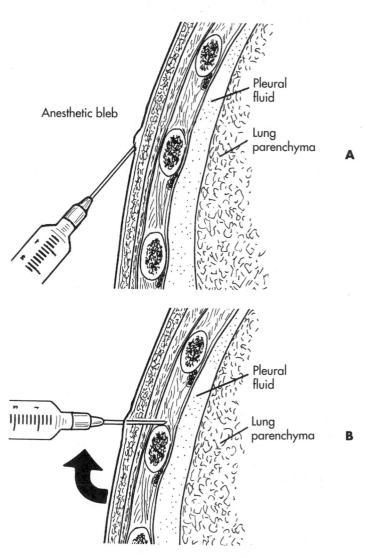

Anesthetic bleb

Pleural fluid

Lung parenchyma

A

Pleural fluid

Lung parenchyma

B

FIG. 99-6 Thoracentesis. **A,** Superficial wheal of local anesthetic. **B,** Infiltration of local anesthetic over the rib into the deeper layers.

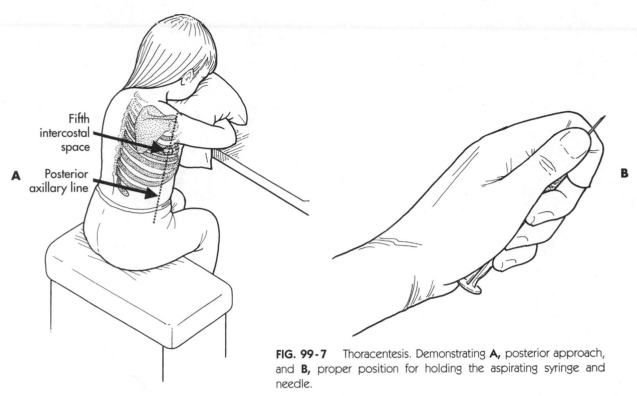

FIG. 99-7   Thoracentesis. Demonstrating **A,** posterior approach, and **B,** proper position for holding the aspirating syringe and needle.

necessary to traverse the chest wall (Fig. 99-7). After injecting local anesthetic, insert the needle through the anesthetic wheal. Slowly advance the tip (commonly described as "walking") up and over the superior margin of the rib through the chest wall to the pleura, aspirating while advancing (Fig. 99-8). Enter the pleural space just over the superior margin of the rib. Aspirate with the syringe to ensure that the needle has indeed reached the fluid. Clamp a hemostat across the needle barrel at the skin surface to prevent further advancement of the needle and to mark the depth of the fluid. Then aspirate fluid into the syringe, rotate the stopcock valve, and eject the fluid through the rubber tube into the specimen tubes or a discard basin.

Alternatively, advance a J-tipped guidewire through the needle into the pleural space (Fig. 99-9). Open the needle only momentarily to prevent pneumothorax. After advancing the guidewire beyond the tip of the needle withdraw the needle and advance an 18-gauge catheter over the guidewire, being sure to hold the end of the guidewire at all times. Then remove the guidewire. Again with minimal exposure to the outside atmosphere connect a syringe to the catheter for removal of fluid. Remove fluid through either the catheter or the needle, depending on available materials. After removing the desired amount of fluid withdraw the needle or catheter and apply a sterile dressing.

Plastic intravenous catheters minimize the chance of the needle's perforating the lung or causing a laceration. "Over the needle" catheters work well for small effusions. Thread "through the needle" catheters into the dependent portions of the pleural space; use a catheter of sufficient caliber to permit withdrawal of the fluid. Position the bevel of the needle superiorly. Once the introducer tip is in the pleural space, elevate the needle hub to direct the needle point inferiorly while advancing the catheter through the needle. Advance the

catheter fully and lock it into the introducer needle hub. Pull the needle out, leaving the catheter in the pleural space. Apply the needle guard to prevent the needle from shearing the catheter, attach the stopcock apparatus, and aspirate the fluid.

Remarks

To differentiate between exudates and transudates obtain the following tests on the pleural fluid: total protein, lactate

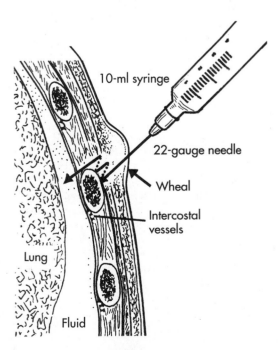

FIG. 99-8   Thoracentesis. "Walking" the needle over the rib into the pleural space.

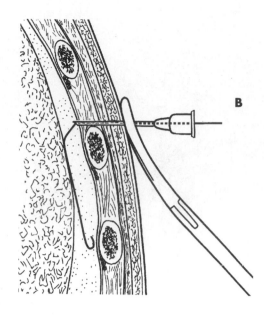

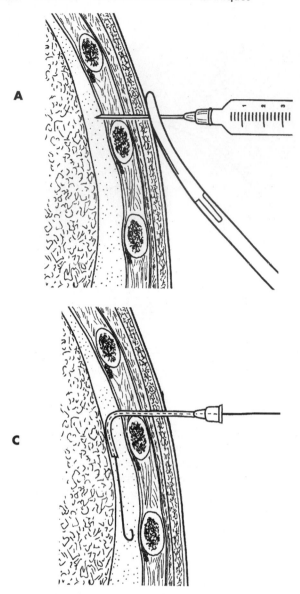

FIG. 99-9 Thoracentesis. **A,** After infiltration of local anesthetic, advance the anesthetic syringe to the pleural space while aspirating. At the point where pleural fluid is first aspirated, mark the depth of needle penetration with a surgical clamp at the level of the skin. Reposition the clamp on the Seldinger needle at the same level and advance it to the pleural space. **B,** Insert the J-tipped guidewire into the pleural space and remove the needle. **C,** Advance the thoracentesis catheter over the guide and remove the guidewire.

(From Boyes RJ, Kruse JA: Selected nonvascular procedures. In Carlson RW, Geheb MA, editors: *Principles and practice of medical intensive care,* Philadelphia, 1993, WB Saunders.)

Table 99-2 Interpretation of Common Laboratory Findings on Pleural Fluid

Tests*	Diseases
pH < 7.2	Empyema, malignancy, esophageal rupture, tuberculosis
Glucose (< 60 mg/dl)	Bacterial infection, tuberculosis, systemic lupus erythematosus
Amylase (> 200 U/dl)	Pancreatic disease, esophageal rupture, malignancy, ruptured ectopic pregnancy
Red blood cells (>5000 RBCs/ml)*	Trauma, malignancy, pulmonary embolus
Chylous effusion	Thoracic duct trauma

*RBC, Red blood cells.

dehydrogenase (LDH), white blood cell (WBC) count and differential, and pH. A glucose level may occasionally be helpful also. Send fluid for routine Gram stain and bacterial culture (both aerobic and anaerobic), KOH and fungal culture, AFB smear and culture, and cytologic analysis. Table 99-2 describes fluid characteristics in some of the conditions encountered in a critical care setting.

Reexpansion pulmonary edema occasionally follows removal of more than 1 liter of fluid at a time (for adults and larger children). A chest roentgenogram after the procedure assesses success in fluid removal and rules out pneumothorax. However, a pneumothorax may rarely occur up to 24 hours after the procedure.

PERICARDIOCENTESIS

Acute inflammation of the parietal pericardium and the underlying pericardium results in acute pericarditis. Frequently this condition produces fever, pain, and a friction

Table 99-3   Causes of Pericarditis

1. Idiopathic (presumed viral cause)
2. Infectious
   a. Viral: coxsackieviruses A and B, echovirus, adenovirus, cytomegalovirus, herpes virus, mumps, influenza virus, Epstein-Barr virus
   b. Bacterial: *Staphylococcus aureus*,[27] *Streptococcus pneumoniae, H. influenzae,* group A *Streptococcus* spp., *Mycobacterium tuberculosis, Salmonella, Legionella* spp.
   c. *Mycoplasma* spp.
   d. Fungal: histoplasmosis, blastomycosis,[43] coccidioidomycosis,[17] *Candida* spp., aspergillosis
   e. Protozoan: toxoplasmosis, amoebae
   f. Rickettsia: *Coxiella burnetii*
3. Physical cause
   a. Chest trauma
   b. Cardiac surgery, myocardial infarction
   c. Radiation therapy to chest wall
4. Vasculitic syndromes: systemic lupus erythematosus, rheumatoid arthritis, rheumatic fever
5. Metabolic disorders: severe hypothyroidism, uremia, gout
6. Tumor
7. Drugs: isoniazid, procainamide, hydralazine, penicillin, phenytoin, heparin
8. Anemias: sickle-cell disease, aplastic anemia, thalassemia
9. Miscellaneous: Kawasaki's syndrome, sarcoid, amyloidosis

From Hoffman JI, Stanger P: Diseases of the pericardium. In Rudolph AM, Hoffman JIE, Rudolph CD, editors: *Rudolph's pediatrics,* ed 19, Newark, Conn, 1991, Appleton & Lange.

rub. Elevation of the S-T segments on electrocardiography is classic in the acute stages.

Pericardial effusions may be purulent, bloody, or serous in nature. The causes of acute pericarditis with effusion are diverse and quite extensive. Table 99-3 summarizes the more common causes.

Techniques

Chapter 110 discusses the procedure for performing pericardiocentesis; the discussion in this section focuses on evaluation of pericardial effusions.[65]

Purulent pericarditis can only be diagnosed through direct examination of the pericardial fluid. Determination of the cause of a pericardial effusion requires proper technique and use of proper media and agents for culture of specific organisms. Place fluid directly into aerobic and anaerobic culture media (broth or blood culture bottles) and perform Gram stain as soon as possible.

Set up fungal stains and cultures with appropriate media. However the frequency of positive fungal culture findings is quite low. This is particularly true with *Histoplasma capsulatum,* but the use of complement fixation titers on the pericardial fluid has been helpful on some occasions.[64] In patients with tuberculous pericarditis the organisms are identifiable on smear in 15% to 42% of patients.[13] Cultures for mycobacterium frequently require a minimum of 2 to 4 weeks for adequate growth of the organism. Therefore send samples for polymerase chain reaction (PCR) analysis for mycobacterium or other organisms, if available. This method usually provides a result in 24 to 48 hours. Submit viral cultures on ice. The time required for successful culture is usually weeks, except in the case of *Herpes* virus infection. Submit the pericardial fluid for specific bacterial antigen tests as directed for *Streptococcus pneumoniae* or staphylococcal techioic acid antibodies.

Also perform blood cultures because frequently the causative organism is recoverable in this manner. Send nasopharyngeal and rectal cultures for analysis of viral causes. Additionally obtain acute and convalescent serum to measure appropriate titers if a virus is isolated. Purulent pericarditis in a child is usually associated with bacteremia or meningitis.

ABDOMINAL PARACENTESIS

Paracentesis is the percutaneous sampling of peritoneal fluid via needle aspiration through the abdominal wall. It allows diagnostic evaluation of ascitic fluid and therapeutic intervention in patients with massive ascites and respiratory compromise or abdominal discomfort. In spontaneous bacterial peritonitis[19] ascitic fluid may become infected via bacteremic seeding, direct extension through the intestinal wall, migration via transdiaphragmatic lymphatics, or the female genital tract. However, in secondary bacterial peritonitis, infection results from an intraabdominal process such as intestinal perforation, intraabdominal abscess, or ruptured appendicitis. Whatever the cause, irritation of the peritoneal membrane triggers an immediate inflammatory response with recruitment of inflammatory cells, increased vascular permeability, and increased production of peritoneal fluid that is rich in fibrinogen and antibodies.[19] This intense inflammatory response produces the clinical manifestations of peritonitis: rigid abdomen with generalized abdominal tenderness and rebound tenderness.

Indications

Paracentesis is indicated for new-onset ascites in patients without a readily identifiable cause; ascites and possible peritonitis, whether chronic or new-onset ascites; suspected spontaneous bacterial peritonitis or secondary bacterial peritonitis; or chronic ascites with patient clinical deterioration or fever without an identifiable source.[44] Therapeutic paracentesis is also indicated for massive ascites that is unresponsive to conservative medical management and is causing respiratory or abdominal distress.[94]

Contraindications

No absolute contraindications exist; however, use caution in patients with moderate to severe coagulopathies. It is safe to perform paracentesis in patients with mild coagulopathies.[71] Avoid puncture through abdominal scars as there may be adhesions and fixation of bowel loops to the abdominal wall.

Complications

Complications with paracentesis are few.[19] Possible complications include introduction of infection into a previously sterile body site with resultant peritonitis,[21] intestinal perforation (although, in most cases, this is probably insignificant[34]), subcutaneous abdominal wall hematoma,[19] blood-streaked fluid from needle penetration of a peritoneal blood vessel, and ascitic fluid leak at the site of puncture. Prevent this last complication by using the Z-track technique for needle insertion. Ascitic fluid can track caudally via Camper's and Scarpa's fascial planes post paracentesis, resulting in scrotal or labial edema.[22]

Equipment

The equipment needed for the procedure includes 1% lidocaine for local anesthesia, 3- or 5-ml syringe and 25-gauge needle, povidone-iodine solution and alcohol preps, sterile 4 × 4 gauze, sterile drapes, sterile latex gloves, and test tubes for fluid analysis and culture. In small children, use a 20- to 22-gauge spinal needle or intravascular catheter; in older children use an 18- to 20-gauge spinal needle or intravascular catheter.

Techniques

First position the patient in the upright sitting position or semierect sitting position with back support.[19,52,71] Then localize the fluid by physical examination. However, if only a small amount of fluid is detectable on physical examination or if the patient has had multiple previous abdominal procedures, localize the fluid by abdominal ultrasound. Ensure that the bladder is completely empty immediately before the procedure by the patient's voiding or via catheterization. The midline approach is most popular; however, determine the best site for needle entry by physical examination or ultrasound localization of the ascitic fluid. The approach can be lower midline, right lower, or left lower quadrant. Using the midline approach, puncture approximately midway between the umbilicus and pubic symphysis (Fig. 99-10). Perform the lateral approach a few centimeters above the inguinal ligament in the right or left lower abdominal quadrant.[52]

Sterilely prepare the entry site with povidone-iodine and then wipe free with 70% alcohol and sterile 4 × 4s. Then place sterile drapes around the entry site. (Note: It is permissible to omit draping in older, cooperative children.) Create a wheal at the site of puncture and infiltrate the area down to the peritoneal lining with 1% lidocaine, using the 25-gauge needle.

Using the appropriate needle for age, insert the needle through the area of infiltration and, in a Z-track fashion, advance it to the level of the parietal peritoneum. Apply traction to the skin in a caudal direction during insertion of the aspiration needle; thus after completing the procedure

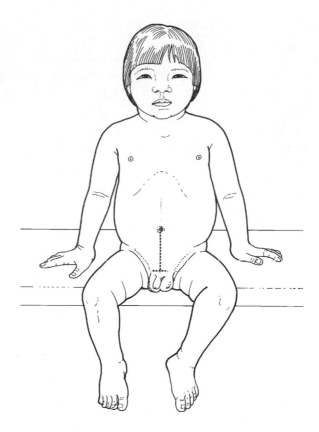

FIG. 99-10 Abdominal paracentesis. The location and technique for puncture when using the midline approach for performing abdominal paracentesis.

and releasing the tension from the skin there is not a direct linear needle track, but a Z-track.[71] Then advance the needle slowly using negative pressure on the syringe until there is return of fluid. If using a spinal needle secure in place with your free hand or with a hemostat and obtain the required amount of fluid (usually 20 to 40 ml if only for diagnostic evaluation). When using an over the needle catheter, advance the catheter forward with removal of the needle on return of ascitic fluid; change the position of the patient if return is sluggish or stops. For performing a therapeutic paracentesis use the over the needle technique with a three-way stopcock connected to a closed intravenous (IV) apparatus and empty IV bag. Although it is possible to perform large-volume paracentesis safely, intravascular fluid shifts may occur, resulting in impairment of effective circulating blood volume; anticipate problems in patients with hypoalbuminemia or cirrhosis. Prevent this impairment in effective circulating blood volume associated with large-volume paracentesis in cirrhosis by concomitant administration of intravenous albumin infusion after each tap.[35] After the procedure remove the needle or catheter and apply direct pressure. Cover the insertion site with a pressure dressing.

Send peritoneal fluid for cell count and differential, protein, glucose, LDH, pH, amylase, and microbiologic evaluation, including Gram stain and routine aerobic and anaerobic cultures. Gram stain detects organisms in ascitic fluid in the majority of patients with secondary bacterial peritonitis[72,73] and in up to 50% to 55% of patients with spontaneous bacterial peritonitis.[21,66] Inoculate 10 ml of ascitic fluid into

Table 99-4   Typical Characteristics of Ascitic Fluid in Spontaneous or Secondary Bacterial Peritonitis

Laboratory tests	Typical values	Comments
Cell count	>500 polymorphonuclear leukocytes (PMNs)	Can be seen in patients with peritonitis, cholecystitis, or pancreatitis
	or 250-500 PMNs and clinical signs of peritonitis	Probable peritonitis
	or >500 WBCs with lymphocyte predominance (usually >70%)	Characteristic of tuberculous peritonitis
Glucose	<50 mg/dl	Levels <30 mg/dl common in tuberculous peritonitis
Protein	>1 g/dl	Often >2.5 g/dl and consistent with an exudate
pH	<7.30	Not a reliable indicator in patients with metabolic acidosis secondary to renal disease
Lactate dehydrogenase (LDH)	Ascitic fluid/serum LDH ratio >0.6	
Amylase	Higher than serum amylase	Consistent with bowel perforation or pancreatic ascites

aerobic and anaerobic blood culture bottles to improve isolation of bacterial pathogens.[74,75] In patients with a history of exposure, immunosuppression, human immunodeficiency virus (HIV), or hematologic malignancies, also send peritoneal fluid for acid-fast bacilli (AFB) and fungal stain and cultures. Do not send peritoneal fluid for AFB and fungal cultures on all patients as the yield of routine AFB and fungal cultures is low; these organisms are rare pathogens in peritonitis in the general pediatric population.

Remarks

Although the incidence of bacterial peritonitis is low in the pediatric population, consider it in the differential diagnosis of the child who has acute abdominal pain, particularly in the presence of chronic ascites. This point is also applicable to the evaluation of the patient with nephrotic syndrome, because of the increased risk for spontaneous bacterial peritonitis. Diagnostic paracentesis is indicated before institution of empiric antimicrobial therapy. Table 99-4 lists typical findings of bacterial peritonitis.

CULDOCENTESIS

Culdocentesis is a rapid and safe method to obtain intraperitoneal fluid for analysis. It involves insertion of a needle through the posterior vaginal vault into the pouch of Douglas. The pouch of Douglas, or cul-de-sac, is the most dependent region of the peritoneal cavity, thus allowing for sampling of free intraperitoneal fluid.

Indications

The primary use of culdocentesis is for diagnosis of ruptured ectopic pregnancies; it has an overall sensitivity of approximately 85% when combined with a positive pregnancy test result.[58] However, with the development of ultrasound and recently with transvaginal probe ultrasound, culdocentesis now has a more limited role. It remains a useful diagnostic tool, especially in early suspected ectopic pregnancies (>6 weeks of gestation), or when ultrasound examination is not readily available, or when findings ultrasound examination are indeterminate. It can also be used for the diagnosis of ruptured corpus luteal cysts and assessment of blunt or pelvic trauma in patients for whom peritoneal lavage is contraindi-

cated. In addition it is an objective diagnostic test in patients with suspected pelvic inflammatory disease[42] and can provide an alternative method of obtaining fluid in the patient with suspected peritonitis.[87]

Contraindications

Contraindications include patients with any of the following: a previous history of salpingitis, which can result in adhesions in the cul-de-sac; fixed mass in the pouch of Douglas; large retroverted uterus; and coagulopathy.[90] Do not perform the procedure on prepubertal girls.

Complications

Complications are uncommon; they include perforation of small or large bowel; intrapelvic hemorrhage; puncture of a pathologic pelvic structure, such as a uterine mass, ovarian mass, or cyst; endometrioma; puncture of a pelvic kidney;[40] and rectal serosal hematoma.[3]

Equipment

Equipment includes an appropriate-size speculum, single-toothed tenaculum, 18-gauge spinal needle, 10- to 20-ml syringes, and appropriate transport media, including aerobic, anaerobic, and gonococcal.

Techniques

Perform a thorough pelvic and bimanual examination to exclude a fixed-retroverted uterus or mass in the pouch of Douglas. Place the patient in the lithotomy position with slight reversed Tredelenberg. Use the largest speculum that the patient can comfortably tolerate, and expose the posterior vaginal vault, gently stretching the mucosa by opening the speculum as widely as tolerated. Use a sterile cotton tip swab and prepare the vaginal vault with povidone-iodine or other suitable antiseptic. Using a single-tooth tenaculum, grasp the lower lip of the cervix to expose the point of reflection of the vaginal mucosa as it crosses over the cul-de-sac.[25,80] The ideal point of insertion of the needle for aspiration is in the midline 1 cm below the point of reflection (Fig. 99-11). Elevate the cervix in the vagina by using the tenaculum with slight traction, thus stretching the mucosa of the posterior vaginal vault.[25,80] Do not use local anesthesia because of the difficulty in achieving adequate anesthesia and the risk of a

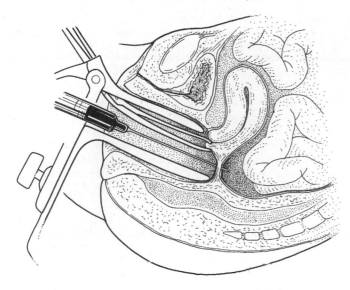

FIG. 99-11 Culdocentesis. Elevate the cervix using the tenaculum, which stretches the mucosa of the posterior vault, exposing the point of reflection. The site of puncture is 1 cm below this point in midline.

Table 99-5 Interpretation of Culdocentesis

Results of aspiration	Interpretation
Dry tap	Nondiagnostic
Clear, serous fluid	Normal cul-de-sac fluid
	Negative tap result
Purulent fluid	Pelvic inflammatory disease
	Tuboovarian abscess
	Intestinal perforation
	Peritonitis
Nonclotting blood	Ruptured or leaking ectopic pregnancy

traumatic tap, which is due to the highly vascular nature of the mucosa. Insert the aspiration needle 3 to 4 cm in a smooth movement through the mucosa and terminate the procedure after obtaining the fluid or after three unsuccessful attempts. If the fluid is purulent or serous, send it for Gram stain and aerobic (including Thayer Martin media for gonococcus) and anaerobic culture. Send the specimen to the laboratory in a sterile syringe with all the air removed; or place it in appropriate aerobic and anaerobic culturettes or transport media. The likely pathogens include *Neisseria gonorrheae, Chlamydia trachomatis,* anaerobic bacteria (primarily *Bacteroides* spp.), *Mycoplasma hominis,* and facultative gram-negative bacilli.[18,56]

Remarks

Pelvic inflammatory disease (PID) is a major public health problem associated with significant morbid conditions, including tubal infertility, chronic pelvic pain, and ectopic pregnancy. Early diagnosis and treatment are imperative to eradicate pathogens and reduce tubal injury. Typically PID is a polymicrobial infection with poor correlation of cervical cultures with causative pathogens. Laparoscopic evaluation remains the gold standard for diagnosis; however, culdocen-

tesis provides a quick, safe alternative for diagnosis and culture evaluation. Cultures obtained via culdocentesis are a reliable indication of microbiologic pathogens in PID.[18] Table 99-5 summarizes the interpretation of fluid obtained by culdocentesis.

AMPHOTERICIN B BLADDER IRRIGATION

Candiduria is a complication of prolonged urinary bladder catheterization and broad-spectrum antimicrobial therapy. Bladder irrigation with amphotericin B is the most effective method to treat this type of infection.[93] Perform irrigation on a continuous or intermittent basis for 2 to 10 days. The basis of the techniques of delivery and dosing of amphotericin B in children is information from adults with candiduria.[23,38,69,91,92]

Indications

There are currently no existing criteria that help the clinician differentiate between fungal colonization and infection.[93] Although a bacterial colony count greater than 100,000/ml of voided urine is indicative of a bacterial urinary tract infection, there is no general agreement for candiduria. Consider bladder irrigation without systemic therapy only in patients with simple cystitis.[29] Candidates for therapy are those who have repeated positive urine culture results for *Candida* despite replacement or removal of the bladder catheter and/or cessation of antibacterial therapy.

Contraindications

Treat patients with systemic or disseminated disease with systemic therapy.[29] In patients with allergy to amphotericin B or in cases in which bladder catheterization is not desirable, consider oral imidazole therapy (i.e., fluconazole). Do not use bladder irrigation in premature infants. The varying sizes of their bladders and their predisposition to disseminated candidal disease make administration of systemic amphotericin B more attractive.

Complications

Side effects attributed to systemic administration of amphotericin B, such as fever, bone marrow suppression, and renal toxicity, do not occur with bladder irrigation because absorption through the bladder mucosa is minimal.[62] The only reported complications are pain and penile cramping associated with the infusion of amphotericin B.[63]

Equipment

The equipment required for bladder irrigation is amphotericin B, sterile water, a urinary catheter, and a clamp.

Techniques

Add amphotericin B (5 to 10 mg) to 1 liter of sterile water for a final concentration of 5 to 10 µg/ml.[77] Connect this solution to a three-way urinary catheter and instill the solution at a rate of 15 to 40 ml/hour. If continuous infusion is inconvenient, instill 75 to 300 ml of solution into the bladder and cross-clamp the urinary catheter for 60 to 90 minutes. Repeat this procedure three or four times per day. If bladder irrigation is successful, urinary cultures usually are sterile by the second day of therapy. Discontinue treatment when urine cultures are sterile or continue treatment for up to 10 days.[33,77]

Remarks

Patients usually respond to bladder irrigation within 48 hours. If a patient is not responding, consider a more invasive illness.

LUMBAR PUNCTURE

Quincke first described the technique of lumbar puncture (LP) and analysis of cerebrospinal fluid (CSF) in 1891.[67] Since the original description LP has become one of the most common nonsurgical, invasive procedures performed in adult and pediatric medicine. It provides valuable diagnostic information.

Indications

LP is primarily indicated for evaluation of patients who have symptoms and signs consistent with meningitis, although it is also useful for evaluation of other neurologic problems, including hemorrhage, malignancy, seizures, and some metabolic or degenerative diseases. The typical manifestations of acute bacterial meningitis include febrile illness with lethargy or irritability, meningeal irritation, and neurologic symptoms, including mental status changes, headache, seizures, and occasional focal neurologic findings. However in the neonate or infant the symptoms and signs may be nonspecific and insidious in onset. LP is indicated as part of the sepsis evaluation in children less than 3 months of age. Consider LP also in febrile children younger than 1 year with suspected bacteremia.[88] Because of the increased incidence of meningitis accompanying or complicating buccal cellulitis (concomitant meningitis in up to 8% of cases)[36] or orbital cellulitis, include LP in the initial evaluation in those children who are too young for accurate clinical evaluation of meningitis. Also consider LP in the evaluation of infants who are less than 1 year of age with apparent febrile seizure. Additionally it may be useful in the evaluation of patients with mental status changes that have no readily identifiable cause. LP is also a therapeutic modality in the management of patients with pseudotumor cerebri and in administration of intrathecal antibiotic therapy or instillation of chemotherapeutic agents.

Contraindications

As a result of the risk of herniation, lumbar puncture is contraindicated in individuals with clinical signs of significantly increased intracranial pressure or a midline shift.[57] Delay LP in patients with clinical findings consistent with significantly increased intracranial pressure or severely ill patients with hemodynamic or pulmonary instability until they are in stable condition and are not at risk for herniation. Also withhold LP in patients with soft tissue infection over the lumbar spine area and in those with severe, unresponsive coagulopathy or severe thrombocytopenia.

Complications

Local pain or backache is the most common side effect of lumbar puncture. Post-tap headaches occur in adults and children over 10 years of age[86] but are uncommon in children less than 10 years. Other complications include vomiting, temporary paralysis, epidermoid tumors,[5] epidural hematomas, subdural or subarachnoid hemorrhage, and acute neurologic or respiratory deterioration. The risk of paralysis is extremely low. Prevent epidermoid tumors by advancing the spinal needle only with the stylet in place. Positioning and manipulation of the sick preterm and term neonate during the LP may result in hypoxemia or apnea and clinical deterioration; however risk of this complication can be lessened by preventing excessive neck flexion, administering preoxygenation to prevent hypoxemia, or using the sitting position.[28,89] Cerebral herniation may occur if one performs a LP in the presence of significantly increased intracranial pressure.[68,81] However, herniation also occurs in patients with severe meningitis, even with no LP. The incidence of introduction of infection with resultant bacterial meningitis, epidural abscess, diskitis, or osteomyelitis is extremely low.[24] Traumatic lumbar punctures occur in 20% to 45% of attempts.[12,78]

Equipment

Most hospitals stock prepackaged lumbar puncture trays that are age-specific and contain all necessary equipment except povidone-iodine and sterile gloves. However, if this is not available the equipment required includes 1% lidocaine for local anesthesia, 25-gauge needle (for local anesthesia) and 3- to 5-ml syringe, 20- or 22-gauge styleted spinal needle with a short bevel (1½ inches for neonates, infants, and young children; 2½ inches for older children or adolescents; or longer for obese patients), povidone-iodine and sterile 4 × 4s, sterile gloves, sterile drapes, and three to four sterile specimen tubes. If the patient is older than 2 years of age, a spinal fluid pressure manometer and three-way stopcock may be desirable to determine opening and closing cerebrospinal fluid (CSF) pressures. For viral cultures include an additional sterile tube as well as a cup of ice in which to place the specimen before laboratory culture.

Techniques

Perform lumbar puncture in either the lateral recumbent or sitting position.[39,53,88] Use the lateral recumbent position for measurement of opening pressure.[82] The sitting position is beneficial in patients with pulmonary disorders and in young infants because it may prevent hyperflexion of the neck that can precipitate respiratory distress with the recumbent technique. With either position maintain proper alignment and adequately restrain the patient. In the critically ill or unstable patient preoxygenate by allowing the patient to breathe FIo_2 = 1.0 at 5 L/min spontaneously via a snug face mask for 3 minutes before positioning for lumbar puncture to prevent hypoxemia during the procedure.[28]

Lateral recumbent approach. Position the patient in the lateral recumbent position near the edge of an examination table with the craniospinal axis parallel to the plane of the examination table. Then flex the patient's knees and torso, preventing excessive flexion of the neck. Locate the iliac crests, imagining a transverse plane between these two points that intersects the spine at approximately the L3-L4 interspace perpendicular to the plane of the table (Fig. 99-12).

Sitting approach. Have an assistant hold the small infant on the edge of the examination table in the sitting position

Iliac crest

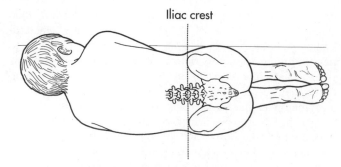

FIG. 99-12 Alignment of the patient for the lateral recumbent approach for lumbar puncture.

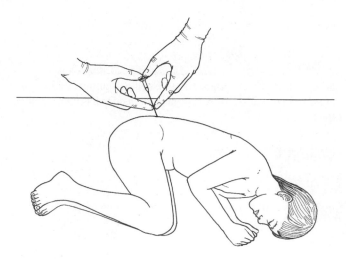

FIG. 99-14 Lumbar puncture. Technique for supporting the spinal needle with two hands and maintaining alignment with the needle directed slightly cephalad.

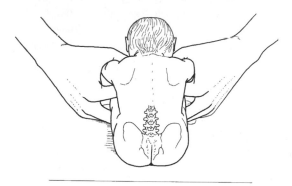

FIG. 99-13 Lumbar puncture. The sitting position.

with hips flexed. Place the thighs against the abdomen and flex the trunk. Have the assistant stabilize the infant by grasping the patient's right elbow and knee with the left hand and the left elbow and knee with the right hand.[52] For the older child perform this technique with the patient voluntarily sitting on the edge of the examination table with the spine flexed by having the patient rest the elbows on the knees. Have an assistant stabilize the patient's position to maintain alignment throughout the entire procedure. In this technique keep the craniospinal axis perpendicular to the plane of the table and keep the transverse plane connecting the iliac crests parallel (Fig. 99-13).

Puncture. After the patient is in proper alignment, locate the site of puncture. The L3-L4 interspace represents the optimal site for performing the LP, since this is below the level of the conus medullaris, even in infants, whose spinal cord terminates at the level of L3. Aseptically put on sterile gloves and prepare the entire lumbar spine with povidone-iodine. Then place sterile drapes around the site of puncture. Use 1% lidocaine for local anesthesia and a 25-gauge needle to raise a wheal over the interspace, then infiltrate the deeper tissue to the level of the paraspinous ligaments. Recheck alignment and ensure that the patient position is secure. Check the spinal needle to ensure that the stylet is firmly in position to prevent implantation of epidermoid tissue; have the stylet in place before advancing the needle. Support the needle between your index fingers and stabilize the hub of the needle with your thumbs. Position the needle in the midline with the bevel up and horizontal to prevent transection of the dural fibers and to lessen the risk of CSF leak.[79,82]

Then, with the needle perpendicular to the vertical plane but held with the bevel pointed slightly cephalad, advance through the skin (Fig. 99-14). Advance it slowly into the deeper structures until detection of slight resistance on penetration of the spinous ligaments. This resistance continues until the needle penetrates the dura, at which time one typically feels a "pop" sensation caused by the change in resistance. This indicates that the needle is in the subarachnoid space. Remove the stylet. CSF should appear from the hub of the needle if it is in the correct position. If there is no return of CSF, rotate the spinal needle 90 degrees in each direction to prevent possible obstruction of the bevel. However, if still unsuccessful, replace the stylet and advance the needle a few millimeters forward, then recheck.[79,82] Should the needle meet resistance, withdraw the needle with the stylet in place and reattempt the procedure, verifying proper position, or attempt a paramedian approach just a few millimeters lateral to midline.

When indicated, attach the three-way stopcock and manometer to the hub of the needle for opening pressure measurement as soon as the spinal needle is in the subarachnoid space and (CSF) is present in the hub (Fig. 99-15). Allow CSF to proceed into the manometer until the level is steady and record this as the opening pressure. There is some fluctuation of the CSF level with the respiratory and cardiac cycles. With the patient in the lateral recumbent position normal CSF opening pressure ranges from 50 to 200 mm. CSF pressures may be artificially elevated in the struggling child or the patient who is unable to relax.[30] Opening pressures are unreliable when the patient is in the sitting position. Obtain a closing pressure immediately before termination of the procedure in a similar fashion.

After obtaining the opening pressure or, in the infant, on appearance of CSF in the hub collect CSF in the sterile tubes. Note the character of the CSF and, if blood-tinged or bloody fluid flows initially, observe the fluid for clearing with subsequent collection. This pattern is typical of a traumatic tap; however, if the fluid does not clear, this may indicate the presence of a subarachnoid hemorrhage. In the premature or full-term neonate limit CSF collection to approximately 2 ml; however, in older children larger volumes (usually 3 to 6

Table 99-6 CSF Manifestations in Common Central Nervous System Infections*

Condition	WBCs/mm³	Protein (mg/dl)	Glucose	Gram stain	Opening pressure
Normal	<6 Cells consisting of lymphocytes and monocytes	<45	60%-70% of peripheral glucose level	Negative	50-200/mm
Acute bacterial meningitis	100-10,000s Occasionally <100; PMN predominance	50-100s	<40 mg/dl or <50% of peripheral glucose level	Positive in up to 80%	Elevated
Partially treated bacterial meningitis	10-100s PMN or lymphocytic predominance	50-100s	<40 mg/dl	Positive or negative	Elevated
Viral meningitis	20-1000; Rarely >1000; early may have PMN predominance, but lymphocytic predominance typical	NL to SL elevated; usually <100	Normal (NL)	Negative	NL or SL elevated
Tuberculous meningitis	20-500; Usually lymphocytic predominance	50-200	<40 mg/dl	Negative	Elevated
Cryptococcal meningitis	NL to 100s; lympho-cytic predominance	100s	<40 mg/dl	Negative	Elevated
Brain abscess	10-100s; PMNs and lymphocytes	50-100s	NL	Negative	Elevated
Epidural abscess	10-100s; lymphocytic predominance	100-1000s	NL	Negative	NL

*NL, Normal; SL, slightly; PMN, polymorphonuclear cells.

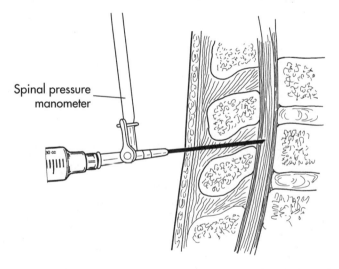

Spinal pressure manometer

FIG. 99-15 Lumbar puncture. Positioning and technique for performing measurement of CSF opening pressure. CSF, Cerebrospinal fluid.

ml) can be safely removed. On completion of CSF collection replace the stylet and remove the needle. Place a bandage over the site and encourage the patient, if able, to lie prone for 3 to 4 hours after the procedure to prevent CSF leakage.

Send CSF for analysis of cell count and differential, protein and glucose determinations, Gram stain, and routine culture. To prevent misinterpretation caused by traumatic red blood cell (RBC) contamination of the CSF send the last tube collected for cell count evaluation. Obtain a peripheral serum glucose level immediately before the LP to determine the CSF serum ratio of glucose.

Refer to Table 99-6 for interpretation of CSF findings. Gram stain evaluation of the centrifuged CSF sediment provides preliminary identification in up to 80% of patients with acute bacterial meningitis.[12] In patients with prior history of antibiotic usage obtain CSF latex particle agglutination for age-appropriate pathogens since prior antibiotics may interfere with Gram stain and culture evaluation. Also send CSF for viral culture in those neonates suspected of having neonatal *Herpes simplex* infection, viral meningitis, or meningoencephalitis; however, the yield of a viral pathogen in this process is low. For viral culture collect CSF in a separate tube and place it in a cup of ice after collection. Restrict acid-fast bacteria (AFB) and fungal studies to patients with history of exposure or clinical findings suggestive of an atypical process, immunocompromised patients including those with HIV, individuals receiving immunomodulatory drugs or receiving myelosuppressive chemotherapy, or comatose patients with unknown history.[1] When considering AFB and fungal evaluation, include stains and cultures, as well as an India ink preparation and cryptococcal antigen in the immunocompromised patient. In suspected cases of tuberculous meningitis send CSF for polymerase chain reaction, which is a rapid and sensitive diagnostic test.[54] Send a CSF Venereal Disease Research Laboratories (VDLR) reagent only from patients with a confirmed positive serum treponemal test result with possible neurosyphilis[2] or from neonates delivered to mothers with positive results for serum VDLR or rapid protein reaction (RPR) (either without history of prior treatment or with treatment failure) in order to exclude congenital syphilis.

Remarks

Computed tomography is indicated before LP in the patient with suspected acute bacterial meningitis who has symptoms or signs suggestive of significantly increased intracranial pressure.[60] Do not delay antibiotic therapy after obtaining

Table 99-7 Age-Specific Causes of Acute Bacterial Meningitis

	Neonates (<2 wk)	Infants (1-3 mo)	Infants (4-24 mo)	Children (2-6 yr)	Older children, adolescents (>6 yr)
Hemophilus influenzae type b*		†	†	†	
Gram-negative bacilli (e.g., *Escherichia coli*, *Klebsiella* spp.)	†	†			
Neisseria meningitidis		†	†	†	†
Streptococcus pneumoniae		†	†	†	†
Group B *Streptococcus*	†	†			
Listeria monocytogenes	†	†			

From Hughes WT, Buescher ES: *Pediatric procedures,* ed 2, Philadelphia, 1980, WB Saunders.
*Incidence declining with institution of *Hemophilus influenzae* type B conjugate vaccines.
†Specific to age range.

blood and urine cultures, as well as culture of any apparent focal site of infection; begin age-appropriate empiric antibiotic therapy. Table 99-7 presents the common causes of acute bacterial meningitis.

While performing LP on infants and children who are critically ill, it is necessary to monitor electrocardiogram, respirations, and pulse oximetry continuously because of the risk of sudden decompensation during the procedure.

In cases of documented bacterial meningitis repeat LP is indicated in those patients with unsatisfactory clinical response after 24 to 72 hours of therapy.[57]

Individuals inexperienced with the technique of spinal puncture should use a transparent hub spinal needle to allow for earlier recognition of penetration into the subarachnoid space by quicker visualization of CSF return in the needle. Also after locating the site of intended puncture mark it by indentation of the skin with a fingernail.

REFERENCES

1. Albright RE Jr, Graham B, Christenson RH, et al: Issues in cerebrospinal fluid management: acid-fast bacillus smear and culture, *Am J Clin Pathol* 95:418-423, 1991.
2. Albright RE, Christenson RH, Emlet JL, et al: Issue in cerebrospinal fluid management: CSF venereal disease research laboratory testing, *Am J Clin Pathol* 95:397-401, 1991.
3. Anasti J, Buscema J, Genadry R, et al: Rectal serosal hematoma: an unusual complication of culdocentesis, *Obstet Gynecol* 65:72S-73S, 1985.
4. Barriga F, Schwartz RH, Hayden GF: Adequate illumination for otoscopy: variations due to power source, bulb, and head and speculum design, *Am J Dis Child* 140:1237-1240, 1986.
5. Batnitzky S, Keucher TR, Mealey J Jr, et al: Iatrogenic intraspinal epidermoid tumors, *JAMA* 237:148-150, 1977.
6. Bluestone CD, Klein JO: Methods of examination: clinical examination. In Bluestone CD, Stool SE, Scheetz MD, editors: *Pediatric otolaryngology,* Philadelphia, 1990, WB Saunders, pp. 111-124.
7. Bluestone CD, Klein JO: *Otitis media in infants and children,* Philadelphia, 1988, WB Saunders.
8. Bluestone CD, Shurin PA: Middle ear disease in children: pathogenesis, diagnosis, and management, *Pediatr Clin North Am* 21:379-400, 1974.
9. Bluestone CD, Klein JO: Otitis media, atelectasis, and eustachian tube dysfunction. In Bluestone CD, Stool SE, Scheetz MD, editors: *Pediatric otolaryngology,* ed 2 Philadelphia, 1990, WB Saunders, pp 320-486.
10. Bluestone CD, Klein JO: Intracranial suppurative complications of otitis media and mastoiditis. In Bluestone CD, Stool SE, Scheetz MD, editors: *Pediatric otolaryngology,* ed 2, Philadelphia, 1990, WB Saunders, pp 537-546.
11. Bluestone CD, Klein JO: Intracranial suppurative complications of otitis media and mastoiditis. In Bluestone CD, Stool SE, Scheetz MD, editors: *Pediatric otolaryngology,* ed 2, Philadelphia, 1990, WB Saunders, pp 487-539.
12. Bonadio WA, Smith DS, Goddard S, et al: Distinguishing cerebrospinal fluid abnormalities in children with bacterial meningitis and traumatic lumbar puncture, *J Infect Dis* 162:251-254, 1990.
13. Boyd GL: Tuberculosis pericarditis in children, *Am J Dis Child* 86:293-300, 1953.
14. Boyes RJ, Kruse JA: Selected nonvascular procedures. In Carlson RW, Geheb MA, editors: *Principles and practice of medical intensive care,* Philadelphia, 1993, WB Saunders, pp 160-177.
15. Cavanaugh RM Jr: Pneumatic otoscopy in healthy full-term infants, *Pediatrics* 79:520-523, 1987.
16. Celli BR: Diseases of the diaphram, chest wall, pleura, and mediastinum. In Wyngaarden JB, Smith LH, Bennett JC, editors: *Cecil textbook of medicine,* ed 19, Philadelphia, 1992, WB Saunders, pp 443-452.
17. Chapman MG, Kaplan L: Cardiac involvement in coccidiomycosis, *Am J Med* 23:87-98, 1957.
18. Chow AW, Malkasian KL, Marshall JR, et al: The bacteriology of acute pelvic inflammatory disease, *Am J Obstet Gynecol* 122:876-879, 1975.
19. Clark HC, Fitzgerald JF, Kleiman MB: Spontaneous bacterial peritonitis, *J Pediatr* 104:495-500, 1984.
20. Collins TR, Sahn SA: Thoracentesis: clinical value, complications, technical problems and patient experience, *Chest* 91:817, 1987.
21. Conn HO: Bacterial peritonitis: spontaneous or paracentetic? *Gastroenterology* 77:1145-1146, 1979.
22. Conn HO: Sudden scrotal edema in cirrhosis: a paracentesis syndrome, *Ann Intern Med* 43:943, 1971.
23. Cuetara MM, Mallo N, Dalet F: Amphotericin B lavage in the treatment of candidial cystitis, *Br J Urol* 44:475-480, 1972.
24. Dripps RD, Vandam LD: Hazards of lumbar puncture, *JAMA* 147:1118-1121, 1951.
25. Eisinger SH: Culdocentesis, *J Fam Pract* 13:95-101, 1981.
26. Feigen RD: Bacterial meningitis beyond the neonatal period. In Feigen RD, Cherry JD, editors: *Textbook of pediatric infectious diseases,* ed 3, Philadelphia, 1992, WB Saunders, p 410.
27. Feldman WE: Bacterial etiology and mortality of purulent pericarditis in pediatric patients: review of 162 cases, *Am J Dis Child* 133:641-644, 1979.
28. Fiser DH, Gober GA, Smith CE, et al: Prevention of hypoxemia during lumbar puncture in infancy with preoxygenation, *Pediatr Emerg Care* 9:81-83, 1993.
29. Fisher JF, Chew WH, Shadomy S, et al: Urinary tract infections due to *Candida albicans, Rev Infect Dis* 4:1107-1118, 1982.
30. Fishman RA: *Cerebrospinal fluid in diseases of the nervous system,* Philadelphia, 1980, WB Saunders, pp 141-167.
31. Fleischer G, Ludwig S, Campos J: Cellulitis: bacterial etiology, clinical features, and laboratory findings, *J Pediatr* 97:591-593, 1980.
32. Fleischer G, Ludwig S: Cellulitis: A prospective study. *Ann Emerg Med* 9:246-249, 1980.
33. Gallis HA, Drew RH, Pickard RH: Amphotericin B: 30 years of clinical experience, *Rev Infect Dis* 12:308-329, 1990.
34. Giacobine JW, Siler VE: Evaluation of diagnostic abdominal paracen-

tesis with experimental and clinical studies, *Surg Gynecol Obstet* 110:676, 1960.

35. Gines P, Arroyo V: Paracentesis in the management of cirrhotic ascites, *J Hepatol* 17(suppl 2):S14-18, 1993.

36. Ginsberg CM: *Haemophilus influenzae* type b buccal cellulitis, *J Am Acad Dermatol* 4:661-664, 1981.

37. Goetz JP, Tafari N, Boxerbaum B: Needle aspiration in *Haemophilus influenzae* type b cellulitis, *Pediatrics* 54:504-506, 1974.

38. Goldman HJ, Littman ML, Oppenheimer GD, et al: Monilial cystitis-effective treatment with installations of amphotericin B, *JAMA* 174:359-362, 1960.

39. Gorelick PB, Biller J: Lumbar puncture, *Postgrad Med* 79:257-268, 1986.

40. Granat M, Gordon T, Isaac E, et al: Accidental puncture of pelvic kidney: rare complication of culdocentesis, *Am J Obstet Gynecol* 138:223-235, 1980.

41. Grogan DR, Irwin RS: Complications associated with thoracentesis, *Arch Intern Med* 150:873, 1990.

42. Hager DH, Eschenbach EA, Spence MR, et al: Criteria for diagnosis and grading of salpingitis, *Obstet Gynecol* 61:113-114, 1983.

43. Herman GR, Marchand EJ, Grur GH: Pericarditis: clinical and laboratory data of 130 cases, *Am Heart J* 43:641-652, 1952.

44. Hoefs JC, Jonas GM: Diagnostic paracentesis, *Adv Intern Med* 37:391-409, 1992.

45. Hoffman JI, Stanger P: Diseases of the pericardium. In Rudolph AM, Hoffman JIE, Rudolph CD, editors: *Rudolph's pediatrics,* ed 19, Norwalk, Conn, 1991, Appleton & Lange, pp 1425-1428.

46. Holmberg K, Axelsson A, Hansson P, et al: The correlation between otoscopy and otomicroscopy in acute otitis media during healing, *Scand Audio* 14:191-199, 1985.

47. Hook EW, Thomas MH, Horton CA, et al: Microbiologic evaluation of cutaneous cellulitis in adults, *Arch Intern Med* 146:295-297, 1986.

48. Howe PM, Fajardo JE, Orcutt MA: Etiologic diagnosis of cellulitis: comparison of aspirates obtained from the leading edge and the point of maximal inflammation, *Pediatr Infect Dis J* 6:685-686, 1987.

49. Hughes WT, Buescher ES: *Pediatric procedures,* ed 2, Philadelphia, 1980, WB Saunders, pp 194-195.

50. Hughes WT, Buescher ES: *Pediatric procedures,* ed 2, Philadelphia, 1980 WB Saunders, pp 196-199.

51. Hughes WT, Buescher ES: *Pediatric procedures,* ed 2, Philadelphia, 1980, WB Saunders, pp 233-235.

52. Hughes WT, Buescher ES: *Pediatric procedures,* ed 2, Philadelphia, 1980, WB Saunders, pp 260-262.

53. Hughes WT, Buescher ES: *Pediatric procedures,* ed 2, Philadelphia, 1980, WB Saunders, pp 178-185.

54. Kaneko K, Onodera O, Tadsahi M, et al: Rapid diagnosis of tuberculous meningitis by polymerase chain reaction (PCR), *Neurology* 40:1617-1618, 1990.

55. Kaplan SL, Feigen RD: Simplified technique for tympanocentesis, *Pediatrics* 62:418-419, 1978.

56. Kirshon B, Sebastian F, Phillips LE, et al: Correlation of ultrasonography and bacteriology of the endocervix and posterior cul-de-sac of patients with severe pelvic inflammatory disease, *Sex Transm Dis* 15:103-107, 1988.

57. Klein JO, Feigen RD, McCracken GH: Report of the task force on diagnosis and management of meningitis, *Pediatrics* 78:959-982, 1986.

58. Krol LV, Abbott JT: The current role of culdocentesis, *Am J Emerg Med* 10:354-358, 1992.

59. Meislin HW: Pathogen identification of abscesses and cellulitis, *Ann Emerg Med* 15:329-332, 1986.

60. Mellor DH: The place of computed tomography and lumbar puncture in suspected bacterial meningitis, *Arch Dis Child* 67:1417-1419, 1992.

61. Newell PM, Norden CW: Value of needle aspiration in bacteriologic diagnosis of cellulitis in adults, *J Clin Microbiol* 26:401-404, 1988.

62. Nix DE, Durrence CW, May JR: Amphotericin B bladder irrigations, *Drug Intell Clin Pharm* 19:299-300, 1985.

63. O'Quinn JR, Lahshminarayan S: Venous air embolism, *Arch Intern Med* 142:2173, 1982.

64. Picardi JL, Kaufmann CA, Schwarz J, et al: Pericarditis caused by *Histoplasma capsulatum, Am J Cardiol* 37:82-88, 1976.

65. Pinsky WW, Friedman RA, Jubelirer DP, et al: Infectious pericarditis. In Fiegen RD, Cherry JD, editors: *Textbook of pediatric infectious diseases,* ed 3, Philadelphia, 1992, WB Saunders, pp 377-386.

66. Pinzello G, Simonetti RG, Craxi A, et al: Spontaneous bacterial peritonitis: a prospective investigation in predominantly nonalcoholic cirrhotic patients, *Hepatology* 3:545-549, 1983.

67. Quincke HI: Ueber hydrocephalus. X. Congress f. innere Medicin, (Wiesbaden) 1891.

68. Richards PG, Towu-Aghantse E: Dangers of lumbar puncture, *Br Med J* 292:605-606, 1986.

69. Rohner TJ, Tuliszewski RM: Fungal cystitis: awareness, diagnosis and treatment, *J Urol* 124:142-144, 1980.

70. Ross DS: In Roberts JR, Hedges JR, editors: *Clinical procedures in emergency medicine,* Philadelphia, 1991, WB Saunders, pp 112-128.

71. Runyon BA: Paracentesis of ascitic fluid: a safe procedure, *Arch Intern Med* 146:2259-2261, 1986.

72. Runyon BA: Ascitic fluid analysis in the differentiation of spontaneous bacterial peritonitis from gastrointestinal tract perforation into ascitic fluid, *Hepatology* 4:447-450, 1984.

73. Runyon BA, Hoefs JC: Spontaneous vs. secondary bacterial peritonitis: differentiation by response of ascitic fluid neutrophil count to antimicrobial therapy, *Arch Intern Med* 146:1563-1565, 1986.

74. Runyon BA, Umland ET, Merlin T: Inoculation of blood culture bottles with ascitic fluid: improved detection of spontaneous bacterial peritonitis, *Arch Intern Med* 147:73-75, 1987.

75. Runyon BA, Canawati HN, Akriviadis AE: Optimization of ascitic fluid culture techniques, *Gastroenterology* 95:1051-1135, 1988.

76. Sachs C: The optimum use of needle aspiration in the bacteriologic diagnosis of cellulitis in adults, *Arch Intern Med* 150:1907-1912, 1990.

77. Sanford JP: The engima of candiduria: evolution of bladder irrigation with amphotericin B for management from anecdote to dogma and a lesson from Michiavelli, *Clin Infect Dis* 16:145-147, 1993.

78. Schreiner RL, Kleinman MB: Incidence and effect of traumatic lumbar puncture in the neonates, *Dev Med Child Neurol* 21:483-487, 1979.

79. Schreiner RL, Stevens DC, Jose JH, et al: Infant lumbar puncture: a teaching simulator, *Clin Pediatr* 20:298-299, 1981.

80. Scott JR: Ectopic pregnancy. In Scott JR, DiSaia PJ, Hammond CB, Spellacy WN, editors: *Danforth's obstetrics and gynecology,* ed 6, Philadelphia, 1990, JB Lippincott, pp 227-228.

81. Sharp CG, Steinhart CM: Lumbar puncture in the presence of increased intracranial pressure: the real danger, *Pediatr Emerg Care* 3:39-43, 1987.

82. Sternbach G: Lumbar puncture, *J Emerg Med* 2:199-203, 1985.

83. Todd J: Office laboratory diagnosis of skin and soft tissue infections, *Pediatr Infect Dis* 4:84-87, 1985.

84. Trapnell DH, Thurston JB: Unilateral pulmonary edema after pleural aspiration, *Lancet* 1:1367, 1970.

85. Uman SJ, Kunin CM: Needle aspiration in the diagnosis of soft tissue infections, *Arch Intern Med* 34:205-217, 1975.

86. Vandam LD, Dripps RD: Long-term follow-up evaluation of patients who received 10,098 spinal anesthetics, *JAMA* 161:586-591, 1956.

87. Veneri RJ, Gordon SC, Ink-Bennett D: Scintigraphic and culdoscopic diagnosis of bile peritonitis complicating liver biopsy, *J Clin Gastroenterol* 11:571-573, 1989.

88. Ward E, Gushurst CA: Uses and technique of pediatric lumbar puncture, *Am J Dis Child* 146:1160-1165, 1992.

89. Weisman LE, Merenstein GB, Steenbarger JR: The effect of lumbar puncture position in sick neonates, *Am J Dis Child* 137:1077-1079, 1983.

90. Wheeler SH, Sornsin SM: Pelvic pain in women. In Schwartz GR, Caytein CG, Mayer T et al, editors: *Principles and practice of emergency medicine,* Philadelphia, 1992, Lea & Febiger, pp 544-545.

91. Wise GJ, Wainstein S, Goldberg P, et al: Candidial cystitis: management by continuous bladder irrigation with amphotericin B, *JAMA* 224:1636-1637, 1973.

92. Wise GJ, Kozinn PJ, Goldberg P: Amphotericin B as an urologic irrigant in the management of noninvasive candiduria, *J Urol* 128:82-84, 1982.

93. Wong-Beringer A, Jacobs RA, Guglielmo BL: Treatment of funguria, *JAMA* 267:780-785, 1992.

94. Wylie R, Arasu TS, Fitzgerald JF: Ascites: Pathophysiology and management, *J Pediatr* 97:167-176, 1980.

Part XIX

SONOGRAPHY TECHNIQUES

100 Diagnostic Ultrasound

David Plummer

Diagnostic ultrasound (US) greatly enhances the evaluation of children with a variety of emergency presentations. The technology has evolved rapidly over the previous decade and is now widely available. Ultrasound has extremely high diagnostic value when done by the physician of first contact.[17] Many Emergency Department (ED) physicians and critical care specialists perform and interpret US.* Understanding these techniques may lead to improved overall use of medical imaging resources.[70] Patients with non-time-critical diagnoses may best obtain ultrasonography in the medical imaging (radiology) suite. However some who have unstable or time-critical diagnoses require bedside diagnosis and intervention in the ED or intensive care unit (ICU). These patients benefit from rapid, goal-directed, limited US performed and interpreted by the emergency physician or critical care specialist.[50] This section describes the indications, contraindications, techniques, and interpretation of ED and ICU US examination for several emergency conditions.

INDICATIONS

Emergency US contributes most to the ED or ICU evaluation for critical presentations. US techniques include, but are not limited to, two-dimensional echocardiography (2-DE); abdominal ultrasound for assessment of hemoperitonum; and bladder ultrasound for detection of urine.

CONTRAINDICATIONS

Contraindications to US are few. The primary contraindication is great urgency for a definitive therapeutic procedure, such as laporotomy, thoracotomy, or pericardiocentesis, in an unstable patient. In children, inability to cooperate because of age, pain, or anxiety is a relative contraindication.

COMPLICATIONS

There are no known complications of US.

EQUIPMENT

There is a broad range of US equipment available. It ranges in cost from approximately ten thousand to several hundred thousand dollars. Higher-cost machines have options and functions not typically used by emergency or ICU physicians. Most physicians performing ED or ICU US require limited functionality and options from their instrument. The components of a US machine that the physician must be familiar with include the display, transducer, image controls, and recording device.

Transducer types that vary in basic configuration and frequency of ultrasound generated are available. Mechanical oscillating heads are less expensive and more durable than linear or curved array models, although image quality is decreased. High-frequency transducers have superior image quality but are unable to image deep structures. A mechanical oscillating head generating 3.5 to 5 MHz US is a cost-effective choice and useful for all the pediatric examinations described here. Each machine must have a recording device such as videotape or hard-copy thermal printer. The image control options on most US machines initially appear overwhelming. However, the physician need only manipulate the overall gain, time gain control (TGC), and depth controls to obtain a limited scan successfully. A clinically useful, limited, goal-directed examination requires knowledge of ultrasonographic principles, anatomic features, and standard examination protocols and minimal experience.[49]

Equipment options that may be excluded include color flow, M-mode, Doppler capabilities, simultaneous electrocardiographic recording, foot pedal control, digital memory, image annotation, and most other software capabilities.

TECHNIQUES
General Considerations

Diagnostic US is an interactive skill and there is a steep initial learning curve. The optimal educational guidelines for these examinations initially proposed by medical imaging colleagues have been modified for a limited emergency examination.[39,46]

Start the examination with the power and depth set to the maximum values. These can then be adjusted appropriately once the goal structure is imaged. Remember the US transducer and therefore US plane have three independent axes of motion (Figs. 100-1 to 100-3). Sweeping of the transducer is motion perpendicular to the scan plane, which changes the plane being imaged. Small changes in the sweep angle markedly change structures seen. Always sweep the scan plane before changing transducer positions. Tilting the transducer moves the beam in the same plane and centers the image. Rotate the transducer by turning on the long axis. When possible obtain the scans on at least two planes by rotating the transducer 90 degrees. Alter the transducer in one plane at a time.

Begin the examination with the child in the supine position; this position alone suffices in most cases. Occasionally moving the patient to a different position augments the examination by moving internal structures relative to the transducer. Alternatives include the lateral decubitus and sitting positions. When possible ask the patient to hold his or her breath in different points of the respiratory cycle. A deep breath can markedly improve the operator's ability to see

---

*References 11, 27, 28, 40, 45, 47, 50, and 64.

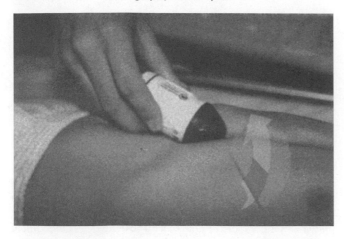

FIG. 100-1 Correct transducer position for obtaining a subxiphoid window. The arrow, perpendicular to the plane of the ultrasound scan, represents the change in the plane with a sweeping motion of the transducer.

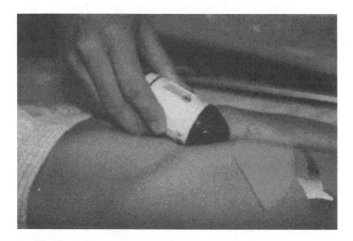

FIG. 100-2 Correct transducer position. The arrow represents the motion of the ultrasound plane if the transducer is tilted. This motion centers images on the ultrasound screen.

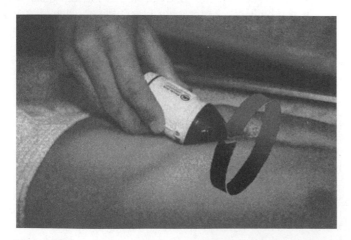

FIG. 100-3 Correct transducer position. The arrow represents the change and the orientation of the ultrasound plane during rotation of the transducer on its long access.

some structures that are otherwise difficult. Apply firm but gentle pressure to enhance image quality. This reduces the distance to the structure, improves skin-transducer contact, and occasionally moves bowel contents away from the image plane. Approach each examination knowing what anatomic landmarks to seek. To help in identifying structures remember that the structures closest to the transducer appear nearest the top of the screen.

ECHOCARDIOGRAPHY

Two-dimensional echocardiography (2-DE) is the application of US technologies to the study of the heart and great vessels. Like the stethoscope and electrocardiogram which preceded it, 2-DE is well suited to bedside ED or ICU use. It is rapid, safe, accurate, and noninvasive and allows for serial examinations. It can be done without interrupting compressions during cardiopulmonary resuscitation.[7] Echocardiography provides a great deal of anatomic and functional information that the physician must then interpret in terms of the patient's clinical condition. Performing the 2-DE examination is more operator-dependent than electrocardiography, but understanding the echocardiographic anatomy is more intuitive than interpreting the electrical vectors of the electrocardiograph. Consequently, physicians outside the traditional medical imaging specialties more routinely use 2-DE.[27,40,64]

Echocardiographic Indications

2-DE may contribute to the evaluation of many different patient presentations:
1. Hypotension (or pulselessness) of unknown cause
2. Suspicion of cardiac trauma, either blunt or penetrating
3. Suspicion of iatrogenic (procedural) complications

Echocardiographic Contraindications

Echocardiography is among the safest imaging tests in medicine. There are no specific contraindications. Relative contraindications relate to the time required for completing ED echocardiography. Do not perform echocardiography when it precludes timely life-saving intervention. There is only one known complication, a breast hematoma in an adult anticoagulated patient.[37]

Standard Examination and Echocardiographic Anatomy

A standard echocardiographic examination consists of viewing the heart from different positions on the chest through echocardiographic windows. The lung does not transmit ultrasonic sound waves; do not interpose lung between the transducer head and the heart (Fig. 100-4). The American Society of Echocardiography defines a series of standard echocardiographic windows normally used in a strict sequential fashion.[29] Most emergency and critical care physicians modify this approach and begin with the window that is most likely to give the needed information rapidly.[40,51]

Echocardiographic Techniques

Begin each examination by orienting the transducer properly. Each transducer has a marker dot that indicates the plane of the US scan (Fig. 100-3). Position the marker dot to face the patient's left side. This dot corresponds to the marker dot indicator on the display.

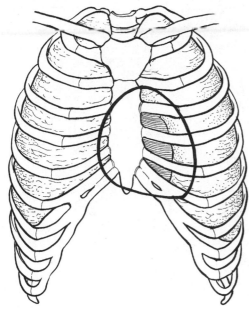

FIG. 100-4 Limited region on the chest wall where the transducer can be placed such that there is no lung interposed between the transducer and the heart. Small deviations in the position of the transducer within this region yield the different echocardiographic windows. This region also extends to the subxiphoid area.

The *subcostal window* (SC) often provides the most significant information for a single-view examination. To obtain this view place the transducer at the left infracostal margin at the level of the xiphoid with the beam aimed at the left shoulder (see Fig. 100-3). Slightly tilt or rotate the transducer to obtain the desired view. The structures closest to the transducer appear nearest the top of the display. With the patient supine the most anterior structure is a small amount of hepatic parenchyma, followed by the right-sided cardiac chambers (Figs. 100-5 and 100-6). The patient can often augment the image by breath holding in maximal inspiration. The anterior and posterior aspects of the pericardium appear as single bright reflecting surfaces. Separation of these bright echoes represents a separation of the visceral and parietal pericardium, usually by fluid (Fig. 100-7). Although a small amount of fluid is normal in the pericardial sac, any separation anteriorly (the nondependent part with the patient supine) represents an abnormal collection, frequently a pericardial effusion or hemopericardium. The SC view has several advantages as a starting point. It quickly screens for mechanical activity, pericardial fluid, and gross assessment of global and regional wall motion abnormalities and provides a four-chamber view to assess the relative size of the ventricles. The physician can readily obtain this view in supine and noncompliant patients, especially critically ill patients. A limited goal-directed examination may be obtained from the subcostal window within 1 minute.

The *left parasternal views* result from placing the transducer in the left parasternal area between the second and fourth intercostal spaces (Fig. 100-8). Rotating the transducer gives either a *left parasternal short axis* (LPSA) or left parasternal long axis (LPLA) view. For the LPLA the plane of the beam is parallel to a line drawn from the right shoulder to the left hip (Figs. 100-9 and 100-10). This view allows

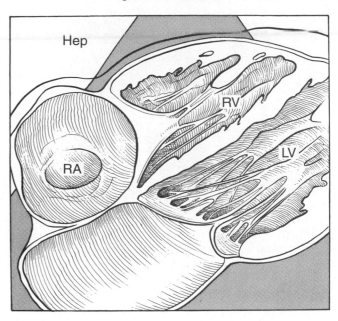

FIG. 100-5 Schematic representation of the heart as seen by the transducer from the subxiphoid window. The structures nearest the transducer appear nearest the top of the screen. *HEP,* Hepatic parenchyma; *RV,* right ventricle; *RA,* right atrium; *LV,* left ventricle.

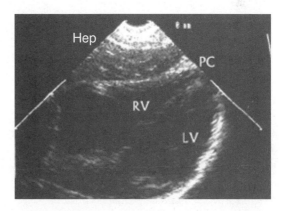

FIG. 100-6 Normal echocardiogram from the subxiphoid window. The structures correspond to those labeled in Fig. 100-5. *HEP,* Hepatic parenchyma; *PC,* pericardial line; *RV,* right ventricle; *LV,* left ventricle.

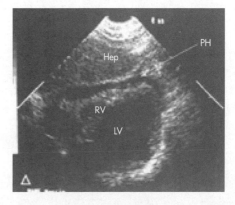

FIG. 100-7 Abnormal black separation of the pericardial line from a pericardial effusion as viewed from the subxiphoid window. *HEP,* Hepatic parenchyma; *PE,* pericardial effusion; *LV,* left ventricle; *PH,* pericardial hematoma (effusion).

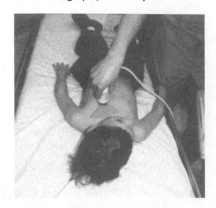

FIG. 100-8 Correct transducer position on the chest wall for obtaining the left parasternal views. Both the short and the long axis views are obtained from the same left parasternal position. Ultrasound plane orientation is consistent with the left parasternal short axis.

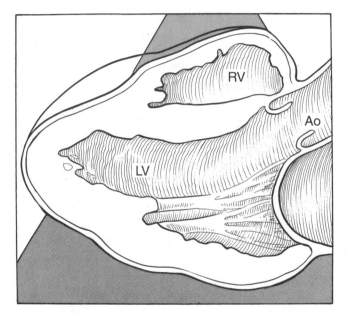

FIG. 100-9 Schematic representation of the left parasternal long axis view. Structures nearest the transducer appear nearest the top of the screen. *RV,* Right ventricle; *LV,* left ventricle; *AO,* aortic cuff flow.

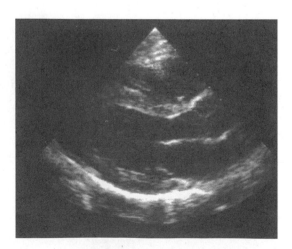

FIG. 100-10 Normal echocardiogram from the left parasternal long position. The cardiac structures correspond to those labeled in Fig. 100-9.

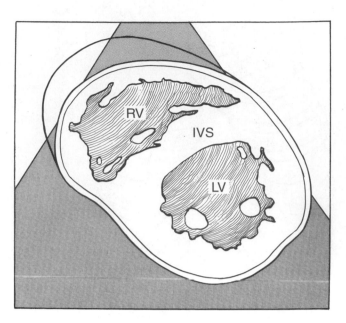

FIG. 100-11 Schematic representation of the heart as seen by the transducer in the left parasternal short axis. The structures nearest the transducer appear nearest the top of the screen. *RV,* Right ventricle; *IVS,* intraventricular septum; *LV,* left ventricle.

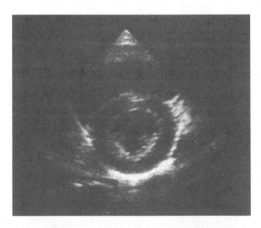

FIG. 100-12 Normal echocardiogram as seen from the left parasternal short axis view. Internal cardiac structures correspond to those labeled in Fig. 100-11.

visualization of the aortic valve and proximal ascending aorta and a good assessment of left ventricular size. Rotating the transducer so the plane of the beam is perpendicular to the long axis of the heart (i.e., toward the left shoulder) reveals the LPSA (Figs. 100-11 and 100-12). By tilting the transducer one can visualize from the apex through the mitral valve to the aortic valve. Both of the left parasternal windows may require positioning the patient in the left lateral decubitus position, which eliminates interposed lung between the transducer and the heart. Attaining these positions may be difficult in noncompliant critically ill patients.

The apical view results from placing the transducer directly over the point of maximum impulse (the apex) with the beam directed to the right shoulder (Fig. 100-13). The operator must tilt and rotate the transducer to get the desired view (Figs. 100-14 and 100-15). The apical view allows assessment of chamber size and location of intracavitary

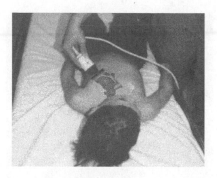

FIG. 100-13   Correct transducer position on the chest wall for obtaining the apical view.

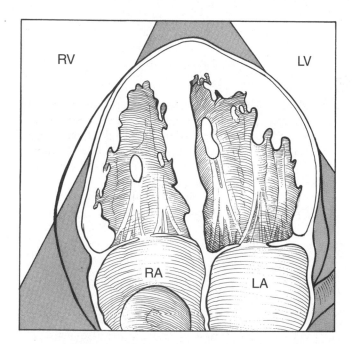

FIG. 100-14   Schematic representation of the heart as seen by the transducer from the apical window. The structures nearest the transducer appear nearest the top of the screen. RV, Right ventricle; RA, right atrium; LV, left ventricle; LA, left atrium.

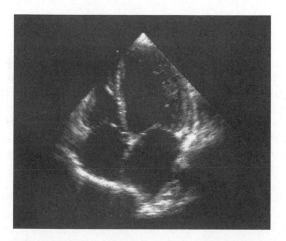

FIG. 100-15   Normal echocardiogram as visualized from the apical window. Internal cardiac structures correspond to those labeled in Fig. 100-14.

masses. It also frequently requires positioning in the left lateral decubitus position.

These four windows and views represent only a sampling of those defined by the American Society of Echocardiography and used in a formal echocardiographic examination. Although it is necessary to know these standard windows, an echocardiographic examination is interactive and the operator must be prepared to adapt the transducer position throughout. Often the emergency physician need not attain each of these windows to answer the limited clinical question. The best window for any examination is the one that gives the desired information.

HYPOTENSION OF UNKNOWN CAUSE

In the ED or ICU hypotension and shock are frequent problems. Successful resuscitation depends on rapid treatment directed at the primary hemodynamic alteration. The physical examination is often both nonspecific and insensitive in detecting the underlying hemodynamic state. Traditional diagnostic methods including intraarterial catheterization, central venous pressure measurements, and pulmonary artery catheterization are invasive, costly, time-consuming, and not easily performed. In this setting bedside 2-DE performed via a single window may rapidly and specifically guide initial resuscitation efforts. By assessing the global motion of the heart and chamber size, the patient can often be quickly assigned to one of four hemodynamic categories:

1. Cardiogenic shock (left ventricular dysfunction)
2. Hypovolemia
3. Cardiac tamponade
4. Right ventricular dysfunction or outflow obstruction

Cardiogenic Hypotension

Patients with cardiogenic shock (resulting from cardiomyopathy or myocarditis) display marked global wall motion abnormalities on 2-DE.[48] In adults this is most often secondary to massive myocardial ischemia.[69] In children the cause is more likely myocarditis, cardiomyopathy, or traumatic myocardial contusion.[1,19,22] Additional aspects of the clinical presentation can help distinguish among these causes. Serial examinations allow immediate feedback about the impact of fluid and drug administration. In the extreme case the patient is erroneously thought to be in electromechanical dissociation (EMD) or pulseless electrical activity (PEA).

Documentation of PEA during cardiac arrest is simple with 2-DE.[7,40,4] Physicians sometimes encounter patients who are clearly alive and rarely awake but ostensibly pulseless. There are also patients who are apneic and nonresponsive in whom a pulse cannot be palpated, yet they are still viable. There are many possible reasons for the failure to palpate a pulse (e.g., inadequate perfusion pressure) and if all these patients are prematurely labeled as having PEA, some potentially salvageable cases are overlooked. Bedside emergency US can eliminate this problem immediately.

As with cardiac tamponade almost any view would probably suffice, but the subcostal view with the transducer directed slightly toward the right shoulder is easiest. CPR must be stopped momentarily while an assessment is made of the presence or absence of wall and valve motion. Critically ill patients often have multiple concurrent chest procedures under way at the time of the echocardiographic examination, with only the subcostal approach available for cardiac imaging. The left parasternal view, in either short or long axis, may be a very good alternative.

As true PEA appears to have a uniformly fatal prognosis, resuscitative efforts are usually futile. Many with suspected PEA are actually exhibiting another condition. Several of these, notably tension pneumothorax, pericardial tamponade, hypovolemia, hypoxia, hyperkalemia, pulmonary embolism, acidosis, or severe hypokinesis, are potentially reversible. Hence a more reliable method of confirming the diagnosis is required. Bedside ultrasonography has the advantage of not only confirming or refuting the diagnosis but often revealing the true diagnosis. The US finding of near-normal or hyperdynamic wall motion immediately suggests the presence of hypovolemia. In such cases, begin massive fluid resuscitation and investigation as to the site of occult blood loss, often by extending the US examination (discussed later). The presence of pericardial tamponade merits immediate drainage, either percutaneously (see Chapter 110) or perhaps more definitively through emergency thoracotomy and pericardiectomy (see Chapter 108). In cases in which wall motion and valvular motion are still noted, although inadequate to produce a pulse pressure, prompt massive inotropic therapy and perhaps balloon pump assistance are indicated. There are no data yet to suggest what subgroup of these patients may be salvaged.

Hypovolemic Hypotension

Patients who are hypovolemic usually display a hyperkinetic heart with small right-sided chambers. This results from either an absolute hypovolemia, as in hemorrhagic shock, or a relative hypovolemia, as in states of reduced afterload, especially early shock with preserved cardiac function. In such cases the initial therapeutic measures must include vigorous fluid resuscitation, and serial 2-DE examinations can help guide therapy. Unexplained hypovolemia of this degree may be due to simple dehydration, but consider unsuspected trauma and occult exsanguination. Rarely a patient has hemodynamically significant valvular disease. In the case of mitral insufficiency the heart's appearance suggests that there is pure afterload reduction with a hyperdynamic profile. This and other valvular disorders can be more accurately imaged with both transesophageal and color flow echocardiography.

Cardiac Tamponade

In the detection of suspected cardiac tamponade, 2-DE has high sensitivity and specificity. The physician has no other practical noninvasive means to confirm this uncommon but lethal diagnosis in the ED setting. Beck's triad of hypotension, elevated neck veins, and muffled heart tones are late and nonspecific. Pulsus paradoxicus is difficult to detect.[16,30] Electrical alternans is specific for tamponade but is uncommon in acute tamponade.[2,21] Kussmaul's sign, the rise of central venous pressure (CVP) on inspiration, occurs only when tamponade is accompanied by constriction.[42] Elevation of the CVP with hypotension is nonspecific and requires invasive, time-consuming catheterization.[25,65] Alternately the CVP may be falsely elevated in hypotensive patients who are placed in Trendelenburg position or have military antishock

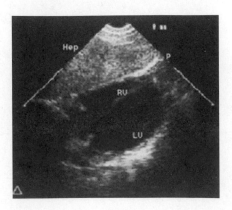

FIG. 100-16 Normal relationship of the pericardium to the hepatic parenchyma and the heart. Note the pericardial line is a single unseparated bright line. *HEP,* Hepatic parenchyma; *PC,* pericardial line; *RV,* right ventricle; *LV,* left ventricle.

trousers (MAST). Traditional anterior-posterior chest roentgenogram studies usually reveal a normal cardiac silhouette with the rapid accumulation of pericardial fluid; an enlarged cardiac silhouette is most commonly the result of cardiomegaly rather than pericardial effusion. Diagnostic pericardiocentesis is also time-consuming and invasive.

The vast majority of patients with cardiac tamponade display pericardial fluid mass on echocardiography. Detection of pericardial fluid does not require specialized knowledge of echocardiographic cardiac anatomic characteristics and standardized cardiac windows or much experience. The demonstration of pericardial fluid in patients with cardiac tamponade is immediate and unequivocal.

The pericardium is a dense fibrous sac that completely encircles the heart and a few centimeters of the proximal aorta and pulmonary artery. The dense pericardial tissue is highly echogenic and it is recognized both anteriorly and posteriorly as the sonographic border of the cardiac image (Fig. 100-16). Under normal conditions a small amount of fluid serves to lubricate the space between the visceral and parietal layers of the pericardium. This fluid is usually less than 30 ml and is usually not visible over the nondependent aspect of the heart. The exquisite sensitivity of US for the detection of pericardial fluid arises from the fact that the effusion appears as an anechoic space separating the echogenic pericardium from the heart. Figs. 100-17 to 100-19 illustrate this appearance. Large pericardial effusions surround the entire heart and are visualized in virtually every view. Small effusions collect first around the more dependent and mobile ventricles. In cases with severe pericardial disease loculated effusions may develop (Fig. 100-20) in regions that are unpredictable. These loculated effusions may result in a regional tamponade syndrome exhibiting atypical signs.[13,59]

When organized blood or fibrin is present, the effusion shows some degree of echogenicity rather than being perfectly anechoic.[6,43] This may provide a clue as to the underlying cause, as in the investigation of a malignancy. Fig. 100-19 shows the echogenic characteristics of organized

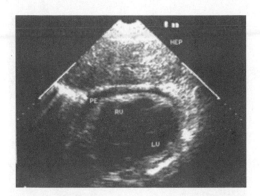

FIG. 100-17   Abnormal separation of the pericardial line as viewed by the subxiphoid window. *HEP,* Hepatic parenchyma; *PE,* pericardial effusion; *RV,* right ventricle; *LV,* left ventricle.

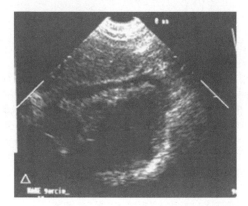

FIG. 100-18   Abnormal separation of the pericardial line from hemopericardium, or pericardial hematoma. Note the extremely small size of the right ventricle. This collapse of the right ventricle throughout the cardiac cycle is an echocardiographic indication of cardiac tamponade.

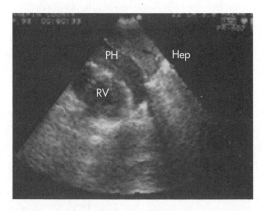

FIG. 100-19   Wide separation of the pericardial line by a large organized pericardial hematoma. This pericardial hematoma is organized and partially echogenic. *RV,* Right ventricle; *PH,* pericardial hematoma.

pericardial blood. With large effusions the heart can develop a remarkable motion as it floats within the distended pericardial sac. This is evident when viewed in real-time sonography but does not correlate with the presence of tamponade physiologic characteristics. The most important 2-DE finding

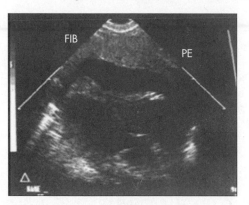

FIG. 100-20   Large separation of the pericardial line from a pericardial effusion secondary to purulent pericarditis. This effusion is partially loculated by dense fibrous adhesions. *PE,* Pericardial effusion; *RV,* right ventricle; *LV,* left ventricle; *FIB,* fibrous adhesion.

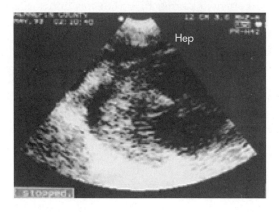

FIG. 100-21   Subxiphoid view of the heart illustrating an abnormal fluid collection. This abnormal collection of fluids separates hepatic parenchyma from the heart. Note that this fluid collection does not follow the contour of the heart and represents free abdominal fluid. *HEP,* Hepatic parenchyma.

is a hyperdynamic heart with diastolic collapse of the right ventricle and atrium (Fig. 100-18).[15,33] This is a sensitive indicator and appears even before paradoxic pulse is present.[15] Other specific findings include right atrial compression, paradoxic motion of the intraventricular septum, and inferior vena cava engorgement.[30] Detecting these latter findings usually requires significant experience.

Occasionally either intraabdominal fluid or pleural effusions may be confused with pericardial effusions. Visualize the hyperechoic image of the pericardium to ensure that the anechoic fluid surrounding the heart is intrapericardial. The subcostal view is often most helpful as there is no pleural reflection between the liver and the heart. A large anechoic space visualized from the subcostal view is fluid in either free abdominal or intrapericardial space (Fig. 100-21). Intrapericardial fluid conforms to the contour of the heart, whereas free intraabdominal fluid does not.

The underlying cause, which may be anything from cardiac rupture to viral pericarditis, may not be evident. In cases in which the only definite finding is the effusion the diagnosis of tamponade is not established and many causes of pericardial fluid (e.g., myopericarditis, severe congestive heart failure [CHF], uremia) may also be associated with hypotension, even without tamponade. Consider hypotensive patients with a hyperdynamic heart and a new or indeterminant-age pericardial effusion to be in cardiac tamponade.[20] In borderline cases in which tamponade is suspected and a pericardial effusion is documented, heart catheterization or diagnostic pericardiocentesis may be required to diagnose tamponade physiologic processes. Right ventricular outflow obstruction is extremely rare in pediatric patients; it is manifested by a vigorously beating left ventricle (LV) with a large, hypodynamic thin-walled right ventricle (RV).[5,57]

CARDIAC TRAUMA: PENETRATING INJURY

Historically most patients with major cardiac injuries die at the scene.[32,38,67] Many factors, including improved emergency medical systems (EMS) and increasing incidence of urban violence, have greatly increased the number of salvageable patients entering EDs with this critical diagnosis. Rapid diagnosis and treatment of cardiac injury, particularly penetrating cardiac injury, are independent determinants of survival of these patients.

Unfortunately the signs and symptoms on physical examination are both nonspecific and insensitive and often are recognized only when catastrophic deterioration occurs. Traditional imaging techniques (computed tomography [CT], angiography) used for diagnosis of penetrating cardiac injury are immediately available to such patients. However a limited 2-DE bedside examination can be performed quite readily in approximately 1 minute, independently of patient compliance.

Hemopericardium is the most common visible feature of penetrating cardiac injury and appears as an echo-free space within the pericardium (Fig. 100-22).[40,51,68] This anechoic appearance results from liquefaction of the pericardial hematoma from defibrination of blood, which regularly occurs in subacute and chronic hemopericardium. However, in acute hemopericardium, there is insufficient time for defibrination to occur; as a result the hemopericardium organizes and partially clots, resulting in a pericardial hematoma. Such hematomas appear diffusely echogenic instead of echo-free (Fig. 100-23) and the hematoma may even be isodense to the

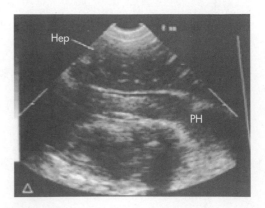

FIG. 100-23 Subxiphoid view of a large organized pericardial hematoma separating the hepatic parenchyma from the heart. Other internal cardiac structures are polyvisualized. *PH*, Pericardial hematoma; *Hep*, hepatic parenchyma.

myocardium, making 2-DE diagnosis very difficult. Consider any intrapericardial collections, whether echo-free or echodense, in cases of penetrating injury to the thorax or upper abdomen to represent penetrating cardiac injury. Rarely a patient with cardiac penetration has a normal appearing echocardiogram if the hemopericardium decompresses into the thorax. Also uncommonly patients may display pneumopericardium, pericardial foreign bodies, or pseudoaneurysm formation.[18,53]

CARDIAC TRAUMA: BLUNT INJURY

Patients who sustain blunt chest injury may suffer cardiac contusion, myocardial hematoma, or cardiac rupture. Cardiac contusion, although variably defined, may lead to arrhythmia, pump failure, or thromboembolism. Concurrent multisystem injury often obscures the early diagnosis. Laboratory diagnosis including standard and right precordial electrocardiogram (ECG), cardiac enzyme fractionation, first-pass radionuclide angiography, technetium-99mm-pyrophosphate, and thallium 201 are technically difficult and/or have insufficient sensitivity or specificity to serve as a standard. However 2-DE, which can be performed at the bedside, is quite sensitive and specific; up to 25% of blunt trauma victims not suspected clinically of cardiac contusion have 2-DE evidence of wall motion abnormalities consistent with the diagnosis, and pericardial effusion accompanies many of these.[54]

There is no gold standard to diagnose a *clinically significant* cardiac contusion. Deceleration injuries most commonly contuse the right ventricle because it is the most anterior aspect of the heart. Therefore 2-DE evidence of right ventricular dilation and dysfunction strongly supports the diagnosis of contusion.[5] This is an important diagnosis in the unstable patient. When RV dysfunction is apparent, it correlates well with the cause of hypotension.[19]

Rarely patients with blunt chest trauma arrive at the ED with cardiac rupture.[9] Blunt cardiac rupture usually results from high-energy impact and accounts for 5% of highway-related deaths. It may also result from relatively minor trauma such as striking the chest with a golf club, or it may

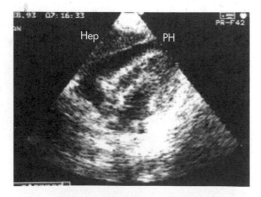

FIG. 100-22 Common appearance of hemopericardium or pericardial hematoma from the subxiphoid window. *Hep*, Hepatic parenchyma; *PH*, pericardial hematoma.

present no external signs of trauma.[12,52] This injury probably has the same time-mortality profile as traumatic aortic rupture, because most patients die at the scene. However, in the patients entering the EMS system alive, survival requires rapid diagnosis and treatment. As many as 20% of patients who sustain blunt cardiac rupture survive at least 30 minutes.[10] Both adult and pediatric patients can be salvaged given a timely diagnosis and intervention.[3,4,9,35,61] Most authors describe the physical signs of cardiac rupture as including hypotension, tamponade, hemothorax exsanguination, and cyanosis.[9] Unfortunately these physical findings are masked by concurrent multisystem injury and are nonspecific. Traditional diagnostic methods include ED thoracotomy, subxiphoid window, and diagnostic pericardiocentesis. Each of these is unnecessarily invasive and time-consuming.

Usually the pericardial sac contains the rupture and these patients have hemopericardium and some degree of cardiac tamponade. Suspect this diagnosis when hemopericardium is present in cases of blunt trauma. Rarely an extrapericardial mediastinal hematoma with cardiac compression has a similar appearance to a ruptured heart.[60]

IATROGENIC (PROCEDURAL) COMPLICATIONS

When a patient decompensates during or after an invasive vascular procedure, the physician can use 2-DE to screen rapidly for inadvertent cardiac penetration or hemopericardium formation with tamponade after CVP, Swan-Ganz catheter, or intravenous pacer placement. The same is true after intracardiac injection or attempted pericardiocentesis. Pneumothorax and hemothorax are other complications that may be suspected or confirmed on the basis of US findings.

ABDOMINAL ULTRASONOGRAPHY

The diagnostic applications of abdominal US have expanded greatly over the last decade. Many of these techniques are sophisticated and time-consuming to learn and perform. Therefore they are procedures for a radiologist. However occasional patients have serious or critical conditions and require immediate diagnostic and therapeutic interventions. Many of these patients may benefit from immediate US performed and interpreted by the emergency or critical care physician. Currently patients suspected of blunt abdominal trauma (or other intraabdominal catastrophe) and those requiring certain invasive procedures may benefit from emergency abdominal US. This examination is a hands-on interactive technical skill similar to 2-DE. There is a learning curve for this procedure and the optimal training guidelines for such proficiency are unknown.

Indications for Abdominal Ultrasonography

1. Blunt abdominal trauma
2. Suprapubic aspiration

Contraindications

There are no absolute contraindications for abdominal US. Do not perform this examination if it impedes lifesaving interventions.

BLUNT ABDOMINAL TRAUMA

Because of the high incidence of blunt and penetrating abdominal trauma and the potentially catastrophic nature of missed injuries, the emergency physician and critical care specialist must be organized and diligent in evaluating these patients. Often the goal in abdominal evaluation is simply to determine whether intraabdominal hemorrhage has occurred. Historically this has been done with physical examination, diagnostic peritoneal lavage, and enhanced CT of the abdomen.

The physical examination, in conjunction with the history, is accurate in only 45% to 50% of children in determining the presence of significant intraabdominal injury.[44] Even in conscious, sober patients with hemoperitoneum there may be no peritoneal signs or guarding. This often leads to a diagnostic delay that increases morbidity and mortality rates. Alternatively mandatory surgical exploration results in an unacceptably high negative laparotomy rate.

Diagnostic peritoneal lavage (DPL) was introduced in 1965 and greatly improved the evaluation of these patients (see Chapter 114). The goal of DPL is detection of hemoperitoneum. The initial studies indicated this technique was 100% accurate. Although subsequent studies failed to validate this initial study, it has proved to be an extremely accurate adjunct and has become a standard procedure in most trauma centers in the United States. DPL however is invasive and time- consuming and may result in a high rate of nontherapeutic laparotomies.[23,31]

Radionuclide liver-spleen scan has the advantage of being noninvasive and it provides information about specific organs. However these scans have been supplanted by the abdominal CT scan, which provides more information.

Abdominal CT scan has certain advantages and disadvantages. It can help identify specific organ injuries as well as the extent of those injuries. In addition it identifies retroperitoneal injury missed by DPL, although not with the same accuracy as it does with intraabdominal solid organs. Most significantly logistic and time requirements to obtain abdominal CT and expertise required for reading preclude this as the test of choice in critical abdominal trauma, and unfortunately many patients continue to undergo hemodynamic decompensation in the radiology suite.[14] Abdominal CT currently provides the most information about the extent and location of intraabdominal injury.

US was first used in blunt abdominal trauma for the detection of hemoperitoneum over 25 years ago, and its use has grown rapidly since 1990. Abdominal US has advantages and disadvantages. It is noninvasive, fast, safe, and portable. It can be applied at the bedside in a serial fashion. This examination has been employed most commonly in European and Japanese trauma centers and is only now undergoing domestic evaluation.[55,63] The limited goal of this examination is the detection of free abdominal fluid, which is interpreted as hemoperitoneum in this clinical setting. Consider any free fluid in the trauma patient to be hemoperitoneum until proved otherwise. US may be the test of choice when rapid diagnosis of hemoperitoneum, irrespective of origin, influences the clinical coarse. The sequence of further medical imaging studies, transfer to the operating room, consultation, referral, or activation of interhospital transfer may all be influenced by the early demonstration of hemoperitoneum.

There are over a dozen prospective controlled series for detection of hemoperitoneum by US.* Among the recent reports sensitivity and specificity range between 90% and 100%. A false-positive examination result occurs when fluid that is not a hemoperitoneum is detected. This occurs with blunt rupture of the bladder or bowel producing free abdominal fluid.[36] Nonsurgical conditions, including congestive heart failure, ascites, or some other transudative conditions, may produce a false-positive result. Fortunately these are not commonly encountered in pediatric trauma. Free intraabdominal fluid collects preferentially in the most dependent portions of the abdomen. When the child is in the supine position fluid collects first in the pelvic recess; with greater amounts the fluid extends to the pericolic gutters. Positioning the patient in Trendelenburg position augments the amount of fluid in the pericolic region and diminishes the amount in the pelvic recess. Each abdominal window described here requires 30 seconds to 1 minute to complete.[56]

TECHNIQUES FOR EXAMINATION FOR HEMOPERITONIUM

Begin the examination by orienting the transducer properly with the marker dot to the patient's left. Adjust the power to maximum, and depth to maximum; adjust both to improve the quality after the goal structure is imaged.[56] Place the transducer in the subxiphoid window (discussed earlier) (Fig. 100-24). Free abdominal fluid must be distinguished from pericardial fluid as discussed (see Fig. 100-21). Next place the transducer in the right lateral intercostal window. Obtain this window by placing the transducer in the midaxial line with the marker dot downward in an inferior intercostal space (Fig. 100-25). The most evident landmark to identify is the kidney, which appears as an oval structure with characteristic hyperechoic medulla (Fig. 100-26). Morison's pouch, a potential space, is a peritoneal reflection bounded by the kidney (Gerota's fascia) and the liver (Glission's capsule).

---

*References 8, 26, 35, 56, 58, 62, and 66.

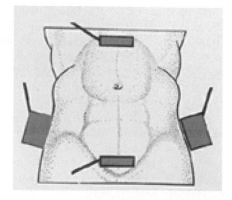

FIG. 100-24 Correct transducer positions for obtaining four abdominal ultrasound windows: subxiphoid, right lateral oblique, left lateral oblique, and superpubic.

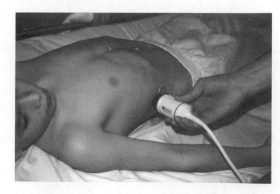

FIG. 100-25 Correct transducer position for obtaining the right lateral oblique window.

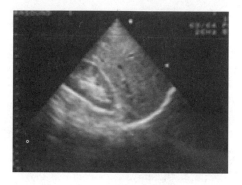

FIG. 100-26 Normal relationship between the kidney and the liver as viewed by the right lateral oblique window. The hepatic parenchyma nearest the top is closely opposed to the renal parenchyma. This close opposition obliterates Morison's pouch.

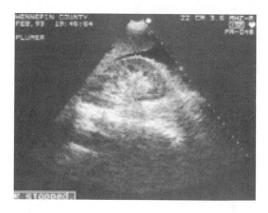

FIG. 100-27 Hemoperitoneum. The hepatic parenchyma nearest the top of the screen is separated from the renal parenchyma by an abnormal collection of fluid that is free-flowing and contains sharp acute angles.

Intraabdominal fluid appears as an anechoic strip within Morison's pouch separating the liver and the kidney (Fig. 100-27). This is the most sensitive window in detecting fluid. Trendelenburg positioning augments this examination. Note that free fluid appears with sharp angles in the recess of the peritoneal reflection. Rarely other intraabdominal contents appear in Morison's pouch; do not mistake fluid-filled loops of bowel for free abdominal fluid (Fig. 100-28). With greater experience the physician can use this view to

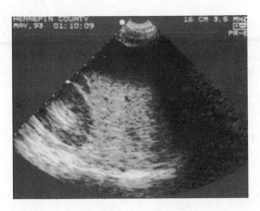

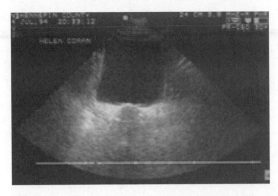

FIG. 100-28   Appearance of a loop of bowel transiently positioned between the liver and the kidney. The fluid within this loop of bowel is not free-flowing and does not result in sharp acute angles. Do not mistake for fluid within Morison's pouch.

FIG. 100-30   Normal suprapubic ultrasound. The large echofree structure nearest the top of the figure is the urine-filled bladder.

males. Reverse Trendelenburg position augments this examination. Unfortunately the bladder must be full for adequate examination. The pouch of Douglas can be imaged without a full bladder with transvaginal or transrectal sonography.

INTERPRETATION

Fresh unclotted blood appears anechoic and, when flowing freely, has sharp acute angles. As clotting begins, the organized blood displays different degrees of echogenicity. Consider the presence of free fluid in the setting of trauma, without preexisting free abdominal fluid, to be hemoperitoneum. Abdominal US does not quantify the amount of free abdominal fluid well. Most authors believe 250 ml of fluid can be detected in adults as a thin strip in Morison's pouch. A strip approaching 0.5 cm in width correlates to 500 ml fluid. The minimal amount of fluid detectable in pediatric patients is not known.

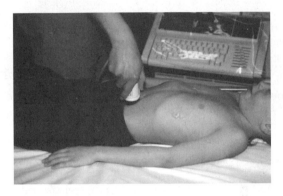

FIG. 100-29   Correct transducer position for obtaining the suprapubic window.

SUPRAPUBIC ULTRASONOGRAPHY

The evaluation of the febrile or septic infant requires collection and culture of different body fluids including urine. Urine can be collected by either bag, bladder catheterization, or suprapubic aspiration. Of these, suprapubic aspiration is the procedure of choice in certain clinical situations. This procedure is described in Chapter 71. Unfortunately blind suprapubic aspiration is often nonproductive and may occur in as many as half of all attempts. The physician may attempt aspiration two or three times before assuming the bladder is empty. This occurs most often when small volumes of urine are in the bladder. This unfortunately is most common in ill children who most urgently need the procedure. US can help increase the yield in these patients by determining the presence of urine before attempted aspiration.[24] This is not a US-guided technique; rather, it is a blind technique but only after the presence of bladder urine has been determined.

detect abnormal pleural subhepatic or perirenal fluid collections.

The next region to examine is the left lateral window. Obtain this view by placing the transducer in the left midaxial line with the marker dot toward the patient's feet (see Fig. 100-24). This is similar to the right lateral window, and the kidney serves as the critical landmark. It is more difficult to detect free abdominal fluid from this approach. This is because the fluid, which layers between the spleen and kidney, is not as well visualized as free fluid layered between the kidney and the liver. However with experience the physician can detect abnormal pleural fluid, intraparenchymal splenic lesions, and perisplenic abnormalities. Like the right lateral view this view can be augmented by the Trendelenburg position.

The most dependent portion of the abdomen can be visualized by using the suprapubic window. Obtain this by placing the transducer in the midline immediately cephalad to the symphysis pubis with the marker dot facing the patient's feet (see Fig. 100-24, Fig. 100-29). A full bladder serves as both an acoustic window and a landmark (Fig. 100-30). This window allows assessment of the pouch of Douglas, a peritoneal reflection and potential space between the posterior bladder and vagina in females and rectum in

Technique

To detect the presence of bladder urine place the transducer in the midline, immediately cephalad to the symphysis pubis with the marker dot toward the patient's feet (see Fig. 100-29). A urine-filled bladder appears as a large anechoic round structure (Fig. 100-30). Demonstrating this structure ensures that urine is present in the bladder and the physician can proceed with suprapubic aspiration. Reconsider the timing of the suprapubic aspiration if unable to demonstrate this structure.

REFERENCES

1. Agarwala BN, Ruschhaupt DG: Complete heart block from mycoplasma pneumoniae infection, *Pediatr Cardiol* 12(4):233-236, 1991.
2. Alcan KE, Zabetakis PM, Marino ND, et al: Management of acute cardiac tamponade by subxiphoid pericardiotomy, *JAMA,* 247(8):1143-1148, 1982.
3. Barrios V, Jimenez-Nacher J, Marin-Huerta E, et al: Successful surgical management of rupture of the left ventricle and interventricular septum due to blunt chest trauma: case report, *Scand J Thorac Cardiovasc Surg* 26(2):157-159, 1992.
4. Baxa MD: Cardiac rupture secondary to blunt trauma: a rapidly diagnosable entity with two-dimensional echocardiography, *Ann Emerg Med* 20(8):902-904.
5. Beggs CW, Helling TS, Evans LL, et al: Early evaluation of cardiac injury by two-dimensional echocardiography in patients suffering blunt chest trauma, *Ann Emerg Med* 16(5):542-545, 1987.
6. Beppu S, Tanaka N, Nakatani S, et al: Pericardial clot after open heart surgery: its specific localization and haemodynamics, *Eur Heart J* 14(2):230-234, 1993.
7. Bocka JJ, Overton DT, Hauser A: Electromechanical dissociation in human beings: an echocardiographic evaluation, *Ann Emerg Med* 17(5):450-452, 1988.
8. Bode PJ, Niezen RA, van Vugt AB, et al: Abdominal ultrasound as a reliable indicator for conclusive laparotomy in blunt abdominal trauma, *J Trauma* 34(1):27-31, 1993.
9. Brathwaite CE, Rodriguez A, Turney SZ, et al: Blunt traumatic cardiac rupture: a 5-year experience. *Ann Surg* 212(6): 701-704, 1990.
10. Bright EF, Beck CS: Non-penetrating wounds of heart: a clinical and experimental study, *Am Heart J* 10:293, 1935.
11. Chang TS, Lepanto L: Ultrasonography in the emergency setting, *Emerg Med Clin North Am* 10(1):1-25, 1992.
12. Chapman TP: Cardiac rupture in blunt trauma without external signs of chest injury, *West J Med* 151(6): 662-663, 1989.
13. Chuttani K, Pandian NG, Mohanty PK, et al: Left ventricular diastolic collapse: an echocardiographic sign of regional cardiac tamponade, *Circulation* 83(6):1999-2006, 1991.
14. Colucciello SA: Blunt abdominal trauma, *Emerg Med Clin North Am,* 11(1):107-123, 1993.
15. Conrad SA, Byrnes TJ: Brief communications: diastolic collapse of the left and right ventricles in cardiac tamponade, *Am Heart J* 115(2):475-478, 1988.
16. Demetriades D: Cardiac penetrating injuries: personal experience of 45 cases, Department of Surgery, Baragwanath Hospital, University of Witwatersrand, Johannesburg, South Africa.
17. Deutchman ME, Hahn RG, Rodney WM: Diagnostic ultrasound imaging by physicians of first contact: extending the family medicine experience into emergency medicine, *Ann Emerg Med* 22(3):594-596, 1993 (editorial).
18. Diaz de la Llera LS, Fernandez-Fernandez J, Garcia de la Llana MA, et al: Topographic diagnosis by two-dimensional echocardiography of an intramyocardial foreign body, *Rev Esp Cardiol* 44(1):62-65, 1991.
19. Eisenach JC, Nugent M, Miller FA Jr, et al: Echocardiographic evaluation of patients with blunt chest injury: correlation with perioperative hypotension, *Anesthesiology* 64(3):364-366, 1986.
20. Eisenberg MJ, Schiller NB: Bayes' theorem and the echocardiographic diagnosis of cardiac tamponade, *Am J Cardiol* 68(11):1242-1244, 1991.
21. Friedman HS, Gomes JA, Tardio AR, et al: The electrocardiographic features of acute cardiac tamponade, *Circulation* 50(2):260-265, 1974.
22. Fujii J, Sato H, Sawada H, et al: Echocardiographic assessment of left ventricular wall motion in myocarditis, *Heart Vessels Suppl* 1:116-121, 1985.
23. Grilliland MG, Ward RE, Flynn TC, et al: Peritoneal lavage and angiography in the management of patients with pelvic fractures, *Am J Surg* 144(6):744-747, 1982.
24. Gochman RF, Karasic RB, Heller MB: Use of portable ultrasound to assist urine collection by suprapubic aspiration, *Ann Emerg Med* 20(6):631-635, 1991.
25. Goldberg SP, Karalis DG, Ross JJ Jr: Severe right ventricular contusion mimicking cardiac tamponade: the value of transesophageal echocardiography in blunt chest trauma, *Ann Emerg Med* 22(4):745-747, 1993.
26. Grussner R, Ruckert K, Klotter HJ, et al: Ultrasonics and lavage in polytraumatized patients with blunt abdominal trauma, *Dtsch Med Wochenschr* 110(40):1521-1526, 1985.
27. Gueret P, Dubourg O, Ferrier A, et al: L'echocardiographie bidimensionnelle dans une unite de soins intensifs cardiologiques (Two-dimensional echocardiography in a cardiac intensive care unit), *Arch Mal Coeur* 79(11):1595-1600, 1986.
28. Hauser AM: The emerging role of echocardiography in the emergency department, *Ann Emerg Med* 18(12):1298-1303, 1989.
29. Henry WL, Demaria A, Gramiak R, et al: Report of the American Society of Echocardiography, Committee on Nomenclature and Standards in Two-Dimensional Echocardiography, *Circulation* 62:212-217, 1980.
30. Himelman RB, Kircher B, Rockey DC, et al: Inferior vena cava plethora with blunted respiratory response: a sensitive echocardiographic sign of cardiac tamponade, *J Am Coll Cardiol* 12(6):1470-1477, 1988.
31. Hubbard SG, Bivins BA, Sachatello CR, et al: Diagnostic errors with peritoneal lavage in patients with pelvic fractures, *Arch Surg* 114(7):844-846, 1979.
32. Ivatury RR, Rohman M, Steichen FM, et al: Penetrating cardiac injuries: twenty-year experience, *Am Surg* 53(6):310-317, 1987.
33. Kochar GS, Jacobs LE, Kotler MN: Right atrial compression in postoperative cardiac patients: detection by transesophageal echocardiography, *J Am Coll Cardiol* 16(2): 511- 516, 1990.
34. Kohlberger EJ, Strittmatter B, Lausen M, et al: Sonographische Akut- und Verlaufsdiagnostik nach stumpfem Bauchtrauma (Sonographic acute and follow-up diagnosis after blunt abdominal trauma), *Helv Chir Acta* 58(1-2):131-136, 1991.
35. Leavitt BJ, Meyer JA, Morton JR, et al: Survival following nonpenetrating traumatic rupture of cardiac chambers, *Ann Thorac Surg* 44(5):532-535, 1987.
36. Le Neel JC, Kohen M, Guiberteau B, et al: Traumatic rupture of the bladder: apropos of 11 cases, *Ann Chir* 44(3):217-225, 1990.
37. Leor J, Livschitz S, Vered Z: Giant breast hematoma requiring blood transfusion: an unusual complication after an echocardiographic study during thrombolytic therapy, *J Am Soc Echocardiogr* 3(6):502-504, 1990.
38. Marshall WG Jr, Bell JL, Kouchoukos NT: Penetrating cardiac trauma, *J Trauma* 24(2):147-149, 1984.
39. Mateer J, Plummer D, Heller M, et al: Model curriculum for physician training in emergency ultrasonography, *Ann Emerg Med* 23(1):95-102, 1994.
40. Mayron R, Gaudio FE, Plummer D, et al: Echocardiography performed by emergency physicians: impact on diagnosis and therapy, *Ann Emerg Med* 17(2):150-154, 1988.
41. McGrath RB: Electromechanical dissociation, *Ann Emerg Med* 18(1):114, 1989 (letter).
42. Meyer TE, Sareli P, Marcus RH, et al: Mechanism underlying Kussmaul's sign in chronic constrictive pericarditis, *Am J Cardiol* 64(16): 1069-1072, 1989.
43. Nasser FN, Giuliani ER: *Clinical two dimensional echocardiography,* Chicago, 1983, Year Book Medical.
44. Olsen WR, Hildreth DH: Abdominal paracentesis and peritoneal lavage in blunt abdominal trauma, *J Trauma* (10):824-829, 1971.
45. Orlando E, Fantini A, Boari C, et al: Ultrasuonocardiografia d'urgenza nelle precordialgie acute di origine cardiovascolare (Emergency ultrasound cardiography in acute precordial pain of cardiovascular origin), *Minerva Med* 78(16):1201-1218, 1987.
46. Pearlman AS, Gardin JM, Martin RP, et al: Guidelines for physician training in transesophageal echocardiography: recommendations of the American Society of Echocardiography Committee for Physician Training in Echocardiography, *J Am Soc Echocardiogr* 5(2):187-194, 1992.
47. Pichler W, Jantsch H, Barton P, et al: The role of sonography at the intensive care unit, *Rontgenpraxis* (12): P 407-411, 1989.

48. Piszczek I, Szyszka A, Ochotny R, et al: Value of echocardiographic examination in determining the etiology of cardiogenic shock: Clinico-echocardiographic correlations, *Kardiol Pol* 31(7):418-427, 1988.

49. Plummer D: Principles of emergency ultrasound and echocardiography, *Ann Emerg Med* 18(12):1291-1297, 1989 (Review).

50. Plummer D: Diagnostic ultrasonography in the emergency department, *Ann Emerg Med* 22(3):592-594, 1993 (editorial).

51. Plummer D, Brunette D, Asinger R, et al: Emergency department echocardiography improves outcome in penetrating cardiac injury, *Ann Emerg Med* 21(6):709-712, 1992.

52. Purdue B, Fernando GC: The mechanism of fatal cardiopulmonary injury caused by a blow from a golf club, *Forensic-Sci-Int* 42(1-2):125-130, 1989.

53. Reid CL, Chandraratna AN, Kawanishi D, et al: Echocardiographic detection of pneumomediastinum and pneumopericardium: the air gap sign, *J Am Coll Cardiol* 1(3):916-921, 1983.

54. Reid CL, Kawanishi DT, Rahimtoola SH, et al: Chest trauma: evaluation by two-dimensional echocardiography, *Am Heart J* 113(4):971-976, 1987.

55. Roscheck H, Marohl K, Freitag H, et al: Poly-, multiple trauma and intra-abdominal injuries, *Unfallchirurg* 93(7):327-330, 1990.

56. Rothlin M, Naf R, Amgwerd M, et al: How much experience is required for ultrasound diagnosis of blunt abdominal trauma? *Langenbecks Arch Chir* 377(4):211-215, 1992.

57. Roudaut R, Dallocchio M: Value of echocardiography in cardiological emergencies in adults. *Ann Cardiol Angeiol (Paris)* 34(9):599-608, 1985.

58. Rozycki GS, Ochsner MG, Jaffin JH: Prospective evaluation of surgeon's use of ultrasound in the evaluation of trauma patients, *J Trauma* 34(4): 516-527.

59. Russo AM, OConnor WH, Waxman HL: Atypical presentations and echocardiographic findings in patients with cardiac tamponade occurring early and late after cardiac surgery.

60. Schabelman SE, Ferdinand K, Poler M: Echocardiographic findings in a patient with tamponade due to anterior mediastinal hematoma, *South Med J* 76(10):1309-1311, 1983.

61. Schiavone WA, Ghumrawi BK, Catalano DR, et al: The use of echocardiography in the emergency management of nonpenetrating traumatic cardiac rupture, *Ann Emerg Med* 20(11):1248-1250, 1991.

62. Schnarkowski P, Brecht-Krauss D, Goldmann A, et al: Sonographic detection of splenic injuries after blunt abdominal trauma, *Ultraschall Med* 12(6):293-296, 1991.

63. Schulz RD, Willi U: Ultrasound diagnosis following blunt abdominal injury in childhood, *Ultraschall Med* 4(3):154-159, 1983.

64. Schwarz KQ, Meltzer RS: TI experience rounding with a hand-held two-dimensional cardiac ultrasound device, *Am J Cardiol* 62(1):157-159, 1988.

65. Shoemaker WC, Carey JS, Yao ST, et al: Hemodynamic monitoring for physiologic evaluation, diagnosis, and therapy of acute hemopericardial tamponade from penetrating wounds, *J Trauma* 13(1):36-44, 1973.

66. Wening JV: Evaluation of ultrasound, lavage, and computed tomography in blunt abdominal trauma, *Surg Endosc* 3(3):152-158, 1989.

67. West RJ, Mangiante EC, Fabian TC: Penetrating cardiac wounds, *J Tenn Med Assoc* 79(1):32-33, 1986.

68. Whye D, Barish R, Almquist T, et al: Echocardiographic diagnosis of acute pericardial effusion in penetrating chest trauma, *Am J Emerg Med* 6(1):21-23, 1988.

69. Widimsky P, Gregor P, Cervenka V, et al: Severe diffuse hypokinesis of the remote myocardium—the main cause of cardiogenic shock? An echocardiographic study of 75 patients with extremely large myocardial infarctions, *Cor-Vasa* 30(1):27-34, 1988.

70. Wilson DB, Vacek JL: Echocardiography: basics for the primary care physician, *Postgrad Med* 87(5):191-193, 196-202, 1990.

TOXICOLOGY TECHNIQUES

101 Gastric Emptying

Marc Gorelick

Each year over 2 million cases of toxic exposures occur in the United States, and the incidence appears to be increasing.[37] Over 70% of these occur in children less than 20 years of age. Although many of these poisonings cause no symptoms, serious morbidity and mortality do occur. In 1991 more than 12,000 pediatric and adolescent poisonings caused moderate to severe effects requiring treatment, with 112 fatalities reported.

The number of toxins with specific antidotes is small. Therefore after initial resuscitation and stabilization the treatment of acute poisoning generally focuses on three objectives: removal of the toxin, prevention of further absorption from the gastrointestinal (GI) tract, and enhanced elimination of substances that have already entered the systemic circulation. Many widely accepted interventions lack evidence supporting their use. More rigorous and systematic evaluation in recent years has engendered controversy and led to continual reassessment of the management of ingestions.[18,19,21,57,62]

One area of debate is the relative effectiveness of ipecac-induced emesis versus lavage in achieving gastric emptying. Several studies have found ipecac to be more effective[1,7,71]; lavage has performed better in others[5,60]; still others have failed to demonstrate clear superiority of either.[12,16,63] Methodologic differences make comparisons of studies difficult, and the best gastric emptying technique is largely dependent on clinical circumstances. More recently experts have called into question the value of any form of gastric emptying and several authors have demonstrated equivalent or better results with activated charcoal alone.* However, because of the small number of critically ill patients (particularly children) in these studies, extrapolation to the clinical situation of a life-threatening pediatric overdose is problematic.

There is at present no single optimal strategy for the treatment of pediatric poisonings.[22,51] In making treatment decisions use an individualized approach based on the timing, nature, and dose of the ingested substance, as well as the child's clinical status.

INDUCED EMESIS

Induction of emesis is the oldest known method of treatment for ingested toxins, with references to various agents found in classical Greek and Latin medical treatises.[51] As doubts about the efficacy of gastric emptying grow[2,34,36,47] and alternative treatment strategies become more widespread, the use of induced emesis has declined in recent years.[37] However, it remains an important part of the emergency management of poisoning under certain circumstances.

Indications

Induction of emesis may be indicated in alert patients who have ingested potentially toxic substances. Emetic agents reduce the amount of toxin in the gastrointestinal tract[1,5,60,63,71] and decrease the absorption of orally administered substances.* The benefit is greatest shortly after an ingestion; there is a significant reduction in effectiveness if administration is delayed.[4,6,50] Thus at present induce emesis primarily for poisoning first aid in the home. Syrup of ipecac is a commonly available over-the-counter emetic agent appropriate for home use.[9] Although administration of ipecac in the hospital setting is becoming less common, potential indications in the Emergency Department include ingestion of toxic compounds that bind poorly to activated charcoal and that would be difficult to remove by gastric lavage (e.g., plant parts, large pills) or patient admission within minutes of exposure.[22]

Contraindications

Box 101-1 lists contraindications to the use of emetics.[9,19,57] Aspiration risk is high in patients who have a depressed level of consciousness or who have ingested a compound with potential to cause rapid neurologic deterioration (e.g., camphor, strychnine, isoniazid, tricyclic antidepressants, nicotine, cocaine). Presume that the risk is also higher in infants less than 6 months of age, although no data exist to support or refute this assumption. Emesis after ingestion of corrosive substances may cause repeated injury to the esophagus.

---

*References 6, 16, 22, 33, 49, 50, and 51.

BOX 101-1 **CONTRAINDICATIONS TO INDUCED EMESIS**

Age less than 6 months
Depressed level of consciousness or seizures
Agents causing rapid neurologic deterioration
    Tricyclic antidepressants
    Camphor
    Strychnine
    Isoniazid
    Nicotine
    Cocaine
Hydrocarbon ingestion
Caustic agents (strong acids or alkali)
Bleeding diathesis
Late stage of pregnancy
Severe cardiac or respiratory disease
Uncontrolled hypertension

---

*References 2, 13, 16, 33, 34, 36, 47, 50, and 63.

Because most hydrocarbons have greater toxicity in pulmonary aspiration than in systemic absorption, emesis is contraindicated. Exceptions are those compounds with greater systemic toxicity indicated by the mnemonic CHAMP (*c*amphor, *h*alogenated and *a*romatic hydrocarbons, heavy *m*etal-containing compounds, *p*esticides).[19] Use caution in patients with a bleeding diathesis, uncontrolled hypertension, severe cardiac or respiratory disease or in late stages of pregnancy. Finally studies have shown that ipecac delays the time to administration of activated charcoal.[34,36] Avoid it when charcoal is the preferred treatment (see later discussion).

Complications

Adverse effects associated with administration of recommended doses of syrup of ipecac are generally mild; they include prolonged vomiting, diarrhea, fever, and lethargy or irritability.[14,67] Chronic misuse of syrup of ipecac or use of the much more potent ipecac fluid extract, a preparation that is no longer commercially available,[3] may produce more serious effects, such as cardiomyopathy, muscle weakness, dehydration, and seizures. Emesis induced by syrup of ipecac has also reportedly caused Mallory-Weiss tears[61] and pneumomomediastinum.[70] Apomorphine, another emetic, may cause typical narcotic effects of respiratory depression, central nervous system depression, and hypotension.[39,57]

Equipment

The most widely used emetic agent is syrup of ipecac, derived from the roots of a plant native to South America. Both central and local mechanisms mediate its emetic effect. It is available in 15-ml and 30-ml unit dose bottles. Another emetic still used occasionally is apomorphine, a narcotic analogue.[39] Because of its potential toxicity and the need for parenteral administration, its use is infrequent at present. Household dish soap is also an effective emetic and a suitable substitute when ipecac is unavailable.[24,56] Copper sulfate[32] and salt water[17,55] have unacceptably high risks associated with their use. Mechanical induction of emesis by gagging, also advocated in the past, is ineffective.[15]

Other supplies include an emesis basin, towels, and extra gowns. Have oxygen and airway equipment, as well as suction, available. Obtain a syringe with a small-gauge subcutaneous needle for administration of apomorphine; also have a narcotic antagonist such as naloxone on hand when using this agent.

Technique

Give syrup of ipecac orally in an age-dependent dose (Table 101-1): 6 to 12 months of age, 10 ml; 1 to 12 years, 15 ml; greater than 12 years, 30 ml.[19,67] Repeat the same dose if no vomiting has occurred within 20 to 30 minutes. Some authors have recommended a higher initial dose of 30 ml for younger children, giving a lower failure rate and shorter time to emesis.[35] The use of expired ipecac does not appear to diminish its effectiveness.[26,30]

Administer fluids with ipecac. Recommended volumes are typically 2 to 4 ounces for young children and 8 to 16 ounces for older children and adults,[19] although studies have shown no effect of the amount of fluid on ipecac's efficacy.[23] Similarly one may give fluids before or after ipecac administration with equivalent results.[8] Alternatively one may use

Table 101-1   Dose of Syrup of Ipecac

Age	Dose
6-12 Months	10 ml
1-12 Years	15 ml
Over 12 Years	30 ml

milk, as it does not alter the effectiveness of ipecac.[27] Finally it is unnecessary to have the child jump or move around after ipecac administration, since this does not affect its action.[46]

A standard dose of ipecac produces emesis in 91% to 100% of children, in an average of 20 minutes (range 14 to 37 minutes),* although time to emesis increases in younger children.[38] The average duration of vomiting is 24 to 56 minutes.[38,67]

An alternative to ipecac is apomorphine in a dose of 0.07 mg/kg subcutaneously.[39] Give fluids orally as described. The time to emesis is generally shorter than with ipecac, approximately 4 minutes. Do not use repeated doses if emesis does not occur. An effective dose of liquid dish soap is 3 tablespoons (45 ml) in 8 ounces of water, yielding similar results to those of the usual dose of ipecac.[24] Liquid detergents intended for laundry or electric dishwashers are toxic; avoid using them.

GASTRIC LAVAGE

Removal of toxic substances from the stomach by means of a hollow tube began in the early nineteenth century with the work of Physick and Dupuytren.[40] An 1869 publication by Kussmaul gained wider popularity for this mode of therapy, which was a mainstay in the management of poisoning for the following hundred years. In recent decades, with continued controversy over its utility (see previous discussion), gastric lavage no longer occupies this central position in the treatment of ingestions. Yet approximately 12% of poisoned patients treated at a health-care facility[37] still undergo the procedure, and it remains an important intervention in selected situations.

Indications

Gastric lavage, in current usage, serves primarily as an adjunct to the administration of activated charcoal, the treatment of choice for most ingestions. Consider several factors in the decision to perform lavage. First critically ill or severely intoxicated patients are more likely to benefit from gastric emptying,[10,22,36,66] and they are usually not candidates for ipecac because of impaired airway protective reflexes. Perform lavage in such patients after adequate airway protection.

Timing is also important. Studies of lavage have shown reduced efficacy after 1 or 2 hours after ingestion[10,36]; however the procedure may yield a substantial return up to 4 or more hours after ingestion of substances that delay gastric emptying (e.g., barbiturates, anticholinergic drugs).[10,66] Sustained-release preparations and poorly soluble compounds (e.g., iron salt, salicylates) are also amenable to delayed lavage.[57,66]

*References 11, 25, 35, 38, 39, and 58.

Consider gastric lavage for known or suspected large quantity ingestions. Recovery increases with the amount of the ingestion.[10] Moreover, massive overdoses exceed the adsorptive capacity of charcoal, and lavage may have added benefit.[49]

Contraindications

Gastric lavage is contraindicated in caustic ingestions, because of the risk of esophageal perforation, and in hydrocarbon ingestions, where the risk of aspiration is great. Obtunded or comatose individuals with an unprotected airway are at high risk for aspiration; perform lavage only after taking adequate steps to protect the airway. Avoid the nasogastric route if there is concomitant head or facial trauma with suspicion of basilar skull fracture, as this may lead to inadvertent intracranial tube placement.[25]

Complications

Placement of a gastric tube is a noxious stimulus and consequently may cause a great deal of discomfort in awake patients (Box 101-2). Gastric tube placement may induce significant tachycardia, generally self-limited, in such individuals.[64] Transient decreases in arterial oxygen saturation may occur during the procedure, but these changes are trivial in younger, nonsmoking patients.[31,64]

Epistaxis is a common, albeit minor, sequela of use of the nasal route. More serious adverse effects arising from mechanical factors include esophageal or gastric tears or perforation, which are rare in otherwise normal individuals.[36,42] In young children electrolyte imbalance may result from the use of large volumes of hypotonic or hypertonic lavage solutions.[69] Older patients are less prone to suffer such effects.[53] Similarly small children may be at risk for hypothermia from unwarmed lavage fluid.[62]

Pulmonary aspiration constitutes the most serious potential risk during gastric lavage; it is reported in 0% to 8.5% of patients undergoing the procedure.[36,43,47] Of note, aspiration may occur even in the presence of an endotracheal tube.[47] However the incidence of serious aspiration events with properly performed gastric lavage appears to be quite low.[18]

Equipment

Basic supplies required for performance of gastric lavage include a gastric tube; a water-soluble lubricant (K-Y Jelly); a cup of water with straw; 60-ml syringes; lavage solution; basins for lavage solution and discarded aspirates; a basin of ice; stethoscope; tape; and towels. In addition prepare for suction and other endotracheal intubation equipment to be immediately available.

BOX 101-2 COMPLICATIONS OF GASTRIC LAVAGE

Epistaxis
Esophageal/gastric tear or perforation
Pulmonary aspiration
Electrolyte imbalance
Hypothermia
Tachycardia
Oxygen desaturation

Table 101-2 *Specialized Lavage Solutions*

Ingested substance	Lavage solution	Resulting compound
Iron	2% Sodium bicarbonate (50 mEq in 150-ml normal saline solution)	Ferrous carbonate (insoluble)
Iodine	75 g Corn starch in 1 L H_2O	Iodide (nontoxic)
Oxalic acid	15-30 g/L Calcium gluconate	Calcium oxalate (insoluble)
Fluorides	15-30 g/L Calcium gluconate	Calcium fluoride (insoluble)
Formaldehyde	10 mg/L Ammonium acetate	Methenamine (nontoxic)

The use of the largest-diameter tube that can be passed is usually recommended.[19,25] A study using an animal model of pediatric ingestion, however, demonstrated no difference in efficacy between No. 16 French and No. 32 French tubes.[20] Although very large–bore tubes more reliably recover large pill fragments, it may be impossible to insert a tube of adequate size for this task in a young child. Prevent unnecessary trauma by selecting a tube that, although large enough to allow aspiration of gastric contents, passes with relative ease. Typical sizes are 14 to 26 French for children and 24 to 40 French for adolescents (see Chapter 62).

Normal saline solution is the preferred lavage solution for most ingestions requiring 2 to 5 liters. Warming the fluid to 40° to 45° C increases the efficacy of emptying,[45] as well as decreasing the risk of hypothermia in very young children. For certain toxins a special lavage solution may act as a neutralizer that converts the ingested substance to one that is less toxic or less soluble.[28,59,62] Examples are listed in Table 101-2.

Technique

Protect the airway of patients with altered consciousness who lack an adequate gag reflex with an endotracheal tube before initiation of gastric lavage. Awake patients and those who are lethargic but have intact airway protective reflexes do not require endotracheal intubation.[19]

Insert the gastric tube via the nasal or oral route; pass very-large-bore tubes through the mouth. Before placement determine the correct length by measuring the distance from the nose to the earlobe and then to the tip of the xiphoid process[68] (Fig. 101-1). Mark the appropriate distance on the tube with tape. Lubricate the end of the tube and insert it into the naris along the floor of the nasal passage. Direct the tip downward and allow it to curve around into the nasopharynx. If excessive resistance is detected, select a smaller tube. A topical vasoconstrictor such as oxymetazoline (Afrin) may be of help.[65] If the tube is too flexible to pass, use a larger size or stiffen the end by chilling it in ice.[54] Facilitate passage of the tube into the esophagus by dropping the child's head forward. Awake, cooperative patients can take sips of water through a straw, advancing the tube with each swallow.[68] If the tube fails to advance, withdraw it as far as the posterior pharynx and repeat the attempt. In awake patients gagging, coughing, and cyanosis are signs of pas-

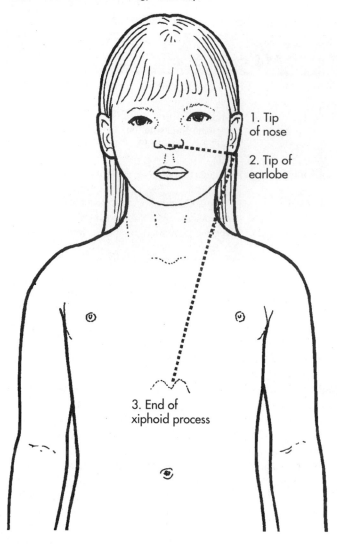

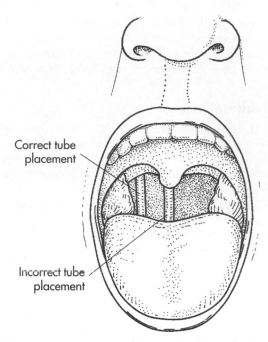

FIG. 101-2 Nasogastric tube in the posterior pharynx, laterally placed.

FIG. 101-1 Nasogastric tube length being measured before insertion.

sage into the trachea; remove the tube immediately. Manual forward displacement of the larynx by gripping the thyroid cartilage may aid in advancing the gastric tube in intubated patients.[52]

After reaching the premeasured distance, use a syringe to aspirate. Recovery of gastric contents indicates placement in the stomach; send the initial aspirate for toxicologic assay if needed. Confirm correct tube placement by auscultation over the stomach while injecting 30 to 60 ml of air. Note a "whooshing" sound immediately; muffling, delay, or absence of such sound indicates malposition of the tube in the esophagus or thorax.[48] Lack of phonation may signal passage

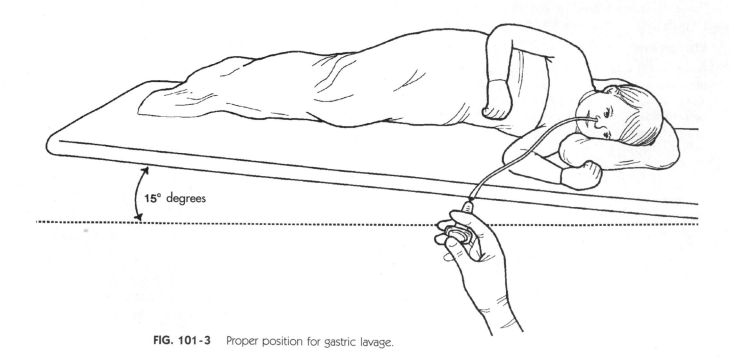

FIG. 101-3 Proper position for gastric lavage.

of the tube into the larynx, as does placement of the tube in a central, rather than lateral, position in the oropharynx[44] (Fig. 101-2). In small children auscultation alone may be misleading. If there is uncertainty about the correct position of the tube in the stomach, obtain a radiograph for confirmation before proceeding.

Perform the lavage with the child in the left lateral decubitus position[62] (Fig. 101-3). This increases the yield of gastric contents and minimizes passage of material beyond the pylorus. In addition, placement of the patient in slight Trendelenburg position, with the head down, decreases the risk of aspiration in the event of vomiting.[29]

Instill small aliquots of lavage fluid—approximately 10 to 15 ml/kg, up to 200 to 400 ml/kg in adolescents and adults[57]—into the stomach and remove after 1 to 2 minutes. Repeat the cycle until the aspirate remains clear. Gentle epigastric massage during this process appears to enhance the recovery of ingested material.[45]

After completion of lavage use the nasogastric tube for administration of activated charcoal. Some authors[28,51] recommend giving a dose of charcoal at the start of the lavage procedure as well.

REFERENCES

1. Abdallah AH, Tye A: A comparison of the efficacy of emetic drugs and stomach lavage, *Am J Dis Child* 113:571-575, 1967.
2. Albertson TE, Derlet RW, Foulke GE, et al: Superiority of activated charcoal alone compared with ipecac and activated charcoal in the treatment of acute toxic ingestions, *Ann Emerg Med* 18:56-59, 1989.
3. Allport RB: Ipecac is not innocuous, *Am J Dis Child* 98:786-787, 1959.
4. Amitai Y, Mitchell AA, McGuigan MA, et al: Ipecac-induced emesis and reduction of plasma concentrations of drugs following accidental overdose in children, *Pediatrics* 80:364-367, 1987.
5. Auerbach PS, Osterloh J, Braun O, et al: Efficacy of gastric emptying: gastric lavage versus emesis induced with ipecac, *Ann Emerg Med* 15:692-698, 1986.
6. Bond GR, Requa RK, Krenzelok EP, et al: Influence of time until emesis on the efficacy of decontamination using acetaminophen as a marker in a pediatric population, *Ann Emerg Med* 22:1403-1407, 1993.
7. Boxer L, Anderson FP, Rowe DS: Comparison of ipecac-induced emesis with gastric lavage in the treatment of acute salicylate ingestion, *J Pediatr* 74:800-803, 1969.
8. Bukis D, Kuwahara L, Robertson WO: Results of forcing fluids: pre- versus post-ipecac, *Vet Hum Toxicol* 20:90-91, 1978.
9. Chafee-Bahamon C, Lacouture PG, Lovejoy FH: Risk assessment of ipecac in the home, *Pediatrics* 75:1105-1109, 1985.
10. Comstock EG, Faulkner TP, Boisaubin EV, et al: Studies on the efficacy of gastric lavage as practiced in a large metropolitan hospital, *Clin Toxicol* 18:581-597, 1981.
11. Corby DG, Decker WJ, Moran MJ, et al: Clinical comparison of pharmacologic emetics in children, *Pediatrics* 42:361-364, 1968.
12. Corby DJ, Lisciandro RC, Lehman RH, et al: The efficiency of methods used to evacuate the stomach after acute ingestions, *Pediatrics* 40:871-874, 1967.
13. Curtis RA, Barone J, Giacona N: Efficacy of ipecac and activated charcoal/cathartic: prevention of salicylate absorption in a simulated ovedose, *Arch Intern Med* 144:48-52, 1984.
14. Czajka PA, Russell SL: Nonemetic effects off ipecac syrup, *Pediatrics* 75:1101-1104, 1985.
15. Dabbous IA, Bergman AB, Robertson WO: The ineffectiveness of mechanically induced vomiting, *J Pediatr* 66:952-954, 1965.
16. Danel V, Henry JA, Glucksman E: Activated charcoal, emesis, and gastric lavage in aspirin overdose, *Br Med J* 296:1507, 1988.
17. DeGenaro F, Nyhan WL: Salt—a dangerous antidote, *J Pediatr* 78:1048-1049, 1974.
18. Easom JM, Lovejoy FH: Efficacy and safety of gastrointestinal decon-

19. Ellenhorn MJ, Barceloux DG: Gut decontamination. In Ellenhorn MJ, Barceloux DG, editors: *Medical toxicology: diagnosis and treatment of human poisoning,* New York, 1988, Elsevier Science, pp 54-63.
20. Fane LR, Combs HF, Decker WJ: Physical parameters in gastric lavage, *Clin Toxicol* 4:389-395, 1971.
21. Fine JS, Goldfrank LR: Update in medical toxicology, *Pediatr Clin North Am* 39:1031-1051, 1992.
22. Fleisher GR, Kearney TE, Henretig F, et al: Gastric decontamination in the poisoned patient, *Pediatr Emerg Care* 7:378-381, 1991.
23. Friday KJ, Powell SH, Thompson WL, et al: Fluid administration in induced emesis: efficacy independent of ingested volume, *Vet Hum Toxicol* 22:365, 1980.
24. Gieseker DR, Troutman WG: Emergency induction of emesis using liquid detergent products: a report of fifteen cases, *Clin Toxicol* 18:277-282, 1981.
25. Glauser JM: Nasogastric intubation. In Roberts JR, Hedges JR, editors: *Clinical procedures in emergency medicine,* ed 2, Philadelphia, 1991, WB Saunders, pp 640-649.
26. Grbcich PA, Lacouture PG, Kresel JJ, et al: Effectiveness of expired ipecac syrup, *Vet Hum Toxicol* 28:317, 1985.
27. Grbcich PA, Lacouture PG, Lewander WJ, et al: Effect of milk on ipecac-induced emesis, *J Pediatr* 110:973-975, 1987.
28. Haddad LM, Winchester JF: A general approach to the emergency management of poisoning. In Haddad LM, Winchester JF, editors: Clinical management of poisoning and drug overdose, ed 2, Philadelphia, 1990, WB Saunders, pp 4-22.
29. Hall AH, Rumack BH: Prevention of absorption in drug overdose. In Callaham ML, editor: *Current therapy in emergency medicine;* Philadelphia, 1987, BC Decker, pp 942-944.
30. Hornfeldt CS, Rogers AA: Efficacy of expired syrup of ipecac, *Vet Hum Toxicol* 26:319, 1984.
31. Jorens PG, Joosens EJ, Nagler JM: Changes in arterial oxygen tension after gastric lavage for drug overdose, *Human Toxicol* 10:221-224, 1991.
32. Karlsson B, Noren L: Ipecacuanha and copper sulphate as emetics in intoxications in children, *Acta Pediatr Scand* 54:331-335, 1965.
33. Kirk MA, Peterson J, Kulig K, et al: Acetaminophen overdose in children: a comparison of ipecac versus activated charcoal versus no gastrointestinal decontamination, *Ann Emerg Med* 20:472-473, 1991.
34. Kornberg AE, Dolgin J: Pediatric ingestions: charcoal alone versus ipecac and charcoal, *Ann Emerg Med* 20:648-651, 1991.
35. Krenzelok EP, Dean BS: Syrup of ipecac failures: a two year review of 4306 cases, *Vet Hum Toxicol* 28:317, 1985.
36. Kulig K, Bar-Or D, Cantrill SV, et al: Management of acutely poisoned patients without gastric emptying, *Ann Emerg Med* 14:562-567, 1985.
37. Litovitz TL, Holm KC, Bailey KM, et al: 1991 Annual report of the American Association of Poison Control Centers National Data Collection System, *Am J Emerg Med* 10:452-505, 1992.
38. Litovitz TL, Klein-Schwartz W, Oderda GM, et al: Ipecac administration in children younger than 1 year of age, *Pediatrics* 76:761-764, 1985.
39. MacLean WC: A comparison of ipecac syrup and apomorphine in the immediate treatment of ingestion of poisons, *J Pediatr* 82:121-124, 1973.
40. Major RH: History of the stomach tube, *Ann Med Hist* 6:500-509, 1934.
41. Reference deleted in proofs.
42. Mariani PJ, Pook N: Gastrointestinal tract perforation with charcoal peritoneum complicating orogastric intubation and lavage, *Ann Emerg Med* 22:606-609, 1993.
43. Matthew H, Mackintosh TF, Tompsett SL, et al: Gastric aspiration and lavage in acute poisoning, *Br Med J* 1:1333-1337, 1966.
44. May M, Nellis KJ: Nasogastric intubation: avoiding complications, *Resid Staff Physician* 30:60-62, 1984.
45. McDougal CB, Maclean MA: Modifications in the technique of gastric lavage, *Ann Emerg Med* 10:514-517, 1981.
46. Meester WD: Emesis and lavage, *Vet Hum Toxicol* 122:225-234, 1980.
47. Merigian KS, Woodard M, Hedges JR, et al: Prospective evaluation of gastric emptying in the self-poisoned patient, *Am J Emerg Med* 8:479-483, 1990.

48. Metheny N: Measures to test placement of nasogastric and nasointestinal tubes: a review, *Nurs Res* 37:324-329, 1988.

49. Neuvonen PJ, Okkola KT: Oral activated charcoal in the treatment of intoxications: role of single and repeated doses, *Med Toxicol* 3:33-58, 1988.

50. Neuvonen PJ, Vartiainen M, Tokola O: Comparison of activated charcoal and ipecac syrup in prevention of drug absorption, *Eur J Clin Pharmacol* 24:557-562, 1983.

51. Olson KR: Is gut emptying all washed up? *Am J Emerg Med* 8:560-561, 1990.

52. Perel A, Ya'ari Y, Pizov R: Forward displacement of the larynx for nasogastric tube insertion in intubated patients, *Crit Care Med* 13:204-205, 1985.

53. Peterson CD: Electrolyte depletion following emergency stomach evacuation, *Am J Hosp Pharm* 36:1366-1369, 1979.

54. Ratzlaff HC, Heaslip JE, Rothwell ES: Factors affecting nasogastric tube insertion, *Crit Care Med* 12:52-53, 1984.

55. Roberts CJC, Noakes MJ: Danger of saline emetics in first-aid for poisoning, *Br Med J* 2:683, 1974.

56. Rodgers GC, Fort P: Use of dish soap as an emetic in the outpatient management of accidental poisonings—an update, *Vet Hum Toxicol* 28 (abstr):321, 1985.

57. Rodgers GC, Matyunas NJ: Gastrointestinal decontamination for acute poisoning, *Pediatr Clin North Am* 33:261-285, 1986.

58. Shirkey HC: Ipecac syrup: its use as an emetic in poison control, *J Pediatr* 69:139-141, 1966.

59. Skoutakis VA: *Clinical toxicology of drugs: principles and practice,* Philadelphia, 1982, Lea & Febiger, pp 12-13.

60. Tandberg D, Diven BG, McLeod JW: Ipecac-induced emesis versus gastric lavage: a controlled study in normal adults, *Am J Emerg Med* 4:205-209, 1986.

61. Tandberg D, Liechty EJ, Fishbein D: Mallory-Weiss syndrome: an unusual complication of ipecac-induced emesis, *Ann Emerg Med* 10:521-523, 1981.

62. Tandberg D, Troutman WG: Gastric lavage in the poisoned patient. In Roberts JR, Hedges JR, editors: Clinical procedures in emergency medicine, ed 2, Philadelphia, 1991, WB Saunders, pp 655-662.

63. Tenebein M, Cohen S, Sitar DS: Efficacy of ipecac-induced emesis, orogastric lavage, and activated charcoal for acute drug overdose, *Ann Emerg Med* 16:838-841, 1987.

64. Thompson AM, Robins JB, Prescott LF: Changes in cardiorespiratory function during gastric lavage for drug overdose, *Human Toxicol* 6:215-218, 1987.

65. Tucker A, Lewis J: Passing a nasogastric tube, *Br Med J* 281:1128-1129, 1981.

66. Value of gastric lavage in treatment of acute poisoning, *JAMA* 133:545-546, 1947 (editorial).

67. Veltri JC, Temple AR: Telephone management of poisonings using syrup of ipecac, *Clin Toxicol* 9:407-417, 1976.

68. Volden C, Grinde J, Carl D: Taking the trauma out of nasogastric intubation, *Nurs' 80* 10:64-67, 1980.

69. Wheeler-Usher DH, Wanke LA, Bayer MJ: Gastric emptying: risks versus benefits in the treatment of acute poisoning, *Med Toxicol* 1:142-153, 1986.

70. Wolowodiuk OJ, McMicken DB, O'Brien P: Pneumomediastinum and retropneumoperitoneum: an unusual complication of syrup of ipecac-induced emesis, *Ann Emerg Med* 13:1148-1151, 1984.

71. Young WF Jr, Bivins HG: Evaluation of gastric emptying using radionuclides: gastric lavage versus ipecac-induced emesis, *Ann Emerg Med* 22:1423-1427, 1993.

102 Gut Decontamination

Marc Gorelick

ACTIVATED CHARCOAL

Given the limitations of gastric emptying techniques, attention has shifted to other strategies of gastrointestinal decontamination that can prevent absorption or hasten elimination of toxins that have already passed the pylorus or even entered the systemic circulation. Activated charcoal, by virtue of its ability to bind a wide variety of chemical compounds, gained attention as a therapeutic agent for ingestions as early as the nineteenth century.[23] However, it has become widely accepted in this country only in the past two decades.[37] A growing body of literature now supports the sole use of activated charcoal for most ingestions.*

Activated charcoal is prepared by pyrolysis of organic material, typically wood pulp, which is then "activated" by treatment with steam. The resulting fine black powder has an extensive network of pores with a tremendous surface area (approximately 1000 m^2/g), accounting for charcoal's adsorptive properties.[43] It is relatively inexpensive, nontoxic, and easy to store and administer, all of which contribute to its current popularity in the emergency management of poisonings.

Indications

The list of substances adsorbed by charcoal is extensive; it is simpler to enumerate the exceptions (Box 102-1).[13,20,24,37] Single-dose charcoal is indicated when a potentially toxic amount of a substance that charcoal can bind has been ingested. Even when a drug known to be poorly adsorbed is involved, the use of charcoal may be appropriate if other coingestants are suspected, as in the case of adolescent self-poisoning. Consider charcoal in the child with signs or symptoms suggestive of an intoxication (e.g., altered mental status, unexplained metabolic acidosis) even in the absence of a known history of ingestion. Although the effectiveness of charcoal is greatest when given shortly after an ingestion, overdose delays absorption of drugs considerably. Thus charcoal can be given even 3 or 4 hours after the event; the upper limit is not known.[39]

Although the main action of a single dose of activated charcoal is to prevent systemic absorption by binding toxins in the gastrointestinal (GI) tract, multiple-dose charcoal may be useful for some drugs by increasing their elimination through a process referred to as *gastrointestinal dialysis*.[31] Charcoal binds compounds with substantial diffusion across the intestinal mucosa, generally those with small volumes of distribution, in the intestinal lumen, preventing back diffusion into the circulation and effectively reducing the elimination half-life. Box 102-2 lists drugs for which multiple doses of charcoal may be effective.† The decision to use

repeated doses of charcoal should take into account the nature and quantity of the substance involved and the toxicity observed or expected.[55]

Contraindications

Do not administer charcoal after ingestion of corrosive substances, as these are not adsorbed and charcoal makes endoscopy difficult. Use charcoal cautiously in patients with an ileus. Box 102-1 lists substances that charcoal adsorbs poorly; however, administration is not harmful and is not specifically contraindicated. Previous recommendations suggest that charcoal be withheld in cases of acetaminophen overdose because of the potential for inactivating N-acetylcysteine (NAC), a specific antidote. Although charcoal binds NAC,[7] the effect on NAC absorption appears to be clinically unimportant.[41,47] Charcoal may therefore be used concomitantly with NAC, although some authors recommend increasing the dose of NAC by 30% to 40%.[16,19]

> ### BOX 102-1 SUBSTANCES POORLY BOUND TO CHARCOAL
>
> Alcohols
> Strong acids and alkali
> Aliphatic hydrocarbons (e.g., kerosene, benzene)
> Boric acid
> Cyanide
> Heavy metals (iron, lead, mercury)
> Lithium
> Mineral acids
> Pesticides

> ### BOX 102-2 DRUGS DEMONSTRATING ENHANCED CLEARANCE WITH MULTIPLE-DOSE CHARCOAL
>
> Carbamazepine
> Digoxin
> Glutethimide
> Nadolol
> Phenobarbital
> Phenylbutazone
> Theophylline
> Tricyclic antidepressants

---

*References 1, 9-11, 26, 29, 30, 35, 40, and 59.
†References 2, 3, 24, 31, 37, 38, 43, 53, and 55.

Complications

The most common side effects of activated charcoal are nausea and vomiting, which are more frequent with rapid administration.[37,39] Constipation may also occur but is usually mild. Rare reports of intestinal obstruction exist.[61] Conversely diarrhea may occur with coadministration of cathartics such as sorbitol,[33] particularly with multiple doses. Repeated doses of a charcoal-sorbitol mixture may also produce hypernatremic dehydration.[15,17] Aspiration of charcoal can cause airway obstruction, bronchospasm, and pneumonitis.[34,45] A minor but frequent practical problem is staining from charcoal spills or vomitus.

Equipment

Commercially available charcoal preparations include unit dose bottles of 15 to 50 grams (60 to 240 ml), either as a plain aqueous suspension or premixed with sorbitol (usually 70% weight/volume [w/v]). In unconscious or uncooperative patients who require charcoal via a nasogastric tube also gather additional supplies for gastric tube placement (see Chapter 101).

Technique

The usual initial dose of charcoal is 1 g/kg, or 50 to 100 g in adolescents and adults.[36] However the effectiveness of charcoal is dependent on the ratio of charcoal to the amount of drug ingested rather than on body weight; a ratio of charcoal/poison of 10:1 is optimal.[37] Since there is no dose-dependent toxicity of charcoal, an estimated initial dose of 25 to 50 g is reasonable for most young children.[54]

Give charcoal orally when possible. Although conventional wisdom holds that cooperation by young children in this endeavor is problematic, investigators have found it to be readily accepted by the majority of young children in whom it was used.[6] The addition of sorbitol appears to enhance charcoal's palatability.[8,44,50] Chocolate or cherry syrup may be added for flavoring, but avoid foods, such as milk and ice cream, that reduce the efficacy of the charcoal.[8] When oral administration is impossible, use a nasogastric tube. If excessive vomiting interferes with the administration of charcoal, give antiemetics parenterally or per rectum.

Cathartic agents may be administered in conjunction with activated charcoal to speed gastrointestinal transit time. More rapid elimination of the charcoal-toxin complex may theoretically enhance the effectiveness of charcoal. Results of clinical studies on this point are conflicting.* Purgatives may not be required routinely, but reserved for cases where charcoal fails to appear in the stool in a timely fashion. With cathartic use monitor the patient closely for excessive fluid loss. Do not use charcoal with sorbitol after the first dose of a repeated-dose charcoal regimen because of the risk of severe osmotic diarrhea.

WHOLE BOWEL IRRIGATION

Whole bowel irrigation (WBI) is one of the newest additions to the emergency treatment of poisoning. Some have advo-

---

*References 18, 25, 33, 38, 44, and 49.

cated mechanical cleansing of the gastrointestinal (GI) tract by means of large volumes of enterally administered fluid, used routinely before colonoscopy and bowel surgery as a method of GI decontamination in cases of toxic ingestion.[56,57,60] The mechanisms of action of WBI include removal of unabsorbed drug from the entire GI tract and possibly increased clearance of toxins via GI dialysis in a fashion similar to that used for activated charcoal.[32,56]

Indications

Consider WBI when traditional techniques of poisoning first-aid may be ineffective or inadequate (Box 102-3), including ingestion of a massive amount of a toxic substance or late presentation after ingestion.[56,60] WBI is successfully used in treatment of toxins poorly adsorbed by charcoal, particularly iron[14,57,58] and other metals.[4,48,52] It may be useful for sustained-release preparations:[56] one study using aspirin found WBI superior to charcoal,[27] whereas there was no difference in another study of theophylline.[5] Finally toxic objects such as mercuric oxide disk batteries[57] and cocaine-filled condoms[22] are removable with this technique. With further use and research the indications for WBI are likely to expand in coming years.

Contraindications

Avoid whole bowel irrigation in patients with mechanical GI obstruction, ileus, perforation, or significant GI hemorrhage.[56] Similarly its safety after ingestion of corrosive substances is unknown. Use WBI cautiously in children with an altered level of consciousness; as with other GI decontamination procedures adequate airway management is essential. Despite a paucity of studies of its safety in infants, one report demonstrates successful use in children as young as 11 months of age.[14]

Complications

Experience with WBI for poisoning and other indications has shown it to be a safe procedure.[42,46,60] The most common adverse effects are abdominal cramping and vomiting,[27,46] which are amenable to reducing the rate of administration temporarily. One study has reported prolonged diarrhea with the use of isotonic saline solution,[51] rather than the standard lavage solutions currently in use. Polyethylene glycol-electrolyte lavage solution (PEG-ELS) decreases the adsorptive capacity of activated charcoal.[21,27,28]

Equipment

The preferred solution for whole bowel irrigation is a polyethylene glycol-containing balanced electrolyte solution (e.g., Golytely, Colyte). It is isoosmotic, and its administration in large quantities produces negligible fluid or electrolyte shifts.[12,46] Irrigation requires approximately 2 to 8 L of solution. Be sure to make available a commode or bedpan. If employing the nasogastric route of administration prepare supplies for nasogastric intubation as well.

Technique

Give PEG-ELS orally or as a nasogastric infusion. The rate of administration is 500 ml/hr for children, and 2 L/hr for adolescents. If vomiting results, slow the rate and gradually increase over 15 to 30 minutes to that recommended. Some patients may require antiemetics. If activated charcoal is indicated, administer a dose before the PEG-ELS. Continue irrigation at the rate indicated until the rectal effluent resembles the clear infusate. This process typically takes 4 to 6 hours.[56]

REFERENCES

1. Albertson TE, Derlet RW, Foulke GE, et al: Superiority of activated charcoal alone compared with ipecac and activated charcoal in the treatment of acute toxic ingestions, *Ann Emerg Med* 18:56-59, 1989.
2. Berg MJ, Berlinger WG, Goldberg MJ, et al: Acceleration of the body clearance of phenobarbital by oral activated charcoal, *N Engl J Med* 307:642-644, 1982.
3. Berlinger WG, Spector R, Goldberg et al: Enhancement of theophylline clearance by oral activated charcoal, *Clin Phamacol Ther* 33:351-354, 1983.
4. Burkhart KK, Kulig KW, Rumack B: Whole bowel irrigation as treatment for zinc sulfate overdose, *Ann Emerg Med* 19:1167-1170, 1990.
5. Burkhart KK, Wuerz RC, Donovan JW: Whole bowel irrigation as adjunctive treatment for sustained-release theophylline overdose, *Ann Emerg Med* 21:1316-1320, 1992.
6. Calvert WE, Corby DG, Herbertson LM, et al: Orally administered activated charcoal: acceptance by children, *JAMA* 215:641, 1971.
7. Chinouth RW, Czajka PA: *N*-acetylcysteine adsorption by activated charcoal, *Vet Hum Toxicol* 22.392-394, 1980.
8. Cooney DO: Palatability of sucrose-, sorbitol-, and saccharin-sweetened activated charcoal formulations, *Am J Hosp Pharm* 37:237-239, 1980.
9. Corby DJ, Lisciandro RC, Lehman RH, et al: The efficiency of methods used to evacuate the stomach after acute ingestions, *Pediatrics* 40:871-874, 1967.
10. Curtis RA, Barone J, Giacona N: Efficacy of ipecac and activated charcoal/cathartic: prevention of salicylate absorption in a simulated ovedose, *Arch Intern Med* 144:48-52, 1984.
11. Danel V, Henry JA, Glucksman E: Activated charcoal, emesis, and gastric lavage in aspirin overdose, *Br Med J* 296:1507, 1988.
12. Davis GR, Santa Ana CA, Morawski SG, et al: Development of a lavage solution associated with minimal water and electrolyte absorption or secretion, *Gastroenterology* 78:991-995, 1980.
13. Ellenhorn MJ, Barceloux DG: Gut decontamination. In Ellenhorn MJ, Barceloux DG, editors: *Medical toxicology: diagnosis and treatment of human poisoning.* New York, 1988, Elsevier Science, pp 54-63.
14. Everson GW, Bertaccini EJ, O'Leary J: Use of whole bowel irrigation in an infant following iron overdose, *Am J Emerg Med* 9:366-369, 1991.
15. Farley TA: Severe hypernatremic dehydration after use of an activated charcoal-sorbitol suspension, *J Pediatr* 109:719-722, 1986.
16. Fleisher GR, Kearney TE, Henretig F, et al: Gastric decontamination in the poisoned patient, *Pediatr Emerg Care* 7:378-381, 1991.
17. Gazda-Smith E, Synhavsky A: Hypernatremia following treatment of theophylline toxicity with activated charcoal and sorbitol, *Arch Intern Med* 150:689-690, 1990.
18. Goldberg MJ, Spector R, Park GD, et al: The effect of sorbitol and activated charcoal on serum theophylline concentrations after slow-release theophylline, *Clin Pharmacol Ther* 41:108-111, 1987.

19. Haddad LM, Winchester JF: A general approach to the emergency management of poisoning. In Haddad LM, Winchester JF, editors: *Clinical management of poisoning and drug overdose,* ed 2, Philadelphia, 1990, WB Saunders, pp 4-22.
20. Harris CR, Kingston R: Gastrointestinal decontamination: which method is best? *Postgrad Med* 92:116-128, 1992.
21. Hoffman RS, Chiang WK, Howland MA, et al: Theophylline description from activated charcoal caused by whole bowel irrigation solution, *Clin Toxicol* 29:191-201, 1991.
22. Hoffman RS, Smilkstein MJ, Goldfrank LR: Whole bowel irrigation and the cocaine body-packer: a new approach to a common problem, *Am J Emerg Med* 8:523-527, 1990.
23. Holt LE, Holz PH: The black bottle: a consideration of the role of charcoal in the treatment of poisoning in children, *J Pediatr* 63:306-314, 1963.
24. Jones J, McMullen MJ, Dougherty J, et al: Repetitive doses of activated charcoal in the treatment of poisoning, *Am J Emerg Med* 5:305-311, 1987.
25. Keller RE, Schwab RA, Krenzelok EP: Contribution of sorbitol combined with activated charcoal in prevention of salicylate absorption, *Ann Emerg Med* 19:654-656, 1990.
26. Kirk MA, Peterson J, Kulig K, et al: Acetaminophen overdose in children: a comparison of ipecac versus activated charcoal versus no gastrointestinal decontamination, *Ann Emerg Med* 20:472-473, 1991.
27. Kirshenbaum LA, Mathews SC, Sitar DS, et al: Whole bowel irrigation versus activated charcoal in sorbitol for the ingestion of modified-release pharmaceuticals, *Clin Pharmacol Ther* 46:264-271, 1989.
28. Kirshenbaum LA, Sitar DS, Tenenbein M: Interaction between whole bowel irrigation solution and activated charcoal: implications for the treatment of toxic ingestions, *Ann Emerg Med* 19:1129-1132, 1990.
29. Kornberg AE, Dolgin J: Pediatric ingestions: charcoal alone versus ipecac and charcoal, *Ann Emerg Med* 20:648-651, 1991.
30. Kulig K, Bar-Or D, Cantrill SV, et al: Management of acutely poisoned patients without gastric emptying, *Ann Emerg Med* 14:562-567, 1985.
31. Levy G: Gastrointestinal clearance of drugs with activated charcoal, *N Engl J Med* 307:676-678, 1982.
32. Mayer AL, Sitar DS, Tenenbein M: Multiple-dose charcoal and whole bowel irrigation do not increase clearance of absorbed salicylate, *Arch Intern Med* 152:393-396, 1992.
33. McNamara RM, Aaron CK, Gemborys M, et al: Sorbitol catharsis does not enhance efficacy of charcoal in a simulated acetaminophen overdose, *Ann Emerg Med* 17:243-246, 1988.
34. Menzies DG, Busuttil A, Prescott LF: Fatal pulmonary aspiration of oral activated charcoal, *Br Med J* 297:459-460, 1988.
35. Merigian KS, Woodard M, Hedges JR, et al: Prospective evaluation of gastric emptying in the self-poisoned patient, *Am J Emerg Med* 8:479-483, 1990.
36. Minocha A, Krenzelok EP, Spyker DA: Dosage recommendations for activated charcoal-sorbitol treatment, *Clin Toxicol* 23:579-587, 1985.
37. Neuvonen PJ: Clinical pharmacokinetics of oral activated charcoal in acute intoxications, *Clin Pharmacokinetics* 7:465-489, 1982.
38. Neuvonen PJ, Olkkola KT: Effect of purgatives on antidotal efficacy of oral activated charcoal, *Hum Toxicol* 5:255-263, 1986.
39. Neuvonen PJ, Okkola KT: Oral activated charcoal in the treatment of intoxications: role of single and repeated doses, *Med Toxicol* 3:33-58, 1988.
40. Neuvonen PJ, Vartiainen M, Tokola O: Comparison of activated charcoal and ipecac syrup in prevention of drug absorption, *Eur J Clin Pharmacol* 24:557-562, 1983.
41. North DS, Peterson RG, Krenzelok EP: Effect of activated charcoal administration on acetylcysteine serum levels in humans, *Am J Hosp Pharm* 38:1022-1044, 1981.
42. Palatnick W, Tenenbein M: Safety of treating poisoning patients with whole bowel irrigation, *Am J Emerg Med* 5:200-201, 1987.
43. Park GD, Spector R, Goldberg MJ et al: Expanded role of charcoal therapy in the poisoned and overdosed patient, *Arch Intern Med* 146:969-973, 1986.
44. Picchioni AL, Chin L, Gillespie T: Evaluation of activated charcoal-sorbitol suspension as an antidote, *J Toxicol Clin Toxicol* 19:433-444, 1982.

45. Pollack MM, Dunbar BS, Holbrook PR et al: Aspiration of activated charcoal and gastric contents, *Ann Emerg Med* 10:528-529, 1981.

46. Postuma R: Whole bowel irrigation in pediatric patients: a comparison of irrigating solutions, *J Pediatr Surg* 23:769-770, 1988.

47. Renzi FP, Donovan JW, Martin TG, et al: Concomitant use of activated charcoal and N-acetylcysteine, *Ann Emerg Med* 14:568-572, 1985.

48. Roberge RJ, Martin TG: Whole bowel irrigation in an acute oral lead intoxication, *Am J Emerg Med* 10:577-583, 1992.

49. Rosenberg PJ, Livingstone DJ, McLellan BA: Effect of whole-bowel irrigation on the antidotal efficacy of oral activated charcoal, *Ann Emerg Med* 17:681-683, 1988.

50. Scholtz EC, Jaffe JM, Colaizzi JL: Evaluation of five activated charcoal formulations for inhibition of aspirin absorption and palatablility in man, *Am J Hosp Pharm* 35:1355-1359, 1978.

51. Senocak ME, Butukpamukcu N, Hicsonmez A: Whole bowel irrigation in children: prolonged post-irrigation diarrhea due to isotonic saline, *Turk J Pediatr* 32:197-200, 1990.

52. Smith SW, Ling LJ, Halstenson CE: Whole bowel irrigation as a treatment for acute lithium overdose, *Ann Emerg Med* 20:536-539, 1991.

53. Swartz CM, Sherman A: The treatment of tricyclic antidepressant overdose with repeated charcoal, *J Clin Psychopharmacol* 4:336-340, 1984.

54. Tenenbein M: General management principles for poisoning. In Barkin RM, editors: *Pediatric emergency medicine: concepts and clinical practice,* St. Louis, 1992, Mosby.

55. Tenebein M: Multiple doses of activated charcoal: time for reappraisal? *Ann Emerg Med* 20:529-531, 1991.

56. Tenebein M: Whole bowel irrigation as a gastrointestinal decontamination procedure after acute poisoning, *Med Toxicol* 3:77-84, 1988.

57. Tenebein M: Whole bowel irrigation for toxic ingestions, *Clin Toxicol* 23:177-184, 1985.

58. Tenebein M: Whole bowel irrigation in iron poisoning, *J Pediatr* 111:142-145, 1987.

59. Tenebein M, Cohen S, Sitar DS: Efficacy of ipecac-induced emesis, orogastric lavage, and activated charcoal for acute drug overdose, *Ann Emerg Med* 16:838-841, 1987.

60. Tenebein M, Cohen S, Sitar DS: Whole bowel irrigation as a decontamination procedure after acute drug overdose, *Arch Intern Med* 147:905-907, 1987.

61. Watson WA, Cremer KF, Chapman JA: Gastrointestinal obstruction associated with multiple-dose activated charcoal, *J Emerg Med* 4:401-407, 1986.

103 Dialysis and Hemoperfusion

Marc Gorelick

DIALYSIS AND HEMOPERFUSION

Extracorporeal methods of drug removal may be useful in certain life-threatening ingestions when substantial absorption of the toxin has already occurred. These methods, discussed in detail elsewhere (see Chapters 67 to 69), include standard hemodialysis and hemoperfusion, which entails passage of blood through a column containing an adsorbing substance such as activated charcoal or an ion-exchange resin.[6] Peritoneal dialysis is occasionally used in acute drug intoxication; however it is far less effective than hemodialysis, which is usually the dialysis procedure of choice.[2,6] Although these techniques may theoretically remove a vast number of poisons,[7] in practice dialysis and hemoperfusion are beneficial for only a small number of substances in selected situations.[1] Of the over 1.8 million toxic exposures reported to the American Association of Poison Control Centers in 1991 extracorporeal techniques were used in only 854 cases; moreover a mere eight drugs accounted for over 60% of these cases.[4,5]

A number of factors relating to the drug itself are important in determining the appropriateness of active detoxification.[2] Table 103-1 lists toxins amenable to hemodialysis or hemoperfusion, along with minimal serum levels above which these techniques should be considered. Levels do not necessarily correlate with symptoms. Base the decision to initiate extracorporeal removal techniques on the clinical features of the poisoning.[6,7] Principally consider dialysis or hemoperfusion when the patient's condition progressively deteriorates despite intensive supportive therapy. Other potential indications include prolonged coma, impairment of normal drug excretory function, toxins with delayed effects, or a significant quantity of circulating substance with toxicity caused largely by metabolites (e.g., methanol, ethylene glycol).[7]

These detoxification techniques are highly invasive, with a number of potential complications. Hypotension, electrolyte imbalance (especially hypocalcemia), and hypothermia may occur.[6] Hemoperfusion frequently induces thrombocytopenia, which is usually transient but may be severe.[3] In addition abnormal bleeding may result from the need for systemic anticoagulation with dialysis and perfusion circuits. Finally symptoms may recur after cessation of dialysis or hemoperfusion in a rebound effect, caused by continued release of drug from binding sites in the body.[2]

Table 103-1 Poisons for Which to Consider Hemodialysis or Hemofiltration

Compound	Severely toxic level	Preferred removal method*
Salicylates	800 µg/ml	HD
Methanol	50 mg/dl	HD
Ethylene glycol	20 mg/dl	HD
Isopropanol	400 mg/dl	HD
Lithium	2.5 mEq/L	HD
Theophylline	60 µg/ml	HP > HD
Phenobarbital	100 µg/ml	HP > HD
Other barbiturates	50 µg/ml	HP > HD
Glutethimide	40 µg/ml	HP > HD
Methaqualone	40 µg/ml	HP > HD

*HD, Hemodialysis; HP, hemoperfusion.

REFERENCES

1. DeBroe ME, Bismuth C, DeGroot G, et al: Haemoperfusion: a useful therapy for a severely poisoned patient? *Human Toxicol* 5:6-11, 1986.
2. Garella S: Extracorporeal techniques in the treatment of exogenous intoxications, *Kidney Int* 33:735-754, 1988.
3. Gelfand MC, Winchester JF, Knepshield JH, et al: Treatment of severe drug overdosage with charcoal hemoperfusion, *Trans Am Soc Artif Intern Organs* 23:599-604, 1977.
4. Litovitz TL, Holm KC, Bailey KM, et al: 1991 annual report of the American Association of Poison Control Centers National Data Collection System, *Am J Emerg Med* 10:452-505, 1992.
5. Litovitz T, Veltri JC: The role of hemoperfusion and hemodialysis in toxicology, *Am J Emerg Med* 5:405, 1987.
6. Winchester JF: Active methods for detoxification. In Haddad LM, Winchester JF, editors: *Clinical management of poisoning and drug overdose*, ed 2, Philadelphia, 1990, WB Saunders, pp 148-167.
7. Winchester JF, Gelfand MC, Knepshield JH, et al: Dialysis and hemoperfusion of poisons and drugs—update, *Trans Am Soc Artif Intern Organs* 23:762-842, 1977.

PART XXI

TRAUMA TECHNIQUES

104 Epidemiology of Pediatric Trauma

Marianne Gausche

Trauma is the leading cause of death in children older than 1 year of age and is a major public health problem in the United States. Trauma accounts for 64% of all deaths among children (Fig. 104-1).[1,3,6,8] In the United States, sixteen million children with trauma are evaluated in Emergency Departments (EDs) each year. Of these children, more than 500,000 are hospitalized and approximately 1.5% die as a result of their injuries.[3,6] The overall yearly morbidity and mortality is high: 50,000 children are disabled and more than 22,000 die from injury.[1,3,6] Injury in children results in more years of potential life lost than all diseases combined.[1,3] The cost of childhood injury in the United States exceeds $8 billion each year.[5]

Eighty-seven percent of all pediatric trauma results from blunt mechanisms.[9] Infants, toddlers, and preschool-age children suffer blunt injury from falls and physical abuse, which results in a higher proportion of head injuries. School-age children (6 to 12 years of age) are injured in motor vehicle collisions, whether as passengers, pedestrians, or cyclists in vehicular collisions. Penetrating trauma accounts for a smaller percentage (10%) of injury in children in comparison with adults (20% to 30%).[4] Drowning and other injuries account for the remaining 3% of pediatric trauma injuries.

Motor vehicle collisions account for the majority of pediatric trauma deaths.[7,9,11] In the United States the average annual death rate from motor vehicle collisions (1986-1992) is 12.8 per 100,000 children: motor vehicle passengers (9.4) and pedestrian (2.5) deaths predominate.[1,11] In their review of childhood injury in the United States, Baker et al.[1] and Waller, Baker, and Szocka[11] reported the following death rates (per 100,000) for nonvehicular mechanisms: homicide (6.4), suicide (3), drowning (2.5), house fire (1.9), suffocation (1.5), unintentional firearm (0.7), fall (0.4), and all other (2.5).

Age, gender, and race are factors in the epidemiology of pediatric trauma. Table 104-1 displays causes of injury-related death by age group. The rates of injury-related deaths decrease with increasing age until adolescence: <1 year, 29.6 per 100,000; 1 to 4 years, 18.9; 5 to 9 years, 9.8; 10 to 14 years, 14; and 15 to 19 years, 67.4. The added mortality risk for infants is related to a number of factors; one factor is the prevalence of abused infants. More than 1.6 million children are abused each year, and child abuse is the leading cause of injury-related death in children under 1 year of age.[1,3,8,11] For every 1000 children, 25 experience abuse or neglect; 60% of these children experience physical abuse.[1,3,8]

The cause of trauma-related deaths in children changes significantly when older adolescents (15 to 19 years) are included. Motor vehicle collisions remain the leading mechanism (49%), but homicide becomes the second leading cause of death (16.6%), followed by suicide (9.9%), drowning (4.2%), suffocation/hanging (3.9%), fire (1.1%), and other causes (12.6%).[1,6]

In all racial groups, children under 5 years of age seem to be at greatest risk for dying from injury (Fig. 104-2). Black and Native American children have the highest risk of dying from injury, with injury-related death rates of 47.2 and 40.7 per 100,000, respectively. The death rate among whites and Asian children is significantly lower—15.7 and 19.1 per 100,000, respectively.[1] Homicide rates in male children are twice that of female children, and the homicide rate in black children is five times that of white children.[4,8] A firearm is the most commonly used weapon in homicides, and a gun in the home markedly increases an adolescent's risk of dying by suicide.[1,3]

The treatment of injuries is a major component of pediatric emergency and critical care services. Slightly more than 50% of all pediatric prehospital calls, approximately 30% of ED

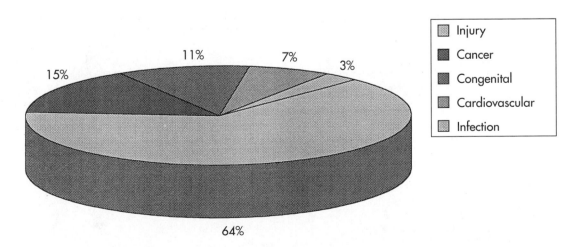

FIG. 104-1 Major causes of death in the pediatric age group, 1992.

Table 104-1   Number of Injury Deaths and Death Rates per 100,000 by Cause and Age, United States, 1992

Injury cause	<1 yrs	1-4 yrs	5-9 yrs	10-14 yrs	15-19 yrs	Total	Rate
Motor vehicle traffic total*	156	721	857	956	4,751	7,441	10.2
Occupant†	144	444	437	574	4,084	5,686	7.8
Motorcyclist†	0	0	2	26	274	299	0.4
Pedal cyclist	0	10	92	145	62	309	0.4
Pedestrian	12	266	325	208	314	1,125	1.5
Nontraffic total‡							
Occupant	0	14	9	13	31	67	0.1
Pedal cyclist	0	0	10	7	6	23	0.0
Pedestrian	4	118	33	26	64	245	0.3
Firearm total	12	105	111	667	4,484	5,379	7.4
Unintentional	1	35	48	132	285	501	0.7
Suicide	0	0	3	172	1,251	1,426	2.0
Homicide	11	69	56	348	2,878	3,362	4.6
Undetermined	0	1	4	15	70	90	0.1
Drowning	101	543	200	220	415	1,479	2.0
Fire/flame	100	607	230	114	111	1,162	1.6
Suffocation/hanging	273	99	65	184	433	1,054	1.4
Choking	103	95	23	16	21	258	0.4
Fall	26	65	20	31	115	257	0.4
Cutting/piercing	8	26	19	42	272	367	0.5
Poison: solid/liquid	18	40	6	41	255	360	0.5
Poison: gas/vapor	3	13	19	14	130	179	0.2
Farm machinery	0	6	17	8	17	48	0.1
Other	382	479	177	199	415	1,652	2.3
UNINTENTIONAL	819	2,467	1,628	1,760	6,234	12,908	17.7
SUICIDE	0	0	10	304	1,847	2,161	3.0
HOMICIDE	326	430	146	441	3,302	4,645	6.4
INTENT UNKNOWN	41	34	12	33	137	257	0.4
ALL INJURY	**1,186**	**2,931**	**1,796**	**2,538**	**11,520**	**19,971**	**27.3**
Rate/100,000/year	**29.6**	**18.9**	**9.8**	**14.0**	**67.4**	**27.3**	

*Includes any motor vehicle traffic deaths not in the categories below.
†See Appendix for details.
‡Nontraffic refers to incidents that occur off public roads.
From Baker SP, Waller AE: *Injury to children and teenagers: state-by-state mortality facts*, Washington, D.C., 1996, National Maternal and Child Health Clearing House.

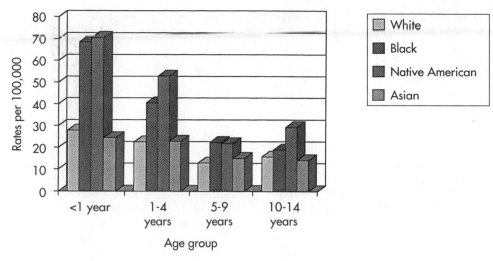

FIG. 104-2   Childhood injury rates by age group and race, 1985.

visits, and approximately 20% of all pediatric critical-care days are related to injuries.

Childhood injury is a public health problem that requires a multidisciplinary approach to effect change. This multidisciplinary approach begins with adequate data regarding the frequency of trauma and its sequelae. The National Pediatric Trauma Registry contains more than 10,000 patients in a multiinstitutional database and is providing the first comprehensive and prospective look at nationwide pediatric trauma care.[10] In addition to data acquisition, public awareness regarding the effects of injury in children must be increased, prevention efforts must be broad-based and realistic, and education of health-care professionals in pediatric trauma care must be improved to further reduce the impact of injury on the nation's children.

REFERENCES

1. Baker SP, Waller AE: *Injury to children and teenagers: state-by-state mortality facts,* Washington, DC, 1996, National Maternal and Child Health Clearinghouse.

2. Brent DA, Perper JA, Allman CJ, et al: The presence and accessibility of firearms in the homes of adolescent suicides: a case-control study, *JAMA* 226(21):2989-2995, 1991.

3. Childhood injuries in the United States, *Am J Dis Child* 144:627-646, 1990.

4. Christoffel KK: Violent death and injury in US children and adolescents, *Am J Dis Child* 144:697-706, 1990.

5. Guyer B, Ellers B: Childhood injuries in the United States: mortality, morbidity, and cost, *Am J Dis Child* 144:649-662, 1990.

6. Holinger PC: The causes, impact, and preventability of childhood injuries in the United States: childhood suicide in the United States, *Am J Dis Child* 144:670-676, 1990.

7. Inaba AS, Seward PN: An approach to pediatric trauma: unique anatomic and pathophysiologic aspects of the pediatric patient, *Emerg Clin North Am* 9(3):523-547, 1991.

8. Peclet MH, Newman KD, Eichelberger MR, et al: Patterns of injury in children, *J Pediatr Surg* 25(1):85-91, 1990.

9. Schafermeyer R: Pediatric trauma, *Emerg Med Clin North Am* 11(1):187-205, 1993.

10. Tepas JJ, Ramenofsky ML, Barlow B, et al: National pediatric trauma registry, *Am J Dis Child* 24(2):156-158, 1989.

11. Waller AE, Baker SP, Szocka A: Childhood injury death rates: national analysis and geographic variations, *Am J Public Health* 79(3):310-315, 1989.

105 Anatomic Distribution of Childhood Injury

Ramon W. Johnson

Recognition of the special anatomic differences and injury patterns in children can facilitate emergency management. Whether the injury is a result of a blunt or penetrating trauma, a child's unique developmental and anatomic differences are strongly correlated with the location and pattern of the injury.

A child is particularly at risk for multisystem injury because kinetic forces are distributed over a smaller area.[13] Multisystem injury occurs most commonly with traffic-related crashes, which account for the majority of pediatric trauma admissions; children younger than 3 years of age have a markedly higher risk of death.[1,17] Response to injury differs between children and adults.

INJURY PATTERNS

Head injury occurs in nearly 50% of Emergency Department (ED) blunt trauma admissions and is followed, in order of decreasing frequency, by extremity fractures, abdominal injuries, chest injuries, pelvis injuries, and spinal injuries (Fig. 105-1).[18,21] Children are susceptible to internal organ injury because of their lack of protective muscle, bone, and subcutaneous tissue mass. This lack of protection permits traumatic forces to be transmitted to the deeper internal structures, sometimes with little or no external evidence of trauma.

Although head and central nervous system trauma carries the highest degree of mortality and morbidity, injuries to the chest and abdomen also account for a significant amount of disability and death.

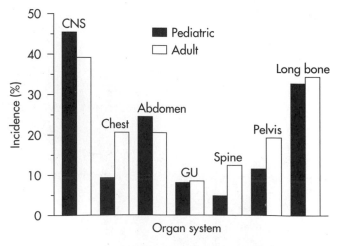

FIG. 105-1 Relative incidence of specific organ injury in adults and children. Significant differences are noted in chest, spinal, and pelvic injuries.

HEAD INJURIES

A child has a relatively large head-to-body ratio and short stature, which results in a high center of gravity that persists until early adolescence.[13] Hence children suffer proportionately more head injuries than adults, and a larger number of children who die as a result of multiple trauma have significant head injuries, with infants having the highest mortality rate.[1]

Other factors that contribute to the pattern of head injuries seen in children include anatomic differences in the neck, skull, and brain. The presence of weaker neck muscles, which are capable of absorbing less force, renders the brain more vulnerable to shearing stress, such as in the shaken baby syndrome. The skull is thinner and provides less protection to the brain, which is less myelinated and therefore more susceptible to severe injury from milder traumatic forces.[11,21] However, children appear to tolerate brain swelling and expanding masses better because of the open sutures, the larger subarachnoid space and cistern area, and greater extracellular space in the brain.[9] Although children with severe head injury have relatively fewer intracranial mass lesions, they are more likely than adults to have intracranial hypertension and to develop brain hyperemia shortly after the injury. The hypertension and hyperemia are distinct from the secondary brain injury that results from cytotoxic edema, which may develop later.[3,9] Children with head injuries may have a more favorable outcome when measures aimed at decreasing hyperemia and brain edema are instituted early.[3]

Finally, children have a better rate of survival after head injury and appear to be more capable than adults in recovering from diffuse brain injury.[1] Children may actually be more vulnerable to long-term disability than adults.[12,20]

NECK INJURIES

Spinal cord and spinal column injuries in childhood are uncommon. Approximately 1% of all seriously injured children have a spinal injury, and childhood spinal cord injury accounts for less than 10% of all spinal cord injuries.[1,15]

There are many anatomic and physiologic differences in the pediatric cervical spine. Children have a larger relative head mass, less nuchal muscular development, and greater flexibility of the ligamentous and joint capsule structures. Vertebral body shape, lack of development of uncinate articulations, and horizontal facet orientation make a child's spine less resistant to sagittal and coronal plane forces.[6,15] Children who do not have head control are at particular risk from sudden forces applied to the cervical spine.[1]

Multiple studies reveal that children younger than 8 to 12 years of age tend to have injuries involving the upper cervical spine (atlantooccipital junction, C1 and C2 regions). Adults and older children tend to have lower-level cervical spine injuries.[14] Because a child's weaker neck muscles offer

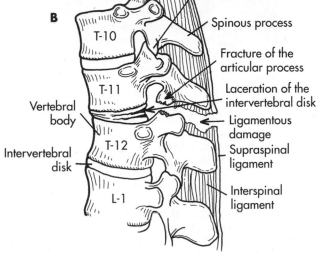

FIG. 105-2   Spinal injuries associated with lap belts. **A,** Avulsion fracture and ligamentous injury. **B,** Articular fracture, disk laceration, and ligamentous injury.

less support, ligamentous injuries without cervical spine injury occur more often, with up to 50% of children with clinical evidence of spinal cord injuries having normal plain x-ray studies.[13,15] Momentary dislocation or subluxation with spontaneous reduction and without fracture or ligamentous injury may also occur because of this intrinsic spinal column elasticity; however, there is much greater elasticity in a child's spinal column than in the spinal cord.[6] Therefore a careful neurologic examination for signs of spinal cord trauma is imperative, even in the presence of normal x-ray studies. Whenever there is a reasonable clinical suspicion of a spinal cord injury, immobilize the neck and obtain additional radiographic studies, computerized tomography, or magnetic resonance imaging.[16]

Finally, there is a strong association between childhood lumbar spine injury and the use of lap-belt restraints by pediatric motor vehicle passengers. These injuries include low thoracic and lumbar spine flexion-distraction injuries in combination with intraabdominal injury (Fig. 105-2).[14]

ABDOMINAL INJURIES

Abdominal injuries are a common cause of death in children, are most commonly a result of blunt trauma, and may be difficult to evaluate. Not only may concomitant multiple injuries divert attention from the abdominal injury, but also the child's inability to communicate because of age, fear, or metabolic/toxicologic causes may reduce the accuracy of the physical examination.

Children are at increased risk for abdominal injuries because of several anatomic features: the relatively large size and anterior location of the abdominal organs in the peritoneal cavity; the decreased protective abdominal muscle, bone, and adipose tissue; and a flexible, thin, and poorly muscularized rib cage.[11] Located more anterior and caudal because of the horizontal orientation of the diaphragm, the liver and spleen are the most commonly injured abdominal organs in children, followed in frequency by the kidney (Fig. 105-3).[8,9,11] Injuries to the pancreas and duodenum occasionally occur, but because of their retroperitoneal location clinical findings are often delayed. In small children, the bladder is an intraabdominal organ and is therefore more vulnerable to injury.

Children with ecchymoses and abrasions over the abdominal or flank regions are at high risk for abdominal injury but may sustain internal organ injury with minimal or no external evidence of trauma.[8,13] Seemingly trivial injury mechanisms may occasionally result in severe intraabdominal injury, especially in children with congenital abnormalities such as hydronephrosis.[11]

THORACIC INJURIES

Thoracic injury in children is a strong marker of severe and multisystem trauma and is associated with a high mortality rate.[1] The pattern of injuries in children with chest trauma is

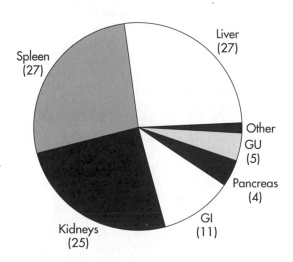

FIG. 105-3   Frequency of intraabdominal organ injury in children by percent.

(From the Pediatric National Registry 1985-1991.)

affected by the greater elasticity and resiliance of the chest wall, which makes fractures of the ribs and sternum less common than in adults.[4,9] Children with rib fractures associated with head or other thoracic injuries have a high mortality rate (71% and 42%, respectively).[17]

The increased compliance of the chest wall permits the transmission of traumatic forces to the deeper thoracic structures, which may cause severe parenchymal injury to the lung with minimal or no signs of external trauma.[10] The greater mobility of the mediastinal structures may produce transection or angulation of the vascular structures, compression of the lungs, and tracheobronchial injury.[11] Great vessel injury following blunt trauma is rare among children, probably because of the greater elasticity of connective tissue that results in increased resistance to shearing forces. Other thoracic injuries in children include pneumothorax, hemothorax, and pulmonary contusions.[1,13] Because of the increased mobility of mediastinal structures, a pneumothorax may rapidly develop into a tension pneumothorax. Hemothorax is associated with a particularly high mortality rate in children.[1]

Death from traumatic asphyxiation occurs almost exclusively in children because of their compliant thorax and the absence of valves in both the superior and inferior vena cava.[19] Any sudden compression of the rib cage against a closed glottis causes a dramatic rise in intratracheal and intrapulmonary pressures and a temporary vena cava obstruction with capillary extravasation and hemorrhaging in the brain and other organs.[11,14]

SKELETAL INJURIES

In children, the density of bone generally is less than in adults, and immature bone is more porous. This porous, compliant bone often responds to stress by buckling rather than fracturing. The periosteum is thicker and less easily disrupted, and the ligaments around major joints are stronger and more resistant to tensile forces than are the adjacent bones.[7]

Despite the elasticity of bones in the pediatric age group, fractures often occur and may be easily missed clinically. Important skeletal injuries include incomplete fractures through the cortex (greenstick, torus, or buckle) and fractures involving the growth plate (Salter-Harris). Although both types of injuries are associated with minimal blood loss, fractures involving the growth plate have the potential to interfere with subsequent normal growth.

Fractures to the femur are more common in children than in adults, whereas fractures to the other extremities appear to occur with equal frequency. Although injuries to the pelvis and extremities can result in life-threatening blood loss and hemodynamic instability, the mortality rate from these injuries is generally lower in children than in adults.[19]

REMARKS

The patterns of injury seen in children are different from that of adults. Effective evaluation and management of pediatric trauma victims requires an understanding of the unique anatomic differences that account for the spectrum of injuries. By studying these patterns of injury, new strategies aimed at prevention can be devised to reduce the severity of trauma.

REFERENCES

1. Allhouse MJ, Rouse T, Eichelberger MR: Childhood injury: a current perspective, *Pediatr Emerg Care* 9:159-164, 1993.
2. Bruce DA, Gennarelli J, Langfit J: Resuscitation from coma due to head injury, *Crit Care Med* 6:254-259, 1978.
3. Bruce DA, et al: Outcome following severe head injuries in children, *J Neurosurg* 48:679-688, 1978.
4. Eichelberger MR, Randolf JG: Thoracic trauma in children, *Surg Clin North Am* 61:1181-1197, 1981.
5. Eichelberger MR, et al: Comparative outcomes of children and adults suffering blunt trauma, *J Trauma* 28:430-434, 1988.
6. Herzenberg JE, Hensinger RN: Pediatric cervical spine injuries, *Trauma Q* 5:73-81, 1989.
7. Hodge D: Musculoskeletal and soft tissue injuries: management principles. In Barkin RA, editor: *Pediatric emergency medicine: concepts and clinical practice,* St Louis, 1992, Mosby.
8. Inaba AS, et al: An approach to pediatric trauma, *Emerg Med Clin North Am* 9:523-548, 1991.
9. Jaffe D, Wesson D: Emergency management of blunt trauma in children, *N Engl J Med* 324:1477-1482, 1991.
10. Kane NM, Cronin JJ, Dorfman GG, et al: Pediatric abdominal trauma: evaluation by computed tomography, *Pediatrics* 82:11-15, 1988.
11. Kisson N, Dreyer J, Walia M: Pediatric trauma: differences in pathophysiology, injury patterns, and treatment compared to adult trauma, *Can Med Assoc J* 142:27-34, 1990.
12. Luerssen TG, Klauber MR, Marshall LF: Outcome from head injury related to patient's age: a longitudinal prospective study of adult and pediatric head injury, *J Neurosurg* 68:409-416, 1988.
13. McCarty DL, Surpure JS: Pediatric trauma: initial evaluation and stabilization *Pediatr Ann* 19:580-596, 1990.
14. Newman KD, Bowman LM, Eichelberger MR, et al: The lap-belt complex: intestinal and lumbar spine injury in children, *J Trauma* 25:1133-1140, 1990.
15. Pang D, Pollack IF: Spinal cord injury without radiographic abnormality in children: the SCIWORA syndrome, *J Trauma* 29:654-664, 1989.
16. Peclet MH, Newman KD, Eichelber MR, et al: Patterns of injury in children, *J Pediatr Surg* 25:85-91, 1990.
17. Rouse TM, Eichelberger MR: Trends in pediatric trauma management, *Surg Clin North Am* 72:1347-1364, 1992.
18. Smyth BT: Chest trauma in children, *J Pediatr Surg* 14:41, 1979.
19. Synder CL, Vivanti NJ, Saltzman DA, et al: Blunt trauma in adults and children: a comparative analysis, *J Trauma* 30:1239-1245, 1990.
20. Tepas JJ, DiScala C, Ramenofsky ML, et al: Mortality and head injury: the pediatric perspective, *J Pediatr Surg* 25:92-96, 1990.
21. Walker ML, Storrs BB, Mayer TA: Head Injuries. In Mayer TA, editor: *Emergency management of pediatric trauma,* Philadelphia, 1985, JB Lippincott.

Kimberly R. Zimmerman

The prompt diagnosis of chest injury is critical but may be difficult because symptoms may not appear for several hours. Because a child's chest wall is very compliant, the transfer of energy to the intrathoracic soft tissues may often occur without evidence of external injury.[1] Pulmonary contusion and pulmonary hemorrhage may occur without overlying rib fractures, especially in young children.[2,4]

A pneumothorax occurs when a one-way–valve air leak develops in the pleural space, either from the lung or through the chest wall. The affected lung is collapsed by air that is forced into and trapped inside the thoracic cavity. When pleural air pressures become high enough on the affected side, the opposite lung is compressed by the displaced mediastinum and trachea, which results in a tension pneumothorax. A tension pneumothorax compromises respiratory status and decreases venous return.

The mobility of mediastinal structures makes the child more sensitive to tension pneumothorax.[4,6] Although the incidence of tension pneumothorax is probably less than 5% of serious injuries, it is a life-threatening condition and requires immediate decompression.

Indications

In a distressed child who has obvious signs of tension pneumothorax, a diagnosis must be made quickly on the basis of clinical findings only; radiologic confirmation is unnecessary.[2,3,5] A child with a tension pneumothorax comes to the hospital with respiratory distress that is poorly relieved by administering oxygen or by opening and clearing the airway; tachycardia, hypotension, a unilateral absence of breath sounds, and neck vein distention (if there is no associated hypovolemia) are also present.[2,3,5] Cyanosis and tracheal deviation are late manifestations.[3,5] The initial management of *tension* pneumothorax is needle thoracostomy.[2,5] It is a quick and effective procedure for pleural air decompression, but not for decompression of hemothorax. Needle thoracostomy does not obviate the need for tube thoracostomy, which is necessary immediately after all needle thoracostomies.

Contraindications

Because needle thoracostomy is a potentially lifesaving procedure, there are no contraindications to performing it when respiratory distress and the appropriate history and physical findings are present. Use caution in patients with known coagulopathies. In some situations, such as in cases of penetrating chest trauma, first consider rapid tube thoracostomy instead of needle thoracostomy to relieve the suspected hemothorax as well as pneumothorax.

Complications

When tension pneumothorax is suspected in a child, the benefits of needle thoracostomy far outweigh the risks.[1,3] Most complications may be avoided by the use of scrupulous

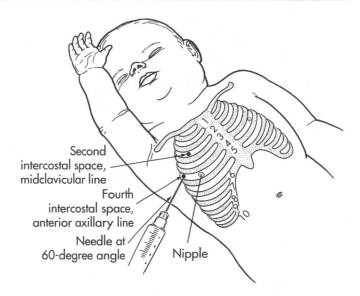

FIG. 106-1 Standard sites for needle thoracostomy.

Second intercostal space, midclavicular line
Fourth intercostal space, anterior axillary line
Needle at 60-degree angle
Nipple

technique. Hemothorax is a possible early complication as a result of placing the midclavicular needle too medially and puncturing the internal mammary artery or as a result of puncturing an intercostal artery because of entry near the inferior rib margin. Proper positioning of the needle averts these complications. Iatrogenic pneumothorax occurs if this technique is performed in a patient who does not initially have a pneumothorax. Needle entry below the nipple line may penetrate the diaphragm, the bowel, or the peritoneum and cause bleeding, viscus rupture, infection, or respiratory compromise. Placing the needle too low in the midclavicular line may puncture the heart or coronary vessels and result in hemopericardium or coronary vessel injury with resultant adverse hemodynamic effects. Although needle thoracostomy must be performed quickly, maintaining sterile technique prevents later infection.

Equipment

The materials necessary for a needle thoracostomy include a 14-gauge over-the-needle catheter, povidone-iodine solution, and a 30-ml syringe.

Techniques

Position the child safely in the supine position; use restraints as needed. Elevate the child's arm behind the head. Prepare the needle entry site with povidone-iodine solution. Either the second intercostal space (midclavicular line) or the fourth intercostal space (anterior axillary line) are acceptable locations to decompress tension pneumothorax (Fig. 106-1).

Before inserting the needle, count the ribs twice. Unless the child is in shock, use a local anesthetic. Place the needle through the skin and onto the rib. Advance the needle at a

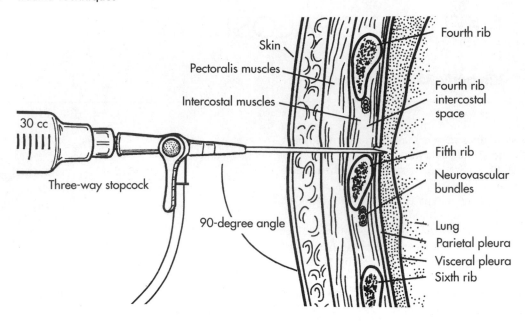

FIG. 106-2 Needle thoracostomy at fourth intercostal space. Puncture the pleura with the needle advanced above the fifth rib.

60-degree angle over the superior aspect of the rib margin until the needle is clearly in the intercostal space. Redirect the needle at a 90-degree angle and push the needle into the pleural space; a "pop" should be felt when the pleura is punctured (Fig. 106-2). Attach a 30-ml syringe to help with needle entry, but remove it to decompress the chest. The sensation of air passing may be felt or heard when the pleural space is entered or if the plunger on the syringe is easily pulled back and the syringe is filled with air. The tension pneumothorax has now been converted to a simple, open pneumothorax. Advance the catheter while withdrawing the needle. If a plain 14-gauge needle is used, there is a risk of puncturing the expanding lung with the needle tip. The use of a soft, pliable catheter reduces this risk.

Monitor the child's vital signs continuously during this procedure. An immediate gush of air and immediate improvement of respiratory status after needle thoracostomy confirm the diagnosis and the success of the procedure. Consider bilateral needle thoracostomy if signs of tension pneumothorax persist after unilateral needle thoracostomy has been performed. Definitive treatment of tension pneumothorax requires the immediate insertion of a chest tube into the fourth intercostal space anterior axillary line (see Chapter 107), after which the needle thoracostomy catheter may be removed.

Remarks

If the patient's condition does not improve after needle thoracostomy, other internal injuries may be present, such as a tracheal-bronchial tear or a significant hemothorax. Also, loculated areas of the lung may be inaccessible to the thoracostomy needle. In such cases a tube or even an open thoracostomy may be necessary to relieve the tension pneumothorax.

REFERENCES

1. Alexander RH, Proctor HJ: *Advanced trauma life support student manual,* ed 5, Chicago, 1993, American College of Surgeons.
2. Bledsoe BE, Porter RS, Shade BR, editors: *Paramedic emergency care,* Englewood Cliffs, NJ, 1991, Brady/Regents/Prentice Hall.
3. Bushore M, Fleisher G, Seidel J, et al, editors: *Advanced pediatric life support,* Elk Grove Village, Ill, 1989, American Academy of Pediatrics, American College of Emergency Physicians.
4. Peclet MH, Newman KD, Eichelberger MR, et al: Thoracic trauma in children: an indicator of increased mortality, *J Pediatr Surg* 25(9):961-966, 1990.
5. Seidel J, Burkett D: *Instructors' manual for pediatric advanced life support,* Dallas, 1988, American Heart Association.
6. Vallee P, Sullivan M, Richardson H, et al: Sequential treatment of a simple pneumothorax, *Ann Emerg Med* 17(9):936-942, 1988.

107 Tube Thoracostomy

Robert H. Winokur

Tube thoracostomy is the insertion of an intrapleural catheter to evacuate air and/or fluid from the pleural space to allow lung reexpansion and improve ventilation. This procedure was first described in the English literature in 1876 as a treatment for empyema.[3] Tube thoracostomy has now become commonplace for the treatment of victims of blunt or penetrating chest trauma and a variety of nontraumatic conditions.

Recent studies in children and adults indicate a good outcome for 76% of patients with blunt and penetrating trauma who have been treated conservatively with tube thoracostomy and observation.[6,8]

Indications

There are two main indications for tube thoracostomy in the pediatric trauma patient: pneumothorax and hemothorax.

Pneumothorax is the most common major consequence of serious thoracic trauma in children.[1] It is often present in the absence of rib fracture or chest wall deformity. With a blunt trauma, sudden increases in intraluminal pressure against a closed glottis may rupture the alveoli and allow air to escape into the pleural space, or a rib fracture may puncture a lung and allow air to escape into the pleural space. With a penetrating trauma, entry of outside air into the pleural space or injury to the lung parenchyma, tracheobronchial tree, or esophagus may also occur. A small, simple pneumothorax may not always require decompression. Observing a small pneumothorax (typically less than 20% by volume) is occasionally acceptable; however, the risk of developing a tension pneumothorax is higher than the risk of complication from tube thoracostomy.[5]

Tension pneumothorax is the accumulation of air outside the lung but within the pleural space. The pleural air is under increased pressure and displaces the mediastinal structures to the contralateral side. The increased pressure diminishes venous return to the heart and thereby decreases cardiac output. This condition is life threatening and most often occurs after tracheobronchial tears, parenchymal lacerations, sucking chest wall defects, and esophageal injuries. Although the clinical triad of hypotension, contralateral tracheal shift, and hyperresonance of the chest may occur along with dyspnea and cyanosis, the tracheal shift and cyanosis are often late findings and are not easily detectable. Treat tension pneumothorax initially with needle thoracostomy of the chest (see Chapter 106); after relieving the tension, immediate tube thoracostomy is imperative. In an unstable patient with chest injury who quickly deteriorates while undergoing positive-pressure ventilation, needle thoracostomy is indicated to relieve suspected tension pneumothorax.

Hemothorax is a collection of blood outside the lung and within the pleural space; it is often a result of injury to vascular structures near or through the pleura. Either the intercostal vessels of the chest wall or the internal mammary vessels are most common bleeding sources; the pulmonary vasculature and the heart are possible but less likely origins. Bleeding may be brisk and, in a child, as much as 40% of the total blood volume can accumulate in the pleural space.[5] Tube thoracostomy allows blood to be evacuated from the pleural space and permits monitoring of the rate of ongoing bleeding. In addition, with patients in shock from massive intrapleural hemorrhage, tube thoracostomy not only corrects major derangements in ventilation and oxygenation but also allows intrapleural blood to be recirculated into the vascular space by autotransfusion.

Immediate tube thoracostomy is needed for the unstable pediatric patient with thoracic injury and clear clinical evidence of a pleural collection of air or blood. Stable patients without clear evidence of a pleural collection may wait for confirmation by chest x-ray. Most pediatric patients with confirmed traumatic pleural collections should undergo tube thoracostomy.

Other nontraumatic indications for tube thoracostomy are spontaneous pneumothorax with respiratory distress and the rapid accumulation of pleural fluid, which also causes severe respiratory distress.

Contraindications

The only contraindication to tube thoracostomy is the need for immediate thoracotomy.[3] In a stable, anticoagulated patient or a patient with a known clotting dysfunction, it may be appropriate to delay tube thoracostomy pending correction if there is no significant respiratory distress. Delaying tube thoracostomy requires close observation and continuous respiratory and cardiovascular monitoring in an intensive care unit.

Complications

Complications of tube thoracostomy include bleeding, persistent pneumothorax, tension pneumothorax, persistent hemothorax, and injury to the internal organs and diaphragm.

Bleeding may occur from the skin incision but is easy to control. Significant bleeding and hemothorax may result from the laceration of intercostal arteries or veins if the physician is not careful in avoiding the neurovascular bundle that lies on the inferior margin of the rib. Laceration of the heart or of the pulmonary artery or vein may also occur when a tube is forcefully placed with a trocar. Therefore avoid the use of trocars.

Persistent pneumothorax may result from the following situations: misplacement of the tube either in the subcutaneous tissue or abdominal cavity; incorrect securing of the tube, with the drainage holes left outside the pleural space; a mechanical problem with blockage or kinking of the tube; a loose tube connection; a malfunction of the drainage system; or a tracheal or bronchial tear or fistula that causes a continuous air leak. Normally, air bubbles through the water

Table 107-1 Chest Tube Size for Children

Age group	Tube size (Fr)
Newborn	8-12
Infant	14-20
Child	20-28
Adolescent	28-36

seal as vacuum drainage evacuates the pneumothorax. With completion of the evacuation, air no longer bubbles through the water seal (without suction). Persistent bubbling of suction indicates a system air leak (if the skin-entry site is airtight), or a tracheobronchial fistula.[2]

Tension pneumothorax may recur, especially when the child is receiving positive-pressure ventilation. Any sudden decline in cardiopulmonary status or significant oxygen desaturation should prompt immediate evaluation of the breath sounds, the chest tube connections, and the drainage system.

Persistent hemothorax may occur secondary to inadequate tube drainage and may require multiple tube placement. Loculations may also contain pockets of fluid and not permit adequate evacuation with a single tube.

A significant complication of tube thoracostomy is organ injury. Intraabdominal trauma with bleeding may elevate the diaphragm, and anatomic landmarks may vary with age. As a result, it is possible to place a tube inadvertently through the diaphragm and into the abdomen and injure the liver, spleen, stomach, colon, small bowel, or diaphragm.[7] Never place a thoracostomy tube below the nipple line, which is the most cephalad location of the diaphragm.

Equipment

The equipment necessary to perform tube thoracostomy includes an organized chest tube tray, chest tubes in sizes 12 to 36 Fr (Table 107-1), dressings, and an adequate suction/drainage setup. Organize the items essential to successful thoracostomy and chest tube placement on a prepared tray (Box 107-1).

The management of children with thoracic trauma requires a basic understanding of chest tube drainage and suction devices. The standard commercial device uses a water-seal mechanism that when attached to the chest tube creates a vacuum and therefore a negative intrathoracic pressure to reexpand a collapsed lung. The pressure within the thoracic cavity normally is lower than the pressure of the atmosphere, and thus air can rush in with any type of penetrating wound. The water-seal vacuum not only creates negative pressure for lung reexpansion but also keeps the outside air from being drawn back into the pleural space. Typically, the apparatus consists of a three-chamber system that attaches at one end to the chest tube and at the other end to a wall suction system. The chamber nearest the chest tube collects blood or fluid from within the chest. The second chamber is the underwater seal chamber and serves two functions: (1) to provide a one-way valve for the escape of air entrapped within the pleural cavity, thus preventing the redevelopment of tension pneumothorax, and (2) with the use of a water siphon, to maintain the normal negative intrathoracic pressure gradient with respect to the surrounding atmosphere. This underwater

BOX 107-1 CHEST TUBE TRAY AND MATERIALS REQUIRED FOR TUBE THORACOSTOMY[2]

Large Kelly clamps (2)
Medium Kelly clamps (2)
Large, curved Mayo scissors (1)
Large, straight suture scissors (1)
Needle holder (1)
No. 4 knife hand and No. 10 scalpel blades (2)
Toothed forceps (1)
Towel clips (4)
0 silk sutures (3)
2-0 silk sutures on cutting needles (2)
Large, free-curved cutting needle (2)
10-ml syringe
1 ½-inch 18-gauge needle
1 ½-inch 22-gauge needle
Sterile towels (4)
4 × 4 gauze pads
High-output vacuum device
Drainage apparatus with water seal
Sterile extension tubing for drainage system
Serrated plastic connectors (straight and Y-type)
Chest tubes (various sizes)
Petroleum jelly gauze
Preparation razor
Local anesthetic
Antiseptic preparation solution
Benzoin tincture
2-inch cloth tape

seal chamber ensures that air, which always enters the lung passively via the path of least resistance, will travel via the natural airways rather than through a hole in the chest wall, thus preventing "paradoxical" respiration.

The third chamber functions as a suction-regulating device that limits the negative pressure by allowing air to be drawn from the atmosphere whenever the force of the vacuum is sufficient to overcome the weight of a water column set at a predetermined height (in centimeters). This last chamber is connected to wall suction at more than 20 cm of water.[2] Again, air bubbles through the water seal until it is removed from the chest. If bubbling persists after the water seal has been removed, look for a system air leak and carefully inspect the chest tube insertion site and all of the drainage connections. Be sure that the entire chest drainage and suction system, from pleural space to vacuum source, is intact before concluding that a pulmonary air leak is present. The more vigorous the bubbling, the larger the leak. In the presence of a large air leak it may be possible to attain more rapid air evacuation by inserting additional larger chest tubes.

Techniques

Identify the side with the suspected pneumothorax or hemothorax. In the presence of abdominal distention, place a nasogastric tube to reduce diaphragmatic elevation. The preferred site of entry is the fourth or fifth intercostal space

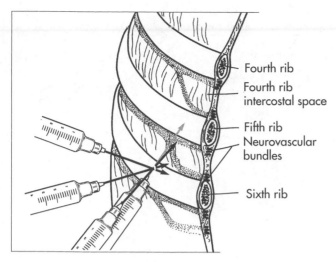

FIG. 107-1   Administration of local anesthetics for tube thoracostomy. Begin at skin incision site and extend superiorly to pleural entry site.

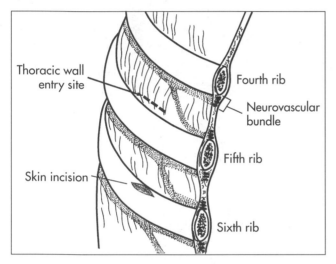

FIG. 107-2   Incision site and pleural entry site for tube thoracostomy.

in the region of the middle-to-anterior axillary line. This area is approximately at the level of the nipple. In the absence of breast development, the nipple lies over the fourth intercostal space. With breast development, the lower margin of the breast originates on the fifth rib.

Place the patient in the supine position with his or her arm restrained over his or her head on the affected side (swimmer's position). Identify the landmarks, prepare the skin with iodine, and drape the area. Along with local anesthetics, the careful use of intravenous analgesics and sedative agents when appropriate markedly reduces the pain of the procedure and reduces the need for physical restraint of pediatric patients. Infiltrate the skin generously with lidocaine (with or without epinephrine) at the level of the incision and in a track one to two rib spaces superiorly above the pleural entry site (Fig. 107-1). In an unstable patient, it may be necessary to proceed without the use of a local anesthetic.

Using the skin scalpel and following the sixth rib contour, make a 1- to 3-cm incision through the skin and into the subcutaneous tissue (Fig. 107-2). Place a curved Kelly clamp into the incision with the tips pointed away from the chest, and dissect a track approximately one to two rib spaces above (Fig. 107-3, *A*). Turn over the Kelly clamp, and using the tip, puncture through the intercostal muscle and into the thoracic cavity (Fig. 107-3, *B*). Be sure to enter the chest cavity on the superior margin of the rib to avoid injuring the intercostal neurovascular (nerve, artery, and vein) bundle. Puncturing the pleural space may require some force, and the patient usually experiences a moderate amount of pain. With entry there typically is a drop in resistance and a gush of air or blood. Widen the hole by opening the Kelly clamp handles, and insert a gloved fingertip to break up any adhesions or loculated areas of the lung and to ensure entry of the chest tube. Avoid injuring the finger on a fractured rib.

Using the gloved finger as a guide, insert an appropriately sized chest tube into the hole and direct it to the proper position (Fig. 107-4). Direct the tube anteriorly for anterior air collections and posteriorly for fluid collections. Air

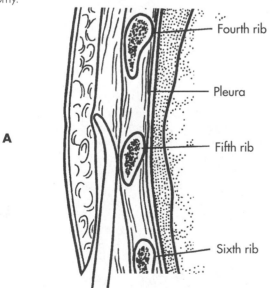

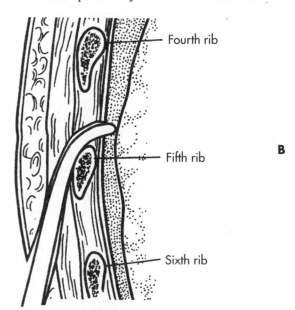

FIG. 107-3   Dissection for tube thoracostomy. **A,** Introduce clamp with tip pointed away from pleura. **B,** Turn clamp and dissect through pleura at point above superior border of fifth rib.

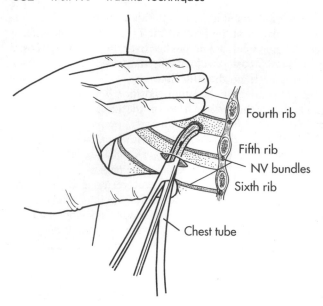

FIG. 107-4 Insertion of chest tube.

usually collects in the nondependent area, and fluid collects in the dependent areas. However, placing a tube posteriorly for pleural air collection is also acceptable. Facilitate insertion of the chest tube by grabbing the distal end of the tube with a long curved Kelly clamp and using it as a guide to insert and direct the tube. Be sure to insert the tube until the last hole is inside the pleural cavity; do not insert the tube too far or the patient may complain of shoulder pain. It is not unusual for the patient to cough as the lung expands.[3]

Finally, secure the tube using 1-0 or 2-0 silk sutures. There are many methods of securing the tube, but it is important that, the technique be understood by whoever is managing and removing the tube. One method of closing the incision around the tube is with a purse-string suture, an adaptation of the horizontal mattress suture technique (Fig. 107-5). This technique leaves equal ends of suture to wrap around the tube before tying the knot and leaves enough suture to pull the purse-string tight and to tie a new knot after removing the chest tube, thus closing the incision. After securing the tube, place a petroleum jelly gauze dressing around the base of the tube at the level of the skin to prevent air moving into the chest cavity with spontaneous breathing. Cover the site with dry sterile gauze and tape securely with benzoin tincture. Avoid taping over the nipple. Be certain to tether the tube to the skin with tape to avoid accidental removal; tape all tube connections. Obtain an x-ray study to check tube placement and efficacy of drainage.[3] Arrange the draining tubes to avoid creating dependent loops; this will obviate the need to routinely strip the chest tube to prevent occlusion by fluid or a blood clot.

Remarks

The thoracic cavity is more elastic and compressible in a child than in an adult. In a child, the chest wall may transmit a large force into the deeper structures of the chest without apparent external injury. Rib fracture and external injury are often absent; however, this absence does not preclude internal damage. A child's lung is more susceptible to laceration;

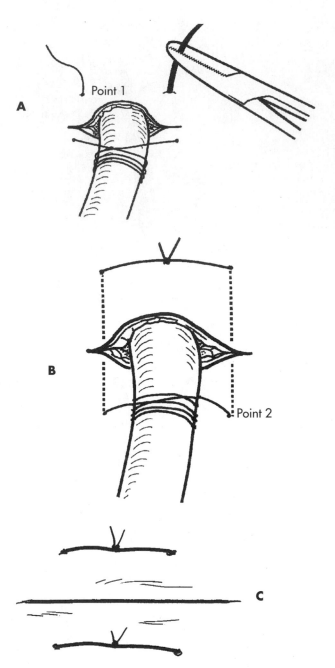

FIG. 107-5 Securing the chest tube with a purse-string suture. **A,** Insert the silk suture into the skin through the subcutaneous tissue at the point marked 1. Come out through the opposite side of the incision. Wrap the suture around the chest tube multiple times and tie it securely in place. **B,** Pass the needle through the skin at the point marked 2 as if to complete the horizontal mattress stitch, and come out through the opposite side of the incision; then tie the suture. This method secures the tube in place while also facilitating removal. **C,** When it is time to remove the tube, cut the suture around the chest tube and tie the ends together. This action closes the incision similarly to the horizontal mattress closure, except that there is a knot at both ends.

therefore avoid the use of trocars. If possible, avoid any anterior approach for tube placement because this approach is inadequate for evacuating fluids and often leaves an unsightly scar.

The correct size for the chest tube varies with age. To obtain a good approximation, use the diameter of the intercostal space as a guide to the diameter of the tube. Other estimations include using the following formulas: 2 × size of the nasogastric tube or urinary catheter, or 4 × size of the endotracheal tube.[4] Tubes ranging from 12 to 20 Fr often are suitable for the smaller child. Use a larger tube to remove blood.

Techniques for decreasing an air leak that cannot be managed by chest tubes alone include the use of jet ventilation, which uses reduced airway pressures; selective intubation of the contralateral bronchus; or occlusion of the ipsilateral bronchus with a small balloon catheter.

REFERENCES

1. Burkle FM, Weibe RA: Pediatric emergencies, *Emerg Med Clin North Am* 9:3, 1991.
2. Cooper A: Critical management of chest, abdomen, and extremity trauma. In Holbrook PR, editor: *Textbook of pediatric critical care,* Philadelphia, 1993, WB Saunders.
3. Dalbec DL, Krome RL: Emergency procedures: thoracostomy, *Emerg Med Clin North Am* 4:3, 1986.
4. Dieckmann RA: Personal communication, January 1994.
5. Golladay ES: Thoracic injuries. In Ehrlich FE, Heldrich FJ, Tepas JJ, editors: *Pediatric emergency medicine,* Rockville, Md, 1987, Aspen.
6. Graham JM, Mattox KL, Beall AC: Penetrating trauma in the lung, *J Trauma* 19:665, 1979.
7. Milikin JS, Moore EE, Steiner E, et al: Complications of tube thoracostomy for acute trauma, *Am J Surg* 140:738, 1980.
8. Reilly JP, Brandt ML, Mattox KL, et al: Thoracic trauma in children, *J Trauma* 34:329-331, 1993.

108 Resuscitative Thoracotomy

Arthur Cooper

Intrathoracic injury is an uncommon event and occurs in approximately 6% of serious pediatric injuries.[4] Nevertheless, the mortality rate is significant and approaches 15%.[4] Most intrathoracic injuries can be managed expectantly or by means of tube thoracostomy. However, for those few children who suffer cardiac arrest from major penetrating thoracic trauma, resuscitative thoracotomy in the emergency department (ED) followed by definitive surgical repair can be lifesaving.[2,5,9-11,14]

Indications

Resuscitative thoracotomy is indicated for the child with penetrating chest trauma *and* one of the following conditions: (1) traumatic cardiac arrest preceded by evidence of cardiorespiratory activity in the field or in the ED (*witnessed arrest*), and (2) suspected *cardiac tamponade* complicated by systolic hypotension or traumatic cardiac arrest.

Indications for immediate transfer to the operating room for emergency thoracotomy following initial resuscitation in the ED include the following: (1) suspected cardiac tamponade not yet complicated by systolic hypotension or traumatic cardiac arrest; (2) intrathoracic hemorrhage that exceeds 20% to 25% of circulating blood volume (approximately 15 to 20 ml/kg) immediately following tube thoracostomy; (3) massive air leak after tube thoracostomy; (4) evidence of gross contamination of the thoracic cavity by esophageal, gastric, or intestinal contents following tube thoracostomy; and (5) destructive injuries of the chest wall, causing open pneumothorax. The salvage rate following resuscitative thoracotomy for penetrating trauma may reach 10%. For blunt trauma the salvage rate is nearly zero, although there have been isolated reports of survival.[2,4,5,9-11] The cost associated with unsuccessful resuscitative thoracotomy is great.[4] Therefore reserve resuscitative thoracotomy for those patients with a reasonable chance for survival.

Contraindications

Limit the use of resuscitative thoracotomy to children with penetrating chest trauma and those with signs of cardiorespiratory activity on arrival at the ED or during resuscitation. Patients who have had an *unwitnessed arrest* are not candidates for the procedure because neurologically intact survival is highly unlikely.

The value of resuscitative thoracotomy after a blunt traumatic cardiac arrest is minimal. The outcome is dismal even among those pediatric patients who have evidence of initial signs of cardiorespiratory activity in the field but no such evidence on arrival in the ED.[2,4,9-11]

Resuscitative thoracotomy for and cross-clamping of the distal thoracic aorta has been occasionally successful in reviving children who arrive at the ED in decompensated hypotensive shock from intraabdominal hemorrhage and subsequently deteriorate into traumatic cardiac arrest.[5] However, do not routinely perform this procedure as part of initial resuscitation in young children as is done in adults,[12] because young children have abundant collateral circulation, which reduces the efficacy; in addition, there is greater potential for avulsion of the intercostal vessels.[3] Thoracotomy offers no significant advantage over emergency laparotomy and direct finger compression of the proximal abdominal aorta, which is the appropriate initial operation in most of these cases.

Complications

Some of the complications of thoracotomy are unavoidable, such as unsuccessful resuscitation. However, improper technique may result in avoidable complications such as air embolism, pneumothorax, hemothorax, hemopericardium, myocardial laceration, coronary artery laceration, phrenic nerve injury, diaphragmatic injury, abdominal perforation into solid or hollow viscera, and injury to the aorta and great vessels, trachea, esophagus, and lung. Infectious complications occur infrequently.

Equipment

Keep the equipment for resuscitative thoracotomy in a sterile, specially marked thoracotomy pack (Box 108-1) that is readily available at all times in the trauma receiving area. Package equipment in such a way that the instrument storage tray fits neatly on a Mayo stand or similar surface for placement directly at the operating physician's side and at a convenient height. Secure disposable items that may be necessary during the procedure (e.g., scalpel blades, Foley catheters, and suture material) to the outside of the pack, which obviates the need to spend valuable seconds locating these supplies at the required moment.

Techniques

Thoracotomy. To prepare for resuscitative thoracotomy, obtain definitive control of the airway with orotracheal intubation and protect the cervical spine as indicated. Continue the resuscitation following current consensus guidelines[1] and rapidly obtain vascular access while the operating physician dons sterile latex gloves, protective eyewear, and a surgical gown.

To perform a resuscitative thoracotomy, place the patient in the supine position, place a small roll beneath the scapula,[9] and prepare the left anterior side of the chest by rapidly pouring a single layer of povidone-iodine solution over the entire left side of the chest. Open the thoracotomy pack (see Box 108-1) and place it adjacent to the operating physician, (who stands at the patient's left side).

Pressing firmly, make an incision directly through the fifth intercostal space (located approximately one finger breadth below the nipple) from the sternal border to the posterior axillary line (Fig. 108-1). Extend the incision through all layers of the chest wall to the level of the parietal pleura. Incise the parietal pleura centrally and extend the incision medially and laterally for the full extent of the surgical wound. Insert an appropriately sized Finochietto rib spreader with the central portion of the U-shaped bracket directed laterally. Separate the ribs using the rotary winch. If exposure is inadequate to see the pericardial sac, transect the fifth costal cartilage (the medial portion of the fifth rib, located just above the incision at the sternal border) in half with a scalpel or heavy scissors (see Fig. 108-1) before completely separating the ribs with the Finochietto rib spreader.[7]

Once the ribs have been separated, the lung will retract by gravity and expose the pericardial sac, which is typically bluish and bulging if there is pericardial tamponade because of myocardial penetration. Identify the phrenic nerve (a narrow whitish band that follows the lateral aspect of the pericardium, roughly parallel to the long axis of the body), and incise the pericardium approximately one finger breadth anterior to (on the sternal side of) the phrenic nerve, taking care not to injure the underlying myocardium (Fig. 108-2). Quickly extend the incision superiorly and inferiorly as far as the respective pericardial reflections to allow rapid egress of entrapped blood. Using the left hand, manually evacuate clotted blood entrapped anterior and posterior to the heart.

Hemorrhage Control. Because the anterior aspect of the right ventricle is fairly well protected by the sternum, most penetrating injuries to the heart involve the left ventricle, which will be readily apparent once the blood contained within the pericardium has been evacuated. Control ongoing hemorrhage from the ventricle by direct digital obliteration of the defect in the ventricular wall. Place a finger or thumb over or into the wound (depending on its size) or insert a Foley catheter through the wound and inflate it with saline (the size of the balloon may limit its utility in small children[8]). Draw back the catheter to occlude the internal opening.

In most cases of penetrating thoracic injury complicated by traumatic cardiac arrest, there is direct injury to the heart regardless of whether cardiac tamponade is clinically evident. However, if after opening the chest and exposing the

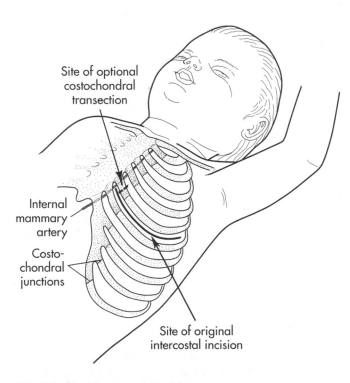

FIG. 108-1   Thoracotomy incision.

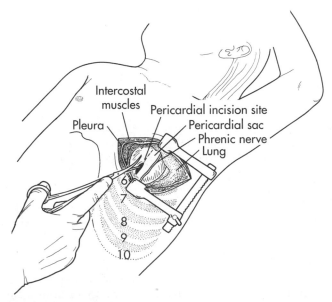

FIG. 108-2   Once the pericardial sac is exposed, identify the phrenic nerve and incise the pericardium.

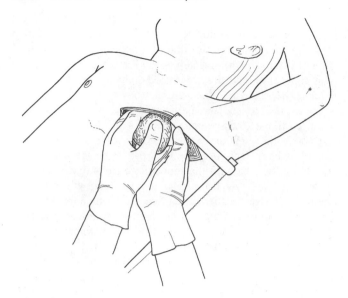

FIG. 108-3 Two-handed technique for cardiac massage in large child.

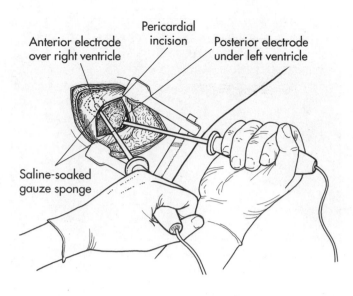

Fig. 108-5 Internal defibrillation.

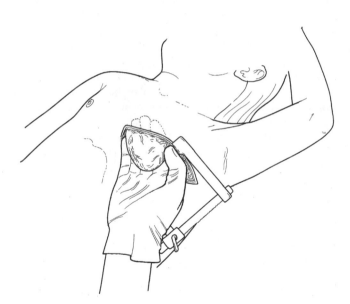

FIG. 108-4 One-handed technique for cardiac massage in small child.

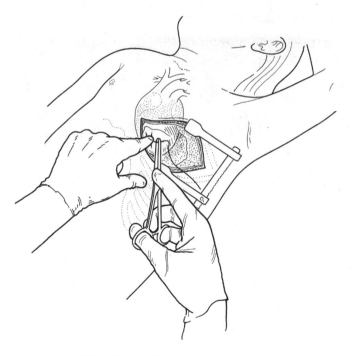

FIG. 108-6 Repair of cardiac wound.

pericardium, massive hemothorax is found in the absence of a bluish, bulging pericardial sac or direct visual evidence of pericardial violation, rapidly attempt to identify and control another source of the bleeding.

Most intrathoracic bleeding is a result of transection (partial or complete) of an intercostal artery or internal mammary artery;[15] control this bleeding by directly compressing the involved artery against the bony elements of the thorax by using a finger or by occluding the defect with a small Foley catheter.

Emergently treat the rare and nearly invariably fatal case of penetrating injury to the thoracic aorta or one of its major branches with direct finger pressure over the arterial defect.

Cardiac Massage and Internal Defibrillation. If the heart is empty and beating in a rapid sinus rhythm, focus on the delivery of intravascular volume, preferably red blood cells while continuing to obliterate the defect. However, if the heart is full and beating in a slow or ineffective rhythm, perform direct manual cardiac massage, again while continuing to obliterate the defect. Administer intravenous, intraosseous, or intracardiac epinephrine (use the intracardiac injection only when there is no reliable intravenous or intraosseous access).

In a large child, use a two-handed technique for cardiac massage (Fig. 108-3). Place the left hand behind the heart as a backboard while intermittently compressing the anterolateral surface of the left ventricle with the right hand. In a small child, use a one-handed technique (Fig. 108-4). Place three or four fingers behind the heart for use as a backboard while intermittently compressing the anterior surface of the left ventricle with the thumb.

Ventricular tachydysrhythmias typically occur when the myocardium becomes hypothermic, hypoxic, and acidotic. Preventive measures include vigorous support of airway, breathing, and circulation, including use of a blood warmer to avoid the reduction in core temperature associated with rapid infusion of refrigerated blood. If ventricular fibrillation or ventricular tachycardia develops in spite of these precautions, defibrillate at a dose of 5 J (increasing to 20 J as necessary), using properly insulated internal paddles of appropriate size (4 cm for the large child, 2 cm for the small child); ensure that other rescuers are clear and that the shafts of the paddles do not touch the retractor or chest wall before discharging the defibrillator. Position one electrode under the left ventricle, below the heart, the other over the right ventricle, above the heart; place a saline soaked gauze sponge should be placed between each electrode and underlying myocardium to maximize electrical conductance and energy transfer (Fig. 108-5). In all cases, administer red blood cells. If type-specific blood is not available, use type O–positive cells in male patients and type O–negative cells in female patients. Control ongoing hemorrhage, continue cardiac massage, and perform internal defibrillation as necessary. Transfer the child to the operating room when the surgical team arrives to assume responsibility for definitive surgical repair and thoracic closure and drainage.

Surgical Repair. If the surgical team is not immediately available, the ED physician may need to repair the cardiac wound. Perform direct suture closure as simply and quickly as possible using nonabsorbable material that is relatively atraumatic, does not require pledgets, and is easy to tie (such as 2-0 silk). The suture must be swaged on moderately large, tapered, semicircular needles (or surgical staples if they are of the appropriate shape and size).[6,13] Accomplish repair by obliterating the defect with the volar surface of the fingertip of the nondominant hand; in the case of a large defect, gently squeeze the edges of the defect together with the tips of the thumb and index finger. While avoiding the coronary arteries, reapproximate the edges of the defect using interrupted simple sutures inserted beneath the occluding fingertip(s) and through both sides of the cardiac wound.

Place the sutures deeply enough to obtain a solid hold of the friable myocardial wall but not so deep that the endocardium is penetrated (Fig. 108-6).[7] Tie the knot with *minimal tension* while withdrawing the occluding fingertip slowly to minimize both myocardial tearing and the potential for air embolism. Repeat the sequence until the wound closure is completed. Begin antibiotic prophylaxis, and cover the open chest wall with a sterile dressing.

REFERENCES

1. American College of Surgeons Committee on Trauma: *Advanced trauma life support student manual,* ed 5, Chicago, 1993, American College of Surgeons.
2. Beaver BL, Colombani PM, Buck JR, et al: Efficacy of emergency thoracotomy in pediatric trauma, *J Pediatr Surg* 22:19-23, 1987.
3. Brotman S, Oster-Granite M, Cox EF: Failure of cross-clamping the thoracic aorta to control intraabdominal bleeding, *Ann Emerg Med* 11:147-148, 1982.
4. Cooper A, Barlow B, DiScala C, et al: Mortality and truncal injury: the pediatric perspective, *J Pediatr Surg* 29:33-38, 1994.
5. Langer JC, Joffman MA, Pearl RH, et al: Survival after emergency department thoracotomy in a child with blunt multisystem trauma, *Pediatr Emerg Care* 5:255-256, 1989.
6. Macho JR, Markison RE, Schecter WP: Cardiac stapling in the management of penetrating wounds of the heart: rapid control of hemorrhage and decreased risk of personal contamination, *J Trauma* 34:711-716, 1993.
7. Maynard AdeL, Cordice JWV, Naclerio EA: Penetrating wounds of the heart: a report of 81 cases, *Surg Gynecol Obstet* 94:605-618, 1952.
8. Pham SM, Johnson R, Durham SJ, et al: Hemodynamic consequences of Foley catheter control in experimental cardiac wounds, *Surg Gynecol Obstet* 169:247-250, 1989.
9. Powell RW, Gill EA, Jurkowich GJ, et al: Resuscitative thoracotomy in children and adolescents, *Am Surg* 54:188-191, 1988.
10. Reilly JP, Brandt ML, Mattox KL, et al: Thoracic trauma in children, *J Trauma* 34:329-331, 1993.
11. Rothenberg SS, Moore EE, Moore FA, et al: Emergency department thoracotomy in children, *J Trauma* 29:1322-1325, 1989.
12. Schwab CW, Adcock OT, Max MH: Emergency department thoracotomy (EDT): a 26-month experience using an "agonal" protocol, *Am Surg* 52:20-29, 1986.
13. Shamoun JM, Barraza KR, Jurkovich GJ, et al: In-extremis use of staples for cardiorrhaphy in penetrating cardiac trauma: case report, *J Trauma* 29:1589-1591, 1989.
14. Sheikh AA, Culbertson CB: Emergency department thoracotomy in children: rationale for selective application, *J Trauma* 34:323-328, 1993.
15. Weil PII, Margolis IB: Systematic approach to traumatic hemothorax, *Am J Surg* 142:692-694, 1981.
16. Wilson SM, Au FC: In-extremis use of a Foley catheter in a cardiac stab wound, *J Trauma* 26:400-402, 1986.

109 HEMORRHAGE CONTROL

Jill M. Baren

Control of hemorrhage is an essential part of comprehensive wound management. Removal of clot material and cessation of active bleeding are necessary for adequate visualization and exploration of a wound. When bleeding is inadequately controlled, hematoma formation occurs and leads to separation of sutured wound edges, establishment of a nidus of infection, and possible progression to wound dehiscence.[3,5] Exsanguinating superficial skin wounds can lead to hypotension, particularly in young children, who have reduced circulating blood volumes. Hemostasis contributes to successful wound healing and to the hemodynamic stability of the pediatric patient.

Attempts to control wound hemorrhage should proceed in a stepwise fashion from the simplest measures to the more advanced techniques. Natural hemostasis normally occurs within 5 to 15 minutes of onset of bleeding and occurs in the majority of patients. In patients who require more aggressive measures to control bleeding, consider the possibility of underlying coagulation disorders or use of anticoagulants such as aspirin.[2]

Indications

All active bleeding requires immediate control techniques to reduce blood loss and possible perfusion abnormalities.

Contraindications

There are no contraindications to controlling hemorrhage, although certain measures are preferred in certain conditions.

Complications

Complications are related to the specific procedure.

Techniques

Simple Methods of Hemorrhage Control

DIRECT PRESSURE AND COMPRESSIVE DRESSINGS. Direct pressure over a wound is the primary method of choice for control of bleeding. Pressure should be continuously applied with a gloved hand and sterile sponges over a broad area for a minimum of 10 to 15 minutes.[5] When combined with elevation of the affected part, this technique is highly effective for the majority of wounds in pediatric patients. If personnel are limited in the emergency department (ED), sterile sponges may be held in place with an elastic bandage, forming a compressive dressing.[4]

TOPICAL VASOCONSTRICTORS. Topical epinephrine (1 ml of 1:1000 solution) may be diluted with 4 to 5 ml of normal saline and applied with a sterile sponge if vasoconstriction is necessary.[5,6] Application of epinephrine solution is absolutely contraindicated for wounds of the fingers, toes, penis, tip of ears, or nose.[6] The benefit of vasoconstriction for standard wound repair may be outweighed by an increase in the risk of wound infection.[3]

ELECTROCAUTERY. Electrocautery is occasionally useful in the ED to control hemorrhage when other simple methods fail, but this technique should be restricted to use on vessels less than 2 mm in diameter. Pinpoint coagulation lessens the chance for surrounding tissue destruction. Bipolar coagulation devices such as Bovie Cautery are better than the monopolar type because they induce less tissue damage. Electrocautery works best in a dry wound field, so sponges and suction should be assembled. Use a small forceps or hemostat to hold the vessel in order to control the application of heat. Electrocautery should not be applied to unbroken skin or skin edges.

PACKING. If bleeding is persistent after standard pressure, it may be necessary to pack the wound cavity. Sponges soaked in sterile saline can be tightly placed in the open wound. When covered with an elastic bandage, they become an extension of a compressive dressing. A variety of synthetic hemostatic agents composed of fibrin or gelatin foams (e.g., Gelfoam, Surgicel, and Avitene) are commercially available and may also be used to achieve hemostasis when they are applied directly on the wound. The mechanism by which they promote coagulation is poorly understood, but they help control oozing when they are used as liners in wound cavities.[3] Once hemostasis is achieved, remove with forceps or by gentle irrigation. These materials are bactericidal and do not interfere with wound healing. They should not be left in wounds or placed against bony structures because they can interfere with callus formation or serve as a nidus for infection.

Control of Hemorrhage with Sutures and Ligatures

LIGATION OF VESSELS. Transection of blood vessels leads to contraction of the cut edge with adequate hemostasis in a few minutes. However, if a vessel is partially transected, it may continue to ooze, or if the vessel is large enough (>2 mm), it may require ligation to control bleeding.[3] It is not prudent to spend a lot of time searching for and ligating vessels while a child slowly exsanguinates. Reserve this technique for easily identifiable bleeding vessels.[3]

Ligation is performed by first identifying and clamping a vessel with a small hemostat. While an assistant lifts the handle of the hemostat, an absorbable suture is passed underneath it around the vessel. Have the assistant release the hemostat after the first knot is tied around the clamped vessel (Fig. 109-1). Three knots are sufficient to anchor the vessel, and the suture material should be clipped close to the knot to decrease the chance of inflammation, fibrosis, or infection in the wound.[2] Clamping and ligation should not be performed on large arteries or on vessels in the hand or wrist.[6] Other vital structures such as nerves often travel with the vasculature, and for this reason, clamping of vessels requires direct visualization.

SUTURING. An effective way to control minor oozing is simply to suture the wound closed. The intrinsic pressure

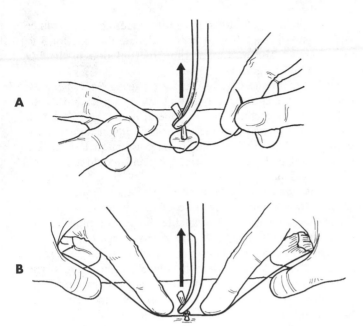

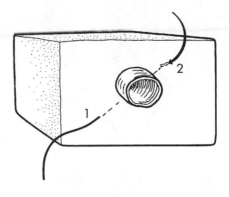

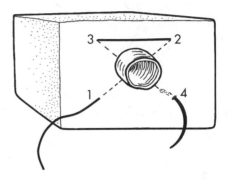

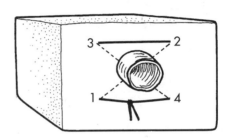

FIG. 109-1 Hemostasis by ligation. **A,** Assistant places gentle, upward traction on vessel with hemostat. **B,** Tighten first knot securely before releasing hemostat.

FIG. 109-2 Hemostasis for retracted, bleeding vessel in deep tissue using figure-of-eight suture technique.

generated within the loops of suture material is often enough to tamponade the bleeding.[6] Scalp wounds in children have the potential to be a major source of blood loss, but they can be well controlled by simple suturing. A figure-of-eight suture can be placed through bleeding tissue in deep wounds as a temporizing measure if the cut edge of the vessel has retracted and cannot be identified for ligation (Fig. 109-2).[3] Use caution, because this technique may cause constriction and devitalization of tissue.[3]

Tourniquets. Failure to control hemorrhage from extremity wounds with direct pressure, topical vasoconstrictors, electrocautery, or ligation is an indication for the application of a tourniquet. Tourniquets also provide the opportunity for exploration of complex extremity wounds in a bloodless field, and they establish rapid control over exsanguinating wounds involving a major vessel.[2]

Tourniquets are capable of causing ischemic and compressive injury to the involved extremity and may further compromise marginally viable tissue.

These deleterious effects can be minimized by observing stringent guidelines for tourniquet times and pressures.[3]

Begin tourniquet application with manual exsanguination of the extremity, which is protected first with smoothened bias or stockinette cloth. Fasten a blood pressure cuff proximally to the upper arm or leg. Have an assistant elevate the extremity while it is wrapped tightly with an elastic or Esmarch bandage in a distal-to-proximal direction (Fig. 109-3). Then inflate the cuff to a pressure approximately 50 to 100 mm Hg greater than systolic blood pressure (BP), and remove the wrapping bandage for wound exploration. Maintain cuff pressure by using a hemostat to clamp the rubber tubing of the sphygmomanometer rather than by tightening its valve. Release of the hemostat facilitates rapid deflation if it becomes necessary.[2,3,5]

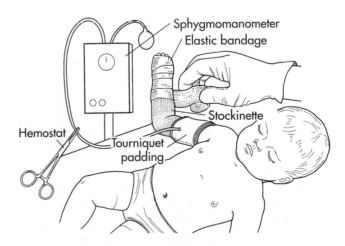

FIG. 109-3 Advanced hemostasis management using tourniquet technique. Protect the extremity with smooth bias or stockinette, apply tourniquet proximally, elevate extremity, wrap with elastic bandage in distal-to-proximal direction, inflate and maintain tourniquet pressure above systolic BP.

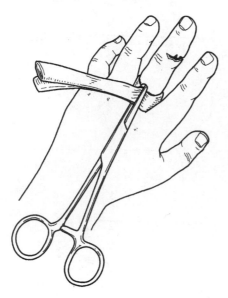

FIG. 109-4 Penrose drain secured with hemostat at base functions as finger tourniquet.

Most patients can tolerate a tourniquet for 30 minutes without anesthesia.[2] If pain occurs, deflate the cuff for 5 to 10 minutes.[2] The maximum time for inflation in the ED should be no longer than 1 hour.[3]

Digital tourniquets are useful for repairing finger wounds, but they have a greater potential for complications.[3] Although several methods are in general use, exercise caution so excessive pressures at the base of the finger do not cause tissue ischemia and necrosis. Finger tourniquet times are much less than those of the arm or leg and should not exceed 15 to 30 minutes.[3]

Penrose drains are used most often as a tourniquet and are secured by a clamp at the base of the finger (Fig. 109-4). There are commercially available finger tourniquets, but these are small enough to be easily forgotten under a dressing. Do not use rubber bands for the same reason.[2,4,5] On an older child or adolescent, place a tight-fitting sterile latex glove over the affected hand. Snip off the tip of the glove over the involved digit, and roll down the latex to the base of the finger. This effectively tamponades bleeding and provides additional sterility to the field (Fig. 109-5, *A* to *C*).[3]

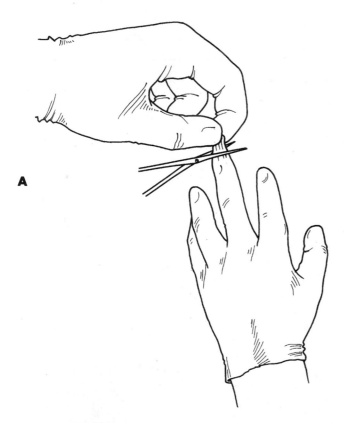

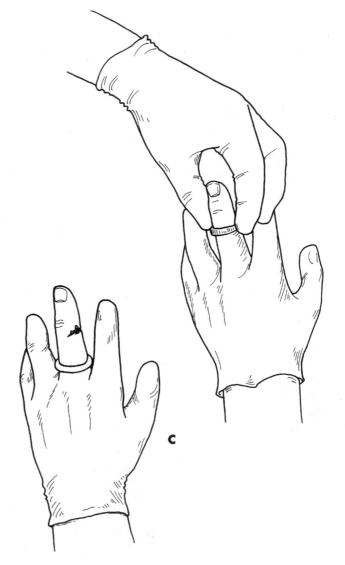

FIG. 109-5 Latex glove serving as "sterile" finger tourniquet. **A,** Snip off fingertip of sterile glove. **B,** Roll down latex to base of digit. **C,** Expose wound.

REFERENCES

1. Finley JM, McConnell RY: Wound management. In *Emergency wound repair,* Baltimore, 1984, University Park Press.
2. Kaplan EN, Hentz VR: Fundamentals of wound management and preoperative preparation. In *Emergency management of skin and soft tissue wounds: an illustrated guide,* Boston, 1984, Little, Brown.
3. Roberts JR, Hedges JR, editors: Principles of wound management. In *Clinical procedures in emergency medicine,* ed 2, Philadelphia, 1991, WB Saunders.
4. Simon RR, Brenner BE, editors: Hemorrhage and hemostasis. In *Emergency procedures and techniques,* ed 2, Baltimore, 1982, Williams & Wilkins.
5. Trott A: Decisions before closure: timing, debridement, and consultation. In *Wounds and lacerations emergency care and closure,* St. Louis, 1991, Mosby.
6. Zukin DD, Simon RR: Precare: patient evaluation, hemostasis techniques, and wound cleansing and antisepsis. In *Emergency wound care principles and practice,* Rockville, Md, 1987, Aspen Publishers.

110 Pericardiocentesis

Stanley H. Inkelis

Pericardiocentesis is the needle aspiration of the pericardial space. In the Emergency Department (ED), reserve pericardiocentesis for patients with life-threatening cardiac tamponade. In the pediatric intensive care unit (PICU), pericardiocentesis may be performed for tamponade and for diagnostic studies of pericardial effusion from other etiologies. If done blindly (without the use of electrocardiographic or echocardiographic monitoring) the morbidity for this procedure is approximately 20%.[2,10,12] If appropriate monitoring and imaging techniques are used, the risk of serious morbidity is approximately 0.5% to 1%.[10] The only indication for the blind approach is in a patient with cardiac tamponade who might die before monitoring can be instituted.[10]

Indications

Pericardiocentesis is indicated for cardiac tamponade of both traumatic and nontraumatic origins when emergent or urgent removal of pericardial fluid is lifesaving. Typically, patients with nontraumatic cardiac tamponade have developed this condition over time, and pericardiocentesis can be performed nonemergently and under controlled conditions. In the PICU, it is also indicated for diagnostic purposes to analyze pericardial fluid for infection or suspected malignancy (see Chapter 99). Because the diagnostic yield is only 25%, perform pericardiocentesis for diagnostic purposes only if the results will alter therapy.[10]

Trauma, particularly penetrating trauma, produces the most acute and rapidly progressive form of cardiac tamponade. As blood (or other fluid) accumulates rapidly, the pericardium has little time to stretch; intrapericardial pressure increases, which produces compression of all cardiac chambers. Initially, normal systolic blood pressure is maintained by an increase in pulse rate and total peripheral vascular resistance. Diastolic pressure rises, which causes a narrowed pulse pressure. As intrapericardial pressure continues to increase, the compensatory mechanisms fail. Diastolic filling is compromised, and central venous pressure increases with a resultant decrease in stroke volume and cardiac output. Systolic blood pressure decreases, and the pulse pressure continues to narrow. Pulsus paradoxus may be clinically evident. At this point the patient demonstrates the classic signs of cardiac tamponade (Beck's triad): distant heart sounds, neck vein distention, and hypotension. Intractable shock, cardiac arrest, and death ensue if intrapericardial pressure is not rapidly reduced.

Contraindications

There are no absolute contraindications to emergency pericardiocentesis. Relative contraindications include unfamiliarity with the procedure and inadequate equipment. In the PICU or in the nonemergent setting, where prophylactic and diagnostic pericardiocentesis may be performed, an uncorrected

---

> **BOX 110-1 COMPLICATIONS OF PERICARDIOCENTESIS***
>
> Puncture or laceration of atrium or ventricle
> Coronary artery laceration
> Cardiac dysrhythmia
> Vasovagal reaction
> Hemopericardium
> Pneumothorax
> Hemothorax
> Perforation of the diaphragm
> Gastric or bowel perforation
> Pneumoperitoneum
> Infection
> Cardiac arrest
> Death

*References 3, 10, 12, 14, and 15.

bleeding diathesis is an absolute contraindication.[3,10,12,14,15] Open thoracotomy is preferred over needle pericardiocentesis if the patient is in cardiac arrest after penetrating trauma and if the equipment and expertise are available.

Complications

A significant complication rate is associated with pericardiocentesis. Box 110-1 lists the complications associated with this procedure.

Equipment

The following equipment is needed to perform a blind pericardiocentesis in the patient with cardiac tamponade who might die before monitoring can be instituted: povidone-iodine solution, sterile gauze and gloves, a 30- to 50-ml syringe, and a 2.5-inch (for infants and small children) or 3.5-inch short-bevel 18- to 20-gauge spinal needle.

In all other cases, the following additional equipment is necessary and may be assembled as a pericardiocentesis tray: sterile drapes, 1% lidocaine, 25-gauge needle, two 5-ml syringes, two 2.5- and 3.5-inch short-bevel 18- and 20-gauge spinal needles, three-way stopcock, 30- and 50-ml syringes, two 18- and 20-gauge intravenous catheter needles, a hemostat, a cable with an alligator clip at each end, and anticoagulant- and nonanticoagulant-containing sterile sample tubes for tests such as culture and cell count. An electrocardiograph (ECG) is mandatory, and a two-dimensional echocardiograph (ECHO) is desirable. Additional equipment to perform the Seldinger technique is necessary in situations in which prolonged drainage is needed. In this case, add a plastic catheter and a flexible guide or J wire to the open tray.

Techniques

Establish vascular access and continuously monitor all patients undergoing pericardiocentesis. The equipment and personnel necessary for intubation and cardiac resuscitation must be immediately available. The use of sedation for this procedure in the ED is unusual because most patients with life-threatening cardiac tamponade are unresponsive. Adequate sedation is essential in situations in which the patient is responsive, such as in the PICU, where the procedure may be elective. In selected cases, premedicate the patient with atropine to prevent a vasovagal reaction.[3]

Subxiphoid, apical, and parasternal approaches have been described for pericardiocentesis.[3,12] The subxiphoid approach appears to be the safest approach and is the only one discussed in this chapter. The subxiphoid approach avoids the pleura, coronary arteries, and internal mammary arteries[10,12] and punctures the pericardium over the right ventricle (Fig. 110-1).

To perform the subxiphoid approach, place the child in a semireclining position (30 to 45 degrees). This position allows fluid to pool inferiorly and anteriorly.[10] Use povidone-iodine (10% solution) to prepare the entire lower xiphoid and epigastric area. Use sterile gloves and, if time permits, drape the area with sterile towels. In patients who are awake, infiltrate 1% plain lidocaine in the area just below and to the left of the xiphoid process and in the area beneath the skin in the direction of the pericardium.

Attach an 18- or 20-gauge spinal needle to a stopcock and a 30-ml syringe. Use the cable with alligator clips at each end to connect the V lead of the ECG to the hub end of the needle. Properly test and ground the ECG machine because small current leaks can cause dysrhythmias.[3,12] Turn the ECG recorder to the V-lead position.

Make a 2-mm incision between the xiphoid process and the left costal margin to facilitate passage of the needle through the skin. Insert the needle through the incision at a 30 to 45 degree angle to the skin. Advance slowly and aim toward the left shoulder while applying continuous gentle suction.[10] The pericardial membrane may be felt to "give" as it is penetrated.[12] The pericardium is no more than 5 cm below the skin in children and 6 to 8 cm below the skin in adult-sized adolescents.[1,3] Constant ECG monitoring is imperative during the procedure to indicate ventricular or atrial puncture. If the needle touches ventricular epicardium, a current of injury pattern occurs with evidence of ST-segment elevation, premature ventricular contractions, or other ventricular dysrhythmias (Fig. 110-2).[3,10,12,14,15] PR-segment elevation, atrioventricular dissociation, or atrial dysrhythmias may occur with atrial contact.[3,8] If any of these patterns are noted, withdraw the needle a few millimeters until the ECG evidence of epicardial contact disappears. Advance the needle at a more medial angle if epicardial contact occurs with the initial attempt and if fluid from the pericardial space is not easily withdrawn.[10]

Once the pericardium has been entered, fluid should flow freely without ECG evidence of myocardial injury. Place a hemostat on the needle at the skin surface to prevent the needle from advancing further than desired. Aspirate until no further fluid is obtained. The child may stabilize as the tamponade is relieved. If a catheter is needed or prolonged drainage is anticipated, use the Seldinger technique to insert a longer and larger-bore catheter with side holes over a flexible guide or J wire.[3]

Two-dimensional echocardiographic (ECHO)-directed pericardiocentesis is the safest and most reliable method of obtaining pericardial fluid in the ED if available.[4,6,13] In the PICU, where pericardiocentesis may be performed under less emergent circumstances, always use two-dimensional ECHO to determine the area of largest effusion and to guide needle entry into the pericardial space.

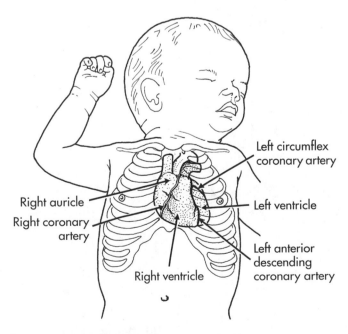

FIG. 110-1   Key anatomic areas of the heart.

Left circumflex coronary artery

Right auricle

Right coronary artery

Left ventricle

Left anterior descending coronary artery

Right ventricle

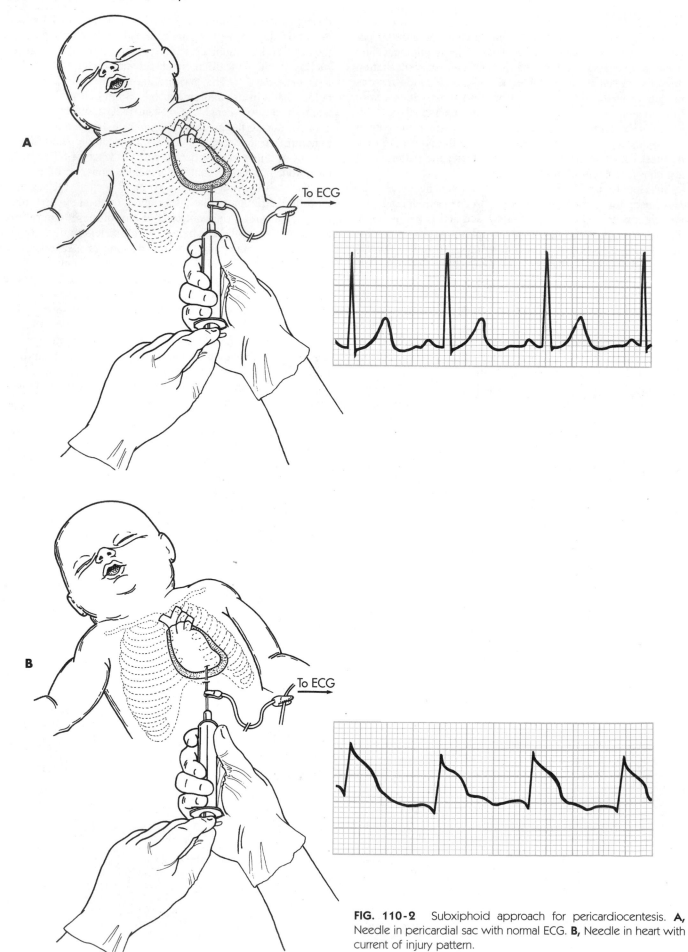

FIG. 110-2 Subxiphoid approach for pericardiocentesis. **A,** Needle in pericardial sac with normal ECG. **B,** Needle in heart with current of injury pattern.

Obtain a chest x-ray study after the procedure to rule out a pneumothorax. Monitor the patient closely in the PICU for 24 hours for evidence of fluid reaccumulation and any complications from the procedure.[3,10,12,14,15] Consider surgical consultation if open drainage is desirable in patients with recurrent pericardial effusion.

Remarks

The most reliable methods of determining the size and distribution of pericardial fluid in patients with pericardial effusion are ECHO, computerized tomography (CT), and magnetic resonance imagery (MRI).[7,10,11] Radiography, fluoroscopy, and radionucleotide imaging are not as reliable.[10]

ECHO is the easiest method in almost all cases because it can be performed at the bedside. Information is obtained rapidly, and the patient does not need to be moved to a CT or MRI scanner. In some situations, such as in postoperative cardiac patients, the fluid distribution is atypical and a CT scan or MRI might provide better definition of the pericardial fluid.[7,10,11] Never obtain a CT scan or MRI for patients who have life-threatening cardiac tamponade.

In most cases it is possible to determine if the blood aspirated during pericardiocentesis is from the pericardial effusion or from cardiac puncture. Bloody pericardial effusion typically does not clot because it is defibrinated by the whipping action of the heart.[10] However, if the bleeding is rapid, bloody pericardial effusion may clot and therefore may be indistinguishable from intracardiac blood. If the bleeding is very fast and pericardial effusion is present, the tap may be dry, which indicates a large clot that must be removed surgically.[10] Other methods of determining the source of the aspirated blood are as follows: (1) the hematocrit of the pericardial effusion is usually lower than that of peripheral blood[10,15]; (2) a drop of intracardiac blood on a gauze pad spreads evenly, whereas bloody pericardial effusion is darker centrally than peripherally[15]; and (3) bloody pericardial effusion usually has a pH that is approximately 0.10 less than arterial blood obtained simultaneously.[3,9]

REFERENCES

1. Baue AE, Blakemore WS: The pericardium, *Ann Thorac Surg* 14:81-106, 1972.
2. Bishop LH, Estes EH, McIntosh HD: The electrocardiogram as a safeguard in pericardiocentesis, *JAMA* 162:264-265, 1956.
3. Callaham ML: Pericardiocentesis. In Roberts JR, Hedges JR, editors: *Clinical procedures in emergency medicine*, ed 2, Philadelphia, 1991, WB Saunders.
4. Callahan JA, Seward JB, Tajik AJ: Cardiac tamponade: pericardiocentesis directed by two-dimensional echocardiography, *Mayo Clin Proc* 60:344-347, 1985.
5. Clarke DP, Cosgrove DO: Real-time ultrasound scanning in the planning and guidance of pericardiocentesis, *Clin Radiol* 38:119-122, 1987.
6. Hanaki Y, Kamiya H, Todoroki H, et al: New two-dimensional, echocardiographically directed pericardiocentesis in cardiac tamponade, *Crit Care Med* 18:750-753, 1990.
7. Hoit BD: Imaging the pericardium, *Cardiol Clin* 8(4):587-600, 1990.
8. Kerber R, Ridges J, Harrison D: Electrocardiographic indications of atrial puncture during pericardiocentesis, *N Engl J Med* 282:1142-1143, 1970.
9. Kindig J, Goodman M: Clinical utility of pericardial fluid pH determination, *Am J Med* 75:1077-1079, 1983.
10. Kirkland LL, Taylor RW: Pericardiocentesis, *Crit Care Clin* 8(4):699-712, 1992.
11. Link KM: Noninvasive evaluation of the pericardium and myocardium, *Curr Opin Radiol* 2:586-594, 1990.
12. Lorell BH, Braunwold E: Pericardial disease. In Braunwold E, editor: *Heart disease: a textbook of cardiovascular medicine,* ed 4, Philadelphia, 1992, WB Saunders.
13. Mayron R, Gaudio FE, Plummer D, et al: Echocardiography performed by emergency physicians: impact on diagnosis and therapy, *Ann Emerg Med* 17:150-154, 1988.
14. Ruddy RM: Procedures (pericardiocentesis). In Fleischer GF, Ludwig S, editors: *Textbook of pediatric emergency medicine*, ed 3, Baltimore, 1993, Williams & Wilkins.
15. Van Heeckeren DW, Moss MM: Pericardiocentesis and pericardial tube insertion. In Blumer JL, editor: *A practical guide to pediatric intensive care,* ed 3, St Louis, 1990, Mosby.

111 Spinal Immobilization

Gail N. Carruthers

Potential spinal injury at any age necessitates spinal immobilization in a neutral position.[1] Spinal injuries are relatively uncommon in children. However when the ligaments or bones of the spine are injured and instability results, neurologic injuries have been shown to occur in up to 29% of cases.[4] Higher cervical locations are more common than middle or lower sites. Although there is no scientific documentation as to what degree of motion is sufficient to cause spinal cord damage in a patient who has an unstable spinal injury, spinal immobilization limits that motion.[1]

In the pediatric patient disproportionate head and chest growth allows for a relative cervical kyphosis in the supine position. Fifty percent of postnatal head circumference growth has occurred by 18 months; in contrast, 50% of the postnatal chest circumference growth has not occurred until age 8 years. As a result, when a young child lies supine, the prominent occiput forces the neck into a flexed position (Fig. 111-1 A and B). This is not only dangerous for an unstable cervical injury but potentially compromises air exchange as well. Spinal immobilization techniques should therefore accommodate the disproportion of the child's head and chest.[6]

Indications

Assume that any child with head, face, neck, or back injury or with multiple traumatic injuries has a spinal cord injury until proved otherwise. Immobilize children with mechanisms of injury that involve blunt or penetrating trauma directly to the spine or forces applied to the spine that involve flexion, extension, or rotation of the head and neck.[3] This includes falls from heights, and sports injuries. Also consider spinal immobilization in children with an altered level of consciousness, neurologic deficit in the arms or legs, and local tenderness or deformity in the cervical, thoracic, or lumbar region. The presence of other injuries may interfere with the child's perception of spine pain. In the infant, because of inability to assess pain accurately, consider the mechanism carefully. Fortunately cervical spine injuries are quite rare in this age group.

Use a rigid cervical collar as the primary adjunct in most cases that involve possible trauma to the head and neck. The purpose of the collar is to splint the head and neck in a neutral position temporarily. Any mechanism capable of injury to the cervical spine should prompt immobilization not only of the head and neck, but of the entire spinal column in order to align the spine in a common plane. Achieve this best by immobilizing the child by using an extrication device or long spine board,[3] in addition to a cervical immobilization device.

Contraindications

There are a few contraindications to spinal immobilization: the presence of a tracheal stoma, which is integral to the

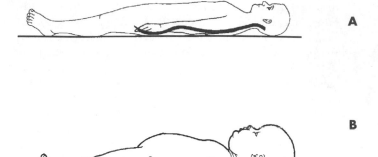

FIG. 111-1 **A** and **B,** Disproportionate head and chest growth in young children allows for relative cervical flexion in infant's supine position.

management of the patient's airway; requirement for any maneuver to ensure adequate oxygenation and ventilation; massive cervical swelling; or any penetrating foreign body to the neck with hemorrhage. Manual in-line immobilization is better in these circumstances.

It is probably unreasonable to attempt to immobilize the crying and fighting child with commercially available immobilization devices; these are usually ineffective in preventing significant movement of the cervical spine and efforts to force placement may result in further manipulation of the spine.[3] Instead enlist the assistance of a parent, caretaker, or friend to hold the child in a position that the child can tolerate that has a neutral effect on the spine and minimizes movement.

Complications

Improper application of a cervical collar generally occurs in one of two ways: by using the wrong size or exercising too little care in its placement. A collar that is too large may push the jaw posteriorly, occluding the airway. A collar that is too small may be too tight, causing airway or circulatory compromise, or too short to provide adequate immobilization.[3]

Spinal immobilization devices with straps may also create problems. Loose straps may fail to prevent excessive sliding of the patient on the spine board, resulting in loss of spinal alignment, whereas tight straps may significantly compromise forced vital capacity, especially in the older severely traumatized child with a distended stomach.[11] In addition strapping patients too firmly in place may cause discomfort and even panic.[4,12]

One adult study evaluated the effect of 30 minutes of standard immobilization on healthy volunteers and concluded that spinal immobilization may cause pain in the absence of any injuries. Keep this in mind while evaluating any trauma patient.[2]

Table 111-1 Efficacy of Spinal Devices and Methods

Collar	Degrees of motion allowed from neutral position in mannequin models					
	Flexion	Extension	Rotation (degrees)	Lateral (degrees)	Summed score*	(%)†
Infant						
Infant car seat, padding, tape with foam collar	8	12	2	3	25	(64)
Head brace	35	38	4	1	78	(205)
with foam collar	11	19	2	2	34	(87)
Half-spine board, tape	1	1	4	6	12	(23)
With foam collar	1	1	2	4	8	(17)
Kendrick's Extrication Device	12	10	19	9	50	(92)
With foam collar	1	1	4	1	7	(11)
Child (Control)						
Head-Immobilizer (foam cushions attached to spine board)	11	18	26	3	58	(122)
With Vertebrace	10	14	1	1	26	(66)
Head brace	16	12	2	1	31	(82)
with Flex-Support	7	9	5	2	23	(58)
Kendrick's Extrication Device	6	8	4	2	20	(53)
with Flex-Support	4	3	1	2	10	(31)
Extriboard Disposable Extrication device	9	7	5	4	24	(73)
with Vertebrace	3	2	2	1	8	(20)
Half-spine board + tape	10	1	4	7	22	(79)
with Flex-Support + tape	2	3	1	2	8	(26)
Full-spine board + tape	4	12	5	3	24	(63)
+ Tape + beanbag + Flex-Support	10	9	3	2	24	(66)
Tape, beanbag	5	5	0	1	11	(31)

From Howell JM: A practical radiographic comparison of short board technique (SBT) and Kendrick Extrication device, *Ann Emerg Med* 18(9): 943-946, 1989.
*Summed score, arithmetic sum of degrees of motion in each direction.
†Summed % score, arithmetic sum of percentage of control motion (degrees of motion allowed/control) × 100 in each direction.

Equipment

Use a properly sized rigid cervical collar in conjunction with one of a variety of spine immobilization devices. Measure the collar so that the front width fits between the point of the chin and the chest at the suprasternal notch. Ideally the collar should be radiographically translucent, easy to apply, and available in a variety of sizes; not interfere with airway structures; and prevent lateral, rotational, and anteroposterior movement of the head.[3]

Use short spine boards and extrication devices (e.g., Kendrick's Extrication Device [KED] board) to stabilize the spine. They are easy to clean and inexpensive. Although there are different types, they also effectively limit the lateral, flexion and extension, and rotational motions of the head, neck, and back.[3]

Radiographic comparisons of various backboard devices indicate that a combination of tape, a rigid-type collar, and either an extrication device or a short board substantially limits cervical motion in adults.[8] A recent analysis of various immobilization devices in children demonstrated that the commercially available pediatric collars fail to provide adequate stabilization of the cervical spine when used alone.[9] Accomplish cervical spine stabilization in the pediatric patient by using a rigid cervical collar in combination with a rigid spinal immobilization device. One study evaluated stability of the various methods using mannequins and concluded that for an infant the addition of an infant cervical collar enhanced the immobilization provided by the half-spine board; for the pediatric mannequin rigid full spine immobilization boards performed better than head immobilization devices designed for attachment to backboards (Table 111-1).[7]

Technique

Any spinal immobilization technique that lowers the young child's occiput or raises the chest is potentially acceptable. A visual landmark to proper cervical spine position is alignment of the external auditory meatus and the shoulders in a single plane.[6]

Use an adjustable cutout backboard to accommodate the occiput (Fig. 111-2, *A*) or a double mattress placed under the back at chest level[12] (Fig. 111-2, *B*). Some investigators have used rectangular expanded rigid polystyrene plastic (Styrofoam) pads to elevate the back to achieve neutral position (defined as normal alignment of the head and neck with gaze straight ahead).[7] Achieve this is by elevating the shoulder blades to a mean height of 25.4 mm; children less than age 4 years require slightly more elevation than their older counterparts.[10] Further confirmatory studies are necessary.

Place the collar around the neck. It should rest on the clavicles and support the lower jaw. If a proper size of collar is unavailable, immobilize the head in a neutral position.

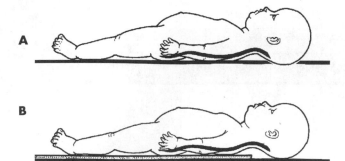

FIG. 111-2 Spinal immobilization methods that accommodate disproportion in the child's head and chest. **A,** Adjustable cutout backboard that accommodates occiput. **B,** Double mattress placed under the back at chest level.

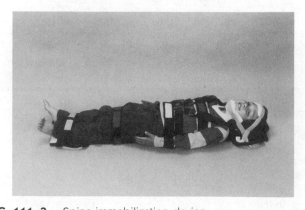

FIG. 111-3 Spine immobilization device.

(Photo courtesy Mr. James Lane, Ferno Pedi-pac immobilization systems, Life-Assist Inc.)

Further stabilize the neck with or without the collar by placing, adjacent to the head, blanket rolls, or pads taped into position with 3-inch adhesive tape placed across the forehead and secured to the spine immobilization device. In adults sandbags further limit lateral movement of the head. However, their weight may actually push the cervical spine out of alignment in the young child and infants.

Pediatric immobilization in neutral alignment necessitates immobilization of entire spinal axis, not just the head and neck. Place blanket rolls or pads on the spine board extending from the axilla to the knees to limit lateral movement of the torso. This ensures that the back remains in alignment with the longitudinal axis of the body. Secure the spine board straps around the chest, pelvis, and legs. Fig. 111-3 demonstrates an effective commercial spine immobilization device for children who are appropriately secured.

After immobilizing the spine pay meticulous attention to maintaining the airway through the use of suctioning, adjunctive airway devices (oropharyngeal or nasopharyngeal airways, described in Chapter 20), or endotracheal intubation.

Remarks

Rigid immobilization allows easy transfer of the patient from one position to another for radiographic procedures, including evaluation of injuries, and for lateral decubitus positioning for suctioning in the event of emesis.

If the immobilized patient's airway becomes compromised, perform a jaw thrust followed by suctioning and placement of an oropharyngeal or nasopharyngeal airway. Assist ventilations with a bag valve mask alone with the collar in place or perform endotracheal intubation after removing the collar, while keeping the neck in neutral position. Studies of manual in-line stabilization during intubation of the adult trauma patient with an unstable cervical spine injury have indicated that orotracheal intubation does not alter neurologic outcome;[13] studies have not been made of the pediatric patient. Orotracheal intubation with an assistant applying in-line stabilization has its advantages in that most physicians are comfortable with the technique (see

Chapter 21). The use of a fibroptic bronchoscope to perform intubation may reduce neck movement in the presence of cervical instability.[5] Limitations of this technique relate to the physician's experience in using the equipment and immediate availability of the device.

Remember that in-line stabilization is not in-line traction. Traction on the spine may result in subluxation or distraction of cervical spine injuries.

REFERENCES

1. American Academy of Orthopedic Surgeons, Committee on Allied Health: *Emergency care and transportation of the sick and injured child,* ed 3, Chicago, 1981, American Academy of Orthopedic Surgeons.
2. Chan D, Goldberg R: The effect of spinal immobilization on healthy volunteers, *Ann Emerg Med* 1:48-51, 1994.
3. Dick T: Prehospital splinting. In Roberts JR, Hedges JR, editors: *Clinical procedures in emergency medicine,* Philadelphia, 1985, WB Saunders.
4. Evans DL: Cervical spine injuries in children, *J Pediatr Ortho* 5:563-568, 1989.
5. Hemmer D: Intubation of a child with a cervical spine injury with the aid of a fiberoptic bronchoscope, *Anaesth Intensive Care* 10:163, 1982.
6. Herzenberg JE, et al: Emergency transport and positioning of young children who have an injury of the cervical spine: the standard backboard may be dangerous, *J Bone Joint Surg* [Am] 71:15-22, 1989.
7. Holley J: Airway management in patients with unstable cervical spine fractures, *Ann Emerg Med* 18:1237, 1989.
8. Howell JM: A practical radiographic comparison of short board technique (SBT) and Kendrick Extrication device, *Ann Emerg Med* 18(9):943-946, 1989.
9. Huerta C, Griffin R, Joyce SM: Cervical spine stabilization in pediatric patients: evaluation of current techniques, *Ann Emerg Med* 16:1121-1126, 1987.
10. Nypaver M, Treloar DM: Neutral cervical spine positioning in children, *Ann Emerg Med* 23(2):208-211, 1994.
11. Schafermeyer RW: Respiratory effects of spinal immobilization in children, *Ann Emerg Med* 20(9):1017-1019, 1991.
12. Sherk, H: Fractures of odontoid process in young children, *J Bone Joint Surg* [Am] 60a:921-924, Oct 1978.
13. Suderman VS: Elective oral tracheal intubation in cervical spine injured adults, Part 1, *Can J Anesth* 39:516-517, 1992.

112 The Pneumatic Antishock Garment

Pamela J. Okada and Roger J. Lewis

The pneumatic antishock garment (PASG), also known as military antishock trousers (MAST), is an inflatable device whose primary purpose is to elevate the blood pressure of patients in uncompensated shock. The PASG was originally thought to increase blood pressure by causing an "autotransfusion" of blood from the legs and abdomen or pelvis into the central circulation, with a resulting increase in central venous pressure, stroke volume, and cardiac output.[14,15] More recent work has shown however that the primary mechanism of action of the PASG is through constriction of vessels in the legs and abdomen (probably through direct mechanical reduction of luminal diameter) with a resulting increase in systemic vascular resistance.[9,12,15,21] A small autotransfusion and rise in central venous pressure probably occur as well.[9,17]

The most common use of the PASG is in patients with posttraumatic hypotension, caused by blood loss.[7,13,14] Since the PASG increases the arterial blood pressure in all patients including those with ongoing blood loss, without providing any direct control at the site of hemorrhage, the application of the PASG may result in an increased rate of hemorrhage in some patients.[3,13] If it does, the application of the PASG in patients with ongoing blood loss, although associated with an increase in blood pressure, may actually lower survival rate. Some animal and human studies have supported this hypothesis.[3,4,5,13]

The most influential study of the PASG in humans was a prospective randomized trial in adults with posttraumatic hypotension, conducted by Mattox, Bickell, Pepe, et al.,[13] who randomized more than 900 patients to treatment with or without the PASG. The investigators found no improvement in survival rate with the PASG when they considered all types of injuries together, and a statistically significant increase in the fatality rate associated with its use in patients with primary thoracic injuries. This suggests that patients with primary thoracic injuries, who are suffering blood loss in an anatomic area not compressed by the PASG, may have an increased rate of exsanguination with the PASG.[3,13] For this reason its use is contraindicated in patients with primary thoracic injury (discussed later).[3,11,13]

Results of some animal studies have suggested that the PASG may be beneficial when the site of hemorrhage is a region directly compressed by the PASG.[1,2] One study in adults with penetrating abdominal trauma found no benefit of the PASG, however.[4] There have been no clinical trials of the PASG in children, and adult and animal data as well as anecdotal experience are the basis of current practice in the pediatric population.

Indications

The PASG may be indicated for the treatment of severe posttraumatic hypotension that is unresponsive to fluid resuscitation and blood replacement, when vascular access is unachievable,[8,19] or when immediate surgical control of hemorrhage is not possible or appropriate. Other possible indications include the stabilization of pelvic or femur fractures and the treatment of spinal shock.[6,10] The PASG may be especially appropriate for the treatment of spinal shock if it covers the denervated area well, as its vasoconstrictive effect may selectively counteract the local vasodilation that occurs in this setting. Another possible indication for the PASG is hypotension caused by anaphylaxis or toxic shock syndrome. In most cases, however, when a general vasoconstrictive effect is desirable and vascular access is available, the use of dopamine, epinephrine, or norepinephrine is preferable to use of the PASG.

Contraindications

The PASG is contraindicated in patients with primary thoracic injury,[3,11,13] uncontrolled hemorrhage of the upper extremities, congestive heart failure or pulmonary edema,[8,15,20] and extrusion of visceral contents or suspected diaphragmatic rupture.[20] Inflation of the abdominal compartment is contraindicated in patients who are pregnant. The PASG is relatively contraindicated in all patients with hypotension and suspected ongoing blood loss, for the reasons outlined.

Equipment

Equipment required for proper use of the PASG are an appropriately sized PASG, a blood pressure cuff, and a stethoscope. PASGs are available in three sizes: toddler size (for ages 2 to 6 years), child size (for ages 7 to 12 years), and adult size.

Complications

Potential complications associated with the use of the PASG include decreased respiratory vital capacity caused by compression of the abdominal organs against the diaphragm, lower extremity compartment syndromes, lower extremity ischemia, metabolic acidosis after prolonged use caused by decreased lower extremity tissue perfusion, decreased glomerular filtration rate and urine output, and skin breakdown (especially at the site of bony prominences). Furthermore because PASG limits physical examination of the abdomen and lower extremities, its use may prevent recognition of other serious injuries.[14,16,18] Minimize complications by preventing prolonged use of trousers and by avoiding intravenous (IV) placement at the ankles if possible.

The most important complication resulting from the deflation of the PASG is hypotension, which may occur with rapid removal of the device before adequate fluid resuscitation. Minimize this problem by vigorous fluid resuscitation and by systematic, slow removal of the PASG.

Techniques

Fig. 112-1 illustrates the technique for the application and removal of the PASG. A description follows.[16]

Positioning of the PASG and the Patient. First unfold the PASG and lay it flat, with each inflation tube easily visible (Fig. 112-1, A). Attach the foot pump and open the stopcock valves. When the valve lever is parallel to the tubing, the valve is open; when it is closed, the valve lever is at a 90-degree angle to the tubing.

Next position the supine patient on the PASG as shown in Fig. 112-1, B, ensuring that you are using the appropriate size of PASG: the top of the garment should be just below the costal margin; the legs should reach the ankles. If the patient is at risk for spinal injuries, stabilize the cervical spine and "log roll" the patient onto the opened trousers. Otherwise elevate the patient's legs and slide the trousers beneath the patient to the buttocks, elevate the hips, and position the top of the garment at the costal margin. Wrap each leg of the garment around the patient's legs and secure with the self-adhesive (Velcro) strips. Finally wrap the abdominal section around the abdomen of the patient and secure with the strips. Decompress the bladder and stomach.

Inflation. To inflate close the stopcock valves to the abdominal compartment and inflate the leg compartments using the foot pump. In children do not inflate the pressure over 50 mm Hg.[20] If a pressure gauge is not available, inflate

the compartments until air escapes through the pressure relief valve. Next close the stopcock valves to both legs, open the valve to the abdominal compartment, and check the blood pressure. If the blood pressure is adequate, do not inflate the abdominal compartment. If the blood pressure is not adequate, inflate the abdominal compartment to a pressure of 50 mm Hg, until air leaks through the relief valves or the blood pressure increases to an acceptable level. Close the valve to the abdominal compartment. Carefully monitor the patient's blood pressure and respiratory status.

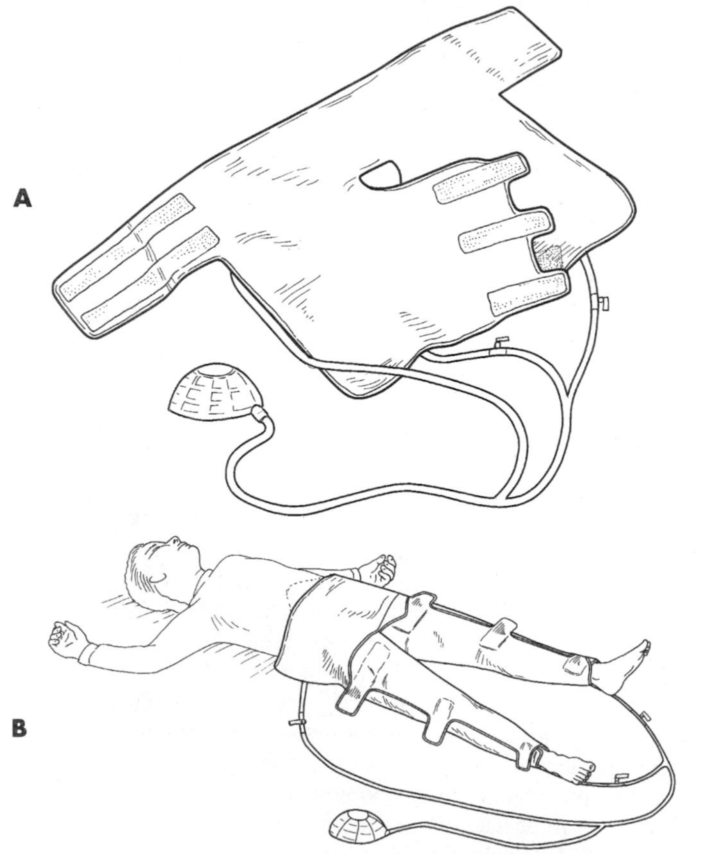

Deflation. Perform deflation and removal of the PASG after the correction of shock. Only deflate the PASG in a hospital setting, after adequate intravenous access is available, and while monitoring the patient continuously. If emergency surgery is indicated, perform deflation in the operating room.

Deflate the PASG gradually and cautiously. Begin by removing the foot pump and tubing. Deflate the abdominal compartment first. Release small amounts of air over several minutes and continuously monitor blood pressure. If the systolic pressure decreases by more than 5 mm Hg, stop deflation and administer fluids or blood until the blood pressure returns to baseline.

Follow deflation of the abdomen by deflation of one leg. Deflate the leg compartment slowly and continuously monitor the patient's blood pressure; deflate the other leg in the same manner. If the patient becomes hypotensive during deflation and vigorous fluid resuscitation is ineffective, it may be necessary to reinflate the garment and postpone removal until the patient is in the operating room.

FIG. 112-1 Technique for application of pneumatic antishock garment. **A,** Unfold the garment and lay flat. **B,** Place the child supine and inflate to 50 mm Hg.

REFERENCES

1. Ali J, Duke K: Pneumatic antishock garment decreases hemorrhage and mortality from splenic injury, *Can J Surg* 34:496, 1991.
2. Ali J, Purcell C, Vanderby B: The effect of intraabdominal pressure and saline infusion on abdominal aortic hemorrhage, *J Cardiovasc Surg* 32:653, 1991.
3. Ali J, Vanderby B, Purcell C: The effect of the pneumatic antishock garment (PASG) on hemodynamics, hemorrhage, and survival in penetrating thoracic aortic injury, *J Trauma* 31:846, 1991.
4. Bickell WH, Pepe PE, Bailey ML, et al: Randomized trial of pneumatic antishock garments in the prehospital management of penetrating abdominal injuries, *Ann Emerg Med* 16:653, 1987.
5. Bickell WH, Pepe PE, Wyatt CH, et al: Effect of antishock trousers on the trauma score: a prospective analysis in the urban setting, *Ann Emerg Med* 14(3):218, 1985.
6. Brunette DD, Fifield G, Ruiz E: Use of pneumatic antishock trousers in the management of pediatric pelvic hemorrhage, *Pediatr Emerg Care* 3(2):86, 1987.
7. Cayten CG, Berendt BM, Byrne DW, et al: A study of pneumatic antishock garments in severely hypotensive trauma patients, *J Trauma* 34:728, 1993.
8. Concannon JE, Matre WM, Verhagen AD: Antishock trousers in pediatrics: a case management report, *Clin Pediatr* 23(2):78, 1984.
9. Gaffney FA, Thal ER, Taylor F, et al: Hemodynamic effects of medical anti-shock trousers (MAST garment), *J Trauma* 21:931, 1981.
10. Garcia V, Eichelberger M, Ziegler M, et al: Use of military antishock trouser in a child, *J Pediatr Surg* 16(4), (suppl 1): 544, 1981.
11. Honigman B, Lowenstein SR, Moore EE, et al: The role of the pneumatic antishock garment in penetrating cardiac wounds, *JAMA* 266:2398, 1991.
12. Jennings TJ, Seaworth JF, Tripp LD, et al: The effects of inflation of antishock trousers on hemodynamics in normovolemic subjects, *J Trauma* 26:544, 1986.

13. Mattox KL, Bickell W, Pepe PE, et al: Prospective MAST study in 911 patients, *J Trauma* 29:1104, 1989.

14. McSwain NE Jr: Pneumatic anti-shock garment: state of the art 1988, *Ann Emerg Med* 17(5):506, 1988.

15. Rubal BJ, Geer MR, Bickell WH: Effects of pneumatic antishock garment inflation in normovolemic subjects, *J Appl Physiol* 67:339, 1989.

16. Shade BR, Bledsoe BE: Pathophysiology of shock. In Bledsoe BE, Porter RS, Shade BR, editors: *Paramedic emergency care,* Englewood Cliffs, NJ, 1991, Brady.

17. Terai C, Oryuh T, Kimura S, et al: The autotransfusion effect of external leg counterpressure in simulated mild hypovolemia, *J Trauma* 31:1165, 1991.

18. Tobias JD, Schlerien CL, Reitz BA: Use of the MAST suit in the postoperative care of patients after the Fontan procedure, *Crit Care Med* 18:781, 1990.

19. Velasco AL, Delgado-Paredes C, Templeton J, et al: Intraosseous infusion of fluids in the initial management of hypovolemic shock in young subjects, *J Pediatr Surg* 26:4, 1991.

20. Ziegler MM, Templeton JM: Major trauma. In Fleisher GR, Ludwig S, editors: *Textbook of pediatric emergency medicine,* ed 3, Baltimore, 1993, Williams & Wilkins.

21. Zippe C, Burchard KW, Gann DS: Trendelenburg versus PASG application in moderate hemorrhagic hypoperfusion, *J Trauma* 25:923, 1985.

113 Helmet Removal

William J. Koenig

In 1980 the American College of Surgeons proposed a standard two-handed technique for the removal of helmets with minimal cervical spine manipulation. Well-designed research in this area is lacking, and it is likely that all techniques cause some cervical spine movement. With increasing interest in mandatory helmet laws, emergency personnel frequently need to use these techniques.

Clinical and epidemiologic studies have led to a few conclusions. First helmets do not appear to be associated with an increased incidence of cervical spine injuries.[1,2] Although contact of the lip of the helmet in forced hyperextension occurs between C6 and T2, this is unlikely to produce high cervical injury.[7] Head injuries occur more frequently and are more severe when motorcyclists do not wear helmets; however, whether they reduce overall crash mortality rate is still a subject of debate.[3,8]

Indications

In many states that have passed laws requiring the wearing of a protective helmet while riding a motorcycle, prehospital and Emergency Department (ED) personnel must be familiar with the mechanisms of helmet removal. This is necessary in order to preserve an open airway, adequately stabilize the head to the backboard, provide in-line stabilization for transporting the patient, examine the patient, or place cervical tongs. Immobilize helmeted injured patients with the helmet in place unless bleeding or airway management necessitates immediate removal. Prehospital personnel can stabilize patients' condition in the field without attempting helmet removal. Use cervical collars for the majority of patients who wear helmets.

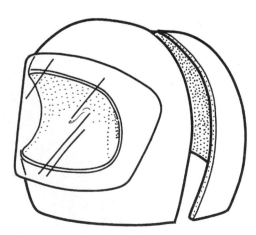

FIG. 113-1   Helmet cut in coronal plane in patients with suspected cervical spine injury.

Contraindications

In patients with a high index of suspicion of cervical spine injury based on clinical or radiographic findings, do not use the technique for helmet removal described in this chapter. Instead bivalve helmets using cast cutters. Use standard cast cutters to cut the helmet in the coronal plane (Fig. 113-1).

Complications

Inappropriate manipulation of the head and/or cervical spine may result in damage to the cervical spinal cord unless there is understanding of the construction of the helmet and the way it conforms to the shape of the head. After removing the helmet, it is imperative to place the child's head into the most suitable alignment to achieve a neutral position of the spine.

Technique

Before beginning the removal of the helmet, examine it for any external signs of trauma. Because the helmet protects the face and head, the only evidence of severity of injury may be on the helmet itself.

Obtain cervical spine radiographs with the helmet in place. Some helmet types contain opaque trim that obscures the lower cervical and thoracic vertebrae; remove the strip before obtaining radiographs.

Although some have proposed a one-person technique,[5] in most emergencies two people are required to accomplish helmet removal (Fig. 113-2, *A* to *D*). This is the preferred technique to minimize cervical spine manipulation in patients when cervical spine fractures are not suspected.[6] One operator applies in-line stabilization by placing the hands on each side of the helmet with the fingers on the victim's mandible. This position prevents slippage if the helmet chin strap is loose. A second operator cuts or loosens the chin strap then places one hand on the mandible at the angle, the thumb on one side and the index and middle fingers on the other mandibular angle. The other hand supports the occipital region while providing additional in-line stabilization (Fig. 113-2, *A*).

The first operator now spreads the helmet by expanding it laterally to clear the ears and, in the case of full facial coverage, may need to tilt it slightly backward to clear the nose (Fig. 113-2, *B*). The second operator has responsibility for in-line stabilization to prevent head tilt (Fig. 113-2, *C*). After removal of the helmet the responsibility for in-line stabilization is transferred to the first operator (Fig. 113-2, *D*), who places his or her hands on each side of the patient's head with the palms over the ears.

Remarks

If the patient wears glasses, remove them through the helmet faceplate before attempting to remove the helmet.

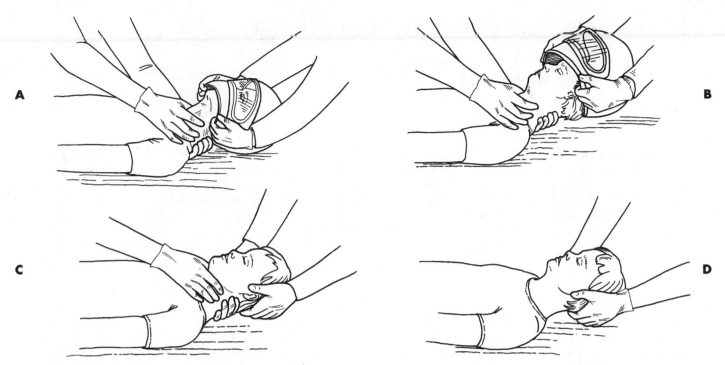

FIG. 113-2   Technique for helmet removal. **A,** While one rescuer applies on-line stabilization, the other begins careful removal. **B,** The helmet is carefully lifted around ears and nose. **C** and **D,** Head-tilt is prevented by good technique and teamwork.

REFERENCES

1. Aprahamian C, Thompson BM, Darin JC: Recommended helmet removal techniques in a cervical spine injured patient, *J Trauma* 24(9):841, 1984.
2. Carr WP, Brandt D, Swanson K: Injury patterns and helmet effectiveness among hospitalized motorcyclists, *Minn Med* 64(9):521, 1981.
3. Heilman DR, Weisbuch JB, Blair RW: Motorcycle related trauma and helmet usage in North Dakota, *Ann Emerg Med* 11(12):659, 1982.
4. Kelly P, Swanson T, Strange G: A prospective study of the impact of helmet usage on motorcycle trauma, *Ann Emerg Med* 10:8, 1991.
5. Maroon JC: Burning hands in football spinal cord injuries, *JAMA* 238(19):2049, 1977.
6. McSwain NE: Techniques of helmet removal from injured patients, *Am Coll Surg Bull* October:19-21, 1980.
7. Meyer RD, Daniel MD: The biomechanics of helmets and helmet removal, *J Trauma* 25(4):329, 1985.
8. Sosin DM, Sacks, Jeffery J: Motorcycle helmet: use laws and head injury prevention, *JAMA* 267(12):1649, 1992.

114 Diagnostic Peritoneal Lavage

Philip L. Henneman

Diagnostic peritoneal lavage (DPL) is a safe, sensitive, and accurate way of diagnosing intraabdominal injuries requiring surgical repair in children and adults with blunt abdominal trauma.[4,6] Root introduced DPL in 1965.[12] It is more accurate than physical examination in children and adults with blunt abdominal trauma.[1] Some authors also recommend DPL for patients with penetrating abdominal trauma, but there is limited experience with the procedure in pediatric patients.

In recent years computed tomography (CT) of the abdomen with gastrointestinal and intravenous contrast has become the primary diagnostic tool in evaluating the stable pediatric patient with blunt abdominal trauma and equivocal abdominal findings or altered mental status.[7] Although CT scanning is less accurate and more expensive than DPL, it is noninvasive and provides organ-specific information that improves the assessment of the need for surgical intervention in the stable pediatric patient. Although DPL is overly sensitive in detecting intraabdominal hemorrhage in children who may not require surgery,[11] it is still indicated in several specific clinical situations.

Indications

DPL evaluation is appropriate for unstable pediatric patients with potential abdominal hemorrhage, unless they are going directly to the operating room (OR). DPL usually requires 15 minutes while the patient is undergoing initial resuscitation in the Emergency Department (ED). Abdominal CT may require a delay of 60 minutes to allow contrast material in the stomach to enter the bowel. Do not take hemodynamically unstable patients to the radiographic suite.

DPL is also ideal when several patients in critical condition arrive in the ED at the same time and the physician must quickly decide who needs to go to the operating room and in what order. DPL may also be indicated when a CT scanner is unavailable or physicians are unable to interpret the films reliably.

Contraindications

Patients with indications for immediate laparotomy should not undergo any diagnostic procedures (e.g., CT or DPL) that delay definitive surgical management. Indications for immediate laparotomy in blunt trauma patients include hypotension unresponsive to initial resuscitation, peritoneal signs, significant gastrointestinal bleeding, pneumoperitoneum, and bowel herniation into the chest. However, it is often prudent to evaluate patients who require immediate surgery for nonabdominal injuries (e.g., epidural hematoma) in the OR with DPL while operating on the nonabdominal injuries.

DPL is contraindicated in the young child who cannot cooperate with the procedure without deep conscious sedation. Evaluate such a patient by abdominal CT. Imaging may be safer in this population, unless instability requires immediate transfer to the OR, where DPL in a controlled setting under general anesthesia is possible.

Complications

The closed technique is the fastest and easiest approach to DPL but is a blind procedure that has a low but definite risk of bowel perforation. Incorrect placement of the lavage catheter results in either inadequate fluid return or false-negative lavage results. The open technique is technically more complicated and lengthy but rarely results in bowel perforation. Use the open technique on patients with prior surgical procedures to prevent bowel perforation and in those patients who have had inadequate return of lavage fluid in another approach.

Inadequate fluid return is a possible complication of any approach but is more common with the closed technique. Incisional hernia is a possible complication of the open technique if one does not properly close the posterior fascia after the procedure. The semiopen technique is a compromise between the closed and open techniques and has a complication rate of bowel perforation of 0.3%.[6] Other less common complications that can occur with any approach include vascular injury and bladder perforation.

Closed technique is probably the ideal approach because the complication rate is very low and the percutaneous procedure requires less time and is better tolerated than the other approaches.[2] Emergency physicians, pediatricians, or surgeon's performing peritoneal lavage, however, should use the technique with which they are most comfortable.

Technique

Ideally sedate the child with benzodiazepines and narcotics (see Chapter 12). Place a nasogastric tube and urinary catheter before performing the lavage to decompress the stomach and bladder.

Perform DPL by using the closed, open, or semiopen technique. The closed technique involves introducing the lavage catheter into the peritoneal cavity over a wire placed through a percutaneous needle (Box 114-1 and Fig. 114-1, *A* to *C*). Perform open and semiopen techniques by locally infiltrating the skin and subcutaneous tissue with lidocaine and epinephrine and then making a 3- to 5-cm incision through the skin, lateral to the umbilicus, and extending the incision in a vertical direction either above or below the umbilicus as indicated. Later, if exploratory laparotomy is needed, this incision can be extended by the surgeon. Bluntly dissect the subcutaneous tissue down to the posterior fascia. When using the open technique, open the posterior fascia and peritoneum (1 to 2 cm) and guide a lavage catheter inferiorly into one of the pelvic gutters.

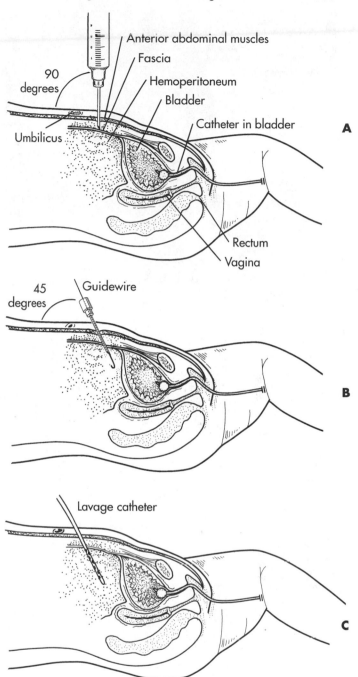

FIG. 114-1   Closed technique for diagnostic peritoneal lavage. **A,** Insertion of needle. **B,** Guidewire passage through needle into peritoneal cavity. **C,** Passage of catheter and dilator over guidewire into abdominal cavity.

(Adapted with permission from Cue JI, Miller FB, Cryer HM, et al: A prospective comparison between open and closed peritoneal lavage techniques, *J Trauma* 30:880-883, 1990.)

The semiopen technique differs from the open technique; make only a small incision (2 to 3 mm) through the posterior fascia. Elevate the posterior fascia with towel clips and poke a lavage catheter through the peritoneum using a trocar. Then slide the lavage catheter over the trocar into one of the pelvic gutters and remove the trocar.[9]

Perform DPL infraumbilically in most patients unless the patient has a pelvic fracture; in this case use a supraumbilical approach. Pelvic fracture increases the likelihood of false-positive lavage results, especially if using an infraumbilical approach.[6] If the patient has had prior abdominal surgery, perform DPL by the open technique. If a midline approach is contraindicated because of prior surgery, perform DPL in the left lower quadrant. Use the left lower quadrant to minimize the possibility of future confusion of the lavage scar with an appendectomy scar.

After introducing the lavage catheter into the peritoneal cavity by whatever technique, attempt aspiration of gross blood. If the lavage result is not positive by aspiration of gross blood, instill 15 ml/kg of warmed normal saline solution, up to 1 L, by gravity into the peritoneal cavity. Applying pressure to the lavage bag either by hand or by pressure bag increases the rate of flow of lavage fluid. After most of the lavage fluid has entered the peritoneal cavity, place the lavage bag below the patient to allow gravity to siphon the fluid from the peritoneum. Ideally 75% of instilled lavage fluid should return, but often less returns. The minimal amount of fluid return to make lavage results reliable is unknown. If less than 25% of instilled fluid returns when using the closed or semiopen technique, then suspect misplacement of the lavage catheter and use the open technique. Once the fluid return has stopped, send a sample to the laboratory for cell count.

Diagnostic Peritoneal Lavage Results

Box 114-2 lists criteria for a positive DPL result; the most common positive result is aspiration of gross blood. The

BOX 114-2 **DIAGNOSTIC PERITONEAL LAVAGE RESULTS**

Positive results

Aspiration of gross blood
Greater than or equal to 100,000 RBCs/mm^3*
Fecal material in lavage fluid
Bacteria present on Gram stain

Equivocal results

Greater than or equal to 50,000 RBCs/mm^3

Controversial results

Greater than or equal to 500 WBC/mm^3
Elevated amylase level
Elevated alkaline phosphatase level

RBC, Red blood cell; *WBC*, white blood cell.

recommended amount of gross blood considered to indicate a positive lavage result ranges from 1 to 20 ml. In adults aspiration of 10 ml of gross blood accounts for approximately 70% of positive lavage results and has a positive predictive value (PPV) of 95% in detecting injury requiring repair.[6] Red blood cell counts greater than 100,000/mm^3 account for the remaining positive lavage results and have a PPV of 89% for adult patients without pelvic fractures and 64% in patients with pelvic fractures; 50,000 red blood cells/mm^3 may indicate a positive result in children.[13] The reported PPV of peritoneal lavage in children ranges from 46% to 100%; the low positive predictive value of lavage in children makes CT scan a valuable adjunctive test in the stabilized pediatric patient with a positive lavage result.[4,13] A hemodynamically unstable pediatric patient with a positive lavage result should undergo prompt laparotomy, as the PPV increases significantly when positive lavage results occur in this clinical setting.[3]

The main value of peritoneal lavage in children is its negative predictive value of 95% to 100%.[3,4,11,13] A negative study result reliably excludes solid viscera as a source of blood loss. When DPL results are negative in hemodynamically unstable pediatric patients, evaluate other sources of shock aggressively.

Recent studies of DPL white blood cell count and amylase level have not found them useful in adults.[6,14] DPL alkaline phosphatase for detection of bowel injury is controversial and inadequately studied in children.[8,10] Consider the presence of bacteria or fecal material in lavage aspirate a positive result; this is a rare finding.

Observe stable patients with a negative lavage result and no other injuries for at least 12 hours before discharge. Consider admission of all patients to a pediatric hospital ward. Occasionally admission to an observation unit within the ED is appropriate as long as the design of the unit accommodates pediatric patients.[5]

Remarks

DPL safely and accurately identifies hemodynamically unstable pediatric patients requiring laparotomy. DPL, however, is not perfect. In one study of adults, DPL missed 7% of solid visceral injuries and 26% of hollow visceral injuries requiring repair.[6] It also does not evaluate the retroperitoneum. It is always important to integrate the patient's clinical picture with the lavage results to determine the most appropriate course.[3] DPL does not replace physical examination or surgical judgment but is a valuable triage tool in the assessment of select pediatric blunt trauma patients. A positive DPL result does not dictate the need for surgery, as one can observe many splenic injuries without operation.

REFERENCES

1. Bivens BA, Sachatello CR, Daugherty ME, et al: Diagnostic peritoneal lavage is superior to clinical evaluation in blunt abdominal trauma, *Am Surg* 44:637-641, 1978.
2. Cue JI, Miller FB, Cryer HM, et al: A prospective comparison between open and closed peritoneal lavage techniques, *J Trauma* 30:880-883, 1990.
3. Day AC, Rankin N, Charlesworth P: Diagnostic peritoneal lavage: integration with clinical information to improve diagnostic performance, *J Trauma* 32:52-57, 1992.
4. Drew RD, Perry JF: The expediency of peritoneal lavage for blunt trauma in children, *Surg Gynecol Obstet* 145:885-888, 1977.
5. Henneman PL, Marx JA, Moore EE, et al: Diagnostic peritoneal lavage: accuracy in predicting necessary laparotomy following blunt and penetrating trauma, *J Trauma* 30:1345-1355, 1990.
6. Henneman PL, Marx JA, Moore EE, et al: The use of an Emergency Department Observation Unit in the management of abdominal trauma, *Ann Emerg Med* 18:647-650, 1989.
7. Jaffe D, Wesson D: Emergency management of blunt trauma in children, *N Engl J Med* 324:1477-1482, 1991.
8. Jaffin JH, Ochsner MG, Cole FJ, et al: Alkaline phosphatase levels in diagnostic peritoneal lavage fluid as a predictor of hollow visceral injury, *J Trauma* 34:829-833, 1993.
9. Markovchick VJ, Elerding SL, Moore EE, et al: Diagnostic peritoneal lavage, *J Am Coll Emerg Phys* 8:326-328, 1979.
10. Marx JA, Bar-Or D, Moore EE, et al: Utility of lavage alkaline phosphatase in detection of isolated small intestinal injury, *Ann Emerg Med* 14:10-14, 1985.
11. Powell RW, Green JB, Ochsner MG, et al: Peritoneal lavage in pediatric patients sustaining blunt abdominal trauma: a reappraisal, *J Trauma* 27:6-9, 1987.
12. Root HD, Hausner CW, Mckinleyt CR, et al: Diagnostic peritoneal lavage, *Surgery* 57:633-637, 1965.
13. Rothenberg S, Moore EE, Marx JA, et al: Selective management of blunt abdominal trauma in children—the triage role of peritoneal lavage, *J Trauma* 27:1101-1106, 1987.
14. Soyka JM, Martin M, Sloan EP, et al: Diagnostic peritoneal lavage: is isolated WBC count >500/mm^3 predictive of intra-abdominal injury requiring celiotomy in blunt trauma patients? *J Trauma* 30:874-879, 1990.

PART XXII

ORTHOPEDIC TECHNIQUES

115 Arthrocentesis

M. Douglas Baker

Arthrocentesis is the puncture and aspiration of a joint. This procedure is useful as both a diagnostic and a therapeutic tool. Fluid obtained via arthrocentesis can be processed for culture, cell count, Gram stain, immunologic studies, chemical analysis, or microscopy. Removal of joint fluid can also result in appreciable reduction in pain and improvement in joint function. When properly performed, arthrocentesis is both informative and safe.

Indications

Arthrocentesis may be indicated in a number of clinical circumstances, including diagnosis of septic arthritis by synovial fluid analysis, diagnosis of systemic illness (i.e., collagen disease) by synovial fluid analysis, diagnosis of ligamentous or bony injury by confirmation of intraarticular blood, relief of pain and improvement of function by removal of joint effusion, and intraarticular instillation of medications in inflammatory arthridites.

Contraindications

Most contraindications to arthrocentesis are relative, not absolute. The most common contraindication to needle puncture is the presence of cellulitis of the area overlying the puncture site.[1,3] In general avoid punctures through infected tissues to prevent introduction of infection into sterile tissues or fluids beneath the infected site. However inflammation can overlie an acutely arthritic joint and mimic cellulitis. Always weigh the risks of performing any procedure against its diagnostic and/or therapeutic benefits.

Arthrocentesis is relatively contraindicated in the child with bacteremia. Hematogenous spread of infection with or without hemorrhage can occur after joint puncture in such a patient.[1] Other relative contraindications include the presence of a bleeding disorder or ongoing anticoagulant therapy. When arthrocentesis is indicated in a child known to have a severe bleeding disorder, it is usually possible to perform it safely after administration of appropriate clotting factors.

Complications

The complications of arthrocentesis are essentially those associated with any needle puncture. As mentioned, infection of originally uninfected joint fluid can result from this procedure. This complication can occur in three ways: deviation from proper sterile technique can allow injection of skin surface bacteria into joint fluid or bone; if, in spite of adherence to proper sterile technique, the needle puncture occurs through infected tissues; and when a patient is bacteremic, regardless of the presence or absence of subsequent intraarticular hemorrhage.

Intraarticular or soft-tissue hemorrhage is the second complication that can result from arthrocentesis.[2] Anticipate such a complication in the child known to have a severe bleeding

disorder. In this setting prior administration of clotting factors permits safe performance of the procedure.

Equipment

Relatively few pieces of equipment are necessary to perform an arthrocentesis (Box 115-1). Assemble sterile gloves, drapes, syringes and needles, skin preparation solutions, and local and/or topical anesthetics. In general, select the largest needle that is practical for aspiration, thus minimizing the possibility of needle lumen obstruction with debris or clot. Other needed equipment includes appropriate laboratory tubes, culture media, and slides for microscopy.

Technique

First identify anatomic structures by palpation of bony landmarks. In general attempt puncture from the extensor surfaces of joints, thereby avoiding neurovascular structures, which tend to be located along flexor surfaces.[3-5]

Perform arthrocentesis using sterile technique. Prepare the skin with antibacterial cleansing solutions, according to institutional standards. Scrub the skin first with a preparation such as povidone-iodine; then paint it with an antiseptic solution and allow it to dry. Before needle puncture remove this solution from the skin surface with alcohol to prevent introduction of iodine into the joint space.

After cleansing of the skin surface administer a local anesthetic. Nerve fibers supply the synovial membrane, articular capsule, and periosteum. Use a vapor coolant to anesthetize the skin surface before needle puncture. This type of anesthesia is, however, short-lived. Alternatively inject 1% lidocaine locally down to the level of the joint capsule.

BOX 115-1 SUGGESTED EQUIPMENT FOR ARTHRO-CENTESIS

Sterile gloves
Sterile drapes
   Plain and fenestrated
Sterile gauze dressings
Sterile syringes
   5 ml, 10 ml, 20 ml
Sterile needles
   25, 21, 18 gauge
Skin-cleansing solution
   Povidone-iodine, alcohol
1% Lidocaine
Vapor coolant
Culture media
Laboratory tubes

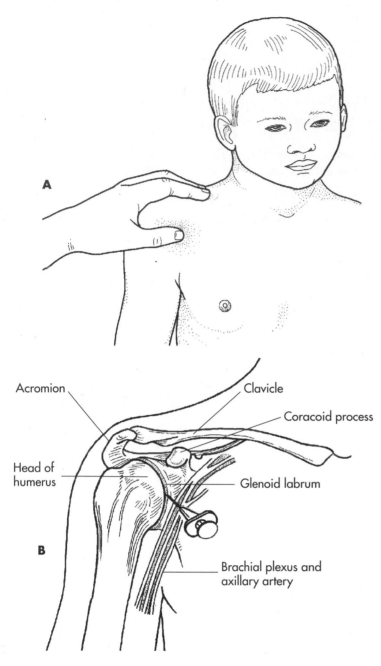

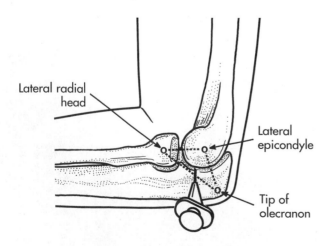

FIG. 115-1 **A** and **B,** Glenohumeral arthrocentesis.

FIG. 115-2 Aspiration of the elbow joint.

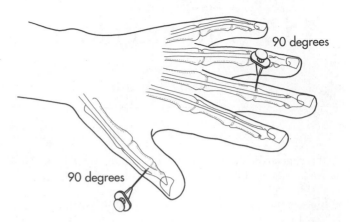

FIG. 115-3 Aspiration of the interphalangeal joint.

Administered in this manner lidocaine has an onset of action of 2 to 5 minutes and lasts 1 to 2 hours.

For all joint aspirations apply suction to the syringe during entry. After obtaining an adequate specimen from the joint, withdraw the needle and place sterile gauze over the puncture site. When possible immobilize the involved joint after aspiration.

Specific Techniques

Shoulder Joint. See Fig. 115-1.

Position. Place the child supine or seated with his/her arm at the side. Restrain the child as needed, with the arm held next to the chest; the hand in the lap, if seated.

Insertion. Palpate the coracoid process below the distal end of the clavicle and medial to the humeral head. Use the anterior approach and puncture just below and immediately lateral to the tip of the coracoid process. Direct the needle perpendicular to the skin surface, angling slightly medially to enter the joint.

Elbow Joint. See Fig. 115-2.

Position. Place the child prone or seated with his/her arm extended and elbow flexed to 90 degrees. Restrain the child as needed, maintaining this arm position. If the child is seated, pronate his/her forearm and place the palm flat on a surface.

Insertion. Use a lateral approach, with the puncture site in the center of the triangle outlined by the radial head, lateral humeral epicondyle, and olecranon. Direct the needle perpendicular to the skin surface. If an elbow effusion is sizable, it may appear inferior to the lateral epicondyle; then aspirate it from a posterolateral approach. To avoid the ulnar nerve and artery do not use a medial approach.

Interphalangeal Joint. See Fig. 115-3.

Position. Place the child prone or seated with his/her forearm extended on a surface. Restrain the child as needed. Slightly flex the finger and apply traction to open the joint.

Insertion. A dorsal approach is best. Direct the needle perpendicular to the skin surface, puncturing it just medial or lateral to the center of the digit, thereby avoiding the extensor tendon, which runs down the midline of the finger, and avoiding the digital vessels, which run peripherally.

Knee Joint. See Fig. 115-4.

Position. Place the child supine with his/her knee actively fully extended. Restrain the child as needed.

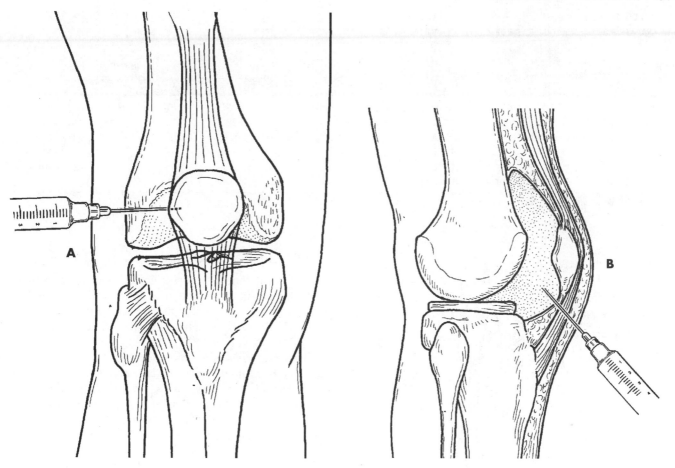

FIG. 115-4 **A** and **B,** Arthrocentesis of the knee joint.

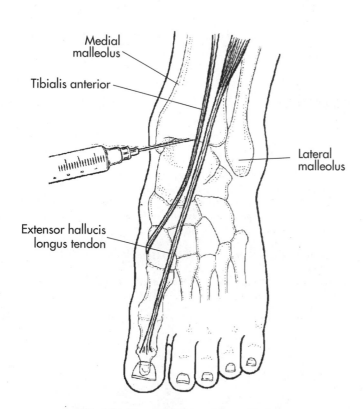

Medial malleolus

Tibialis anterior

Lateral malleolus

Extensor hallucis longus tendon

FIG. 115-5 Aspiration of the ankle joint.

Insertion. A lateral approach to aspiration is preferable, thereby avoiding the vastus medialus muscle. Puncture the skin midway down the patella (cephaladcaudad) at its posterior margin. Angle the syringe 15 degrees above horizontal.

Ankle Joint. See Fig. 115-5.

Position. Place the child supine with his/her foot held in slight plantar flexion. Further restrain the child as needed.

Insertion. Use the medial malleolus as the medial landmark and the anterior tibial tendon as the lateral landmark, and palpate the medial malleolar sulcus. The tendon can be easily identifiable through active dorsiflexion of the foot. Puncture the skin of the sulcus with the needle angled slightly inferiorly. Often it is necessary to advance the needle 2 to 3 cm to reach the joint.

Wrist Joint. See Fig. 115-6.

Position. Seat the child with his/her hand held prone on a surface with the wrist flexed approximately 25 degrees. Apply traction and restrain the child further as needed.

Insertion. Palpate the dorsal radial tubercle, which is the dorsal elevation of the center of the distal end of the radius. The extensor pollicis longus tendon lies in the groove on the radial side of this structure and is most easily identifiable with the wrist and thumb actively extended. Insert the needle dorsally immediately distal to the dorsal tubercle on the ulnar side of the extensor tendon. Avoid the anatomic snuffbox located on the radial side of this tendon.

Table 115-1 Characteristics of Synovial Fluid*

Disease	Appearance	Viscosity mucin clot string test	WBC/ml	PMN (%)	Serum glucose (%)	Crystal
Normal	Clear, straw colored, transparent	Good	≤200	<20	95-100	None
Traumatic arthritis	Bloody, straw colored, opaque	Good	<2000	<25	95-100	None
Aseptic inflammatory arthritis	Turbid, translucent	Fair to poor	2000-50,000	50-75	75	Needlelike (gout), rhomboid (pseudogout)
Septic arthritis	Purulent, turbid, opaque	Poor	>50,000	>75	20-50	None

*WBC, White blood cell; PMN, polymorphonuclear.

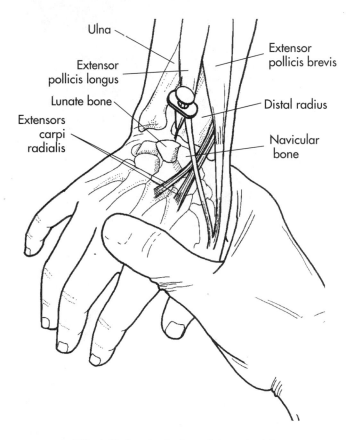

FIG. 115-6 Aspiration of the wrist joint.

Labels:
Ulna
Extensor pollicis longus
Lunate bone
Extensors carpi radialis
Extensor pollicis brevis
Distal radius
Navicular bone

Joint Fluid Interpretation

Normal joint fluid is straw colored, clear enough to read through, free-flowing, and nonclotting. Normal fluid produces a positive string sign finding and forms a good mucin clot. The glucose concentration of joint fluid is usually 80% that of serum.[5]

The *string sign* is a simple test that helps the physician judge synovial fluid viscosity. Perform this test by measuring the length of the string formed by a falling drop of fluid released from a syringe. Normal fluid produces a string of 5 to 10 cm. Inflammation reduces viscosity (via hyaluronate degradation) and causes the synovial fluid to form shorter strings or to fall in drops.[2,4]

The *mucin clot test* also correlates with fluid viscosity. Good mucin clot formation occurs with normal joint fluid and indicates a high degree of hyaluronate polymerization. Inflammatory states reduce mucin clot formation. Generate mucin clots by mixing four parts of 2% acetic acid with one part joint fluid.

Table 115-1 presents a summary of joint fluid analysis. Most of these parameters are variable for any given disease entity.

REFERENCES

1. Doughty RA, Rose C: Pain-joints. In Fleisher GR, Ludwig S, editors: *Textbook of pediatric emergency medicine,* ed 3, Baltimore, 1993, Williams & Wilkins, pp 377-381.
2. Ezell SL, Kubernick ME, Benjamin GC: Arthrocentesis. In Roberts JR, Hedges JR, editors: *Clinical procedures in emergency medicine,* ed 2, Philadelphia, 1991, WB Saunders, pp 847-859.
3. Ruddy RM: Procedures, arthrocentesis. In Fleisher GR, Ludwig S, editors: *Textbook of pediatric emergency medicine,* ed 3, Baltimore, 1993, Williams & Wilkins, pp 1663-1667.
4. Steinbrocker O, Newstadt DH: *Aspiration and injection therapy in arthritis and musculoskeletal disorders,* Hagerstown, Md, 1972, Harper & Row.
5. Thompson GR: Arthrocentesis: do's and dont's, *Hosp Med* pp 123-142.

116 Splinting

Dennis R. Durbin

Children frequently enter Emergency Departments for illnesses and injuries that benefit from temporary immobilization with splinting. Immobilization is the mainstay of fracture management and contributes to the recovery from soft tissue trauma such as sprains and contusions. At the very least proper immobilization provides comfort and protects the injured part from further trauma.

Emergency physicians often provide short-term immobilization for minor sprains, contusions, and other soft tissue conditions. In addition, splints constitute temporary therapy for fractures or more significant sprains until placement of definitive circumferential casts. For most indications splints provide adequate short-term immobilization equal to that of casts. Accomplish effective splinting by using either premade commercial immobilizing devices or custom-tailored splints made from either plaster of Paris, fiberglass, or splinting preparations that incorporate the padding and splint material into a single product. Splints allow for continued swelling without the risk of ischemic injury that circumferential casts carry.[32] In addition it is possible to remove splints for bathing, exercise of the injured part, or wound care if indicated.[5]

Indications

Splinting is indicated in a variety of musculoskeletal injuries or conditions that may benefit from short-term immobilization (Box 116-1). When splinting is indicated, it should relieve pain and protect the injured part from further trauma. Additional benefits are specific to the type of injury being treated. Splinting of fractures helps maintain alignment of the bony fragments, thus promoting proper healing and minimizing the potential for subsequent neurovascular injury. Splinting deep lacerations that cross joints can relieve tension on the wound and prevent wound dehiscence. Immobilization provides comfort in acute or chronic inflammatory disorders such as tenosynovitis, chronic arthritis, and joint infections. Deep space infections of the hands and feet or a cellulitis that crosses a joint similarly benefits from immobilization.

BOX 116–1 **CONDITIONS THAT BENEFIT FROM SPLINTING**

Fractures and sprains
Contusions and abrasions
Acute or septic arthritis
Lacerations that involve tendons or cross joints
Puncture wounds (especially animal bites) of hands, feet
Deep space infections of hands, feet
Tenosynovitis

The duration of immobilization varies, depending on the specific injury or condition. Immobilize contusions and abrasions for patient comfort for 1 to 3 days and lacerations that cross joints for 5 to 7 days. Immobilize for infectious conditions 3 to 5 days until swelling decreases and the involved part can move without significant pain.[5] Immobilize mild sprains for approximately 1 week; fractures have variable periods of immobilization, depending on the site and type of fracture. Determine the exact length and type of immobilization in consultation with the physician who sees the child in follow-up evaluation.

Contraindications

Since even serious or complicated fractures can benefit from initial immobilization before definitive treatment, there are rarely circumstances for which a temporary splint would be contraindicated, assuming correct application. Certain fractures require the evaluation of an orthopedic surgeon before discharge from the Emergency Department; do not manage these injuries with initial splinting and delayed follow-up evaluation. These include open fractures, femur or supracondylar humerus fractures, and fractures with suspected neurovascular compromise.

Complications

In general the complications of splints are similar to, but not as common as, the complications seen with the use of circumferential casts. The most worrisome complications of use of a circumferential cast are soft tissue compression, venous obstruction, and continued swelling of the injured extremity leading to *ischemic injury* and a compartment syndrome.[8,17,32] Although the risk of ischemic injury is much lower with splints, the elastic bandage used in making splints (Webril) can cause significant constriction. If continued swelling after splint application is a concern, cut the bandage lengthwise before applying the splint material. In addition carefully consider how tightly to place the elastic bandage over the splint. Instruct patients with injuries that have the potential for development of significant swelling (e.g., crush injuries, forearm and lower leg fractures) to seek follow-up evaluation within 24 to 48 hours. Tell the child and parents to monitor for the signs of vascular compromise.

As a result of the exothermic chemical reaction that occurs when plaster of Paris combines with water, use of plaster of Paris may result in *thermal injury* to the patient. Significant burns can occur with either circumferential casts or splints.[15] Temperatures in excess of 50° C have been reported to develop after the placement of plaster of Paris splints.[3] Skin exposure to this temperature for 12 minutes results in second-degree burns.[30] Temperatures generally peak between 20 and 30 minutes after wetting.[28] There are a number of factors that can affect the amount of heat produced during plaster formation (Box 116-2). To decrease the risk of thermal injury use as few sheets of plaster as necessary to achieve adequate splint strength, avoid extra fast-drying plaster, use fresh dip water as close to 24° C as possible, and never wrap the splint with a sheet or towel during the drying phase.[5] Alternatively use one of the prefabricated splint materials described later, which create less heat during drying.

Pressure sores can develop after splinting and are usually due to wrinkles in the stockinette or bandage or to splint motion over improperly padded bony prominences.[32] Minimize these by applying a smooth covering of stockinette and bandage, particularly over flexed joints and by using extra padding over bony prominences. In addition when molding the splint during its setting time, use the palms of the hands rather than the fingertips, to prevent making ridges or indentations in the plaster.

Bacterial or fungal *infections* can occur under a splint and are due either to contamination of the splint material or to an underlying wound.[5,13,14] The risk of infection is higher in the presence of an open wound or abrasion beneath the splint, but infection can occur even with intact skin. Clean all wounds and abrasions properly and cover them before the application of the splint. Since one of the distinct advantages of splinting is ease of removal of the device, encourage patients to inspect and clean underlying wounds each day.

Equipment

Plaster of Paris. The source of plaster of Paris is gypsum (calcium sulfate dihydrate), a naturally occurring substance that forms a powder when heated and dehydrated.[32] Water added to plaster of Paris incorporates into the crystalline lattice of the calcium sulfate dihydrate molecules, converting the powdery plaster into a firm mass. While plaster of Paris sets, there is a critical period during which any movement of the plaster interferes with the proper formation of the crystalline lattice, thus weakening the splint.[28] Plaster reaches its peak strength when its water content has decreased through evaporation to 21% of its initial level, generally about 24 hours after application.[32] During this time protect the splint from undue stress, such as weight bearing.

Modern-day plaster of Paris is available impregnated onto strips of a crinoline-type material that helps keep the plaster molded into the desired form during curing. It is commercially available in widths of 2, 3, 4, or 6 inches. There are two general types of plaster, based on setting time: fast-drying plaster sets in 5 to 8 minutes; extra-fast-drying plaster sets in 2 to 4 minutes.[28] For most Emergency Departments regular fast-drying plaster is sufficient and preferable to

extra-fast-drying because it is easier to work with and more comfortable to the patient because it produces less heat during setting.

Prefabricated Synthetic Splints. Prefabricated splint rolls that combine padding and splint material in one product have gained popularity for Emergency Department use. The splint material used varies among products from plaster of Paris to fiberglass and plastic sheets (e.g., OCL, Orthoplast, Ortho-glass). In general no one synthetic material is superior to another, though some may have advantages (weight, ease of application or removal) for specific uses.[4] The primary advantages of using a prefabricated splint roll as opposed to a custom-made plaster of Paris splint are time saved and ease of application of the splint. On the other hand plaster is generally less expensive than the prefabricated splint materials and is more modifiable to individual anatomic characteristics. Plaster is heavier and bulkier and delays weight bearing significantly compared to the synthetic materials.[4] If these factors are important in an individual splint, opt for synthetic materials. Otherwise plaster of Paris custom-made splints are generally preferable for Emergency Department use.

Stockinette. Use a single layer of cotton stockinette under circumferential casts and plaster of Paris splints. It functions to protect the skin and, when folded over the ends of the splint or cast, creates a padded rim to prevent pressure sores. It is commercially available in 2-, 3-, 4-, 8-, 10-, and 12-inch widths.

Soft Cotton Bandage. Apply a layer of cotton roll (We-bril) over the stockinette to provide padding and protection of the skin and bony prominences. It is available in widths of 2, 3, 4, and 6 inches.

Elastic Bandage. Use elastic (Ace) bandages to secure the splint to the extremity. They are available in 2-, 3-, 4-, and 6-inch widths.

Orthopedic Felt. Employ half-inch-thick felt to pad bony prominences such as the olecranon, radial and ulnar styloids, patella, fibular head, and medial and lateral malleoli.

Utility Knife. Use a utility knife or plaster scissors to cut and shape dry plaster or to cut prefabricated splint rolls to the desired length.

Bucket. Use a stainless steel bucket to dip splint material for moistening. Plaster can clog drains so do not prepare it directly in a sink. In addition replace the water in the bucket between splints and discard residual plaster since reusing dip water accelerates setting time and increases heat production during setting.

Protective Clothing. Wear protective gowns, gloves, and safety glasses, particularly when using plaster of paris, to protect clothing and prevent skin or eye injury from plaster dust or wet plaster.

Techniques

The following section provides *general* information about application of custom-made plaster of Paris splints. If using a prefabricated splint roll, omit stockinette and Webril since the splint material already incorporates the necessary padding. For unique or additional steps required in the placement of individual splints see the sections that describe individual anatomic regions

Patient Preparation. Applying a splint to a moving target in the form of an anxious toddler or preschool-age child significantly alters the effectiveness of the final result. When-

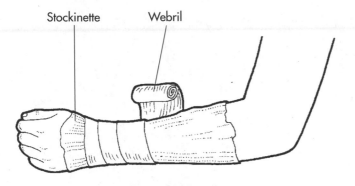

Stockinette   Webril

FIG. 116-1   Padding beneath a splint.

ever possible place splints with the child sitting in a parent's lap or distracted by a small toy. Idle distracting conversation using a calm, soothing tone of voice can also be beneficial. Before the child enters the room prepare all necessary equipment to minimize the time required to make the splint.[20] Before application of the splint, debride, cleanse, repair, and dress any wounds or abrasions in the usual manner.

Padding. If a splint involves the digits, pieces of Webril or gauze should be placed between the toes or fingers to prevent maceration. Then apply stockinette as the first layer of skin padding in custom-made splints. In general extend the stockinette 2 to 3 inches beyond each end of the planned length of the splint and fold it back to provide a padded rim. Take care to remove wrinkles from the stockinette, particularly in areas of joint flexion such as the elbows and ankles. Failure to produce a smooth, even layer of stockinette may lead to pressure sores in the wrinkled areas.

After placement of the stockinette apply additional cotton padding using Webril and wrap it around the extremity in a distal to proximal direction, taking care to overlap each turn by 50% (Fig. 116-1). Layer the Webril at least two to three layers thick and also extend 2 to 3 inches beyond each end of the splint to incorporate it into the padded rims. Place extra padding over bony prominences. Prevent wrinkles in the Webril by gently stretching and tearing the roll during application. To immobilize a joint in flexion, place it in the proper position before application of Webril. If necessary, use short, overlapping pieces of padding to prevent wrinkling around the joint. If there is risk of significant swelling, reduce the possibility of ischemic injury caused by the constriction of Webril by cutting it along the side of the extremity opposite to the plaster splint.

Plaster Preparation. The required length and width of the splint depend on the body part involved and the strength of stabilization desired. The easiest way to determine proper splint length is to lay the dry plaster sheets next to the involved extremity. Always err on the side of cutting the splint too long because it is possible to fold excess plaster back onto itself, if necessary. In general make the width of the splint at least 50% of the circumference of the involved extremity. The upper extremity typically requires 8 to 10 layers of plaster, the lower extremity, 12 to 14 layers.[5] Note specific size recommendations in the sections describing individual splints. Immerse the plaster sheets in fresh, room-temperature water until the bubbling stops. Remove the plaster slab and spread it on a smooth, hard surface to remove excess moisture and wrinkles and to spread the plaster evenly throughout the layers.

Splint Application. Position the splint on the extremity and fold the exposed Webril and stockinette back over the ends of the splint. One can apply an optional layer of Webril or gauze over the splint to prevent the elastic bandage from being incorporated into the drying plaster. Once the splint is in proper position (it is frequently helpful for an assistant to hold it in place), wrap an elastic (Ace) bandage around the splint and extremity from distal to proximal. Put sufficient tension on the elastic to secure the splint in place without causing unnecessary constriction of the swollen extremity. With the elastic bandage secured use the palms of the hands to mold and contour the splint to the extremity. Avoid using fingertips to mold the splint as this may lead to indentations that can cause pressure sores. Complete any manipulation of the plaster before it reaches a thick, creamy consistency. After this time any movement of the plaster weakens the ultimate strength of the splint as a result of incomplete crystal lattice formation

Discharge Instructions. Give all patients both verbal and written discharge instructions concerning splint care and monitoring for complications. In general provide slings for upper extremity injuries, and if necessary, crutches to children over 7 years of age for lower extremity injuries. Instruct patients and their parents about proper rest and elevation of the injured extremity to relieve pain and swelling. If the injury is less than 24 hours old and the patient or parents can easily remove and reapply the splint, apply ice packs for at least 30 minutes during the first 24 to 48 hours after the injury.[5]

If using plaster of Paris as the splinting material, tell patients not to stress the splint (e.g., with weight bearing) for at least 24 hours until the splint has had adequate time to dry fully. Synthetic splinting materials do not require this and typically harden before discharge from the Emergency Department. Keep the splint dry at all times. Remove it for bathing as needed. Give patients and their parents guidelines about the proper length of immobilization and where to seek follow-up evaluation in the event the splint prematurely breaks or significantly weakens.

Instruct patients and their parents to monitor for signs of developing neurovascular compromise. Tell them to take seriously any increase in pain after splint placement and arrange for a physician to evaluate promptly, not over the telephone. Symptoms of numbness or tingling, pallor, or decreased capillary refill of the distal extremity should also prompt a repeat evaluation in the Emergency Department. Finally arrange proper referral and follow-up evaluation for every patient.

Specific Techniques

Clavicle Splints

REMARKS. The clavicle is the most frequently broken bone in children. It has a double curve shape in the horizontal plane, with the two curves joining at the junction between the middle and lateral thirds of the bone. This point is the weakest part of the bone and consequently is the most common site of fracture.[24] In infants and small children the

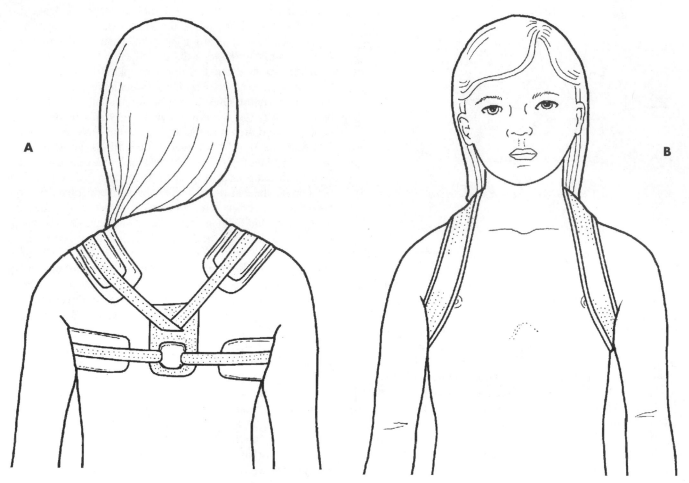

FIG. 116-2 Figure-of-eight clavicle harness **A,** Anterior view. **B,** Posterior view.

fracture is typically a greenstick type; in older children and adolescents a complete fracture is more common.

The usual cause of a clavicle fracture is a fall, onto an outstretched hand, the elbow, or the shoulder. Occasionally direct force applied to the clavicle from an anterior and superior position may force it onto the upper ribs, resulting in fracture. Open fractures of the clavicle are very rare because of the mobility of the overlying skin and the more common indirect mechanism of injury.

SPLINTING TECHNIQUE. Conservative management with immobilization is generally all that is required for pediatric clavicle fractures. In children below age 6 years the fracture virtually never warrants reduction.[24] Complete healing and remodeling of even grossly malaligned fractures are typical. In older children and adolescents markedly displaced fractures may require closed reduction before immobilization.

Splinting of clavicle fractures provides more comfort than immobilization.[24] Splint with a simple triangular sling or a figure-of-eight harness. Studies comparing the effectiveness of the two methods demonstrate no difference in the functional or cosmetic results.[1,23] Figure-of-eight harnesses produce a higher rate of complications, most commonly patient discomfort from chafing or axillary pressure.[1] There are also reports of subsequent neurovascular compromise or fracture nonunion as complications of figure-of-eight harnesses.[29]

Figure 116-2 outlines application of a figure-of-eight harness. For maximum ease stand behind the patient and ask the patient (or an assistant) to hold the patient's arms up. Place the harness through each axilla and adjust by tightening the straps in the back. The buckle for the straps should hang in the midline of the back. Tighten the harness and move the shoulders up and back into a position of comfort. Remove the harness for bathing; it should remain in place for 3 weeks. Forewarn parents about the "bump" of callus that forms, which remodels and disappears over a period of 6 to 9 months.

Rib Splints

REMARKS. Rib fractures are relatively rare in childhood; always consider significant intrathoracic injury after chest trauma even in the absence of rib fracture. The compliance of the pediatric chest may result in underlying cardiac or pulmonary contusion even if there is no overlying rib fracture. Suspect child abuse when rib fractures are present without an adequate explanation of cause.

SPLINTING TECHNIQUE. Recognition and prompt management of the serious complications associated with rib fractures (pneumothorax, hemothorax, cardiac or pulmonary contusion) are more important than treatment of the fracture itself. Satisfactory healing of rib fractures typically occurs in 3 weeks, even after significant angulation or overriding of the fracture fragments.[6] Otherwise uncomplicated rib fractures do not warrant immobilization. Methods of immobilization

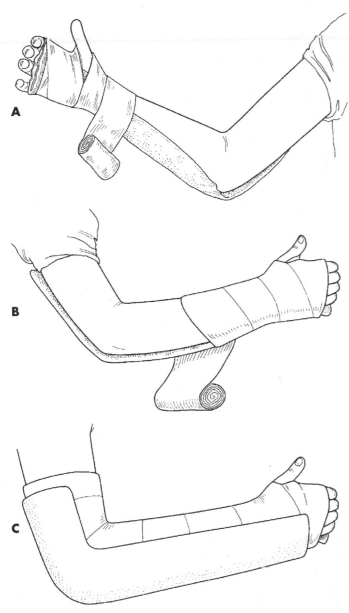

FIG. 116-3 **A** to **C,** Long arm posterior splint.

to the elbow, assessment of their function after elbow injury is mandatory. Likewise assessment of vascular integrity of the distal extremity is part of every evaluation of elbow trauma.

A variety of conditions warrant immobilization of the elbow. The supracondylar humerus fracture is the most common elbow fracture in childhood, accounting for up to 60% of elbow fractures.[27] It usually results from a fall onto an outstretched hand with the elbow in extension. Fractures of the lateral humeral condyle are the second most common (20%), and medial epicondylar fractures account for about 10%.[16] Splint these fractures while awaiting immediate orthopedic evaluation, with frequent assessment of distal neurovascular integrity.

Elbow dislocations may occur alone or in combination with fractures, most commonly of the medial epicondyle, proximal radius, radial head, coronoid process, or olecranon.[16] A uniquely pediatric condition, the "nursemaid's" or "pulled" elbow, represents subluxation of the radial head, typically caused by pulling on an outstretched and pronated arm.[22] (Chapter 118 details management of this entity.)

Nontraumatic conditions of the elbow that may benefit from immobilization include infectious or inflammatory arthritis, cellulitis, and overuse syndromes such as tendonitis and bursitis.

SPLINTING TECHNIQUE. Immobilize the elbow for any cause with either a long arm posterior splint or a double sugar tong splint. The long arm posterior splint extends from the distal metacarpals to the proximal humerus (Fig. 116-3). Immobilize the elbow in 90 degrees of flexion with the forearm in a neutral (thumb up) position.[5] Slightly dorsiflex the wrist. The patient should actively assume this position without assistance. Use the techniques outlined for general splint preparation; have the splint form a gutter along the ulnar surface of the hand and forearm and extend along the posterior surface of the elbow and humerus. Cut a notch in the splint to ensure a smooth contour around the elbow. Once the splint is in place, assess the patient for any signs of neurovascular compromise before discharge from the Emergency Department.

An alternative to the posterior long arm splint is the double sugar tong splint (Fig. 116-4). As with the posterior splint, make this splint extend from the distal metacarpals to the proximal humerus. Fashion it in two pieces, a forearm segment and a humerus segment. Have the forearm segment extend from the distal metacarpals up to and around the elbow and back to the posterior aspect of the hand. The proximal segment includes most of the humerus and likewise encircles the elbow. Keep the elbow, forearm, and wrist in the same positions as with the long arm posterior splint. Hold the two pieces together with the elastic wrap. If management of the injury requires regular removal of the splint, the posterior splint may be preferable because of its ease of removal and reapplication. Otherwise there are no significant differences between these two splinting techniques.

Wrist Splints

REMARKS. Forearm fractures are among the most common bony injuries of childhood. The usual mechanism of injury is a fall onto an outstretched hand, with most of the force absorbed by the radius.[25] Unlike in adult wrist fractures, this mechanism typically does not result in an intraarticular

such as strapping and binding, which have been advocated in the past, produce a number of complications, most significantly the development of atelectasis or pneumonia caused by the constriction of chest excursion. Effective management of rib fractures involves adequate analgesia with either systemic narcotic or nonnarcotic pain relievers, or intercostal nerve block with a long-acting local anesthetic.

Elbow Splints

REMARKS. The elbow joint has complex anatomic relationships that provide for both flexion/extension and rotation. The elbow comprises three articulations (1) between the ulna and the trochlea of the humerus, (2) between the radial head and the capitellum of the humerus, and (3) between the proximal ulna and radius.[18] Injury to the elbow typically results from a fall, either onto an outstretched arm (with the elbow in extension) or directly onto the elbow. Upper extremity fractures account for approximately 70% of pediatric fractures.[12] The elbow is second only to the distal forearm in frequency of upper extremity fractures. Because of the close proximity of the ulnar, radial, and median nerves

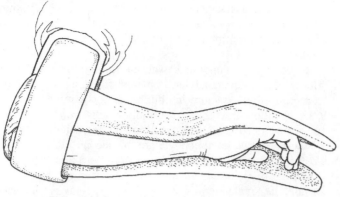

FIG. 116-4 Double sugar tong arm splint.

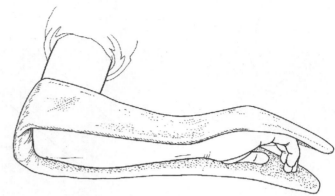

FIG. 116-6 Sugar tong arm splint.

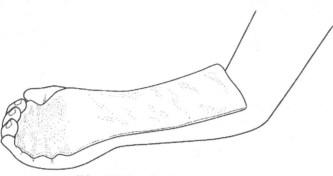

FIG. 116-5 Simple volar splint.

fracture in children. A distal forearm fracture is usually either a buckle (torus) or a simple fracture. The fracture usually occurs in the distal one-third of the forearm either at the junction of the diaphysis and metaphysis or at the physis.[7] This region becomes particularly vulnerable to injury during the growth spurt of early adolescence. The peak incidence of distal forearm fractures in boys and girls mirrors the age at which peak velocity of growth in height occurs (12 years for girls, 14 years for boys).[2] In about 50% of patients a fracture of the distal ulna accompanies the radius fracture.[7,25] Isolated ulnar fractures are very uncommon.[25]

Distal forearm fractures generally heal well after 2 to 3 weeks of immobilization. If desired, splint for a few days before definitive treatment with a circumferential cast. Complications related to distal radius or ulna fractures are very uncommon because of the tremendous ability to remodel.[24]

SPLINTING TECHNIQUE. There are two basic splints that immobilize the wrist. The simple volar splint (Fig. 116-5) is best for wrist sprains, contusions, or other soft tissue injuries (cellulitis, synovitis, etc.). Make the splint to extend from the proximal forearm to the metacarpal heads. Ascertain that the fingers and thumb are free to move. Splint the wrist in a neutral (thumb up) position and slightly extended. Fold back the distal end of the splint onto itself, providing a "shelf" on which the fingers can rest in a position of function.

Another effective forearm splint is the sugar tong short arm splint (Fig. 116-6). This splint may be preferable to the simple volar splint for initial management of wrist and forearm fractures because it also immobilizes the elbow, eliminating supination and pronation. Place the elbow (actively) in 90 degrees of flexion with the wrist neutral and

slightly extended. After measuring the appropriate length of splint material wrap the splint from the volar aspect of the metacarpal heads, down the forearm, around the elbow, and up to the dorsal aspect of the metacarpal heads. Wrap the elastic bandage in a distal to proximal direction. Take care to maintain proper position of the elbow and wrist during the molding of this splint. It is preferable to provide a simple sling for the patient to use in conjunction with the sugar tong splint before orthopedic referral.

Hand and Finger Splints

REMARKS. Children frequently injure the hand, and management of pediatric hand injuries presents some unique challenges. Use hand splints to manage carpal, metacarpal, and phalange fractures; infections; burns; lacerations; or contusions.[9,11,31] The general aim of management is, by the most conservative means possible, to obtain the best *functional* result.[6,31] Hand injuries, no matter how benign they may appear on initial clinical or radiographic evaluation, should always receive appropriate follow-up evaluation after initial Emergency Department management to ensure proper recovery of function.

There are significant potential pitfalls to the Emergency Department management of hand fractures. Even subtle degrees of residual *rotational malalignment* after initial closed reduction of metcarpal and phalangeal fractures can create significant functional impairment after establishment of full range of motion.[19,31] Assess rotational alignment best by examining the planes of the fingernails with the interphalangeal joints in flexion[31] (Fig 116-7, *A*). Ensure that all fingernails are in the same plane; with full flexion of the fingers, they should all point to the tubercle of the trapezium (Fig. 116-7, *B*). Rotational malalignment manifests itself in abnormal angulation of the fingers in flexion (Fig. 116-8).

Simply splinting the hand in a position of function produces a good initial reduction and immobilization of most metacarpal and phalangeal fractures.[31] Avoid the "rest-injury" position, the one patients naturally assume after significant injury to the hand, at all costs[31] (Fig. 116-9). A hand that becomes stiff in this position is relatively nonfunctional. Avoid this position by splinting the wrist in extension, the metacarpophalangeal joints in 90 degrees of flexion, and the proximal interphalangeal joints in about 15 degrees of flexion (Fig. 116-10). This is the "safe" or "intrinsic-plus" position.[31] In addition, to prevent rotational malalignment after reduction of a finger fracture, never splint fingers

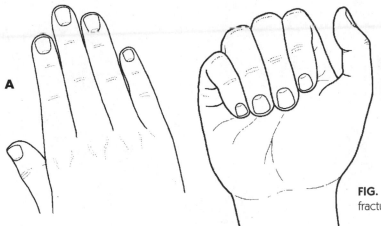

FIG. 116-7   **A** and **B,** Normal alignment of fingers after hand fracture reduction.

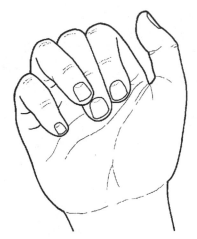

FIG. 116-8   Malrotation of fingers after hand fracture reduction.

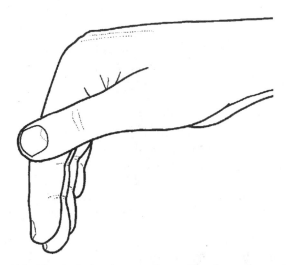

FIG. 116-10   Intrinsic-plus or safe position for metacarpal and phalangeal fractures.

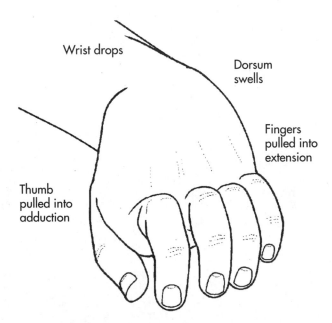

Wrist drops

Dorsum swells

Fingers pulled into extension

Thumb pulled into adduction

FIG. 116-9   Avoid the rest-injury position for metacarpal and phalangeal fractures.

individually; "buddy tape" or splint them to an adjacent finger to maintain normal alignment.

SPLINTING TECHNIQUES

Gutter Splints. Immobilize uncomplicated fractures of the fifth metacarpal (boxer's fracture) or the fourth or fifth phalanges using an ulnar gutter splint; make the splint to extend along the ulnar surface of the forearm from the distal fingers to the proximal forearm (Fig. 116-11, *A*). Incorporate the fourth and fifth fingers into the splint together after placing a piece of gauze or bandage between them (Fig. 116-11, *B*). Make the splint wide enough to cover both the volar and dorsal surfaces of the fourth and fifth metacarpals (Fig. 116-11, *C* and *D*).

Use a radial gutter splint to immobilize second and third metacarpal or phalangeal fractures (Fig. 116-12). As in preparing the ulnar gutter splint, separate the fingers by a piece of gauze before incorporation into the splint, which extends along the radial surface of the forearm. Cut a hole in the splint material to accommodate the thumb, but do not incorporate it into the splint. Make the splint material wide enough to cover both the volar and dorsal surfaces of the second and third metacarpals.

Pay attention to the position of the fingers within the

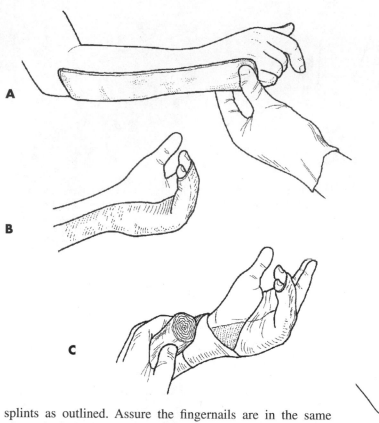

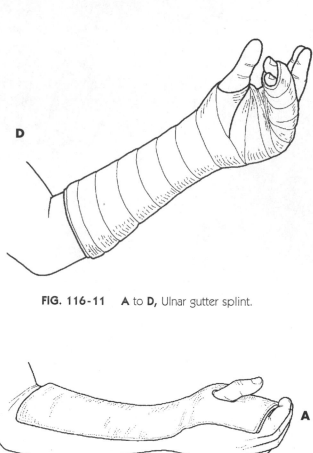

FIG. 116-11 **A** to **D,** Ulnar gutter splint.

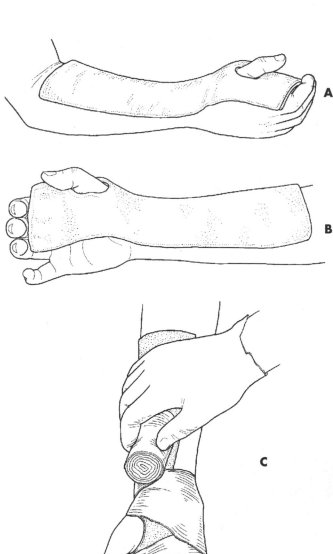

splints as outlined. Assure the fingernails are in the same plane, the interphalangeal joints in 15 degrees of flexion, the metacarpophalangeal joints in 90 degrees of flexion, and the wrist in approximately 30 degrees of extension.

Thumb Spica Splint. Use the thumb spica splint to immobilize nonrotated, nonangulated, nonarticular fractures of the thumb metacarpal or phalanx (Fig. 116-13). In addition, immobilize ulnar collateral ligament injuries (gamekeeper's thumb) properly using this splint. Extend the splint along the radial surface of the forearm from the tip of the thumb to the proximal forearm. Keep the wrist in 30 degrees of extension, with the thumb abducted and the interphalangeal joint in slight flexion. An alternative method of making a thumb spica splint is to incorporate a thumb extension into a simple volar short arm splint.

Finger Splints. Immobilize most isolated finger sprains adequately with buddy taping to an adjacent normal finger (Fig. 116-14). The most common site sprained is the proximal interphalangeal (PIP) joint. Obtain a good anteroposterior (AP) and lateral radiograph to rule out a subtle fracture, place gauze between the fingers, and apply tape across the middle and proximal phalanges. One to two weeks of immobilization is typically sufficient before beginning range of motion exercises.

Immobilize finger lacerations, tendon repairs, and nonrotated, nonangulated phalangeal fractures effectively with a dorsal extension block (Fig. 116-15). This simple finger splint incorporates foam padding and an aluminum strip into a single product customizable by bending the aluminum into the desired position. Extend the finger splints from the distal phalanx to the dorsum of the wrist. It is usually preferable to place these splints on the dorsum of the finger because it provides the most effective immobilization without interfering with the tactile surface of the digit. As with the gutter

FIG. 116-12 **A** to **C,** Radial gutter splint.

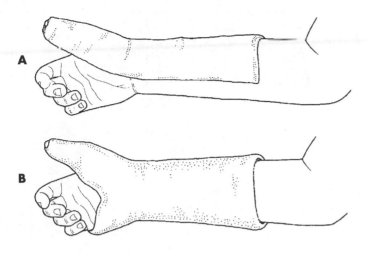

FIG. 116-13   **A** and **B,** Thumb spica splint.

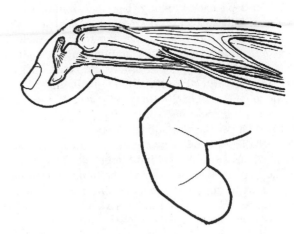

FIG 116-16   Mallet finger deformity. Note extension at proximal interphalangeal joint, flexion at distal interphalangeal joint.

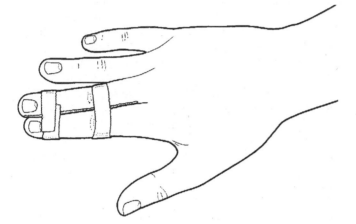

FIG. 116-14   Buddy taping of fingers.

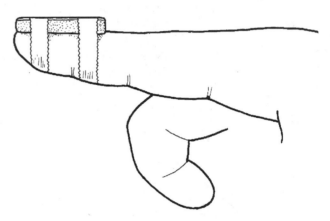

FIG 116-17   Mallet finger splint.

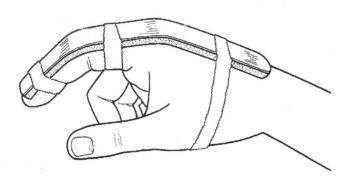

FIG. 116-15   Dorsal extension block.

splints, the metacarpophalangeal (MCP) joint is flexed 90 degrees, and the interphalangeal joints are flexed about 15 degrees. Use ½-inch or 1-inch tape to secure the splint over the middle and proximal phalanges and the dorsum of the hand.

Effective immobilization of mallet and boutonnière finger deformities requires specialized splints. In adults mallet finger deformities typically result from a rupture of the extensor tendon inserting into the distal phalanx, causing a flexion deformity of the distal interphalangeal (DIP) joint[6,9]

(Fig. 116-16). In children a more typical injury producing a mallet finger deformity is a physeal injury of the distal phalanx. Treat this by applying a splint over the dorsum of the distal interphalangeal joint, and allow use of the rest of the finger (Fig. 116-17). Complete healing requires 3 weeks of immobilization.

The common extensor tendons form a structure called the central slip that inserts into the base of the middle phalanx and extends the PIP joint.[6] Rupture of the central slip results in a boutonnière deformity, characterized by loss of extension of the PIP joint and hyperextension of the DIP joint (Fig. 116-18). This may be an acute rupture after a laceration over the dorsum of the PIP joint or a gradual rupture after a closed injury to the joint. Immobilize with splinting of the PIP joint in extension while allowing free movement of the MCP and DIP joints (Fig. 116-19). Because of the risk of recurrence of this deformity all boutonnière injuries require follow-up evaluation by an orthopedist.

Knee Splints

REMARKS. In many Emergency Departments the knee immobilizer has virtually replaced plaster or fiberglass splints for immobilization of mild to moderate knee sprains and soft tissue injuries.[5] The advantages of the knee immobilizer are that it is lightweight, is easy to apply and remove, and can be placed over a patient's clothing. Use it to immobilize relatively minor injuries that do not require immediate orthopedic evaluation, traction, or casting. For more unstable knee sprains or fractures of the tibia or fibula a more effective method of immobilization is a custom-made plaster or fiberglass splint. Effective knee splints include the long leg posterior splint (Fig. 116-20), long leg sugar tong splint (Fig. 116-21), and bilateral knee splint (Fig. 116-22), made with medial and lateral slabs of splint material.

SPLINTING TECHNIQUE. Knee immobilizers are available in a variety of sizes (small, medium, large, extra large). Determine the proper size by placing the immobilizer on the stretcher next to the injured leg, aligning the patellar cutout area with the knee (Fig. 116-23). Extend the immobilizer from a few inches above the malleoli to just beneath the crease of the buttocks. Place the immobilizer around the knee with the metal supports along the medial and lateral aspects of the knee and hold in place by securing the self-adhesive (Velcro) straps. Give patients crutches to prevent weight bearing and arrange appropriate orthopedic follow-up evaluation.

Choice of which custom-made splint design to use depends on the degree of immobilization desired and the specific nature of the injury. For instance the bilateral knee

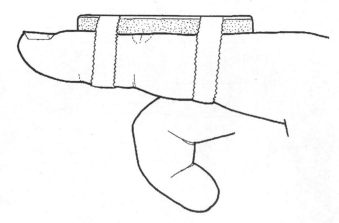

FIG. 116-19 *Boutonnière deformity splint.*

splint provides excellent immobilization of the medial and lateral collateral ligaments and is the best choice to immobilize injuries to these structures. Immobilize fractures of the tibia and fibula with a long leg sugar tong splint, which limits inversion and eversion of the ankle. The easiest to apply is the posterior (gutter) splint. If an assistant is available, he/she can elevate the leg during application of the stockinette, bandage, and splint material. If an assistant is not available, place the patient in the prone position with the splint laid along the posterior aspect of the leg until secured in place. Because of its fairly easy application the posterior gutter splint is a frequent choice for a temporary splint for injuries planned for immediate operative intervention.

Ankle Splints

REMARKS. Ankle injuries in children primarily involve the epiphyseal plate and are of particular concern because of the risk of growth disturbance with resultant leg length discrepancy. Since in children the major ligaments about the ankle (as well as other joints) are stronger than the adjacent epiphyseal plate, ligamentous injuries (sprains) are extremely rare.[12] Inversion or eversion injuries that might typically

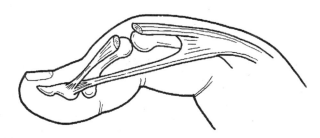

FIG. 116-18 *Boutonnière deformity. Note flexion at proximal interphalangeal joint, extension at distal interphalangeal joint.*

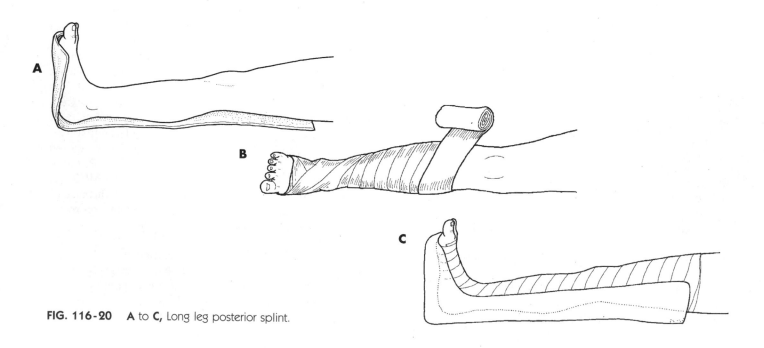

FIG. 116-20 **A** to **C,** *Long leg posterior splint.*

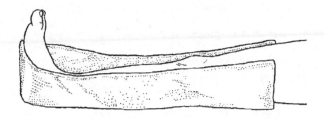

FIG. 116-21   Long leg sugar tong splint.

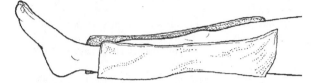

FIG. 116-22   Bilateral knee splint.

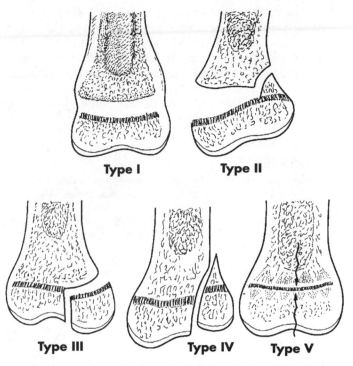

Type I   **Type II**

Type III   **Type IV**   **Type V**

FIG. 116-24   Salter-Harris classification of physeal injuries.

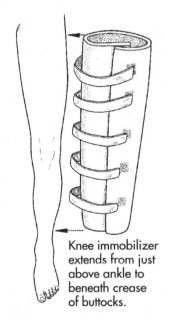

Knee immobilizer
extends from just
above ankle to
beneath crease
of buttocks.

FIG. 116-23   Aligning a knee immobilizer.

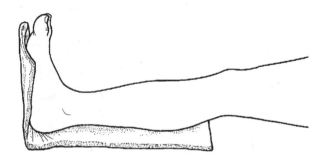

FIG. 116-25   Short leg posterior splint.

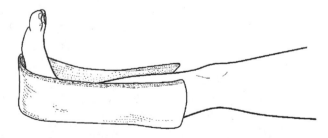

FIG. 116-26   Short leg sugar tong splint.

result in ligamentous sprains in adults are more likely to result in a fracture of the epiphyseal plate in a child. A classification system designed by Salter and Harris has proved useful in determining the prognosis of a particular epiphyseal plate fracture-separation[21] (Fig. 116-24). Evaluate any significant ankle injury accompanied by localized tenderness and swelling by radiography. In a child with open growth plates assume a normal ankle radiograph result in the face of point tenderness and swelling over the distal end of the fibula or tibia to be a Salter-Harris type I epiphyseal plate injury, not an ankle sprain. The prognosis for normal growth after type I to III injuries is generally excellent. Ideal treatment consists of a plaster walking cast for 3 weeks. Accomplish initial immobilization with one of a number of ankle splint designs.

SPLINTING TECHNIQUE. The short leg posterior (gutter) splint is among the most common splints used in the Emergency Department[26] (Fig. 116-25). Use this to immobi-

lize distal tibia and fibula fractures, ankle sprains, reduced ankle dislocations, tarsal and metatarsal fractures, and other medical conditions requiring ankle immobilization. In a study comparing the effectiveness of a number of ankle splint designs the short leg sugar tong splint (Fig. 116-26) was found to prevent ankle plantar flexion most effectively and to break less frequently than the posterior splint.[10] For temporary (a few days) immobilization before definitive casting either design is acceptable.

Extend the short leg posterior splint from the metatarsal

heads to the proximal lower leg. Apply this splint with the patient lying prone and the leg elevated in the air. During drying mold the splint to hold the ankle at an angle of 90 degrees. Pass the sugar tong splint beneath the foot from the calcaneus to the metatarsal heads and extend up the medial and lateral aspects of the lower leg to the level of the fibular head. Make a particularly effective ankle splint by combining a posterior and a sugar tong splint.

REFERENCES

1. Andersen K, Jensen PO, Lauritzen J: Treatment of clavicular fractures: figure-of-eight bandage versus a simple sling, *Acta Orthop Scand* 57:61, 1987.
2. Bailey DA, et al: Epidemiology of fractures of the distal end of the radius in children as associated with growth, *J Bone Joint Surg* 71:1225, 1989.
3. Becker DW: Danger of burns from fresh plaster splints surrounded by too much cotton, *Plast Reconstr Surg* 62:436, 1978.
4. Bowker P, Powell ES: A clinical evaluation of plaster-of-Paris and eight synthetic splinting materials, *Injury* 23:13, 1992.
5. Chudnofsky CR, Otten EJ, Newmeyer WL: Splinting techniques. In Roberts JR, Hedges JR editors: *Clinical procedures in emergency medicine,* ed 2, Philadelphia, 1991, WB Saunders.
6. Connolly JF, editor: *DePalma's the management of fractures and dislocations, an atlas,* ed 3, Philadelphia, 1981, WB Saunders.
7. Dicke TE, Nunley JA: Distal forearm fractures in children, *Orthop Clin North Am* 24:333, 1993.
8. Foisie PS: Vokmann's ischemic contracture: an analysis of its proximate mechanism, *N Engl J Med* 226:671, 1942.
9. Green DP: Hand injuries in children, *Pediatr Clin North Am* 24:903, 1977.
10. Halvorson G, Iserson KV: Comparison of four ankle splint designs, *Ann Emerg Med* 16:1249, 1987.
11. Hausman MR, Lisser SP: Hand infections, *Orthop Clin North Am* 23:171, 1992.
12. Hodge D, et al: Trauma to elbows, knees, and ankles, *Pediatr Emerg Care* 7:188, 1991.
13. Houang ET, et al: Outbreak of plaster-associated pseudomonas infection, *Lancet* 1:728, 1981.
14. Huoang ET, et al: Survival of *Pseudomonas aeruginosa* in plaster of Paris, *J Hosp Infect* 2:231, 1981.
15. Kaplan SS: Burns following application of plaster splint dressings, *J Bone Joint Surg* 63:670, 1981.
16. Karasick D, Burk DL, Gross GW: Trauma to the elbow and forearm, *Semin Roentgenol* 26:318, 1991.
17. Linson MA, Lewinnek G, White AA: Ischemic complications of femoral cast-bracing: Report of two cases, *Clin Orthop* 162:189, 1982.
18. Murphy WA, Siegel MJ: Elbow fat pads with new signs and extended differential diagnosis, *Radiology* 124:659, 1977.
19. Rang M, editor: *Children's fractures,* ed 2, Philadelphia, 1983, JB Lippincott.
20. Rang MC, Willis RB: Fractures and sprains, *Pediatr Clin North Am* 24:749, 1977.
21. Salter RB: Injuries of the ankle in children, *Orthop Clin North Am* 5:147, 1974.
22. Schunk JE: Radial head subluxation: epidemiology and treatment of 87 episodes, *Ann Emerg Med* 19:1019, 1990.
23. Stanley D, Norris SH: Recovery following fractures of the clavicle treated conservatively, *Injury* 19:162, 1988.
24. Tachdjian MO, editor: *Pediatric orthopedics,* vol 4, Philadelphia, 1990, WB Saunders.
25. Tredwell SJ, Peteghem KV, Clough M: Pattern of forearm fractures in children, *J Pediatr Orthop* 4:604, 1984.
26. Waickerle JF: Ankle injuries. In Tintinalli JE, Rothstein RJ, Krome RL, editors: *Emergency medicine: a comprehensive study guide,* New York, 1985, McGraw-Hill.
27. Webb AJ, Sherman FC: Supracondylar fractures of the humerus in children, *J Pediatr Orthop* 9:315, 1989.
28. Wehbe MA: Plaster uses and misuses, *Clin Orthop* 167:242, 1982.
29. Wilkins RM, Wiedel JD: Ununited fractures of the clavicle, *J Bone Joint Surg* 65:773, 1983.
30. Williamson C, Scholtz JR: Time-temperature relationships in thermal blister formation, *J Invest Dermatol* 12:41, 1949.
31. Wood VE: Fractures of the hand in children, *Orthop Clin North Am* 7:527, 1976.
32. Wu KK: *Techniques in surgical casting and splinting,* Philadelphia, 1987, Lea & Febiger.

117 Cast Problems

John P. Dormans

Emergency physicians often evaluate and treat children with problems related to casts. This chapter identifies problems that may occur in conjunction with casting and outlines tools and techniques to solve these problems.

Indications and Contraindications

Children with casts may experience several different problems, ranging from broken, wet, or tight casts to compression complications resulting from irritation of soft tissues over bony prominences to neurovascular complications (Fig. 117-1). Cast removal may be indicated if a cast is tight, wet, or broken or if neurovascular complications or local pressure phenomena occur. Splitting or spreading the cast may be indicated if the cast is too tight; windowing a cast may be indicated to inspect a surgical wound or to look for signs of pressure irritation. Repair or reinforcement of a cast is indicated if the cast is broken or weak.

Complications

If the cast is tight circumferentially, neurovascular problems may occur. Initially, there is venous compression with venous stasis and edema distally. With time or more severe constriction, arterial compression can occur with true ischemia of the distal part. Compartment syndromes can ultimately occur with Volkmann's ischemic contracture.[2,2a]

If a cast is broken, fracture reduction may be lost, or skin and soft-tissue irritation may occur. If a cast gets wet, the padding of the cast remains wet for a long time, and maceration of the skin may result. Additionally, children often place objects inside their casts. This again can result in skin irritation, ulceration, infection, and full-thickness skin loss. Local pressure on the soft tissues overlying a bony prominence can lead to erythema, blistering, or a partial or full-thickness skin necrosis (Fig. 117-2). A careful history should be taken, a physical examination should be performed to identify these problems and address them according to the techniques outlined below.

Equipment

Most procedures for cast problems require only a short list of tools.[1,5] Fig. 117-3 shows these tools. The most important tool for dealing with these problems is a cast saw. Most cast saws consist of an electric motor that drives a serrated circular blade in an oscillating fashion. The arc of oscillation is such that rigid structures (e.g., casts) are readily divided, whereas soft tissues (e.g., skin), which are less rigid and fixed, are spared. However, skin lacerations can occur, especially over a bony prominence where the soft tissues are "bound down" to the underlying bone (i.e., less subcutaneous soft tissue). Several types of cast saws are available. Cast saws that are quiet and compact are currently available and are especially advantageous for the pediatric population.

A spreader tool is useful once the cast has been split. Insert the blades of the spreader device into the longitudinal split created by the cast saw. Spread a cast by compressing the handles. This is a useful tool for removing, univalving, bivalving, or windowing casts.

Bandage scissors are useful for cutting the padding underneath the cast. An assortment of various sized bandage scissors is needed to cut different sizes of casts and different thicknesses of padding. The scissors should be sharpened often.

Cast shears may be used instead of a cast saw.[4] These are occasionally used for the removal of small casts, such as a clubfoot cast. They are safe but require care and precision in use.

Techniques

Cast Removal. The cast saw should be used with care that skin laceration does not occur. The finger or thumb may be used as a guide to prevent inadvertent diving of the blade beyond the plaster and padding into the soft tissues (Fig. 117-4). The cast saw should be moved in an "up-and-down" or "in-and-out" movement rather than a longitudinal gliding movement.[1,5] The loss of resistance encountered at the inner surface of the plaster can be felt by the person removing the cast. Once the cast is bivalved, the underlying padding may be divided and the cast may be removed. Care should be exercised over bony prominences, because the soft tissues are relatively fixed in these areas and are more easily injured. With the advent of synthetic casting material, cast complications have become more common. The use of a cast saw for the removal of synthetic casting material can generate excessive amounts of heat, which can cause skin burns. Heat-resistant blades are commercially available to help lessen the chances of this complication.[4]

Soaking Off a Cast. Cast removal with a cast saw may be difficult on an infant or child who has a clubfoot or metatarsus adductus cast. If cast removal is indicated in this situations, the cast can be soaked off. This can be accomplished by soaking the cast in 1 to 2 L of warm water with a small amount of vinager for approximately 30 minutes until the cast is soft. When this is anticipated, the physician who applied the cast usually leaves a small ball of plaster exposed on the surface of the cast. After soaking, this ball of plaster can be used to find the end of the roll of plaster, and the plaster material can be unrolled in such a way that the cast saw is not needed.

Splitting and Spreading of a Cast. If a cast is too tight circumferentially, it can be split by univalving or bivalving.

UNIVALVING. Fig. 117-5 illustrates univalving. A longitudinal mark is made from one end of the cast to the other. Use the cast saw to divide the plaster or fiberglass and the spreader bar to spread the casting material. Once this is done,

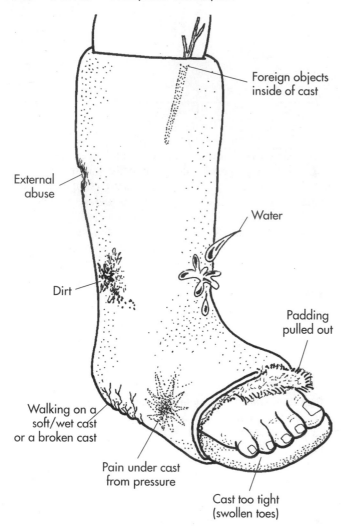

FIG. 117-1 What can go wrong.

Labels on figure:
- Foreign objects inside of cast
- External abuse
- Water
- Dirt
- Padding pulled out
- Walking on a soft/wet cast or a broken cast
- Pain under cast from pressure
- Cast too tight (swollen toes)

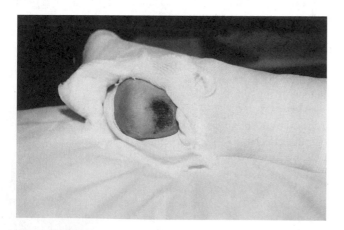

FIG. 117-2 Heel ulcer resulting from unrecognized pressure over the bony prominence of the calcaneus.

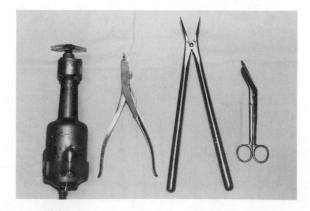

FIG. 117-3 Tools needed for doing cast work, from left to right: cast saw, two types of cast spreaders, and bandage scissors.

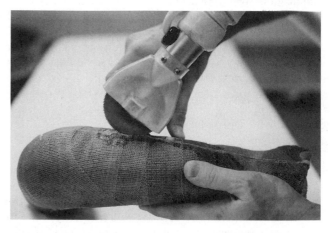

FIG. 117-4 Thumb is used to prevent inadvertent plunging of the cast saw blade after dividing casting material with cast saw. Without this prevention technique, skin lacerations may occur when removing, windowing, or splitting casts.

the underlying padding is exposed and the cast can be divided longitudinally with a pair of sharp bandage scissors. Some physicians recommend "splitting to the skin" (i.e., dividing all of the plaster and underlying padding, thus exposing the skin). This is the safest method of relieving circumferential compression and preventing complications.

Fiberglass has a tendency to be more elastic than plaster. If a fiberglass cast is univalved and subsequently spread, it has a tendency to spring back into its original shape, which may cause further compression of the limb. Plaster, on the other hand, tends to remain in the spread position once it has been split and spread. For this reason, fiberglass casts, once univalved, may need to be bivalved or held open with a spacer to prevent further compression.

BIVALVING. The cast is split longitudinally along the length of the cast on two sides, which are usually 180 degrees from each another. The underlying cast padding is split if indicated. Bivalving of a cast additionally allows the removal of one half of the cast, so the skin or surgical incisions can be inspected. This process leaves the cast loose and somewhat unstable; it should be secured with tape to avoid this problem. These casts usually need to be "snugged up" and repaired with additional rolls of plaster or fiberglass once the swelling has subsided.

Windowing a Cast. Windowing a cast may be indicated if there are complaints of pain underneath the cast or if there are signs of infection of a surgical wound.[3] Fig. 117-6 illustrates the technique. The window is accomplished by

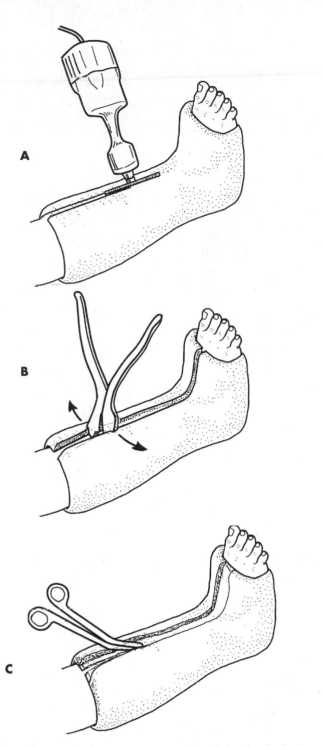

FIG. 117-5   Univalving a cast. **A,** Cast is split longitudinally from one end to the other with cast saw. **B,** Spreader bar is inserted, and cast is spread. **C,** Bandage scissors are used to divide cast padding to skin.

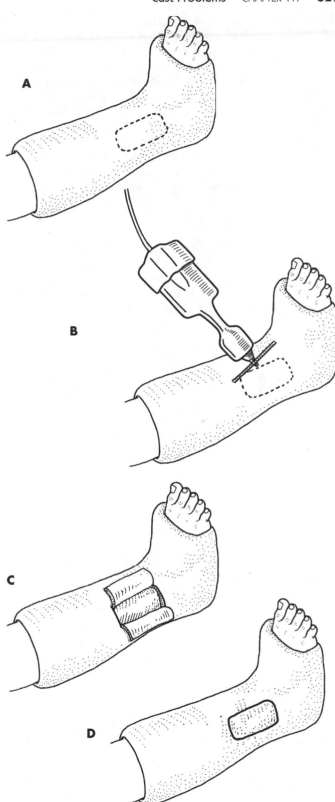

FIG. 117-6   Windowing a cast: **A,** Mark the area to be windowed on the cast using a marker. **B,** Use a cast saw to make the window. Remove and save the window. **C,** Split the cast padding longitudinally to the skin. **D,** Always replace the window to avoid window edema. Hold the window in place with either tape or casting material.

first using a marker to outline the portion of the cast that needs to be removed. Use the cast saw next to remove the plaster or fiberglass portion. Then use bandage scissors to open the underlying padding. Heel pain in particular is always a reason for concern. If it is present, window the cast to look for signs of pressure or ischemia of the soft tissues of the heel. Replace and secure the cast window to prevent window edema.

Reinforcing a Cast. Cast reinforcement or repair is occasionally indicated if a cast is broken or has been previously split. To make this repair, an additional roll or two of plaster or fiberglass material should be wrapped around the broken portion of the cast. The plantar, or foot, portion of a lower extremity cast is an area where this commonly occurs if the patient walks on the cast when it is not dry or set, or if the plantar portion of the cast is not strong enough. When this occurs, there are two options: the cast must be replaced or repaired. If the damage is minimal and there are contraindications to removing the cast, the broken portion of the cast may simply be reinforced with an additional roll of plaster or fiberglass. If the damage is more severe and beyond repair, replace the cast.

Remarks

Patient and family education is paramount in avoiding cast problems. If a patient has a broken cast, it is often because he was not properly instructed in proper cast care rather than that he is being uncooperative. To prevent cast problems, give written instructions that include directions for showering and bathing to all patients who have casts applied. Ideally, a child with a plaster or fiberglass cast should use a washcloth for bathing and not take a tub bath or shower. Although commercially available plastic or rubber bag devices can be obtained, they are often unsuccessful in keeping the cast dry, and problems result, often necessitating a cast change.

REFERENCES

1. Hilt NE, Cogburn SB: Cast and splint therapy. In Hilt NE, Cogburn SB, editors: *Manual of orthopaedics,* St. Louis, 1980, Mosby.
2. Rang M: *Children's Fractures,* ed 2, Philadelphia, 1983, JB Lippincott.
2a. Rockwood CA Jr, Williams KE, King RE: *Fractures in children,* vol 3, Philadelphia, 1991, JB Lippincott.
3. Spearman PW, Barson WG: Toxic shock syndrome occurring in children with abrasive injuries beneath casts, *Pediatr Orthop* 12:169-172, 1992.
4. Wenger DR: Casts in children. In Wenger DR, Rang M: *The art and practice of children's orthopaedics,* New York, 1993, Raven Press.
5. Wu KK: *Techniques in surgical casting and splinting,* Philadelphia, 1987, Lea & Febiger.

118 Dislocations, Subluxations, and Diastasis

Stephen Ludwig

Reduction is the repositioning of bones that have moved out of their normal anatomic alignment. A bone may be completely absent from its regular articulation in a joint, as in a dislocation. There may be partial loss of relationship with a joint, as in a subluxation. Diastasis refers to the disruption of a ligamentous connection between adjacent bones, such as in the relationship between the radius and the ulna (Fig. 118-1).

This chapter covers a number of common malposition situations, and it also provides specifics about the following conditions common to pediatric patients:

- Finger dislocation
- Patella dislocation
- Knee dislocation
- Shoulder dislocation
- Acromioclavicular separation
- Elbow dislocation
- Radial head subluxation

Indications

Significant displacement of a bone from its anatomic location causes a risk of soft-tissue bleeding, injury to surrounding blood vessels and nerves, and injury to adjacent bony structures. Thus any dislocated bone should be returned to its anatomic position.

Dislocations should be returned to their anatomic positions as promptly as possible, because progressive swelling and hemorrhage from tissue injury may make it more difficult to affect a relocation. After a joint is returned to its functional position, the healing and rehabilitation process begins. In some cases (e.g., in the dislocated radial head), a return to the normal anatomic position brings immediate return of function.

Contraindication

The only contraindication to relocation of a joint is uncertainty that a dislocation has occurred or concern about making a major fracture worse. A relocation should not be attempted if the technique is not known or if the patient cannot tolerate the procedure. Contaminated, open fractures must be reduced cautiously. In many cases, if open fractures do not have associated distal ischemia, an orthopedist should be consulted first. Any emergency orthopedic procedure should be managed in the context of an overall trauma resuscitation plan, prioritizing airway, breathing, and circulation.

Complications

Forces that lead to dislocation may also cause bone fracture. Fracture may accompany all true dislocations. The process of relocation may also lead to fractures. Thus all relocations should be checked radiographically. The only exceptions to this are dislocated radial heads or patellas where immediate

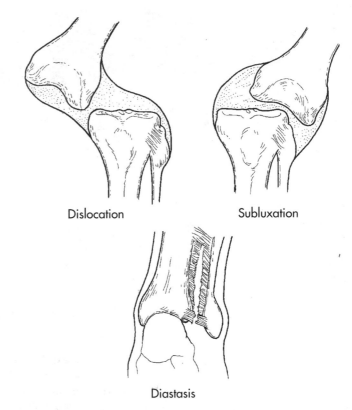

Dislocation   **Subluxation**

Diastasis

FIG. 118-1   Displacement of bones from normal anatomic position.

return of function signals correct position and lack of fracture.

Other complications include sensorineural injury produced by dislocation. It is important to carefully check and document sensorineural status.

Equipment

Basic equipment needs pertain to specific injuries. In general, splinting and bandaging supplies are necessary to rest the injured body parts after achieving relocation. In some cases, conscious sedation and analgesia may be used (Chapters 12 to 14) to diminish anxiety and pain.

Techniques

Finger Dislocation. Finger dislocations are interphalangeal and metacarpal phalangeal dislocations. Children most often dislocate the proximal joints. Sometimes it is not possible to reduce a dorsal dislocation because of the interposition of the volar plate (often in thumb dislocation). Before attempting relocation, obtain anteroposterior and lateral radiographs to check the position of the volar plate, and document any fractures (Fig. 118-2, A).

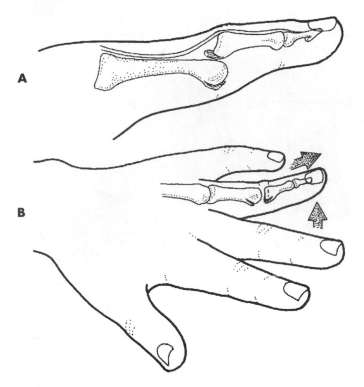

FIG. 118-2   A, Finger dislocation with interposition of volar plate. **B,** Relocation of finger.

A digital block may provide good analgesia (Chapter 16). Hold the hand proximal to the dislocation and at the tip of the finger. Apply steady, firm traction along the long axis of bone by pulling the distal segment (Fig. 118-2, *B*). If this does not work, pull in the same direction, but increase the angle of deformity (hyperextension) by a few degrees at the same time. The phalanx should move back into place. Immobilize the digit for 3 to 4 weeks. Obtain postreduction radiographs to document the location of all fracture fragments. If relocation is unsuccessful because of interposition of the volar plate or another factor, consult an orthopedic surgeon for open reduction.

Patella Dislocation. The patella usually jumps laterally outside the tibiofemoral tract along which it normally glides (Fig. 118-3, *A*). Patellar dislocations are usually sports injuries or the result of a fall.[6]

Check radiographs for possible fracture fragment. Hold the hip in 30-degree flexion. Extend the knee while applying steady, firm, medial pressure to the lateral aspect of the patella (Fig. 118-3, *B*).[1,3] The patella should immediately move into position, and function should return. When the patella has been returned to anatomic locale, check other knee ligaments and tendons. Obtain radiographs, including anteroposterior, lateral, and sunrise views. A knee immobilizer may be necessary for 2 to 4 weeks.

Dislocation of Knee. Knee dislocations have a high incidence of popliteal artery compromise, so take prompt action. Both anterior and posterior dislocations can occur. Anterior dislocations are more common. Perform a complete neuromuscular assessment, and document this before and after the relocation.

Apply traction longitudinally along the line of the limb with the knee extended while an assistant applies counter-

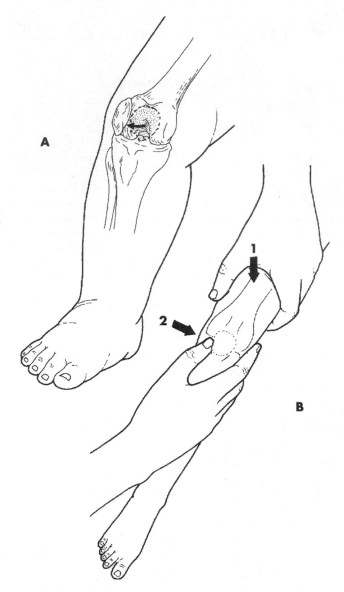

FIG. 118-3   A and **B,** Relocation of patella.

traction (Fig. 118-4, *A*). With posterior dislocation, apply similar traction. After disengaging the articular surface, place a hand under the tibia and push it anteriorly into place (Fig. 118-4, *B*). If there is question of popliteal artery injury, perform a postreduction arteriogram.

Shoulder Dislocations. Shoulder dislocations occur to the glenohumeral joint. The head of the humerus usually dislocates anteriorly; however, reports exist of posterior, inferior, and superior dislocations (Fig. 118-5). The possibility of injury to the axillary nerve or artery requires checking and rechecking the neurovascular integrity.[10] Sensation to pinprick over the lateral deltoid tests the axillary nerve. Descriptions of three shoulder relocation techniques follow. Before using these techniques, give the patient a combination of a narcotic and a sedative. Muscle relaxation is important, so use sedative combinations before the procedures.

The easiest method is the traction-countertraction method. With this technique, place a folded sheet around the child's chest (Fig. 118-6, *A*). One person pulls in countertraction while another pulls the humerus laterally and down (Fig.

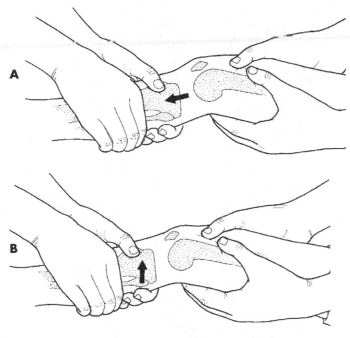

FIG. 118-4   **A** and **B,** Relocation of knee.

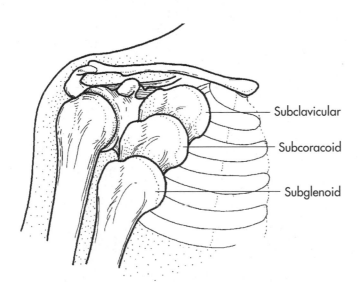

Subclavicular

Subcoracoid

Subglenoid

FIG. 118-5   Dislocation of shoulder, three positions.

118-6, *B*). After relocating the shoulder, apply a sling and swathe to hold the position. Sometimes another force producing lateral traction is necessary after freeing the humeral head from contact with the inferior glenoid vein (Fig. 118-6, *C*).

To use the Stinson technique, place the patient prone on an examining table with the affected arm hanging toward the floor. Place a towel or pillow under the arm. A wrist strap holds weight around the distal forearm (Fig. 118-7). Use 10 to 15 lb over 20 to 30 minutes. The combination of the weight and muscle relaxation will ease the humerus back into position.

With the third technique, the Hennepin method, keep the patient sitting in an upright position of 45 degrees. Support the patient's elbow with the right hand, and with the left hand slowly and gently externally rotate the arm (Fig. 118-8).

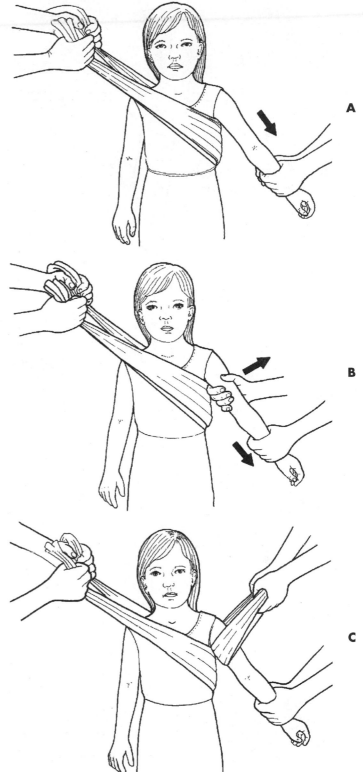

FIG. 118-6   **A** to **C,** Relocation of shoulder, traction-countertraction technique.

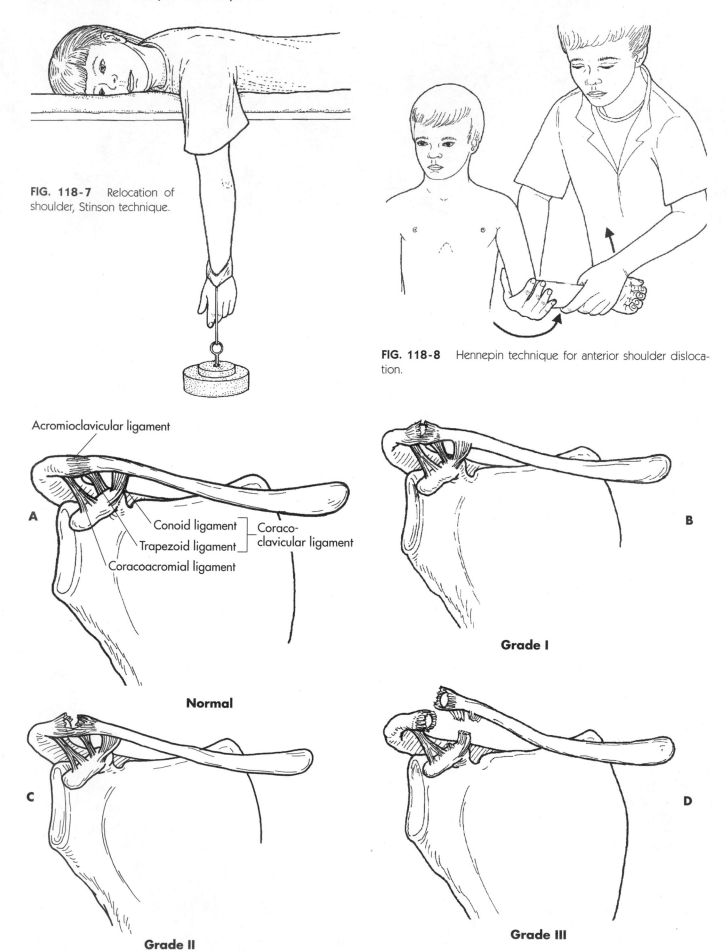

FIG. 118-7 Relocation of shoulder, Stinson technique.

FIG. 118-8 Hennepin technique for anterior shoulder dislocation.

Acromioclavicular ligament

Conoid ligament $\Big]$
Trapezoid ligament $\Big]$ Coraco-clavicular ligament

Coracoacromial ligament

A

Normal

B

Grade I

C

Grade II

D

Grade III

FIG. 118-9 **A** to **D,** Classification of acromioclavicular tears.

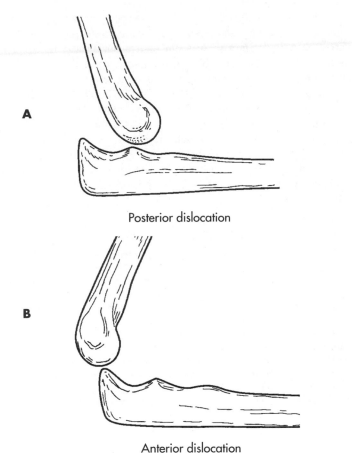

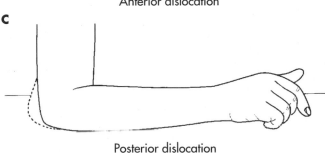

FIG. 118-10 A to C, Anterior and posterior elbow dislocation.

Rotate the arm to a 90-degree external rotation. When the patient feels pain, stop and allow the muscles to relax. If the shoulder has not returned to its proper position, elevate the arm, and reduction should occur.[4,5]

Acromioclavicular Separation. Acromioclavicular separations in shoulder separation are not common in childhood. They occur with falls directly onto the tip of the shoulder.[2] The three grades of injury classification are (Fig. 118-9):

Grade I: capsular tear but no displacement

Grade II: tear of the acromioclavicular capsule and mild upward clavicle displacement

Grade III: disruption of both the acromioclavicular joint and the coracoclavicular ligaments, resulting in marked superior displacement of the distal end of the clavicle.

The acute management involves putting the arm to rest by placing it in a sling. Maintain the arm in a sling until pain ceases in grade I or grade II injuries. Grade III injuries may require surface repair. No immediate relocation techniques are necessary.[9]

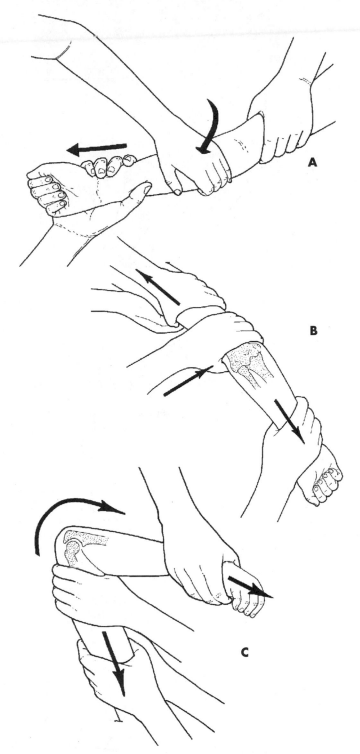

FIG. 118-11 A to C, Relocation of elbow dislocation.

Elbow Dislocation. Elbow dislocations occur most often in the posterior position with displacement of the ulnar olecranon posteriorly. Prolonged delays in treatment may damage articular cartilage and compromise circulation to the arm (Figure 118-10). After administration of analgesics and sedatives, apply gentle traction with the elbow in a position of comfort with the wrist supinated. Have an assistant apply countertraction (Fig. 118-11). Pull the olecranon forward by applying pressure on the forearm, disengaging it from under the humerus. After relocation, apply a splint with the elbow

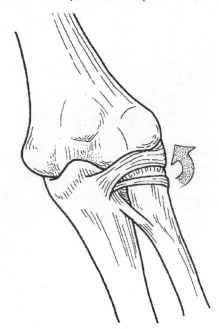

FIG. 118-12 Anatomy of radial head subluxation.

flexed at 90 degrees. Reassess neurovascular status and a postprocedure radiograph.[8]

Radial Head Subluxation. Radial head subluxation, or "nursemaid's elbow," is a common occurrence in young children. Pulling the arm along its long axis with the wrist pronated traps the radial head distal to the annular ligament and produces subluxation (Fig. 118-12).[7]

Most children with this injury are around 2 years of age. The typical history is of someone pulling the arm or of the child falling with the distal arm held in a fixed position. At presentation, the arm usually hangs limply by the child's side or the other hand supports it.

Once the examiner has a good history consistent with the mechanism of injury noted above, no radiographs are necessary. Carefully attempt to rule out pain around the wrist or shoulder. If radial head subluxation is suspected, the examiner should place one hand supporting the elbow with the thumb over the radial head. The examiner's other hand is placed on the child's wrist. Externally rotate the forearm while flexing at the elbow (Fig. 118-13). In most cases, the examiner will appreciate a crack or popping sensation over the radial head. Within 10 to 15 minutes, the child should regain full use of the arm. No follow-up radiographs are indicated with this injury. Neither splinting nor a sling is necessary.

REFERENCES

1. Dunmire S, Paris PM: *Atlas of emergency procedures,* Philadelphia, 1994, WB Saunders.
2. Eldman DK, Siff SJ, Tullos HS: Acromioclavicular lesions in children, *Am J Sports Med* 9:150-154, 1981.
3. Fleisher G, Ludwig S: *Textbook of pediatric emergency medicine,* ed 3, Baltimore, 1993, Williams & Wilkins.
4. Jastremski MS, Dumas M, Pennalver L: *Emergency procedures,* Philadelphia, 1992, W.B. Saunders.
5. MacEwen GD, Kasser JR, Heinrich SD: *Pediatric fractures: a practical approach to assessment and treatment,* Baltimore, 1993, Williams & Wilkins.
6. Nsouli AZ, Nahabedran A: Intra-articular dislocation of the patella, *J Trauma* 28:256-258, 1988.
7. Shunk JE: Radial head subluxation: epidemiology and treatment of 87 episodes, *Ann Emerg Med* 19:1019-1023, 1990.
8. Simon RE, Brenner BE: *Emergency procedures and techniques,* ed 2, Baltimore, 1987, Williams & Wilkins.
9. Tolo V, Wood B: *Pediatric orthopedics in primary care,* Baltimore, 1993, Williams & Wilkins.
10. Wagner KT, Lyne ED: Adolescent traumatic dislocation of the shoulder, *J Pediatr Orthop* 3:61-62, 1983.

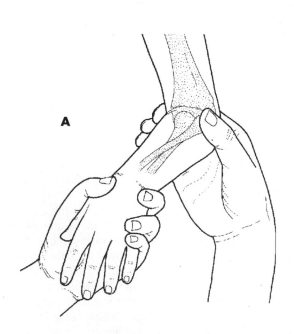
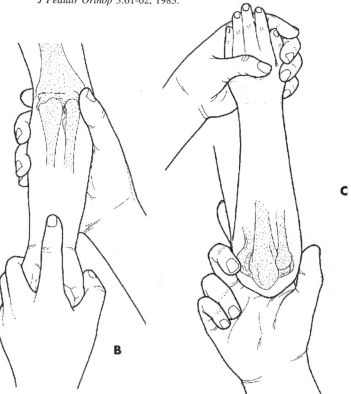

FIG. 118-13 **A** to **C,** Reduction of radial head subluxation.

119 Crutch Walking

Stephen Ludwig

Many conditions require that a child avoid bearing weight on one of the lower extremities. In such cases, the child needs crutches. Evaluate children for their ability to use crutches, carefully fit them for properly sized crutches, and teach both children and caretakers how to use the crutches correctly. As with any other medical equipment or device, incorrect use may do more harm than good.

Indications

Crutches are indicated for any condition that requires limited weight bearing. Such conditions may be traumatic, infectious, or rheumatologic in origin. The prevention of pain and stress on the body part is the main reason that crutches are used. Train patients in either partial weight-bearing or non–weight-bearing techniques according to the condition being treated.

Contraindications

If crutches of the correct size are unavailable, it is better not to use improperly fitted equipment. Evaluate whether the patient is too young, lacks the mental competence to follow instructions, or lacks the needed coordination to use crutches. In general, do not give crutches to a patient younger than 4 years of age. Check the patient's overall neuromuscular strength and coordination before giving crutches. Do not give them to a child who is too weak or too ill to use them correctly. Have patients demonstrate competence on straight, smooth surfaces before releasing them from the Emergency Department.[1]

Complications

The use of incorrectly sized crutches may result in secondary problems. Crutches that are too long will hurt a patient's axilla, causing abrasions, contusions, or open skin defects. Crutches that are too short will be unstable. Incorrect use of crutches may result in falls and more serious trauma. Crutches that do not have rubber tips may slip on smooth (e.g., tile) surfaces.

Equipment

Adjustable wooden or aluminum axillary crutches with adjustable handles should be used. Make sure that there are rubber tips for the bottom of the crutches to provide nonskid contact with floors. The crutches also need to have rubber pads for the top ends and rubber pads for the handle grips.

Techniques

Fitting the Crutches. With the patient standing, place the crutch 6 inches anterior and 6 inches lateral to the patient (Fig 119-1). Make sure that the top of the crutch is at least 2 to 3 inches below the axilla. Adjust the handle so that the elbow is flexed 10 to 15 degrees when the hand is holding the

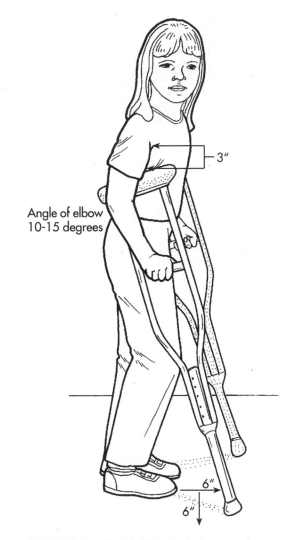

Angle of elbow 10-15 degrees

3"

6"

6"

FIG. 119-1   Crutch-fitting techniques and use.

handle. Adjust both crutches to the same height.[2] Table 119-1 shows the appropriate crutch sizes for children.

Teaching the Patient

PARTIAL WEIGHT BEARING. When teaching partial weight-bearing techniques, teach the patient how to walk on a flat surface.[1] Have the child place both crutches forward and to the side of the body. Instruct him or her on the amount of weight to put on the injured foot. Ask the child to push down on the handpiece of the crutches. Have the child move the crutches ahead and move the injured foot into line with the crutches. Tell him or her to take a normal step by moving the uninjured foot forward between the crutches and past the point at which the rubber tips touch the floor.

To teach the child to walk upstairs, instruct him or her to stand as close to the step as possible. Have him or her place

Table 119-1 Appropriate Crutch Size by Patient Height

Patient size	Crutch size (inches)
6'10"	65
6'8"	64
6'6"	62
6'4"	60
6'2"	58
6'0"	56
5'10"	54
5'8"	52
5'6"	50
5'4"	48
5'2"	46
5'0"	44
4'10"	42
4'8"	40
4'6"	38
4'4"	36
4'2"	34
4'0"	32
3'10"	30
3'8"	28
3'6"	26
3'4"	25

Courtesy Baxter Health Care Corporation, McGraw Park, Ill.

the crutches under one arm and place the free hand on the handrail. If there is no handrail, instruct the child to keep one crutch in each hand and to push down on the handpiece of each crutch. Have the child place the crutch tips not on the first step but as close as possible to the first step. Have the child push down on the handpiece and railing and hop up onto the first step with the uninjured foot. The crutches and injured foot are then brought up to the step on which the uninjured foot is now standing.

To teach the child to walk downstairs, instruct him or her to stand as close to the step as possible. Have him or her place both crutches onto the center of the stair below and extend the injured foot forward. Have the child bend the hip and knee and slowly lower his or her body down the step. The child should then move the uninjured foot to the lower step.

NON–WEIGHT BEARING When teaching non–weight-bearing techniques, have the child stand on the uninjured leg while flexing the injured leg. Have the child put the crutches 8 to 12 inches forward. Tell her to place her weight onto the hands and to pick up and swing forward to the uninvolved leg in front of the crutches. The crutch tips and the uninvolved leg should form a triangle. Tell the child to hold the upper end of the crutches against the chest wall and not to rest them in the axilla.

Remarks

Make sure that the patient is wearing the proper footwear. A loose-fitting pair of slippers may result in another injury. If there is any doubt about a child's competence, it is better to use a wheelchair or to carry the child.

REFERENCES

1. Children's Hospital of Philadelphia: *ED nursing procedure manual,* Philadelphia, 1995, Children's Hospital of Philadelphia.
2. Lohr JA: *Pediatric outpatient procedures,* Philadelphia, 1991, JB Lippincott.

120 Compartment Syndrome

Stephen Ludwig

Compartment syndrome is a condition in which swelling and pressure occur within a closed osteofascial compartment and cause elevation of tissue pressure and resultant myoneural necrosis. Compartment syndromes occur in both adults and children and require a high index of suspicion to diagnose. Compartment syndromes occur after mechanical trauma, burns, surgery, and with toxin-induced tissue damage. Tight casts, dressings, splints, or intraosseous lines may also contribute to the problem.[1,3]

The cardinal feature of a compartment syndrome is pain that is out of proportion to the injury. Certain fractures are also more likely to produce the syndrome, including supracondylar fractures, radius and ulnar fractures, and fractures of the tibia. Figs. 120-1 and 120-2 show the compartments of upper and lower extremities, but compartment syndrome may affect any closed osteofascial compartment.

Indications

Maintain a high index of suspicion for compartment syndrome. Pain usually subsides after splinting fractures and administering a mild analgesic. Therefore suspect compartment syndrome in children who complain of increasingly severe and unrelenting pain. This pain may occur within hours to days after the injury. As the pain continues, numbness and tingling ensue. Finally, even passive movement of the muscles in the compartment exacerbates the pain, and muscle strength diminishes. There may be sensory and motor nerve dysfunction. Because arterial pulses may still be palpable distal to the compartment syndrome, their presence is not a reliable sign that compartment syndrome is not present.

If there is suspicion of increased compartment pressure, obtain measurements of the pressure. Obtain prompt orthopedic consultation to determine the need for fasciotomy. Act promptly because permanent damage may occur within 6 to 12 hours.

Contraindications

There are no known contraindications to measuring tissue pressure. Use care in interpreting the reading. Rely on clinical signs and symptoms of compartment syndrome more than on tissue pressure readings. If the child has clinical signs and symptoms of compartment syndrome, obtain an orthopedic consultation regardless of the tissue pressure reading.

Complications

There are no known complications to obtaining a tissue pressure measurement if sterile technique is used and if the patient does not have a bleeding diathesis. If there is a question of superficial cellulitis, it is best not to advance the needle through the infected skin. Use strict aseptic technique

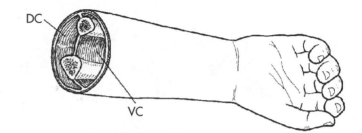

FIG. 120-1 Two compartments of the forearm. *DC*, Dorsal compartment; *VC*, volar compartment.

(Redrawn from Matsen FA: *Compartmental syndromes*, New York, 1980, Grune & Stratton.)

throughout the procedure to avoid infection. Pain is a complication when needles are inserted into muscle.

Equipment

Two common techniques are used in tissue pressure measurement: (1) a needle manometer, and (2) a Solid State pressure monitor.[1] Other techniques of tissue pressure measurement are less favorable because of unreliability. For the needle manometer method obtain 18-gauge needles, a 20-ml syringe, and a 3-way stopcock. A mercury manometer, intravenous extension tubing, and normal saline are also useful. The Solid State pressure monitor unit is self-contained except for the saline and an 18-gauge needle.

Techniques

Pressure Readings. Whiteside et al. first described the standard needle manometer technique of tissue pressure measurement.[5] Connect an 18-gauge needle to a 20-ml syringe via saline/air-filled tubing and a 3-way stopcock. On the third limb of the stopcock, connect the system to a mercury manometer (Fig. 120-3). Clear the skin site and insert the needle into the compartment. Increase the pressure in the syringe until the air/saline interface moves, and record the pressure on the manometer.

If using the Solid State pressure monitor technique, attach a saline-filled needle to the device. Insert the needle into the appropriate compartment. After a brief period of equilibration time, record a measurement.

Interpretation. The average pressure in most compartments is 8.5 mm Hg with a standard deviation of 2 to 6 mm Hg.[4] Some experimental subjects report pain when pressures exceed 30 mm Hg.[4] False-positives occur with the placement of needles into solid structures, and false-negatives occur because of equipment problems or placement in the incorrect compartment.

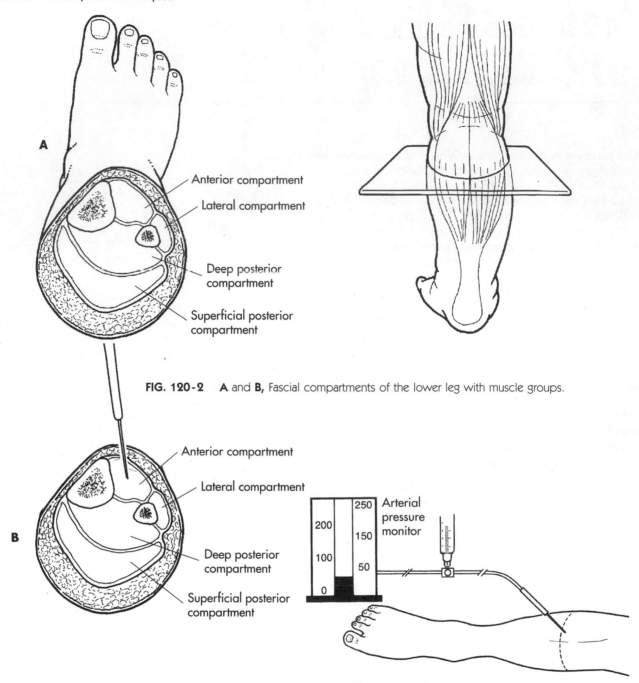

FIG. 120-2 **A** and **B,** Fascial compartments of the lower leg with muscle groups.

A

Anterior compartment

Lateral compartment

Deep posterior compartment

Superficial posterior compartment

B

Anterior compartment

Lateral compartment

Deep posterior compartment

Superficial posterior compartment

250 · Arterial pressure monitor

200

150

100

50

0

FIG. 120-3 Direct measurement of pressures within the muscles of each of the four lower leg compartments.

Treatment

When treating compartment syndrome, take the initial steps necessary to increase limb perfusion. Aid perfusion by loosening pressure dressings, bandages, and casts and by supporting arterial blood pressure if the patient is hypotensive. If edema is present, diuretics may help to relieve the resultant tissue pressure.[2] Fasciotomy is indicated when noninvasive techniques fail.

Remarks

Compartment syndromes can also occur in the hands and feet, but these sites are less common.[3] Infiltrated intravenous or intraosseous lines or pneumatic antishock trousers may also produce compartment syndrome iatrogenically (see Chapter 37).[1,3]

REFERENCES

1. Christianson JT, Wulff K: Compartment pressure following leg injury: the effect of diuretic treatment, *Injury* 16:591, 1985.
2. Gelberman RH, Garfin SR, Wergenroeder PT, et al: Compartment syndromes of the forearm: diagnosis and treatment, *Clin Orthop* 161:252, 1981.
3. Rimar S, Westry JA, Rodriquez RL: Compartment syndrome in an infant following emergency intraosseous infusion, *Clin Pediatr* 27:259, 1988.
4. Van Ryn D: Compartment syndromes. In Roberts JR, Hedges JR, et al: *Clinical procedures in emergency medicine,* Philadelphia, 1991, WB Saunders.
5. Whiteside TE, Hancy TC, Morimoto K, et al: Tissue pressure measurements: a determinant for the need of fasciotomy, *Clin Orthop* 113:43, 1975.

121 Dressings, Slings, and Wrappings

Stephen Ludwig

The purposes of dressings, slings, and compression wrappings are to: (a) control swelling and bleeding, (b) limit motion, (c) provide support and anatomic positioning, (d) protect against contamination and infection, and (e) decrease pain.[3] A dressing must be comfortable and acceptable to the patient so it will be worn. It is important that the dressing does not create its own trauma (e.g., when an elastic bandage is too tight). The healing power of most pediatric patients is great. Appropriate dressings allow nature to take its course.

Chapter 116 discusses splinting, which may be useful in conjunction with dressings.

Indications

Any injured body part may require a special dressing to limit the extent of injury and protect against reinjury. Open wounds should be dressed with sterile technique. Dressings come in different materials with these common indications (Table 121-1). Taping techniques may be employed for athletic competition to prevent injury by stabilizing a ligament or muscle group. Taping limits movement.

Contraindications

There are no contraindications to dressings, slings, or wrappings, with the exception of idiosyncratic reactions to certain materials.

Dressings in contact with open wounds must be sterile. If they are not sterile, their use is also contraindicated. With these two rare cautions in mind, most dressings, slings, and wrappings are safe and easy to use.

Complications

The complications that result from dressings, slings, and wrappings are caused by improper application. For example, an elastic roller bandage that is too tight may cause ischemia or edema distal to its application. Other applications may leave body parts fixed in nonphysiologic positions, making return of function more difficult. Other complications come with idiocyncratic reactions to certain materials and dressings that are are too occlusive for the clinical situation and do not allow sufficient air in or the elimination of wound moisture.

Techniques

Universal Hand Dressing. The universal hand dressing is used for lacerations, sprains, or tendon injuries of the hand. To apply it, position the wrist at 15 degrees of extension with fingers flexed 50 degrees at the metacarpal phalangeal joint. There should be 20 to 30 degrees of flexion at the interphalangeal joint, with the thumb in 10- to 15-degree flexion (Fig. 121-1).[5] Place fluffs of gauze between the fingers and thumb. Extend these down beyond the wrist. Use a gauze roll to encircle the hand, and place it between finger spaces. Then

Table 121-1 Dressings

Layer	Function
Contact layer dressing	
Dry	
Cotton gauze	Absorption of blood, serum, wound exudates
	Adheres to wound
	Allows drying
Semiocclusive	
Adaptic	Less wound adherence
Telfa	Allows drainage
Xeroform	Some débridement when removed
Occlusive	
Petrolatum	Nonstick
Tegaderm	Prevents drying
Duoderm	No air penetration
Absorbent layer	
Gauze pads	Absorption of secretion
	Protection from trauma
Outer layer	
Cotton (Webril)	Soft, conforms to surface
	Protective but nonsupportive
Cling roller bandage	Holds contact and absorbent dressing
	Loose dressing
	Allows air penetration
	Flexible
Rubberized roller (Ace)	Provides compression
	Less flexible force

wrap the hand with an elastic bandage with finger holes cut out for digits. Elevate the hand.

Dynamic Finger Dressing. The dynamic finger dressing is used for finger injuries to both protect and stabilize. It provides proper support. Position the injured finger adjacent to a noninjured mate. Place a piece of felt (e.g., an eye patch) between the digits and then tape the digits, first circumferentially, then in a figure-of-eight pattern around the wrist (Fig. 121-2).[2]

Sling. A sling places any part of the upper extremity at rest and allows elevation of the hand. To use a triangle bandage, place one point of the bandage over the shoulder of the noninjured arm. Keep the central point of the triangle at the elbow. Bring the third point over the ipsilateral shoulder. Flex the patient's elbow at 90 degrees or greater. The edge of the sling must support the hand at the level of the metacarpal phalangeal joint (Fig. 121-3).[6] Commercially applicable slings are also available and function in the same way (Fig. 121-4).

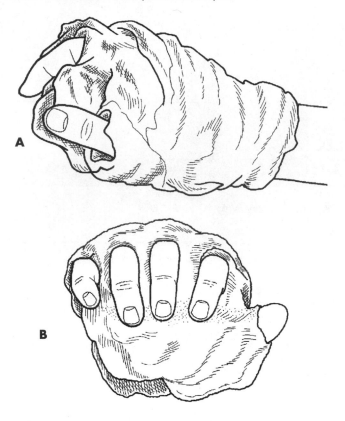

FIG. 121-1 **A** and **B,** Universal hand dressing (cock-up splint). Note 15-degree dorsiflexion at wrist.

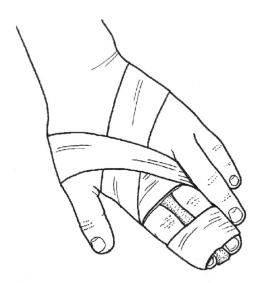

FIG. 121-2 Dynamic finger splint.

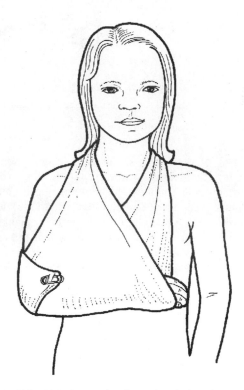

FIG. 121-3 Basic sling, triangle bandage.

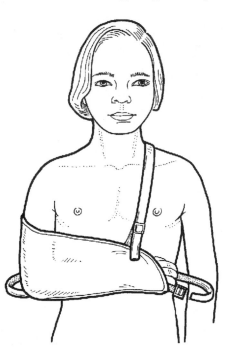

FIG. 121-4 Sling, commercial.

Sling and Swathe. The addition of the swathe supports the arm against the body and limits shoulder rotation. This dressing is used after shoulder dislocation or after a fracture of the upper humerus (Fig. 121-5).[2,6]

Ankle Compression Wrap (Taping). Ankle taping is used to achieve ankle support. Ligaments should always be supported in the shortened position; for example, the patient's ankle should be dorsiflexed and elevated.

Dry the foot and ankle, and apply tincture of benzoin to skin. Apply the tape in strips, not in one continuous ribbon.

Apply five or six strips first. Begin laterally, cross anteriorly over the distal tibia (Fig. 121-6, *A*), continue across the heel cord, pass distal to the lateral malleolus onto the lateral calcaneus and under the sole of the foot, and end on top of the medial forefoot (Fig. 121-6, *B*). Apply additional strips in figure-of-eight style around the ankle (Fig. 121-6, *C*).[4]

Plantar-Bar Dressing. For injury to the proximal one third to one half of the sole of the foot use a plantar bar. After caring for and dressing the plantar wound or foreign body, have the patient put on his shoe. Using a small block of wood

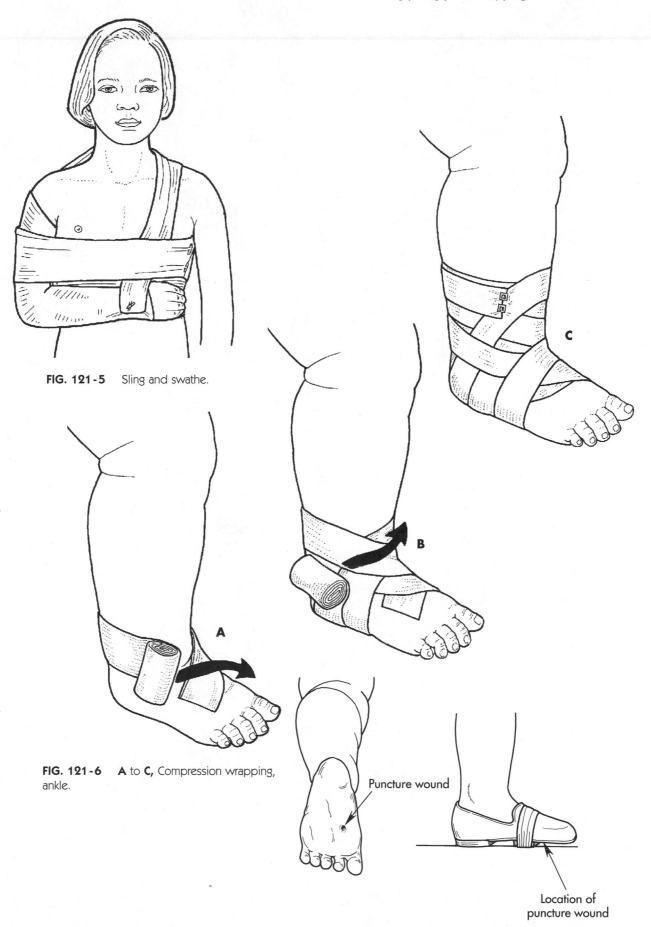

FIG. 121-5   Sling and swathe.

FIG. 121-6   **A** to **C,** Compression wrapping, ankle.

Puncture wound

Location of puncture wound

FIG. 121-7   Plantar-bar dressing.

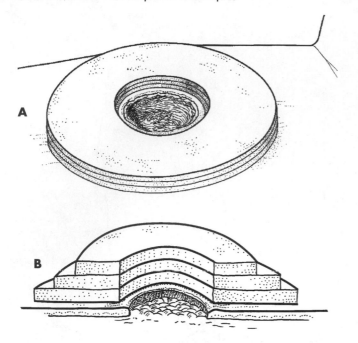

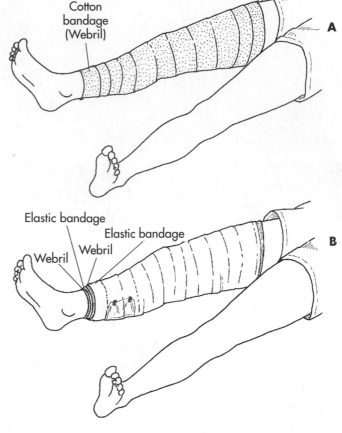

FIG. 121-8   **A** and **B,** Relief padding (doughnut or pyramid dressing).

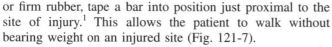

FIG. 121-9   **A** and **B,** Jones compression dressing, knee.

or firm rubber, tape a bar into position just proximal to the site of injury.[1] This allows the patient to walk without bearing weight on an injured site (Fig. 121-7).

Pyramid or Doughnut Dressing.   This dressing is also used for small lacerations, puncture sites, or ulcerative lesions. It allows pressure to be distributed around a lesion while protecting it and keeping it clear (Fig. 121-8).[1]

Jones Compression Dressing.   The Jones compression dressing is used for soft-tissue injuries of the knee. The dressing limits swelling from edema or hematoma formation while permitting flexion and extension at the joint.

Apply cotton along the leg from ground to ankle. Next apply an elastic bandage in a distal-to-proximal direction. Apply a second layer of cotton and a second elastic wrap (Fig. 121-9).[5]

REFERENCES

1. Chisholm CD, Schlesser JF: Plantar puncture wounds: controversies and treatment recommendation, *Ann Emerg Med* 18:1352, 1989.
2. Fleisher G, Ludwig S: *Textbook of pediatric emergency medicine,* ed 3, Baltimore, 1993, Williams & Wilkins.
3. Roberts JR, Hedges JR: *Clinical procedures in emergency medicine,* ed 2, Philadelphia, 1991, WB Saunders.
4. Simon RE, Brenner BE: *Emergency procedures and techniques,* ed 2, Baltimore, 1987, Williams & Wilkins.
5. Simon RR, Koenigshnecht SJ: *Emergency orthopedics: the extremities,* ed 2, Norwalk, Conn, 1987, Appleton and Lange.
6. Tola V, Wood B: *Pediatric orthopedics in primary care,* Baltimore, 1993, Williams & Wilkins.

PART XXIII

HAND/FOOT TECHNIQUES

122 Amputations

Douglas Yoshida

Although the overall incidence of amputations in the pediatric population is unknown, the U.S. Consumer Product Safety Commission estimates that exercise bicycles alone have amputated fingers of over 1200 children in the past few years.[3] With few exceptions consider all amputated parts in children for replantation. Advances in microsurgical technique over the last 25 years have enabled surgeons to replant digits of children with up to a 70% to 96% success rate.[3,8] Historically success rates of major limb replantation with children have not been as good as with adults; however, more recent series document limb survival rates that are comparable.[9,33]

Indications

Replantation. Box 122-1 summarizes the indications and contraindications for replantation. *Replantation* is reattachment of a completely amputated part. Although it is possible for an experienced microsurgeon to replant almost any part, a viable replant may not have useful function. However, since children demonstrate better nerve regeneration and generally have better functional outcomes than adults, indications for replantation are more extensive than they are for adults.

Mechanism of injury is an important factor in replant success. Sharp, guillotine-type injuries have the best chance for successful replantation, whereas crush injuries carry a

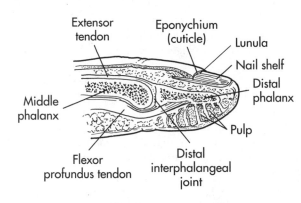

FIG. 122-1 Amputation proximal to lunula of nail bed.

poorer prognosis.[29] The level of the injury is also important. For example replants of amputations through the proximal phalanx function much more poorly than replants of amputations through the midmetacarpal level, because the structure of the tendons is much more complex at the proximal phalanx level ("no man's land").[1]

Ischemia time is another important factor in the success of the replant. The more proximal the replant, the less tolerant it is of ischemia. Warm (ambient temperature) ischemia is in general poorly tolerated after 6 hours. Cold ischemia (4° C) is tolerable for up to 24 hours with distal amputations.[1,10,29,33] Digital replants have been successful up to 33 hours after amputation.[30] The final factors in replantation success are the technical skill and experience of the surgeon.

The replantation team must make the decision to replant on a case-by-case basis with consideration of not only the technical and aesthetic factors, but also the psychosocial profiles of the patient and parents.

Fingertip Amputations. Primary treatment of distal fingertip amputations by the nonhand surgeon is appropriate if the amputation is distal to the lunula of the nail bed (Fig. 122-1).

Contraindications

Replantation. The absolute contraindications to replantation are associated life-threatening injuries, severe medical problems that would preclude the long operative time necessary for replantation, and severe multilevel injury to the amputated part.[1,10,29,33]

Fingertip Amputations. There are no contraindications to the treatment of fingertip amputations. Consider all amputations proximal to the lunula of any digit, and especially of the thumb, for possible replantation.*

BOX 122-1   **INDICATIONS AND CONTRAINDICATIONS TO REPLANTATION** [1, 10, 29, 33]

Indications

All pediatric amputations
Multiple digits
Thumb amputations
Proximal amputations (hand, wrist, and forearm)

Absolute contraindications

Associated life threats
Severe crush injuries or multilevel amputation
Inability to withstand prolonged surgery

Relative contraindications (generally ignored in children)

Single digit, unless thumb
Heavily contaminated amputations
Prolonged warm ischemia
Lower extremity
Avulsion injuries

---

*References 7, 8, 13, 14, 22, 33, and 35.

Complications

Replantation. Complications of the initial treatment of the patient with an amputation are rare. Further damage to the amputated part or stump can occur if attempts at hemostasis, débridement, or cleansing are overaggressive. Improper storage of the amputated part can damage the stump because of freezing or maceration, which decreases replantation success.[10,23,29]

Complications after the replantation itself are common. There are risks associated with surgery and prolonged anesthesia. Additionally patients often require repeat surgeries for fasciotomies, skin grafts, and evaluation of muscle viability. A course of two or three repeat operations for arterial or venous thrombosis is common,[10,34] as well as prolonged hospital stays for wound care and rehabilitation. Up to 41% of cases of digital replantation require blood products that subject the child to transfusion risks.[3] Depending on the replanted part and the surgeon's expertise, approximately 20% to 40% of replants fail and require reamputation.[33] Late complications include cold intolerance, limited range of motion and sensation, anesthesia, parasthesias, chronic pain, nonunion, and malunion.[10]

Fingertip Amputations. There are no well-controlled studies of complications of fingertip amputations in children. However it appears that early complications, such as infection, are rare and occur at a rate of 0% to 7% with conservative management of the fingertip.[15,17,19] Higher infection rates may occur if using skin grafts or flaps. Necrosis or partial necrosis of an amputated part, graft, or flap often occurs. Treat such complications expectantly until demarcation of viable tissue has occurred.[13,21]Osteomyelitis of the distal phalanx is a rare event.[12]

Long-term complications of fingertip amputations occur commonly in adults but appear to be less troublesome in children. Abnormal sensation of the fingertip occurs in 30% to 50% of adults, most often with cold intolerance.[20] Diminished two-point discrimination, hypersensitivity, and tenderness also can result. These complications can occur with any technique the surgeon uses to repair the fingertip and "are the consequence of the injury and not of the treatment."[20] One comparative study in children found that conservative treatment resulted in better sensation and function than either split-thickness skin grafts or local flaps. Nail and fingertip deformities can occur, but deformities appear to be less frequent with conservative treatment.[11]

Equipment

Replantation. Equipment for the storage and preservation of the amputated part before possible replantation includes: a sterile plastic bag, normal saline solution, sterile dressing material, and ice. To care for the stump splinting material and sterile dressing material suffice in most cases. Occasionally a tourniquet or blood pressure cuff is necessary to control hemorrhage.[5]

Fingertip Amputations. Perform basic wound care and secure laceration equipment (Chapter 131), primarily 5-0 or 6-0 (nylon and Vicryl) suture material, a Penrose drain to function as a tourniquet, a nonadherent dressing (e.g., Xeroform), and a small bone ronguer to manage fingertip amputations.

Techniques

Replantation. Evaluate and stabilize patients sustaining major amputations according to basic resuscitation principles. Restrain a child who is unable to cooperate (Chapter 11). Control hemorrhage with direct pressure. If direct pressure fails to control bleeding, temporarily use a tourniquet to help identify the bleeding vessels. Then apply point pressure to the isolated vessel to achieve hemostasis. Prolonged use of a tourniquet can result in ischemic damage to the stump. Attempt to minimize ischemia time with tourniquets to less than 20 to 30 minutes, although a specific maximum inflation time is not known. Avoid blind ligation or clamping as it can cause further damage to nerves or vessels.[5,10,29] Remove all jewelry. As soon as feasible contact the replantation surgeon. Consider sedation and analgesia (see Chapters 12 and 13) after ascertaining hemodynamic stability and evaluating other potentially serious injuries.

Obtain plain radiographs of both the stump and amputated part. Gently cleanse both the stump and amputated part of foreign material with normal saline or lactated Ringer's solution. Reserve vigorous irrigation or débridement of devitalized tissue for the operating room. Give antitetanus prophylaxis, if indicated (see Table 130-1), and administer a first-generation cephalosporin intravenously.[10,29] Treat grossly contaminated or human bite amputations with broad-spectrum antibiotics (e.g., cefoxitin or ampicillin/sulbactam).

After controlling bleeding cover the stump with a saline-solution moistened dressing and splint and elevate it. Wrap the amputated part in a saline solution moistened dressing and then place in a sterile plastic bag or collection cup. Place the bag or cup in an ice-filled container, which should cool the part to a temperature of about 4° C (Fig. 122-2). Do not allow the amputated part to have direct contact with the ice. Do not use dry ice or freezing.[5,10,29]

Handle partial amputations as complete amputations. Perform neurologic and vascular examinations. Do not divide any remaining tissue bridges because they may contain adequate collateral circulation.[8] Splint the extremity; take care to prevent malrotation of any neurovascular structures. If there is evidence of arterial insufficiency, cool the distal part as for a complete amputation.[29]

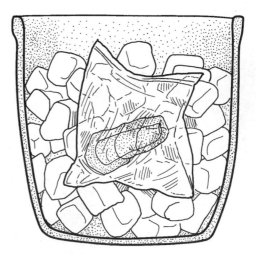

FIG. 122-2 Management of stump and amputated part of finger. Avoid direct contact of amputated part with ice.

Fingertip Amputations: General Treatment. There are numerous methods to manage fingertip amputations, ranging from conservative methods of allowing the wound to heal by secondary intention, to complex pedicle flaps.* In general children demonstrate remarkable wound healing and regenerative capabilities; therefore manage most fingertip amputations conservatively.[20,32] However since opinions on management vary, discuss the case with a hand surgeon before treating a child who has considerable tissue loss or exposed bone.

First determine the mechanism and time of injury. Factors to consider in the repair are the child's hand dominance, the child's avocations, and the parents' ability to care for the wound. Allowing the wound to heal by secondary intention may require more wound care than primary closure, grafts, or flaps. Next address the size and configuration of the defect, presence or absence of bone exposure, and determination of nail bed injury. Chapter 126 discusses nail bed repair. Obtain radiographs for significant crushing injury and for partial amputations with possible fracture of the distal phalanx.

Initial management consists of adequate sedation, analgesia, and immobilization of the young child. A digital block suffices for the majority of cases (Chapter 15), although no anesthetic may be necessary for clean, relatively superficial amputations.[15] If bleeding continues, use direct pressure or tourniquet. The patient tolerates the tourniquet better after anesthesia and/or analgesia and sedation. Then irrigate the wound with normal saline solution; do not place antiseptics directly into the wound. Splints are not usually necessary. If a splint is desired to protect the finger and dressing, assure that it does not inhibit motion of the distal interphalangeal joint. Consider prescribing an oral antibiotic such as dicloxacillin, cephalexin, or erythromycin for 5 to 7 days, although there are no data that indicate decreased infection rate among children on antibiotics.

Fingertip Amputations: Specific Treatment

AMPUTATIONS WITHOUT BONE EXPOSED. Allow fingertip amputations in children involving only soft tissue to heal by secondary intention.† After irrigation with normal saline solution and débridement of obviously nonviable tissue apply a nonadherent dressing to the wound, and then apply a two-layer absorbent dressing. Refer the patient for follow-up evaluation by the pediatrician, primary physician, or hand surgeon within 48 hours. Thereafter prescribe warm soaks and dressing changes on a periodic basis. Recommendations for the frequency of dressing changes vary from four times a day to once every 2 weeks.[15,16] Once a day is reasonable because it can coincide with the child's bathing.[15,16]

The time to complete healing depends on the amount of tissue avulsed; but healing generally occurs within 10 to 30 days.[11,12,16] Functional and cosmetic results are usually excellent; regeneration of a normal or near-normal appearing nail, skin, and pulp is the norm, especially in younger children.[6,11,12,16,27] One group reports excellent results using a semi-occlusive dressing (Opsite), placed over the fingertip and changed once a week.[24]

Other methods for managing amputations without bone exposure are primary closure and skin grafting. Perform primary closure of amputated fingertips if the defect is small and if it is possible to close it without tension and without

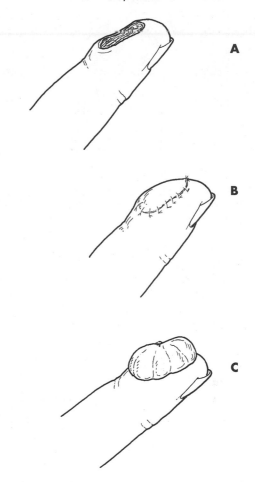

FIG. 122-3 Partial fingertip amputation without bone exposed. **A,** Clean defect. **B,** Reapply amputated part after cleaning and defatting. Suture in place. **C,** Hold graft in place with cotton stent secured with long ends of wound suture.

further shortening of the fingertip.[28] This situation is unusual. Consider composite skin grafting if the child is over 12 years of age or has the amputated part, and if the area of defect is over 1 cm.[2] Cleanse the amputated part, defat with an iris scissors or scalpel, and then suture in place with 5-0 nylon or silk. Construct a stent of either cotton or nonadherent dressing (Xeroform) to improve contact of the graft (Fig. 122-3).[21] One study indicated that conservative treatment may yield better results than replacement of the severed tip.[11] Reserve the use of harvested full- or split-thickness skin grafts for the specialist. *Never discard any available amputated tissue.*

AMPUTATIONS WITH BONE EXPOSED. The management of pediatric fingertip amputations with exposed bone is controversial. Although there is ample evidence that conservative treatment alone results in excellent outcomes, some authors still advocate the use of advancement flaps or skin grafts with exposed bone.*

If the conservative method is chosen, another controversy arises as to whether or not to ronguer back the exposed bone. If the amputation reveals only a relatively small amount of bone exposure, or the exposed bone is flush with the soft tissue, do not remove any bone.

For larger amounts of exposed bone some authors have

---

*References 2, 11, 12, 15, 17, and 19-21.
†References 1, 4, 20, 26, 28, 31, and 32.

*References 2, 4, 6, 11, 12, 16, 17, 19-21, 24, 26, 27, 28, 31, and 32.

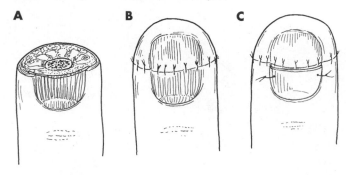

FIG. 122-4 Amputation with bone exposed. **A,** Clean part and stump. **B,** Suture into perfect anatomic location. **C,** Secure by suturing fingernail over wound.

reported excellent results with regeneration of soft tissue and nail over exposed bone that is left alone.* Others have advocated trimming the bone flush with the soft tissue.[17,20,4] Consider leaving exposed bone alone in younger children and ronguering the phalanx only in older children; substantial soft tissue regeneration appears to occur most readily among children less than 12 years of age.[12,16,6,27] Involve the hand surgeon in planning the Emergency Department (ED) approach.

In patients who have the retrieved amputated part and a clean, noncrushing amputation distal to the lunula consider reattaching the fingertip as a composite graft.[13,21] One may do this in the ED if the patient is cooperative and the physician has adequate time and suturing expertise. Older children with proximal lesions may require K-wire fixation of the phalanx. After digital anesthesia débride and irrigate the stump and fingertip, and suture the tip with 5-0 or 6-0 nylon. Repair the nail bed and replace the nail, if possible, as it acts as a splint (Fig. 122-4). Satisfactory revascularization and nerve regeneration often result. However, partial necrosis is common.[13,21]

The use of local advancement flaps such as the Atasoy-Kleinert Volar V-Y flap, the Kutler lateral V-Y flap, and the Moberg volar flap, serves to cover the exposed bone immediately and may allow for more rapid healing than conservative methods.[2,18,25] However, it usually requires time and high technical expertise that are sometimes not available among ED physicians. Reserve these procedures for the hand surgeon. Two comparative studies in children concluded that conservative treatment produced a superior cosmetic outcome and better sensation and function to either split-thickness skin grafts or local flaps, including those in which bone was exposed.[11,12]

PARTIAL AMPUTATIONS. Do not remove a partial amputation of the fingertip, even if it is dangling from a narrow skin bridge, because collateral circulation may be present and the tissue may provide valuable venous drainage.[4] After evaluating circulation (color, capillary refill) and neurologic status (two-point discrimination), repair the fingertip as described in the preceding section. Consider the use of metacarpal or wrist block anesthesia in partial amputations (Chapter 16), because this may cause less compromise on venous outflow than a digital block.[21,28]

*References 6, 11, 16, 19, 24, and 27.

Remarks

Replantation. In children attempt to replant amputated parts; however, consult a hand surgeon before advising patients and parents about long-term treatment and prognosis. Evaluate every amputation on a case-by-case basis. Do not create false expectations.

When it is necessary to refer a patient to another facility with specialized expertise for possible replantation, do not apply a bulky dressing as significant unrecognized blood loss may occur during transport.[29]

Fingertip Amputations. Management of fingertip amputations with bone exposed is somewhat controversial. Therefore consult a hand specialist.

REFERENCES

1. American Society for Surgery of the Hand: Major injuries requiring urgent treatment. In *The hand, primary care of common problems,* ed 2, New York, 1990, Churchill Livingstone.
2. Atasoy E, Ioakimidis E, Kasdan ML, et al: Reconstruction of the amputated finger tip with a triangular volar flap: a new surgical procedure, *J Bone Joint Surg* 52A:921-926, 1970.
3. Baker GL, Kleinert JM: Digit replantation in infants and young children: determinants of survival, *Plast Reconstr Surg* 94:139-145, 1994.
4. Beatty E, Light Tr, Belsole RJ, et al: Wrist and hand skeletal injuries in children, *Hand Clin* 6:723-738, 1990.
5. Beger A, Millesi H: Technique and results of digital and upper limb replantation. In Tubiana R, editor: *The hand,* vol 3, Philadelphia, 1988, WB Saunders.
6. Bossley CJ: Conservative treatment of digit amputations, *NZ Med J* 82:379-380, 1975.
7. Chen C, Wei F, Chen H, et al: Distal phalanx replantation, *Microsurgery* 15:77-82, 1994.
8. Cheng G, Pan D, Yang Z et al: Digital replantation in children, *Ann Plast Surg* 15:325-331, 1985.
9. Daigle JP, Kleinert JM: Major limb replantation in children, *Microsurgery* 12:221-231, 1991.
10. Dalsey, WC: Management of amputations. In Roberts JR, Hedges, JR, editors: *Clinical procedures in emergency medicine,* ed 2, Philadelphia, 1991, WB Saunders.
11. Das SK, Brown HG: Management of lost finger tips in children, *Hand* 10:16-27, 1978.
12. Douglas BS: Conservative management of guillotine amputation of the finger in children, *Aust Pediatr J* 8:86-89, 1972.
13. Elsahy NI: When to replant a fingertip after its complete amputation, *Plast Reconstr Surg* 60:14-21, 1977.
14. Golder RD, Stevanovic MV, Nunley JA, et al: Digital replantation at the level of the distal interphalangeal joint and the distal phalanx, *J Hand Surg* 14A:214-220, 1989.
15. Farrell RG, Disher WA, Nesland RS, et al: Conservative management of fingertip amputations, *JACEP* 6:243-346, 1977.
16. Illingworth CM: Trapped fingers and amputated finger tips in children, *J Pediatr Surg* 9:853-858, 1974.
17. Ipsen T, Frandsen PA, Barfred T: Conservative management of fingertip injuries, *Injury* 18:203-205, 1987.
18. Kutler W: A new method for fingertip amputation, *JAMA* 133:29-30, 1947.
19. Lamon RP, Cicero JJ, Frascone RJ, et al: Open treatment of fingertip amputations, *Ann Emerg Med* 12:358-360, 1983.
20. Louis DS: Amputations. In Green DP, editor: *Operative hand surgery,* ed 2, New York, 1988, Churchill Livingstone.
21. MacDonald CJ, Tountas CP: Fingertip injuries in children. In Serafin D, Georgiade NG, editors: *Pediatric plastic surgery,* St. Louis, 1984, Mosby.
22. May JW, Toth BA, Gardner M: Digital replantation distal to the proximal interphalangeal joint, *J Hand Surg* 7:161-166, 1982.

23. McGee Dl, Dalsey WC: The mangled extremity compartment syndrome and amputations, *Emerg Med Clin North Am* 11:739-753, 1993.

24. Mennen U, Wiese A: Fingertip injuries management with semi-occlusive dressing, *J Hand Surg* 18B:416-422, 1993.

25. Moberg E: Aspects of sensation and reconstructive surgery of the upper extremity, *J Bone Joint Surg* 36A:817-825, 1964.

26. Rosenthal EA: Treatment of fingertip and nail bed injuries, *Orthop Clin North Am* 14:675-697, 1983.

27. Rosenthal LJ, Reiner MA, Beicher MA: Nonoperative management of distal fingertip amputations in children, *Pediatrics* 64:1-3, 1979.

28. Sandzen SC: Management of the acute fingertip injury in the child, *Hand* 6:190-197, 1974.

29. Schlenker JD, Koulis CP: Amputations and replantations, *Emerg Med Clin North Am* 11:739-753, 1993.

30. Sixth People's Hospital, Shanghai: Reattachment of traumatic amputations: a summing up of experience, *Chin Med J* 1:392, 1967.

31. Stevenson TR: Fingertip and nailbed injuries, *Orthop Clin North Am* 23:149-159, 1992.

32. Tubiana R: Finger tip injuries. In Tubiana R, editor: *The hand,* vol 3, Philadelphia, 1988, WB Saunders.

33. Urbaniak JR: Replantation in children. In Serafin D, Georgiade NG, editors: *Pediatric plastic surgery*, St. Louis, 1984, Mosby.

34. Urbaniak JR: Replantation. In Green DP, editor: *Operative hand surgery*, ed 2, New York, 1988, Churchill Livingstone.

35. Yamano Y: Replantation of fingertips, *J Hand Surg* 18B:157-162, 1993.

123 Felon

Thomas A. Scaletta

A felon is a subcutaneous infection involving the distal pulp space of a digit. It most commonly occurs after innocuous trauma during the child's manipulation of her paronychial fold and eponychium (Fig. 123-1). A felon sometimes develops after an overt injury such as a puncture wound or bite. In immunosuppressed patients felons can occur after minor punctures such as fingersticks for glucose determination.[8] *Staphylococcus aureus* is the most frequent organism; however, an anaerobic organism or *Candida albicans* is an occasional isolate.

The distal pulp space of the affected digit is painful, throbbing, swollen, tense, warm, and erythematous. Lymphangitis may be present. Sensation and capillary refill remain normal until advanced necrosis occurs. Laboratory data are not helpful. However, a radiograph of the finger may screen for osteomyelitis.

Indications

Incise and drain all felons.

Contraindications

There are no contraindications to draining a felon.

Complications

Osteomyelitis of the distal phalanx causing bony-tuft necrosis may occur concurrently with a felon or may be a complication of an inadequately treated felon. If there is radiographic evidence of osteomyelitis, then initiate antibiotic therapy for at least 6 weeks in consultation with a hand surgeon or orthopedist.

Suppurative tenosynovitis or septic arthritis of the distal interphalangeal joint can occur with inadequately drained felons. Infection can rapidly spread through the synovium-lined spaces of the digit and hand.[5]

Equipment

In addition to equipment for a digital block and irrigation the following are necessary for incision, drainage, and packing a felon:
No. 11 scalpel
Narrow, small hemostat
Forceps
Pickups
¼-inch cotton ribbon

Techniques

As illustrated in Fig. 123-1 the tangential, fibrous septae that bind the skin to the distal phalanx and contribute to fingertip stability during grasping also compartmentalize the digital pad. Do not incise these septae to drain loculated areas of infection, because it may result in excessive mobility of the digital pad. The goal is to achieve an adequate incision and

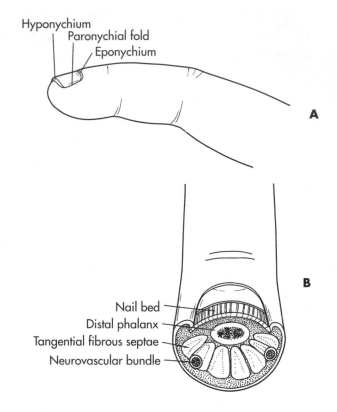

FIG. 123-1 Fingertip anatomy. **A,** Surface structures. **B,** Cross-sectional anatomic characteristics.

drainage while maintaining maximal stability of the fingertip and avoiding the neurovascular bundle.

Remove any rings from the affected digit. Administer conscious sedation if needed (Chapters 12 and 13). Position the child supine with the arm extended. Using sterile technique perform a digital anesthetic block, drape the finger, and make *one* of the two following incisions.

In general make a unilateral longitudinal incision from 5 mm distal to the distal interphalangeal joint (DIP) crease extending to the free edge of the nail at the hyponychium, as depicted in Fig. 123-2, *A*. Incise the finger dorsal (posterior) to the path of the neurovascular bundle, which travels along the volar one-third of the digit (Fig. 123-2, *B*).[2,7] Whenever possible avoid incision of pincer surfaces such as the ulnar surface of the thumb or the radial surface of the index finger.

If the abscess "points" over the pad (i.e., if there is a maximally tense and tender area that reaches a peak), then instead of the longitudinal technique, perform a limited volar midline incision across the "point" (Fig. 123-3, *A* and *B*).[1-3]

Open loculations of pus by gently spreading a hemostat within the incision and avoid the flexor tendon sheath.

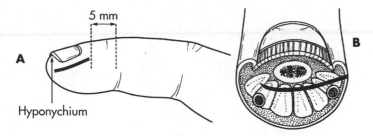

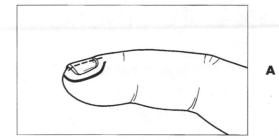

FIG. 123-2   A, Lateral view of longitudinal incision. **B,** Cross-sectional view of longitudinal incision.

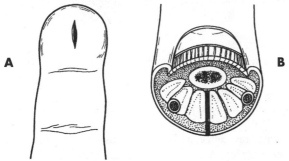

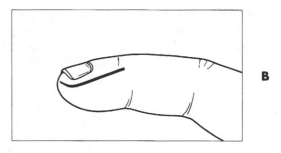

FIG. 123-4   A, "Fish mouth" incision. **B,** "Hockey stick" incision.

FIG. 123-3   A, View of the volar incision over the "point." **B,** Cross-sectional view of the volar incision.

Afterward irrigate the open space copiously and pack loosely with gauze. Recheck and remove the packing 48 hours later and then begin warm soaks. Completely immobilize the hand (Chapter 116) and instruct the patient to keep it elevated. Prescribe oral antistaphylococcal antibiotic coverage for the common skin pathogens (e.g., dicloxacillin, cephalexin, or erythromycin) for a 5- to 7-day course.[2,4] Arrange follow-up evaluation with a hand surgeon.[6]

Remarks

Extended incisions such as the "hockey stick" and the "fish mouth" incisions (Fig. 123-4), or the bilateral longitudinal incision adequately treat the infection but often create a painful scar, impaired fingertip sensation, or inadequate circulation, causing permanent limitation of function.[2,4] Reserve these approaches for severe abscesses.[6]

REFERENCES

1. Canales FL, Newmeyer WL, Kilgore ES: The treatment of felons and paronychias, *Hand Clin* 5(4):515-523, 1989.
2. Kilgore ES, Brown LG, Newmeyer WL, et al: Treatment of felons, *Am J Surg* 130(2):194-198, 1975.
3. Lammers RL, Freemyer BC: Hand. In Rosen P, Barkin RM, et al, editors: *Emergency medicine—concepts and clinical practice,* ed 3, St. Louis, 1993, Mosby.
4. Lewis RC: Infections of the hand, *Emerg Med Clin North Am* 3(2):263-274, 1985.
5. Milford L: Infections of the hand. In Crenshaw AH, editor: *Campbell's operative orthopaedics,* ed 8, vol 1, St. Louis, 1992, Mosby.
6. Moran GJ, Talan DA: Hand infections, *Emerg Med Clin North Am* 11(3):608-609, 1993.
7. Neviasser RJ: Infections. In Green DP, editor: *Operative hand surgery,* ed 2, New York, 1988, Churchill Livingstone.
8. Perry AW, Gottlieb LJ, Zachary LS, et al: Fingerstick felons, *Ann Plast Surg* 20(3):249-251, 1988.

124 Paronychia

S. Marshal Isaacs

A paronychium is an infectious inflammatory process of the lateral and/or proximal soft tissue folds of the fingernail. It is a relatively common finding in children, and the most common hand infection.[12,14] A paronychium develops after direct trauma to the nail fold, often secondary to splinters, minor abrasions, or picking and biting.[6] This trauma, often combined with suboptimal hygiene, allows a small localized infection (abscess) to form around the nail root at the side and/or base of the fingernail. The infection can also extend under the nail (subungual abscess), between the nail root and the periosteum of the phalanx.

Paronychium is a clinical diagnosis, established by a bulging tender region usually with a central white area (pus) along the base or the side of the fingernail, often surrounded by erythema. Distinguish this condition from a felon, which is an infection of the pulp of the distal finger (Chapter 123), and from a herpetic whitlow (Chapter 124), an infection of the distal phalanx characterized by the presence of herpetic vesicles, absence of frank pus, and slow response to treatment.[8,10,11] This differentiation may be difficult in a young child with small fingers.

Mild paronychia without frank pus may resolve simply with frequent warm soaks and oral antibiotics, but many require surgical intervention. Bacterial culture most often reveals mixed anaerobic and aerobic pathogens, with either pure aerobic or pure anaerobic bacteria found in approximately 24% of all cases.[2,3,12] One study has implicated *Candida albicans* infrequently as a cause of paronychia.[3] Definitive treatment of a paronychium involves incision and drainage and use of concomitant oral antibiotics. Nail removal is seldom necessary.

Indications

Incision and drainage of a paronychium are indicated in a child whose clinical examination demonstrates pus or abscess formation at the nail fold.[14] Incise all immature paronychia involving erythema without fluctuance that do not resolve with simple warm soaks. In addition if the abscess dissects beneath the dorsal root of the nail fold (subungual abscess) or continues around the base of the nail or eponychium to the lateral fold on the opposite side of the fingernail, a more extensive drainage procedure is indicated, including possible nail removal (Chapter 128).[4]

Contraindications

There are no absolute contraindications to incision and drainage of a paronychium.

Complications

Complications after incision and drainage of a paronychium are rare and most often relate to a persistent infection. In addition there are reports of formation of a chronic paronychium, injury to or infection of the nail bed, extension of the infection to the fat pad (felon), tenosynovitis, and osteomyelitis.[1,7,9,13]

Equipment

Treatment of a paronychium is usually simple. Equipment includes normal saline and povidone-iodine solutions for soaking, 1% lidocaine (without epinephrine), a 5-ml syringe with a 20- to 25-gauge needle, a scalpel with a No. 11 blade or an 18-gauge needle, a straight hemostat, scissors, sterile ¼-inch plain gauze, polymyxin/neosporin ointment, nonadherent dressing, and sterile bandages. Not all of this equipment is needed in every case requiring incision and drainage.[5]

Technique

Have the child soak her finger in a 1:1 solution of normal saline and povidone-iodine solutions. Soaking softens the eponychium and cleanses the outer surface of the finger. Administer conscious sedation (Chapters 12 and 13) and restrain the child if necessary (Chapter 11). Ensure adequate lighting and position the child supine with the arm extended. Consider a digital block using 1% lidocaine without epinephrine; some patients with small pus collections do not require local anesthesia at all. Drape the area and use a No. 11 blade or an 18-gauge needle to lift the skin edge off the nail at the site of maximal swelling (Fig. 124-1). This allows the pus to drain and prevents an actual skin incision.

If the pus collection is more extensive, or the paronychium recurs after the procedure described, a more definitive procedure is indicated. After digital block advance the scalpel blade and iris scissors or 18-gauge needle into the lateral nail fold or hyponychium. Keep the instrument parallel to the nail. Sweep the hemostat from side to side to break up any loculations (Fig. 124-2). Irrigate the wound and then place a wick of sterile gauze in the nail fold. Dress the wound and instruct the patient to begin warm soaks in 24 hours. Arrange for a wound check in 24 to 48 hours.

If pus dissects beneath the dorsal root of the nail fold or continues around to the proximal fold to the lateral fold on the opposite side of the fingernail, partial or total nail removal is indicated to ensure complete drainage. After digital block lift the eponychium on the affected side off the nail. Using a hemostat dissect under the nail, taking care not to injure the nail matrix. Use scissors to resect one-fourth to one-half the nail (Fig. 124-3). Occasionally the entire nail must be removed (see Chapter 128). Place a piece of sterile gauze under the eponychium. Provide a nonadherent sterile dressing. Instruct the patient to begin warm soaks 24 to 48 hours after a revisit to reevaluate the wound.[9,10]

Remarks

There are no controlled studies comparing different approaches to indicate when to be conservative and when to be aggressive in children. Although no true contraindications exist, there may be difficulties related to anesthesia, patient restraint, immunosuppression, or antibiotic choice.

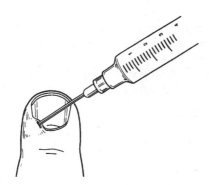

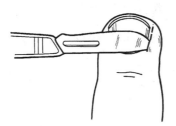

FIG. 124-1   Simple paronychia: lift skin fold off nail at site of maximal swelling.

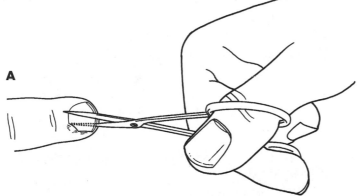

FIG. 124-2   More extensive paronychium: incise and loosen the hyponychial or lateral nail fold with a scalpel held parallel to the nail.

There is no need to culture the drainage from simple uncomplicated paronychia, and there is no clear cut evidence to support the use of oral antibiotics, although most physicians tend to treat the surrounding erythema with a short course (5 days) of oral penicillin, dicloxacillin, erythromycin, or cephalosporin. Further testing, imaging studies, cultures, and fungal scrapings may be appropriate in the immunocompromised patient or for the patient who has a poor response to therapy or suffers recurrences.[9] Finally consider children who do not respond to aggressive management to have an atypical offending organism or herpetic infection; refer such children to a hand surgeon.

REFERENCES

1. Baran R, Bureau H: Surgical treatment of recalcitrant chronic paronychias of the fingers, *J Dermatol Surg Oncol* 7:106, 1981.
2. Brook I: Aerobic and anaerobic microbiology of paronychia, *Ann Emerg Med* 19:994, 1990.
3. Brook I: Bacterilogic study of paronychia in children, *Am J Surg* 68:422, 1981.
4. Daniel CR: Paronychia, *Dermatol Clin* 3:461, 1985.
5. Lee TC: The office treatment of simple paronychias and ganglions, *Med Times* 109:49, 1981.
6. Neviaser RJ: Infections. In Green DP, editor: *Operative hand surgery*, ed 2, New York, 1988, Churchill Livingstone.
7. Roberts JR: Fingernail avulsion and injury to the nail bed, *Emerg Med News* March:7, 15, 34, 1993.
8. Roberts JR: Herpetic whitlow: an unusual paronychia, *Emerg Med News* May:9-10, 26, 1993.
9. Roberts JR: The clinical approach to paronychia, *Emerg Med News* April:4, 22-23, 1993.
10. Roberts JR, Hedges JR, editors: *Clin Proc Emerg Med* 1991, pp 604-605.
11. Rosato FE, Rosato EF, Plotkin SA: Herpetic paronychia: an occupational hazard of medical personnel, *N Engl J Med* 283:804, 1970.
12. Whitehead SM, Eykyn SJ, Phillips I: Anaerobic paronychia, *Br J Surg* 68:422, 1981.
13. Zook EG: Nail bed injuries, *Hand Clin* 1(4): 1985.
14. Zook L: The paronychium. In Green DP, editor: *Operative hand surgery*, ed 2, New York, 1988, Churchill Livingstone.

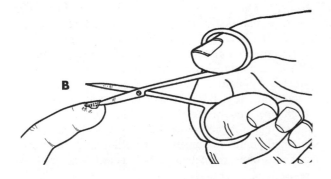

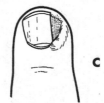

FIG. 124-3   Paronychium involving proximal and lateral nail folds. **A,** Insert scissors under nail through pus collection. **B,** Do not injure nail matrix. Hold instrument perpendicular to nail bed. **C,** Resect portion of nail.

125 Subungual Hematoma

Russell U. Braun

Subungual hematoma (SUH), a blood collection contained under the nail, is common with hand and foot injuries. It usually arises from an injury to the nail bed.[1] Box 125-1 demonstrates the wide spectrum of possible nail bed injuries.

A SUH can be very painful as a result of pressure. An additional concern is possible nail bed injury and sequelae of nail deformities. The management of SUH has changed over the last 5 years. Treatment of hematoma greater than 25% of the nail surface area has historically been nail removal.[3] However several newer studies challenge this practice; there is now literature supporting less aggressive management with equally good results.[2,5,6] Antibiotics for SUH with associated open distal phalangeal fractures with antibiotic coverage also may not be necessary.[5]

Indications

Hematoma Evacuation. Pain is the only indication for evacuation of SUH. Nail trephination alleviates pressure discomfort from expanding hematoma. This procedure is generally painless and leads to immediate relief of pain. SUH drainage within 24 to 36 hours of injury provides pain relief, although after a longer interval the pressure pain subsides spontaneously.

Nail Removal. Nail removal may be indicated for determination and treatment of nail bed injuries associated with SUH. A classic article on nail bed injuries[2] emphasized poor outcomes without nail removal and nail bed repair. Other investigators, in contrast, found an association with occult nail bed laceration only when SUH involved more than 50% of the nail surface.[6] Nail growth occurs at the nail root (germinal matrix or lunula), as shown in Fig. 123-1 but is dependent on the full nail bed for proper nail development. Disruption of any part of the nail bed may lead to a permanent deformity of the nail. Therefore assessing probability of nail bed injuries establishes whether nail removal is indicated (see Chapter 128).

Definitive evaluation and repair of nail bed injuries associated with a violated nail prevent subsequent nail deformities. *A violated nail is an absent, deformed, or split/lacerated nail. Proper repair requires meticulous anatomic realignment, minimal debridement, and maintenance of skin folds including the eponychium. Other indications for nail bed repair include complex nail lacerations such as partial amputations, avulsion injuries, stellate lacerations, and crush injuries.

Contraindications

Conservative management, such as nail trephination, is usually adequate for SUH. Consider trephination regardless of SUH size or presence of a distal phalanx fracture, as long as the nail is not violated and remains intact.[5] One prospective study performed nail trephination as the sole mode of treatment on SUH; patients with disruption of the nail/nail border or preexisting nail deformity were excluded. Follow-up evaluation was available on 45 of 48 adult patients (94%), for a total of 47 SUHs. Patients reported an average nail regrowth period of 4 ± 2.6 months. Regardless of the relative size of the SUH or the presence of underlying fracture no patients experienced infection, osteomyelitis, or major nail deformity with conservative management by trephination alone.

Therefore nail trephination is usually adequate treatment for SUH if the nail is intact. Do not remove the nail; it can serve as a natural splint for the underlying healing nail bed. Moreover antibiotics are usually not necessary for SUH after nail trephination, even in the presence of multiple nail hematoma drainage holes or a phalyngeal fracture.[2] However, antibiotics may still be useful but have unproven benefit with nail disruption or laceration in the setting of a fracture.

Complications

Removal of the nail and primary repair of a disrupted nail bed run the risk of nail bed scarring with subsequent nail deformity. Patients with a large SUH ultimately lose the nail as the digit heals; forewarn children and parents of this complication.

Electrocautery can cause painful burns if employed too aggressively.

Equipment/Technique

Perform nail trephination at the base of the nail using either electrocautery (hand-held battery-powered cautery unit), an 18-gauge needle, or a heated paper clip. Cleanse the injured digit with providone-iodine solution and consider digital anesthesia. Anesthesia is usually not necessary if the child is cooperative and penetration of the nail can be accomplished without touching the nail bed. Next ballot the SUH for blood evacuation from underneath the nail. Make the hole in the nail large enough for prolonged drainage of the hematoma.[7] Pierce the nail gently to prevent penetration of the nail bed. Fig. 125-1 illustrates the technique with a electrocautery unit.

BOX 125–1 **NAIL BED INJURIES**

Simple laceration
Crush injury with laceration
Avulsion laceration
Laceration with associated fracture
Laceration with loss of skin and pulp tissue
Laceration with partial amputation

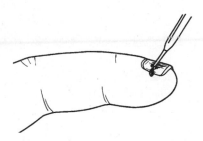

FIG. 125-1 Evacuation of a subungual hematoma. Pierce the nail at the base with the electrocautery unit by using gentle pressure.

Remarks

Consider conservative management for SUH without nail violation in the pediatric patient. Nail removal can be a very tedious project and potentially more traumatic than the injury itself. In the setting of nail violation, including nail laceration and avulsions, use the combination of a digital regional block and conscious sedation before nail removal and nail bed repair.

Soak the removed nail in hydrogen peroxide while repairing the nail bed injury; this almost effortlessly cleans the nail, which can then be reapplied.

Destruction or disruption of the nail bed significantly limits normal nail growth. Always warn the child and parents of this complication.

Refer fingertip injuries involving displaced open fractures, significant soft tissue injury, and severe nail bed disruption to a hand surgeon for formal repair in the operating room.

REFERENCES

1. Hart RG, Kleinert HE: Fingertip and nail bed injuries, *Emerg Clin North Am* 11:755-765, 1993.
2. Hedges JR: Subungual hematoma, *Am J Emerg Med* 6:85, 1988.
3. Kleinert HE, Putcha SM, Ashbell TS, et al: The deformed finger nail: a frequent result of failure to repair nail bed injuries, *J Trauma,* 7:177-190, 1967.
4. Roberts JR: Fingernail avulsion and injury to the nail bed, *Emerg Med News* March: 7-35, 1993.
5. Seaberg DC, Angelos WJ, Paris PN: Treatment of subungual hematomas with nail trephination: a prospective study, *Am J Emerg Med* 9:209-210, 1991.
6. Simon RR, Wolgin M: Subungual hematoma: association with occult laceration requiring repair, *Am J Emerg Med* 5:302-304, 1987.
7. Zook L: The paronychium. In Green DP, editor: *Operative hand surgery,* ed 2, New York, 1988, Churchill Livingstone.

126 Subungual Splinter

Russell U. Braun

The subungual foreign body is a common yet troublesome pediatric problem. Frequent offenders include wood splinters, thorns, and metallic foreign bodies.

Indications

There are no contraindications. If the splinter is tiny and superficial, and the child is young and/or uncooperative, consider warms soaks alone first; ensure follow-up evaluation to assess for pain or infection.

Complications

Removal of a foreign body underneath a nail can be a tedious and time consuming process. The patient or other family member may have pushed the foreign body deeper during unsuccessful attempts at removal before seeking medical attention, increasing the technical difficulties and the possibility of infection.

Equipment/Techniques

Complete nail removal is rarely necessary for complete removal of the foreign body (see Chapter 128). Partial nail removal may be adequate for foreign bodies lodged distally that a hemostat or splinter forceps can grip securely. First anesthetize the digit; then lift the nail with a forceps, grip the foreign body, and remove. Trimming the fingernail with a horizontal cut may facilitate localizing the object.

For foreign bodies inserted more deeply under the nail remove a wedge of fingernail to provide better access (see Fig. 124-3, A to C).[1] After wedge resection of the nail grasp the foreign body and remove with splinter forceps.

A third technique involves using a needle hook to snare the foreign body. Make the hook by carefully bending a 25- or 27-gauge sterile hypodermic needle with a needle holder. Introduce this instrument carefully along the same tract created by the foreign body underneath the nail.[2] Withdraw the needle and foreign body without damaging the nail bed (Fig. 126-1).

Remarks

Several authors have recommended scraping the nail to extract the foreign body. Avoid this technique, which is painful and time consuming.

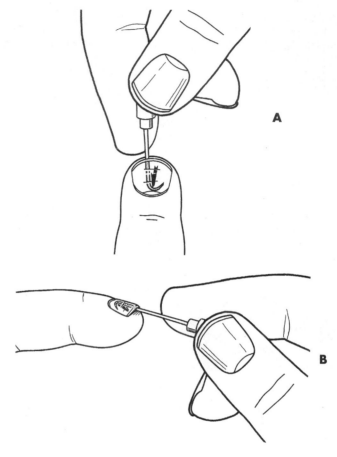

FIG. 126-1 Technique of using bent needle to extract subungual splinter. **A,** Insert needle under nail and proximal to foreign body. **B,** Withdraw snared foreign body with needle bend held horizontally to nail bed.

REFERENCES

1. Barnett RC: Soft tissue foreign body removal. In Roberts JR, Hedges JR, editors: *Clinical procedures in emergency medicine,* Philadelphia, 1991, WB Saunders.
2. Davis LJ: Removal of subungual foreign bodies, *J Fam Prac* 11:714, 1980.

127 Herpetic Whitlow

Alan Gelb

Herpetic whitlow is an infection of the fingers or thumb caused by type 1 or type 2 herpes simplex virus. Other terms used to describe this condition are herpes febrilis of the fingers, recurrent traumatic herpes, herpetic paronychia, and aseptic felon.[1-4]

Autoinoculation from primary herpetic gingivostomatitis most often causes this infection in children. It can sometimes result from kissing of the child's fingers by an adult with herpes labialis or occasionally from autoinoculation or transmission from genital herpetic infection.[1]

After an incubation period of 2 days to 2 weeks thin-walled, tender, pruritic vesicles or papules with slightly erythematous borders appear in the paronychial, eponychial, and subungual regions of a single phalanx. These vesicles may then coalesce and contain turbid fluid that comprises necrotic epithelial cells. Axillary or epitrochlear adenopathy and lymphangitis are present in 15% to 20% of patients.[1]

The lesions and pain usually progress over a period of 12 days. Viral shedding is present during this time.[3] The lesions then crust over and resolve over an additional 2 to 3 weeks.

Usually the diagnosis is clinical. Confirm it by Giemsa or methylene blue stain on cells scraped from the base of an intact vesicle that reveals multinucleated giant cells (Tzank test)[1] (see Chapter 97 for technique). A viral culture of vesicular fluid is also confirmatory but requires at least 24 hours.

Twenty to fifty percent of patients have recurrence less intense and of shorter duration than the primary infection.[4] One or 2 days of burning, itching, or tingling over a previously involved phalanx often precedes recurrences.

Indications

Cleaning and basic wound care (see Chapter 130), along with a dry sterile dressing, are always indicated to decrease spread of infection. *There are no indications for incision and drainage of a herpetic whitlow.*

Contraindications

Do not perform any procedure on the infected area, except simple wound care. Manipulation of the area does not improve healing. There are no contraindications to placing a dry sterile dressing.

Complications

Incision and drainage of lesions prolong disability, allow bacterial secondary infection, and may increase retrograde neural or systemic spread of herpes infection to the central nervous system.[1]

Equipment/Technique

Use equipment and technique for wound care of a whitlow as described in Chapter 130. Dress the wound as described in Chapter 136.

Remarks

The primary differential diagnosis is a felon (Chapter 123). This is important because felons require incision and drainage. Herpetic whitlow usually causes deep and severe pain out of proportion to the more mild external clinical appearance. The pulp of the finger or thumb remains soft, as opposed to that in a bacterial felon or pulp abscess. Also herpetic vesicles are usually present in the mouth of children with whitlow. Inflammatory cells in vesicular fluid also suggest bacterial infection.

Involvement of more than one finger suggests coxsackie viral infection.[3]

Acyclovir is effective, but reserve the drug for patients with recurrent infections or immunocompromise.[3]

REFERENCES

1. Hurst LC, Gluck R, Sampson SP, et al: Herpetic whitlow with bacterial abscess, *J Hand Surg* 16A:311-314, 1991.
2. Kohl S: Postnatal herpes simplex virus infection. In Feigin RD, Cherry JD, editors: *Textbook of pediatric infectious diseases,* Philadelphia, 1992, WB Saunders.
3. Moran GJ, Talal DA: Hand infections, *Emerg Med Clin North Am* 11(3):601-619, 1993.
4. Weisman E, Trancale JA: Herpetic whitlow: a case report, *J Fam Pract* 33:516-517, 1991.

128 · Fingernail Removal

Beth C. Kaplan

Any injury to the nail bed may result in growth of a deformed nail since the entire nail bed is responsible for generation and migration of the nail. When a nail bed injury occurs, remove the nail and repair the nail bed as soon as possible.[6] Delayed repairs are often unsuccessful and are likely to produce a suboptimal outcome.[3]

Traumatic nail bed disruptions are common in children, especially in the older age group.[10,11] The typical mechanism resulting in nail bed injury is compression of the nail and the distal phalanx, in situations such as closing of a door onto the fingertip or crushing between two objects.[10] The most common nail bed injuries are simple lacerations, followed by stellate lacerations, crush injuries, and avulsion injuries (see Box 125-1).[10]

Nail regrowth occurs at a rate of 0.1 mm/day; a new nail takes approximately 6 months to grow.[4,5] Regrowth is slow in children less than 3 years. A completely normal nail never grows back in a child who has sustained a destroyed nail bed.[7]

Indications

Removal of the nail, exploration, and repair of the nail bed injury are indicated in any child with a probable nail bed injury. Suspect serious nail bed disruption with injuries involving laceration, crushing, loosening, avulsion, or amputation of the nail. Kleinert classifies acute nail bed injuries as (1) simple lacerations, (2) crushing lacerations, (3) avulsive lacerations, (4) lacerations with associated fractures, (5) lacerations with loss of skin and pulp, and (6) fingertip amputations.[3] In addition, a subungual hematoma of significant size (generally defined as greater than 50%) and a smaller hematoma with nail violation (absent, deformed, or split/lacerated nail) suggests nail bed laceration and are indications for nail removal and nail bed repair.[2,7] Subungual hematomas result from a crush or blunt trauma to the fingernail, leading to injury and bleeding from the vascular nail bed (see Chapter 125).

Contraindications

There are no absolute contraindications to nail removal. Avoid removing a nail for a subungual hematoma alone without a violated nail unless the hematoma is more than 50%.

Complications

Deformity of the regenerated nail occurs without meticulous repair of the nail bed. Ischemia, scar contracture, adhesions, paronychia, and osteomyelitis are other possible complications.[2,7]

Equipment

Use providone-iodine solution, normal saline solution, and sterile gauze to establish a sterile field. Anesthetize the digit with 1% lidocaine delivered with a 5-ml syringe and a 25-gauge needle. Use a hemostat and iris scissors to remove the nail plate. Repair the nail bed with fine absorbable sutures, and close the skin with 5-0 nylon suture. Dress with a nonadherent dressing (e.g., Xeroform) and apply splint.

Techniques

Prepare the digit and perform a digital block (see Chapter 15). After adequate anesthesia, elevate the nail plate by gently opening and closing the iris scissors inserted under the distal edge of the nail and work proximally until the nail is free.[6,10] Once the nail is elevated from the nail bed firmly grasp the length of the nail with the hemostat and apply gentle pressure until the nail is removed from the finger. The nail can also be gently elevated from the nail bed with the

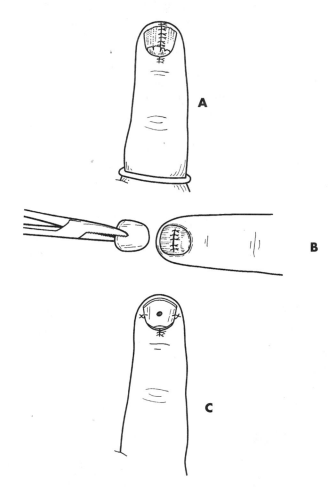

FIG. 128-1 Repair of nail bed laceration and replacement of nail. **A,** Repair nail bed and eponychium precisely. **B,** Clean and debride nail for replacement. **C,** Put hole in nail and reattach with sutures.

proximal nail left in place.[2] Then explore the nail bed laceration, accurately appose, and repair with a fine absorbable suture.[8] Use a finger tourniquet to provide a bloodless field[4,9,10] (Fig. 128-1, *A*). In order for normal regrowth to occur the nail bed must be smooth; inaccurate approximation of the nail bed may result in scar formation and deformed regrowth. Entirely remove the nail plate when it is necessary to expose the nail bed fully or if the plate needs débridement.[2] If it is necessary to remove the nail entirely, clean and trim the edges, assuming there is enough tissue to sacrifice.[1,10]

Principles of nail bed repair are as follows: use minimal débridement, preserve tissue when possible, and maintain patency of the nail fold for optimal regrowth.[3,5,7] If the nail plate is intact, replace it to serve as a dressing and splint and to preserve patency of the nail fold (Fig. 128-1, *B*).[4,9] Place a hole in the nail to allow drainage (Fig. 128-1, *C*). Hold the nail in place with a 5-0 nylon suture placed distally or on each side of the nail.[4,10] Use nonadherent gauze packing molded to the margins when there is damage to the nail. Dress the fingertip with a nonadherent gauze and a gauze dressing, and splint the distal interphalangeal; dress the entire hand in young children (see Chapter 136).[5,10] The new nail pushes the old one out.[6] Check the wound 24 to 48 hours after repair. Keep the splint in place for 2 to 3 weeks, and remove the anchoring suture in 2 weeks.[4,5]

Remarks

Consider a radiograph to rule out fractures and foreign bodies.[6] When a distal phalanx fracture accompanies a nail bed injury, treat it according to the type of fracture. Treat a nondisplaced fracture with nail bed repair and splinting with the nail plate; a displaced fracture requires Kirschner wire.[8,9] Consider all of these to be open fractures; use antibiotics accordingly.[1]

Advise the patient and parents that complete nail regrowth may require 6 to 12 months and that a cosmetic defect or deformity may occur.[7,9]

REFERENCES

1. Ditmars DM: Finger tip and nail bed injuries, *Occup Med* 4:449-461, 1989.
2. Hart RG, Kleinert HE: Fingertip and nail bed injuries. In Uehara DT, editor: *Emergency medicine clinics of North America,* Philadelphia, 1993, WB Saunders.
3. Kleinert H, Putcha S: The deformed fingernail, a frequent result of failure to repair nail bed injuries, *J Trauma* 7:177-190, 1967.
4. Lammers RL: Soft tissue procedures. In Roberts JR, Hedges JR, editors: *Clinical procedures in emergency medicine,* Philadelphia, 1991, WB Saunders.
5. Rosenthal EA: Treatment of fingertip and nail bed injuries, *Orthop Clin North Am* 14:675-697, 1983.
6. Russell RC, Casas LA: Management of fingertip injuries, *Clin Plast Surg* 16:405-424, 1989.
7. Simon RR, Brenner BE: Plastic surgery principles and techniques. In Retford DC, editor: *Emergency procedures and techniques,* Baltimore, 1994, Williams & Wilkins.
8. Stevenson TR: Fingertip and nailbed injuries, *Orthop Clin North Am* 1:149-159, 1992.
9. Van Beek AL, Kassan MA, Adson MH, et al: Management of acute fingernail injuries, *Hand Clin* 6:23-35, 1990.
10. Zook EG: The perionychium. In Green DP, editor: *Operative hand surgery,* New York, 1988, Churchill Livingstone.
11. Zook EG: Nail bed injuries, *Hand Clin* 1:701-716, 1985.

129 Tendon Lacerations

Karl A. Sporer

Hand injuries make up 1.7% of all pediatric Emergency Department (ED) visits, and lacerations make up 38% of this group.[1] In all pediatric hand lacerations consider tendon and other deep space injuries to nerves and arteries. The superficial location of extensor tendons on the dorsum of the hand predisposes them to injury. Flexor tendons are less frequently involved. Fig. 129-1 divides the hand into anatomic zones. Box 129-1 summarizes extensor tendon laceration treatment guidelines and possible complications by zone.

Indications

Many extensor tendon lacerations not at the wrist are easy to repair in the ED. Repair partial extensor tendon lacerations that involve more than 50% of the tendon as though they were full tendon injuries.[2] Splint any lacerations less than 50% after primary repair and refer to a hand surgeon. *Do not repair flexor tendons in the ED.*

Contraindications

Extensor tendon lacerations at the wrist and all flexor tendons require repair under general anesthesia by a qualified hand surgeon.

If small size of the structures, gross wound contamination, lack of patient cooperation, or physician confusion about anatomic characteristics precludes full visualization, consult with a hand surgeon and anticipate operative exploration.

Complications

Extensor tendon adhesions are a rare complication of primary repair because of lack of tendon sheath on the extensor surface. Infection is a potential complication of any open wound of the hand. Tenosynovitis, osteomyelitis, and pyarthrosis can be especially devastating to hand function. Mallet finger and boutonnière deformities can result from zone I and II injuries.

Partial tendon lacerations can be misleading because they usually have normal function and are detectable only by direct inspection. The several backup systems in the digit (junctura tendinea, extensor hood, and intrinsic muscles) often account for a paradoxic full range of digital motion even with complete laceration of an extensor tendon.

Equipment

The equipment needed is that described for lacerations (Chapter 131). A blood pressure cuff is necessary to create a clean bloodless field. Use a nonabsorbable monofilament nylon suture of 4-0 or 5-0 size,[3] because of its longer duration of strength and its relative nonreactivity. Other nonabsorbable materials may also be suitable.

Techniques

Obtain local anesthesia of the wound margins with 1% lidocaine infiltration. Use analgesia and conscious sedation

---

BOX 129–1 **EXTENSOR TENDON ZONES** (SEE FIG. 129–1)*

Zone I:	Mallet finger
Zone II:	Boutonnière deformity
Zone III:	Area between the MCP and PIP and between the PIP and DIP. There is often joint involvement.
Zone IV:	Tendons are discrete structures with no fibrous sheath. Even trivial-appearing lacerations are often associated with tendon injuries.
Zone V:	Area of the dorsal retinaculum
Zone VI:	Dorsal forearm

Treat zones I and II by splinting. Arrange for zone V and VI injuries to be repaired under general anesthesia. Zones III and IV are amenable to ED repair, if conditions are optimal.

*MCP, Metacarpophalangeal; PIP, proximal interphalangeal; DIP, distal interphalangeal; ED, Emergency Department.

---

when indicated (see Chapters 12 and 13). Restrain the child if necessary and place supine. Elevate the arm for 1 minute to exsanguinate the limb with a blood pressure cuff inflated and clamped at one and one half the normal systolic pressure. This is usually well tolerated by a conscious patient for 15 to 20 minutes.

Clean the wound with a high-pressure normal saline solution irrigation for 5 to 10 minutes. Direct inspection of the wound is necessary to visualize any partial tendon lacerations or any other proximate injuries such as joint or nerve involvement. Exposure of the wound must be adequate; extend with an incision if necessary.

To repair the tendon use the modified Kessler suture, which is essentially two horizontal sutures placed so that the knot lies between the cut tendon ends[4] (Fig. 129-2).

Splinting is crucial to a good outcome. Position the wrist in the splint at 45 to 50 degrees of wrist extension and with the interphalangeal joints of the fingers in almost complete extension. Prophylactic antibiotics are indicated for any significantly contaminated wound. Also consider tetanus immunization. (see Table 130-1).

Mallet Finger

Disruption of the extensor tendon at its attachment to the distal phalanx causes this zone I injury. Make the diagnosis by observing the characteristic flexion of the distal interphalangeal (DIP) joint with free passive range of motion and an avulsion fracture noted on radiograph at the DIP joint (Fig. 129-3). To treat splint the finger in full extension for 6 to 8 weeks and refer to a hand surgeon.

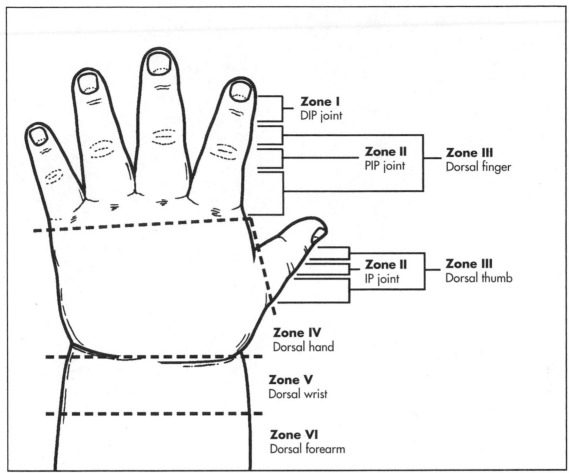

FIG. 129-1   Extensor tendon zones. *DIP, Distal interphalangeal; IP, interphalangeal; PIP, proximal interphalangeal.*
(Redrawn from Newmeyer WL: *Primary care of hand injuries,* Philadelphia, 1979, Lea & Febiger.)

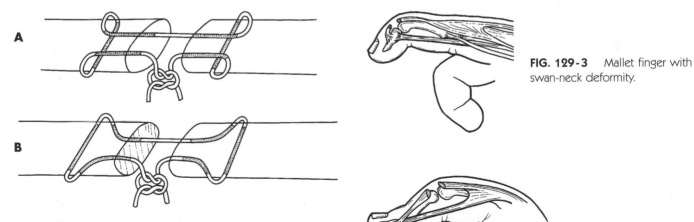

FIG. 129-2   **A,** Longitudinal sutures cross plane of horizontal sutures. **B,** Longitudinal sutures are placed more proximally to wound than horizontal sutures. Modified Kessler suture for repair of extensor tendon injury.

FIG. 129-3   Mallet finger with swan-neck deformity.

FIG. 129-4   Boutonnière deformity.

Boutonnière Deformity

Disruption of the central slip of the extensor hood causes this zone II injury. This allows the lateral slips of the extensor tendon to slip toward the palm, causing the characteristic deformity of PIP flexion and DIP hyperextension (Fig. 129-4). Make the diagnosis by the distinctive physical examination findings. Treat by splinting the finger in full extension for 6 to 8 weeks.

REFERENCES

1. Bhende MS, Dandrea LA, Davis HW: Hand injuries in children presenting to a pediatric emergency department, *Ann Emerg Med* 22:1519-1523, 1993.
2. Blair WF, Steyers CM: Extensor tendon injuries, *Orthop Clin North Am* 23:141-148, 1992.
3. Ketchum LD: Suture materials and suture techniques used in tendon repair, *Hand Clin* 1:43, 1985.
4. Wray RC, Weeks PM: Experimental comparison of techniques of tendon repair, *J Hand Surg* 5:144, 1980.

PART XXIV

Wound Care

130 Principles of Wound Healing

Jonathan Grisham

By their nature and physiology, children are prone to injuries. Lacerations alone account for as many as 40% of all injuries seen in Emergency Departments (EDs). This section describes the treatment of a wide variety of common, "minor" wounds in children, such as lacerations, punctures, burns, abrasions, and other miscellaneous injuries. This chapter reviews the general approach to injured patients, the anatomy of skin, mechanisms of soft tissue injury, and general principles of wound healing. Chapter 131 provides an overview of the techniques required to repair both simple and complex lacerations. Chapter 132 deals with wounds produced by thermal or abrasive mechanisms, including debridement, healing, and dressings. Chapters 133 and 134 focus on mammalian bites and envenomation injuries, with an emphasis on more common and clinically important bites. Chapter 135 addresses miscellaneous wound management techniques, including treatment of puncture wounds of the foot, the incision and drainage of abscesses, the treatment of epistaxis and septal hematomas, and problems associated with various ostomy sites. Chapter 136 illustrates several techniques for bandaging and dressing wounds in children.

GENERAL APPROACH

Approach children with apparently minor and localized wounds with care. Address the ABCs, perform a brief primary survey, and then perform a more detailed, focused physical examination. Before administering local anesthetics or sedative/analgesic agents that may impair subsequent examinations, evaluate the wound and the surrounding structures meticulously, including circulation, motor function, and

Table 130-1   Tetanus Prophylaxis

	Immunization history	Tetanus toxoid	Tetanus immune globulin
Clean wounds*	≥3, third within 10 years	–	–
	≥3, third within >10 years	+	–
	<3, or unknown	+	–
High-risk wounds†	≥3, third within 5 years	–	–
	≥3, third within >5 years	+	–
	<3, or unknown	+	+

From Zukin DD, Simon RR: *Emergency wound care: principles and practice,* Rockville, Md, 1987, Aspen.
*Examples of clean wounds include simple lacerations and noncontaminated abrasions.
†Examples of high-risk wounds are dirty or contaminated wounds, wounds with a crush component or tenuous vascularity, certain animal bites, and deep puncture wounds.

sensation. In addition, attend to the emotional state of the child. Injured children often experience significant pain and anxiety, and the environment of a doctor's office or ED may aggravate these feelings.

Obtain a pertinent history from the patient or caregiver, and place special emphasis on the significant past medical history, allergies, last meal, immunization status, and injury mechanisms. Ascertain the child's tetanus status and immunize him or her when appropriate (Table 130-1).[12] Finally, give the child nothing by mouth until it is clear that he or she does not require a sedative or general anesthetic.

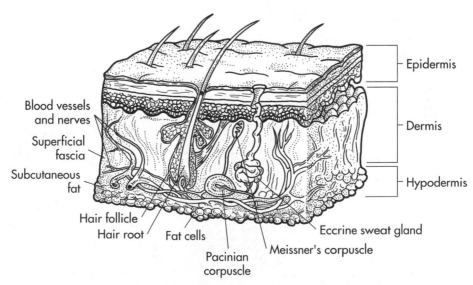

Blood vessels and nerves
Superficial fascia
Subcutaneous fat
Hair follicle
Hair root
Fat cells
Pacinian corpuscle
Meissner's corpuscle
Eccrine sweat gland
Epidermis
Dermis
Hypodermis

FIG. 130-1   Cross-section of skin and subcutaneous tissues.

ANATOMY OF SKIN

A cross-section of the skin (Fig. 130-1) demonstrates the two layers of the skin, the epidermis and the dermis, as well as the subcutaneous tissues and skin appendages. The primary function of the epidermis is to protect the dermis by keeping in moisture and keeping out infection. In commonly used areas the stratum corneum epidermis hypertrophies and forms a callus, which provides even more protection for underlying dermal tissues. The dermis provides tensile strength because of its high collagen content; dermal capillaries branch throughout this layer and provide nutrients to the skin. Below the dermis lies subcutaneous fat, through which course the large vessels and nerves that supply the skin. The relative size of each of these elements changes from one body region to another. For example, the depth of subcutaneous tissue varies from extremely thin on the dorsum of the hand to plentiful on the buttocks or abdomen. The organized arrangement of collagen fibers in the dermis creates specific lines of skin tension throughout the body, termed *Langer's lines* (Fig. 130-2). Being aware of these lines and understanding the variability in skin structure is important in selecting appropriate techniques of wound repair and predicting eventual cosmetic outcome. A laceration that runs parallel to skin tension lines heals with a finer scar than one that crosses these lines and is subject to greater tension during wound healing.[3]

MECHANISMS OF TISSUE INJURY

The primary mechanisms of soft tissue injury are mechanical or thermal.[10] Shearing, tension, and compression forces each produce distinct types of mechanical injury.[12] A *shear* laceration is caused when a sharp object, such as a knife, cuts through tissue. Such lacerations usually heal well because there is little damage to adjacent tissues. *Tension* lacerations occur when the force of an impact overcomes inherent tensile strength and results in a bursting of the skin.

Compression injuries occur when tissue is caught between underlying bone and a hard object. These injuries often result in stellate-type lacerations with varying degrees of crush injury to surrounding tissue. Because of this damage to adjacent tissue, compression injuries heal more poorly than other types of injuries.

Similar to thermal (burn) injuries, abrasions are produced by frictional forces and are characterized by a loss of variable depths of skin. Such thermal injuries can be produced by convection, conduction, radiation, cold, or electricity. Various source and host factors influence the severity of the injury (see Chapter 132).

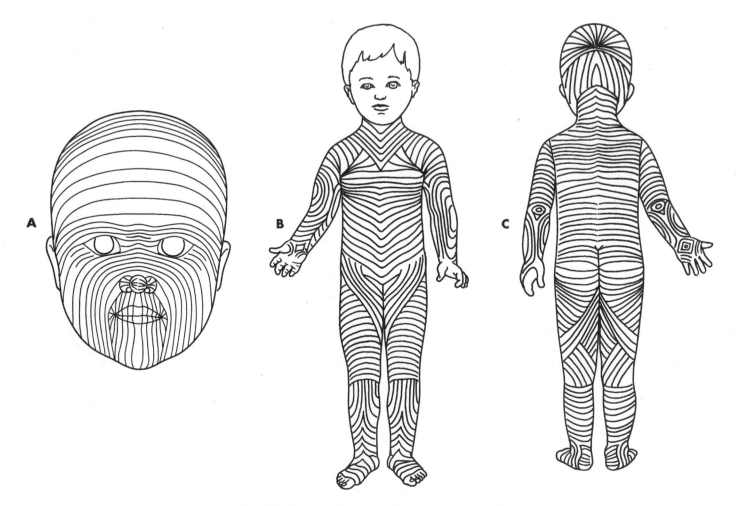

FIG. 130-2 A to C, Langer's lines of the face and body.

WOUND HEALING

Categories

Wounds such as lacerations that are repaired by approximating the wound edges with sutures heal by primary intent. Close such wounds before significant bacterial contamination of the tissue occurs. This time limit has been described as the "Golden Period" of wound repair. Close most wounds within 8 hours of injury, but in children there is much variability in wound infection risk. For example, clean facial wounds that are repaired after 24 hours may have outcomes as good as those closed much earlier.[1] Even many wounds in more vulnerable tissues can be repaired up to 12 hours after the injury with a high probability of success. Assess each wound individually to determine whether primary closure is appropriate. Anatomic location and appearance of the wound, the mechanism of injury, and the health status of the host are key factors.

Burns and abrasions generally heal by the development of healthy granulation tissue, or the process of secondary intent. This type of wound healing is typified by the healing process of a partial-thickness burn, which is initially cleaned, debrided, and dressed to prevent contamination and infection.

Tertiary intent occurs when wounds are managed with delayed primary closure.[2] For example, a contaminated wound is first evaluated 36 hours after injury. The wound is cleaned, dressed, and allowed to form granulation tissue. The wound is reevaluated in 3 to 5 days, and if there is no sign of infection, the wound is closed at that time in the usual manner.

Physiology

Unless impaired by infection or immunodeficiencies, all wounds heal by some combination of the same basic mechanisms. Although there may be considerable overlap and sometimes an absence of specific stages of wound healing, such healing follows a generally linear sequence of the following stages: (1) vasoconstriction and coagulation, (2) inflammation, (3) fibroplasia, (4) deposition of collagen matrix, (5) angiogenesis, (6) epithelialization, and (7) wound contraction. A more general classification of wound healing includes three phases: the inflammatory phase, the repair phase, and the maturation phase. These phases correspond well to the more specific stages outlined previously.[4,5,8]

Inflammatory Phase. Immediately following an injury, blood vessels in the injured area undergo intense vasoconstriction, which helps to decrease blood loss and facilitates hemostasis and clot formation. Platelets are activated, become sticky, and are enmeshed in a web of fibrin. Intrinsic and extrinsic coagulation cascades are activated, which further decreases bleeding. A variety of vasoactive amines and prostaglandins are produced, and fibronectin appears. Fibronectin is very abundant 1 to 2 days after the injury and serves as a "glue" to hold cells and matrix elements together. As the initial vasoconstriction gives way to local vasodilation, a complex cellular response ensues with the arrival of polymorphonuclear cells and monocytes, which rapidly give way to invading macrophages. The macrophage is central to the modulation of wound repair because it contributes to angiogenesis and to the production of various growth factors and because it functions as a scavenger, phagocytizing bacteria, necrotic tissue, clotted blood, and other material that can increase inflammation and slow wound healing.

Repair Phase. The essential activity during the repair phase of healing is the laying down of immature collagen and ground substance by fibroblasts. This activity begins approximately 3 days after the injury. The wound gradually gains some tensile strength as these collagenous materials increase. Within 3 weeks, sufficient collagen is present, and the number of fibroblasts decreases. This immature collagen matrix provides the substrate for the next phase of healing, the maturation phase.

Maturation Phase. During the maturation phase of healing, the disorganized embryonic collagen is reformed with much stronger bonds and is reoriented to align along mechanical lines, thus greatly increasing the tissue tensile strength. The formation of collagen into stronger, more compact bundles causes wound contraction, which in most wounds is beneficial because it shrinks the ultimate scar size. However, in certain situations this contraction of tissue can actually worsen the shape and appearance of the final scar tissue.

Epithelialization

With loss of the epidermis, eschar or a scar is formed when serous fluids combine with the necrotic, desiccating cells of the upper dermis. Within minutes of tissue injury, the process of epithelialization begins. The regeneration of epithelial tissue occurs from viable tissue in the wound edges and from surviving squamous cells in the hair follicles and glands. Dividing epithelial cells migrate across the tissue defect, whether it is a narrow gap between wound edges or a large area of burned tissue. Cellular migration is most effective in a moist environment, such as when the wound is covered with ointment and an occlusive dressing. Granulation tissue is composed of fibroblasts, inflammatory cells, blood vessels, and epithelial cells, and it represents a healthy, healing wound.

The complex pattern of wound healing explains why wounds regain their tensile strength so slowly. A typical laceration regains only approximately 5% of its previous strength 2 weeks after the injury, 30% at 1 to 2 months, and full tensile strength 6 to 8 months after the original injury.[11] This progression may be delayed by any factor that adversely affects normal wound healing. Even with the best outcomes, injured tissue never has the same strength as normal tissue.

FACTORS AFFECTING WOUND HEALING

The physiology of wound healing can be easily disrupted by a variety of factors[5] such as low tissue oxygen tension, tissue edema, poor nutrition, vitamin deficiency, the presence of a foreign body, certain medications such as steroids, or infection. Infection is the most common reason for poor wound healing. The risk of infection is increased in badly contaminated wounds such as animal bites, deep puncture wounds, poorly vascularized areas, and wounds with significant crush injury. Proper wound healing is greatly augmented by proper cleansing, irrigation, debridement, antisepsis of the wound, and skillful and timely repair. In addition, occlusive dressings and an antibacterial ointment may speed healing by keeping the upper dermal layers moist. However, totally occlusive dressings may actually promote bacterial growth around the wound. Antibiotics have unproven value in preventing wound infection; decide to use an antibiotic on the basis of the type and appearance of the wound, the degree of contamination, the time from injury to presentation, and various host factors.

PAIN CONTROL

With the exception of some full-thickness injuries in which sensory enervation is destroyed, most wounds are painful, and the manipulation necessary for evaluation and treatment may cause additional pain. The humane care of injured children requires a thorough understanding of physical restraint, sedation and analgesia, and local and regional anesthesia; these topics are discussed in detail in Chapters 11 to 16.[7,9]

REFERENCES

1. Berk WA, Osbourne DD, Taylor DD: Evaluation of the "golden period" for wound repair: 204 cases from a third world emergency department, *Ann Emerg Med* 17:496, 1988.
2. Dimick AR: Delayed wound closure: indications and techniques, *Ann Emerg Med* 17:1303, 1988.
3. *Gray's anatomy,* ed 13, Philadelphia, 1985, Lea & Febiger.
4. Hunt TK: The physiology of wound healing, *Ann Emerg Med* 17:1265, 1988.
5. Hunt TK: Basic principles of wound healing, *J Trauma* 30:S122, 1990.
6. Robson MC: Disturbances of wound healing, *Ann Emerg Med* 17:1274, 1988.
7. Selbst SM: Sedation and analgesia. In Fleisher GR, Ludwig S, editors: *Textbook of pediatric emergency medicine,* Baltimore, 1993, Williams & Wilkins.
8. Sinkinson CA, Zitelli JA: Maximizing a wound's potential for healing, *Emerg Med Rep* 10:83, 1989.
9. Terndrup TE: Pain control, analgesia, and sedation. In Barkin RM, editor: *Pediatric emergency medicine: concepts and clinical practice,* St Louis, 1992, Mosby.
10. Trott A: Mechanisms of surface soft tissue trauma, *Ann Emerg Med* 17:1279, 1988.
11. Trott A: *Wounds and lacerations: emergency care and closure,* St Louis, 1991, Mosby.
12. Zukin DD, Simon RR: *Emergency wound care: principles and practice,* Rockville, Md, 1987, Aspen.

131 Laceration Repair

Jonathan Grisham and Michelle Perro

Pediatricians and emergency physicians must often evaluate and manage a wide variety of wounds in children, including simple and complex lacerations. The vast majority of these lacerations can be repaired in the emergency department (ED) by using a few basic principles. Refer complex or severe wounds to a plastic or other qualified surgeon. This chapter outlines the needed equipment, discusses the basics of wound care, and reviews several techniques for laceration repair. The approach to specific types and locations of lacerations are covered elsewhere in this text, and discussions of more advanced techniques are also available.[18,20]

Indications/Contraindications

Repair any laceration that meets the criteria for primary closure as soon as possible. If the wound requires techniques beyond that of the treating physician, refer the patient to a qualified specialist. Relative contraindications to closure include old (e.g., >6 to 8 hours on the hand) or severely contaminated wounds, some animal bites, and wounds with embedded foreign bodies that cannot be removed.

Complications

Serious complications of laceration repair are unusual when wounds are repaired with proper technique. Although uncommon, wound infection is probably the most frequent complication and is more likely with contaminated lacerations, with inadequate irrigation and antisepsis, in anatomic areas after less vascular supply (e.g., hands and fingers), and with certain types of suture material (e.g., gut or silk). Giving proper attention to these factors reduces the chance of infection. Another potential complication is a cosmetically bad result because of poor technique or unavoidable host factors such as a hypertrophic scar. Although the vast majority of wounds heal with an acceptable scar, some injuries inevitably lead to an unattractive result. Poor cosmetic outcomes can often be revised in the future by a plastic surgeon. Infections of deeper structures, including tenosynovitis, pyarthrosis, abscess formation, and osteomyelitis, also may complicate laceration repair. Bacteremia and sepsis may occur in rare cases.

Equipment

Prepackaged suture trays are commonly found in hospitals, offices, and emergency departments (EDs) and generally contain standard (and often disposable) instruments, including a needle holder, hemostat, scissors, forceps, drapes, and syringes. These instruments are sufficient for most laceration repairs. However, when repairing an extensive or difficult laceration, select a plastic surgery tray with a higher grade and wider variety of instruments.

The needle holder is an essential piece of equipment that is specifically designed to securely grasp a suture needle. It is easier to control the suture when the needle is grasped at the

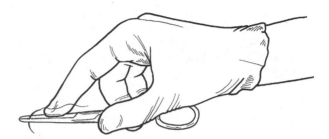

FIG. 131-1 Proper technique for using the needle holder.

junction of the proximal and middle third of the metal needle arc. Also, if the needle holder is "palmed" (Fig. 131-1) rather than held like scissors, fine control is enhanced.

Use the clamp or hemostat for ligating small vessels, for probing and for dissecting. *Do not* use this instrument as a needle holder because it is ineffective for adequately grasping the needle.

Both smooth and toothed forceps are available to grasp and control tissue during suturing. Use the toothed forceps for most repairs because they require less force to grasp the skin and cause less tissue damage.

Use a pair of small Iris scissors for trimming wound edges, debriding tissue, and cutting the suture after tying. When doing large amounts of tissue revision, use blunt-tipped Metzenbaum dissection scissors.

Suture needles come in a variety of sizes and forms; most come preattached to the suture. Select a ⅜ circle-curved needle for most repairs and a ½ circle when sewing in the web spaces of the hands or feet. In general, the best configuration to use is a "reverse cutting" type of needle, which has a triangular cross-section and the sharp cutting edge on the outer perimeter to minimize the cutting of skin where suture tension is greatest. A tapered needle has a circular cross-section and is more difficult to pass through the tough dermis; use this needle for special tasks such as tendon repair. For most pediatric repairs, especially on the face, use a high-grade needle such as a plastics needle (designated P or PS), even though these needles are more expensive than the cuticular (C) grade. To aid in selection, suture packets contain a picture of the enclosed needle in the actual size and cross-section. If the repair requires fine cosmesis, select a small needle, such as P3.

Suture materials are classified as absorbable or nonabsorbable and are made from a variety of naturally occurring and synthetic materials. Table 131-1 outlines the characteristics of commonly used suture material. Table 131-2 lists the chemical and trade names.[8] All suture materials induce a host inflammatory response and can increase the risk of infection. Synthetic and monofilament sutures generally cause much less tissue reactivity and have a lower incidence of wound infection than those that are braided or made from natural

Table 131-1 Common Suture Materials and Their Characteristics

Suture	Fiber type	Absorption pattern	Infection potential	Ease of handling
Absorbable				
Gut	Natural multifilament	Rapid	High	Good
Chromic gut	Natural multifilament	Rapid to intermediate	High	Good
Fast-absorbing gut	Natural multifilament	Very rapid	High	Good
Dexon (polyglycolic acid)	Synthetic multifilament	Intermediate to long	Low	Good
Vyeril (polyglactin)	Synthetic multifilament	Intermediate to long	Low	Good
Polydioxinone (PDS)	Synthetic monofilament	Prolonged	Very low	Very good to excellent
Glycolide trimethylene carbonate (GTMC)	Synthetic monofilament	Prolonged	Very low	Very good to excellent
Nonabsorbable				
Silk	Natural multifilament	N/A	High	Excellent
Nylon	Synthetic monofilament	N/A	Very low	Very good in finer sizes
Polypropylene	Synthetic monofilament	N/A	Very low	Fair
Polybutester	Synthetic monofilament	N/A	Very low	Very good

From Grisham JE, Zukin DD: Suture selection for the pediatrician, *Pediatr Emerg Care* 6: 301, 1990.

Table 131-2 Chemical and Trade Names of Synthetic Suture Materials

Chemical name	Trade name
Polyglycolic acid	Dexon
Polyglactin	Vicryl
Polydioxanone	PDS
Glycolide trimethylene carbonate	Maxon
Nylon	Ethilon or Dermalon
Polypropylene	Prolene
Polybutester	Novafil

From Grisham JE, Zukin DD: Suture selection for the pediatrician, *Pediatr Emerg Care* 6: 301, 1990.

fibers. A synthetic monofilament suture causes the least amount of tissue reactivity.

Sutures are sized inversely; therefore a 6-0 suture is smaller than a 3-0 suture. Generally, a 4-0 or 5-0 size is best for absorbable sutures placed below the epidermis. For skin closure, use a small suture (and needle) such as 5-0 or 6-0 nylon on the face and larger 3-0 or 4-0 sizes on the scalp, trunk, or extremities. Table 131-3 suggests which materials best serve various anatomic areas and the time course for suture removal. In the pediatric patient, suture removal can be as difficult as the initial procedure; therefore obviate the need for suture removal by closing clean, fine facial lacerations in young children with a rapidly absorbable material such as fast-absorbing gut.

Use stainless steel staples to close certain simple lacerations that do not involve deeper structures; staples can also be used for small scalp lacerations or to speed repair of long wounds on the trunk and extremities. With good technique, stapling is as effective as traditional suturing in terms of cosmetic results and offers savings in cost and time.[3] Some companies now market a small, disposable staple gun (Precise, 3M Company, Inc., St. Paul, Minn.), with 5 to 25 staples each. It is important to remove the staples with a special staple remover because using other instruments to bend the staples may damage tissue and deter healing.

Use skin tape, such as a "Steri-Strip" (3M Company, Inc., St. Paul, Minn.), to close superficial lacerations in areas not under tension. When used properly, skin tape can produce excellent cosmetic results, and the advantages are numerous. It is painless, has a decreased risk of infection compared with sutures, may be applied quickly, and requires minimal technical expertise. Skin tape is impractical for use on small children who may inadvertently remove it and is not adequate for areas under tension or movement, moist areas, or wound edges that do not remain everted after tape placement. When tissue tensile strength is in question after suture removal, place skin tape to maintain approximation of the wound edges, which decreases the eventual width of the scar by minimizing tension across the healing wound. One specific indication for skin tape is for the loose approximation of old or contaminated wounds, such as a dog bite on an extremity.

To maximize the effectiveness of skin tape, apply it to clean and dry wounds. Before tape placement, wipe the skin edges with an alcohol swab to remove skin oils, and apply benzoin tincture to the skin around the wound to improve adhesion. Exercise care when applying benzoin because it causes pain when applied directly to a wound and is toxic to tissues.

If a tissue adhesive, or skin glue, is approved for use in the United States, use it to repair some types of traumatic and surgical wounds, especially when health-care facilities may not be accessible, such as on wilderness expeditions. Histoacryl Blau is the agent most widely used. The burning sensation with application is reduced by adequate hemostasis and slow application.[12] The obvious advantage of a skin glue for the pediatric patient is the avoidance of injections, and cosmetic results can equal those produced by the suture technique. Wound research is exploring ways of decreasing infections while providing easy, rapid, and atraumatic closure

Table 131-3   Suture Selection and Removal by Anatomic Region

Region	Suture	Suture removal
Face	Skin: 6-0 nylon or polypropylene P3 needle or	4 days
	5-0 or 6-0 fast-absorbing gut	Absorbs in <5 days if area is kept moist
	Deep: 5-0 Vicril, Dexon, Maxon, or POS	Absorbable
Scalp	3-0, 4-0, or 5-0 nylon or polypropylene FS-2 needle or larger	5-7 days
	Galea: 2-0 Vicril, Dexon, Maxon, or POS	Absorbable
Hand	5-0 or 6-0 nylon or polypropylene FS-2 needle	Joint 10-14 days; other areas 7-10 days
	No deep sutures	
Extremities	Skin: 4-0 or 5-0 nylon or polypropylene FS-2 needle	Joint 10-14 days; other areas 7-10 days
	Deep: 4-0 Vicril, Dexon, Maxon, or POS	Absorbable
Trunk	Skin: 4-0 or 5-0 nylon or polypropylene FS-2 needle	7 days
	Deep: 4-0 Vicril, Dexon, Maxon, or POS	Absorbable
Oral mucosa and tongue	5-0 to 6-0 Vicril, Dexon, Maxon, or POS or 4-0 or 5-0 plain gut	Absorbable

in the pediatric patient. Tissue growth factor[15] or proteolytic enzymes[13] may be used to manage wounds in the future.

Techniques

Precare: Wound Preparation. Hemostasis is necessary before adequate evaluation and wound closure can occur. In most cases, local direct pressure and elevation of the injured part quickly and effectively stops the bleeding.[6] Before applying pressure, remove all clots and place the tissue in its original position to avoid ischemia. Control refractory bleeding from an extremity by using a sphygmomanometer that is placed proximal to the wound and inflated to a pressure just one and one half times the patient's systolic pressure. Do not inflate the cuff for more than 20 to 30 minutes. This technique can be uncomfortable; sedate children if necessary to improve their tolerance (see Chapters 12 and 13).

If hemostasis is problematic in a digit, use a sterile surgical drain as a tourniquet, and clamp a hemostat to the drain as a reminder to remove it at the end of the procedure. An alternate method involves placing a tight sterile glove on the affected hand, cutting off the tip of the glove on the digit receiving the tourniquet, and rolling the remaining glove finger down to the base of the digit. The maximum tourniquet time is 20 to 30 minutes. As a rule, do not ligate bleeding arteries anywhere in the extremities because they may require microsurgical repair, and clamps may damage adjacent nerves. Pending consultation with a surgical specialist, use direct pressure or the previously mentioned techniques to stem the bleeding.

If a wound continues to bleed despite these measures, several additional techniques are available. Epinephrine (1:1000) administered directly on the wound stops small dermal bleeding temporarily but should not be used in any area with end-arterial perfusion (e.g., fingers, toes, penis, ears, nose). Place 1 ml diluted with 5 ml of saline on a 4 × 4 gauze pad and hold it on the bleeding region for approximately 5 minutes. Another modality for attenuating bleeding is to pack the wound with a hemostatic material such as Surgicel or Gelfoam and reapply pressure. Suturing the wound closed often controls bleeding, especially in vascular areas such as the scalp. Check for hematoma formation after wound closure and before bandaging the wound because a hematoma may become a nidus for infection and prevent wound healing. Evacuation of the hematoma may be necessary.

Before manipulating the wound any further, ensure that the environment is appropriate (see Chapters 6 to 10), and administer a local or regional anesthetic. In many cases, children also need an oral or parenteral sedative/anxiolytic agent to control behavior, minimize negative psychologic effects, and maximize amnesia for the procedure. Always monitor and prepare for possible complications such as apnea. Sedation and analgesia are discussed in Chapters 11 to 16.

Wound irrigation is the most important procedure for decreasing wound infection rates. When held 2 cm above the wound, firm pressure on the plunger of a 35-ml syringe and a 19-gauge needle or angiocatheter delivers 8 pounds of pressure per square inch,[16] which effectively removes particulate matter and bacteria. Although high-pressure irrigation is crucial in preventing wound infections, it can itself cause tissue trauma.[19] Prevent dissection of solution into the tissue by keeping the catheter tip above and not in the wound. Irrigate the wound with 100 to 1000 ml of normal saline, depending on the size, location, and contamination of the wound, and use a splash guard such as the Zerowet Splashshield (Zerowet, Inc., Redondo Beach, Calif.) or other such device instead of an angiocatheter to prevent splashing. In addition, wear a protective mask and eyewear to prevent further cross-contamination.

After irrigation, provide topical antisepsis before suturing. In every case, good handwashing before donning sterile gloves is mandatory. If the gloves have talc, wipe gloved hands with a sterile wet towel to avoid getting tissue-toxic talc into the wound.[2]

The key to antisepsis is to prepare the wound with the least toxic yet most potent antibacterial agent. Do not use agents such as alcohol, hydrogen peroxide, and detergent scrubs, which are very toxic to the exposed tissue in an open wound. Table 131-4 reviews antiseptic agents and their relative toxicities. Achieve an optimal balance between antibacterial efficacy and low tissue toxicity with a 1% povidone-iodine solution (Betadine preparation solution). This preparation comes as a 10% solution and is diluted 1:10 with saline to produce a 1% concentration. Do not confuse the Betadine preparation solution with Betadine surgical scrub, which is a

Table 131-4 Characteristics of Antiseptic Agents

Antiseptic	Antibacterial activity	Tissue toxicity
Saline	0	0
Sterile water	0	0.5
Shur-Clens (plurionic F-68)	1	0.5
Povidone-iodine preparation solution	9	1
Hexachlorophene solution	8	2
Hydrogen peroxide	3	5
Betadine surgical scrub (detergent)	9	8
Alcohol	10	10

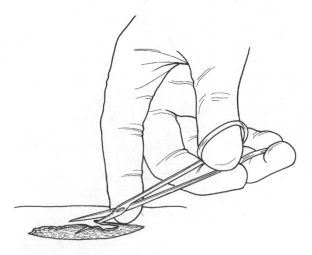

FIG. 131-2 Facilitate wound healing and improve cosmetic results by trimming a 1-mm rim of tissue from the wound edge using Iris scissors.

detergent and very toxic to tissues. Other cleansers are available (nonionic surfactants, pluronic F-68 [Shur-Clens], or polaxemer 188 [PharmaClens]; these cleansers lift the bacteria off the site surface but do not have the bactericidal activity of povidone-iodine solution.

Prepare the wound and the surrounding skin with the 1% povidone-iodine solution, and after repairing any open fascia, place a povidone-iodine–soaked gauze pad directly on the wound for approximately 1 minute. Do not irrigate the solution from the wound before closure. Avoid scrubbing the wound unless it is heavily contaminated.[14] If mechanical scrubbing is required, a high-porosity sponge such as the Optipore (Calgon Vestal, St Louis, Mo.), is less damaging to tissues than one with a low porosity. In general, do not use topical antibiotics in antisepsis unless there is a contraindication to using povidone-iodine.

Wound-edge debridement and revision is often necessary to facilitate healing and to maximize cosmesis, especially in contaminated wounds or those with a surrounding crush injury. Devitalized tissue impairs the ability of the wound to resist bacterial invasion by serving as a culture medium and by inhibiting leukocyte functions. Excise any devitalized tissue in or around the wound to decrease the risk of infection, expedite healing, and yield the best cosmetic result. Even straight, shear lacerations often have a fine rim of jagged tissue that can be trimmed with an Iris scissors or excised with a scalpel before closure (Fig. 131-2). Removal of a 1-mm margin of tissue before closure often improves the final result. Whenever wounds are trimmed, ensure that the angle of the resulting wound edge is 90 degrees from the plane of the skin.

Wounds with small irregularities in their configuration can be converted into a simple ellipse before closure. After outlining the desired ellipse with a skin pencil or with stab marks from a No. 11 scalpel (Fig. 131-3, *A*), excise the tissue with a No. 15 scalpel blade (Fig. 131-3, *B*) or with an Iris scissors (Fig. 131-3, *C*). To achieve proper closure without undue tension, make the length of the ellipse exceed the width by at least a 3-to-1 ratio, and always attempt to align the long axis of the ellipse with the skin tension (Langer's) lines, if possible. The difference between viable and devitalized tissue often is not immediately recognized; therefore spare as much tissue as possible to minimize tension on the wound after closure and to allow for revisions that may be required later.

Remove any foreign material that has not been washed

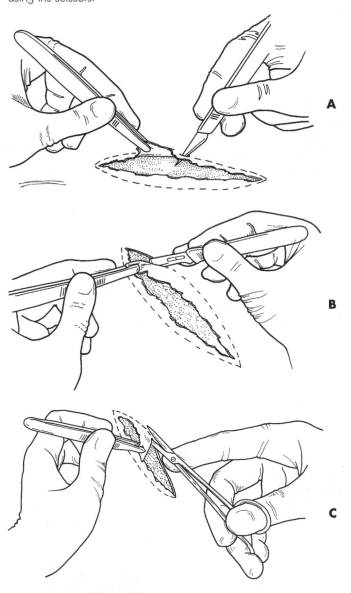

FIG. 131-3 Creating an ellipse to improve wound closure. **A,** Mark the desired ellipse using a No. 11 scalpel blade. **B,** Cut the premarked ellipse with forceps and a No. 15 scalpel blade or Iris scissors. **C,** Alternatively, use an Iris scissors.

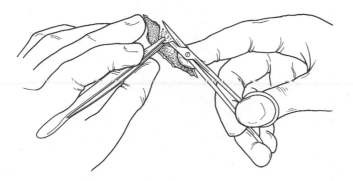

FIG. 131-4   Excision of retained foreign material.

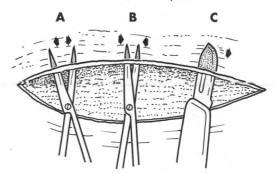

FIG. 131-5   Three techniques for undermining the wound edge. **A,** Insert Iris scissors to desired depth and spread, bluntly dissecting the tissue planes. **B,** Use the tips of the Iris scissors in a cutting fashion for more rapid dissection. **C,** Use a No. 15 scalpel for even faster and more precise dissection. With all techniques, undermine to a width equal to the gape of the wound (*shaded area*).

away by irrigation or excised with initial debridement to minimize the risk of infection and to avoid "tattooing" the skin with retained material. Pluck large particles with a fine forceps or excise them as shown (Fig. 131-4); rub away small adherent particles with a sponge and nonionic surfactant as previously described. This process is very painful in unanesthetized wounds; therefore use systemic analgesia and sedation when adequate local anesthesia cannot be achieved.

Lacerations closed under significant tension tend to produce wider and more unattractive scars. Minimize the extrinsic tension on a healing wound by undermining the edges of the laceration before closure and by closing the deep tissue layer as well as the skin. Undermining allows the skin to stretch by breaking the connection between the dermis and subcutaneous tissues. This technique can permit wound edge apposition with minimal tension even in gaping lacerations.[11] Using one or more of the techniques shown in Fig. 131-5, undermine the laceration at different levels depending on anatomic location; generally it should be undertaken in the plane of subcutaneous fat or fascia. Use a No. 15 scalpel or a pair of Iris scissors to perform sharp dissection. Alternatively, bluntly dissect the tissues by inserting the same Iris scissors (closed) into the desired tissue plane and opening them to tear fibrous connections. Although time consuming, this technique of blunt dissection is preferred because there is less risk of injuring an underlying vital structure such as a tendon or nerve and because it causes much less bleeding than sharp dissection. To avoid damaging hair structures, do not undermine in areas with hair follicles, such as the scalp or the eyebrows; use caution to avoid vital structures when undermining in an extremity.

Although hair removal is occasionally necessary to keep a clear surgical field, close the majority of lacerations without shaving. If hair removal is required, trimming with clippers or scissors causes less tissue injury than shaving and is associated with less risk of infection. *Never* shave the eyebrows because they are slow to grow back and can serve as valuable landmarks during suturing. For lacerations in or around the scalp, tape back the hair with paper tape, clip it back with hair clips, or grease it with an antibacterial ointment or a bacteriostatic surgical lubricant to keep it out of the wound during suturing.

Make the decision to administer antibiotics to prevent wound infection on the basis of several variables. Antibiotics have not been shown to prevent wound infection in most uncomplicated wounds[17]; but grossly contaminated wounds; wounds involving penetration into a joint, tendon, or bone;

animal bites (including through-and-through oral lacerations); or wounds to certain body areas such as the hands have a significant risk of infection and *may* benefit from prophylactic antibiotics. If an antibiotic is to be given, administer a first-generation cephalosporin parenterally at the earliest opportunity (within 3 hours of injury),[9] and for most wounds continue oral therapy with a similar agent or an antistaphylococcal penicillin such as dicloxacillin. Certain types of wounds require specific antibiotic coverage and are discussed elsewhere (Chapters 133 to 135).

Wound Closure.   Closure by primary intent occurs when any technique (sutures, skin tapes, staples) is used to close a laceration soon after the injury. Rapid healing and excellent cosmetic results are generally produced with primary closure, and this type of closure is the treatment of choice for uninfected or uncontaminated wounds. Current practice dictates that this type of repair be accomplished within 24 hours for clean facial and scalp lacerations or within 8 to 16 hours for most wounds in other regions.[1,10] Determine whether a primary closure can be performed on the basis of age and location of the wound, the mechanism of injury, degree of contamination, and various host factors.

Allow certain types of wounds, such as those with decreased vascular supply, a debilitated host, or a crush component to heal by the formation of granulation tissue (secondary intent). Other types of injuries that heal better by secondary intent include abscess cavities, puncture wounds, some animal bites, and partial-thickness tissue loss. For example, fingertip amputations have better functional and cosmetic outcomes if allowed to heal by this method instead of by closure or grafting.[4,7] For all of these types of injuries, clean and prepare the wound in the same manner as for those that are to be closed, and pack or dress it with a sterile dressing that will be changed at regular intervals.

Manage contaminated or infected wounds with delayed primary closure, which allows healing by the process of tertiary intent. Prepare the wound for delayed primary closure by irrigating, cleansing, and debriding in the usual fashion; pack any wound cavity with a bulky, absorbent dressing, and cover the entire wound with a layer of petrolatum- or antibiotic-impregnated gauze. Leave most wounds undisturbed for 3 to 5 days; some may require an interim wound check. If there is no sign of tissue infection at

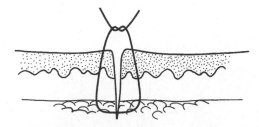

FIG. 131-6 Achieve wound edge eversion by creating a suture loop that is widest at the base.

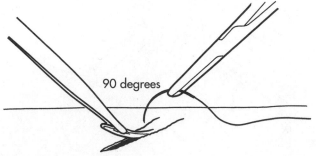

FIG. 131-7 Entering the skin at a 90-degree angle and everting the wound edge with forceps creates a loop of suture that is widest at the base.

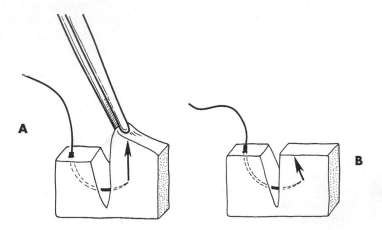

FIG. 131-8 Exiting the skin to create a broad-based suture loop. **A,** Use a skin hook or fine-toothed forceps to evert the wound edge as the needle exits the tissue. **B,** Alternatively, advance the needle an additional 2 to 3 mm across the wound, then rotate back up and out of the skin along the track shown.

follow-up, irrigate and prepare the wound and close it with a minimum number of monofilament sutures in a single layer. This technique allows for acceptable closure of most contaminated or old wounds.

Basic Techniques

THE SIMPLE INTERRUPTED STITCH. The simple interrupted stitch is both the easiest and the most versatile for closing wounds. Mastery of this technique allows closure of the majority of lacerations encountered in the pediatric population. Select a needle size and suture material appropriate to the task as previously discussed. Grasp the needle with the needle holder. To improve control of the wound, place the sutures approximately 2 mm apart and 2 mm from the wound edge on delicate areas (such as the face). More frequent and closer sutures decrease wound tension and leave a less prominent scar. Use larger "bites" for other parts of the body in which cosmesis is less crucial, such as the trunk or extremities.

Enter the skin on the opposite side of the laceration so that the clinician is suturing toward himself or herself. The interrupted stitch forms a loop through the tissue with the knot sitting on top of the wound. To encourage wound edge eversion, make the suture loop larger at the base than at the top (Fig. 131-6). Create the broad base of the loop by entering the skin at a 90-degree angle (Fig. 131-7) rather than tangentially. In addition, creating a broad-based suture loop is further facilitated by exiting the wound with the techniques illustrated (Fig. 131-8). If the two sides of the wound are uneven, it may be necessary to pass through each wound edge separately. Bring the needle out through the skin on the near side of the laceration; remember to follow the natural curve of the needle as it is pulled through the tissue. Leave the short end of the suture approximately 2 cm long so that it stands upright to facilitate knot tying.

For most individuals the instrument tie is the simplest way to create a secure knot (Fig. 131-9). To prevent unraveling, make the first throw a surgeon's knot. The first and second throws must be snug enough to lightly approximate the wound edges without strangulating the tissue. Properly square all subsequent knots to maintain the closure. For monofilament synthetic materials such as nylon, four to five throws may be required for each knot to avoid unraveling, and pull all knots to the side of the wound to avoid entrapment during healing.

Use the interrupted stitch to close small lacerations with one of two techniques. Close the wound by starting at one end and working in a stepwise fashion to the other end; this approach is best for simple, linear lacerations with equal sides. If the sutures are placed unevenly or if the sides of the

wound are unequal, this technique can result in a bunching of tissue on one side of the wound, or a *dog-ear deformity*. For larger, wider, and uneven lacerations, use the "halving" method, in which the wound is bisected with the first stitch, followed by a similar bisecting of progressively smaller lengths of the laceration on either side of the first, central suture.

THE RUNNING SUTURE. The running suture (Fig. 131-10) is a series of simple interrupted sutures except that the suture is not cut and tied with each stitch. Place the first loop at one end of the wound (preferably the end nearest the hand with the needle holder); tie the knot in the usual manner but do not cut the suture. Place the next loop a few millimeters down the laceration and continue making loops down the wound until the defect is closed. When all of the stitches are in place, adjust the tension of each loop so that the wound edges are gently approximated. On the final loop, do not pull the suture completely through so that a small loop remains on the opposite side of the wound. Complete the repair by tying the suture to the preceding loop of suture.

The advantage of the running suture is speed. The disadvantage is that the entire suture line can unravel if the suture breaks anywhere along the repair. In addition, if care is not taken to keep the two sides of the laceration equal while

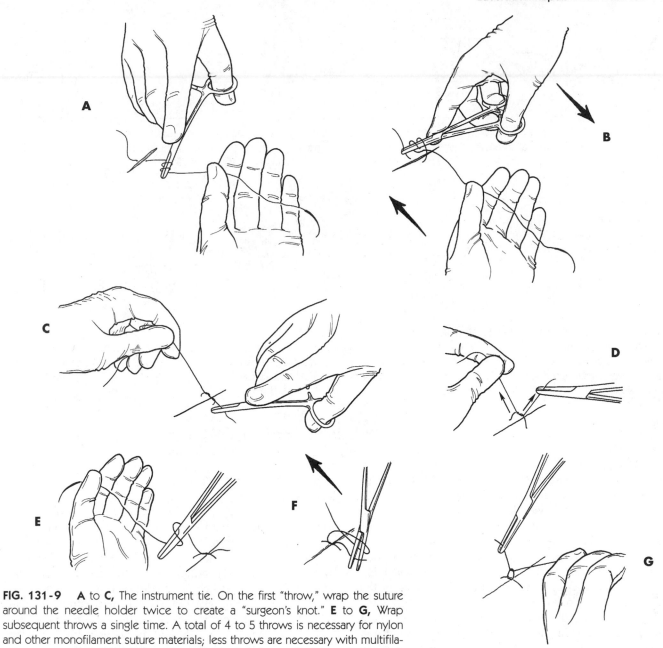

FIG. 131-9 **A** to **C,** The instrument tie. On the first "throw," wrap the suture around the needle holder twice to create a "surgeon's knot." **E** to **G,** Wrap subsequent throws a single time. A total of 4 to 5 throws is necessary for nylon and other monofilament suture materials; less throws are necessary with multifilament sutures and natural fibers. Crisscross the hands over the wound with each throw as shown by the arrows in **B** and **F.**

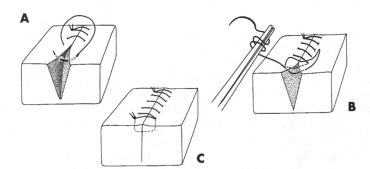

FIG. 131-10   The running suture. **A,** After tying the initial simple suture, place consecutive loops along the length of the laceration. **B,** After the final pass through tissue, tie the free end against a loop left free on the opposite side of the wound. **C,** Orientation of suture loops.

suturing, a dog-ear deformity results. The running suture is best for long, straight lacerations, not for stellate or irregular wounds.

THE VERTICAL MATTRESS SUTURE. The vertical mattress suture (Fig. 131-11) exaggerates wound edge eversion and is useful in body areas such as the dorsum of the hand, the flexor surface of the wrist, or the web spaces of the digits, where skin edges tend to invert. This stitch consists of a double line of suture across the wound. Begin the same as with a simple skin suture, entering and exiting the skin at least 3 mm from the wound edge (Fig. 131-11, *A* and *B*). With a backhand technique, make another pass across the wound, placing this suture in line with the first approximately 1 to 2 mm from the wound edge (Fig. 131-11, *C* to *E*). Tie the knot in the usual fashion; if this knot is tied too tightly, excessive puckering of the wound occurs. For longer lacera-

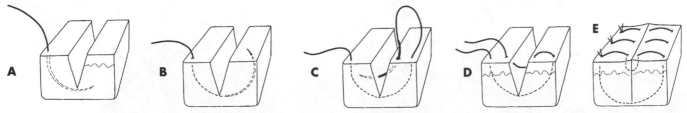

FIG. 131-11 **A** to **E,** The vertical mattress suture. After initially placing a simple interrupted stitch with a somewhat larger bite, make a backhand pass across the wound, taking small, superficial bites. When the knot is tied, the edges of the laceration should evert slightly.

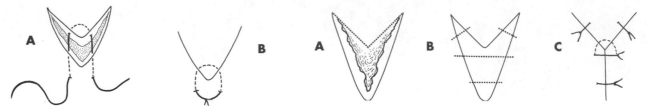

FIG. 131-12 **A** and **B,** The corner stitch. Also known as the half-buried horizontal mattress stitch, this technique allows repair of flap-type lacerations without further compromising blood flow. Place additional simple interrupted sutures along the sides of the flap if necessary.

FIG. 131-13 **A** to **C,** Technique for repairing a flap with a necrotic tip. After debridement, use a combination of simple sutures and a corner stitch, which converts a V-shaped wound into a Y-shaped wound.

tions, alternate simple sutures with vertical mattress sutures to ensure edge eversion.

Advanced Techniques

THE CORNER STITCH AND REPAIR OF FLAP LACERATIONS. Use the corner or half-buried horizontal mattress stitch (Fig. 131-12) to repair wounds with devascularized tissue, such as simple flaps or stellate wounds. With this technique the suture remains above the dermal blood vessels to avoid compromising the remaining blood supply. With the needle, enter the intact skin across from the apex of an angulated flap and exit the wound edge just below the skin surface in the subcuticular plane. Course the needle through the tip of the flap, again in the subcuticular plane. Never allow the needle to exit through the skin surface while coursing through the tip of the flap. Direct the needle back into the edge across from the flap, again in the subcuticular plane, and exit the skin approximately 3 mm from the initial entry site. As the suture is tied in the usual manner, the tip of the flap should come to rest in the apex of the wound. Use 5-0 or 6-0 nylon sutures for this stitch.

Many lacerations have a flap configuration. A flap with a proximal base (closer to the heart) has better perfusion than a flap with a distal base. Flaps in well-perfused areas of the body such as the face, survive better than those in poorly perfused areas such as the hand or the shin. To repair simple flaps with intact perfusion, suture the tip into place using the corner stitch. Suture in place the two sides of the flap; take very small, shallow bites from the flap edge and normal-size bites from the intact edge. Use as few sutures as possible and be certain not to cinch the sutures too tightly.

To repair long, narrow flaps with necrotic tips, first trim enough of the tip to yield a flap with a length-to-width ratio of approximately 1:1. Use simple sutures to repair the top part of the wound. Suture the flap into place using the corner stitch for the tip and small bites for the flap edges (Fig. 131-13). The final appearance of the wound will be Y-shaped.

REPAIR OF WOUNDS WITH BEVELED EDGES. Unlike the neat, 90-degree wound edges of simple lacerations, many lacerations are at a tangent and yield beveled edges. If beveled wounds are sutured with a standard skin suture, an unsightly tissue ledge often results. To repair these beveled wounds, take a normal-to-generous bite from the broad edge, followed by a very small bite (1 to 2 mm from the edge) from the thin edge. This technique usually yields a level wound repair without ledges (Fig. 131-14). A second, more difficult method of repair involves excising the beveled edges entirely; this method leaves a slightly larger wound, but the edges are 90 degrees to the skin plane. Repair the laceration in the usual fashion. Excision is the method of choice when the thin edge appears necrotic.

REPAIR OF STELLATE WOUNDS. Compression-type injuries, such as striking the forehead against the pavement, often lead to stellate lacerations with multiple converging flaps of skin. With conventional suturing, the tips often invert into the center of the wound. To prevent this inversion, use a single corner stitch to bring together the tips of all of the flaps. Once the tips have been approximated, place simple interrupted sutures to close the linear parts of the wound (Fig. 131-15).

THE DOG-EAR DEFORMITY. A dog-ear deformity occurs when a laceration with unequal sides is sutured from one end to the other, leaving a small pucker of tissue at the end. The best way to deal with a dog-ear deformity is to prevent it from developing by making fine adjustments while suturing, gathering slightly more tissue between sutures on the longer side of the laceration. Some wounds are best closed by the "divide and conquer," or "halving" technique of multiple

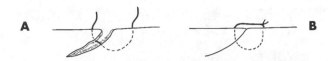

FIG. 131-14   **A** and **B,** Repair of a wound with beveled edges. Taking a large bite from the large side and a small bite from the thin flap yields a level repair.

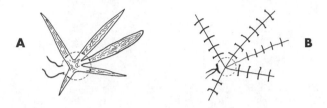

FIG. 131-15   **A** and **B,** Repair of a stellate wound with a combination of simple sutures and an extended half-buried horizontal mattress stitch.

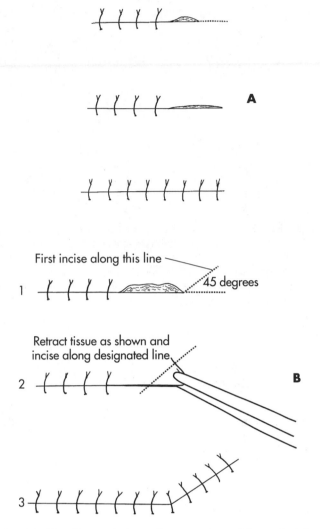

First incise along this line

45 degrees

1

Retract tissue as shown and incise along designated line

2

3

FIG. 131-16   Two techniques for managing a "dog-ear" deformity. **A,** The simplest technique involves extending the laceration and gathering small portions of the excess tissue between each suture loop. **B,** Larger deformities. *1,* Excise to extend wound; *2,* do angled incision; excise a wedge of tissue to equalize the sides of the laceration; *3,* use simple sutures to complete the closure.

bisecting stitches; this technique allows the same type of adjustments to be made and prevents a deformity on the end of the wound. If faced with a dog-ear deformity, take one of two approaches to deal with the redundant tissue. The easiest alternative involves simply extending the laceration and completing the closure, gathering excess tissue with each stitch as described previously (Fig. 131-16, *A*). For larger defects, excise a small triangle of tissue to create wound edges of equal length (Fig. 131-16, *B*). Then close the wound in standard fashion.

Layered Closures.   In the layered closure use deep, buried sutures in addition to the skin sutures previously described. Closing the deep layer of a laceration improves the final cosmetic outcome of the repair by providing additional support to the wound during the interval between the removal of skin sutures and the development of adequate tensile strength. Deep-layer closure also decreases hematoma formation and minimizes infection risk. In addition, in the repair of facial wounds the deep layer ensures alignment of the muscles of facial expression.

Place the deep sutures in collagen-containing tissue, such as the dermis or the fascia overlying muscles. Do not attempt to suture fat or muscle tissue itself. For most buried repairs use a synthetic material, which carries a lower potential for infection than traditional plain or chromic gut sutures.[5,8] Avoid placing deep sutures in infection-prone wounds such as animal bites and lacerations to the extremities. Never put deep sutures in the hand, where vital tendons and nerves lie beneath the skin and where a deep-space infection can be devastating.

For facial repair the best deep stitch is the buried knot suture, which leaves the surface on which the skin rests smooth and flat. An alternate technique is the buried horizontal mattress suture.

THE BURIED KNOT SUTURE.   The buried knot suture keeps the knot buried at the bottom of the suture loop. Enter the deep portion of the wound with the needle and come out just below the skin surface by grasping the fibrous tissue of the dermis as the needle exits (Fig. 131-17, *A*). Enter the opposite side at the same level just beneath the skin; course deeply, exiting just across from the initial deep entry point (Fig. 131-17, *B*). Before tying the knot, ensure that both strands of the suture pass out on the same side of the loop (Fig. 131-17, *C*). Tie the knot while an assistant approximates the wound edges. Tuck the knot down to the base of the loop and well away from the skin surface (Fig. 131-17, *D*).

THE BURIED HORIZONTAL MATTRESS SUTURE.   To place a buried horizontal mattress suture, take equal bites of tissue from either side of the laceration (Fig. 131-18). Course the suture parallel to the skin surface. Avoid cinching the knot too tightly because doing so causes the skin to pucker. This stitch is easier to master than the buried knot stitch and is especially useful when deep repair is needed in a shallow wound or in areas with little subcutaneous tissue. The major disadvantage of the technique is that the knot lies close to the surface, which risks extrusion during wound healing.

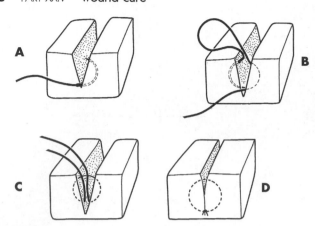

FIG. 131-17 **A** to **D,** The buried-knot stitch for closing the deep tissue layer. The absolute depth (vertical plane) of the suture loop is not as important a factor as ensuring that a good amount of fibrous tissue is grasped under the wound edge (in the horizontal plane). Note that the knot lies at the base of the wound, which prevents the risk of extrusion during healing.

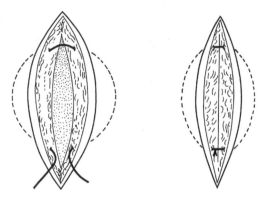

FIG. 131-18 The horizontal mattress stitch is useful for closing the deep layer in shallow lacerations and in body areas with little subcutaneous tissue. Certain dyed suture materials may cause a tattooing of the skin if placed in such a shallow position.

Aftercare. After the wound has been repaired, clean and dress it and splint it if needed as described in Chapter 136. Reexamine all wounds at high risk for infection within 36 to 72 hours. Remove sutures at the appropriate times (see Table 131-3), and place adhesive strips across the wound to reduce tension in areas such as the face or over joints. Advise all patients of the importance of good aftercare in maximizing the potential for an optimal outcome.

Remarks

Box 131-1 lists some general caveats for repairing lacerations or other wounds in children.

REFERENCES

1. Berk WA, Osbourne DD, Taylor DD: Evaluation of the "golden period" for wound repair: 204 cases from a third-world emergency department, *Ann Emerg Med* 17:496, 1988.
2. Bodiwalia GG, George TK: Surgical gloves during wound repair in the accident-and-emergency department, *Lancet* 2(8289):91, 1982.

3. Brickman KR, Lambert RW: Evaluation of skin stapling for wound closure in the ED, *Ann Emerg Med* 18:1122, 1989.
4. Douglas BS: Conservative management of guillotine amputations of the finger in children, *Aust Paediatr J* 8:80, 1972.
5. Edlich RF, et al: Physical and chemical configuration of sutures in the development of surgical infection, *Ann Surg* 177:679, 1972.
6. Edlich RF, et al: Initial management of the multiple trauma patient, *Compr Ther* 7:31, 1981.
7. Farrell RG, et al: Conservative management of fingertip amputations, *J Am Coll Emerg Phy* 6:243, 1977.
8. Grisham JE, Zukin DD: Suture selection for the pediatrician, *Pediatr Emerg Care* 6:301, 1990.
9. Lammers RL: Principles of wound management. In Roberts JR, Hedges JR, editors: *Clinical procedures in emergency medicine,* Philadelphia, 1985, WB Saunders.
10. Lindsey D: The 6-hour golden period is 22-karat brass. In *Simple surgical emergencies,* New York, 1983, Arco.
11. McGuire MF: Studies of the excisional wound. I. Biomechanical effects

of undermining and wound orientation on closing tension and work, *Plast Reconstr Surg* 66:419, 1980.

12. Quinn JV, Drzewiecki A, Li MM, et al: A randomized controlled trial comparing a tissue adhesive with suturing in the repair of pediatric facial lacerations, *Ann Emerg Med* 22:1130, 1993.

13. Rodeheaver GT, et al: Proteolytic enzymes as adjuncts to antimicrobial prophylaxis of contaminated wounds, *Am J Surg* 129:537, 1975.

14. Rodeheaver GT, et al: Mechanical cleansing of contaminated wounds with a surfactant, *Am J Surg* 129:241, 1975.

15. Ross R: Platelet-derived growth factor, *Lancet* 1:1179, 1989.

16. Stevenson TR, et al: Cleansing the traumatic wound by high-pressure syringe irrigation, *J Am Coll of Emerg Phy* 5:17, 1976.

17. Thirlby R, Blair A: The value of prophylactic antibiotics for simple lacerations, *Surg Gynecol Obstet* 156:212, 1983.

18. Trott A: *Wounds and lacerations: emergency care and closure,* St Louis, 1991, Mosby.

19. Wheeler CB, et al: Side effects of high pressure irrigation, *Surg Gynecol Obstet* 243:775, 1976.

20. Zukin DD, Simon RR: *Emergency wound care: principles and practice,* Rockville, Md, 1987, Aspen.

132 Management of the Burn Patient

Susan B. Kirelik and William H. Hawk

EPIDEMIOLOGY

Burn injuries account for approximately 20,000 hospitalizations each year; many times this number of children are burned and managed on an outpatient basis.[8,12] In the United States, burns, fire-related injuries, and smoke inhalation constitute the third leading cause of death in children.[12] Scalds from hot water or foods are the leading cause of burn morbidity in children less than 4 years of age.[8,12,13]

PATHOPHYSIOLOGY

Significant burn injuries result in a myriad of systemic changes, including hypovolemia from third-space and evaporative fluid losses, immune system dysfunction, generalized edema, and gastrointestinal dysmotility.

Burned tissue sustains varying degrees of injury depending on the type and temperature of the burning agent and the duration of contact with the burning agent. In general, the hotter the temperature of the material, the less time needed to produce a full-thickness injury (Table 132-1).[11] In children, less time is required to produce a full-thickness burn because of their thinner stratum corneum epidermis.

EMERGENCY DEPARTMENT EVALUATION AND MANAGEMENT

Assessment

After evaluating the ABCs and performing primary and secondary surveys, establish intravenous (IV) access in children who have greater than 10% body surface area (BSA) burns and in adolescents or adults with greater than 20% BSA burns; ideally place these IVs through normal skin.[20] If possible, avoid cutdown lines and central lines to minimize the risk of infection.[4,20]

Assess the patient's burn, including depth (Table 132-2), extent (percentage BSA), and location. Burn depth is often impossible to determine in the Emergency Department (ED) and is easily underestimated. Detailed classification of burn depth becomes useful later in the patient's course, but for ED purposes distinguish burns as either full thickness or partial thickness.

Estimate the percentage BSA covered by second- and third-degree burns. Use the patient's palm (generally 1% BSA) as a reference. For a more accurate measurement use a Lund-Browder chart to indicate the location and depth of the patient's burns (Fig. 132-1). This method takes into account the changing distribution of BSA at various ages.

Document the location of the burns, and recognize that the same thermal insult may produce deeper injuries in areas with thinner skin. Burns of the hands, face, and perineum, as well as burns over joints, may require hospitalization and

Table 132-1 Time Required to Produce Full-Thickness Injury in Adults from Contact with Hot Water.

Temperature (° F)	Time
120	10 min
122	5 min
127	1 min
130	30 sec
140	5 sec

From Katcher ML: Scald burns from hot tap water, *JAMA* 246 (1): 1219-1222, 1981.

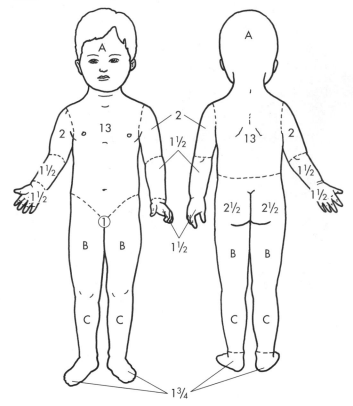

Relative percentages of areas affected by growth (age in years)

Area	0	1	5	10	15	Adult
A: half of head	9-1/2	8-1/2	6-1/2	5-1/2	4-1/2	3-1/2
B: half of thigh	2-3/4	3-1/4	4	4-1/4	4-1/2	4-3/4
C: half of leg	2-1/2	2-1/2	2-3/4	3	3-1/4	3-1/2

FIG. 132-1 Lund-Browder burn-size chart.

(Modified from Lund CC, Browder NC: The estimate of areas of burn, *Surg Gynecol Obstet* 79:352, 1944.)

Table 132-2   Depth of Burn Wounds

Burn injury	Injury depth	Appearance	Healing
First degree	Epidermis only	Erythematous Painful Blanches easily	Heals very well without scarring
Superficial second degree (superficial partial thickness)	Entire epidermis Superficial portion of the dermis Dermal elements remain (hair follicles, nerve endings, sebaceous glands)	Blistered and erythematous Painful	Heals with some scarring Healing from remaining dermal elements
Deep second degree (deep partial thickness)	Entire epidermis Significant portion of the dermis is destroyed Few remaining dermal elements	Blistered and erythematous or white and dry May be difficult to distinguish from full thickness	Slow healing with significant scarring Healing from few remaining dermal elements
Third degree (full thickness)	Entire epidermis Entire dermis	White, dry, leathery, no blanching Insensate	Very slow healing occurs only from wound edges Requires grafting if larger than 4 cm^2
Fourth degree	Entire epidermis Entire dermis Underlying structures (bone, muscle, tendon)	Visible injury to underlying structures	Requires extensive surgical care

specialized care.[19] As described later in this chapter, circumferential burns may need immediate escharotomy.

Intravenous Fluids

Patients with significant burns have enormous fluid requirements. Give 20-ml/kg boluses of isotonic fluid to those patients with evidence of hypovolemia or shock until the vital signs stabilize, then calculate ongoing fluid needs using the formula in Box 132-1.[7,10] Diligently monitor volume status by using urine output, heart rate, and capillary refill as guides. Invasive hemodynamic monitoring occasionally is necessary.[3] Because of the capillary leak, avoid colloidal solutions during the first 8 to 24 hours after the burn injury; add them after this time to replace lost serum protein.[9,19]

TREATMENT OF THE BURN WOUND
Debridement

Partial- and full-thickness burns often need debridement. Leave all intact blisters alone and cover them with a protective dressing such as gauze. Provide systemic analgesia and sedation for the patient with significant burns, and use topical or local anesthetics for small burns (see Chapters 12 to 16). Gently rub saline-soaked gauze over more superficial partial-thickness burns to remove necrotic tissue, ruptured blisters, and any foreign material; take care not to injure viable tissue. Use forceps and scissors to remove larger pieces of necrotic tissue. Cleanse the wound with a diluted povidone-iodine solution or saline.

Dressings

The goal of a burn-wound dressing is to maintain hydration and minimize bacterial proliferation, which helps prevent further tissue damage.

BOX 132-1   **RESUSCITATION FLUIDS FOR BURNED CHILDREN**

Formula using BSA

First 24 hours (starting at time of injury)

5000 ml/m^2 burned area + 2000 ml/m^2 maintenance fluid given as lactated Ringer's solution (LR) or normal saline (NS)

Give one half over the first 8 hours and the second half over the next 16 hours

Second 24 hours

3750 ml/m^2 burned area + 1500 ml/m^2 maintenance fluid given as D5 ⅓ NS with 1-2 mEq K$^+$/kg/day

Parkland formula*

First 24 hours

4 ml/kg/% BSA burn given as LR or NS

Give one half over the first 8 hours and the second half over the next 16 hours

Add maintenance fluids for children under 30 kg

From Herndon DN, et al: Management of burn injuries. In Eichelberger M, editor: *Pediatric trauma: prevention, acute care, rehabilitation*, St. Louis, 1993, Mosby.

*This formula may greatly underestimate fluid requirements in very young children.

Simple superficial partial-thickness burns (first degree) can easily be treated by the primary physician on an outpatient basis. Gently clean these wounds with saline and regularly apply a mild emollient cream.[16] Generally no further medical

Table 132-3 Burn Dressings

Dressings	Indications	Advantages	Disadvantages
Bismuth-impregnated petrolatum gauze (Xeroform)	Clean, fresh partial-thickness burn	Inexpensive Protects healing skin during dressing change Less pain with dressing change	
Silver sulfadiazine	Burns at risk for infection(older burns, burns with early evidence of infection) Burns in which biosynthetic dressings fail to adhere	Antibacterial activity; helps prevent burn-wound infection	Messy Requires BID dressing changes Damage to healing epithelium with cleansing at each dressing change Dressing changes painful Temporary side effect (e.g., leukopenia, thrombocytopenia, rash, mild interference with reepithelialization)
Mefanamide acetate	Burns at risk for infection and those with an eschar	Penetrates eschar Antibacterial activity	Side effects (carbonic anhydrase inhibitor) limit use to inpatient basis
Biosynthetic dressings	Clean, fresh partial-thickness burns free of eschar and with prompt capillary refill Do not use with burns likely to be full-thickness burns (chemical or contact burns)	Less pain and less frequent dressing changes when compared to silver sulfadiazine Physical barrier against bacteria helps prevent infection Prevents wound desiccation Protects healing skin during dressing change	Requires medical personnel familiar with use of the dressing Risk of complications if burn depth is misdiagnosed

care is required. Cover facial burns with a topical antibiotic ointment only.

A large variety of burn-wound dressings have been studied and described. The indications for and the advantages and disadvantages of some of the more commonly used dressings are outlined in Table 132-3.

When using Xeroform gauze, cut it to the appropriate size, apply it to the clean and debrided wound, and cover with a bulky gauze dressing. Change the outer gauze portion of the dressing 2 days after the injury and assess the wound for infection. Leave the Xeroform gauze in place if it is adherent. If the Xeroform is slippery and nonadherent, remove it for wound care and either reapply it or apply an alternate dressing. Once adherent, the Xeroform separates as the wound reepithelializes. Have the parent or patient change the outer gauze daily and trim the drying edges of the Xeroform with scissors. Reevaluate the burn in 5 to 7 days.

Silver sulfadiazine is a topical chemotherapeutic agent. Apply it in a thin layer to a cleaned and debrided burn wound and cover with several layers of fine mesh gauze followed by several layers of roll gauze. With a large wound, apply the cream to the gauze and apply the gauze to the wound. With burns to the fingers or toes, dress each digit individually. Cut tube gauze to form a vest to keep dressings in place on the trunk. Change the dressings twice a day, and clean and debride the wound each time. If the regimen is too difficult for family members to perform, admit the patient or arrange daily follow-up visits.

Biobrane (Winthrop Pharmaceuticals) and DuoDERM (ConvaTec) are recently developed biosynthetic dressings. Biobrane is a semipermeable bilayer dressing that adheres to the wound until spontaneous separation occurs with wound reepithelialization; it allows fluid to escape without letting wound become desiccated.[17] Although there are several types of Biobrane available with different pore sizes, use the regular porous Biobrane for partial-thickness burns.[22] Debride the burn wound and remove intact blisters. Cut the dressing to an appropriate size and apply it under some tension; take care to apply it without wrinkles. For areas with difficult topography, mesh the dressing before application.[18] Secure the dressing with Steri-Strips if needed and cover it with a bulky gauze dressing. The following day, change the outer gauze and inspect the Biobrane for adherence. Adherence is essential to the function of the dressing and usually occurs within 24 to 36 hours.[22] If fluid collections are noted at this first dressing change, aspirate them with a needle. Apply a new Biobrane dressing if the current dressing is nonadherent and the wound is without infection or eschar.[6] Follow the patient closely until complete adherence is documented, and then monitor the wound for signs of infection every other day.[5,6,16] If the dressing fails to adhere by the second day, remove it and apply a different type of dressing. Once the dressing is completely adherent, remove the bulky gauze dressing and apply net gauze. The patient may now bathe and shower normally. As the wound reepithelializes, the dressing becomes detached at the periphery; trim away loose portions of the dressing with scissors.

DuoDERM is an occlusive biosynthetic dressing that interacts with the wound exudate to form a gel, which helps to prevent wound desiccation and helps to protect the wound during dressing changes.[21] Apply the dressing to the debrided wound with a margin of 2 to 3 cm over the normal surrounding skin. Change the dressing every 7 to 10 days or sooner if the dressing leaks or an excessive amount of gel is formed underneath.[1] The patient may bathe and shower normally after the DuoDERM dressing has been applied. Assess the wound at frequent intervals for signs of infection.

Biologic dressings are an alternate type of dressing for clean burns without evidence of infection. Such dressings include cadaveric allografts, porcine skin and cultured skin replacements, and autologous cultured epithelium. These dressings are generally not used in the ED or in an outpatient setting.

Immobilization

During the early part of wound healing, splint wounds over joints in the position of function to protect the new tissue, and elevate the burned extremities between dressing changes to minimize swelling. Later, incorporate passive range-of-motion exercises to prevent contractures. Include physical therapy early in the child's healing process.

Escharotomy

Indications for escharotomy include circumferential burns of the chest or extremities with evidence of vascular or respiratory compromise. The equipment required includes a No. 11 scalpel, gauze to provide pressure for bleeding, and Xero-

form gauze for dressing. Because an escharotomy is performed through insensate full-thickness burns, generally no anesthetics are required. Provide conscious sedation in the awake patient (see Chapters 12 to 16). Make incisions with a scalpel into the subcutaneous tissue only (Fig. 132-2). Usually the devitalized tissue falls aside easily with the knife cut. Extend the incision throughout the burn and a small way into normal tissue; use caution to avoid underlying vascular or neuromuscular structures. Use pressure to control bleeding. After the procedure, observe the patient for signs of improved circulation or ventilation. Apply Xeroform gauze to the wounds.

Excision and Grafting

Excision and grafting is often necessary for full-thickness burns to provide viable tissue for wound healing and to treat bacterial invasion.[4] An obvious full-thickness injury needs grafting within 24 hours to prevent colonization of the eschar. Treat wounds of an indeterminate depth with conservative management for 7 to 10 days.[10] Arrange for excision and grafting by a surgeon skilled in burn-wound management.

Antibiotics and Tetanus

Prophylactic antibiotics are not recommended for burn wounds. Select the appropriate antibiotics on the basis of the results of cultures or wound biopsies.

Because burn wounds are at high risk for tetanus, update the patient's tetanus immunizations when required, as described in Table 130-1, p. 665.[15]

DISPOSITION FROM THE EMERGENCY DEPARTMENT

The American Burn Association's criteria for admission and transfer to a burn center are listed in Box 132-2. The American Burn Association classifies burns as minor, moderate, or major (Box 132-3).[2,18]

FOLLOW-UP CARE

Base the type and frequency of follow-up care on the size, depth, and location of the burn and on the family's resources in dealing with the required treatment regimen. Reevaluate burns that are at high risk for infection or of indeterminate depth within 1 to 2 days. Follow-up the more minor burns within 5 to 7 days. Watch diligently for the development of wound infection, which may be heralded by increasing wound pain, increasing erythema, induration surrounding the wound, or a foul-smelling odor. Refer seriously infected burns to a skilled surgeon because aggressive treatment, including excision and grafting, may be required.

During the healing phase, itching may be intense and scratching may damage the delicate healing wound. Prescribe diphenhydramine or hydroxyzine to help control pruritus. Use moisturizers generously because burn wounds tend to be dry as a result of the destruction of sebaceous glands.[19]

Because healing burn wounds may develop keloids in susceptable patients, refer those with a history of hypertrophic scars for specialized care. For several months after

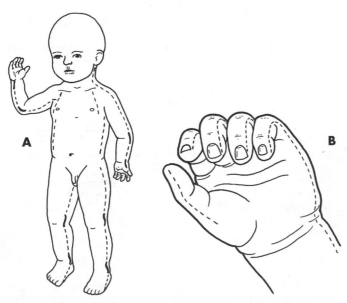

FIG. 132-2   A, Perform escharotomy along the lines indicated. **B,** In the hand, make incisions along the medial and lateral aspects of each digit.

BOX 132-2 AMERICAN BURN ASSOCIATION BURN CENTER REFERRAL CRITERIA

1. Second- and third-degree burns greater than 10% total body surface area (TBSA) in patients under 10 or over 50 years of age
2. Second- and third-degree burns greater than 20% TBSA in other age groups
3. Second- and third-degree burns that involve the face, hands, feet, genitalia, perineum, and major joints
4. Third-degree burns greater than 5% TBSA in any age group
5. Electrical burns, including lightning injury
6. Chemical burns
7. Burn injury with inhalation injury
8. Burn injury in patients with preexisting medical disorders that could complicate management, prolong recovery, or affect mortality
9. Any patients with burns and concomitant trauma (e.g., fractures), in which the burn injury poses the greatest risk for morbidity or mortality In such cases, if the trauma poses the greater immediate risk, the patient may be treated initially in a trauma center until stable before being transferred to a burn center. Physician judgment is necessary in such situations and should be in concert with the regional medical control plan and triage protocols
10. Hospitals without qualified personnel or equipment for the care of children should transfer children with burns to a burn center with these capabilities
11. Burn injury in patients who require special social, emotional, or long-term rehabilitative support, including cases involving suspected child abuse or substance abuse

---

From American Burn Association: Hospital and prehospital resources for optimal care of patients with burn injury: guidelines for development and operation of burn centers, *J Burn Rehabil* 11:97-104, 1990.

BOX 132-3 AMERICAN BURN ASSOCIATION BURN SEVERITY CLASSIFICATION

Minor pediatric burns

First- or second-degree burns less than 10% BSA
Third-degree burns less than 2% BSA and not involving the eyes, ears, face, or perineum

Moderate pediatric burns

Second-degree burns 10% to 20% BSA
Third-degree burns 2% to 10% BSA

Major pediatric burns

Second-degree burns greater than 20% BSA

From Punch JD, Smith DJ, Robson MC: Hospital care of major burns, *Postgrad Med* 85(1): 205-214, 1989.

the injury, the healed wound will be sensitive to trauma, including sunburn; therefore apply sunscreens diligently for at least 1 year after the injury.

REFERENCES

1. Afilalo M, et al: DuoDERM hydroactive dressing versus silver sulphadiazine/Bactigras in the emergency treatment of partial-thickness skin burns, *Burns* 18(4):313-316, 1992.
2. American Burn Association: Hospital and prehospital resources for optimal care of patients with burn injury: guidelines for development and operation of burn centers, *J Burn Rehabil* 11(2):97-104, 1990.
3. Dries DJ, Waxman K: Adequate resuscitation of burn patients may not be measured by urine output and vital signs, *Crit Care Med* 19(3):327-329, 1991.
4. Finkelstein JL, et al: Pediatric burns: an overview, *Pediatr Clin North Am* 39(5):1145-1163, 1992.
5. Gerding RL, Imbembo AL, Fratianne RB: Biosynthetic skin substitute vs 1% silver sulfadiazine for treatment of inpatient partial-thickness thermal burns, *J Trauma* 28(8):1265-1269, 1988.
6. Gerding RL, et al: Outpatient management of partial-thickness burns: biobrane versus 1% silver sulfadiazine, *Ann Emerg Med* 19(2):121-124, 1990.
7. Graves TA, et al: Fluid resuscitation of infants and children with massive thermal injury, *J Trauma* 28(12):1656-1659, 1988.
8. Hazinski MF, et al: Pediatric injury prevention, *Ann Emerg Med* 22(2):456-467, 1993.
9. Herndon DN, Rutan RL, Rutan TC: Management of the pediatric patient with burns, *J Burn Care Rehabil* 14(1):3-8, 1993.
10. Herndon DN, et al: Management of burn injuries. In Eichelberger M, editor: *Pediatric trauma, prevention, acute care, rehabilitation*, St Louis, 1993, Mosby.
11. Katcher ML: Scald burns from hot tap water, *JAMA* 246(1):1219-1222, 1981.
12. McLoughlin E, Mcguire A: The causes, cost, and prevention of childhood burn injuries, *Am J Dis Child* 144:677-683, 1990.
13. McLoughlin E, Brigham PA: Stop carelessness? No, reduce burn risk, *Pediatr Ann* 21(7):423-428, 1992.
14. Peate WF: Outpatient management of burns, *Am Fam Physician* 45(3):1321-1330, 1992.
15. Peter G, editor: *Report of the committee on infectious diseases*, ed 22, Elk Grove, Ill, 1991, American Academy of Pediatrics.
16. Phillips LG, Robson MC, Heggers JP: Treating minor burns: ice, grease, or what? *Postgrad Med* 85(1):219-222, 1989.
17. Phillips LG, et al: Uses and abuses of a biosynthetic dressing for partial–skin thickness burns, *Burns* 15(4):254-256, 1989.
18. Punch JD, Smith DJ, Robson MC: Hospital care of major burns, *Postgrad Med* 85(1):205-214, 1989.
19. Schonfeld N: Outpatient management of burns in children, *Pediatr Emerg Care* 6(3):249-253, 1990.
20. Williams RJ, Porvaznik J: Initial resuscitation of major burn patients, *J Fam Pract* 28(1):42-50, 1989.
21. Wyatt D, McGowan DN, Najarian MP: Comparison of a hydrocolloid dressing and silver sulfadiazine cream in the outpatient management of second-degree burns, *J Trauma* 30(7):857-865, 1990.
22. Yang JY, Tsai YC, Noordhoff MS: Clinical comparison of commercially available Biobrane preparations, *Burns* 15(3):197-203, 1989.

133 Animal Bites

Mary Workman Rutherford

Human and animal bites are common pediatric complaints in Emergency Departments (EDs). Although the complications of bites are relatively well understood, many aspects of their treatment remain controversial.

Approximately 1% of ED visits involve bites, and each year in the United States approximately 10,000 patients require hospitalization for complications of animal bites.[21] The large majority of bites brought to medical attention are dog bites (80% to 85%), followed by cat (5% to 10%), human (5% to 10%), and rodent (1% to 2%) bites.[5,33] The majority of these patients are between 10 and 30 years of age, and the second greatest number are under 5 years of age.[1,25]

Indications

All animal bites require basic wound management. Table 133-2 lists the indications for antibiotic prophylaxis. Table 130-1 provides indications for tetanus prophylaxis. Table 133-1 lists the indications for rabies prophylaxis, and Box 133-1 lists the indications for hospitalization.[18]

Contraindications

There are no contraindications to wound management of animal bites. However, management of airway, breathing, and circulation, as well as evaluation and treatment of intracranial hemorrhage, take precedence over wound care if the bite is severe, especially if there is massive tissue avulsion (e.g., pit bull or exotic animal bites) or if there is a potential penetrating skull injury (e.g., crush injury of an infant's head).

Primary wound closure is relatively contraindicated for deep puncture wounds, including most cat bites, wounds in immunocompromised hosts, hand wounds in general, human bites other than superficial wounds, and wounds more than 24 hours old at presentation. Primary closure is absolutely contraindicated for wounds already clinically infected at presentation and for closed-fist injuries.

Complications

Dog bites most commonly involve the lower extremities, followed by the hands, arms, face, and trunk. Cat bites usually involve the hands, followed by the arms, lower extremities, face, and trunk.[21,33] Bites to infants and young children often occur on the face,[7,11,20] especially with dogs, rodents, and (rarely) pet ferrets.[28,30] Bite injuries to the face are most common in infants; complications, especially those involving infection, can be severe and involve the nose, lips, ears, eyelids, skull, or orbits.[20,34] Human bites can and do occur in young children and, although often inflicted by siblings, can be a sign of child abuse.[22] In older children, human bites most often are the result of fights with other children and can typically involve the hands and face.

> **BOX 133-1   INDICATIONS FOR HOSPITALIZATION FOR ANIMAL BITES**
>
> Intravenous antibiotic treatment required for wound infection
> Rapidly progressive cellulitis, lymphangitis, lymphadenitis, tenosynovitis, or septic arthritis
> Major trauma from large animals
> Craniofacial injuries in infants
> Fever or other signs of systemic infection

Table 133-1   Rabies Postexposure Prophylaxis

Animal type	Evaluation and disposition of animal	Postexposure prophylaxis recommendations
Dogs and cats	Healthy and available for 10-day observation	Do not begin prophylaxis unless animal develops symptoms of rabies*
	Rabid or suspected rabid	Immediate vaccination
	Unknown (escaped)	Consult public health officials
Skunks, raccoons, bats, foxes, and most other carnivores; woodchucks	Regard as rabid unless geographic area is known to be free of rabies or until animal proven negative by laboratory tests†	Immediate vaccination
Livestock, rodents, and lagomorphs (rabbits and hares)	Consider individually	Consult public health officials; bites of squirrels, hamsters, guinea pigs, gerbils, chipmunks, rats, mice, other rodents, rabbits, and hares almost never require antirabies treatment

From Immunizations Practices Advisory Committee: Rabies prevention—United States, 1991, *MMWR* 4D[RR3]:1, 1991.
*During the 10-day holding period, begin treatment with HRIG and HDCV or RVA at first sign of rabies in a dog or cat that has bitten someone. The symptomatic animal should be killed immediately and tested.
†The animal should be killed and tested as soon as possible. Holding for observation is not recommended. Discontinue vaccine if immunofluorescence test results of the animal are negative.

Human-bite injuries to the hands are often sustained over the metacarpophalangeal joints (closed-fist injuries),[22,23] and human bites to the face typically include lacerations, puncture wounds, and avulsions of the tip of the nose, earlobes and, in the case of falls or seizures, the tongue.[22]

The most common infectious complication of a bite is bacterial infection; the predominant species of bacteria is a function of the oral flora of the biting animal. For human bites, most infections are a result of mixtures of oral and skin flora (Table 133-2), including *Staphylococcus* spp., *Streptococcus* spp., *Eikenella corrodens,* gram-negative enterics, and other aerobic and anaerobic oral flora.[3,15,31]

Most infections that result from animal bites are polymicrobial, with between 2.8 and 3.6 bacterial species isolated per wound culture.[16,33] In general, the bacterial oral flora inoculated into the wound by the bites of most mammalian species is similar to human flora (see Table 133-2).[3,12] However, there are important exceptions to this generalization. *Pasteurella multocida* infection is a relatively common sequela of cat bites and usually occurs within the first 24 hours; although less common, this infection can also occur following bites by dogs and other species.[3,12,33] Other significant aerobic pathogens not found in human bites are *Capnocytophaga canimorsus*[9] and *Staphylococcus intermedius.*[32] Additionally, *Streptobacillus moniliformis* and *Spirillum minus,* the agents of rat-bite fever, can complicate the bites of several small rodents.[8,27] However, in one large Los Angeles study that reviewed 50 rat bites in children, Ordog, Balasubramamium, and Wasserberger[28] were unable to isolate these organisms from any case. In addition to the more common pathogens listed in Table 133-2, there have been reports of unusual systemic infections after animal and human bites, including rat-bite fever, tularemia, plague, cat-scratch fever, leptospirosis, brucellosis, syphilis, tuberculosis, and hepatitis B.[33,35]

Less common bacterial complications of both human and animal bites are septic arthritis, tenosynovitis, osteomyelitis, meningitis, brain abscess, disseminated intravascular coagulopathy, and endocarditis. Closed-fist injuries, especially those involving penetration of the metacarpophalangeal capsule, can lead to deep space infections, septic arthritis, and osteomyelitis; *E. corrodens* can be isolated in approximately 25% of these injuries, and anaerobic bacteria are present in more than half of these infections.[12] Bites can be puncture wounds, crush injuries, or both. Dog bites typically result in crush injuries, which appear clinically as avulsions and lacerations, whereas cats, whose jaws are not as strong, produce puncture wounds that can involve deeper structures such as tendons and joint capsules.[10] The pathology of bites results from not only the direct injury but also, and often more importantly, from contamination of the site with oral flora from the saliva and teeth of the biting animal. Various clinical series and case reports have documented the microbiology of infections associated with dog and cat bites,* human bites,[2,15,23,31] and bites of more exotic animals[33] (see Table 133-2). In addition, skin flora and environmental debris can further contaminate the wound.

---

*References 3, 10, 12-16, 24, 29, and 33.

Equipment

The equipment required for wound care is outlined in Chapter 131. For irrigation use an 18- to 20-gauge needle or intravenous catheter and a 15- to 20-ml syringe. For immobilization, use splints, bulky gauze dressings, and slings.

Techniques

Techniques for the management of bites include three separate therapeutic decisions: management of the wound, including consideration of primary closure; prophylaxis for bacterial infection and tetanus; and consideration of postexposure prophylaxis for rabies (Box 133-2).

Wound Management

GENERAL MANAGEMENT. The general management of human and animal bites is copious irrigation and, wherever anatomically possible, meticulous debridement both to decrease the risk of infection and to improve cosmetic outcome (Box 133-3).[5] In one study, irrigation decreased the risk of infection following a dog bite from 69% to 12%;[4] cat bites tend to be deeper puncture wounds and are associated with a higher infection rate, partly because of difficulty in adequately irrigating a narrow, deep wound.[10] Examine wounds carefully for damage to underlying structures; if damage is present, evaluate these injuries clinically and radiographically. Evaluation is especially important for closed-fist injuries, where fractures, disruption of the joint capsule, and retained foreign bodies can occur.[22] Additional important steps in wound management are immobilization and elevation of injured extremities;[28] these steps are especially important for closed-fist injuries.[23] Because of the potential for infection, patients need close follow-up, especially if they are being treated as outpatients.

PRIMARY WOUND CLOSURE. The long-standing controversy surrounding primary closure of bites has not been resolved. There has been a trend toward primary closure, especially of dog bites, where data from controlled trials indicate lower rates of wound infection following careful wound toilet and primary closure.[4,6,36] Cat bites usually cannot be closed because of the difficulty in cleaning the puncture wounds adequately. However, large lacerations or severe facial injuries inflicted by cats can be adequately irrigated and debrided; in such cases perform either primary closure or delayed primary closure.[35] Noninfected human bites, especially those involving the face and those less than 12 hours old, can sometimes be sutured.[22,26] If in doubt, do not suture, and close the wound with Steri-Strips or skin closure tapes. For human bites with signs and symptoms of infection, allow healing by secondary intention and recommend scar revision at a later date if necessary.[22] However, in any therapeutic scheme observe all bite wounds for signs of cellulitis; if the wound begins to suppurate, remove the sutures and further irrigate and debride the wound as described in Box 133-3.

Antibiotic Prophylaxis. Antibiotic prophylaxis of adequately irrigated and debrided and clinically uninfected bites has not been substantiated.[11,17] However, most practitioners continue to use antibiotics to prophylactically treat bites that are at higher risk of infection (Box 133-4).[11,12,19,33] Large, fresh lacerations that can be thoroughly irrigated and debrided; bites to the face, scalp, and mouth (except in infants); and most dog and rodent bites pose a lower risk of

Table 133-2   Management of Common Bites

Animal	Main pathogens	Anatomic sites	Primary wound closure	Antibiotic prophylaxis	Tetanus prophylaxis	Rabies prophylaxis	Comments
Dogs	Staphylococci	Face	+	−	+	Rarely; consider if stray, unprovoked attack, ill-appearing, or uncaptured	In infants, antibiotics may be indicated for facial wounds
	Streptococci	Hands, feet	−	+	+		
	Pasteurella spp.						
	Gram-negative organisms						
	Anaerobes	Trunk, extremities	+	−	+		
Cats	*Pasteurella* spp.	Face	±	+	+	Rarely; same as above for dogs	Wound closure suggested for large or disfiguring wounds; prophylaxis less necessary for superficial wounds
	Staphylococci	Hands, feet	−	+	+		
	Streptococci						
	Gram-negative organisms						
	Anaerobes	Trunks, extremities	±	+	+		
Humans	*Eikenella* spp.	Face	±	± +	+	No	Consider admission for IV antibiotic prophylaxis for closed-fist injuries; consider delayed primary closure of older or very dirty wounds
	Staphylococci	Hands, feet	−	+	+		
	Streptococci						
	Gram-negative organisms	Trunk, extremities	±	±	+		

BOX 133-2 SCHEMATIC MANAGEMENT BITES

Wound management
    Anesthesia
    Irrigation
    Debridement
    Irrigation
    Closure (if indicated)
    Immobilization and elevation (if indicated)
Prophylaxis for bacterial infection
    Antibiotic prophylaxis
    Tetanus prophylaxis
Rabies prophylaxis
Close follow-up and observation

---

coverage. Various regimens that have been advocated include dicloxacillin plus penicillin (especially for human bites), amoxicillin/clavulanic acid, penicillin alone (especially for cat bites), third-generation cephalosporins and, for patients who are allergic to penicillin, erythromycin (which does not provide particularly good coverage for *P. multocida* or *E. corrodens*) or tetracycline. If a decision is made to treat with prophylactic antibiotics, administer the first dose in the ED. Treat for 3 to 5 days. For treatment of clinically infected bites, establish a specific bacteriologic diagnosis. Pending culture results, include coverage for *Staphylococcus aureus*, penicillin-sensitive oral flora, *E. corrodens* in human bites, *P. multocida* in cat and dog bites, and gram-negative enterics for immunocompromised hosts. Ordinarily, dicloxacillin is a good first choice.

Tetanus is a possibility with any mammalian bite. Admin-

BOX 133-3 SURGICAL MANAGEMENT OF BITES

1. To avoid the inoculation of organisms, anesthetize the wound by injecting through intact skin at the edge of the wound rather than through the wound.
2. Irrigate the wound with several hundred milliliters of sterile normal saline solution under pressure. To achieve approximately 20 pounds per square inch of pressure, use an 18- to 20-gauge needle on a 15- to 20-ml syringe. Alternatively, for a bacteriocidal effect, use a 9:1 dilution of 10% povidine-iodine solution in normal saline to make a 1% solution for irrigation.[19] This solution does not kill the rabies virus. To avoid further tissue damage, do not irrigate the wound with solutions such as benzalkonium chloride, ethyl alcohol, quaternary ammonium compounds, chlorhexidine, and hydrogen peroxide.[19]
3. Explore the wound. Inspect for deep structure injury or penetration into areas such as the joint space and synovial sheath.
4. Debride the wound. Surgically debride all devitalized tissue and remove any foreign matter from the wound. Surgically excise wound margins in areas where anatomically and cosmetically possible.[4] This procedure decreases the risk of infection, facilitates repair, and leads to a better cosmetic outcome.
5. Reirrigate following debridement.
6. Consider wound closure (see text). When closure is indicated, use as few subcutaneous sutures as possible and occlude the wound with a pressure dressing to minimize dead space.[19] Wound tapes (e.g., Steri-Strips or skin closure tapes) may be used to reinforce the sutured wound.
7. Immobilize and elevate the wound. For closed-fist injuries, use a molded plaster splint in the position of greatest function, and dress it with a bulky gauze dressing. Begin range-of-motion exercises early in the follow-up period.

BOX 133-4 HIGH-RISK ANIMAL BITES REQUIRING ANTIBIOTIC PROPHYLAXIS

Bites to the hand, wrist, or foot in all age groups and to the face and scalp in infants
Puncture wounds and crush injuries that cannot be adequately debrided
Bites involving immunocompromised hosts
Human bites to the hand and full-thickness cat and nonhuman-primate bites
Bites more than 8 to 12 hours old at presentation

---

ister postexposure tetanus prophylaxis for any penetrating wound in a patient who has not been adequately immunized (see Table 130-1, p. 665).

Rabies Prophylaxis. Rabies is the single most important complication of animal bites. Consider postexposure prophylaxis carefully for every animal bite. Rabies is an almost uniformly fatal viral disease and is transmitted by the saliva of infected mammals. Animals most likely to be rabid in the United States are skunks, bats, raccoons (currently limited to the eastern states), and foxes.[18] Although extensive rabies vaccination and animal control programs have dramatically reduced the risk in urban areas, rabies does occur in domestic and peridomestic animals, including dogs, cats (especially feral cats), horses, and cattle.

Make decisions regarding rabies postexposure prophylaxis on the basis of the animal species involved, the vaccination status of the animal, the behavior of the animal at the time of the attack, whether the attack was provoked or unprovoked, and the epidemiology of rabies in the area the exposure occurred.[18] Table 133-1 outlines the approach to postexposure rabies prophylaxis currently recommended by the Cen-

infection and typically do not require prophylactic antibiotics. The choice of antibiotics for prophylaxis remains controversial.* Because most human and animal bite–wound infections are polymicrobial, use broad-spectrum antibiotic

---

*References 3, 6, 12, 13, 16, 24, and 33.

ters for Disease Control and Prevention. In general, postexposure prophylaxis is indicated when bites involve wild mammals (e.g., skunks, foxes, raccoons in the eastern United States, bats) and either the animal cannot be captured or, if the animal is captured, there is pathologic evidence of rabies infection.[18] In addition, use postexposure prophylax is for patients when bites involve dogs, cats, or livestock that either showed abnormally aggressive behavior and subsequently escaped or develop clinical signs of rabies while quarantined (see Table 133-1). Rabies prophylaxis is generally not indicated for bites from rodents and lagomorphs (e.g., rabbits).

When a dog, cat, or other domestic animal is in quarantine, do not start prophylaxis as long as the animal's clinical state remains normal (see Table 133-1).[18] Questions about the need for postexposure rabies prophylaxis can be directed to local and state health departments, who generally maintain 24-hour consultation services. Treatment for rabies includes both active immunization with human diploid cell vaccine (HDCV) and passive immunization with rabies immune globulin (RIG) at a dose of 20 IU/kg of body weight.[18] For bites up to 1 week old, give both RIG and HDCV if the possibility of a rabies exposure exists; for the treatment of older bites, consult local and state health departments or an infectious disease consultant regarding the use of RIG. Administer HDCV in six doses at 0, 1, 3, 7, 14, and 28 days after exposure. Where anatomically possible, infiltrate half of the RIG dose around the wound site and the remainder in a site distant from the vaccine site (HDCV).[18]

Remarks

Indications for the hospitalization of children are outlined in Box 133-1. Use aerobic and anaerobic wound and blood cultures to guide antibiotic therapy. The presence of deep bites to an infant's skull requires a cranial computed tomography scan to exclude intracranial injury.

REFERENCES

1. Avner JR, Baker MD: Dog bites in urban children, *Pediatrics* 33:55, 1991.
2. Baker MD, Moore SE: Human bites in children: a six-year experience, *Am J Dis Child* 141:1285, 1987.
3. Brook I: Microbiology of human and animal bite wounds in children, *Pediatr Infect Dis J* 6:29, 1987.
4. Callaham M: Treatment of common dog bites: infection risk factors, *J Am Coll Emerg Phys* 7:83, 1978.
5. Callaham M: Dog bite wounds, *JAMA* 244:2327, 1980.
6. Callaham M: Prophylactic antibiotics in common dog bite wounds: a controlled study, *Ann Emerg Med* 9:410, 1980.
7. Chun YT, Berkelhamer JE, Herold TE: Dog bites in children less than 4 years old, *Pediatrics* 69:119, 1982.
8. Cole JS, Stoll RW, Bulger RJ: Rat-bite fever: report of three cases, *Ann Intern Med* 71:979, 1969.
9. Danker WM, Davis CE, Thompson MA: DF-2 bacteremia following a dog bite in a 4-month-old child, *Pediatr Infect Dis J* 6:695, 1987.
10. Dire DJ: Cat bite wounds: risk factors for infection, *Ann Emerg Med* 20:973, 1991.
11. Dire DJ: Emergency management of dog and cat bite wounds, *Emerg Clin North Am* 10:719, 1992.
12. Goldstein EJC: Bite wounds and infection, *Clin Infect Dis* 14:633, 1992.
13. Goldstein EJC, Citron DM, Finegold SM: Dog bite wound and infection: a prospective clinical study, *Ann Emerg Med* 9:508, 1980.
14. Goldstein EJC, Citron DM, Finegold SM: Role of anaerobic bacteria in bite wound infections, *Rev Infect Dis* 6(suppl 1):S177, 1984.
15. Goldstein EJC, Citron DM, Wield B, et al: Bacteriology of human and animal bite wounds, *J Clin Microbiol* 8:667, 1978.
16. Goldstein EJC, Reinhardt JF, Murray PM, et al: Outpatient therapy of bite wounds: demographic data, bacteriology, and a prospective, randomized trial of amoxicillin/clavulanic acid versus penicillin +/− dicloxacillin, *Int J Dermatol* 26:123, 1987.
17. Guy RJ, Zook EG: Successful treatment of acute head and neck dog bite wounds without antibiotics, *Ann Plast Surg* 17:45, 1986.
18. Immunizations Practices Advisory Committee: Rabies prevention—United States, 1991, *MMWR* 40(RR 3):1, 1991.
19. Karkal SS, Tandberg D, Talan DA: Minimizing morbidity and mortality from mammalian bites, *Emerg Med Rep* 11:1, 1990.
20. Karlson TA: The incidence of facial injuries from dog bites, *JAMA* 251:3265, 1984.
21. Kizer KW, Town M: Epidemiologic and clinical aspects of animal injuries, *J Am Coll Emerg Phys* 8:134, 1979.
22. Leung AKC, Robson WLM: Human bites in children, *Pediatr Emerg Care* 8:255, 1992.
23. Mann RJ, Hoffeld TA, Farmer CB: Human bites of the hand: twenty years of experience, *J Hand Surg* 2:97, 1977.
24. Marcy SM: Special series: management of pediatric infectious diseases in office practice: infections due to dog and cat bites, *Pediatr Infect Dis* 1:351, 1982.
25. Marr J, Beck A, Lugo J: An epidemiologic study of the human bite, *Public Health Rep* 94:514, 1979.
26. Martin LT: Human bites: guidelines for prompt evaluation and treatment, *Postgrad Med* 81:221, 1987.
27. McGill RC, Martin AM, Edmunds PN: Rat-bite fever due to *Streptobacillus moniliformis*, *Brit Med J* 1:1213, 1966.
28. Ordog GJ, Balasubramamium S, Wasserberger J: Rat bites; fifty cases, *Ann Emerg Med* 14:126, 1985.
29. Ordog GJ: The bacteriology of dog bite wounds on initial presentation, *Ann Emerg Med* 15:1324, 1986.
30. Paisley HW, Lauer BA: Severe facial injuries to infants due to unprovoked attacks by pet ferrets, *JAMA* 259:2005, 1988.
31. Schmidt DR, Heckman JD: *Eikenella corrodens* in human bite infections of the hand, *J Trauma* 23:478, 1983.
32. Talan DA, Goldstein EJC, Staatz D, Overturf GD: *Staphylococcus intermedius:* clinical presentation of a new human dog bite pathogen, *Ann Emerg Med* 18:410, 1989.
33. Weber DJ, Hansen AR: Infections resulting from animal bites, *Infect Dis Clin North Am* 5:663, 1991.
34. Wilberger JE Jr, Pang D: Craniofacial injuries from dog bites, *JAMA* 249:2685, 1983.
35. Wiley JF Jr: Mammalian bites: review of evaluation and management, *Clin Pediatr* 29:283, 1990.
36. Zook EG, Miller M, van Beek AL, et al: Successful treatment protocol for canine fang injuries, *J Trauma* 20:243, 1980.

134 Envenomations

Jonathan Grisham

Stings and envenomations by animals, insects, and reptiles are a common occurrence but usually cause little harm and do not usually require medical attention. However, each year as many as 1 million individuals come to the emergency department (ED) with illnesses or injuries caused by stings and envenomations; children are especially vulnerable. Although other creatures may be more frightening, inflict more severe injuries, or have more potent toxins, the bee is responsible for the majority of fatalities as a result of bee-sting anaphylaxis.

Venomous animals possess specific venom-producing glands and an apparatus for injecting the toxic materials, which are used for offensive (killing prey) or defensive purposes. Venoms vary widely in their actions and potencies, causing tissue necrosis, allergic reactions, and toxic effects on virtually any organ system of the victim. The severity of an envenomation depends on the potency and volume of the venom injected and on a variety of host factors. For all envenomations, basic wound-care principles and general supportive care are the mainstays of initial treatment. Although antivenins are available for the bites of certain species, they are usually derived from horse serum and often cause serum sickness or hypersensitivity reactions. Generally reserve the use of antivenin for severe envenomations that are causing systemic symptoms or for those occurring in small children or debilitated hosts.

Chapter 131 describes the management of soft tissue injuries from bites. This chapter discusses emergency procedures to treat envenomations. With the exception of antivenin, no special equipment or materials are required in the treatment of envenomations.

INVERTEBRATE BITES AND STINGS

Although most bug bites are relatively harmless, some can result in serious morbidity and even mortality.[3,6,10] Envenomation can cause local tissue toxicity (e.g., brown recluse spider[7]), systemic toxicity (e.g., black widow spider[9]), or allergic or anaphylactic reactions (e.g., Hymenoptera). Table 134-1 lists the characteristics and management of the most clinically important bites and stings.

Indications. Basic first aid measures, cool compresses, and analgesics are indicated for any bite or sting. In the ED, also consider tetanus prophylaxis. Provide supportive care and appropriate drug therapy for patients who develop any allergic or systemic reactions. Administer antivenin for patients with severe systemic reactions to black widow spider envenomations.

Contraindications. There are no specific contraindications to caring for invertebrate envenomation injuries with simple wound care. Avoid surgical incision of lesions and intralesional steroid injections because none of these procedures have any proven value and may cause disfigurement.

Complications. The careless use of ice directly on bite wounds may worsen the local tissue injury. Excisional or injection procedures on the lesion may result in cosmetic problems or wound complications. Certain methods of tick removal may increase the likelihood of local cellulitis, retention of foreign bodies (tick body parts), or enhanced transmission of tickborne illnesses. The administration of antivenin can lead to both immediate and delayed hypersensitivity reactions.

Techniques. Regardless of the animal involved, provide local wound care, including gentle cleansing of the area, debridement, and removal of embedded stingers.[5,11] Treat mild pain with cold compresses, but use ice with caution to avoid excessive vasoconstriction. Consider tetanus prophylaxis. If needed, infiltrate a local anesthetic around the wound but not into the lesion. Treat persistent or severe pain with analgesics. Administer antipruritics to control pruritis.[9,11]

Because allergic reactions to *Hymenoptera* stings cause the greatest mortality,[6] be prepared to manage such reactions. The normal response to a bee sting is a small, painful, pruritic lesion that resolves within a few hours. Treat such local inflammation from a single sting with a cool compress and possibly diphenhydramine if itching is pronounced; discharge the patient after a brief period of observation.

Administer subcutaneous epinephrine (1:1000 concentration at 0.01 ml/kg) (maximum subcutaneous dose = 0.3 mg) or intravenous epinephrine (1:10,000 concentration) at 0.10 ml/kg (maximum dose = 1 mg) to any child with a sting accompanied by bronchospasm, stridor, or urticaria. Add an inhaled β-agonist, oxygen, and steroids for bronchospasm. Consider administering diphenhydramine (1 mg/kg) intramuscularly or intravenously. If symptoms resolve and there are no respiratory findings, discharge the patient with careful instructions and 3 to 5 days of oral diphenhydramine. With persistent urticaria, wheezing, or other systemic signs, hospitalize the child and continue therapy with antihistamines, epinephrine, and hydrocortisone. Continue to treat wheezing with an inhaled β-agonist as needed. Aggressively manage the respiratory and cardiovascular effects of anaphylaxis with appropriate ventilatory and fluid support.

SNAKE BITES: GENERAL PRINCIPLES

As many as fifty thousand snake bites occur in the United States each year; most are caused by nonvenomous snakes and are generally innocuous.[2,8] However, thousands of bites by venomous species do occur each year; many of these bites occur in children and adolescents. The results of such envenomations can range from no or minimal symptoms to severe toxicity and death.* As many as 50% of the bites from

---

*References 2, 3, 6, 8, 10, and 11.

Table 134-1   Characteristics of Important Invertebrate Bites and Stings

Organism	Effects	Management	Comments
Black widow spider (*Latrodectus mactans*)	Latrodectism Neuromuscular toxicity No local symptoms except pain, which can radiate Wide variety of nonspecific symptoms; nausea/vomiting Generalized pain and muscular rigidity Mild-to-severe hypertension Respiratory distress	Antivenin (2.5 ml IV over 30 min) if under 40 kg or if larger with respiratory distress or hypertension Opiates and a muscle relaxant (diazepam) PRN 10% calcium gluconate solution, 0.5 ml/kg/dose IV over 5 min for severe muscular cramping	Female is shiny black with red hourglass on abdomen Found throughout United States Potential reactions to antivenin; thus use only with more severe symptoms and skin test beforehand Calcium infusions are only minimally effective
Brown recluse spider	Loxoscelism Systemic symptoms occur only in small children Spectrum of reaction from minor local inflammation to severe tissue necrosis Local pain within hours, then erythema and central blister Enlarging area of discoloration over a few days, then rupture of blister and ulceration	No approved antivenin available yet Supportive care for systemic symptoms General principles of wound care If enlarging area of necrosis, aggressive debridement or excision Dapsone may be useful for adults but is contraindicated in children	Small, shy spider with violin-shaped mark on back Some wounds may need eventual skin grafting
Tarantula	Mild venom produces only minimal local reactions	General wound care	Rarely bite unless provoked
Scorpion (*Centruroides* spp.)	Excitatory neurotoxicity affects autonomic and neuromuscular systems Local pain, autonomic hyperactivity, seizures, respiratory distress	General supportive care Local anesthetic for pain Antivenin available for severe symptoms only Phenobarbital for agitation and seizures	Many species not harmful *C. sculpturatus* (southwest US) is potentially lethal Use of narcotics for pain may increase risk of arrhythmias
Centipede	Bites are painful, but mild toxin produces only local symptoms	General wound care Systemic analgesic or local anesthetic for pain	Millipedes are harmless but secrete a toxin that causes dermatitis
Hymenoptera (bee, hornet, wasp, yellow jacket)	Painful stings Reactions are primarily allergic and vary from local inflammation to mild systemic symptoms (itch, urticaria, wheezing) to severe anaphylaxis	Local wound care; avoid squeezing embedded stingers during removal Treatment based on severity of symptoms and includes cool compresses, antihistamines, IV fluids, epinephrine, hydrocortisone	This class causes 50% of all mortality from venomous bites and stings Children with significant systemic reactions should carry an emergency insect sting kit (with epinephrine) and consider hyposensitization
Fire ant	Inflicts multiple stings Toxin affects mast cells Immediate wheal and flare then central vesicle Local pain, erythema, and induration can last 10 days	Routine local wound care Antihistamines for pruritis	Primarily in southern United States Painful sting, but systemic reactions are uncommon
Tick	Bites are painless Can transmit wide variety of infectious diseases and cause tick paralysis	Complete removal of tick without injecting saliva or leaving head embedded Pull out with fine forceps, grasping the mouth part and pulling upward[5]	Painless bites necessitate careful skin surveys in endemic areas Repellent to prevent bites Many popular methods of removal; mostly ineffective

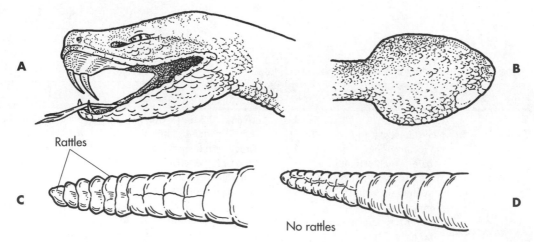

FIG. 134-1   Physical characteristics of venomous pit vipers. Pit vipers have a characteristic pit located midway between the eye and nostril (**A**), a triangular head and elliptic pupils (**B**), and a single row of subcaudal plates that may end with a rattle in some species (**C** and **D**). Note that the color and pattern of the snake's skin are not reliable in identifying species.

venomous snakes result in little or no envenomation. Many variables influence the severity of a particular bite.

The vast majority of reptile envenomations in this country involve snakes of the Crotalidae (pit viper) family, which includes rattlesnakes, water moccasins, and copperheads. The remaining few percent of bites are inflicted by the coral snake (family Elapidae) and various imported exotic snakes.[2,3]

Indications. Perform simple first aid measures and local wound care for all snake bites. Transport all suspected envenomation injuries to a medical center for definitive care. Provide supportive and symptomatic care, and consider antivenin when patients demonstrate systemic reactions. Consider tetanus prophylaxis.

Contraindications. There are no specific contraindications to simple wound care of snake bites. Fasciotomy or wound excision is contraindicated except in rare instances. Cryotherapy and electrical shock treatments are absolutely contraindicated because of their lack of efficacy and demonstrated harmful effects.

Complications. The inappropriate or incorrect use of tourniquets, the incision or excision of bites, and the application of cryotherapy or shock treatment can worsen local and regional tissue injury and may lead to amputation. The side effects of antivenin therapy include immediate and delayed reactions of variable severity. The injudicious use of fasciotomy can result in infection, scarring, and long-term limb disabilities.

Techniques. When a snakebite occurs, first assess whether a venomous species is responsible. Some venomous snakes have certain features (Fig. 134-1) and generally leave identifiable fang marks. Institute management in the field if the snake is a venomous species or if there are clinical signs of envenomation. Separate the patient from the snake and keep

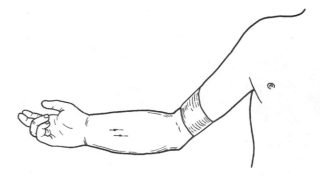

FIG. 134-2   Procedure for field management of pit-viper bites. If definitive care is more than 1 hour away, the wound is less than 5 minutes old, and the wound is on an extremity, apply a constriction band as shown. Place a band that is at least 1-inch wide circumferentially around the affected extremity just proximal to the bite or any area of swelling. Wrap the band tightly enough to obstruct venous and lymph drainage but not arterial blood flow. Consider incision and suction of the bite wound; to do this, make a single, straight, shallow incision through the fang mark and always along the long axis of the extremity. Apply suction with a syringe or a commercial devise such as The Extractor. Use oral suction only if there are no oral sores or cavities. Continue suction for at least 30 to 60 minutes.

him or her warm and calm; give the patient nothing by mouth. Remove all jewelry, cleanse the wound, and keep the affected limb immobile and at the level of the heart. If close to definitive care, transport the patient rapidly to an ED. For Crotalidae bites only, consider applying a lymphatic constriction band and performing incision and suction of the bite wound (Fig. 134-2) within 5 minutes of the injury; perform this procedure only if definitive care is not immediately available. These measures are of equivocal value; do not delay transport to an ED. Do not apply ice or administer electric shock treatments.

In the ED, institute or continue general supportive care

(Box 134-1), local wound care, and pain management. Obtain baseline laboratory studies and administer broad-spectrum antibiotics for all severe envenomations. Immediately obtain antivenin; it is the mainstay of therapy. Most local poison control centers and many zoos keep an index of available stocks. Because of the potentially severe reactions to equine serum, perform a preliminary skin test as described in the package insert before administering antivenin. Perform skin testing *only* if antivenin is to be used. Such tests may be a poor predictor of a patient's reaction to antivenin; the results should be weighed in relationship to other factors in deciding whether to administer antivenin treatment.

SNAKE BITES: SPECIFIC MANAGEMENT TECHNIQUES
Pit Vipers

The Crotalidae family of snakes causes the vast majority of problematic snakebites in the United States. Although each species may have different effects on the victims, the basic approach to management is fairly uniform, and a single antivenin is effective against all members of this family.

Bites initially produce prominent local effects, including pain and erythema, which are followed by edema that may rapidly progress up the extremity. Within hours, signs of tissue necrosis appear with blisters or hemorrhagic bullae. Edema can be severe enough to jeopardize perfusion. Without definitive therapy, these findings can rapidly progress to tissue necrosis.

The magnitude of local symptoms may or may not correspond to the severity of the envenomation. Bites by certain species such as the Mojave rattlesnake produce little local reaction but potentially deadly systemic effects.[2] Crotalid venom can cause dysfunction in virtually any organ system, but most prominent are the effects on the hematologic, neurologic, and cardiovascular systems. Early systemic symptoms include numbness, weakness, nausea, sweating, and paresthesias. Without treatment, the patient may progress to shock, coagulopathy, hemorrhage, nervous system dysfunction, and death. Provide supportive measures while preparing to administer antivenin.

Definitive therapy of pit viper bites sometimes requires the use of specific antivenin. A polyvalent Crotalidae antivenin (Wyeth-Ayerst Laboratories) is available and is effective against rattlesnake, copperhead, and water moccasin venoms.

Indications. Administer antivenin as soon after the bite as is feasible and ideally within 4 hours.[2] After 24 hours antivenin is ineffective, and between 12 and 24 hours the benefits are unclear. Make the decision to treat with antivenin and determine the amount to be given on the basis of the severity of the envenomation (Table 134-2) and the vulnerability of the victim. Use scoring systems such as the one in Table 134-2 only as a general guide; remember that bites by certain species (Mojave rattlesnake) may produce minimal local reactions initially and be followed by severe life-threatening systemic effects.

Contraindications. There are no absolute contraindications to the administration of antivenin except for a history of prior anaphylaxis. When hypersensitivity to antivenin is expected or emerges during treatment, manage the allergic symptoms aggressively to allow the continuation of antivenin therapy whenever possible.

Complications. True allergic or anaphylactic reactions occur commonly with antivenin administration; less serious anaphylactoid-type reactions also occur. Additionally, delayed reactions such as serum sickness occasionally occur following therapy.

Techniques. The dosage of antivenin is *not* based on a patient's weight; children generally require larger amounts than adults. Dilute the antivenin in a volume of fluid appropriate to the size of the child. Start the infusion slowly, and monitor closely for evidence of anaphylaxis. If no reactions occur, increase the rate of infusion and give the balance of the antivenin over 2 hours. If mild allergic symptoms occur, stop or slow the infusion, give diphenhydramine, and resume administration at a slower rate. If allergic symptoms persist, weigh the severity of envenomation and the need for antivenin against the risks of anaphylaxis. If the infusion must be continued, aggressively treat allergic manifestations with antihistamines, steroids, and epinephrine. The package insert provides detailed directions for skin testing and antivenin administration.

Monitor the response to antivenin therapy for 3 to 5 hours after the initial infusion. If clinically indicated by the progression of symptoms, administer additional vials of antivenin every 30 to 60 minutes. Extremity edema is caused by the actions of the venom, not by tissue necrosis, and improves with antivenin; therefore the dangerous and disfiguring procedure of fasciotomy is almost never indicated. Consider performing a fasciotomy only if there is objective evidence

Table 134-2 Severity Scoring and Initial Antivenin Therapy for Crotalidae Envenomations

Grade	Severity	Clinical and laboratory findings	Initial therapy*
0	None	Less than 1 inch of edema or erythema around fang mark Minimal pain No systemic signs or laboratory changes	Wound care only No antivenin
1	Mild	Less than 5 inches of edema and erythema around wound Moderate pain No systemic signs or laboratory changes	Usually no antivenin 5 vials if small child or debilitated patient
2	Moderate	History of more than one bite or of being bitten by a large snake Edema progressing toward trunk Ecchymoses only in area of edema Widely distributed pain Mild systemic symptoms: nausea, vomiting, paresthesias Mild laboratory abnormalities	5-10 vials, depending on size and condition of patient
3	Severe	History of more than one bite or of being bitten by a large or toxic snake Rapidly progressive edema Generalized petechiae/ecchymoses Prominent systemic effects: shock, hypothermia, coagulopathy Laboratory abnormalities	10-15 vials, depending on size and condition of patient
4	Critical	Very rapid progression of edema, reaching the trunk within few hours Early ecchymoses and signs of tissue necrosis Severe pain Early onset of systemic effects: paresthesias, fasciculations, cramping, shock, coagulopathy, seizures, coma, death	15-20 vials, depending on size and condition of patient

*For smaller children, these antivenin doses may need to be increased by as much as 50%.

of compartment pressures of at least 30 mm Hg that are sustained for more than 1 hour.[2] Perform minor debridement of necrotic tissue at the wound site 3 to 5 days after the injury.

Coral Snake

Although lacking the identifying features of the pit vipers, coral snakes have distinctive markings. The nose is always black, followed by a yellow ring and a black band. Red and black bands alternate along the length of the animal and are always separated by a yellow ring ("red on yellow, kill a fellow"). There are two species of coral snake, the Eastern and the Western coral snake; most problems are caused by the former.[3] This snake is found in many states east of the Mississippi.

Envenomations by the coral snake cause minimal local reaction but can produce profound neurotoxicity.[2,3] The onset of symptoms occurs within several hours and may begin with malaise and weakness and progress to nerve palsies (dysphagia, diplopia). Worsening neurologic function and pronounced weakness may lead to respiratory failure.

Indications, Contraindications, and Complications. The indications, contraindications, and complications of coral snake envenomation are the same as for crotalidae envenomations.

Techniques. First aid measures for coral snake envenomations are the same as for Crotalidae envenomations except that constriction bands and wound incision are ineffective in preventing absorption of elapid venom. Aggressively support the patient as described in previous sections.

Once coral snake envenomation has been confirmed, acquire antivenin and perform skin testing. Antivenin (Wyeth-Ayerst Laboratories) is available for only the Eastern coral snake, *Micrurus fulvius*. Initially give three to five vials by intravenous infusion over 2 hours. Titrate the need for additional antivenin to the patient's clinical response. As many as ten vials may be needed for severe envenomations or if treatment has been delayed. Serum sickness commonly occurs, especially when larger amounts of antivenin are given.

MARINE ENVENOMATIONS

A few venomous marine animals are found along the U.S. coasts and pose a threat to people swimming or wading in these waters. Envenomations by these animals are rarely fatal but can cause painful local reactions and various systemic toxicities.[1,4,6] The characteristics of common marine envenomations are outlined in Table 134-3.

Indications. Initiate treatment for any local or systemic signs of marine envenomation.

Contraindications. There are no specific contraindications to the treatment of marine envenomations.

Complications. The potential complications of treating marine envenomations include a worsening of local tissue injury by using inappropriate techniques of wound care, as well as reactions to antivenin administration.

Techniques. As with all envenomations, initiate general and first aid measures in the field. If possible, remove the patient from further exposure to venom. Keep the patient calm, warm, and give nothing by mouth. Initiate basic wound care principles as appropriate. Provide definitive care as needed on the basis of exposure and symptoms. Be prepared to provide general supportive care and to administer specific antivenin when indicated and available. Table 134-3 provides a brief overview of the management of envenomations from specific marine animals.[1,3,4,6]

Table 134-3   Characteristics of Common Marine Envenomations

Animal	Effects	Management	Comments
Coelenterata (jellyfish, corals, anemones)	Nematocysts discharge toxin Local pain, burning, wheals, paresthesias, ulcerations Systemic reactions in severe envenomations Cramping, weakness, nausea Paresthesias to seizures to coma Arrhythmias, respiratory failure are rare Multisystem collapse can occur	Immediately wash the area with seawater or vinegar to deactivate nematocysts Remove adherent material by applying shaving cream or a paste of baking soda and scraping with a knife or razor Topical steroids or antihistamines for inflammation Analgesics for pain	Supportive care PRN No specific antivenins except for box jellyfish Fresh water and attempts to rub away adherent material cause nematocysts to discharge Corals can cause severe wounds at high risk for infection
Echinodermata (starfish, sea urchins)	Severe pain that may spread Erythema and edema may progress up the extremity Systemic signs primarily neurologic, with paresthesias and paralysis	Control pain with hot-water immersion (45° C) and analgesics Remove embedded spines if easily accessible Antibiotics only PRN	Retained spines can cause granuloma formation Spines may be radiopaque and can cause tatooing of skin
Elasmorbranch (stingrays)	Injury from trauma and venom Bad lacerations with embedded barb fragments Severe local pain that may last for days Systemic symptoms range from mild and nonspecific to arrhythmias, shock, death Paresthesias may persist for weeks	Hot-water immersion to relieve pain and inactivate venom Analgesics Vigorous irrigation and debridement of the wound Loose primary or delayed closure of lacerations as needed	Common cause of marine envenomations Injury usually occurs when a wader steps on the back of this bottom dweller
Scorpaenidae (scorpionfish, lionfish, stonefish)	Immediate, intense spreading pain Central ischemia followed by cyanosis Surrounding edema and erythema Systemic toxicities can affect any organ system and range from mild to fatal	Hot water immersion to relieve pain and inactivate venom Analgesics and wound care, including irrigation and debridement Polyvalent antivenin is available for use with severe stonefish injuries	Found in coastal waters off the southern parts of the United States Antivenin available through Sea World or the Steinhart Aquarium in San Francisco

REMARKS

For a patient who has suffered any type of envenomation injury, the general approach is the same. Remember that the best first aid possible is timely transport to an ED for evaluation and definitive care. Many venomous animals, both vertebrate and invertebrate, have specific antivenins available. Early and aggressive use of these antivenins when appropriate can save life and limb, but their use is fraught with potential and serious complications.

The most effective approach to envenomation injuries is, of course, prevention by instructing children about the identification and avoidance of potentially venomous animals in the local environment.

REFERENCES

1. Auerbach PS: Stings of the deep, *Emerg Med* 21:26, June 1989.
2. Gold BS, Wingert WA: Snake venom poisoning in the United States: a review of therapeutic practice, *South Med J* 87:579, 1994.
3. Hodge D, Tecklenburg FW: Bites and stings. In Fleisher GR, Ludwig S, editors: *Textbook of pediatric emergency medicine,* ed 3, Baltimore, 1993, Williams & Wilkins.
4. Kizer KW: Marine envenomations: not just a problem of the tropics, *Emerg Med Rep* 6:129, 1985.
5. Needham GR: Evaluation of five popular methods for tick removal, *Pediatrics* 75:997, 1985.
6. Otten EJ: Venomous animal injuries. In Rosen P, Barkin RM, editors: *Emergency medicine: concepts and clinical practice,* ed 3, St. Louis, 1992, Mosby.
7. Russell FE: Arachnid envenomations, *Emerg Med Serv* 20:16, 1991.
8. Russell FE, et al: Snake venom poisoning in the United States: experiences with 550 cases, *JAMA* 233:341, 1975.
9. Stewart C: Emergency management of arachnid envenomations: spider bites and scorpion stings, *Emerg Med Rep* 14:75, 1993.
10. Tully SA, Wingert WA: Venomous animal bites and stings. In Barkin RM, editor: *Pediatric emergency medicine: concepts and clinical practice,* St Louis, 1992, Mosby.
11. Wasserman GS: Wound care of spider and snake envenomations, *Ann Emerg Med* 17:1331, 1988.

135 Miscellaneous Wounds

Stephanie A. Walton, James Hopkins, Gayle Garvin, and Jonathan Grisham

SKIN ABSCESS

Skin abscesses are often encountered in children and are often the result of minor trauma that alters the local environment and allows normal flora to establish a local infection. In children, these infections are most often caused by staphylococcal or streptococcal organisms.[1]

Equipment

The equipment commonly needed to incise and drain a skin abscess is listed in Box 135-1.

Techniques

Appropriate management of an abscess requires drainage, occasionally irrigation, wound care, and follow-up.[7]

The most important step in management is drainage of the abscess. Use standard sterile technique and prepare the area with an iodinated cleanser and sterile drapes. Anesthetize the area with a local nerve block, circumferential block, infiltrative anesthetic, or ethyl chloride spray. Use a No. 15 scalpel to open the abscess, and make an incision parallel to local skin lines to the depth of the superficial fascia. Make the opening large enough to allow complete drainage of purulent material (Fig. 135-1, *A*). Suction, irrigate, or manually express purulent material from the cavity. To allow drainage of the entire abscess, insert a hemostat or gloved finger into the lesion to break septa or adhesions that may be present (Fig. 135-1, *B* and *C*). If a pathogen other than *Staphylococcus aureus* is suspected, culture the material that drains when the abscess is first opened. Flush the abscess cavity with a dilute antiseptic solution such as povidone-iodine and saline, and complete the irrigation process with a volume of normal saline that is at least ten times the abscess volume. This procedure reduces the bacterial load and helps prevent recurrence.

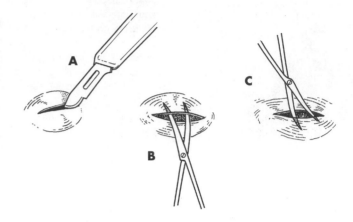

FIG. 135-1 Technique for incision (**A**) of an abscess and breaking of septa or adhesions (**B** and **C**).

Pack the wound with iodoform gauze or place a drain to prevent reaccumulation of the abscess. For small wounds, use the corner of a 2″ × 2″ gauze. Loosely approximate the wound borders and allow the wound to heal by secondary intent. Dress the wound with dry gauze and cover with a gauze bandage. Recheck the wound and change the packing on a daily basis until the cavity is small enough that it no longer requires packing.

Although most abscesses that are incised and drained heal without antibiotics, certain clinical situations warrant their use. If antibiotics are necessary, use a semisynthetic penicillin such as dicloxacillin for coverage of staphylococci and streptococci. Provide broader antibiotic coverage for special circumstances such as an immunocompromised or diabetic patient. Amend antibiotic coverage on the basis of the results of initial wound cultures. Close follow-up is essential to good patient care. Monitor the wound closely to ensure proper healing.

EPISTAXIS AND SEPTAL HEMATOMA

Epistaxis, or nose bleeding, is a common complaint in the pediatric population. Although nasal bleeding is rarely a serious condition, it is frightening to children and their parents. Epistaxis may occur at any age, at any time, or during any season, but it is more common during the winter months.

Etiology

The vast majority of nosebleeds in children originate from the anterior portion of the nasal septum in a vascular anastomosis called Kiesselbach's area (Fig. 135-2). Disruption of this rich vascular plexus results in nasal bleeding. Box 135-2 lists both the common and uncommon causes of epistaxis. Epistaxis in children is most commonly a result of

---

BOX 135–1	**EQUIPMENT FOR INCISION AND DRAINAGE OF AN ABSCESS**

Local anesthetic (lidocaine buffered with a 1:10 dilution of bicarbonate, or ethyl chloride)
5- or 10-ml syringes
25- to 27-gauge needles
Povidone-iodine solution
Sterile drapes and gloves
No. 15 scalpel
Saline irrigation solution
Hemostat
Bulb syringe
Variety of gauze pads
Drain

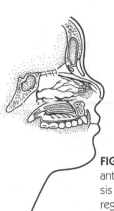

FIG. 135-2   Blood supply to the nose. The anterior septum has a rich vascular anastomosis called Kiesselbach's area. The posterior region is supplied by the sphenopalatine artery.

BOX 135–3   FOCUSED HISTORY FOR PATIENTS WITH EPISTAXIS

Medications, especially aspirin, anticoagulants, or elicit drugs?
Prior history of epistaxis and other bleeding or bruising?
Was there an inciting event such as trauma, or was the onset spontaneous?
Concurrent illness such as an upper respiratory tract infection?
From which naris is the bleeding coming?
What has been tried to stop the bleeding?
How long has the bleeding continued?

BOX 135–2   CAUSES OF EPISTAXIS IN CHILDREN

Common
Inflammation

Upper respiratory infections
Allergic rhinitis

Trauma

Physical injury: nose picking, repeated hard blowing, blunt trauma with or without fracture
Foreign body
Dry air, low humidity

Uncommon
Bleeding dyscrasias

Disorders of platelets
Hemophilias
Drug-induced: aspirin and anticoagulant drugs (e.g., warfarin [Coumadin])

Vascular

Telangiectasia, hemangiomas
Hypertension (rare)

Neoplasms

Leukemias, benign polyps

BOX 135–4   RISK FACTORS HELPFUL IN DETERMINING THE LIKELIHOOD OF A BLEEDING DISORDER

Bilateral or posterior nasal bleeding
Duration of bleeding longer than 10 minutes or volume of blood loss more than 30 ml
More than 25 episodes each year
The occurrence of episodes over the majority of a child's life

---

BOX 135–5   EQUIPMENT FOR EVALUATING AND TREATING EPISTAXIS

Light source and head mirror or head lamp
Papoose or other restraint device as needed
Suction apparatus, including Frazier and Yankauer suction tips and a variety of catheters
Nasal speculum
Topical anesthetics/vasoconstrictors
Cautery device: silver nitrate sticks or battery-powered electrocautery pen
Petrolatum gauze for packing
Nasal sponge or nasal tampon
Foley or pneumatic catheters if a posterior bleeding site is suspected

---

either the dried, inflamed nasal mucosa seen with upper respiratory tract infections or the local trauma of rubbing or picking the nose.

Bleeding arising from the sphenopalatine artery (see Fig. 135-2) in the posterior nasal regions may be extensive and life threatening as a result of blood loss and risk of aspiration. Such bleeding is extremely uncommon in children and is usually associated with coagulopathy or other systemic disorders.

In addition to the usual general history, elicit certain relevant information (Box 135-3) from patients with nasal bleeding.

Rarely are any laboratory studies necessary in the child with brief and isolated episodes of epistaxis. If there is suspicion of a concurrent systemic disorder or protracted bleeding, obtain a complete blood count, platelet count, and type and cross match. Obtain coagulation studies in patients who are taking anticoagulants or are suspected of having a clotting disorder.

Katsanis et al.[6] developed a scoring system using risk factors, which is helpful in determining the likelihood that a patient has a bleeding disorder (Box 135-4).

Equipment

Before initiating the ear, nose, and throat examination, prepare and have ready all equipment that may be required. Box 135-5 lists the equipment commonly needed. In addition to these items, have an emesis basin ready because swallowed blood often produces gastric irritation, and vomiting is common.

Techniques

Identify and aggressively treat any cardiovascular compromise resulting from the blood loss. After a general evaluation of the patient, focus the examination on the nose and nasopharynx while simultaneously beginning treatment. After initial stabilization of this child, refer him or her to an otolaryngologist for definitive therapy.

To examine older children and adolescents, place them in a seated upright position with the head slightly forward and in the sniffing position. Restrain younger children with a commercial restraint device or a wrapped sheet if needed to allow an adequate examination. Initiate hemostasis by pinching the nose to apply direct pressure.

The primary goal of the examination is to locate the site of bleeding. The evacuation of clotted blood is necessary before the source of bleeding can be found; evacuation may also lead to a diminution of the bleeding. If there is active bleeding, use a suction device to evacuate clotted and fresh blood. Instruct the older patient to blow his or her nose to clear out clotted blood.

If the source of bleeding is anterior, attempt to achieve hemostasis with simple measures before resorting to cauterization. The simplest and safest approach involves packing the bleeding naris with topical thrombin and applying gentle pressure by squeezing the anterior portion of the nose for 10 minutes. If bleeding continues, try a topical anesthetic and vasoconstrictor. Excellent anesthesia and vasoconstriction is provided by 4% cocaine solution, but it has the potential to produce toxicity because of its rapid absorption across the mucous membranes. Exercise caution in its use. Other topical alternatives include 0.5% neosynephrine or epinephrine (1:1000). Either of these agents can be combined with topical lidocaine to achieve anesthesia and vasoconstriction.

If hemostasis is not achieved by these measures, prepare to cauterize. After isolating the area of bleeding by suctioning old and new blood, apply a silver nitrate stick directly to the point of bleeding. To avoid soaking the silver nitrate stick with blood, it may be helpful to first cauterize a small ring around the site to decrease incoming blood flow and then to roll the tip onto the site from above. Exercise caution to prevent the silver nitrate from being washed into the rest of the nasal passages by free-flowing blood.

If bleeding continues, pack the anterior nose, preferably with a nasal sponge or nasal tampon. After being inserted into the nose, these devices expand and tamponade as they absorb blood and mucus. A variety of these devices are available, including smaller sizes for pediatric patients. If necessary, trim larger sizes to fit before insertion.

Immediately refer patients with posterior bleeding to an otolaryngologist and arrange for hospital admission. Begin temporizing measures to stop the bleeding until an otolaryngologist arrives. To tamponade posterior bleeding sites, use a specially made nasal catheter if available or insert a Foley catheter into the nasopharynx, inflate the balloon, and apply anterior traction to the catheter. The placement of posterior nasal packs is difficult, very uncomfortable, and not without attendant risks; leave this procedure to specialty consultants or others with comparable experience.

An aggressive search for a bleeding source is unnecessary for children whose bleeding was brief and uncomplicated and has ceased by the time of the examination.

To prevent recurrence of epistaxis, recommend the use of a humidifier. Regularly applying petroleum jelly to the anterior mucosa is an effective and simple way to keep the tissues moist. Treat allergic or infectious rhinitis with the appropriate medications. Show patients and parents how to properly apply pressure by squeezing the nose should bleeding recur.

SEPTAL HEMATOMA
Etiology

The extensive vascular plexus of the nose can be easily injured by even minor trauma. Most commonly, the superficial vessels are injured, which results in epistaxis. Occasionally nasal trauma can cause bleeding directly into the nasal septum and result in a septal hematoma (Fig. 135-3). This collection of blood lies in the potential space created when the mucoperichondrium is torn away from the cartilage. Failure to identify and drain a septal hematoma before ischemic necrosis of the cartilage occurs may have serious consequences, including deformity of the nasal bridge, nasal obstruction, and infections such as chondritis, meningitis, and cavernous sinus thrombosis.

Techniques

In any patient with nasal trauma, perform a careful search for a septal hematoma regardless of whether a nasal fracture occurs. Carefully inspect each nasal passage and confirm the patency of both sides. Although the hematoma will look purple or ecchymotic later, initially it may be the color of nasal mucosa. Palpate with a small, blunt instrument whenever there is significant concern to evaluate for fluctuance.

After administering an effective topical anesthetic such as 4% cocaine solution, incise and drain the hematoma. Make a vertical and horizontal incision across most of the mass in an L-shaped or hockey-stick configuration (Fig. 135-4, A). Completely evacuate the hematoma with suction or irrigation to allow approximation of the mucoperichondrium and cartilage. Place a small drain to facilitate drainage of any ongoing bleeding, and pack the anterior nose (Fig. 135-4, B). Except certain older adolescents, admit to the hospital most children with septal hematomas for ongoing care and specialty

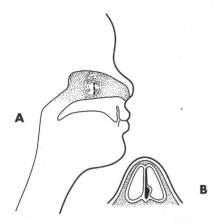

FIG. 135-3 Septal hematoma. **A,** Position of hematoma on septum. **B,** Hematoma lies next to septum and may look like bulge of pink mucosa.

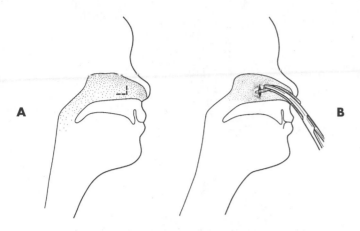

FIG. 135-4   Incision of a septal hematoma (**A**) and insertion of a drain (**B**).

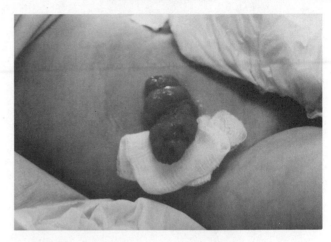

FIG. 135-5   Prolapsed colostomy with healthy viable mucosa (no intervention necessary).

consultation with an otolaryngologist. Any sign of suppuration requires aggressive treatment, including additional drainage and parental antibiotics.

OSTOMY COMPLICATIONS IN PEDIATRICS

Infants and children may have gastrointestinal or genitourinary stomas for short-term management of a variety of conditions. A permanent ostomy may be required for more serious disorders. Younger children generally have a standard diverting ostomy, whereas an older child may have a permanent continent diversion. The history should include the time, character, and quantity of the last effluent, as well as a determination of the type of intestinal or urinary diversion present. Perform a complete physical examination and pay careful attention to the stoma and the surrounding skin.

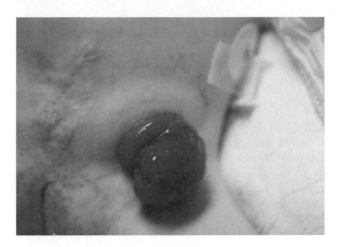

FIG. 135-6   Prolapsed stoma with circulatory compromise. Note the dusky color change.

Mechanical Complications

Mechanical complications of a stoma include stomal stenosis, prolapse, retraction, peristomal herniation, and bowel obstruction secondary to adhesions. Stomal stenosis may or may not be recognized on visual inspection and may occur with reduction of output, diarrhea, or crampy abdominal pain. Perform a careful digital examination of the stoma to reveal a skin-level stenosis. In smaller stomas pass a catheter or perform dye studies to identify the stenosis. The process of the examination may temporarily relieve the obstruction but may cause an eventual worsening of the stenotic state. Refer the patient for surgical correction when a stoma causes gastrointestinal obstruction.

Prolapse of the stoma may occur (Fig. 135-5) and by itself is not an indication for immediate intervention. Attempt to reduce the mass if the prolapse is associated with abdominal pain, decreased output, or a change in the color of the stoma (Fig. 135-6). Reduce the prolapse by gently working with both hands; start from the distal portion and make sure that the portion of the bowel eased back into the abdomen does not slide out again as the reduction progresses.

Retraction of the stoma below the skin layer (Fig. 135-7) may cause problems because it becomes difficult to get an appliance to stick and collect drainage. No immediate intervention is necessary for stoma retraction unless there is partial or complete detachment of the stoma from the skin layer. For superficial detachment at skin level, prescribe

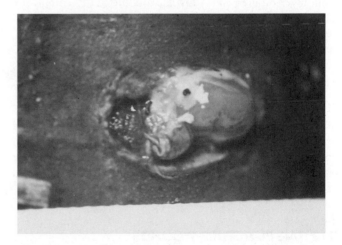

FIG. 135-7   Stomal recession and partial separation of the functional stoma below the level of the skin. The mucous fistula to the right is at the skin level. Close observation is necessary because the stoma is very prone to stenosis and obstruction.

antibiotics and observe closely for spread into the subcutaneous tissue, which may cause a necrotizing cellulitis. The risk of peritonitis is high if the detachment reaches the fascial layer; in this case refer the patient for surgical intervention.

Peristomal herniation, or a protrusion of colon or ileum

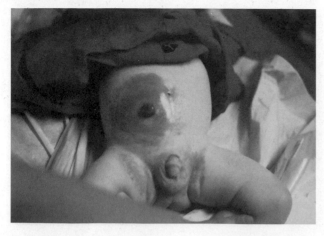

FIG. 135-8 Peristomal and groin *Candida albicans*. Treatment involves using antifungal powder.

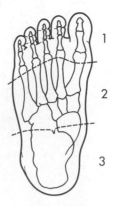

FIG. 135-9 Puncture zones of the foot. Zone 1 overlies the metatarsal neck and extends distally to the toes. This zone carries the highest risk of bone or joint penetration and infection because of its primary weight-bearing surface and scant amount of overlying soft tissue. Zone 2 comprises the distal end of the calcaneus to the neck of the metatarsals. This region overlies all tarsal bones and joints as well as the shaft of the metatarsals. Zone 3 overlies the calcaneus.

into the subcutaneous layers of skin surrounding the stoma, may cause problems with pouch adherence but is not a surgical emergency.[1]

Cutaneous Complications

The peristomal skin is subject to a loss of integrity associated with recurrent disease and with repeated contact with stool and urine. These problems are aggravated by improperly fitted appliances. Generally avoid antibiotics because they are rarely necessary and can cause diarrhea that further impairs adherence of the appliance and aggravates the peristomal dermatitis.

Infection by *Candida albicans* is a commonly occurring dermatitis in the peristomal area (Fig. 135-8). Apply antifungal medication topically in the powder form to maximize effectiveness. Mix it with a small amount of water and paint a thin layer on the rash. Allow the mixture to dry completely before placing an appliance. Avoid using creams or ointments in the peristomal area because they prevent pouch adherence.

Treat contact dermatitis by removing the offending agent; often adhesive tapes are responsible.

Metabolic Complications

Infants and children are especially at risk for ostomy-related metabolic imbalances. Diarrhea or a mechanical obstruction may lead to excessive sodium, potassium, and bicarbonate losses, and metabolic acidosis may quickly follow.[11] Obtain electrolytes if warranted by the history or physical examination.

PLANTAR PUNCTURE WOUNDS
Etiology and Complications

Puncture wounds are common in children and are often viewed as unimportant because of their sometimes benign appearance. Puncture wounds to the foot have a peak incidence between May and October and are more common in boys than in girls.[3] The most common penetrating objects are nails (98%). Infectious complications occur in 0.6% to 14.8% of all puncture wounds and include cellulitis, soft

tissue abscesses, osteomyelitis, osteochondritis, and pyarthrosis.[2] Cellulitis is the most common complication.

The location of the wound is an important risk factor for the development of infectious complications. The foot can be divided into three regions or zones (Fig. 135-9).[9] Deeper wounds that penetrate plantar fascia or those with a retained foreign body are more prone to infection than are superficial punctures. Foreign bodies are found in more than 3% of wounds. Common foreign bodies are bits of shoe, sock, rust, dirt, wood, and glass.[3]

Techniques

Perform a detailed history, examination, and wound classification for all patients with puncture wounds (Box 135-6). Obtaining appropriate historical information is invaluable. Be sure to address the important historical questions listed in Box 135-7.[4]

When examining the injured foot, assess the vascular and neurologic status as well as the depth and location of the wound. Pain along the plantar aspect of the foot with active flexion and extension of the toes is suggestive of deeper tissue penetration.[5]

To help direct management decisions, classify the puncture wound into one of four categories on the basis of severity and appearance of the wound (see Box 135-6).

Cleanse the wound and remove debris with a dilute povidone-iodine solution.[10] Although it may not reduce the risk of infection, soak the injured foot to help remove dried blood, dirt, or other foreign material from around the wound. Because all puncture wounds are regarded as tetanus-prone, assess the patient's tetanus status and provide immunizations when needed (see Chapter 130). Obtain x-ray examinations whenever a retained foreign body is suspected and for deep wounds that may have penetrated plantar fascia, bone, or a joint.

Enlarge the puncture site by coring (Fig. 135-10) to allow for better visualization of the wound tract, easier irrigation, and improved drainage.[12]

BOX 135–6   **SUMMARY OF PUNCTURE-WOUND MANAGEMENT CATEGORIES**

Category 1

Clean, superficial wounds with no suspicion of a retained foreign body
  Tetanus prophylaxis as indicated
  Requires only cleansing of the puncture site
  X-ray examinations and prophylactic antibiotics not indicated
  Follow-up as needed

Category 2

Grossly contaminated wounds, deep wounds, or wounds with a high suspicion of a retained foreign body
  Tetanus prophylaxis as indicated
  Cleanse puncture site
  Local anesthetic or posterior tibial nerve block
  Coring procedure to enlarge puncture site and to search for the foreign body (see Fig. 135–10)
  Irrigation and packing
  X-ray examination if suspicious of deep penetration or a retained foreign body
  Discharge with close follow-up
    Prophylactic antibiotics of no proven value
    No weight bearing for 3 to 4 days
    Return for first wound check within 48 hours
    Patient instructed to return for foot pain, swelling, or a decreased ability to bear weight on the affected foot
(If cellulitis develops, proceed with the treatment in Category 3)

Category 3

Wounds presenting with cellulitis or soft tissue abscesses but no evidence of underlying deeper tissue infection
  Tetanus prophylaxis as indicated
  Puncture-site cleansing
  Coring procedure if not already done
  Culture of cellulitic area via needle aspiration

X-ray examination to rule out foreign body or early, deeper tissue infection
Discharge with close follow-up
  Antibiotic regimen to cover staphylococci and group A streptococci
  No weight bearing for 3 to 4 days
  Return for first wound check in 48 hours
  Return if foot pain, erythema, and swelling do not improve with oral antibiotics
(If patient fails to respond to oral antibiotics, begin IV antibiotics and consider the possibility of a retained foreign body or deeper tissue infection.)

Category 4

Wounds presenting with a high suspicion of an underlying deep tissue infection, (e.g., osteomyelitis, osteochondritis, or pyarthrosis)
  Tetanus prophylaxis as indicated
  X-ray examination to evaluate for early changes of osteomyelitis or a bone scan if plain x-ray films are negative
  Complete blood count and erythrocyte sedimentation rate (ESR)
  Combined surgical/medical approach
    Surgical debridement of necrotic tissue, irrigation, and search for foreign body
    Obtain intraoperative wound cultures
  Initial antibiotic regimen should cover for both *Staphylococcus* spp. and *Pseudomonas* spp.
  Consider serial ESR measurements to monitor response
  Modify antibiotic regimen on the basis of culture and sensitivity results
  Duration of IV antibiotics is debatable
  Consider bone scan, CT scan, or MR of foot
(If no response with postoperative antibiotics, consider the possibility of a missed foreign body, additional necrotic tissues that require further debridement, or missed pyarthrosis)

Modified from Inaba AS, et al: An update on the evaluation and management of plantar puncture wounds and *Pseudomonas* osteomyelitis, *Pediatric Emerg Care* 8(1):38–44, 1992.

BOX 135–7   **PUNCTURE WOUNDS: IMPORTANT HISTORICAL INFORMATION**

When did the injury occur and how long has the patient waited before seeking medical care?
Did the injury occur indoors or outdoors?
What was the penetrating object, and what was the condition of that object?
Approximately how deep did the object penetrate into the foot, and was the object intact on removal?
What type of footwear was the patient wearing at the time of the injury and what was the condition of the footwear?

What region of the foot sustained the penetrating injury?
If there was a delay in seeking medical care, what type of wound care was performed at home by the caretaker?
What symptoms has the patient experienced since sustaining the injury?
What is the patient's tetanus immunization status?
Does the patient have any medical conditions that may increase his or her risk for potential infectious complications?

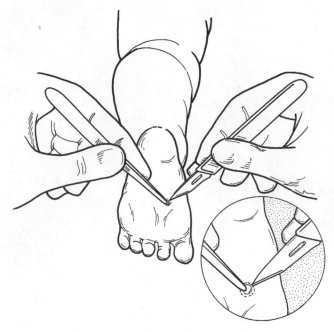

FIG. 135-10 Coring of a puncture wound.

Anesthetize the area surrounding the puncture site using a local anesthetic or a posterior tibial nerve block. Using a No. 11 scalpel blade and forceps, excise a 2- to 3-mm full-thickness rim of skin around the puncture site. Alternatively, use a 4-mm disposable skin biopsy punch to core out tissue surrounding the wound.

Perform high-pressure irrigation with normal saline using a large syringe, angiocatheter, or splashguard. Direct the stream over the puncture site with the tip of the catheter approximately 1 cm above the wound. Do not place the catheter tip inside the wound because doing so may force debris further into the wound cavity or cause the deep tissues to balloon with saline.[12]

Dress the wound, provide antibiotics, perform additional procedures, and arrange follow-up care as outlined in Box 135-6.

REFERENCES

1. Broadwell DC, Jackson BS: *Principles of ostomy care,* St Louis, 1982, Mosby.
2. Chisholm CD, Schlesser JF: Plantar puncture wounds: controversies and treatment recommendations, *Ann Emerg Med* 18(12):1352-1357, 1989.
3. Fitzgerald RH, Cowan JDE: Puncture wounds of the foot, *Orthop Clin North Am* 6:4, 1975.
4. Inaba AS: The rusty nail and other puncture wounds of the foot, *Contemp Pediatr* 10(3): 138-156, March 1993.
5. Inaba AS, et al: An update on the evaluation and management of plantar puncture wounds and *Pseudomonas* osteomyelitis, *Pediatr Emerg Care* 8(1):38-44, 1992.
6. Katsanis E, et al: Prevalence and significance of mild bleeding disorders in children with recurrent epistaxis, *Pediatr* 113:73, 1988.
7. Lohr JA: *Pediatric outpatient procedures,* Philadelphia, 1991, JB Lippincott.
8. Reference deleted in galleys.
9. Patzakis MJ, et al: Wound site as a predictor of complications following deep nail punctures to the foot, *Western J Med* 150(5): 545-547, 1989.
10. Resnick CD, Fallat LM: Puncture wounds: therapeutic considerations and a new classification, *Foot Surg* 29(2): 147-153, 1990.
11. Schwarz KB, et al: Sodium needs of infants and children with ileostomy, *J Pediatr* 102(4): 509-513, 1983.
12. Zukin DD, Simon RR: *Emergency wound care,* Rockville, Md, 1987, Aspen.

136 Dressings

Susan B. Kirelik

Wound dressings serve several important functions that promote wound healing. Dressings that prevent wound desiccation have been shown to promote wound healing by creating a moist environment and preventing the formation of an eschar that would otherwise delay the migration of new epithelial cells.[3] Wound dressings protect the healing tissue from trauma by providing both padding and partial immobilization; semiocclusive wound dressings may provide a physical barrier to decrease bacterial contamination of the wound. In addition, dressed wounds are less painful than those left uncovered.[3] A well-dressed wound promotes both patient and parent satisfaction.

Indications

In general, dress most partial-thickness wounds (including sutured wounds, minor burns, and abrasions) with a nonadherent dressing. Adherent dressings offer several advantages for certain wounds, particularly burns and abrasions; these dressings are discussed in Chapter 132.

Contraindications

Most facial wounds do not require layered dressings and may be covered with only an antibacterial ointment.[4] Never dress wounds before appropriate debridement and cleansing.

Complications

Although generally benign, wound dressings have many potential complications. Circulatory compromise and tissue necrosis may occur from tape, gauze, or bandages that are placed circumferentially or too tightly on a digit or extremity. The improper use of certain dressing materials or splints may cause injury as a result of pressure or friction. Maceration of underlying tissue may result from a dressing that permits an environment that is too moist. Damage to the delicate new epithelium may occur when an adherent plain-gauze dressing is removed. The removal of tape placed over an eyebrow may result in permanent hair loss. Stiffness may occur if a dressing results in joint immobilization over a long time period.

Equipment

Although an enormous variety of dressing materials are now available, treat most wounds in the Emergency Department with a few basic materials (Table 136-1). Some of the newly developed biosynthetic dressing materials offer several advantages over the more traditional dressing materials. However, these biosynthetic materials are generally not appropriate for the Emergency Department because they are fairly expensive and require that wounds be followed closely by health-care professionals who are skilled at recognizing potential complications. The use of biosynthetic materials for burns is discussed in Chapter 132.

Techniques

Dress most wounds with two to three layers of material.[2] Use a nonadherent material for the first layer; cut it to size and place it over the wound. Use a layer of plain gauze or gauze roll to help secure the nonadherent dressing; use several layers if the wound requires pressure or hemostasis or will have a significant amount of exudate. Secure the gauze in place by applying the tape in strips or in a spiral instead of circumferentially (Fig. 136-1). To improve tape adherence, apply the tape to clean, dry skin; follow skin-tension lines.[1] On the trunk of an infant or toddler, cover the entire dressing with a vest that is cut from tube gauze. If the wound is over a joint, apply a splint to provide partial immobilization.

With most wounds, keep the dressing in place for approxi-

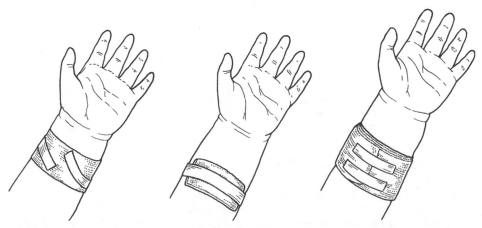

FIG. 136-1 Secure gauze with tape; place the tape in strips or a spiral (not circumferentially).

Table 136–1   Wound Dressing Materials

	Examples	Uses	Comments
Nonadherent materials			
Impregnated materials	Petrolatum gauze Bismuth-impregnated gauze (Xeroform)	Initial layer of most wounds	Plain petrolatum gauze may inhibit wound healing; therefore Xeroform is preferred[5]
Nonimpregnated materials	Telfa		Use with antibacterial ointment to provide moist environment
Absorbent/protective layers			
Plain gauze	4" × 4" 2" × 2"		
Roll gauze	Conform Kerlix	Several layers on the digit provide partial immobilization Used on the trunk, extremities, scalp	
Securing materials			
Tape			
Elastic bandage			Use only in verbal children who are able to inform parents of increasing pain if too tight
Tube gauze	Stockinette	Cut to form a vest on the trunk for an infant or toddler Secure on digit by tying ends cut longitudinally around wrist	Use with care on the digit; may cause vascular occlusion if improperly applied
Miscellaneous			
Wound-packing materials	Packing Strip Iodoform gauze	Packing abscess	
Splints		Partial immobilization of wounds over joints	
Scissors			

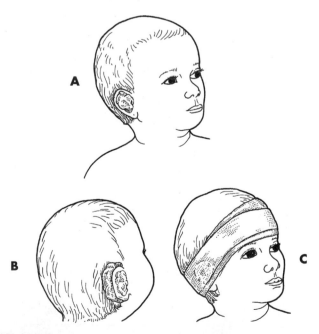

FIG. 136-2   Dressing ear wounds. **A,** Use moistened cotton to pack the anterior aspect of the ear, and **B,** fluffs of gauze to bolster the posterior aspect. **C,** Apply a circular bandage around the head. Place a gauze tie anterior to the ear to tighten the bandage and to apply pressure to the wound. Use a similar dressing for scalp wounds, but avoid the ear when applying this bandage.

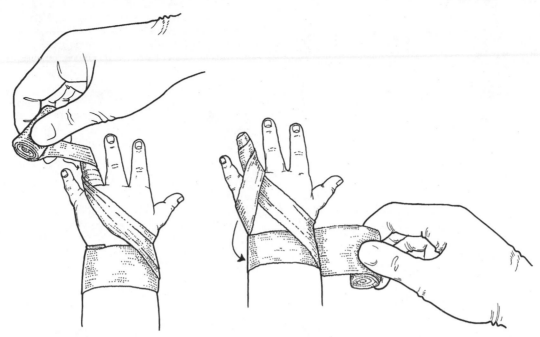

FIG. 136-3   Finger bandage. Begin with a circular wrap around the wrist; cross the dorsal hand and ascend the finger with a spiral wrap. Spiral down the finger and angle back over the hand to end with a circular wrap at the wrist. This pattern may be repeated several times to provide a bulky dressing and partial immobilization of the digit.

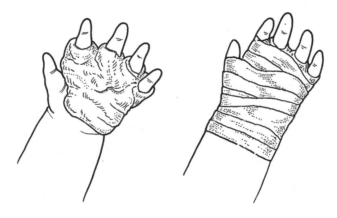

FIG. 136-4   Bulky hand dressing for injuries to the palm, dorsal hand, and proximal phalanges. Place fluffs of plain gauze between the fingers. Gauze is used to hold the dressing in place.

mately 24 hours. After this time the parent or patient may change the dressing, taking care to gently cleanse the wound and remove any crusted blood or exudate. The parent or patient should redress the wound and keep it covered until adequate wound healing has occurred. Keep most simple lacerations covered for approximately 7 days.[3] Inspect the wound for signs of infection at follow-up visits.

Remarks

With any small wound, always consider using a simple adhesive-strip bandage (Band-Aid) in place of a layered dressing. Such bandages are excellent, inexpensive dressings that are well appreciated by children and therefore usually left in place. Use only a topical antibiotic ointment for wounds on the face or scalp unless a pressure dressing is needed.

Several anatomic locations (ear, finger, and hand) provide a challenge, especially in the infant or toddler. Tips for securing dressings in these areas are illustrated in Figs. 136-2 through 136-4.

REFERENCES

1. Caruso R: Why do bandages fall off?, *Dermatol Nurs* 2(5):275-277, 1990.
2. Cuzzell JZ: Choosing a wound dressing: a systematic approach, *AACN* 1(3):566-577, 1990.
3. Krasner D: Resolving the dressing dilemma: selecting wound dressings by category, *Ostomy Wound Manage* 35:62-69, 1991.
4. Trott A: Wound dressing and bandaging techniques. In *Wounds and lacerations: emergency care and closure,* St. Louis, 1991, Mosby.

FOREIGN BODY REMOVAL

137 Foreign Bodies

Eustacia Su

Older infants and toddlers are very curious about their world and their bodies. Therefore their explorations often involve placing objects in various orifices. These incidents are usually uncomplicated and self-limited, but when the child or caregiver is unable to remove the foreign body or when there is a complication (bleeding or pain), a trip to the Emergency Department (ED) usually follows.

These unintended problems are a complication of the same exploratory behavior that results in ingestions of drugs or toxins. By the time a child is 5 years of age, enough experience and admonitions have usually accrued to extinguish most of this behavior and the resulting complications. Sometimes an older child's peers may dare him or her into putting a foreign body into an orifice, usually the ear. When treating school-age and older children who come to the ED with retained foreign bodies, consider the possibility of a developmental delay or emotional disturbance. Infants less than 6 months of age are usually not physically able to put an object into a specific orifice; although in such a case the most likely culprit is an older sibling, rule out the possibility of child abuse or neglect under the guise of inadequate supervision.

Certain presentations are suspicious by their very nature. Children do not put foreign bodies into their rectums; such a presentation demands evaluation for abuse. Vaginal foreign bodies can be innocuous, especially soft foreign bodies such as toilet paper or facial tissue paper in a young toddler. Maintain a high index of suspicion when dealing with more phallic foreign bodies or those that must have caused a significant amount of pain on insertion, especially in a child at an unusual age for such a presentation, (i.e., young infants or preadolescent girls).

A child may also come to the ED with a complaint that does not mention a foreign body but is actually a complication of foreign-body retention. Therefore halitosis or purulent rhinorrhea may be the presenting complaint of a forgotten but retained nasal foreign body; malodorous vaginal discharge may be the result of a vaginal foreign body. Persistent cellulitis may result from a retained soft tissue splinter.

Such visits to the ED provide an opportunity for caregiver education to prevent future injuries. Remind the caregivers that small objects such as buttons, peanuts, miniature marshmallows, and disk batteries can be lethal to preschoolers and younger children. If the child is not up-to-date on his or her immunizations, take this opportunity to improve the nation's dismal record of childhood immunizations.

138 Nasal Foreign Bodies

Eustacia Su

Infants explore their environment by putting everything into their mouths. As their awareness of their bodies increases, they put objects into other orifices such as the nose. Nasal foreign bodies (FBs) may be tolerated for years and appear only as a chronic nasal discharge or a rhinolith. Suspect a nasal FB in a child with halitosis or unilateral, suppurative, mucopurulent, or blood-tinged and fetid nasal discharge.[13] It may be difficult to find the FB because it is not obvious (e.g., a small piece of rubber sponge) and because the child may deny or have forgotten placing an FB in the nose.[1] The FB may even be discovered incidentally.[10]

Nasal FBs that are particularly difficult to remove include impacted FBs (e.g., swollen or germinating seeds or beans), encrusted FBs that have been present for a long time, FBs inserted with force, and live FBs. A loose FB also poses a risk of aspiration (Box 138-1).[10]

Differential Diagnosis

Sinusitis, malignancy, polyps, unilateral choanal atresia, and osteoma may present a similar clinical picture.

Indications

Prompt removal of all nasal FBs prevents many complications, especially if the FB contains any corrosive or other potentially destructive material, such as with button batteries.[12] In some cases, perform removal in the operating room (OR) for optimal patient control, lighting, sterility, and precise instrumentation. Many removals can be performed safely and effectively in the Emergency Department. Considerations include the age and cooperativeness of the child and the nature and location of the FB.

Contraindications

Complicated cases need the help of a general anesthetic and the facilities available in the OR:

1. FBs that have penetrated the cranial vault
2. FBs that have already caused significant tissue damage that requires further debridement and repair[7]
3. FBs that are likely to fall apart and cause aspiration

Complications

Aspiration of the nasal FB is a potentially fatal complication of both the FB itself and the attempt at removal. True glottic FBs carry a mortality rate of 45% and result in anoxic encephalopathy in 21% of the cases.[11] Intracranial penetration and subsequent infection of the meninges and intracranial contents are also serious complications of intranasal FBs.[6]

Tissue damage may occur as a result of electrolysis during attempts to irrigate out button batteries by using electrolyte solutions; tissue damage may also result from the leakage of corrosive chemicals if the battery is crushed during removal.[2,7]

Trauma to the intranasal structures may destroy the nasal septal cartilage or the turbinates and may cause sinusitis if the ostia become closed.[5] Epistaxis is a common result of intranasal trauma but is usually not serious.

Equipment

Box 138-2 lists the equipment needed to remove a nasal FB.[5]

Techniques

Sedation. Adequate sedation and restraint are essential when removing a nasal FB. Consider the need for a general anesthetic in more difficult cases. Place the patient in the head-down or Trendelenburg position to avoid aspiration.

BOX 138–1 **TYPES OF NASAL FOREIGN BODIES**

Animate

Screw-worm fly (*Cochliomyia hominivorax*); eats healthy, living tissue
Cochliomyia macellaria; eats living or dead tissue
Ordinary maggot (blowfly)
Fungi

Inanimate

Trauma: bone spicules or cartilage
Supernumerary teeth may erupt into floor of nose, resembling osteomas
Beans, peas, chalk, beads, and similar objects
Stone, wood, plasticene, rubber, door handle, washers
Batteries, thimbles, bullets

BOX 138–2 **EQUIPMENT FOR REMOVAL OF NASAL FOREIGN BODIES**

Head lamp
Nasal specula (all sizes)
Bayonet forceps
Right-angle blunt hook
Cerumen spoon (wire loop)
Ear curette
Alligator forceps
Self-made cotton-tip applicator
No. 4 Fogarty catheter or No. 8 Foley catheter
Suction tubes: Yankauer, tonsil tip 10–12 and, if available, a suction catheter with a soft, flexible, funnel-shaped tip (e.g., Richards Co. Memphis, TN)
Additional medications (to anesthetize or shrink the nasal mucosa)
Chemicals to kill live FB (e.g., 25% chloroform to kill larvae of *C. hominivorax*)
Nasopharyngoscope or nasopharyngeal mirror

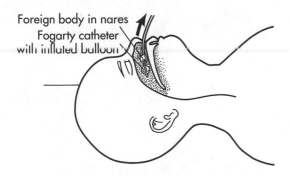

FIG. 138-1   Use of a Fogarty catheter to remove a nasal foreign body.

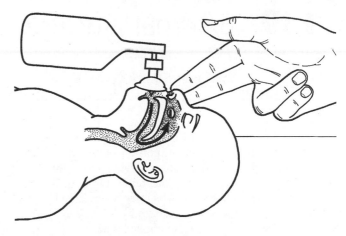

FIG. 138-2   Removal of a nasal foreign body by forceful exhalation. Cover mouth with mask, but leave nose clear. Place Ambu bag or mouth-to-mouth mask. Use finger pressure to occlude unobstructed naris. Apply cricoid pressure.

Preparation. Ensure that good lighting and all of the required equipment are working properly and are immediately available. The head lamp is the optimal lighting system because it leaves both hands free to perform the procedure. Ensure that the suction equipment is working well and that spare suction tips are immediately available. Have emergency airway equipment immediately at hand in case of dislodgment and aspiration of the FB during the procedure. Position the bed to minimize physician fatigue.

If the FB is radiopaque, an x-ray study delineates its size, shape, and location; this information is useful when planning how to remove the FB and minimize complications.[6]

Procedure. Shrink the nasal mucosa to facilitate visualization and removal of the FB. Use either 4% topical lidocaine with 0.25% phenylephrine chloride or cocaine hydrochloride (4% solution, maximum dose 3 mg/kg). Palpate with the tip of a small bayonet forceps; make sure that the object to be removed is not intrinsic soft tissue.

Choose the appropriate instrument ahead of time if the nature of the FB is known (e.g., a firm, smooth FB may be easily removed with a soft funnel-tipped catheter, whereas a disk may be more easily removed with bayonet forceps if its flat profile is seen). Remove a disk battery with a blunt, right-angle hook to avoid crushing the battery and releasing caustic chemicals. A soft wax crayon tends to disintegrate, and its irregular surface is not conducive to removal by suction; a cerumen curette is usually more useful. Wrap petrolatum gauze around the sharp end of an FB to protect the nares from trauma during extraction.[8]

Kill live FBs before removal because any movement of the animal complicates an already difficult procedure. Kill screw-worm larvae with a 25% solution of chloroform. If the patient is still awake and cooperative, he or she may expel most of the larvae by blowing his or her nose. Administer piperazine or hexylresorcinol orally followed by an $MgSO_4$ purge to eradicate the intestinal infestation.

If there is a significant risk of the FB falling into the posterior pharynx, stabilize the posterior portion by passing the Fogarty catheter behind the FB, inflating the balloon posterior to the FB, and retracting the balloon against the FB (Fig. 138-1).

In small children (between ages 1 and 4), attempt removal as follows: achieve local vasoconstriction, restrain the child if necessary, place the child in the Trendelenburg position, place an Ambu bag over the mouth, and squeeze the bag forcefully while obstructing the uninvolved naris with an external finger press (Fig. 138-2).[3] Forceful mouth-to-mouth or mouth-to-mask exhalation may be used in place of the Ambu bag.[14]

After the FB has been removed, examine the nares carefully for the presence of any residual or unsuspected FBs, and check for damage caused by the FB (abrasions, lacerations, fractures, and burns). If needed, perform posterior rhinoscopy with a nasopharyngoscope[9] or a nasopharyngeal mirror to rule out the presence of any further FB.

Postprocedure Care

Antibiotics are not necessary. Some patients may require nasal packing for epistaxis (see Chapter 135).

REFERENCES

1. Baluyot, Sabino T Jr: Foreign bodies in the nasal cavity. In Paparella MM, Shumrick DA, editors: *Otolaryngology*, Philadelphia, 1980, WB Saunders.
2. Cannon CR: The miniature battery: a new foreign body hazard, *J Miss State Med Assoc* 29:41-42, 1988.
3. Cohen HA, Goldberg E, Horev Z: Removal of nasal foreign bodies in children (letter), *Clin Pediatr* 32:192, 1993.
4. DeWeese DD, Saunders WH, editors: *Textbook of otolaryngology*: acute and chronic diseases of the nose, St Louis, 1993, Mosby.
5. Abelson TI, Witt WJ: Ear, nose and throat. In Roberts JR, Hedges JR, editors: *Clinical procedures in emergency medicine*, ed 2, Philadelphia, 1991, WB Saunders.
6. Fallon MJ, Plante DM, Brown LW: Wooden transnasal intracranial penetration: an unusual presentation, *J Emerg Med* 439-443, 1992.
7. Fosarelli P, Feigelman S, Pearson E, et al: An unusual intranasal foreign body, *Pediatr Emerg Care* 4:117-118, 1988.
8. Harun S, Montgomery P, Ajulo SOP: An unusual oronasal foreign body, *J Laryngol Otol* 118-119, 1991.
9. Hocutt JE, Corey GA, Rodney WM: Nasolaryngoscopy for family physicians, *Am Fam Physician* 42(5):1257-1268, 1990.
10. Kittle PE, Aaron GR, Jones HL, et al: Incidental finding of an intranasal foreign body discovered on routine dental examination: case report, *Pediatr Dent* 13:49-51, 1991.
11. Lima JA: Laryngeal foreign bodies in children: a persistent, life-threatening problem, *Laryngoscope* 99:415-420, 1989.
12. McRae D, Premachandra DJ, Gatland DJ: Button batteries in the ear, nose, and cervical esophagus: a destructive foreign body, *J Otolaryngol* 18:317-319, 1989.
13. Ross EV: *Proteus mirabilis* isolation as a sign of nasal foreign body (letter), *Clin Pediatr* 29:514-515, 1990.
14. Shapiro RS: Foreign bodies of the nose. In Bluestone CD, Stool WE, Scheetz MD, editors: *Pediatric otolaryngology*, ed 2, Philadelphia, 1990, WB Saunders.

Eustacia Su

The external auditory canal (EAC) has its narrowest point at the isthmus, which is the bony portion of the canal. Most firm foreign bodies (FBs) do not progress beyond this point. Other FBs may be pushed to, but rarely through, the tympanic membrane. Live FBs such as insects may crawl beyond the isthmus and cause severe distress by beating their wings or their legs against the tympanic membrane.[1]

The skin of the EAC is exquisitely sensitive (especially over the bony portion of the canal, where the skin is thin), bleeds easily, and forms subepithelial hematomas from very trivial trauma. The external auditory canal is not an area in which a local anesthetic can be used effectively or easily because a circumferential wheal of anesthetic is required.[2] When the volume of local anesthetic is sufficient, the soft tissue swelling reduces the effective working orifice diameter to a point at which the procedure becomes even more challenging if not impossible (Fig. 139-1).

The patient's cooperation is essential for the success of this procedure. Because cooperation is not typical of the age group most affected by FBs in the ear, adequate conscious sedation and analgesia are crucial to ensure successful removal and to avoid propulsion of the FB through the tympanic membrane as an undesired complication. Consider using conscious sedation (see Chapters 12 and 13).

Indications

Remove any FB in the external auditory canal. The only decision is whether it is feasible to remove the FB in the Emergency Department or whether the patient needs to be under general anesthesia before any attempt at removal is made. Indications for a nonoperating-room attempt include the following:
1. FB in the outer portion of the EAC (external to the bony portion)
2. Easily visible FB
3. FB that is accessible to available instruments

Contraindications

For FBs that have been pushed beyond the isthmus or are lying against the tympanic membrane, refer the patient to a specialist, who would probably prefer not to deal with iatrogenic complications resulting from previous attempts at removal (e.g., EAC completely occluded by blood or swollen from trauma).[3] Other contraindications include a patient with severe hemophilia or other bleeding diathesis and the inability to adequately restrain the patient either physically or chemically.

Complications

Several complications can occur as a result of the removal of FBs from the external auditory canal:
1. Otitis externa
2. Perforation of the tympanic membrane

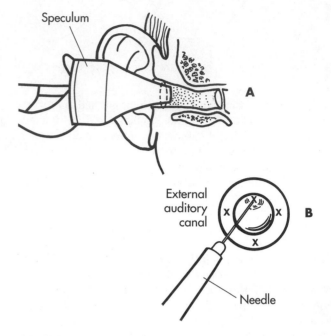

FIG. 139-1 Technique for four-quadrant field-block anesthesia in the external auditory canal. **A,** Withdraw, then tilt the speculum slightly in both the vertical and horizontal planes. **B,** Direct injections in all four quadrants (x), and inject 0.25 ml of local anesthetic to produce a perceptible bulge in the soft tissue.

3. Significant trauma to the EAC, which may cause stenosis and may require operative correction and grafting to restore patency
4. Necrosis of the tissues of the EAC as a result of electrolysis from an impacted button battery[4]

Equipment

Use immobilization devices such as a sheet or papoose board to minimize any potential or undesired movement by the child (see Chapter 11). Medications for conscious sedation or light anesthesia mandate the immediate availability of airway equipment and neuromuscular blocking agents in case the child develops apnea.

An adequate light source is crucial; an operating microscope is optimal but is generally not available in most Emergency Departments. The binocular vision provided by the microscope permits depth perception and allows more accurate placement of the instruments. A headlamp with separate specula is the next best choice, followed by an otoscope with an operating head.

Assemble the following instruments before starting the procedure: alligator or Hartmann forceps, suction apparatus and catheters of different sizes, suction heads (No. 3 and No.

5), wire loops and blunt hooks of various sizes, and a No. 8 Foley or No. 4 Fogarty catheter.

Techniques

The first attempt at removal has the best chance for success.[3] Explain the procedure to the parents and to the child in an age-appropriate manner. Do not violate the child's trust if at all possible. Immobilize the child by physical restraint or chemical sedation to minimize any potential, undesired, or unanticipated movement. Mummy wrap the child in a sheet before placing him or her on a papoose board. This position provides the most effective physical restraint but still requires an assistant to hold the head. Instrumentation of the EAC may produce a reflex cough in older children.[2]

In young children and infants, apply traction in a direction that is purely posterior to the EAC; this procedure straightens the EAC for better visual assessment. In older children, as in adults, traction in a superior, lateral, and posterior direction provides better visualization.

Use mineral oil to kill a live FB such as an insect. Ether and alcohol have also been recommended, but if the EAC is already excoriated either by the movement of the insect or by the patient's attempts to remove it, the instillation of either substance will be very painful. Irrigation is probably the best means of removal after the insect is no longer moving because dead insects tend to fragment easily. If a part of the insect is embedded into the EAC wall, forceps removal is necessary.

The most common FB is a bead or an eye from a stuffed toy. These objects are smooth and polished and are difficult to grasp. If there is enough of a gap between the edge of the object and the canal wall, pass a blunt, right-angle hook beyond the FB. Turn the hook 90 degrees and withdraw it with the FB (Fig. 139-2). A smooth, rounded FB may be easier to remove by using a plastic suction catheter with a soft funnel tip. If the suction of the vacuum between the FB and the tympanic membrane is too great, the Fogarty catheter might be useful; it can be passed beyond the FB, inflated, and withdrawn, pulling the FB with it. Be careful not to puncture the tympanic membrane.

A metal cerumen curette may also be used to remove impacted FBs if the loop can be passed behind the FB. Another method for removing a smooth, firm FB such as a bead, which does not peel or disintegrate, is to apply glue (such as cyanoacrylate) to the wooden end of an applicator and place the glue-laden end against the FB.[6] When the glue has set, gently pull back on the applicator and remove the FB. There is a significant risk that the Super-Glue will bond to the skin of the external auditory canal on contact, further complicating the situation.

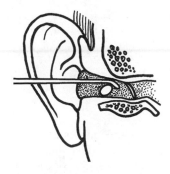

FIG. 139-2   Removal of foreign body from the external auditory canal. Using a small, blunt, right-angled hook, rotate the tip behind the foreign body. Withdraw the hook and foreign body.

Irrigation with water at body temperature is a gentler and less invasive way to remove small, hard objects; seeds or beans cannot be removed in this manner because these organic objects may swell and become impacted. Do not irrigate when attempting to remove a button battery because electrolysis will cause necrosis of the surrounding tissues, especially if an electrolyte solution is used.[5]

Postprocedure Care

Examine the ear for residual FBs and for damage to the canal wall and tympanic membrane. Determine whether the child's immunization status is current, particularly against tetanus and especially if there are any lacerations or abrasions of the canal wall. Caution the parents that there may be some residual bleeding. Prescribe a steroid-antibiotic suspension if there is significant inflammation.

REFERENCES

1. Paparella MM, Meyerhoff WL, et al: Surgery of the external ear. In Paparella MM, Shumrick DA, Gluckman JL, et al, editors: *Otolaryngology*, ed 3, Philadelphia, 1991, WB Saunders.
2. Abelson TI, Witt WJ: Otolaryngologic procedures. In Roberts JR, Hedges JR, editors: *Clinical procedures in emergency medicine*, ed 2, Philadelphia, 1991, WB Saunders.
3. Bresler K, Shelto C: Ear foreign body removal: a review of 98 consecutive cases, *Laryngoscope* 104 (4 Pt 1): 367-370, 1993.
4. McRae D, Premachandra DJ, Gatland DJ: Button batteries in the ear, nose and cervical esophagus: a destructive FB, *J Otolaryngol*, 18: 317-319, 1989.
5. Cannon CR: The miniature battery: a new foreign body hazard, *J Miss State Med Assn* 29:41-42, 1988.
6. Hanson RM, Stephens M: Cyanoacrylate-assisted foreign body removal from the ear and nose in children, *J Paediatr Child Health* 30(1): 77-78, 1994.

140 Rectal Foreign Bodies

Eustacia Su

Children rarely place foreign bodies (FBs) in the rectum. Despite the commonly held fear that a glass mercury thermometer may either break off or become "lost" in the rectum, sexual abuse or molestation is the most common cause of rectal foreign bodies. The physician must rule out exploitation or abuse even in the adolescent who states that he or she willingly placed the FB in his or her rectum.

The "body packer," who transports cocaine by concealing it in the rectum, is a rather difficult exception because the history is often evasive and because the complications of releasing cocaine in the rectum during the course of removal can be dire.[6,11]

Unintentional injuries can occur, such as in a child who sits down while riding a bicycle without a seat or a child who jumps into the water while waterskiing and impales himself or herself on a submerged branch.[2] Ingested FBs eventually reach the rectum but do not usually present a problem because they have already traversed the gastroesophageal junction and the pylorus; these FBs usually pass through the rectum without difficulty.[5]

The indications for x-ray studies are controversial, but if there is any significant amount of pain, particularly abdominal pain, obtain an abdominal x-ray series or computerized tomography to rule out a perforation.[3] If the history is unreliable, an x-ray study may be helpful in detecting and locating radiopaque FBs. A voiding cystourethrogram may be necessary before the rectal examination if there is a question of penetration.

If the child has been chronically abused, removal of the rectal FB is technically easier, but adequate sedation and analgesia are absolutely imperative.

Indications

Remove any FB in the rectum because a delay may result in obstruction, perforation, or infection.[14] The patient who comes to the Emergency Department (ED) with a rectal FB has probably exhausted all ordinary means in attempting removal. The FB will not pass spontaneously. The majority of rectal FBs can be removed safely and successfully in the ED.[4,14]

Contraindications

If there is any question that a perforation or tear has occurred, consult a general surgeon to have the procedure performed with a general anesthetic.

The operating room is the place to remove objects that are too large to remove without major dilation, too high in the colon, or those that have been retained for a long time (depending on the clinical circumstances, usually 1 week). Consult a surgeon to remove objects with large, spiky projections or other features that pose a significant risk for perforation. Give patients who are immunosuppressed optimal antimicrobial prophylaxis and have the procedure performed in the operating room under the most sterile conditions possible despite the anatomic circumstances.

Complications

The most serious complication of removal of a rectal FB is bowel perforation; perforation is more likely with a sharper object or a greater force of introduction.[7] Perforation may also occur during removal. When the perforation occurs above the peritoneal reflection, it results in free air under the diaphragm and peritonitis. Perforation below the peritoneal reflection manifests in a more insidious manner; signs of pelvic abscess or sepsis may not appear for several days.

Other complications include bleeding, mucosal laceration, a torn anal sphincter, and retention or fragmentation of the foreign body.[13]

Equipment

For removal of rectal FBs, use a private, well-lit room equipped with a proctosigmoidoscopy table, lubricant, rubber gloves, an examining light, a local anesthetic with appropriate syringes and needles, and parenteral narcotics and sedatives. If digital extraction is unsuccessful, an operative anoscope or proctoscope, a Parks retractor (Fig. 140-1, *A*), a Deaver retractor, or vaginal speculum will be needed for visualization; grasping tools will also be necessary (Table 140-1).

Techniques

If a proctosigmoidoscopy table is available, place the patient in the prone position with the hips and knees flexed. If no table is available, place the patient in the Sims position (lying on the side) on the most comfortable examining table possible.

Use adequate sedation and analgesia (see Chapters 12 and 13). Muscle relaxation is crucial to the success of the procedure. A local anesthetic in a field block may also be needed for optimal dilation of the anal sphincter.[13] After a povidone-iodine preparation, inject 1% lidocaine with epinephrine 1:200,000 (unless contraindicated) radially around the anal sphincter. Inject the anesthetic anteriorly and posteriorly into the submucosal tissue.

At this time, set a time limit (e.g., 30 minutes). If FB removal is not accomplished in this time, refer the patient to a consultant for treatment or hospital admission.[8]

Gentle suprapubic pressure helps move the FB into the distal rectum, where the examining finger guides the FB toward the anus. The FB may lodge against the sacrum posteriorly and need gentle redirection.

If digital extraction is unsuccessful, select a specific technique on the basis of the nature, size, shape, and orientation of the FB. Each technique requires speculum visualization and a means of grasping the FB (see Table 140-1). Because the FB most often has a diameter greater

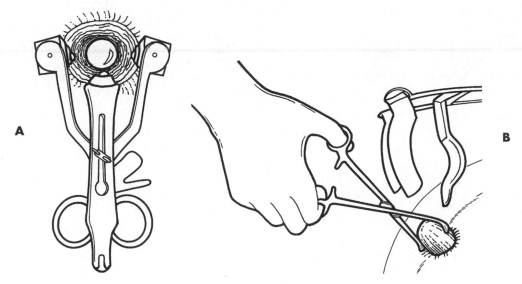

FIG. 140-1   **A,** Parks retractor used to visualize a rectal foreign body. **B,** Tenaculum forceps used to remove a foreign body. When the foreign body is too large to remove through the retractor, remove the retractor as the foreign body emerges.

Table 140–1   Grasping Tools for Removing a Rectal Foreign Body

Grasping tools	Nature of object
Tenaculum forceps	Nonfriable, elongated object (e.g., dildo, cucumber)
Ring forceps	Banana or friable, elongated FB
Tonsil snare	Pencil
Obstetrical forceps	Ball, orange
Spoons	Vibrator, light bulb
Foley catheters	FB with distal portion narrower than proximal portion
Endotracheal tube	Glass jar

than that of the speculum, remove the speculum and grasping tool together (Fig. 140-1, *B*).

If available, a flexible sigmoidoscope with a polypectomy snare provides several advantages: the ability to distend the bowel around the FB, convenience of outpatient management, and the reported ability to retrieve high-lying objects.[12] The patient may not need to be as deeply sedated with this technique.

Glass FBs present their own peculiar problems. Glass is slippery, difficult to grasp, and may shatter during attempted removal. There may also be a vacuum effect in the distal colon when traction is applied; this effect may be circumvented by inserting a Foley catheter or endotracheal tube past the FB to allow air to enter behind the FB and release any suction forces. The inflated balloons also serve as traction devices.[9,10]

Catharsis with a nonabsorbable polyethylene glycol solution (GoLytely or Colyte) has gained in popularity for expelling foreign bodies from the gastrointestinal tract.[11] This technique usually applies to ingested foreign bodies, particularly cocaine packets. Instill 2 to 3 L/hr into the stomach via a nasogastric tube (see Chapters 101 and 102). It may be desirable to add a contrast material to the electrolyte solution to outline the bowel and identify the number of FBs to be expelled. This technique is often used even with button batteries and other orally ingested FBs; it is obviously contraindicated if there is any suspicion of perforation.

Initiate appropriate antibiotic coverage immediately if a perforation is suspected. Bowel anaerobes are the predominant contaminants. Select a broad spectrum drug regimen; clindamycin or metronidazole with an aminoglycoside is one regimen; ticarcillin-clavulanic acid, imipenem, or cefoxitin is another regimen.[1]

Postprocedure Care

After removal of the rectal FB and regardless of the technique used, perform proctosigmoidoscopy to look for perforation, bleeding, or mucosal trauma. The presence of abdominal pain, deep mucosal lacerations, significant bleeding, or suspicion of perforation mandates admission. Perforation most commonly occurs at the first rectosigmoid angulation, approximately 15 cm from the anus. Perforation may have occurred before the procedure, which may complicate even the most atraumatic removal.

REFERENCES

1. Abramowicz M, Rizack MA, Hirsch J, et al, editors: The choice of antimicrobial drugs, *Med Lett Drugs Ther* 30:35, 1988.
2. Ashcraft KW, Holder TM: *Acquired anorectal disorders in pediatric surgery,* ed 2, Philadelphia, 1993, WB Saunders.
3. Barone J, Sohn N, Nealon T: Perforations and foreign bodies of the rectum, *Ann Surg* 184:601, 1976.
4. Barone J, Yee J, Nealon T: Management of foreign bodies and trauma of the rectum, *Surg Gynecol Obstet* 156:453, 1983.
5. Bloom RR, Nakano PH, Gray SW, et al: Foreign bodies of the gastrointestinal tract, *Am J Surg* 52:618, 1986.
6. Carvana D, Weinbach B, Goerg D, et al: Cocaine packet ingestion: diagnosis, management and natural history, *Ann Intern Med* 100:73, 1983.
7. Crass RA, Tranbaugh RF, Kudsk KA, et al: Colorectal foreign bodies and perforation, *Am J Surg* 142:85, 1981.

8. Davis SM: Management of rectal foreign bodies. In Roberts JR, Hedges JR, editors: *Clinical procedures in emergency medicine,* ed 2, Philadelphia, 1991, WB Saunders.

9. Diwan V: Removal of 100-watt electric bulb from rectum (letter), *Ann Emerg Med* 11:643, 1982.

10. Garber H, Rubin R, Eisenstat T: Removal of a glass foreign body from the rectum, *Dis Colon Rectum* 24:323, 1981.

11. Jonsson S, O'Meara M, Young JB: Acute cocaine poisoning: importance of treating seizures and acidosis, *Am J Med* 75:1061, 1983.

12. Kentarian JC, Riether RD, Sheets JA, et al: Endoscopic retrieval of foreign bodies from the rectum, *Dis Colon Rectum* 30:902, 1987.

13. Sohn N, Weinstein M: Office removal of foreign bodies in the rectum, *Surg Gynecol Obstet* 140:209, 1978.

14. Wigle R: Emergency department management of retained rectal foreign bodies, *Am J Emerg Med* 6:385, 1988.

141 Vaginal Foreign Bodies

Eustacia Su

Preschool-aged girls sometimes insert foreign bodies (FBs) into the vagina during self-exploration. The most common type of vaginal FB seen in this age group is toilet paper or other wadded up pieces of newspaper, paper towel, or bits of cloth.[7] This behavior is probably normal and probably not indicative of sexual abuse. Other FBs removed from the vaginas of prepubertal girls include safety pins, pieces of crayon, beans, glass beads, coins, plastic toys, and small buttons. Postpubertal girls sometimes insert objects of some phallic significance, but the most common FB in this age group is a retained menstrual tampon.

A common presenting complaint is that the child has a profuse, foul-smelling, purulent, and sometimes blood-stained discharge; vulvovaginal inflammation is sometimes present. The child rarely admits placing the FB in her vagina, and the adolescent has usually forgotten that the tampon was inserted and not removed. Because the history is often not helpful, detection of the FB may require rectal palpation, vaginoscopy, or x-ray examination.[7]

The physician must maintain a high of suspicion for sexual abuse, particularly if the FB is likely to have caused pain during insertion or has a particularly phallic or religious/satanic significance and if the patient is not at an age at which she is likely to have spontaneously placed an FB in her vagina.

Indications

Remove all detected vaginal FBs because the resultant vulvovaginitis will not otherwise resolve. The age and likelihood of cooperation from the child is a significant determinant of whether this procedure can be accomplished in the Emergency Department (ED). Another significant factor is the availability of the appropriate equipment. Most EDs do not have a vaginoscope or hysteroscope. In general, remove vaginal FBs from prepubertal girls and virgins in the operating room and with the use of a general anesthetic and a vaginoscope or hysteroscope.[2]

Contraindications

Remove the FB in the operating room when any of the following conditions exist: (1) there is a suspected perforation or significant tear; (2) the child is too young or too agitated to undergo the procedure without the use of a deep sedative or general anesthetic, or (3) the FB is of a size or configuration such that removal might result in serious injury. If child abuse is suspected, perform the procedure to protect the evidence collected.

Complications

The most common complication of a retained vaginal FB is a self-limited vaginitis that resolves spontaneously after removal of the FB. The inflammation may be so extensive that it results in polyp formation.[1] A fistula may form if the FB has been present for a long time.[8] A tear or perforation may occur during the removal of an FB of an unusual size or configuration. Minimize psychologic trauma in these patients with the generous use of a sedative or anesthetic. Failure to immediately place a long-retained tampon in a hermetically sealed container instead of an open wastebasket results in the room being unusable for hours until the stench clears.

Equipment

For a postpubertal girl, the following equipment is necessary for removal of a vaginal FB: several sizes of vaginal specula, ring forceps, Bozeman forceps, a tenaculum, obstetric forceps, and a vacuum. For a prepubertal, virginal girl, a

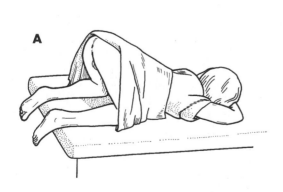
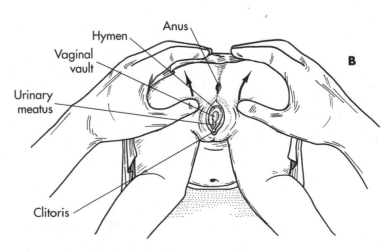

FIG. 141-1 **A,** Knee-chest position with "sway-backed" posture. **B,** Lifting the perineum in the knee-chest position (with anatomic landmarks).

vaginoscope, hysteroscope, or resectoscope (if available) is also necessary. Because the vaginoscope or hysteroscope is generally not available without an attached consultant, the use of this instrument is not covered in this chapter.

Procedure

Placing a prepubertal girl in the knee-chest position (Fig. 141-1) permits visualization of the vagina and cervix with minimal manipulation.[5] Postpubertal girls, particularly those who already use tampons or have been sexually active, may be examined in the usual dorsal lithotomy position with a vaginal speculum of the appropriate size.

An examination of the vagina, either with direct visualization using a speculum or vaginoscope or indirectly with a rectal or bimanual examination, will reveal the presence and nature of the FB. If the FB is known to be radiopaque, an x-ray examination may also help define its position, shape, and orientation.

Remove the FB with the ring or Bozeman forceps if the FB can be seen and easily grasped and if no further injury will result from the procedure. If the exudate is too thick to permit visualization of the FB, a lavage should help to remove enough of the exudate. If there is any suspicion that the FB may be a battery, use water rather than an electrolyte solution for irrigation to prevent electrolysis. If the FB is partially or completely hidden by the cervix, move the cervix with the tenaculum.

Make sure that what the examiner is extracting is an FB and not a tumor or unidentified portion of the normal anatomy. If the FB is particularly large and round, obstetric forceps may provide better traction.[3,4] Another method that has had reported success uses the soft vacuum cup.[6]

Postprocedure Care

After removal of the vaginal FB, exclude the possibility of any residual FB, tears, lacerations, fistulae, or other tissue damage.

REFERENCES

1. Aridogan N, Cetin MT, Kadayifci O, et al: Giant cervical polyp due to a foreign body in a "virgin," *Aust N Z J Obstet Gynaecol* 28(2):1466-1467, 1988.
2. Bacsk'o G: Use of the hysteroscope in pediatric gynecology for diagnosis of vaginal hemorrhage and injury, *Zentralbl-Gynakol* 115:1129-1130, 1993.
3. Emge KR: Vaginal foreign body extraction by forceps: a case report, *Am J Obstet Gynecol* 167:514-515, 1992.
4. Escamilla JO: Vaginal foreign body extraction by forceps: case report (letter), *Am J Obstet Gynecol* 169:233-234, 1993.
5. McCann J, Wells R, Simon M: Genital findings in prepubertal girls selected for nonabuse: a descriptive study, *Pediatrics* 86(3):428-439, 1990.
6. Pelosi MA, Giblin S, Pelosi MA: Vaginal foreign body extraction by obstetric soft vacuum cup: an alternative to forceps (letter; comment), *Am J Obstet Gynecol* 168(6 Pt 1):1891-1892, 1993.
7. Pokorny S, Pokorny W: Benign gynecology. In Ashcraft KW, Holder TM, editors: *Pediatric surgery*, ed 2, Philadelphia, 1993, WB Saunders.
8. Unda-Urzaiz M, Prieto-Ugidos N, Iriate-Soldevilla I, et al: Vesicovaginal fistula in an 8-year-old girl, *Arch Esp Urol* 42:473-475, 1989.

142 Soft Tissue Foreign Bodies

Eustacia Su

A crawling or playing child encounters many types of foreign bodies (FBs). A thorough history may provide pertinent information about the soft tissue FB, which helps plan its removal. Assess the risk and timing of a potential infection: some soft tissue FBs produce infection in a few days, whereas others may cause an infection to flare up after weeks or months and for no apparent reason.

Remove organic material immediately because it carries microbial contaminants and provokes a much greater chemical inflammatory response than inorganic FBs. Sea urchin spines, for example, are covered with slime and marine organisms; thorns provoke an intense inflammatory response even with no microbial contamination.[27] Chronic inflammation may not manifest as purulence but as disability from pain.

Glass or plastic may be removed electively. Inert metallic FBs (e.g., BBs) may be left in place if no vital structures are threatened and if the FB is too deeply embedded to allow easy removal. The inert FB may have carried dirt, pieces of clothing, or other contaminated material into the wound; these materials mandate exploration and debridement even when the FB itself does not.

Wounds that bleed excessively, are painful, or heal poorly should provoke suspicion of a retained FB; also consider an FB with recurrent abscesses or poorly healing cellulitis.[17] Embedded FBs in the patient with multiple trauma may seem to be an overlying artifact on routine x-ray examinations; these objects must be proven to be extrinsic or otherwise extracted.

Indications

Remove any easily accessible FB. A reasonable goal is a maximum of 30 to 60 minutes for the removal procedure, which is the maximum period for effective local anesthesia. If the best assessment suggests that more time is required for the process, the operating room is a more appropriate location for the procedure. Consider elective scheduling for glass, plastic, or non-toxic, metal FBs.[2]

Contraindications

Soft tissue FBs requiring removal in the operating room include the following:
1. FBs in the deep spaces of the hands or feet or in otherwise inaccessible locations
2. Greasy or oily FBs or the suspicion that grease or oil has entered the hand or forearm from a machinery mishap
3. FBs that may have caused neurovascular disruption in their course through the soft tissues

Leave FBs that are inert, have caused little injury in the course of penetration, are inaccessible, and unlikely to cause further complications.

Imaging

Radiopaque FBs can be localized on x-ray studies that can guide the removal of the FBs. Visibility on x-ray studies depends on the relative density, configuration, size, and orientation of the FB. Even large pieces of wood are often not seen on standard x-ray studies unless they have been painted, whereas most glass FBs larger than 2 mm are readily visible.[7,26] Soft tissue (underpenetrated) x-ray films may improve the identification of some FBs. Xerography is not significantly more sensitive in detecting splinters[15] (Box 142-1).

The radiopaque FB may be best localized by placing markers on the entrance wound or by inserting needles (at approximately 90 degrees to each other) close to the FB and with the patient under local anesthesia. X-ray examinations at different angles guide three-dimensional localization and removal.[1,4]

Obtain a postprocedure x-ray study after removal of a radiopaque FB to document its complete removal; this procedure can be omitted if the object was single and unlikely to fragment (e.g., a needle).

High-resolution ultrasound, computed tomography, and magnetic resonance imaging may better identify FBs (particularly wood) and delineate the surrounding anatomy; however, these methods are rarely used until complicated wound healing suggests the presence of a retained FB that was not detected on initial plain x-ray studies or exploration.[3,5]

Complications

Infection and FB reaction are the two most common complications of FBs and attempted removal. Staphylococcal infections are the most common infections associated with soft tissue wounds and FBs. *Pseudomonas* osteomyelitis is a rare

---

BOX 142-1   TYPES OF SOFT TISSUE FOREIGN BODIES

Radiopaque FBs

Metallic FBs (e.g., aluminum, lead, iron, steel)
Most glass FBs
FBs containing calcium, barium and similar substances
Pencil graphite
Painted FBs that would otherwise be radiolucent (e.g., wood)

Radiolucent FBs

Wood
Plastic
Rubber
Paper

complication (approximately 1%) and is specific to plantar wounds caused by a sharp object usually going through a rubber-soled shoe.[12]

Neurovascular damage is a complication of both the initial injury and blind exploration and groping. A retained FB may cause poor healing, recurrent cellulitis and abscesses, and chronic pain and disability.

Traumatic tattooing may occur if ground-in dirt or graphite particles (from an embedded pencil) are not completely removed. These marks are permanent, and the tissue must be completely excised.

Underestimating the degree of difficulty and the amount of time required for the removal procedure results in a dissatisfied patient and caregiver and a frustrated physician.

Equipment

A standard suture tray with a scalpel usually suffices for most simple FB removal procedures. Special pickups, splinter forceps, tissue retractors, and other equipment may be selected as needed. Good direct light, perhaps even a head lamp, is essential. Magnification may be required. If fluoroscopy is available, use it to facilitate the removal of a deeply embedded radiopaque FB.

A bloodless field greatly facilitates the removal of a soft tissue FB in an extremity. Elevate the extremity and wrap an elastic bandage from the distal to the proximal end to drain the extremity before applying an arterial tourniquet (usually a blood pressure cuff). A Penrose drain may be used at the base of the digits. Alternatively for a finger site on an older child, snip the fingertip of a tightly-sized sterile glove and roll the material to the base of the digit. This technique provides hemostasis and a sterile field. Circulation to the extremity can be stopped safely for 20 to 30 minutes.

Provide adequate local anesthesia. Using lidocaine with epinephrine in wounds to the trunk or head also results in a nearly bloodless field, but its use is contraindicated in wounds on the appendages, tip of the nose, ears, and penis. Select the appropriate syringes, needles, and drugs for use before the procedure and have extras available during the procedure.

Young children probably need sedation and parenteral analgesia (see Chapters 12 and 13). Make sure that the appropriate monitoring devices, drugs, antagonists, and airway equipment are close at hand.

Techniques

The specific techniques for removal of an FB in soft tissue vary depending on the situation and are discussed in the following sections.

General Principles. Establish adequate sedation and analgesia that is appropriate to the duration and complexity of the procedure as well as to the age of the child.

The usual principles of wound management apply (see Chapter 130). Prepare the area around the wound in the usual aseptic manner. After inducing adequate local anesthesia, remove ground-in dirt with a scrub brush or sterile toothbrush.

The entrance wound often needs to be enlarged with an adequate skin incision. Blind grasping into a wound through an inadequate skin incision or puncture is not only frustrating and self-defeating but also may result in damage to crucial structures, especially on the face, hands, or feet. Spread the sides of the enlarged wound with a hemostat. If the end of the FB is easily found either by direct visualization or by "feeling" with a hemostat, extract it by gentle traction and follow the longitudinal axis of the FB. This technique minimizes the possibility of splintering or breaking the FB.

Following the entrance tract of the FB is not easy, especially when the FB traverses muscle or fat. Injecting methylene blue into the entrance wound may delineate the FB tract,[12] but unfortunately this tract is often closed.

Consider excising a block of tissue that contains the palpable but not visualized FB; this procedure is more effective and removes devitalized, contaminated, or tattooed tissues; it may also be face-saving if attempts at removing dirt or graphite have not been successful.

Easily Palpable Foreign Body. An easily palpable FB may seem deceptively simple to remove. When the wound is enlarged, the scalpel may push the perpendicularly oriented FB (e.g., splinter or thorn) to one side. In this case it may be more effective to make a small elliptical incision around the FB, grasp the block of skin and subcutaneous tissue (including the closest end of the FB), undermine the sides of the block of tissue until the FB is reached, grasp the FB with forceps, and remove the block of tissue with the FB (Fig. 142-1). Alternatively, an ellipse of skin overlying the FB may be excised and pressure may be put on the sides to push the FB into view for removal.

A tangentially embedded, palpable wood splinter requires careful debridement. Grasping and pulling the splinter may be adequate if the end protrudes, but care must be taken not to leave any shards in the wound. The best approach in this case is to cut along the length of the splinter, remove it, and assiduously irrigate the length and depth of the wound. Suture the wound when debridement and irrigation are adequate and the FB has not been in place for too long (less than 6 hours). If there is any increased risk of infection, leave the wound open and arrange follow-up for secondary repair.

Foreign Bodies in the Sole of the Foot. Foreign material is carried into the soft tissues when a child wearing a tennis shoe steps on a sharp object that penetrates the sole of the foot. Some physicians advocate routinely enlarging the wound by excising a 2-mm rim of skin around the entrance wound; this procedure allows better visualization and irrigation. Explore these puncture wounds, but do not blindly probe because doing so might drive foreign material farther into the soft tissues and fascial planes. Any trace of pigmentation or discoloration should prompt thorough debridement of the wound, usually by excising the ellipse of tissue that contains the tract. Rubber shreds, sock material, and wood splinters have been found in these wounds. Irrigate the wound thoroughly, leave it open, soak it at frequent intervals in warm water, and allow it to heal secondarily.[6,10-12]

Subungual Foreign Bodies. Digital block anesthesia must precede any manipulation of a nail or nail bed. If the FB is deeply embedded in the nail bed, remove a portion of the nail to gain access to the FB, and remove the FB with splinter forceps.[8] Sometimes the nail may need to be completely removed (especially for wood splinters) because the entire, intact FB must be extracted to prevent subungual infection and osteomyelitis of the underlying distal phalanx.

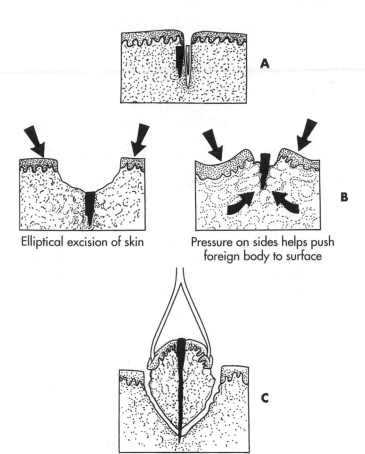

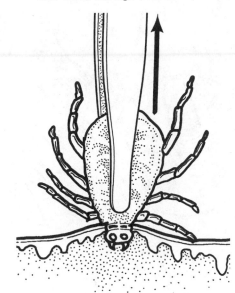

FIG. 142-2   Removal of an embedded tick. Apply axial traction perpendicular to the skin surface.

FIG. 142-1   A, Cutting down on top of the foreign body may push it into the side of the incision, where it will be difficult to locate. **B,** Removal of a deeply embedded foreign body. **C,** Excision or undermining of a block of tissue containing the foreign body. After undermining, grasp the foreign body at the subcutaneous position and remove it with the block of excised tissue.

Plant and Animal Spines. Cactus spines enter the soft tissues most often when a child runs into a cactus. The spines vary in size and number; generally the smaller the spines, the more that are embedded in the skin and soft tissues. Manage larger spines in the same manner as wood splinters; remove individually using forceps and gentle, axial traction. Small (glochid) spines are much more difficult to manage because they tend to be numerous. Several techniques have been suggested for removal, and all involve the application of a liquid (depilatory wax, adherent facial-mask gel, and household glue) that dries to form a firm layer and that when peeled back pulls the glochids with it.[14,16,18,24,25] If the cactus spines are deeply embedded, especially in sensitive areas, carefully weigh the risk to benefit ratio of deep exploration. Leaving the spines in place stimulates a granulomatous reaction, but infections are rare.

Sea urchin spines are intrinsically reactive and are often contaminated with slime, debris, and calcareous material. They cause an intense FB reaction and may produce significant morbidity when retained.[27] Attempts at removal are complicated by the fact that the spines are nearly colorless and very brittle.[19,22] If removal does not seem feasible, it may be better to allow the body enough time to react before opening and draining the wound and curetting out all of the foreign material. Allow the wound to heal by secondary intention.

Tick Removal. Remove ticks as soon as possible to prevent the transmission of tickborne diseases. Ixodid ticks cement their mouth parts to the skin of the host; traditional methods of forcing disengagement are ineffective. Mechanical removal requires a hemostat, and gloves prevent the infection from being transmitted to the person removing the tick. To free the tick, grasp it as close to the patient's skin surface as possible and apply steady axial traction from the mouth to the caudal end (Fig. 142-2). Do not squeeze, puncture, or crush the tick. Excise any remaining mouth parts and use a local anesthetic if the removed tick appears to be incomplete. Twisting the tick in a counterclockwise direction may facilitate removal because ticks screw themselves into the skin in a clockwise direction.[21]

Ring Removal. It is sometimes necessary to remove a ring to prevent laceration of tissue or vascular compromise. For the first attempt, use thorough lubrication and circular traction on the ring. If this attempt fails, wrap a 15- to 20-inch piece of umbilical tape, thick silk suture, or string around the base of the finger; start proximal to the ring and pull the end under the ring.[20] Wrap the string snugly, and place each loop immediately adjacent to the next to compress the soft tissue swelling and to prevent bulging between the loops. Continue this process beyond the proximal interphalangeal joint, which usually is the greatest obstacle to ring removal (Fig. 142-3). Unwind the proximal end of the wrap and force the ring over the distal, wrapped portion of the finger. If this method fails or is too painful for the patient despite optimal local anesthesia, use a ring cutter. Minimize the amount of metal dust that falls into any open wound; technically this consequence is impossible to avoid. An FB granuloma may result from retained metal dust.[9] Spread the cut ends of the ring using large hemostats (e.g., Kelly clamps). A cast splitter may be able to accomplish this task if the ring is made of a base metal and is too thick for the hemostat to spread.

Zipper Entrapment. The most common childhood prepu-

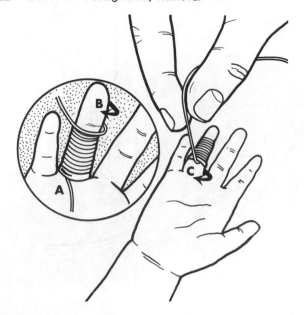

FIG. 142-3 String technique for ring removal from a swollen finger. **A,** Pass the proximal end under the ring and hold securely. **B,** Wind string in a tight spiral with loops abutting. **C,** Unwind string from proximal end. Slide ring forward over loops of string while unwinding proximal end.

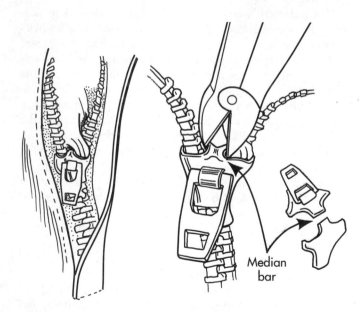

FIG. 142-4 Release of entrapped foreskin from zipper.

tial injury is entrapment in a zipper.[28] Local anesthesia is painful to achieve, and unzipping the zipper may lacerate the skin or worse, may increase the amount of tissue trapped in the mechanism. Cutting the median bar of the zipper with a bone cutter or wire clippers causes the teeth to fall apart and frees the skin (Fig. 142-4).[23] If the clothing can be sacrificed, cut the zipper away from the clothing, and cut off the bar at the bottom of the rows of teeth; this procedure also causes the teeth to fall apart and allows the diamond or bridge to pull off easily. If the appropriate cutting device is not available or if the median bridge is not accessible, use a local anesthetic and liberally apply mineral oil. This may allow the

skin to be pulled free after waiting for the oil to soak in for at least 10 minutes.[13]

Postprocedure Care

With all soft tissue FBs, leave the wound open and repair it secondarily if the following concerns exist: extensive exploration, possible contamination, penetration through fascial planes, a retained FB, or too long an interval since the injury.

Give a tetanus booster (or diphtheria-tetanus booster) to all patients with soft tissue FBs when there is any question regarding the completeness of the patient's tetanus-immunity status.

Close follow-up is imperative. Arrange for a wound-check visit within 48 hours to screen for infectious complications. The routine administration of antibiotics is controversial and depends on the nature of the FB, the extent of contamination, the length of time since the injury, and the amount of manipulation that occurred during extraction.

REFERENCES

1. Ariyan S: A simple stereotactic method to isolate and remove foreign bodies, *Arch Surg* 112:857, 1977.
2. Barnett RC: Soft tissue foreign body removal. In Roberts JR, Hedges JR, editors: *Clinical procedures in emergency medicine,* ed 2, 1991, Philadelphia, WB Saunders.
3. Bauer AR: Computed tomographic localization of wooden foreign bodies in children's extremities, *Arch Surg* 118:1084, 1983.
4. Bhavsar MS: Technique of finding a metallic foreign body, *Am J Surg* 141:305, 1981.
5. Bodne D, Quinn SF, Cochran CF: Imaging foreign glass and wooden bodies of the extremities with CT and MR, *J Comput Assist Tomogr* 9:1135, 1985.
6. Chisholm CD, Schlesser JF: Plantar puncture wounds: controversies and treatment recommendations, *Ann Emerg Med* 18:1352-1357, 1989.
7. Courter BJ: Radiographic screening for glass foreign bodies: what does a "negative" foreign body series really mean? *Ann Emerg Med* 19:997-1000, 1990.
8. Davis LJ: Removal of subungual foreign bodies, *J Fam Pract* 11:714, 1980.
9. Fasano FJ Jr, Hansen RH: Foreign body granuloma and synovitis of the finger: a hazard of ring removal by the sawing technique, *J Hand Surg* 12A:621-623, 1987.
10. Fitzgerald RH, Cowan DE. Puncture wounds of the foot, *Orthop Clin North Am* 6:965-972, 1975.
11. Inaba AS, Zukin D, Perro M: An update on the evaluation and management of plantar puncture wounds and *Pseudomonas* osteomyelitis, *Pediatr Emerg Care* 8:38-44, 1992.
12. Johanson PH: *Pseudomonas* infections of the foot following puncture wounds, *JAMA* 204:262-264, 1968.
13. Kanegaye JT, Schonfeld N: Penile zipper entrapment: a simple and less threatening approach using mineral oil, *Pediatr Emerg Care* 9:90-91, 1993.
14. Karpman RR, Sparks RP, Fried M: Cactus thorn injuries to the extremities: their management and etiology, *Ariz Med* 37:849, 1980.
15. Kuhns LR, Borlaza GS, Seigel RS, et al: An in-vitro comparison of computed tomography, xeroradiography, and radiography in the detection of soft tissue foreign bodies, *Radiology* 132:218, 1979.
16. Lindsey D, Lindsey WE: Cactus spine injuries, *Am J Emerg Med* 6:362, 1988.
17. MacDowell RT: Unsuspected foreign bodies in puncture wounds, *J Musculoskel Med* 7:33, 1986.
18. Martinez TT, Jerome M, Barry RC, et al: Removal of cactus spines from the skin: a comparative evaluation of several methods, *Am J Dis Child* 141:1291, 1987.
19. McWilliam LJ, Curry A, Rowland PL, et al: Spinous injury caused by a sea urchin, *J Clin Pathol* 44:428, 1991.

20. Mizrahi S, Lunski I: A simplified method for ring removal from an edematous finger, *Am J Surg* 151:412, 1986.
21. Needham GR: Evaluation of five popular methods for tick removal, *Pediatrics* 82:925, 1988.
22. Newmeyer WL: Management of sea urchin spines in the hand, *J Hand Surg* 13:455-457, 1988.
23. Nolan JF, Stilwell TJ, Sands JP: Acute management of the zipper-entrapped penis, *J Emerg Med* 8:305-307, 1990.
24. Putnam MH: Simple cactus spine removal, *J Pediatr* 98:333, 1981.
25. Schunk JE, Corneli HM: Cactus spine removal, *J Pediatr* 110:667, 1987.
26. Tandberg D: Glass in the hand and foot, *JAMA* 248:1872-1874, 1982.
27. Wilson GE, Curry A, Kennaugh JH, et al: Severe granulomatous arthritis due to spinous injury by a "sea mouse" annelid worm, *J Clin Pathol* 43:291-294, 1990.
28. Yip A, Ng SK, Wong WC, et al: Injury to the prepuce, *Br J Urol* 63:535-538, 1989.

143 Eye Foreign Bodies

Eustacia Su

Eye injuries are feared by the layperson. Children are more prone to eye injury and foreign bodies (FBs) than are adults because they have not yet learned to be as careful or protective of their own or their playmates' eyes (e.g., throwing sand at each other). The child's judgment and movements are not finely tuned, and he or she is less able to avoid a playmate's eye with a stick when playing. Because a young child's eyes are at the height of an adult's hands, the child may run into an object held by the adult (e.g., the burning end of a cigarette).

In one study, children under 10 years of age accounted for 4% of the patients seen by a busy eye emergency department (ED) but accounted for more than 18% of those admitted and 26% of all ocular penetrations. Although most eye injuries do not threaten sight, they do so disproportionately in children.[10]

A "lost" or retained contact lens is an increasing problem, especially because children are now being fitted with these devices at a younger age and even in infancy.[3,5,9] The physician must be able to recognize the different types of contact lenses, locate them in the extraocular structures, know the complications, and remove them with the least amount of trauma.

Indications

Remove all extraocular FBs. The nature of the injury and the patient's clinical status dictates how and when the FB is removed.

Indications for removal of a patient's contact lens include an altered level of consciousness in the patient, eye trauma with the lens in place, and the inability of the wearer and caregivers to remove the contact lens.

Contraindications

A suspicion of globe penetration mandates immediate ophthalmologic consultation. Maintain a high index of suspicion while taking a careful history; look for risk factors (e.g., hammering while splitting wood and not wearing proper eye protection),[11] and perform the physical examination (loss of visual acuity that does not correct after application of a topical anesthetic, or an irregular, "keyhole" shape to pupil) (see Chapters 86 to 90). Be aware that iris tissue that has prolapsed through the cornea may resemble a superficial corneal FB.[4] Suspected intracranial penetration through the orbit mandates neurosurgical consultation, appropriate imaging studies, and exploration in the operating room if indicated.[6]

A deeply embedded FB or other complicating circumstances may result in inadvertent penetration of the globe or significant trauma to adjacent uninjured tissue during attempted FB removal. Consult an ophthalmologist promptly if there is concern for such an injury.

A patient who is uncooperative because of youth, mental deficiency, or intoxication may require a general anesthetic to prevent iatrogenic trauma or other complications.

The main contraindication to removal of a contact lens is the presence of corneal perforation either de novo or in the past because the contact lens functions as a bandage for the corneal repair site.[1]

Complications

It is extremely rare for the entire depth of the cornea to be perforated during extraction of a corneal FB.

Undetected remnants of a removed FB may result in FB reactions and granulomas.[2] The epithelium has difficulty healing over such remnants; as a result the epithelium either sloughs, which results in persistent eye inflammation, or grows over and encloses the remnant, which may or may not be resorbed. Some scarring results from such an occurrence, but a small lesion, even in the optical center of the cornea, does not significantly affect vision.

Remove residual rust rings using a slow-speed ocular drill and appropriate burr. These lesions usually do not cause scarring or affect vision and can wait for elective removal by an ophthalmologist.

Infection rarely occurs even with large corneal defects, but most infections can be prevented with the instillation of ophthalmic antibiotic drops or ointment after the procedure.

Enucleation is a devastating but unfortunately not a rare complication of a penetrating injury to the globe. Evisceration of the globe contents may occur during overzealous examination of an eye that has sustained a penetrating injury.

Equipment

The equipment needed for the management of FBs in the eye includes a topical anesthetic (e.g., proparacaine 0.5%), sterile cotton-tipped applicators, fluorescein strips, a slit lamp or other form of magnification (e.g., loupes) and ultraviolet light, an eye spud or 25-gauge needle attached to the wooden end of a cotton-tipped applicator or 3-ml syringe, a slow-speed drill and burrs, a plunger for hard–contact lens removal, mydriatic agents (e.g., homatropine 5% or cyclopentolate 1%), an antibiotic ointment (e.g., sulfacetamide 10%), eye patches, and tape (preferably nonallergenic).

Techniques

General. Carefully evaluate the eye and establish the integrity of visual acuity, the globe, and the ciliary structures and function.

If the child is too small or too uncooperative to sit still for a slit-lamp examination, some other form of magnification must be used. Otherwise, if possible, place the child in a seat that allows use of the slit lamp (see Chapter 87).

Cooperation is essential and sedation may be required

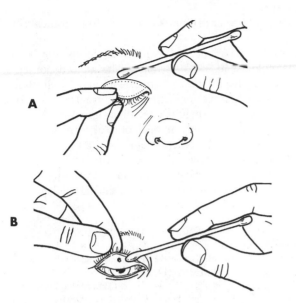

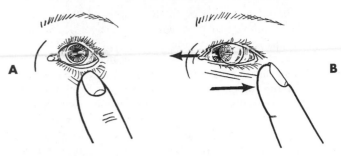

FIG. 143-2   Rigid contact lens removal. **A,** Pull the edge of the lower lid down so that it can slide under the edge of the contact lens. **B,** Retract the lid tissue laterally while the patient looks medially and blinks.

FIG. 143-1   Eversion of upper lid for foreign body removal. **A,** Pull eyelashes and upper lid downward and forward. Place applicator above tarsal plate and push down on it. Pull lid up against applicator to evert. **B,** Hold edge of upper lid against superior orbital rim. Remove foreign body with an applicator or other appropriate instrument.

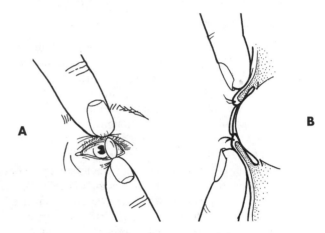

FIG. 143-3   **A,** "Tiddlywinks" technique for rigid contact lens removal. Push edge of lower eyelid under edge of contact lens. Push upper lid down onto upper edge of contact lens. Contact lens should "flip" out. **B,** Lateral view.

because the examination becomes significantly more difficult and fraught with complications if the child is struggling and clenching the eyelids shut.

Examine the bulbar conjunctival surfaces for any obvious lesions; then inspect the tarsal conjunctival surfaces. The lower tarsal conjunctiva is easily seen, but evert the upper lid for a thorough examination of the upper tarsal conjunctiva (Fig. 143-1). To evert the upper lid, place the cotton tip of an applicator on the outer surface of the upper lid and above the tarsal plate; apply traction to the eyelashes to evert the tarsal plate over the applicator tip. Remove any FB by brushing it off with another cotton-tip applicator (see Chapter 86).

Examine the bulbar conjunctiva and cornea. Use a form of magnification to examine this area. The slit lamp provides the optimal means of magnification, but it is difficult to use in the young, uncooperative child. Examine the eye without applying fluorescein because it may obscure an FB. Remove the FB if it is visible and readily removable. If no FB is detected, dampen the end of the fluorescein strip with a small drop of water or saline and apply the dampened area to the edge of the lower tarsal conjunctiva. Abrasions may reveal the presence of an FB by their pattern or location. A corneal FB usually has a fluorescein-positive ring around it. Vertical linear scratches reveal the presence of a tarsal FB.

A superficial FB can usually be irrigated off the cornea and then removed from the conjunctiva with a cotton-tipped applicator. Do not use the cotton tip to remove a corneal FB because it removes a significant area of epithelial cells wherever it contacts the cornea.

Extract the embedded FB with a spud (if available) or a 25-gauge needle attached to the wooden end of an applicator. Hold the spud or bevel *tangentially* to the surface of the cornea and scoop out the foreign body.

Reexamine the eye and look for any residual FB or rust

ring. Drill out any residual rust ring if the child is cooperative enough to make this procedure feasible and if the correct equipment is available.

Contact Lens Removal

SOFT (HYDROPHILIC) LENSES. A soft contact lens that requires removal in the ED has usually been in the eye for a long time and has resisted removal efforts by the patient and caregivers. If the lens appears or feels dry to the patient, irrigate it with sterile saline. Using the index finger, pull the lens inferiorly so that a portion of it is now off the cornea, and "pinch" the lens off the surface of the eye. The lens may tear and leave remnants in the eye; however, this rarely happens, especially if the lens is well moistened. If the lens is still intact, immerse it immediately in sterile saline.

HARD OR GAS-PERMEABLE LENSES. Remove hard or gas-permeable lenses using three different techniques:

1. If the lens is situated on the cornea or can be easily manipulated back onto the cornea, the patient or the examiner may be able to remove the lens by retracting the lids at the lateral canthus while the patient looks medially. The edge of the lower lid should catch the lower edge of the contact lens and flip it off the cornea as the lids narrow (Fig. 143-2).

2. If the lens is too adherent, try gently pushing on the

lower lid just inferior to the margin of the lens and bringing the upper lid down onto the superior margin of the lens (the "tiddlywinks" method) (Fig. 143-3).

3. If the lens is adhered to the conjunctiva to such an extent that it cannot be manipulated onto the cornea or is on the cornea and cannot be removed by either of the previous methods, push a simple plunger with a small suction cup very gently onto the lens to extract it by suction. A drop of honey on the fingertip also causes the lens to adhere to the finger strongly enough to allow removal; this method is useful if no suction-tipped device is available. The honey is easily washed off the lens.

After the contact lens has been removed, place it in sterile saline in a sealable container.

Postprocedure Care

After the FB has been removed, thoroughly reexamine the eye for residual FBs, abrasions, ulcerations, penetration, and any other complications. If there is no evidence of any of these problems (other than abrasions), instill a dilator drop (cyclopentolate 1% or homatropine 5%) into the eye to relieve ciliary spasm, if present; although infection is rare, also instill an antibiotic ointment (e.g., sulfacetamide ophthalmic ointment 10%).[7]

Pressure patching the lids shut may facilitate epithelial healing by minimizing the relative movement of the lids over the cornea; it also keeps light away from the photosensitized eye, which decreases patient discomfort. Pressure patching is indicated in all injuries resulting in corneal abrasions but is contraindicated if the corneal ulcer results from an active infection.[12] A pressure patch is also contraindicated if there has been a penetrating injury to the globe. Be sure the patch is tight enough so that the lids cannot open under it; a tight fit also ensures that the lashes are not inverted toward the cornea and do not cause further corneal abrasions (see Chapter 90).[4]

The patient must keep both eyes closed for patching. Hold the first patch in vertical orientation and fold down the middle, and place the doubled patch on the patient's closed lids. Hold the second patch in a horizontal orientation and place over the doubled patch. Tape the patches in place, and orient the tape from the cheek superomedially to the medial end of the eyebrow (see Chapter 90).

Update the child's tetanus immune status if it is not current because scattered case reports of tetanus from corneal FBs do exist.

Instruct the patient and parents to follow up with an ophthalmologist in 24 to 48 hours. The majority of superficial abrasions heal within this time without complications. A possible long-term complication is recurrent erosion, which may occur weeks or months after the original injury appears to have healed completely. A small area of corneal epithelium fails to bond to the basement membrane[4] and usually comes off in the morning when the patient first opens his or her eyes. This area may heal before an examination can take place; 5% sodium chloride ointment and a bandage contact lens may be required for healing.[8]

REFERENCES

1. Aiello LP, Iwaoto M, Taylor HR: Perforating ocular fishhook injury, *Arch Ophthalmol* 110:1316-1317, 1992.
2. Ainbinder DJ, O'Neill KP, Yagci A, et al: Conjunctival mass formation with unexpected foreign body, *J Pediatr Ophthalmol Strabismus* 28:176-177, 1991.
3. Amos CF, Lambert SR, Ward MA: Rigid gas-permeable contact lens correction of aphakia following congenital cataract removal during infancy, *J Pediatr Ophthalmol Strabismus* 29(4):243-245, 1992.
4. Barr DH, Samples JR, Hedges JR: Ophthalmologic procedures. In Roberts JR, Hedges JR, editors: *Clinical procedures in emergency medicine,* ed 2, Philadelphia, 1991, WB Saunders.
5. Epstein RJ, Fernandes A, Gammon JA: The correction of aphakia in infants with hydrogel extended-wear contact lenses: corneal studies, *Ophthalmology* 95(8):1102-1106, 1988.
6. Kazarian EL, Stokes NA, Flynn JT: The orbital puncture wound: intracranial complications of a retained foreign body, *J Pediatr Ophthalmol Strabismus* 17:247, 1980.
7. King JWR, Brison RJ: Emergency department management of traumatic corneal epithelial injuries without topical antibiotic prophylaxis, *J Emerg Med* 8:373, 1990.
8. Laibson PR: Epithelial basement membrane dystrophy and recurrent corneal erosion. In Fraunfelder FT, Roy FH, editors: *Current ocular therapy,* Philadelphia, 1980, WB Saunders.
9. Levin AK, Edmonds SA, Nelson LB, et al: Extended-wear contact lenses for the treatment of pediatric aphakia, *Ophthalmology* 95(8):1107-1113, 1988.
10. MacEwen CJ: Eye injuries: a prospective survey of 5671 cases, *Br J Ophthalmol* 73(11)888-894, 1989.
11. Owen P, Keightley SJ, Elkington AR: The hazards of hammers, *Injury* 18:61-62, 1987.
12. Sexton RR: Superficial keratitis. In Wilson LA, editor: *External diseases of the eye,* Hagerstown, Md, 1979, Harper & Row.

144 Removal of a Barbed Fishhook

Eustacia Su

A barbed fishhook that is embedded in the skin is quite difficult to remove because it is designed not to slip out of the soft tissue of a fish's mouth. There are several techniques for removing the single, barbed hook; the choice of technique depends on the prevailing conditions.[2] The choices are very limited when dealing with a multiple-barbed hook (most often a triple hook), especially if the patient wants to use the hook again.

Indications

The presence of the hook in an accessible area is indication for removal.

Contraindications

Arrange a subspecialty consultation and removal in the operating room for the rare instances in which the removal of embedded hooks may cause serious complications (e.g., penetration of the cornea or globe),[1,6] tearing through the edge of the eyelid, or a situation in which there is a possibility of GI mucosal penetration (e.g., esophagus or rectum). The techniques for removal remain essentially the same.

Procedure

The use of an adequate local anesthetic is essential in the young child. The older child or adolescent who can tolerate a certain degree of pain may prefer to take the chance that the procedure will cause less pain than would the administration of a local anesthetic.

The traditional method for removing small fishhooks is to advance the hook in an antegrade direction, which forces the barb through the skin; clip off the end of the hook, including the barb, and remove the rest of the hook in a retrograde direction. Infiltrate the overlying skin with 1% lidocaine to obtain local anesthesia over the point of the hook.[3]

If the hook is so large that pushing the hook through the skin in an antegrade direction would result in too much trauma or a defect that is too large, insert an 18-gauge needle through the entrance wound and along the hook to cover the barb while the hook is pulled out in a retrograde direction (Fig. 144-1). Alternatively, a No. 11 blade may be inserted parallel to the shank of the hook and down to the barb. Free the subcutaneous tissue from the barb with the point of the blade, and using the blade as a guide along which to slide out the barb, back the hook out of the wound.

One technique may be used in the field or in cases in which the use of a local anesthetic is either refused or contraindicated (Fig. 144-2).[4] This technique requires tying a piece of string or umbilical tape around the belly of the hook where it enters the skin. To provide strong traction, wrap a significant length (approximately 1 foot) around the dominant hand of the person performing the extraction. Another technique involves wrapping the ends around a tongue

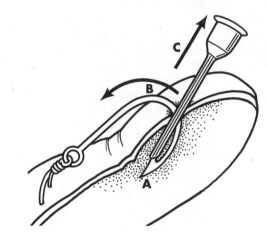

FIG. 144-1 Removal of barbed fishhook (needle-cover method). **A,** Cover the barb with the bevel of a needle. **B,** Rotate hook and **C,** remove needle and hook together.

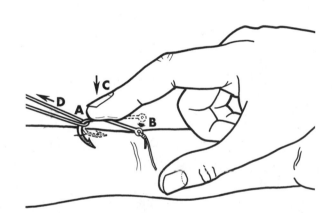

FIG. 144-2 Removal of barbed fishhook (string method). **A,** Tie string around belly of hook and wrap the ends around hand or tongue blade. **B,** Depress shaft of hook using thumb and middle finger. **C,** Disengage barb from subcutaneous tissue using index finger to press downward. **D,** Pull sharply; hook should exit easily through entry wound.

blade.[7] The hook is held parallel and close to the skin by the nondominant index finger while the thumb and middle finger stabilize and depress the barb, which helps the index finger to disengage the barb from the subcutaneous tissue. The dominant hand then gives a *sharp* pull to remove the hook through the entry wound. The hook "surfs" and usually exits very rapidly; keep the expected path of the hook clear of other potential victims.

Remarks

The least traumatic method of fishhook removal is the simple retrograde method; unfortunately, this method tends to be useful only with barbless hooks. The needle-cover technique is the next preferred method but is limited to use with larger hooks. Both the needle-cover and string techniques are adjuncts to the retrograde technique. When these techniques have failed, use the advance-and-cut technique, which traumatizes previously undamaged skin and for this reason is not the first-line technique. If the hook is already through the skin, use the advance-and-cut technique first.

In general, there seems to be a very low risk of infection in fishhook injuries. Therefore antibiotic prophylaxis seems to have no detectable advantage in reducing the already infinitesimal infection rate that results from these injuries, even when these injuries involve deep structures.[5]

REFERENCES

1. Aiello LP, Iwamoto M, Taylor HR: Perforating ocular fishhook injury, *Arch Ophthalmol* 110:1316-1317, 1992.
2. Barnett RC: Editorial: a few ways to unsnag a fishhook, *Emerg Med* 13:22, 1981.
3. Barnett RC: Three useful techniques for removing imbedded fishhooks, *Hosp Med* vol 72, July 1982.
4. Barnett RC: Soft tissue foreign body removal. In Roberts JR, Hedges JR, editors: *Clinical procedures in emergency medicine,* ed 2, Philadelphia, 1991, WB Saunders.
5. Doser C, Cooper WL, Ediger WM, et al: Fishhook injuries: a prospective evaluation, *Am J Emerg Med* 9:413-415, 1991.
6. Temel A, Gunay M: Corneal perforation due to a fishhook, *Injury* 22(4):327-328, 1991.
7. Terrill P: Fishhook removal (letter), *Am Fam Physician* 47(6):1372, 1993.

145 Gastrointestinal Foreign Bodies

Jacalyn S. Maller

The ingestion of foreign bodies (FBs) is a common occurrence in children. The majority of ingestions occur during the toddler and preschool years (6 to 48 months).[2] During this time, innate curiosity, use of the mouth as a third "hand" for exploration, poor oral motor-sensory coordination, and the lack of back molars to adequately chew food predispose these children to the risks of ingestion or aspiration. Coins, particularly pennies, are the most commonly ingested items, followed by toys, buttons, marbles, pen caps, and button batteries.[2,17]

Clinical presentations range from an absence of symptoms to clear signs of esophageal impaction (vomiting, drooling, pain, dysphagia) or respiratory complaints related to compression of the trachea by the esophagus, which has been distended by the ingested FB. A history of ingestion may not be forthcoming from a preverbal child, and the caregiver may not have noticed the episode. Therefore the emergency physician must maintain a high index of suspicion for FB ingestion in the child who comes to the Emergency Department with acute stridor, drooling, refusal to feed, or a recent onset of failure to thrive. Less common presentations include esophageal perforation, esophageal-aortic fistula, tracheoesophageal fistula, breathholding spells, and an altered level of consciousness.

Indications

Fortunately, the majority (80% to 90%) of FBs traverse the gastrointestinal (GI) tract without complications and do not require any procedural intervention.[12]

Remove all FBs that are lodged in the esophagus. Fig. 145-1 illustrates the three anatomic sites of relative narrowing, where FBs are most likely to lodge: (1) cricopharyngeal muscle, (2) aortic arch crossing, and (3) gastroesophageal (GE) junction. Weak peristalsis below the striated cricopharyngeal muscle accounts for the majority (75% to 90%) of esophageal impactions occurring at this site.[6,8] Complications of esophageal impaction depend on the object involved and on the duration of impaction and may include respiratory compromise (from tracheal compression, aspiration, or atelectasis), esophageal perforation (from acute laceration, prolonged pressure necrosis, or corrosive damage), mediastinitis, retropharyngeal abscess, pneumothorax, or tracheal or aortic fistula formation.[8]

In most cases, simply observe coins in the esophagus (especially those initially seen at the GE junction) for several hours but for no longer than 12 to 24 hours in the asymptomatic child; the length of this observation period is controversial. Consider factors such as age of the child, ability to tolerate oral fluids, and reliability of the caregiver. Remove the FB by endoscopy or Foley balloon catheter when passage into the stomach does not occur or if the patient becomes symptomatic.[9-11]

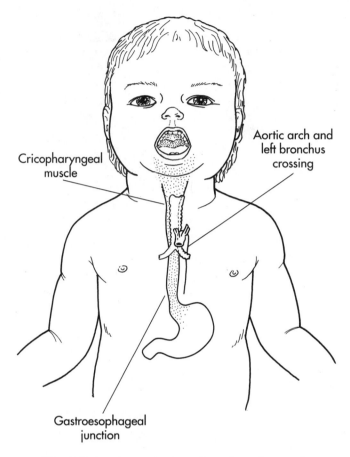

FIG. 145-1 Anatomic sites of esophageal narrowing.

Sharp, pointed, or elongated FBs such as open safety pins, toothpicks, and sewing needles may become impacted at various levels of the GI tract, including the esophagus and small bowel, and cause perforation, infection, or hemorrhage that is manifested clinically as an acute abdomen. Promptly remove sharp esophageal FBs by endoscopy. Management of an asymptomatic patient who has a sharp object in the stomach or in the small or large bowel is controversial. Many gastroenterologists advocate endoscopic removal of sharp objects in the stomach that are longer than 5 cm to avoid the subsequent need for surgery if the object becomes impacted in the bowel.[17]

Immediately remove button batteries, most commonly from hearing aids and other small electronic devices, that are in the esophagus or are causing GI symptoms.[7] Mucosal damage can occur from alkali produced by an electrochemical current when the battery reacts with fluid in the GI tract. This current, in turn, can dissolve the battery's seal and cause leakage of alkali (which plays a lesser role in tissue injury).

*See text for indications for removal of coins in esophagus. Obtain GI consultation to determine need for removal.

Toxicity from the systemic absorption of the heavy metal (e.g., mercury) contained in the battery may occur with the ingestion of mercuric oxide batteries. In practice, clinical symptoms of mercury poisoning do not occur, even with toxic blood levels, because the mercuric oxide is converted to less toxic metabolites in the GI tract.

Patients with a history of esophageal disease (e.g., tracheoesophageal fistula, esophageal web) are more likely to sustain repeated episodes of esophageal impaction of food and other objects and are less likely to have a successful nonendoscopic removal. In such a patient, arrange immediately for FB removal by endoscopy when the patient presents with a history or physical examination that is compatible with esophageal impaction. In addition, use endoscopy to look for anatomic abnormalities in patients without a known history of esophageal abnormalities but with a second episode of esophageal impaction. Box 145-1 lists GI FBs that may require removal.

Contraindications

Generally do not attempt FB removal for asymptomatic patients in whom the object is in or past the stomach radiographically. However, even in an asymptomatic patient it may be necessary to remove long (>5cm) or sharp objects that fail to progress on two X-ray studies, as well as button batteries.

Techniques

There are many excellent techniques for FB removal (Box 145-2).

ENDOSCOPY
Equipment

Arrange for an endoscopy to be performed in the operating room by a specialist skilled in the technique and with the use of a general anesthetic. Advantages include the ability to (1) visualize directly the object being removed, (2) search for multiple FBs that may not be visible radiographically, (3) visualize anatomic abnormalities (webs, strictures) that may predispose the patient to impaction, and (4) to evaluate the site of impaction for mucosal damage caused by the foreign body.[6] Direct examination and FB removal with a rigid or flexible endoscope is the oldest and safest method available.

Techniques

Control the airway and administer an anesthetic (preferably general) to ensure a cooperative patient. Use endoscopy rather than alternative methods of blind extraction to remove sharp or pointed objects or esophageal button batteries, as well as for patients with repeated episodes of impaction.

Advantages of the flexible endoscope include built-in suction and magnification and the ability to examine the stomach and duodenum. However, with an over-tube it is safe to use the flexible endoscope for sharp or pointed objects. Rigid endoscopy may be preferable over flexible endoscopy for the removal of sharp or pointed esophageal FBs, for acutely symptomatic patients, and for button batteries and objects that have been lodged for a prolonged (>2 week) time period.

Complications

Complications of endoscopy include esophageal perforation with secondary mediastinitis and risks associated with general anesthesia (aspiration, laryngospasm, death). Esophageal perforation associated with endoscopy is rare during blunt FB removal.[6]

FOLEY CATHETER EXTRACTION

The Foley catheter is useful for the removal of blunt esophageal FBs, particularly coins, that have been present for less than 48 to 72 hours. One recent retrospective study of the fluoroscopic Foley catheter technique documented an overall success rate of 91% in 415 cases of esophageal FBs; however, the success rate dropped to 83% in children with underlying esophageal disease. The mean age of the patients was 29 months, with children under 24 months accounting for 45% of the cases. All FBs in the series were blunt except one.[11]

Equipment

The equipment necessary for Foley catheter extraction includes a mouth gag, a 10-ml syringe, a water-soluble contrast agent, and a 14- or 16-French Foley catheter.[5] Keep airway equipment, including oxygen, suction, a bag-valve-mask, endotracheal tubes, and McGill forceps immediately available in case complications occur. Immobilize or sedate a younger or uncooperative patient.

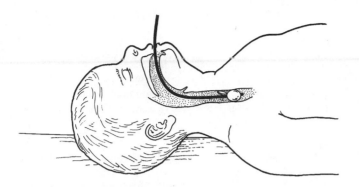

FIG. 145-2 Use of Foley catheters for esophageal foreign body removal.

Techniques

Arrange for an experienced physician (often a radiologist or surgeon) to perform a Foley catheter extraction in the radiology suite and with fluoroscopy; this procedure avoids the costs and risks of the operating room, general anesthetic, and hospitalization. After anesthetizing the oropharynx with a local anesthetic spray, insert the catheter through the nose or mouth. Once the tip is beyond the FB, use fluoroscopy to visualize the tip of the catheter by inflating the balloon with 3 to 5 ml of contrast medium. Leave the syringe on the balloon port (Fig. 145-2). Put the fluoroscopy table in a steep Trendelenburg position and place the child prone to avoid aspiration while pulling the object out with gentle, steady traction. In some cases, it is easier to use the distended balloon to push the object into the stomach. The oral approach, instead of the nasal approach avoids FB reimpaction in the nasopharynx. Avoid numerous attempts at extraction.[5] One sign that may predict unsuccessful balloon extraction is esophageal edema or tracheal narrowing as seen on a lateral chest X-ray examination. This sign indicates prolonged FB retention and is more common in younger patients (no more than 1½ years of age).[14]

Complications

Complications associated with the use of the Foley catheter are uncommon and occur in 0.5% to 2% of patients.[4,10,11] Complications include nasal cavity impaction, epistaxis, vomiting, esophageal mucosal injury, tracheal intubation, and laryngospasm. The most feared complication, irreversible airway obstruction, is rare. The availability of airway equipment and the presence of physicians skilled in resuscitation best prevent this tragic outcome. Other complications are the psychologic and emotional effects this procedure may have on the young patient.[13] The use of intravenous sedation may avert this complication but may increase the risk of airway complications.

ESOPHAGEAL BOUGIENAGE

Esophageal bougienage using an appropriately sized bougie dilator is an alternative technique for the removal of FBs from the GI tract. This method is useful for esophageal coins in asymptomatic children with no prior history of esophageal disease or FB impaction. The ingestion must be acute (<24 hours), with a single coin documented radiographically.

Techniques

To perform an esophageal bougienage, pass a lubricated and appropriately sized bougie dilator into the mouth and to the esophagus in an upright patient; this procedure will dislodge the coin into the stomach. Surgeons experienced in this technique have used it without the need for sedation or intravenous access.

Complications

Complications with an esophageal bougienage are rare with careful patient selection. Patients with known esophageal disease or prior manipulation are at increased risk for esophageal perforation because of alterations in esophageal distensibility, wall strength, or diameter. Patients with a FB present for longer than 24 to 48 hours may develop pressure necrosis from chronic impaction and also have a higher risk of perforation with blind techniques.[3]

GLUCAGON

Glucagon sometimes hastens the passage of FBs from the distal esophagus into the stomach. Glucagon relaxes the smooth muscle of the distal esophagus and decreases lower esophageal sphincter pressure. It is effective less than 50% of the time in adults with esophageal meat impaction[15,16] but theoretically may be useful in children with distal esophageal coins.

Techniques

Use glucagon in a dose of 0.03 to 0.1 mg/kg/dose intravenously; the maximum pediatric or adult dose is 1 mg.

Contraindications

Contraindications to the use of glucagon include a known drug allergy, insulinoma, or pheochromocytoma.[15]

Complications

The side effects of intravenous glucagon include nausea and vomiting.

MAGNET

The use of fluoroscopy to remove metallic FBs, including button batteries, with an orogastric tube magnet (OGTM) has been successful in a very limited patient sample.[15,17] Children with metallic FBs that have been lodged in the esophagus, stomach, or duodenum for less than 24 to 30 hours are candidates for this technique.

Techniques

Obtain an X-ray study of the entire GI tract to document the position of the FB. Pass the OGTM through the mouth and into the midesophagus. Place the patient in a left lateral decubitus position on a fluoroscopy table. If the object is in the stomach, use fluoroscopy to advance the OGTM through the cardia of the stomach; direct the magnet toward the fundus of the stomach, where the object generally will lodge. When the magnet makes contact with the FB, remove the unit and obtain an X-ray study to document complete removal of the object. In the reported series the entire procedure took less than 3 minutes.[15,16]

Complications

No complications have been reported using the OGTM technique. However, because of the limited patient sample and availability of other techniques, do not use this technique as a first-line procedure.

Remarks

During the past 10 years, many new techniques have emerged for GI FB removal. Although the Foley catheter and esophageal bougienage obviate the need for an anesthetic or the operating room, optimal control of the airway remains of paramount importance. Airway control may be accomplished most safely and effectively with the endoscopic removal of GI FBs. Fortunately, most children who ingest GI FBs remain asymptomatic and pass them spontaneously.

REFERENCES

1. Bendig DW: Removal of blunt esophageal foreign bodies by flexible endoscopy without general anesthesia, *Am J Dis Child* 140:789-790, 1986.
2. Binder L, Anderson WA: Pediatric gastrointestinal foreign body ingestions, *Ann Emerg Med* 13:112-117, 1984.
3. Bonadio WA, Jona JZ, Glicklich M, et al: Esophageal bougienage technique for coin ingestion in children, *J Pediatr Surg* 23:917-918, 1988.
4. Campbell JB, Condon VR: Catheter removal of blunt esophageal foreign bodies in children, *Pediatr Radiol* 19:361-365, 1989.
5. Campbell JB, Quattromani FL, Foley LC: Foley catheter removal of blunt esophageal foreign bodies: experience with 100 consecutive children, *Pediatr Radiol* 13:116-119, 1983.
6. Hawkins DB: Removal of blunt esophageal foreign bodies from the esophagus, *Ann Otol Rhinol Laryngol* 99:935-940, 1990.
7. Litovitz, J, Schmitz BF: Ingestion of cylindrical and button batteries: an analysis of 2382 cases, *Pediatrics* 89(4):747-757, 1992.
8. Nandi P, Ong GB: Foreign body in the aesophagus: review of 2394 cases. *Br J Surg* 65:5-9, 1978.
9. Savitt DL, Wason S: Delayed diagnosis of coin ingestion in children, *Am J Emerg Med* 6:378-381, 1988.
10. Schunk JE, Corneli H, Bolte R: Pediatric coin ingestions: a prospective study of coin location and symptoms, *Am J Dis Child* 143:546-548, 1989.
11. Schunk JE, Harrison AM, Corneli HM, et al: Fluoroscopic Foley catheter removal of esophageal foreign bodies in children: experience with 415 cases, *Pediatrics* 94(5):709-714, 1995.
12. Taylor RB: Esophageal foreign bodies, *Emerg Med Clin North Am* 5(2):301-311, 1987.
13. Tenebein M: Commentary on catheter removal of blunt esophageal foreign bodies in children, *Pediatr Trauma Acute Care* 3(2):7-8, 1990.
14. Towbin R, Lederman HM, Dunbar JS, et al: Esophageal edema as a predictor of unsuccessful balloon extraction of esophageal foreign body, *Pediatr Radiol* 19:359-360, 1989.
15. Volle E, Beyer P, Kaufmann HJ: Therapeutic approach to ingested button-type batteries: magnetic removal of ingested button-type batteries, *Pediatr Radiol* 19:114-118, 1989.
16. Volle E, Hanel D, Beyer P, et al: Ingested foreign bodies: removal by magnet, *Radiology* 160:407-409, 1986.
17. Webb WA: Management of foreign bodies of the upper gastrointestinal tract, *Gastroenterology* 94:204-216, 1988.

PART XXVI

DENTAL TECHNIQUES

146 Dental Emergencies

Robert L. Sweeney

Dental emergencies are a common reason for children's visits to the Emergency Department (ED). By the age of 14 years, 30% of all children have sustained injuries to primary teeth, and 22% have injured permanent teeth.[1]

Predisposing factors to dental injuries include gait unsteadiness in toddlers, contact sports, normal childhood rough-and-tumble play, and bicycle and auto crashes.[4] Common mechanisms of teeth trauma include falls, sports injuries, and domestic violence. Injuries may include soft tissue injuries as well as injuries to teeth, teeth structures, and bone. Teeth have the lowest potential of any tissue for returning to a healthy and normal state after injury.[2,4]

Teeth Anatomy and Development

The management of dental emergencies depends on the age of the patient and the type of tooth involved. Primary teeth begin to erupt from the gums sometime during the first 3 months of life. These deciduous teeth shed throughout the first 2 decades of life and are replaced completely by permanent teeth by the age of 20. Table 146-1 lists the normal eruption patterns for primary and permanent teeth. Fig. 146-1 presents the anatomy of a tooth and dentoalveolar structures.

All teeth have a tough outer matrix of enamel that surrounds an inner dentin layer and central pulp. The enamel is a rigid structure that is not vascular and has no nerve supply, whereas the dentin is a softer composite of microtubules, nerve processes, and fluid.[5] The pulp contains the nerves and blood supply of a tooth; the nerves and blood supply originate from the marrow of the alveolar bone of the maxilla or mandible. The crown or coronal portion of the tooth projects above the gingiva; the root or apex is the region below the gum line. Periodontal ligaments and cementum hold the teeth in place and anchor the root to the surrounding alveolar bone.

Fig. 146-2 presents the specific nomenclature of the teeth. The different surfaces of the crown are defined by their relation to the tongue and mouth. The biting surface of the molars and premolars is the occlusal surface; for the incisors, the biting surface is the incisal surface.

Indications

Treat all injuries to teeth on the basis of the specific injury or fracture classification and the age of the patient (see the Techniques section later in this chapter).

Contraindications

The only absolute contraindication to dental procedures is the presence of other more serious injuries or infections (especially of the airway) that require more immediate treatment. A relative contraindication is an uncooperative child who cannot open the mouth voluntarily and participate in the procedure. If appropriate sedation and analgesia (see

Table 146-1 Eruption Schedule for Teeth

	Primary teeth			
	Eruption at age (months)		Shedding at age (years)	
	Lower	Upper	Lower	Upper
Central incisor	6	7 ½	6	7 ½
Lateral incisor	7	9	7	8
Cuspid	16	18	9 ½	11 ½
First molar	12	14	10	10 ½
Second molar	20	24	11	10 ½
Incisors	Range ±2 months		Range ±6 months	
Molars	Range ±4 months			

	Permanent teeth*	
	Age (years)	
	Lower	Upper
Central incisors	6-7	7-8
Lateral incisors	7-8	8-9
Cuspids	9-10	11-12
First bicuspids	10-12	10-11
Second bicuspids	11-12	10-12
First molars	6-7	6-7
Second molars	11-13	12-13
Third molars	17-21	17-21

Modified from Massler M, Schour I: *Atlas of the mouth and adjacent parts in health and disease,* 1946, The Bureau of Public Relations Council on Dental Health, American Dental Association.
*The lower teeth erupt before the corresponding upper teeth. The teeth usually erupt earlier in girls than in boys.

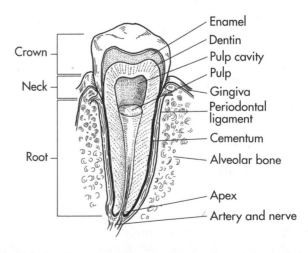

FIG. 146-1 Normal dental anatomy showing relations of dentoalveolar structures.

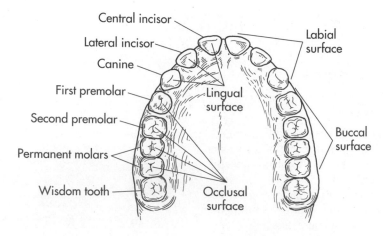

FIG. 146-2 Nomenclature of teeth showing positional arrangement and names of dental surfaces.

BOX 146-1 **COMPLICATIONS OF DENTAL INJURIES AND UNSUCCESSFUL REPAIR PROCEDURES**

Primary teeth

Color change
Infection or abscess
Pulp necrosis
Loss of space
Injury to erupted secondary dentition

Permanent teeth

Color change
Infection or abscess
Pulp necrosis
Loss of space

BOX 146-2 **CONTENTS OF A DENTAL BOX**

Anesthetics
  Lidocaine 2% with 1:100,000 epinephrine
    Amide
    Length of action: 1-1.5 hours
  Procaine 2% with 1:300,000 norepinephrine (Levophed)
    Ester
    Length of action: 1-1.5 hours
  Bupivacaine 0.5% with 1:200,000 epinephrine
    Amide
    Length of action: 8 hours
Copalyte
Cotton rolls
Dental aspirating syringe
Dental explorer
Dental floss
Drains (Penrose)
Dycal and applicator
Eugenol-based medication
Gauze (2 × 2)
Hemostat
Iodoform gauze
Irrigating syringe
Mouth mirror
Periodontal probe
Scissors
Sterile No. 15 scalpel

Chapters 12 and 13) together with parent or caretaker assistance does not work, consult a dentist or oral or maxillofacial surgeon.

Complications

Complications of dental injuries occur when there is a treatment delay or when the procedures used to repair teeth are unsuccessful (Box 146-1).

Equipment

Keep dental supplies in a dental box. Box 146-2 lists the equipment required for the treatment of dental injuries.

Techniques

To determine the appropriate dental procedure for treating acute trauma to the teeth, obtain a history of the mechanism and a past medical history. Important points to address during the child's medical history are congenital cardiac disease (consider prophylaxis for endocarditis), bleeding history, allergies, medications, and tetanus-immunization status. Make note of prior dental conditions.

Conduct an organized examination of the mouth and teeth. This examination includes the following procedures:[3]

1. Inspect the shape and contour of the maxilla and mandible. Suspect a condylar injury and injury to the body of the mandible whenever a patient has struck his or her chin.

2. Evaluate occlusion. Have the child open and close his or her mouth. Teeth displacement or facial bone fractures may lead to malocclusion. Occlusion is a sensitive way for the child and physician to determine if teeth have moved. The child with a temporomandibular joint dislocation cannot shut his or her mouth (see Chapter 149).

3. Assess mobility. Teeth that move singly may identify a fracture or subluxation. En bloc movement may be a result of alveolar bone fractures.[3]

4. Assess soft tissues. Treat intraoral and extraoral lacerations with standard wound care (see Chapter 131) after

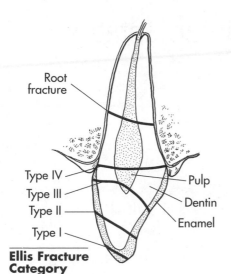

Ellis Fracture Category

FIG. 146-3 Dental fractures may occur through any of the components of the teeth. Descriptions are anatomic or by classification.

subluxed or avulsed teeth have been stabilized.[4] Check for the involvement of glands, ducts, and nerves.

5. Identify and locate missing teeth or tooth fragments. Missing teeth may be embedded in soft tissue or intruded into the alveolar bone or secondary teeth; the patient may have also aspirated them. Do not assume an apparently empty socket means that the tooth is avulsed. An x-ray study may be necessary.

6. Examine teeth carefully for fractures. Facial trauma commonly injures the teeth or their bony anchorage. Inspect teeth that are still in place for disruption of the alveolar attachments.

Fractures. A dental x-ray examination is often an important part of the dental assessment. A panoramic (Panorex) x-ray examination is optimal for bony visualization but may be unavailable in many EDs. In this situation, defer a panoramic x-ray examination to the dental consultant and obtain standard mandible or maxilla (facial) x-ray films.

The Ellis classifications (Fig. 146-3) categorize fractures of the teeth. Establish the fracture classification on the basis of direct inspection and sometimes together with the x-ray study. Class I fractures through only the enamel require no acute ED intervention. Soften sharp edges with an emery board and refer the patient for elective repair.

Class II fractures through the dentin and Class III fractures into the pulp require ED treatment for preservation of the tooth and prevention of infection, as well as for symptomatic pain relief. Cover exposed dentin as soon as possible for thermal and chemical protection and to prevent infection and pulp necrosis. Prepare a protective paste from a commercial preparation of calcium hydroxide (Dycal). Apply this paste to the tooth at the site of injury. After the paste has dried, coat this area with dental varnish (Copalyte). Clear nail polish is an optional substitute for Copalyte. Cover the entire preparation with metal foil and refer the patient for definitive repair in the next 24 hours.[5]

If calcium hydroxide paste is unavailable, pack fracture pockets with small cotton pledgets soaked in eugenol. This technique also works well for acute loss of fillings or fractures into large caries.

Table 146-2   Recommended Antibiotic Regimens for Dental/Respiratory Tract Procedures

Antibiotic	Dosage
Oral route	
Amoxicillin	50 mg/kg up to 3 g 1 hr before procedures, then half that dose at 6 hr after procedure
Penicillin-allergic (oral)	
Erythromycin *or* clindamycin	20 mg/kg up to 800-1000 mg 2 hr before procedure, then half that dose 6 hr after procedure
Unable to take by mouth (parenteral)	
Ampicillin	50 mg/kg IV or IM up to 2 g 30 min before procedure, then half that dose at 6 hr after procedure
Unable to take by mouth (parenteral) penicillin-allergic	
Clindamycin	10 mg/kg IV up to 300 mg 30 min before procedure, then half that dose at 6 hr after procedure
Erythromycin ethylsuccinate *or* stearate	800 mg 2 hr before and 400 mg 6 hr after procedure (ethylsuccinate) 1 g 2 hr before and 500 mg at 6 hr after procedure (stearate)

Modified from Dajani AS, Bisno AL, Chung KJ, et al: Prevention of bacterial endocarditis: recommendations by the American Heart Association, *JAMA* 264:2920-2921, 1990, American Medical Association. (Amended)

Pulp is distinguished from the yellow or pink dentin by a darker, bloody appearance when the fracture site is wiped clean. Treat Class III fractures with pulp exposure with calcium hydroxide and in the same manner as for Class II fractures. Refer the child to a dentist or oral or maxillofacial surgeon to perform pulp treatment within 24 hours.

Remarks

Dental procedures produce a transient bacteremia. Administer antibiotics to patients who are at risk for endocarditis or the seeding of indwelling medical devices. Table 146-2 presents the current American Heart Association recommendations for prophylaxis for the endocarditis that can result from dental procedures.

REFERENCES

1. Andreasen JO, Ravn JJ: Epidemiology of traumatic dental injuries to primary and permanent teeth in a Danish population sample, *Int J Oral Surg* 1:235, 1972.
2. Castaldi C: Injuries to the teeth. In Vinger PF, Hoerner EF, editors: *Sports injuries: the unthwarted epidemic,* Littleton, Mass, 1981, PSG Publishing.
3. Dembo J: Tooth avulsion and fracture. In Schwartz GR, Clayton CG, et al, editors: *Principles and practices of emergency medicine,* Philadelphia, 1992, Lea & Febiger.
4. Josell SD, Abrams RG: Managing common dental problems and emergencies, *Pediatr Clin North Am* 38:1325, 1991.
5. Kokkevold P: Common dental emergencies: evaluation and management for emergency physicians, *Emerg Med Clin North Am* 7:29, 1989.

147 Tooth Stabilization and Replantation

Robert L. Sweeney

In addition to fractures of the teeth, a dental injury may cause concussion, subluxation, displacement, or avulsion. A concussion is a traumatic injury to the tooth and its supporting structure without displacement or mobility. Subluxation injuries simply loosen the tooth in place; periodontal ligaments and alveolar attachments remain intact and the tooth rests in its original socket.

Tooth displacement partially disrupts ligaments and alveolar attachments, and the tooth shifts from its normal location in the socket. Displacement may be intrusive (i.e., the injury has pushed the tooth deeper into the alveolar bone or into a secondary tooth) or extrusive (i.e., the tooth is partially out of its socket) (Fig. 147-1). Displaced teeth may shift anteriorly, posteriorly, or laterally. Teeth may also be avulsed out of the socket.

Indications

Indications for tooth stabilization are displacement or avulsion.

Contraindications

Tooth concussions and subluxations do not require stabilization. Prescribe a soft diet and refer the patient to a dentist or oral or maxillofacial surgeon within 24 hours. The only absolute contraindication to tooth stabilization for displacements or avulsions is the presence of other serious injuries or infections that require more urgent treatment. Another contraindication is an uncooperative child, who may require immediate consultation from a dentist or oral or maxillofacial surgeon in the Emergency Department (ED). First consider conscious sedation and analgesia (see Chapters 12 and 13). Do not proceed if a young age, severe pain, or intolerance to the procedure render precise stabilization impossible.

Complications

Dental trauma and inadequate tooth stabilization can compromise patients both cosmetically and functionally by causing malocclusion. Functional problems may affect mastication or speech.

Complications of inadequate tooth stabilization include the embedding of tooth fragments into soft tissue, persistent bleeding, tooth aspiration, dentoalveolar abscess, and death of the tooth with tooth loss and damage of the tooth bud. If there is an associated alveolar bone fracture, inadequate tooth stabilization delays or complicates fracture healing.

Equipment

Box 146-2 lists the equipment needed for tooth stabilization.

Techniques

Repositioning of Displaced Teeth. Unless the injury has caused intruded teeth, displaced teeth are repositioned to their normal alignment and stabilized in place.

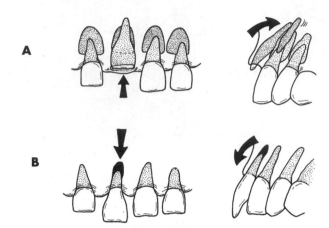

FIG. 147-1 Displacement may involve intrusion (**A**) and extrusion (**B**). Intrusion may encroach on unerupted secondary teeth or on alveolar bone. Extrusion may occur in any direction.

Reposition the teeth after administering a good local anesthetic to the involved tooth, such as a supraperiosteal infiltration (Fig. 147-2), or after a dental nerve block. A dental nerve block to the upper teeth, the infraorbital nerve block (Fig. 147-3), anesthetizes the maxillary teeth as well as the lower eyelids, side of the nose, and upper lip. The dental nerve block to the lower teeth, the inferior alveolar nerve block (Fig. 147-4), anesthetizes the mandibular teeth, lower lip, and chin. In children, a supraperiosteal infiltration is often adequate, especially if only one tooth has been displaced.

After adequate anesthesia has been obtained, manipulate the teeth back into place with gentle pressure. Do not dislodge the teeth during the movement. Once the teeth are in place, stabilize them as explained in the following section. Obtain a dental consultation if there is difficulty in getting the teeth back into their proper place or if there is uncertainty regarding precise alignment.

Stabilization. After replacing an avulsed or displaced tooth, stabilize it into position. In the ED there are several good methods to stabilize the tooth. The easiest but most temporary method involves immobilizing the tooth with a periodontal pack. These packs are commercially available and are composed of a puttylike substance that the physician forms around the affected tooth and the teeth on either side. The pack is prepared by mixing a predetermined amount of resin and catalyst and kneading the subsequent paste until the

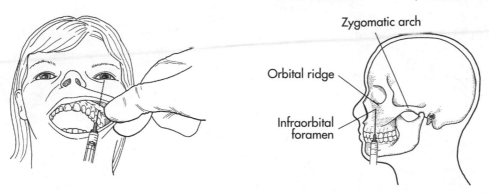

Fig. 147-2   Supraperiosteal infiltrations. Retract lip with dry gauze to expose the mucobuccal fold over the identified tooth or tooth socket. After applying a topical anesthetic and with the bevel facing the bone, advance the needle to the level of the tooth apex; inject 1 to 2 ml of local anesthetic.

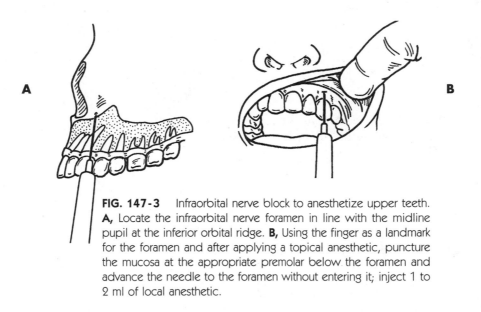

FIG. 147-3   Infraorbital nerve block to anesthetize upper teeth. **A,** Locate the infraorbital nerve foramen in line with the midline pupil at the inferior orbital ridge. **B,** Using the finger as a landmark for the foramen and after applying a topical anesthetic, puncture the mucosa at the appropriate premolar below the foramen and advance the needle to the foramen without entering it; inject 1 to 2 ml of local anesthetic.

proper consistency is obtained.[1] Periplast is a commercial preparation for periodontal packs. Apply the pack to both sides of the teeth (Fig. 147-5). These packs provide only temporary stabilization until a more permanent apparatus is available.

Arch bars and wiring provide the most definitive stabilization of avulsed teeth and alveolar bone fractures (Fig. 147-6). However, these techniques are considerably more complicated, and precise alignment in a preschool child is sometimes difficult in the ED. Arch bars consist of ribbons of flexible metal alloy with tabs for the attachment of anchoring wires. The bars stretch between a set of stable teeth on each side and bridge the loose tooth. Wire all teeth to the bar; anchor the bar to the stable teeth and the loose tooth to the bar.

To place arch bars, anesthetize the area with a supraperiosteal infiltration or with one of the dental nerve blocks. Stretch the appropriate length of bar across the buccal surface of the selected teeth, and wire the bar into position by passing the wire under the arch bar, around the tooth, and over the bar. Twist the wires with a heavy-duty needle holder or wire holder. Curve the loose end of the wire back onto itself to prevent injury to the patient.

A technique that is intermediate between arch bars and a periodontal pack involves suturing loose teeth in place. Using a 1-0 or 2-0 silk suture, weave a figure-of-8 between the stable tooth and the avulsed tooth. Anchor the tooth in place by tightening and knotting the suture.

When other associated injuries prevent the perfect realignment of displaced teeth in the ED, attempt a best approximation. Do not forcibly relocate teeth that are not loose in their displaced position; leave them in place and refer to a dental consultant.

Avulsion.   An injury may avulse teeth completely from their sockets. Avulsion of a primary tooth requires no specific treatment beyond dental evaluation for other associated injuries, local wound care, and mild analgesics. On the other hand, avulsion of a permanent tooth requires replacement of the tooth. The successful treatment of avulsed teeth is very time-dependent; delays of longer than 30 minutes often result in complete loss of the tooth and of periodontal ligament viability.

The goal of treatment of an avulsed tooth is rapid replacement of the tooth into the original socket to preserve key tooth attachments. The tooth pulp is devascularized and therefore requires pulp treatment (root canal); therefore

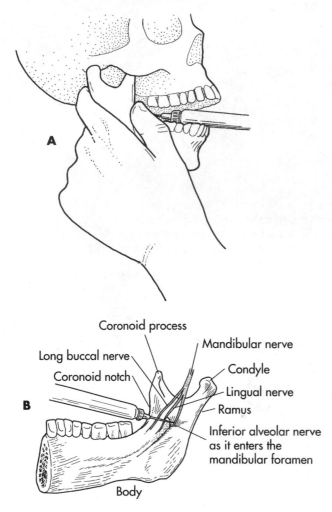

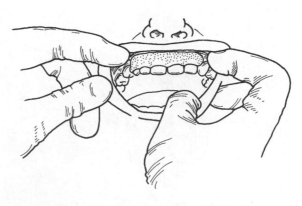

FIG. 147-5 After replacing the tooth, stabilize it with a periodontal pack.

Coronoid process

Long buccal nerve

Coronoid notch

Mandibular nerve

Condyle

Lingual nerve

Ramus

Inferior alveolar nerve as it enters the mandibular foramen

Body

Fig. 147-4 The inferior alveolar nerve block (intraoral approach). **A,** Identify the anterior border of the ramus of the mandible, the coronoid notch, with the left index finger and the left thumb. Grasp the ramus between an intraorally placed thumb and extraorally positioned index finger, with the thumb positioned on the coronoid notch. **B,** Aim the needle at the mandibular foramen, which is slightly posterior to the thumb tip, at its inferior border, just above the surface of the molars. Advance until the needle tip hits bone, then withdraw a few millimeters, aspirate, and inject.

(Redrawn from Roberts JR, Hedges JR: *Clinical procedures in emergency medicine*, Philadelphia, 1991, WB Saunders.)

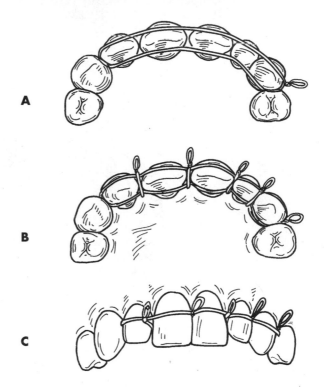

FIG. 147-6 **A** to **C,** Arch bars and metal wiring provide maximum stabilization but are technically difficult to use in young children (see text).

replantation aims to preserve the tooth's ligamentous connections to the alveolar bone and the tooth's other important attachments to surrounding support structures.

Preparation for tooth replantation begins immediately. Handle the tooth by the crown only and immerse it as soon as possible into a preservation solution.[1,4]

Place the avulsed tooth under the tongue of an older child or, for a young child, under the tongue of a parent during transport to the hospital. Cold milk is also an effective transport/preservation medium for avulsed teeth. One excellent tooth salvage solution is a commercially available preparation of a cell culture medium (Hanks solution), which is the active component of the tooth preservation kit marketed as "Save a Tooth." Emergency Medical Services

systems, children's sports teams, and schools have begun using such transport media for avulsed teeth.

Hanks solution markedly extends the 30-minute replantation window up to at least 6 and possibly 24 hours. In the ED, this solution permits the emergency physician to address all of the patient's injuries and conduct a more controlled preparation of the socket before tooth replacement.

Socket Preparation/Replantation. Preparation of the socket requires first anesthetizing the area with either a supraperiosteal infiltration or one of the dental nerve blocks. After anesthetizing the socket, suction any clot and irrigate the socket with normal saline. Clean dirt from the tooth itself with gentle irrigation or agitation of the tooth-preservation solution. Avoid scrubbing because doing so may remove any adherent bone spicules on the root of the tooth. Once the socket has been prepared, orient the tooth and gently place it into the socket. Apply firm pressure on the tooth to fully seat it back into the proper position. If the tooth does not fit back into position completely, remove it and inspect the socket for obstruction. A fragment of the alveolar ridge may occasionally be the source of the obstruction. If possible, leave the bone in place and position it out of the path of the tooth so that the bone fragment is forced into position when the tooth is replaced. After replantation, stabilize the tooth using the previously described stabilization techniques.

Remarks

Use dental protective devices for the prevention of dental injuries. These injuries can occur in any sport, but not all sports require protectors. Advise participants to wear protectors at all times when dental injury is a possibility. Mouth guards also reduce the risk of concussion and neck injuries.[2,3]

REFERENCES

1. Amsterdam JD: General dental emergencies. In Tintinali JE, Krome RL, Ruiz E, editors: *Emergency medicine: a comprehensive study guide,* New York, 1992, McGraw-Hill.
2. Castaldi C: Injuries to the teeth. In Vinger PF, Hoerner EF, editors: *Sports injuries: the unthwarted epidemic,* Littleton, Mass, 1981, PSG Publishing.
3. Josell SD, Abrams RG: Managing common dental problems and emergencies, *Pediatr Clin North Am* 38:1325, 1991.
4. Nelson LP, Neff JH: Dental emergencies. In Fleisher GR, Ludwig S, et al, editors: *Textbook of pediatric emergency medicine,* Baltimore, 1988, Williams & Wilkins.

148 Dental Infections and Extractions

Robert L. Sweeney

INFECTIONS

Dental infections generally originate from either cavities (dental caries), a tooth fracture, or a gingival infection. The most common infection is a periapical abscess. Although the abscess may originate in the alveolar bone surrounding the tooth, osteomyelitis is rarely present. The abscess usually extends toward the buccal side of the tooth and usually to the gingival buccal reflection. On physical examination the abscess appears as soft tissue swelling, tenderness, and fluctuance at the gingival reflection of the infected tooth.[1]

Indications

All periapical abscesses require incision and drainage.

Contraindications

If pus cannot be aspirated, treat the infection with an antistaphylococcal antibiotic and refer the patient to a dentist or oral or maxillofacial surgeon. Do not attempt an incision. In addition, obtain immediate consultation in the Emergency Department if the child cannot cooperate with the procedure after appropriate analgesia and sedation.

Complications

Complications of incision and drainage are pain and bleeding. The incision may also lacerate nerves, arteries, or veins.

Equipment

See Box 146-2.

Techniques

Incision and drainage of a periapical abscess is similar to the drainage of any other abscess. First place the patient in a sitting position. Have a rigid large-bore suction catheter immediately available, and enlist at least one assistant to help with the procedure. Apply a topical anesthetic, then obtain local anesthesia either through a dental nerve block or direct infiltration over the site (see Figs. 147-2 to 147-4).

Confirm the presence of the abscess by needle aspiration of pus. If unable to localize an area of pus through aspiration, postpone the procedure and manage the patient medically until a more localized infection develops. If pus aspiration is successful, note the location but do not aspirate more than one or two drops from the abscess. Leave the abscess as large as possible to make it easier to find during the dissection.

After anesthetizing the area, make an incision directly at the gingival reflection overlying the abscess site. Using a pair of mosquito hemostats, carry the dissection along the alveolar bone to the abscess (Fig. 148-1). If unable to find the abscess, use probing needle aspirations to relocalize it. After encountering pus, widen the entrance to the abscess by spreading the hemostat. Instruct an assistant to suction actively any pus to prevent gagging or aspiration. After draining the abscess, irrigate the area with 50 to 100 ml of saline. The packing of periapical abscesses is generally not necessary.

Little data exist to support postdrainage antibiotics. However, penicillin and erythromycin are reasonable choices.

TOOTH EXTRACTIONS
Complications

The two most common complications following a tooth extraction are postextraction hemorrhage and the formation of a dry socket.

Bleeding following extraction generally occurs as a result of an incomplete thrombus formation in the evacuated socket. Ironically, the cause of the bleeding is secondary to the excessive clot contained in the socket itself. The first step in evaluating these patients involves suctioning this clot from the socket. The use of direct pressure by having the patient bite on a gauze pad often controls this type of bleeding. If the bleeding persists despite this maneuver, inject the surrounding gingiva with an epinephrine-containing anesthetic. Irrigate the socket with a warm saline solution and pack it firmly with a thrombotic matrix such as Surgicel or Avitene to resolve any additional bleeding. If this degree of therapy is necessary, oversew the socket with 4-0 silk sutures. Persistent bleeding requires an evaluation of the patient's coagulation status and a consultation with the surgeon who removed the tooth.

A dry socket, or acute alveolar osteitis, results from inflammation of the evacuated tooth socket. This condition generally occurs secondary to incomplete adherence of the original clot with secondary inflammation. Pain results from exposure of the alveolar bone and can be relieved by irrigating the socket and packing it with eugenol-soaked iodoform gauze.

REFERENCE

1. Kokkevold P: Common dental emergencies: evaluation and management for emergency physicians, *Emerg Med Clin North Am* 7:29, 1989.

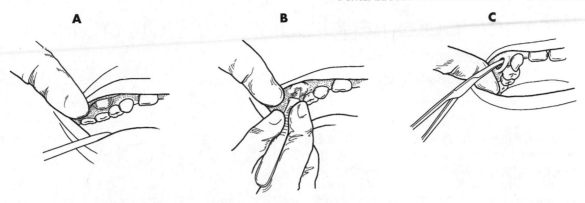

FIG. 148-1   Incision and drainage of periapical abscess. **A,** Identify abscess. **B,** Make a stab incision. **C,** Open it with a hemostat.

149 Temporomandibular Joint Dislocation

Alfred D. Sacchetti and Robert L. Sweeney

The temporomandibular joint (TMJ) (Fig. 149-1) is unique in that its motion involves both rotating around the condyle and sliding forward in the mandibular fossa. Dislocation occurs when the condyle slides too far forward and slips anterior to the articular eminence of the temporal bone. At this point the muscular attachments of the mandible pull the condyle superiorly and trap it. This phenomenon explains why patients with a mandibular dislocation have a fixed, open-mouth malocclusion.

Indications

All TMJ dislocations require reduction.

Contraindications

The only contraindication to reduction of a TMJ dislocation is the presence of other severe injuries that have a higher priority for treatment.

Complications

Attempts to reduce the TMJ dislocation may cause increased pain if they are not successful.

Equipment

No special equipment is required to reduce a TMJ dislocation.

Techniques

To relocate a dislocated mandible, place the patient in the sitting position and administer a pretreatment narcotic and benzodiazepine (see Chapters 12 and 13). Wrap both thumbs heavily with gauze or tongue depressors to prevent operator injury during the reduction. To perform the reduction, grasp the mandible with the thumbs on the posterior molars and exert a firm, steady, downward pressure. It is the fatiguing of the masseter muscle that allows relocation. This procedure requires steady pressure, not a rapid jerking motion.

Perform this maneuver while facing the patient; have an assistant hold the patient's forehead to prevent head flexion. This maneuver can also be performed from the back of the patient by using body weight to lean down onto the molars. As the condyle is displaced interiorly to the articular eminence of the temporal bone, the muscle naturally pulls the condyle backwards into the mandibular fossa (Fig. 149-1). Because this process naturally closes the patient's mouth, be careful to remove the thumbs quickly to avoid being bitten.

Placing the thumbs to the buccal side of the molars avoids the reflex biting that occurs when the mouth closes. The

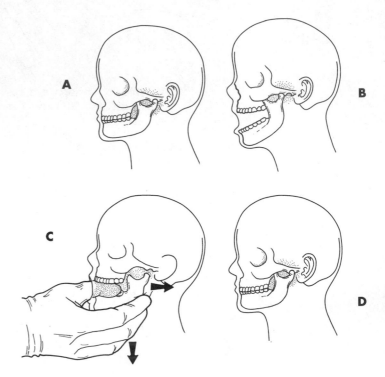

FIG. 149-1 Temporomandibular joint. **A,** Condyle rests normally in the mandibular fossa. **B,** The dislocated condyle locks anterior to the articular eminence. **C,** Reduction requires steady, firm, downward and backward pressure. **D,** The masseter muscle snaps the mandible in place.

disadvantage of this approach is that it limits the amount of downward pressure that can be placed on the mandible to clear the articular eminence of the temporal bone. After relocating the jaw, prescribe a soft diet for 1 week and instruct the patient to restrain from excessive wide opening of the mouth.[1] Place a Barton's bandage to prevent wide opening of the mouth. A Barton's bandage can be made by wrapping an elastic wrap or Ace wrap around the top of the head and under the chin. Make several wraps over the chin to prevent the chin from opening.

REFERENCE

1. Loyk NH, Larsen PE: The diagnosis and treatment of the dislocated mandible, *Am J Emerg Med* 7:329, 1989.

PART XXVII

BLOOD COMPONENT THERAPY

150 Blood Component Transfusion

Stephen M. Schexnayder and Kimo C. Stine

The management of critically ill and injured children requires blood and its various components. It is important for the clinician in the Emergency Department (ED) and intensive care unit (ICU) to understand the derivation of these components, the advantages and disadvantages of each particular product, and the primary indications for the use of each product.

The use of individual blood components rather than whole blood is the therapy of choice in the vast majority of clinical situations. The blood bank usually initially separates donated whole blood into packed red blood cells and platelet-rich plasma. The platelet-rich plasma is centrifuged again, and the plasma and platelets are separated. The blood bank stores platelets in a gas-permeable bag at room temperature; the platelets have a shelf life of 5 days. The blood bank may then freeze the plasma and use it as fresh frozen plasma or may thaw it under refrigeration and separate it into plasma and cryoprecipitate. Plasma that has had the cryoprecipitate removed is used for the production of biologic products such as albumin or plasma protein fraction, as well as for some individual clotting factors.

The blood bank collects most blood from human donors into a sterile plastic bag system using citrate-phosphate-dextrose-adenine (CPDA-1) as an anticoagulant. A typical whole-blood donation contains 450 ml of donor blood with approximately 63 ml of CPDA-1.[102] Within 8 hours of donation, the blood bank typically fractionates the whole blood into specific components, with red blood cells having a shelf life of 35 days in CPDA-1. Red blood cells are often collected into an anticoagulant mixture of citrate-phosphate-dextrose (CPD), which gives them a storage life of 21 days. After separation into red blood cells and plasma, a nutrient solution such as Adsol (Baxter Healthcare Corporation, Fenwal Division, Deerfield, IL) or Nutricel (Cutter Biological, Division of Miles Laboratories, Inc., Berkeley, CA) is added to the red blood cells to prolong the storage life to 42 days. Di(2-ethylhexyl)-phthalate (DHEP) is a plasticizer present in the blood-storage bags and slowly leaches out to help preserve membrane integrity of the red blood cell.[71]

RED BLOOD CELL–CONTAINING PRODUCTS

All stored red blood cells undergo progressive deterioration over time, which results in the loss of flexibility and membrane surface area (the "storage lesion")[174] and impairs oxygen delivery. During storage at 4° C, there is a slow depletion of intracellular adenosine triphosphate (ATP) and 2,3 diphosphoglycerate (DPG). ATP depletion results in dysfunction of the sodium-potassium pump, causing cellular swelling. Loss of 2,3 DPG increases the oxygen affinity of the red blood cell, thereby inhibiting oxygen unloading in the tissues.[153] Table 150-1 summarizes red blood cell–containing products.

Whole Blood

Indications. Whole blood is not generally available; the most efficient use of resources involves separating the com-

Table 150-1 Red Blood Cell–Containing Products

Product	Shelf life	Unit volume	Advantages	Disadvantages
Whole blood	CPDA-1: 35 days CPD + nutrient solution: 42 days	450 ml + 63 ml anticoagulant	1. Provides RBC mass 2. Provides volume	1. Rarely available 2. Exposure to WBC and platelet antigens 3. WBC, platelets nonfunctional unless fresh
Packed RBCs	Same as whole blood	250 ml	1. Widely available 2. Efficient use of blood resources	1. Less volume expansion
Frozen packed RBCs (deglycerolized)	10 years frozen; 24 hours after thawing	Variable	1. Maintains ATP, 2, 3 DPG concentrations well 2. Most WBCs are removed 3. Allows storage of rare blood types or extended storage for autologous blood	1. Expensive
Washed RBCs	24 hours after washing	Variable	1. Removes 70% of WBCs 2. Removes K+, platelets 3. Decreases febrile reactions 4. Decreases viral infection transmission	1. Time consuming to prepare 2. WBC removal less efficient than third-generation WBC filters

ponents. The indications for the use of whole blood are few and remain controversial. After 24 hours of storage, whole blood has no functional granulocytes and only 50% of the functional activity of platelets and factor VIII.[11,113] If available, whole blood may be indicated in rapid and acute exsanguination when volume restoration is as critical as improvement in oxygen-carrying capacity. For children undergoing cardiac surgery, especially neonates, some centers provide a unit of whole blood less than 36 hours old.[80] Reconstituted whole blood, which is made by mixing packed red blood cells with fresh frozen plasma, is used for exchange transfusions.

Contraindications. Because specific blood components are indicated in most situations, whole blood is contraindicated except in the few situations previously described.

Complications. Because whole blood involves the administration of a greater blood volume than packed red blood cells, volume overload may result. In addition to the risk of infectious disease transmission, the administration of whole blood carries the risk of exposing the patient to donor white blood cell and platelet antigens and associated reactions, which are discussed in the next section. As blood ages, lactate, ammonia, and potassium accumulate in the stored product, which results in the transfusion of deleterious compounds into an already compromised patient.

REACTIONS

Immediate Hemolytic Reactions. The most feared of all transfusion reactions, the immediate hemolytic reaction occurs when there is an antigen-antibody response that destroys the transfused red blood cells, generally as a result of blood group (ABO) mismatch. Because this mismatch usually arises from a clerical error[69] and may be rapidly fatal, take extreme care in even life-threatening situations in the ED or ICU to ensure that the blood is for the intended recipient. Rapid hemolysis releases free hemoglobin, which causes hemoglobinemia and hemoglobinuria. This hemolysis also consumes haptoglobin, a protein that binds free hemoglobin, which results in a low plasma haptoglobin level. The most common symptoms of a hemolytic reaction are fever, chills, pain at the infusion site, back pain, shortness of breath, and shock.[125]

Disseminated intravascular coagulation, as well as renal failure secondary to the hemoglobinuria, may also result from a hemolytic transfusion reaction. Direct therapy toward immediately stopping the transfusion, supporting intravascular volume, and administering diuretics to promote renal perfusion. The choice of a loop diuretic vs. mannitol is controversial. Maintaining urine pH above 6.5 with intravenous bicarbonate may be helpful in reducing renal injury.[178]

Febrile Reactions. Febrile reactions are the most common transfusion reactions and are usually the result of recipient antibodies to the antigens present on donor lymphocytes, granulocytes, or platelets.[121] Because fever may also be the first sign of a hemolytic reaction, these reactions require investigation. These reactions are generally treated with antipyretics such as acetaminophen. More severe febrile reactions are treated with meperidine.[26] The use of a leukocyte filter may decrease the incidence of these reactions.

Allergic Reactions. Although rare, severe allergic hypersensitivity reactions or anaphylaxis may present with flushing, laryngeal edema, and hypotension, and they are most likely to occur in transfusion recipients who have an IgA deficiency.[124] Milder allergic reactions, such as those characterized by urticaria, erythema, or pruritus, are treated with antihistamines. Severe reactions require epinephrine, corticosteroids, and fluid resuscitation.[81]

Delayed Hemolytic Reactions. Occasionally a hemolytic transfusion reaction may occur several days after transfusion; a delayed reaction is manifested primarily by extravascular hemolysis and results in anemia. Delayed reactions probably result from a secondary immune response against the donor red blood cells in patients who have either previously received transfusions or have experienced a previous pregnancy.[81]

TRANSFUSION-TRANSMITTED DISEASES

Hepatitis. Blood banks currently screen for antibodies to hepatitis B and C. Although blood is tested for hepatitis B surface antigens and antibodies to the hepatitis B core antigen, these serologic tests may be negative during the incubation period of the disease when the patient is viremic;[138] therefore a small risk for the transmission of hepatitis B persists.

Hepatitis C is responsible for approximately 90% of all transfusion-associated hepatitis.[1] In 1990, blood banks initiated routine testing for antibodies to hepatitis C in the United States. Preliminary evidence indicates that screening has reduced the incidence of transfusion-acquired hepatitis C.[43] Because hepatitis C is not responsible for all cases of non-A, non-B hepatitis and because the antibody test is not 100% effective in identifying all cases, blood banks also perform "surrogate" testing for elevated levels of alanine aminotransferase and antibodies to the hepatitis B core antigen.

Human Immunodeficiency Virus. Human immunodeficiency virus–1 (HIV-1) is the primary etiologic agent for acquired immune deficiency syndrome (AIDS) in the United States and is of major concern to most transfusion recipients. Since 1985, U.S. blood banks have screened all blood products for antibodies to HIV-1 in addition to extensive donor screening in an attempt to exclude anyone in a high-risk group. Blood banks also encourage confidential donor self-exclusion after the screening interview. In addition, blood banks screen blood for antibodies to HIV-2, which are found primarily in West Africa.[5] As with other viral infections, a "window" period exists with HIV. This window period occurs between the time HIV infects a person and the time he or she is antibody positive, which makes the transmission of HIV possible despite a negative antibody test. The estimated window is approximately 45 days.[27] The risk of transmission of HIV from a unit of transfused blood is between 1 in 450,000 and 1 in 660,000.[42]

Screening for the p24 antigen of HIV-1 in donated blood began in early 1996, reducing the risk of HIV infection to an estimated 1 in 750,000.

Human T-Cell Lymphotrophic Viruses. Blood transfusions may also transmit the retroviruses human T-cell lymphotrophic viruses (HTLV) type I and II. HTLV-I carries an association with adult T-cell leukemia and with a neurologic syndrome known as tropical spastic paraparesis, or HTLV-I–associated myelopathy.[15] HTLV-II is a retrovirus found in many intravenous drug abusers.[85] Blood banks currently screen for antibodies to HTLV-I and HTLV-II. The prevalence of infection by HTLV-I and HTLV-II in the U.S. blood supply is low[66] and, of those infected, there is a lifetime risk of approximately 4% of contracting the clinical diseases associated with HTLV-I.[42]

Cytomegalovirus. Cytomegalovirus (CMV) is a herpes virus carried by lymphocytes. Many adults have serologic evidence for a past infection with CMV.[164] In the immunocompetent or older child, CMV causes a mild or even subclinical viral illness that is similar to infectious mononucleosis. However, in the unborn child, young infants, and immunocompromised patients, the infection may produce devastating or even fatal results.[98,154] CMV infection exists as three types: primary for the unexposed, and either reactivation or reinfection for those previously exposed to CMV. CMV causes pneumonitis, hepatitis, ulcerative gastritis, retinitis, encephalitis, leukopenia, thrombocytopenia, and hemolytic anemia.[89] Therefore CMV seronegative blood products are used in neonates and the immunocompromised, but leukofiltered products are also effectively used to prevent CMV disease in susceptible patients.[39,50]

Other Infections. A blood transfusion may transmit the Epstein-Barr virus (EBV), [89] *Yersinia enterocolitica,* malaria, *Trypanosoma cruzi,* brucellosis, toxoplasmosis, and babesiosis, but U.S. blood banks do not screen for these agents.[42,111] Blood may also transmit syphilis, and U.S. blood banks screen all blood with a nontreponemal test. Bacterial infection from a unit of blood contaminated with either grampositive or gram-negative organisms is uncommon[109]; however, the administration of contaminated units, especially those with gram-negative organisms, can produce a fatal reaction.[108] Platelet transfusions more commonly produce bacteremia, especially with platelets that have been stored for more than 4 days; therefore there is a 5-day limit for platelet storage.[104,105]

OTHER ADVERSE EFFECTS OF TRANSFUSIONS

Microembolization. Microaggregates of the degradation products of leukocytes, platelets, and fibrin accumulate during the first week of blood storage.[130] Most of these aggregates are smaller than the filter pore size of 170 microns typically used in red blood cell transfusion and therefore may pass into circulation. These microaggregates may cause pulmonary dysfunction and possibly contribute to adult respiratory distress syndrome, but this possibility is controversial.[151] Filters with smaller pore sizes effectively remove these aggregates but slow the transfusion rates considerably. Recent additions of high-flow 40-micron filters allow the use of microaggregate filters in situations that require rapid transfusion.

Immunosuppression. A pretransplantation blood transfusion enhances renal transplant graft survival,[120] but in recent years Smith[150] has described a general immunomodulatory effect of blood transfusion in other patients. Recent work has suggested that the beneficial effect of pretransplantation transfusion is waning, possibly because of superior immunosuppressive regimens.[24] Investigators have suggested a possible adverse effect of transfusion in many malignancies[120] and postoperative patients.[17] A retrospective comparison has shown a decreased incidence of infection in postoperative patients who received autologous blood vs. those who received homologous blood.[99]

Equipment. Transfuse all red blood cell–containing products through a filter. The most widely used filter is 170 microns, but some authorities recommend giving all transfusions through 40-micron filters.

Techniques. Infuse blood either by gravity, under pressure using a pressure-bag apparatus, or via an infusion pump.

Packed Red Blood Cells

Indications. Packed red blood cells (PRBCs) are the component of choice for most red blood cell transfusions, including replacement during surgery, red blood cell loss, and sporadic transfusion therapy. The average hematocrit of PRBCs is 75% or, with a nutrient solution added, 50% to 60%.[80] Transfuse PRBCs to increase oxygen transport to the tissues. PRBC transfusion in combination with crystalloid resuscitation is standard therapy for hemorrhagic shock.[86] The advantages of PRBC transfusions over whole-blood transfusions include a decrease in the amount of citrate, ammonia, and organic acids in the product.

The level of hemoglobin or hematocrit on which to base the decision to transfuse is controversial, and this level has significantly declined in the past 2 decades. The National Institutes of Health Consensus Development Conference on perioperative red blood cell transfusion concluded that "otherwise healthy patients with a hemoglobin of 10 g/dl or greater rarely require perioperative transfusion, whereas those with acute anemia with resulting hemoglobin values of less than 7 g/dl will frequently require red cell transfusions. It appears that some patients with chronic anemia, such as those with chronic renal failure, tolerate hemoglobin values of less than 7 g/dl. The decision to transfuse red cells will depend on clinical assessment aided by laboratory data, such as arterial oxygenation, mixed venous oxygen tension, cardiac output, the oxygen extraction ratio, and blood volume, when indicated."[119,p.2701]

Critical values derived from animal studies indicate marginal oxygen reserve and the need for transfusion in the patient with anemia (Box 150-1).[58] Although these numbers are useful in patients who are undergoing hemodynamic monitoring, clinical assessment remains necessary because many critically ill or injured children require transfusion at higher hemoglobin levels. Because such measurements are almost never available in the ED, clinical judgment is still the cornerstone of the decision to transfuse.

Red blood cell transfusion in neonates has historically occurred at much higher hemoglobin or hematocrit levels than in older children and adults. A recent survey of neonatal intensive care units found that the median "transfusion trigger" for a neonate with respiratory distress was a hematocrit of 40% with a range of 23% to 45%; the transfusion trigger for a stable neonate without respiratory distress was a hematocrit of 20% to 45% with a median of 30%.[88] Some authors have recommended transfusion after the removal of 5% to 10% of the neonate's blood volume over a few days,[70,155] but this recommendation is controversial.[48,135] Some authors have suggested deciding to transfuse on the basis of restoring the neonate's red blood cell mass rather than on the hematocrit.[122] Despite some available methods, few clinicians determine red blood cell mass routinely. Other clinicians have suggested that elevated lactic acid levels predict the need to transfuse infants with anemia of prematurity,[72] but oxygen delivery is more efficient in acidosis because of the Bohr effect.[153]

Complications. Complications of PRBC transfusion are the same as for whole-blood transfusions, except that there is a reduced risk of volume overload.

Techniques. Numerous formulas exist for determining the volume of PRBCs for transfusion, but most often clinicians transfuse red blood cells in aliquots of 10 to 15 ml/kg. A transfusion of 10 ml/kg of PRBCs generally raises a child's hemoglobin level by 2.5 to 3 g/dl; likewise a 15 ml/kg transfusion elevates the hemoglobin concentration by 3.5 to 4.5 g/dl. Most clinicians consider 15 ml/kg of PRBCs to be the maximum for a single simple transfusion. A commonly used formula is as follows[73]:

$$\text{Volume of cells (ml)} = \frac{\text{(Estimated blood volume [ml])} \times \text{(desired change in hematocrit)}}{\text{Hematocrit of PRBCs}}$$

Estimated blood volumes are 85 to 100 ml/kg for premature infants, 85 ml/kg for term newborns, and 75 ml/kg for children more than 1 month old, adolescents, and adults.[110]

Because the full crossmatch procedure may require 30 to 60 minutes, the practitioner may occasionally need to transfuse red blood products before completing the full crossmatch. Most trauma centers use uncrossmatched type O-negative packed cells[87] for girls and type O-positive cells for boys in shock.[86] Many centers now use type-specific PRBCs. If a technologist is immediately available, the blood bank can usually provide type-specific PRBCs in 5 minutes.

Frozen Packed Red Blood Cells

Using glycerol as a protectant, blood banks may freeze PRBCs and store them for up to 10 years. The blood bank deglycerolizes frozen PRBCs by defrosting and washing them with an automated cell washer. If frozen within hours of collection, the PRBCs contain high levels of ATP and 2,3 DPG but have a 24-hour expiration once they have been thawed and washed.

Indications. Deglycerolized PRBCs are used primarily for patients who require an antigen-matched transfusion because of preexisting red blood cell antibodies or for the prevention of antibody formation in children who require transfusions at frequent intervals.[80] Deglycerolized PRBCs are also used for patients with IgA deficiency to prevent anaphylaxis related to anti-IgA antibodies in the recipient (see Table 150-5).

Complications. Complications of deglycerolized PRBC transfusion are the same as for whole blood except that freezing destroys the leukocytes and may lessen the transmission of intracellular viruses.

Washed Red Blood Cells

Indications. Washing PRBCs reduces the number of leukocytes by 70% and may prevent febrile nonhemolytic and allergic transfusion reactions in patients who have a history of such reactions.[54] Washed red blood cells are used for transfusions in patients who have an IgA deficiency. The shelf life of the washed unit is only 24 hours. However, third-generation leukocyte filters are more efficient at leukocyte removal than either washed PRBCs or frozen deglycerolized PRBCs (see Table 150-5).[152]

Complications. Complications of washed PRBC transfusion are the same as for whole blood. A theoretical advantage to using washed cells is the reduced risk of transmission of intracellular viruses such as CMV.[2]

Leukocyte-Filtered Red Blood Cells

Current leukocyte filters (so-called "third-generation filters") are 99.9% effective in removing white blood cells from a unit of PRBCs.[148] Two filters currently being marketed are the Sepacell (Baxter Healthcare, Fenwal Division, Deerfield, IL) and the Pall RC (Pall Corporation, Glen Cove, NY). These filtration devices effectively prevent transfusion-acquired CMV infection in infants and in patients with hematologic malignancies.[39,50] Filtration is most effective in removing leukocytes within the first 24 hours of storage of the blood product.

Indications. Because of the efficiency in removing blood that potentially is infected with CMV, many blood banks now use leukocyte-filtered PRBCs in place of CMV seronegative products.[34] These filters also reduce the transmission of other lymphocyte-transmitted viral diseases, such as HTLV-I, HIV-1, and EBV,[83] and they may also reduce febrile nonhemolytic transfusion reactions (see Table 150-5).

Irradiated Red Blood Cells

The proliferation of transfused lymphocytes may cause transfusion-associated graft vs. host disease (TAGVHD) in an immunodeficient host.[3] Irradiation of cellular blood products renders the lymphocytes contained in the product incapable of proliferating.

Indications. The irradiation of blood cellular components is appropriate for many patients (Box 150-2). Immunocompetent patients may develop TAGVHD if they receive partially human leukocyte antigen (HLA)– identical, HLA-homozygous lymphocytes, such as might occur when they receive a directed donation from a blood relative such as a sibling or a parent.[31,74] Because TAGVHD carries a 90% fatality rate in children,[167] prevention is of paramount importance (see Table 150-5).

Complications. The storage of PRBCs after irradiation may cause an increase in the potassium of the plasma contained in the unit[128]; therefore irradiate the PRBCs just before transfusion.

NON–RED BLOOD CELL CONTAINING PRODUCTS

Table 150-2 summarizes the non–red "blood" cell containing products.

Table 150-2   Non–Red Blood Cell Containing Products

Product	Shelf life	Unit volume	Advantages	Disadvantages
Fresh frozen plasma	1 year frozen; 6 hours thawed	250 ml	1. Provides all coagulation factors 2. Readily available	1. Requires ABO compatibility 2. Requires 30 minutes to thaw
Cryoprecipitate	1 year frozen	10 ml	1. Provides factors VIII, IX, XIII, VWF, fibrinogen	
Platelet concentrates	5 days (store at room temperature)	50-70 ml	1. Contains approximately 5.5×10^{10} platelets	1. Contains some RBCs, WBCs, plasma
Platelet apheresis	5 days (store at room temperature)	200-400 ml	1. Contains $3\text{-}5 \times 10^{11}$ platelets from a single donor	1. Expensive
Buffy coat transfusion	None	30-50 ml	1. Contains $0.35\text{-}0.5 \times 10^{9}$ WBC 2. Generally available	1. May be insufficient number of WBCs to meet demands 2. Must be transfused as soon as possible to ensure WBC survival 3. Requires freshly donated blood
Leukophoresis	None	200-400 ml	1. Contains $1\text{-}4 \times 10^{11}$ WBC from a single donor (if stimulated with corticosteroids) 2. Contains sufficient RBCs to cause a hemolytic reaction	1. Requires time to prepare donor and perform apheresis

---

> **BOX 150-2   PATIENTS WHO SHOULD RECEIVE IRRADIATED CELLULAR BLOOD COMPONENTS**
>
> Patients in the neonatal intensive care unit or infants less than 4 months old
> Fetuses receiving intrauterine or periumbilical transfusions
> All patients with immunodeficiency (congenital or acquired)
> Patients undergoing solid-organ transplantation (organs containing lymphoid tissue)
> Candidates for bone marrow transplantation
> Patients receiving immunosuppressive chemotherapy
> Patients receiving directed blood donations from partially HLA-identical, HLA-homozygous donors

From Kevy, SK: Red cell transfusion. In Nathan DG, Oski FA, editors: *Hematology of infancy and childhood,* ed 4, Philadelphia, 1993, WB Saunders.

Fresh Frozen Plasma

Fresh frozen plasma (FFP) contains all the clotting factors present in whole blood. Blood banks prepare FFP by separating the plasma from the red blood cells within 6 hours of collection and freezing it at $-18°$ C.[90] FFP is not cross-matched but is ABO matched to the patient's blood group. As a rule it is necessary to transfuse FFP within 6 hours of thawing. However, if the patient needs only stable coagulation factors (factors V and VIII), FFP may be transfused for as long as 24 hours after thawing.

Indications. FFP is the most overused of all blood products.[117] True indications for FFP are few because specific therapy is preferable for specific coagulation defects.[117] Use FFP to reverse the anticoagulant effects of warfarin when there is not time to wait for the effect of vitamin K (6 to 12 hours), such as with bleeding or emergency surgery.[117] FFP is also indicated when a specific factor concentrate is unavailable, such as for deficiencies of factors II, V, VII, X, XI, or antithrombin III.[90] FFP is also often appropriate in the therapy of thrombotic thrombocytopenic purpura, usually in combination with plasmapheresis.[139] Consider using FFP for the child with hepatic failure and serious hemorrhage.[20]

Contraindications. FFP is not generally appropriate for routine use during massive transfusion, for the treatment of immunodeficiencies, for increasing intravascular volume, or for nutritional support.

Complications. Febrile and allergic reactions, as well as the transmission of transfusion-related infections, are potential complications of FFP administration and have been described previously.

Equipment. FFP is transfused using a standard 170-micron filter.

Techniques. Transfuse FFP in volumes of 10 to 15 ml/kg.[143] The frequency of transfusion depends on the half-life of the factor needed (Table 150-3). For instance, replacement of factor VII may require transfusions every few hours, whereas treatment for factor XI deficiency may require therapy only every few days.

Cryoprecipitate

Blood banks produce cryoprecipitate by thawing FFP at $4°$ C. This process precipitates a small amount of protein that is rich in fibrinogen, von Willebrand's factor (VWF), factor VIII, fibronectin, and factor XIII.

Indications. Although historically used primarily for the

Table 150-3 Characteristics of Coagulation Factors Important in Transfusion Therapy

Factor	Minimum hemostatic level (U/dl)	Increase in plasma level with dose of 1 U/kg (U/dl)	Half-life
Prothrombin (II)	15-40	1	3 days
V	10-25	1.5	12-36 hours
VII	5-10	1	4-6 hours
VIII	30-50	2	12-15 hours
IX	20-50	1	18-30 hours
X	10-20	1	36-60 hours
XI	10-30	2	1-3 days
XIII	1-5	1-3	3-10 days
VWF	30-50	2	12-15 hours
Fibrinogen (1)	75-150 mg/dl	*	4-5 days

From Gill, JC, Montgomery RR: Principles of therapy for hemostasis factor deficiencies. In Nathan DG, Oski FA, editors: *Hematology of infancy and childhood,* ed 4, Philadelphia, 1993, WB Saunders.
*1 unit of cryoprecipitate/5 kg will raise the fibrinogen 50-100 mg/dl.

treatment of factor VIII deficiency, indications for cryoprecipitate include the treatment of bleeding associated with von Willebrand's disease, as well as deficiencies in the quantity or function of fibrinogen. In the critical care and ED setting, this condition occurs most often in the face of disseminated intravascular coagulation (DIC). Although correction of the underlying stimulus for DIC is the primary therapy, in this situation many intensivists use cryoprecipitate as supportive therapy for associated acute bleeding.

Complications. Febrile and allergic reactions, as well as the transmission of transfusion-related infections, are potential complications of cryoprecipitate administration.

Equipment. Transfuse cryoprecipitate using a standard 170-micron filter.

Techniques. Each unit of cryoprecipitate contains approximately 100 units of factor VIII and 250 mg of fibrinogen. The dose for the treatment of hypofibrinogenemia is one bag per 5 to 7 kg body weight.[51,143] For DIC, repeat this dose for ongoing hemorrhage until the fibrinogen level reaches 150 to 200 mg/dl. For the topical control of bleeding, mix cryoprecipitate with thrombin and paint it on the bleeding sites to form a strong clot known as "fibrin glue."[133]

Specific Factor Deficiency and Replacement

Factor VIII deficiency, or hemophilia A, constitutes approximately 85% of all congenital coagulation deficiencies.[156] Factor IX deficiency, also known as hemophilia B or Christmas disease, is the second most common coagulation protein deficiency.[96] Patients with factor levels of 15% to 25% of normal have "mild deficiency," whereas those with 5% to 15% of the normal level are "moderately deficient." Children with levels of less than 5% are "severe." Patients with levels above 25% rarely bleed except during major surgery or trauma.[77]

Indications. Specific factor replacement therapy is the preferred treatment of any coagulation disorder when a specific factor concentrate is available. Patients with factor VIII deficiency have received factor replacement most often.

HIV transmission from factor replacement was first reported in 1982,[6] and the HIV epidemic caused a major evolution in factor replacement during the 1980s with the introduction of recombinant factor VIII in the 1990s. Currently all factor replacements (except recombinant agents) undergo some method of viral inactivation such as affinity chromatography or solvent-detergent treatment.[8,55]

Complications. Inhibitors develop in 10% to 15% of all patients with severe factor VIII deficiency.[173]

Equipment. Factor concentrates come with filter needles for reconstitution and administration. Because individual factors vary in their preparation technique, use the information supplied with each product.

Techniques

FACTOR DEFICIENCY. Treatment of factor deficiencies requires the knowledge of not only the particular factor missing but also of the volume of distribution of the factor and its functional half-life (see Table 150-3). FFP contains one unit of each of the coagulation factors in each milliliter of plasma, but because of the doses required, the treatment of some factor deficiencies with FFP would induce volume overload. Monitor specific factor levels during treatment, or measure the partial thromboplastin time when specific factor levels are not available. The best indicator for treatment is the clinical status of the patient.

Treatment of hemorrhage in factor VIII deficiency depends on the location of the hemorrhage. In the United States there are currently eight human and three recombinant factor VIII products on the market.[8] The preparations vary by viral inactivation or production methods. Consult a hematologist regarding the choice of a particular factor VIII preparation.

Joint or muscular bleeds are the most common locations of hemorrhage; treat these bleeds with 20 U/kg of factor VIII concentrate.[51] For epistaxis or dental bleeding, generally use antifibrinolytic therapy such as Amicar and pressure plus 20 U/kg of factor if bleeding continues. For major surgery or a life-threatening hemorrhage (central nervous system, airway, gastrointestinal, or retroperitoneal hemorrhage), give 50 U/kg followed by 25 U/kg every 12 hours for 5 to 7 days. Factor VIII may be administered as a continuous infusion in these situations by giving the 50 U/kg loading dose followed by 2 to 3 U/kg/hour.[18] In some cases, the clinical condition may warrant increasing the infusion rate.

Because of a larger volume of distribution, use a higher dose of factor IX. For minor bleeding such as hemarthrosis or muscle hemorrhage, give 20 to 30 U/kg. For more serious hemorrhages or major surgery, give 80 to 100 U/kg followed by 20 to 40 U/kg every 12 to 24 hours. Treat hematuria accompanied by either factor VIII or IX deficiency with vigorous hydration.

Desmopressin (DDAVP), a synthetic analogue of vasopressin, increases factor VIII and VWF in patients with a mild-to-moderate deficiency.[40,94] DDAVP may work by promoting the release of factor VIII and VWF from storage sites.[94] Patients should undergo a trial with laboratory evaluation of the response to the drug because the response is variable.[51] For patients who are known responders, give 0.3 µg/kg as an intravenous infusion over 20 to 30 minutes when bleeding occurs or before a procedure.

The treatment of hemorrhage in patients who develop antibodies to factor VIII varies with the degree of inhibitor

Table 150-4 Therapy for von Willebrand's Disease

Type	Pathogenesis	Therapy
I	Mild to moderate VWF deficiency	Desmopressin; Humate-P;* cryoprecipitate
IIa	Small, abnormal multimers	Humate-P;* cryoprecipitate
IIb	Abnormal molecule binding to platelets	Humate-P;* cryoprecipitate
III	Severe VWF deficiency	Humate-P;* cryoprecipitate
Pseudo von Willebrand's disease (platelet type)	Defect in glycoprotein receptor on platelet	Platelet transfusion

*Humate-P is preferred if available because of a decreased risk of transfusion-associated infections compared with cryoprecipitate; Humate-P dose: 15-30 U/kg.

produced. Patients who are "low responders" have inhibitor titers less than 10 Bethesda units and are treated by using higher doses of factor VIII.[91] For life-threatening hemorrhages, administer a bolus of 100 U/kg followed by an infusion of 20 U/kg per hour. Because this treatment may induce an anamnestic response in 4 to 5 days, reserve it for patients with life-threatening bleeding.[173]

For patients known to be "high responders" (inhibitor titers above 10 Bethesda units), use prothrombin complexes (factor IX, 50 to 100 U/kg every 12 hours)[92] or activated prothrombin complexes (activated factor IX, 75 U/kg every 12 hours for a maximum of three doses).[149] Potential problems with activated prothrombin complexes include the development of DIC or even myocardial infarction, and antifibrinolytic therapy is generally contraindicated with the use of activated prothrombin complexes.[162] Porcine factor VIII concentrate may also be used in patients with inhibitors.[22] Preliminary experience with activated factor VII indicates that patients who have not responded to other therapies may benefit from the administration of this substance.[65]

VON WILLEBRAND'S DISEASE. Von Willebrand's disease is a group of disorders characterized by either a deficiency of VWF, the presence of an abnormal factor, or an abnormal interaction with platelets. Von Willebrand's disease is the most commonly inherited hemorrhagic disorder.[59] Correctly diagnosing the specific type of disorder is of paramount importance because treatment varies with the specific type of disease. Type I disease, the most common type, involves a deficiency of VWF. It is generally easy to manage this type with desmopressin as described previously.[93] In refractory cases use cryoprecipitate or Humate-P, a factor VIII preparation containing a high titer of VWF.[7] Type III disease, a severe deficiency of VWF, always requires VWF infusion. Because Humate-P is safer in terms of potential infectious complications, use cryoprecipitate only if Humate-P is not readily available (see Table 150-3 for dosing).

The presence of a functionally abnormal protein characterizes type II von Willebrand's disease. There are two types: Type IIa in which the multimers are abnormally small, and Type IIb in which the molecule binds spontaneously to platelets, resulting in mild thrombocytopenia. Type IIa may respond transiently to but generally requires infusion of VWF as previously described.[179] Desmopressin may actually worsen type IIb; treat it with an infusion of VWF.[68]

Platelet-type von Willebrand's disease, also known as pseudo von Willebrand's disease, involves a defect in the glycoprotein receptor on the platelet and is treated with platelet transfusion.[101]

Table 150-4 summarizes therapies for the various types of von Willebrand's disease.

Platelet Transfusion

Platelets constitute an important component of the coagulation system through their interaction with vascular endothelium and plasma coagulation factors. When a disruption in vascular endothelium occurs, the exposure of platelets to collagen promotes the adhesion of platelets to the exposed surface in the presence of VWF.[171] The platelets swell and adhere and then release granules that lead to irreversible aggregation. Thromboxane A_2 promotes irreversible aggregation and vasoconstriction. Cyclooxygenase inhibitors such as low-dose aspirin oppose the aggregation and vasoconstriction.

Indications. Hemostatic disorders from platelets may be a result of either defective platelet function or thrombocytopenia. Thrombocytopenia may result from the inadequate production or consumption of platelets.[4] Normal platelet counts are between 150,000 and 400,000/µl, but normal neonates may have as few as 100,000/µl.[56] The absolute number at which to transfuse a patient depends on the clinical scenario. In patients with normal platelet function, active bleeding is usually not a risk until platelet counts fall below 10,000/µl; life-threatening hemorrhage generally occurs only when levels fall below 5,000/µl.[106] Patients with coagulation defects such as platelet dysfunction or coagulation-factor deficiencies may require more aggressive support to prevent bleeding. In patients with active bleeding, many sources recommend maintaining the platelet count above 50,000.[118] Box 150-3 lists the disorders in which platelet dysfunction is present.

A recent study tested an algorithm in which the clinician prophylactically transfused platelets to adults with acute leukemia only if the platelet count fell below 5000/µl.[53] If fever or minor hemorrhagic manifestations were present, the clinician gave platelets for a count below 10,000/µl. Clinicians transfused platelets at levels above 10,000 only if the patient was receiving heparin, was to undergo a minor surgical procedure, or had another coagulation disorder. The investigators found this strategy safe and effective, but it is controversial among experts in the field.

If platelet function is normal, reserve platelet transfusions before most surgery for levels below 30,000 to 60,000/µl.[145,146] Assess platelet function by using the template bleeding time; do not give platelets if the bleeding time is less than twice normal.[118] For operations in which a small amount of hemorrhage could have a devastating effect (i.e., central nervous system or ocular), maintain the level above 100,000/µl despite little available scientific evidence for this practice.[146] Because the transfused platelets depart rapidly from circulation, do not transfuse platelets for patients with

BOX 150-3 **CONDITIONS ASSOCIATED WITH PLATELET DYSFUNCTION**

Drugs
    Aspirin
    Dipyridamole
    Nonsteroidal antiinflammatory agents
    Valproic acid
    Beta-lactam antibiotics
        Penicillin, ampicillin, extended-spectrum penicillins
        Cephalosporins
    Antihistamines
    Phenothiazines
    Radiographic contrast agents
Uremia
Cardiopulmonary bypass
Down's syndrome
Infections
Disseminated intravascular coagulation
Vitamin deficiencies (B_{12}, C)
Myeloproliferative disorders
Cirrhosis

antibody-mediated thrombocytopenia (e.g., alloimmune neonatal thrombocytopenia or idiopathic thrombocytopenic purpura) despite severe thrombocytopenia unless life-threatening hemorrhage occurs.

Complications. Complications associated with red blood cell transfusions as previously described may also occur with platelet transfusion.

Equipment. Transfuse platelets using a standard 170-micron filter, or use a white cell filter to reduce the leukocyte content.

Techniques. One unit of random donor platelets contains the platelets from a single unit of donated whole blood, or approximately 5 to 10×10^{10} platelets suspended in 50 to 70 ml of plasma.[142] Apheresis units obtained from a single donor contain 3 to 5×10^{11} platelets suspended in approximately 200 to 400 ml of plasma. If the volume required for transfusion would overload the patient, centrifuge the platelets with a reduction of the plasma component to approximately 10 ml; however, this process takes between 1 and 2 hours, which may be unacceptable in critical situations.[144] Another strategy involves splitting an apheresis unit into smaller aliquots; however, after entering the unit, the entire unit must be used within 4 hours or discarded unless a special sterile connection device is used.

The dose for platelets may be calculated from several formulas, most of which originated for adult patients. One unit of random donor platelets per 10 kg of body weight should raise the platelet count to a hemostatic level (50,000 to 100,000/μl),[146] or one unit of platelet apheresis should raise the platelet count of a 70-kg patient to a hemostatic level. For an apheresis unit, the most common dose is 10 ml/kg.

Many patients who require multiple platelet transfusions develop alloimmunization, which results in decreased platelet survival. Alloimmunization results from the patient's exposure to allogeneic blood, which causes the formation of antibodies that compromise the recovery and survival of transfused cells. Multiple strategies advocated for the prevention of alloimmunization include the use of single-donor platelet products,[52] leukocyte filtering,[134] ultraviolet-irradiated platelets,[75] and HLA matching of platelet donors.[176]

For patients with alloimmunization, use the "corrected count increment" (CCI) to determine the effectiveness of a particular platelet transfusion. It is calculated by the following formula:

$$CCI = \frac{(\text{Posttransfusion count} - \text{pretransfusion count}) (\text{BSA m}^2)}{\text{Platelets given} (\times 10^{11})}$$

with the posttransfusion platelet count measured 1 hour after transfusion.[49] However, some evidence indicates that an accurate count is obtained 10 to 15 minutes after completion of the infusion.[57,116] CCI values of at least 10,000 indicate a satisfactory response, whereas a count of less than 7000 indicates either alloimmunization or an autoantibody.[115]

Because ABO antigens are present on the platelets, ABO matching is desirable but not mandatory.[64] If transfusing a large volume of ABO-incompatible plasma with platelets into an infant or small child, volume-reduce the product to prevent the development of a positive direct Coombs' test or hemolysis.[103] Red blood cells may contaminate platelet concentrates, particularly random donor platelets, and Rh sensitization may occur if an Rh-negative patient receives Rh-positive cells. This situation is primarily of concern with Rh-negative female patients; if such contamination is present, give Rh immunoglobulin (Rhogam) to prevent alloimmunization.[90]

Granulocyte Transfusion

Blood banks obtain granulocytes by harvesting the buffy coat from a fresh unit of whole blood (less than 6 hours old)[30] or through leukopheresis. Although the buffy coat preparation is generally available quickly, the apheresis product takes hours to collect and deliver. Achieve optimal leukopheresis after administering corticosteroids[67] or a granulocyte colony-stimulating factor[13] to the donor. The buffy coat from one unit of donated whole blood contains approximately 0.35 to 0.5×10^9 leukocytes,[172] whereas the leukopheresis products contain between 1 and 4×10^{11} platelets from corticosteroid-stimulated donors.

Indications. Granulocyte transfusions for patients with neutropenia are controversial.[159] The most common scenario in pediatrics for granulocyte transfusion is the neonate with overwhelming sepsis and neutropenia (absolute granulocyte count [{% polymorphonuclear leukocytes + % band forms} × total white blood cell count] <500 to 1000/μl). Many clinical trials have examined bone marrow neutrophil storage pools for depletion before transfusion, but storage pool depletion may be identified by the presence of more than 75% immature neutrophils in the white blood cell differential count.[33] Two randomized, prospective studies showed questionable efficacy in neonatal sepsis and leave unanswered the question regarding the routine use of such transfusions.[12,172]A more recent comparison of granulocyte transfusions (obtained from leukopheresis), intravenous immunoglobulin, and supportive care showed no difference in survival among the groups,[29] but because of a limited number of patients, the study may have had insufficient power to detect the difference. A recent survey of neonatal transfusion practices found that only 35% of the responding hospitals were using such transfusions.[161]

Studies of patient survival in adults with sepsis and neutropenia have yielded mixed results but have shown an overall trend toward increased survival in patients who received granulocytes.[30,159] There are no studies in older children to assess the efficacy of granulocyte transfusions in sepsis.

Complications. Potential adverse effects from granulocyte transfusions include worsening pulmonary status and deoxygenation. Despite an initial report of severe pulmonary reactions[175] with the concomitant administration of amphotericin B and granulocytes, this finding has not been substantiated.[158] Because leukocytes are the mediators of febrile transfusion reactions, fever is common with transfusions. Emergency granulocyte transfusion with incomplete donor testing often occurs and may increase the risk of transfusion-associated infection.

Equipment. Transfuse granulocytes through a standard 170-micron filter. Do not use leukocyte filters.

Techniques. Because granulocyte products often contain a significant amount of red blood cell contamination, ideally a crossmatch should be performed.[126] Because leukopheresis products contain between 200 and 400 ml of plasma,[76] volume overload often results if the full unit is transfused in a neonate or small child. In a small child, use a volume of 10 to 20 ml/kg. Transfuse granulocytes as soon as possible after collection and preferably within 4 to 8 hours.

SPECIAL TOPICS IN BLOOD-COMPONENT THERAPY

Massive Transfusion

Massive transfusion is defined as the replacement of more than one blood volume in a 6-hour period and may cause citrate toxicity, electrolyte disturbances, acid-base abnormalities, hypothermia, and coagulopathy.

Citrate toxicity is the most serious concern regarding massive transfusion in pediatrics. Citrate binds divalent cations and thereby causes transient hypocalcemia[44] and hypomagnesemia[97] when a large amount of blood is given within a short time period. Citrate toxicity is most common in patients with hepatic or renal disease.[44] Hypocalcemia is treated with intravenous calcium chloride (10 to 20 mg/kg) only for symptomatic patients, documented hypocalcemia, or electrocardiographic abnormalities such as a prolonged QT interval.[28]

Thrombocytopenia generally causes the coagulopathy that may occur after massive transfusion. Most abnormal bleeding occurs with platelet counts below 100,000 in children, but bleeding correlates poorly with prothrombin times and partial thromboplastin times.[36] The results of a randomized, blind study using prophylactic platelet administration suggests that this approach neither reduces bleeding nor diminishes transfusion requirements.[129] However, other authorities advocate prophylactic platelet usage,[123] particularly with the high mortality rate (77% in one series) associated with the

Table 150-5   Unique Transfusion Issues for Special Situations

Situation	Issue
Neonates	Use irradiated cells
	Consider excluding paternal donation (particularly paternal cells or maternal plasma)
	Use CMV seronegative products or leukodepleted products
Sickle-cell anemia	Use leukodepleted or washed cell products
	Consider race-specific transfusion
Unusual antibody	Frozen deglycerolized RBCs
Immunocompromised patients (or candidates for transplantation)	Use irradiated cells
	Use CMV seronegative products or leukodepleted product
Directed donations from blood-related donors	Use irradiated cells
IgA deficiency	Frozen deglycerolized RBCs

coagulopathy of massive transfusion in adults.[19] Recently, the use of red blood cells containing the nutrient solution Adsol has produced a higher incidence of coagulation abnormalities (elevated prothrombin times) than previously reported.[45]

Hypothermia is another important cause of altered hemostasis and necessitates the use of a blood warmer; however, most devices restrict the flow of blood and thus require a longer transfusion time. Microwave blood warmers may be used, but only commercial devices designed for warming blood, not commercial cooking microwaves, can be used because of excessive hemolysis.[9] High-flow blood warmers are now commercially available.

Several electrolyte disturbances may occur with massive transfusion. Although hyperkalemia may occur because of the leakage of the red blood cells' potassium into the plasma during storage, hypokalemia is more common.[71] Hypokalemia occurs as a result of the metabolism of citrate to bicarbonate and produces alkalosis and an intracellular shift of potassium ions. This hypokalemia also relates to the process of the transfused cells regaining metabolic function and taking up potassium.[71] Hypocalcemia resulting from the binding of calcium by citrate has been discussed previously.

Autologous Donation

Because of the concern regarding transfusion-associated infection (primarily HIV), autologous donation has increased greatly in this country, even in pediatrics.[41] Children as young as 8 years of age have donated blood for planned surgical procedures, primarily orthopedic.[114,147] Because the donations must be planned well in advance of the anticipated surgery, they are not useful in emergency medicine; however, intensivists often use such donations in the management of postoperative patients. The technique is safe and eliminates the need for homologous blood in the vast majority of cases.[141]

Patients generally donate at weekly intervals and receive iron supplementation (6 mg/kg/day).[114] They make no donations the week before surgery. Some information suggests that recombinant erythropoietin may be useful in autologous donation,[82] but little information is available from clinical studies.

Because even autologous donations present some risk of transfusion reactions and clerical error, give autologous transfusions only when a transfusion is indicated and not merely because autologous blood is available.[147]

Directed Donations

Recent concern regarding transfusion-associated infection has also stimulated interest in directed donations of blood for patients. This practice presumes that blood from family and friends poses less risk of disease transmission than blood from the general donor supply. However, directed donation generally entails *increased* risk because individuals are unlikely to reveal high-risk behaviors to other family members and friends. Several groups have found a higher rate of positive infectious disease markers in directed vs. standard donors, which implies that such donations carry a greater risk than standard donors.[35,165] Because of the risk of transfusion-associated graft vs. host disease, irradiate all blood products from blood relatives.[157]

Blood from parents may pose some special problems for neonates because of the presence of maternal-paternal-neonatal incompatibilities. Do not transfuse maternal plasma to the neonate because the maternal plasma may contain antibodies that react with the neonate's erythrocyte, leukocyte, platelet, and HLA antigens.[157]

Paternal erythrocytes, leukocytes, and platelets may express antigens to which the mother has passively immunized the neonate. Some authorities advise against transfusing cellular elements from the father, but if there is no alternative, perform a major antiglobulin crossmatch (not a routine procedure in neonatal crossmatching).[160]

Autotransfusion

Autotransfusion has a long tradition in medicine, but as the concern over homologous transfusion increases, its use has likewise increased. Autotransfusion may exist in several forms: intraoperative salvage, intraoperative normovolemic hemodilution, or collection and autotransfusion in the ED or ICU. Blood salvage has occurred during orthopedic or cardiac procedures[87] or as part of a major trauma resuscitation when a child comes to the ED with massive hemothorax.

Indications. Intraoperative blood salvage is the most commonly used form of autotransfusion. Blood may either be collected and reinfused without processing, or it may be collected into a cell washer and returned after concentration. Because the blood salvaged from a serosal cavity is generally deficient in fibrinogen and platelets,[163] it is possible to transfuse the salvaged blood with minimal or no anticoagulants.

If the scavenged blood is being returned without washing, remove it via suction into a plastic bag and add an anticoagulant (citrate). Reinfuse the contents of the bag through a standard or microaggregate blood filter. This system is attractive because of its simplicity but carries the risk of infusing free hemoglobin,[21] surgical field debris, and tissue proteins that may initiate coagulation.[84]

A number of commercial products are available for the

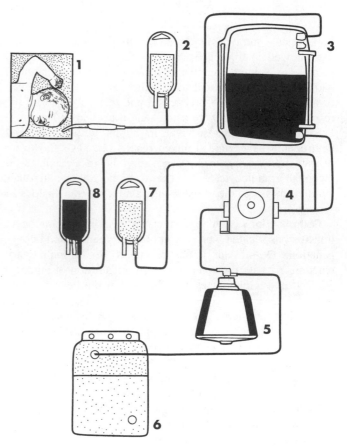

FIG. 150-1 Autotransfusion. Suction shed blood (1) from the patient and anticoagulate (2). A reservoir (3) serves to filter out tissue, clots, and other debris; it stores the blood until the next cycle of processing. The processor pumps blood (4) into a spinning centrifuge bowl (5), which captures the red blood cells. Plasma overflows into a waste bag (6), removing free hemoglobin, activated clotting factors, and other fluids. When the hematocrit reaches approximately 50%, the processor adds sterile saline (7) to wash the cells. After washing is complete, the processor resuspends the cells in saline and pumps them from the centrifuge bowl into a reinfusion bag (8) for return to the patient.

(Courtesy Haemonetics Corp.)

intraoperative salvage and washing of blood. The process includes removing blood, adding anticoagulant, filtering, pumping it into a centrifuge bowl to allow plasma removal and saline washing of the red blood cells, returning red blood cells to a bag, and reinfusing them into the patient. Combined with preoperative autologous donation, this technique can eliminate homologous transfusions in as many as 80% of well-planned cases.[114]

A recent case report has documented two cases of coagulopathy after the reinfusion of scavenged blood, but the exact origin of the coagulopathy was uncertain.[107] These systems require expensive equipment and trained personnel but are used by many centers throughout the country (Fig. 150-1).

Another autotransfusion technique being used by some centers with increased frequency is intraoperative normovolemic hemodilution. With this procedure, a predetermined amount of blood is withdrawn and replaced with either crystalloid or colloid solution just after the induction of an anesthetic. The blood initially withdrawn is reinfused to provide both volume and red blood cell mass. A potential advantage of this technique is that a hemorrhage that occurs

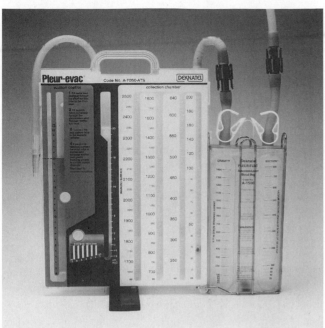

FIG. 150-2 The Pleur-Evac Autotransfusion System. The autotransfusion bag (*right*) attaches to the thoracostomy drainage device and serves as the reinfusion bag.

(Courtesy Deknatel, Inc.)

during the procedure loses blood that has a lower hematocrit. Anesthesiologists have used this technique successfully in children undergoing cardiac[78] and orthopedic procedures.[63]

Contraindications. The major contraindication to autotransfusion is disseminated infection or malignancy involving the operative site,[41] because this procedure could promote the spread of infection or tumor. A potential contraindication to autotransfusion is infection from within the cavity from which the blood is obtained (such as a perforated bowel).

Complications. All complications of massive transfusion may occur with autotransfusion but can be minimized by reinfusing less than 3500 ml into an adult.[127] Prevent microemboli by using a 40-micron filter. Air embolism has occurred when an air-filled bag infused air under pressure after it was empty[23]; therefore evacuate all air from bags.

Equipment. Both in the ED and critical care unit, a number of systems may be used to scavenge blood from a hemorrhage within a body cavity. The most common use of such systems involves the management of hemothorax, where a rapid hemorrhage can be evacuated through a thoracostomy tube into a closed system.[177] Simple systems such as the Sorenson Autotransfusion System[38,168] or Pleur-Evac Autotransfusion System (Fig. 150-2) are available.

Techniques. Collect the blood from a sterile cavity into a sterile bag and add anticoagulant (usually citrate-phosphate-dextrose). When filled, either reinfuse the bag directly through a 40-micron filter or transport it to the blood bank for washing and concentration. Such a system also allows the collection of blood from postoperative hemorrhage in the ICU with a minimal amount of equipment. Reinfusion systems are safe for use in children for up to 15% of total blood volume without washing before reinfusion.[16]

Exchange Transfusion

Exchange transfusion is a technique that may be necessary in the management of hyperbilirubinemia in the neonate. However, after the neonatal period, intensivists most often perform this procedure for the management of complications of sickle cell anemia[170] or for the management of hyperleukocytosis of acute leukemia.[25]

Because of the lack of randomized trials, the basis of the need for exchange transfusion in sickle cell anemia is anecdotal evidence that exchange transfusion offers the potential advantage of increasing hematocrit and reducing the hemoglobin S (HbgS) while minimizing changes in blood volume and viscosity. A reduction in HbgS can result in improvements in oxygen delivery[100] and viscosity.[137]

Indications. The most common indications for exchange transfusion in sickle-cell disease are severe, progressive acute chest syndrome;[170] acute cerebrovascular events such as infarction, hemorrhage, or ischemia;[32] and refractory priapism.[131] Additional indications for exchange transfusion include selected cases of eye surgery, retinal arterial vasoocclusion, hepatic failure, septic shock, and before cerebral angiography and surgery.[170]

Another use for exchange transfusion occurs with children with acute leukemia who have leukocyte counts above 200,000/μl or who have symptoms of leukostasis such as a visual disturbance, mental status change, respiratory distress, or priapism.[25] Vigorous hydration alone may be sufficient to lower the white blood cell count below 200,000/μl in the asymptomatic patient. Another alternative therapy is leukopheresis for children in whom adequate venous access can be obtained.[95]

Techniques. Exchange transfusions are generally performed with either whole blood or, most commonly, with reconstituted whole blood (PRBCs and FFP). Numerous recommendations for the volume of exchange transfusion range from the transfusion of one-half to twice the blood volume. A number of formulas exist for calculating the volumes,[14,112] and Table 150-6 lists some recommendations.

Historically, exchange transfusions are laborious procedures performed by withdrawing blood, discarding it, and then infusing the same volume of blood. A single-lumen catheter may be used (generally in a large central vein) if the withdrawal and transfusion cycles are alternated. However, this technique lengthens the procedure considerably. Alternatively, use an arterial catheter for blood withdrawal and a venous catheter for transfusion. A double-lumen venous catheter such as those designed for hemodialysis can also be used, but take care to use the proximal port for withdrawal and the distal port for transfusion to decrease recirculation through the system.

Some centers use automated exchange transfusion with a machine capable of erythrocytapheresis, but this procedure requires expensive equipment and specialized personnel.[79,169] Another less costly automated method uses standard volumetric intravenous infusion pumps.[136]

Use leukocyte-depleted blood to minimize alloimmunization.[132] In sickle cell anemia, an extended antigen match and the use of blood from African-American donors may further reduce the risk of alloimmunization.[166]

Assess and record vital signs at frequent intervals. Check

Table 150-6 Volumes for Exchange Transfusion

Indication	Volume to be exchanged	Desired end point
Rapid correction of anemia	Double-volume exchange* of reconstituted whole blood, or the formula:[113] $$\frac{\text{Weight (kg)} \times \text{Blood volume (ml/kg)} \times \text{Hgb desired (g/dl)}}{22 \text{ g/dl}\dagger - ([\text{Hgb observed \{g/dl\}} + \text{Hgb desired \{g/dl\}}]/2)}$$	Desired end point Hgb >5 g/dl, no clinical evidence of congestive heart failure
Hyperleukocytosis associated with acute leukemia (WBC over 200,000 or CNS symptoms [blindness, nerve palsy, headache])	Double-volume exchange* (blood volume/kg × weight in kg) of reconstituted whole blood	WBC <200,000 or resolution of CNS symptoms
Sickle cell anemia with acute cerebrovascular accident, acute chest syndrome, or refractory priapism	Double-volume exchange* of reconstituted whole blood	HgbS of <20% to 30% and hemoglobin <14 g/dl
Hyperbilirubinemia	Double-volume exchange* of reconstituted whole blood	Fall in serum bilirubin to desired level

*Estimated blood volumes for premature infants are 85 to 100 ml/kg, 85 ml/kg for term newborns, and 75 ml/kg for children over 1 month old, adolescents, and adults.[110]
†Average Hgb of packed red blood cells.

serum calcium (or ionized calcium), potassium, hematocrit, and platelet count at the midpoint and at the end of the transfusion. Keep calcium readily available (10 to 20 mg/kg of calcium chloride) should symptomatic hypocalcemia occur.

Perform neonatal exchange transfusion for hyperbilirubinemia using the same technique and most often a double-volume exchange (twice the calculated blood volume). Perform this procedure with a single-lumen umbilical venous catheter or a combination of arterial and venous umbilical catheters.

Extracorporeal Life Support

Extracorporeal life support (ECLS) is a technique used increasingly for the management of infants and children with severe respiratory or cardiac failure (see Chapter 27). The blood bank is an integral part of the ECLS team because these patients require significant blood-product support at the initiation of and throughout ECLS support. ECLS protocols vary substantially between centers, but most centers use fresh (less than 3 to 5 days old) red blood cells for priming the circuit, as well as for emergency transfusions. Another suggested priming mixture is a combination of heparin, THAM (tromethamine), 5% albumin, sodium bicarbonate, and PRBCs.[46] If time permits, check electrolytes and ionized calcium on the circuit. After initiating support, rapidly infuse one-half to one unit of platelet apheresis.

Indications. Indications for transfusion are also variable among centers, but to maximize oxygen delivery most centers transfuse PRBCs to maintain the hematocrit at 40% to 45%.[140] However, a small study recently questions this practice. Investigators maintained one group of infants at a hematocrit of 35% and another group at a hematocrit of 45%.[62] The group with the lower hematocrit had significantly lower donor exposure and significantly less clotting in the circuit.

The circuit and membrane oxygenator consume platelets;

transfuse platelets to keep the platelet count above 80,000 to 150,000.[37] To prevent volume overload, platelets often undergo plasma volume reduction for transfusion to infants.

Patients receive heparin for anticoagulation to prevent clot formation in the circuit; the ECLS staff monitors activated clotting times to provide a global index of hemostasis that is typically in the range of 180 to 240 seconds.[61] In a child with bleeding complications, maintain the activated clotting time at lower levels, typically 160 to 180 seconds. Transfuse FFP to help prevent or treat hemorrhage, but specific indications are unclear.[60] Monitor fibrinogen levels; if such levels are low (less than 150 mg/dl), give cryoprecipitate.[47]

REFERENCES

1. Aach RD, et al: Serum alanine aminotransferase of donors in relation to the risk of non-a, non-b hepatitis in recipients: the transfusion-transmitted viruses study, *N Engl J Med* 304:989-994, 1981.
2. Adler SP: Transfusion-associated cytomegalovirus infections, *Rev Infect Dis* 5:977-993, 1983.
3. Anderson KC, Weinstein HJ: Transfusion-associated graft-versus-host disease, *N Engl J Med* 323:315-321, 1990.
4. Andrew M, Barr RD: Increased platelet destruction in infancy and childhood, *Semin Thromb Hemost* 8:248-262, 1982.
5. Anonymous: Update: HIV-2 infection in the United States, *MMWR* 38:572-580, 1989.
6. Anonymous: *Pneumocystis carinii* pneumonia among persons with hemophilia A, *MMWR* 31:365-367, 1982.
7. Anonymous: *Med Letter* 35:51-52, 1993.
8. Anonymous: *Med Letter* 35:78, 1993.
9. Arens JF, Leonard GL: Danger of overwarming blood by microwave, *JAMA* 218:1045-1046, 1971.
10. Reference deleted in proofs.
11. Baldini M, Costea N, Dameshek W: The viability of stored human platelets, *Blood* 16:1669-1693, 1960.
12. Baley JE, et al: Buffy coat transfusions in neutropenic neonates with presumed sepsis: a prospective, randomized trial, *Pediatrics* 80:712-720, 1987.
13. Bensinger WI, et al: The effects of daily recombinant human granulocyte colony-stimulating factor administration on normal granulocyte donors undergoing leukapheresis, *Blood* 81:1883-1888, 1993.

14. Berman B, Krieger A, Naiman JL: A new method for calculating volumes of blood required for partial exchange transfusion, *J Pediatr* 94:86-89, 1979.

15. Blattner WA, Saxinger CW, Gallo RC: HTLV-I, the prototype human retrovirus: epidemiologic features, *Prog Clin Biol Res* 139:223-243, 1985.

16. Blevins FT, et al: Reinfusion of shed blood after orthopaedic procedures in children and adolescents, *J Bone Joint Surg* 75-A:363-371, 1993.

17. Blumberg N, Heal JM: Transfusion and host defenses against cancer recurrence and infection, *Transfusion* 29:236-245, 1989.

18. Bona RD, et al: The use of continuous infusion of factor concentrates in the treatment of hemophilia, *Am J Hematol* 32:8-13, 1989.

19. Boyan CP, Howland WS: Immediate and delayed death associated with massive transfusion, *Surg Clin North Am* 49:217-222, 1969.

20. Braunstein AH, Oberman HA: Transfusion of plasma components, *Transfusion* 24:281-286, 1984.

21. Brener BJ, Raines JK, Darling RC: Intraoperative autotransfusion in abdominal aortic resection, *Arch Surg* 107:78-84, 1973.

22. Brettler DB, et al: The use of porcine factor VIII concentrate (Hyate:C) in the treatment of patients with inhibitor antibodies to factor VIII, *Arch Intern Med* 149:1381-1385, 1989.

23. Bretton P, Reines HD, Sade RM: Air embolization during autotransfusion for abdominal trauma, *J Trauma* 25:165-166, 1985.

24. Brunson ME, Alexander JW: Mechanisms of transfusion-induced immunosuppression, *Transfusion* 30:651-658, 1990.

25. Bunin NJ, Kunkel K, Callihan TR: Cytoreductive procedures in the early management of leukemia and hyperleukocytosis in children, *Med Pediatr Oncol* 15:232-235, 1987.

26. Burks LC, et al: Meperidine for the treatment of shaking chills and fever, *Arch Intern Med* 140:483-484, 1980.

27. Busch MP, et al: Evaluation of screened blood donations for human immunodeficiency virus type 1 infection by culture and DNA amplification of pooled cells, *N Engl J Med* 325:1-5, 1991.

28. Buskard NA, Varghese Z, Wills MR: Correction of hypocalcemic symptoms during plasma exchange, *Lancet* 2:344-345, 1976.

29. Cairo MS: Neutrophil transfusions in the treatment of neonatal sepsis, *Am J Pediatr Hematol Oncol* 11:227-234, 1989.

30. Cairo MS: The use of granulocyte transfusions in neonatal sepsis, *Transfus Med Rev* 6:14-22, 1990.

31. Capon S, et al: Transfusion-associated graft-versus-host disease in an immunocompetent patient, *Ann Intern Med* 114:1025-1026, 1991.

32. Charache S, Luban B, Reid CD: Management and therapy of sickle-cell disease, Washington, DC, US Department of Health and Human Services, Public Health Service, National Institutes of Health Publication 92-2117, 1991.

33. Christensen RD, Bradley PP, Rothstein G: The leukocyte left shift in clinical and experimental neonatal sepsis, *J Pediatr* 98:101-105, 1981.

34. Collins MB: Personal communication, August 18, 1993.

35. Cordell RR, et al: Experience with 11,916 directed donors, *Transfusion* 26:484-486, 1986.

36. Cote CJ, et al: Changes in serial platelet counts following massive blood transfusion in pediatric patients, *Anesthesiology* 62:197-201, 1985.

37. Dalton HJ, Thompson AE: Extracorporeal membrane oxygenation. In Fuhrman BP, Zimmerman JJ, editors: *Pediatric critical care,* St Louis, 1992, Mosby.

38. Davidson SJ, Emergency unit autotransfusion, *Surgery* 84:703-707, 1978.

39. De Grann-Hentzen YC, et al: Prevention of primary cytomegalovirus infections in patients with hematologic malignancies by intensive white-cell depletion of blood products, *Transfusion* 29:757-760, 1989.

40. de la Fuente B, et al: Response of patients with mild and moderate hemophilia A and von Willebrand's disease to treatment with desmopressin, *Ann Intern Med* 103:6-14, 1985.

41. De Palma L, Luban NLC: Autologous blood transfusion in pediatrics (editorial), *Pediatrics* 85:125-128, 1992.

42. Lackritz EM, et al: Estimated risk of transmission of the human immunodeficiency virus by screened blood in the United States, *N Engl J Med* 333:1721-1725, 1995.

43. Donahue JG, et al: The declining risk of post-transfusion hepatitis C virus infection, *N Engl J Med* 327:369-373, 1992.

44. Dzik WH, Kirkley SA: Citrate toxicity during massive blood transfusion, *Transfus Med Rev* 2:76-94, 1988.

45. Faringer PD, et al: Blood component supplementation during transfusion of AS-1 red cells in trauma patients, *J Trauma* 34:481-487, 1993.

46. Faulkner S: Personal communication, September 23, 1993.

47. Faulkner SC, et al: Techniques utilized for extracorporeal membrane oxygenation support of the postoperative pediatric cardiac patient, *Proc Am Acad Cardiovasc Perfus* 13:32-35, 1992.

48. Fetus and Newborn Committee, Canadian Pediatric Society: Guidelines for transfusion of erythrocytes to neonates and premature infants, *Can Med Assoc J* 147:1781-1786, 1992.

49. Galel SA, Grumet FC: Platelet alloimmunization. In Rossi EC, Simon TL, Moss GS, editors: *Principles of transfusion medicine,* Baltimore, 1991, Williams & Wilkins.

50. Gilbert GL, et al: Prevention of transfusion-acquired cytomegalovirus infection in infants by blood filtration to remove leukocytes, *Lancet* 1:1228-1231, 1989.

51. Gill JC, Montgomery RR: Principles of therapy for hemostasis factor deficiency. In Nathan DG, Oski FA, editors: *Hematology of infancy and childhood,* ed 4, Philadelphia, 1993, WB Saunders.

52. Gmur J, et al: Delayed alloimmunization using random single-donor platelet transfusion: a prospective study in thrombocytopenic patients with acute leukemia, *Blood* 62:473-479, 1983.

53. Gmur J, et al: Safety of stringent prophylactic platelet transfusion policy for patients with acute leukemia, *Lancet* 338:1223-1226, 1991.

54. Goldfinger D, Lowe C: Prevention of adverse reactions to blood transfusion by the administration of saline-washed red blood cells, *Transfusion* 21:277-280, 1981.

55. Gomperts ED: Procedures for the inactivation of viruses in clotting factor concentrates, *Am J Hematol* 23:295-305, 1986.

56. Gordon JB, Bernstein ML, Rogers MC: Hematologic disorders in the pediatric intensive care unit. In Rogers MC, editor: *Textbook of pediatric intensive care,* Baltimore, 1992, Williams & Wilkins.

57. Gorgone BC, Anderson JW, Anderson KC: Comparison of 15 minute and 1 hour post–platelet counts in pediatric patients (abstract), *Transfusion* 26:555, 1986.

58. Gould SA, Moss GS: Administration of red cells: the transfusion trigger and red cell substitutes. In Rossi EC, Simon TL, Moss GS, editors: *Principles of transfusion medicine,* Baltimore, 1991, Williams & Wilkins.

59. Green D: Von Willebrand's disease. In Rossi EC, Simon TL, Moss GS, editors: *Principles of transfusion medicine,* Baltimore, 1991, Williams & Wilkins.

60. Green TP, Payne NR, Steinhorn RH: Indications for transfusion of fresh-frozen plasma during extracorporeal membrane oxygenation (letter), *Transfusion* 31:477, 1991.

61. Green TP, et al: Whole blood activated clotting time in infants during extracorporeal membrane oxygenation, *Crit Care Med* 18:494-498, 1990.

62. Griffin MP, et al: Benefits of a lower hematocrit during extracorporeal membrane oxygenation, *Am J Dis Child* 46:373-374, 1992.

63. Haberkern M, Dangel P: Normovolemic haemodilution and intraoperative autotransfusion in children: experience with 30 cases of spinal fusion, *Eur J Pediatr Surg* 1:30-35, 1990.

64. Heal HJ, Blumberg N, Masel D: An evaluation of crossmatching HLA and ABO matching for platelet transfusions to refractory patients, *Blood* 70:23-30, 1987.

65. Hedner U, et al: Clinical experience with human plasma-derived factor VIIa in patients with hemophilia A and high titer inhibitors, *Haemostasis* 19:335-343, 1989.

66. Herr V, et al: Transfusion-associated transmission of human t-lymphotrophic virus types I and II: experience from a regional blood center, *Transfusion* 33:208-211, 1993.

67. Hinckley ME, Huestis DW: Premedication for optimal granulocyte collection, *Plasma Ther* 2:149-152, 1981.

68. Holmberg L, et al: Platelet aggregation induced by 1-desamino-8-D-arginine vasopressin (DDAVP) in type IIB von Willebrand's disease, *N Engl J Med* 209:816-821, 1983.

69. Honig CL, Bove JR: Transfusion-associated fatalities: review of Bureau of Biologics reports 1976-1978, *Transfusion* 20:653-661, 1980.

70. Hume H: Pediatric transfusions: quality assessment and assurance. In Sacher RA, Strauss R, editors: *Contemporary issues in pediatric transfusion medicine,* Arlington, Va, 1989, American Association of Blood Banks.

71. Isbister JP: Haemotherapy for acute hemorrhage, *Anaesth Intensive Care* 12:217-228, 1984.

72. Izraeli S, et al: Lactic acid as a predictor for erythrocyte transfusion in healthy preterm infants with anemia of prematurity, *J Pediatr* 122:629-631, 1993.

73. Johnson KB, editor: *The Harriet Lane Handbook,* ed 13, St Louis, 1993, Mosby.

74. Jugi T, et al: Post-transfusion graft-versus-host disease in immunocompetent patients after cardiac surgery (letter), *N Engl J Med* 321:56, 1989.

75. Kahn RA, Duffy RF, Rodey GG: Ultraviolet irradiation of platelet concentrate abrogates lymphocyte activation without affecting platelet function in vitro, *Transfusion* 25:547-550, 1985.

76. Kalmin ND, Grindon AJ, Comparison of two continuous-flow cell separators, *Transfusion* 23:197-200, 1981.

77. Kasper CK, Dietrich SL: Comprehensive management of hemophilia, *Clin Haematol* 14:489-512, 1985.

78. Kawamura M, et al: Safe limit of hemodilution in cardiopulmonary bypass: comparative analysis between cyanotic and acyanotic heart disease, *Jpn J Surg* 10:206-211, 1980.

79. Kernoff LM, et al: Exchange transfusion in sickle cell disease using a continuous flow cell separator, *Transfusion* 17:269-271, 1977.

80. Kevy SK: Red cell transfusion. In Nathan DG, Oski FA, editors: *Hematology of infancy and childhood,* ed 4, Philadelphia, 1993, WB Saunders.

81. Kevy SV: Current concepts in pediatric transfusion medicine. In Summers SH, Smith DM, Agranenko VA, editors: *Transfusion therapy: guidelines for practice,* Arlington, Va, 1990, American Association of Blood Banks.

82. Kickler TS, Spivak JL: Effect of repeated whole blood donation on serum immunoreactive erythropoietin levels in autologous donors, *JAMA* 260:65-67, 1988.

83. Klapper EB, Goldfinger D: Leukocyte-reduced blood components in transfusion medicine: current indications and prospects for the future, *Clin Lab Med* 12:711-721, 1992.

84. Kruskall, MS: Intraoperative autotransfusion. In Rossi EC, Simon TL, Moss GS, editors: *Principles of transfusion medicine,* Baltimore, 1991, Williams & Wilkins.

85. Lee H, et al: High rate of HTLV-II infection in seropositive IV drug abusers in New Orleans, *Science* 244:471-474, 1989.

86. Lefebre J, McLellan BA, Coovadia AS: Seven years' experience with group O unmatched red cells in a regional trauma unit, *Ann Emerg Med* 16:1344-1349, 1987.

87. Leveque CM, Yawn DH: Limiting homologous blood exposure, *Clin Lab Med* 12:771-785, 1992.

88. Levy GJ, et al: National survey of neonatal transfusion practices. I. Red blood cell therapy, *Pediatrics* 91:523-529, 1993.

89. Luban NLC, Sacher RA: Transfusion-transmitted cytomegalovirus and Epstein-Barr diseases. In Rossi EC, Simon TL, Moss GS, editors: *Principles of transfusion medicine,* Baltimore, 1991, Williams & Wilkins.

90. Luban NLC, DePalma L: Transfusion therapy in the pediatric intensive care unit. In Holbrook P, editor: *Textbook of pediatric critical care,* Philadelphia, 1993, WB Saunders.

91. Lusher JM: Management of patients with factor VIII inhibitors, *Trans Med Rev* 1:123-130, 1987.

92. Lusher JM, et al: Efficacy of prothrombin-complex concentrates in hemophiliacs with antibodies to factor VIII, *N Engl J Med* 303:421-425, 1980.

93. Mannucci PM: Desmopressin (DDAVP) for the treatment of disorders of hemostasis, *Prog Hemost Thrombo* 8:19-45, 1986.

94. Mannucci PM, et al: 1-desamino-8-D-arginine vasopressin: a new pharmacologic approach to the management of hemophilia and von Willebrand's disease, *Lancet* 1:869-872, 1977.

95. Maurer HS, et al: The effect of initial management of hyperleukocytosis on early complications and outcome of children with acute lymphoblastic leukemia, *J Clin Oncol* 6:1425-1432, 1988.

96. McGraw RA, et al: Structure and function of factor IX: defects in hemophilia B, *Clin Haematol* 14:359-383, 1985.

97. McLellan BA, Reid SR, Lane PL: Massive blood transfusion causing hypomagnesemia, *Crit Care Med* 12:146-147, 1984.

98. Meyers JD, et al: Risk factors for cytomegalovirus infection after human marrow transplantation, *J Infect Dis* 153:478-488, 1986.

99. Mezrow CK, Bergstein I, Tartter PI: Postoperative infections following autologous and homologous blood transfusion, *Transfusion* 32:27-30, 1992.

100. Miller DM, et al: Improved exercise performance after exchange transfusion in subjects with sickle cell anemia, *Blood* 56:1127-1131, 1980.

101. Miller JL: Platelet-type von Willebrand's disease, *Clin Lab Med* 4:319-331, 1984.

102. Moore GL, et al: Some properties of blood stores in anticoagulant CPDA-1 solution: a brief summary, *Transfusion* 21:135-137, 1981.

103. Moroff G, et al: Reduction of the volume of stored platelet concentrations for neonatal use, *Transfusion* 24:144-146, 1984.

104. Morrow, JF, Braine HG, Kickler TS: Septic reactions to platelet transfusions: a persistent problem, *JAMA* 266:555-558, 1991.

105. Muder RR, et al: *Staphylococcus epidermidis* bacteremia from transfusion of contaminated platelets: application of bacterial DNA analysis, *Transfusion* 32:771-774, 1992.

106. Murphy S, et al: Indications for platelet transfusion in children with acute leukemia, *Am J Hematol* 12:347-356, 1982.

107. Murray DJ, Gress K, Weinstein SL: Coagulopathy after reinfusion of scavenged red blood cells, *Anesth Analg* 75:125-129, 1992.

108. Myhre BA: Fatalities from blood transfusion, *JAMA* 244:1333-1335, 1980.

109. Myhre BA: Bacterial contamination is still a hazard of blood transfusion (editorial), *Arch Pathol Lab Med* 109:982-983, 1985.

110. Nathan DG, Oski FA, editors: *Hematology of infancy and childhood,* ed 4, Philadelphia, 1993, WB Saunders.

111. Ness PM: Bacterial and protozoal transmission by transfusion. In Rossi EC, Simon TL, Moss GS, editors: *Principles of transfusion medicine,* Baltimore, 1991, Williams & Wilkins.

112. Nieburg PI, Stockman JA: Rapid correction of anemia with partial exchange transfusion, *Am J Dis Child* 131:60-61, 1977.

113. Nilsson L, et al: Shelf-life of bank blood and stored plasma with special reference to coagulation factors, *Transfusion* 23:377-381, 1983.

114. Novak RW: Autologous blood transfusion in a pediatric population: safety and efficacy, *Clin Pediatr* 27:184-187, 1988.

115. Nugent DJ: Platelet transfusion. In Nathan DG, Oski FA, editors: *Hematology of infancy and childhood,* ed 4, Philadelphia, 1993, WB Saunders.

116. O'Connell B, Lee EJ, Schiffer CA: The value of 10-minute posttransfusion platelet counts, *Transfusion* 28:66-67, 1988.

117. Office of Medical Applications of Research, National Institutes of Health: Fresh frozen plasma: indications and risks, *JAMA* 253:551-553, 1985.

118. Office of Medical Applications of Research, National Institutes of Health: Platelet transfusion therapy, *JAMA* 257:1777-1780, 1987.

119. Office of Medical Applications of Research, National Institutes of Health: Perioperative red cell transfusion, *JAMA* 260:2700-2703, 1988.

120. Opelz G: Identification of unresponsive kidney-transplant recipients, *Lancet* 1:868-871, 1972.

121. Perkins HA, et al: Nonhemolytic febrile transfusion reactions, *Vox Sang* 11:578-600, 1966.

122. Phillips HM, et al: Determination of red-cell mass in assessment and management of anaemia in babies needing blood transfusion, *Lancet* 1:882-884, 1986.

123. Phillips TW, Soulier G, Wilson RF: Outcome of massive transfusion exceeding two blood volumes in trauma and emergency surgery, *J Trauma* 27:903-910, 1987.

124. Pineda AA, Taswell HF: Transfusion reactions associated with anti-IgA antibodies: report of four cases and review of the literature, *Transfusion* 15:10-15, 1975.

125. Pineda AA, Brzica SM Jr, Taswell HF: Hemolytic transfusion reaction: recent experience in a large blood bank, *Mayo Clin Proc* 53:378-390, 1978.

126. Price TH: Plateletpheresis and leukapheresis. In Rossi EC, Simon TL, Moss GS, editors: *Principles of transfusion medicine,* Baltimore, 1991, Williams & Wilkins.

127. Raines J, et al: Intraoperative autotransfusion: equipment, protocol, and guidelines, *J Trauma* 16:616-623, 1976.

128. Ramirez AM, et al: High potassium levels in stored irradiated blood (letter), *Transfusion* 27:444-445, 1987.

129. Reed RL II, et al: Prophylactic platelet administration during mass

transfusion: a prospective, randomized double-blind clinical study, *Ann Surg* 203:40-48, 1986.

130. Reynolds LO, Simon TL: Size distribution measurements of microaggregates in stored blood, *Transfusion* 20:669-678, 1980.

131. Rifkind S, et al: RBC exchange pheresis for priapism in sickle cell disease, *JAMA* 242:2317-2318, 1979.

132. Rosse WF, et al: Transfusion and alloimmunization in sickle cell disease, *Blood* 76:1431-1437, 1990.

133. Rousou JA, et al: Fibrin glue: an effective hemostatic agent for nonsuturable intraoperative bleeding, *Ann Thorac Surg* 38:409-410, 1984.

134. Saarinen UM, et al: Effective prophylaxis against platelet refractoriness in multitransfused patents by use of leukocyte-free blood components, *Blood* 75:512-517, 1990.

135. Sacher RA, Luban NLC, Strauss RG: Current practice and guidelines for the transfusion of cellular blood components in the newborn, *Transfus Med Rev* 3:39-54, 1989.

136. Schexnayder SM, et al: A technique for automated exchange transfusion in children and young adults (abstract), *Clin Research* 41:738A, 1993.

137. Schmalzer EA, et al: Viscosity of mixtures of sickle and normal red cells at varying hematocrit levels: implications for transfusion, *Transfusion* 27:228-233, 1987.

138. Seefe LB: Transfusion-associated hepatitis B: past and present, *Trans Med Rev* 2:204-214, 1988.

139. Sennett ML, Conrad ME: Treatment of thrombotic thrombocytopenic purpura: plasmapheresis, plasma transfusion, and vincristine, *Arch Intern Med* 146:266-267, 1986.

140. Short BL: Clinical management of the neonatal ECMO patient. In Arensman RM, Cornish JD, editors: *Extracorporeal life support,* Boston, 1993; Blackwell Scientific.

141. Silvergleid AJ: Safety and effectiveness of predeposit autologous transfusions in preteen and adolescent children, *JAMA* 257:3403-3404, 1987.

142. Simon TL: Platelet transfusion therapy. In Rossi EC, Simon TL, Moss GS: *Principles of transfusion medicine,* Baltimore, 1991, Williams & Wilkins.

143. Simon TL: Evolution in indications for blood component transfusion, *Clin Lab Med* 12:655-667, 1992.

144. Simon TL, Sierra ER: Concentration of platelet units into small volumes, *Transfusion* 24:173-175, 1984.

145. Simpson MB: Prospective-concurrent audits and medical consultation for platelet transfusion, *Transfusion* 27:192-195, 1987.

146. Simpson MB: The clinical use of platelet preparations. In Summers SH, Smith DM, Agranenko VA, editors: *Transfusion therapy: guidelines for practice,* Arlington, Va, 1990, American Association of Blood Banks.

147. Simpson MB, et al: Autologous transfusions for orthopaedic procedures at a children's hospital, *J Bone Joint Surg* 74A:652-657, 1992.

148. Sirchia G, et al: Removal of leukocytes from red blood cells by a transfusion through a new filter, *Transfusion* 30:30-33, 1990.

149. Sjamsoedin LJM, et al: The effect of activated prothrombin-complex concentrate (FEIBA) on joint and muscle bleeding in patients with hemophilia A and antibodies to factor VIII, *N Engl J Med* 305:717-721, 1981.

150. Smith DN: Immunosuppressive effects of blood transfusion, *Clin Lab Med* 12:723-741, 1992.

151. Snyder EL, Bookbinder M: Role of microaggregate blood filtration in clinical medicine, *Transfusion* 23:460-470, 1983.

152. Snyder EL, Stack G: Febrile and nonimmune transfusion reactions. In Rossi EC, Simon TL, Moss GS, editors: *Principles of transfusion medicine,* Baltimore, 1991, Williams & Wilkins.

153. Sohmer PR, Dawson RB: The significance of 2,3 DPG in red blood cell transfusions, *CRC Crit Rev Clin Lab Sci* 11:107, 1979.

154. Stern H, Tucker SM: Prospective study of cytomegalovirus infection in pregnancy, *Br J Med* 2:268-270, 1973.

155. Stockman JA III: Anemia of prematurity: current concepts in the issue of when to transfuse, *Pediatr Clin North Am* 33:111-128, 1986.

156. Storer DL: Blood and blood component therapy. In Rosen P, Barkin RM, editors: *Emergency medicine: concepts and clinical practice,* ed 2, St Louis, 1992, Mosby.

157. Strauss RG: Directed and limited-exposure donor programs for children. In Sacher RA, Strauss R, editors: *Contemporary issues in pediatric transfusion medicine,* Arlington, Va, 1989, American Association of Blood Banks.

158. Strauss RG: Granulocyte transfusions. In Rossi EC, Simon TL, Moss GS, editors: *Principles of transfusion medicine,* Baltimore, 1991, Williams & Wilkins.

159. Strauss RG, Therapeutic granulocyte transfusions in 1993 (editorial), *Blood* 81:1675-1678, 1993.

160. Strauss RG, et al: Directed and limited-exposure blood donations for infants and children, *Transfusion* 30:68-72, 1990.

161. Strauss RG et al: National survey of neonatal transfusion practices. II. Blood component therapy, *Pediatrics* 91:530-536, 1993.

162. Sullivan DW, et al: Fatal myocardial infarction following therapy with prothrombin-complex concentrates in a young man with hemophilia A, *Pediatrics* 74:279-281, 1984.

163. Symbas PN: Autotransfusion for hemothorax: experimental and clinical studies, *J Trauma* 12:689-695, 1972.

164. Tegtmeier GE: Postransfusion cytomegalovirus infection, *Arch Pathol Lab Med* 113:236-245, 1989.

165. Toy P, et al: Higher non-A, non-B hepatitis surrogate marker rates in designated donor units (abstract), *Transfusion* 28:17S, 1988.

166. Vichinsky EP, et al: Alloimmunization in sickle cell anemia and transfusion of racially unmatched blood, *N Engl J Med* 322:1617-1621, 1990.

167. Von Fliedner V, Higby DJ, Kim U: Graft-versus-host reaction following blood transfusion, *Am J Med* 72:951-961, 1982.

168. Von Koch L, Defore WW, Mattox KL: A practical method of autotransfusion in the emergency center, *Am J Surg* 133:770-772, 1977.

169. Wayne A, et al: Automated red cell exchange in sickle cell disease. The Joint Congress of International Society of Blood Transfusion and American Association of Blood Banks, November 1990.

170. Wayne AS, Kevy SV, Nathan DG: Transfusion management in sickle-cell disease, *Blood* 81:1109-1123, 1993.

171. Weiss HJ: Platelet physiology and abnormalities of platelet function: II, *N Engl J Med* 293:580-588, 1975.

172. Wheeler JG, et al: Buffy coat transfusions in neonates with sepsis and neutrophil storage-pool depletion, *Pediatrics* 79:422-425, 1987.

173. White CG II, et al: Factor VIII inhibitors: a clinical overview, *Am J Hematol* 13:335-342, 1982.

174. Wolfe LC: The membrane and lesions of storage in preserved red cells, *Transfusion* 25:185-203, 1985.

175. Wright DG, Robichaud KJ, Pizzo PA: Lethal pulmonary reactions associated with the combined use of amphotericin B and leukocyte transfusions, *N Engl J Med* 304:1185-1189, 1981.

176. Yankee RA, et al: Selection of unrelated compatible platelet donors by lymphocyte-HLA matching, *N Engl J Med* 288:760-764, 1973.

177. Young GP, Purcell TB: Emergency autotransfusion, *Ann Emerg Med* 12:180-186, 1983.

178. Zager RA, Gamelin LM: Pathogenetic mechanisms in experimental hemoglobinuric renal failure, *Am J Physio* 256:F446-455, 1989.

179. Zimmerman TS, Ruggeri ZM: von Willebrand's disease, *Prog Hemost Thrombo* 6:203-236, 1982.

PART XXVIII

MEDICOLEGAL PROCEDURES

151 Sexual Abuse

Jane M. Lavelle

Child-adolescent sexual abuse is an exploitive sexual act that is imposed by an older, dominant perpetrator onto a child or adolescent who lacks emotional and cognitive maturity.[4,11,33,43] A common theme in cases of sexual misuse includes the use of power, age, and position in relation to the child; the inability of the child to consent, which leads to helplessness; and an attempt on the child's part to please the adult. These acts incorporate a broad spectrum of acts that range from nontouching abuses such as genital viewing to fondling, kissing, masturbation, vulvar or gluteal coitus, and digital or genital penetration. Incest refers to the specific situation in which sexual abuse occurs between individuals who cannot marry; this term includes those having a family role, regardless of blood relationship. The true incidence of sexual misuse is unknown and remains largely underreported. An estimated 250,000 to 300,000 cases occur yearly in the United States, but only 50,000 of these cases are reported. Girls are the victims twice as often as boys.[1,4,20,33]

Children and adolescents may also be victims of sexual assault. Sexual assault includes any type of contact by the offender with the genitalia of the victim and is characterized by physical force and violence. Rape is defined as the introduction of the penis within the labia without consent. The perpetrator is fulfilling no sexual needs via the act. The average annual frequency of rape is 37 cases per 100,000 population; however, only an estimated 10% to 20% of these cases are reported. Adolescents and young adults have the highest incidence of sexual assault.[5,6]

Such complaints are common in the Emergency Department (ED), and there are many ways by which a child/adolescent may come to the ED. Law enforcement officers may bring a patient for medical evaluation. Disclosure by the child to the caretaker or worries of the caretaker may precipitate a visit. The child/adolescent may also present with genital or nongenital complaints in which sexual abuse is part of the differential diagnosis. Nongenital complaints include physiologic symptoms such as headache, abdominal pain, or constipation. Conversely, the child/adolescent may have behavioral or psychologic symptoms such as stylized or provocative sexual behavior, sleep disturbance, school failure, substance abuse, depression, anxiety, or suicidal ideation. Genital complaints include such things as vaginal pain, discharge, bleeding, or urinary-related symptoms. The emergency physician must become familiar with the medical issues, examination skills, local laws, and practices of the crime laboratory.[3,14,20,33,39,43]

Evaluation includes obtaining a detailed history of events followed by a complete physical examination and the collection of medical and forensic evidence. These cases usually represent social and mental health emergencies rather than the rare physical emergency and thus deserve a multidisciplinary approach. A routine plan or department policy should be in place for this type of emergency such as with other clinical emergencies. The purpose of the evaluation is to collect information, record it accurately and legibly, treat medical problems and, most important, protect the patient from further harm. The purpose is not to determine whether a crime has occurred. Box 151-1 summarizes the evaluation and management of the sexually abused child.

Indications

If the history suggests that an abusive episode has occurred within the preceding 72 hours or if the patient has any abdominal/pelvic/perineal symptoms, perform the evaluation immediately in the ED because the potential to detect injury and to collect seminal products and other body fluids and debris decreases with time.[5,11,20,33] If this is not the case, refer the patient and family to the appropriate clinical setting for nonemergent evaluation. Minimize reexamination and interviewing. The average time from the first episode of abuse to disclosure is 3 years; therefore sexual abuse is a chronic problem, and it may be difficult to ascertain the timing of the last abusive episode.[11,20,39,43] In this case, the physician may choose to delay the evaluation and refer the patient to a sexual abuse clinic, if possible. On the other hand, an adolescent is more likely to be the victim of date rape or an acute assaultive episode; therefore immediate evaluation is appropriate and indicated.[5,6] Remember that the manner in which the team handles the medical, legal, and psychosocial matters influences the future impact of the abusive episode on the victim.

Contraindications

Evaluation of the sexual abuse victim may be contraindicated if the patient refuses to cooperate. Do not repeat the abuse or violence, and do not make promises that cannot be kept. In most cases, someone whom the patient trusted has betrayed him or her (perpetrators usually know their victims); therefore it is important to explain the reason for the examination and how it will proceed. Adolescents may be victims of force and violence. If the child or adolescent is unable to cooperate, postpone the examination. In the rare case that the patient has come to the hospital with worrisome signs and symptoms such as significant abdominal pain or profuse vaginal or rectal bleeding, an examination performed with the patient under general anesthesia is indicated.

Complications

There are no specific complications associated with the physical examination or collection of specimens.

Equipment

The equipment necessary for the evaluation of sexual abuse or assault includes a good light source, a comfortable examination table, a sheet, materials for specimen collection, and a handheld magnifying glass or an otoscope (Box 151-2).

BOX 151-1 **CHECKLIST FOR EVALUATION AND MANAGEMENT OF SEXUAL ABUSE**

History (in the patient's own words)

Consent
Time/date/place of event/others present
Force, threats, restraints
Description of the assault (vaginal, oral, anal penetration, ejaculation, condom, foreign body)
Bathing, urination, defecation, douche, mouthwash, oral hygiene
Past medical history
Sexual history
Gynecologic history

Physical examination

General description of patient, including mental status and development
Complete physical examination
Genital examination; Tanner staging
Speculum examination

Sexually transmitted diseases

Cultures
    Neisseria gonorrhoeae
    Chlamydia trachomatis
    Herpes simplex virus
    Trichomonas vaginalis
Wet mount
    Trichomonas vaginalis
    Gardnerella vaginalis
    Whiff test
    pH
Serum
    Hepatitis B
    Human immunodeficiency virus
    Treponema pallidum

Forensic evidence

Samples for sperm, acid phosphatase, P-30 and mouse anti-human semen-5
Serum for blood-group antigens
Nail scrapings
Scalp and pubic hair specimens
Photographs

Management considerations

Sexually transmitted diseases
Pregnancy
Scheduled follow-up
Crisis intervention/social work and psychiatry
Child protective services
Police report

BOX 151-2 **EQUIPMENT NECESSARY FOR THE EVALUATION OF THE ABUSED CHILD/ADOLESCENT**

Quiet, private room	Red-topped tubes
Gowns, sheets	Glass slides
Camera	Venipuncture equipment
Cotton-tipped swabs	Wood's lamp
Dacron-tipped swabs	Paper bags/envelopes/wooden sticks
Eye dropper	
Nonbacteriostatic saline	Comb
	Labels
Light source	Otoscope/magnifying glass

BOX 151-3 **THE RAPE KIT**

Cotton-tipped swabs	Envelopes for specimen storage
Brown paper bag	Wooden sticks
Labels	Eye dropper
Collection box	Glass tubes for specimen storage
Tamperproof seal	Glass slides
Victim consent form	Combs
Specimen checklist	
Form for "chain of evidence"	

A rape kit organizes the material needed for the collection of forensic evidence (Box 151-3).

Techniques

The diagnosis of sexual abuse or assault depends primarily on the history obtained from the patient. Physical and laboratory findings merely supplement the history.* The procedure consists of obtaining consent and a history, performing a physical examination, screening for sexually transmitted disease and pregnancy, collecting forensic evidence, administering acute medical treatment, documenting the evaluation, determining disposition, notifying the appropriate agencies, and scheduling follow-up.

Consent. Become familiar with the local laws. Obtain consent from the patient or parent for the examination and collection of forensic specimens or photographs. Rape victims have the right to limit consent to a confidential report and may limit the collection of evidence.[5,6,37,46] Minors can consent to the evaluation and treatment of sexual assault, but legislation may obligate the physician to at least attempt to contact the parent or legal guardian if that person is not the alleged perpetrator. To identify an adult figure who can assist the patient through the procedure and during the next few weeks and months, ask the adolescent with whom he or she would like to share the information.

History. The history obtained during the interview with the patient is the most important piece of evidence.[11,18,39,43]

---

*References 4, 11, 18, 33, 37, 39, and 41.

A history thoughtfully taken by the physician is often admissible in court as an exception to the hearsay rule.[37] The essentials to be accomplished during the history include the recording of the facts, validation of the child's complaints, reassurance, assessment of the extent of physical and laboratory examination needed, and assessment of the child's safety.[20,33,43] Contact the hospital's child abuse experts and, when possible, include them in the first interview or schedule the interview to take place in their clinic.

The interview requires some experience and knowledge of normal child development and behavior. Prepare the child/adolescent by discussing what the evaluation entails. Remember that control and power are central to abuse; avoid exerting power. Demonstrate patience, exhibit a calm, nonjudgmental demeanor, and allow the patient to make choices during the evaluation. Be cognizant of the feelings that the historical information can invoke in an interviewer, and avoid projecting these feelings toward the patient or the patient's family. The environment in which the interview takes place should be comfortable, warm, safe, and quiet, and the interviewer should be free from interruption. Interview the child alone if possible or in the presence of a second trusted person, such as a counselor or social worker. If a family member is present, instruct him or her to allow the child to talk freely, to be supportive, and to not answer for the child. Establish rapport and trust; introduce all of the team members. Continually reassure the child by expressing the knowledge that this is scary and is very hard for him or her. Allow digression and gently get the child back on course. Do not forget that the child often cares a great deal about the perpetrator; therefore do not tell the child that "Uncle Joe is bad." Do reinforce that the child did nothing wrong and that sharing this information with other loved ones and the doctor is a good thing to do.

Conduct the interview with *nonleading* questions (e.g., "Tell me what happened to you. Where were you? and What else happened?" instead of "Did John put his pee-pee there?"). Try to work at the developmental and cognitive level of the child (e.g., "Gee, I don't understand. Could you tell me that again?"). Use the child's nicknames for various body parts. Ask the child to draw the room in which the abusive episode occurred or to draw himself or herself with the perpetrator. This tactic often facilitates history taking by serving as a diversion for the child, and it may help him or her through the difficult disclosure. The use of anatomic dolls can also help the child explain what happened.

Ascertain the child's name, age, legal guardian, developmental age, school grade, address, telephone number, the identity of the perpetrator, date of last contact, and previous episodes of abuse. Obtain family information, including parent's and sibling's names, ages, and place of residence, as well as frequent caretakers.

Explore the nature of the event, including the details of who, where, when, how often, and what happened. Determine whether there was a use of force, threats, or the presence of any weapons. The police may choose to investigate the scene of the event.

Observe the demeanor and physical condition of the child/adolescent during the interview; note spontaneous statements and try to use the *exact words* given by the patient. Explore whether there are any incentives to fabricate

the event. Obtain the perpetrator's name, age, address, and relationship to the child. If the perpetrator is a family member or friend, be cognizant of the degree of pressure placed on the victim. Ask if there were any witnesses to the event and get their names, addresses, and telephone numbers.*

Collect the same information from an adolescent victim. For all victims, inquire about clothing changes, defecation, urination, bathing, or douching following the attack. A brief review of the patient's past medical history is also important. From postpubertal patients obtain a brief gynecologic and sexual history, including last menstrual period, gravity and parity, last consensual intercourse, sexual preference, and history of sexually transmitted diseases.

After finishing the interview of the child/adolescent, interview the caretaker. Occasionally it is impossible to obtain any history from the child because of age or emotional or physical state. In this instance, obtain the history from the caretaker or reschedule a second visit.[5,6]

Physical Examination. The physical examination is a therapeutic and diagnostic procedure and serves to provide further information and to document normalcy for the victim. The physical examination addresses three purposes: (1) identification of pertinent physical findings and conditions that need treatment, (2) collection of specimens for evidence, and most important (3) the reassuring of the patient that he or she is well or "undamaged." The presence of a normal physical examination is common (26% to 73% of the children who have been allegedly sexually abused)[11,20,39] and *is consistent* with sexual abuse. Examine the genitalia only in the context of a full physical assessment; the extent of the examination depends on the history. Continue to allow the patient to have some control during the evaluation. For example, allow him or her to choose which gown to wear and whether or not to have the parent/guardian present during the examination. Continually reassure the patient that he or she is doing the right thing and that it is understandable that this event is difficult and frightening for him or her. Remember, it is not necessary to decide whether a crime has occurred; just collect the evidence carefully and record the data.

Begin by noting the emotional state of the child or adolescent and proceed with recording the weight, height, and vital signs. Follow this initial assessment with a head-to-toe examination. Search carefully for bruises or abrasions. Carefully examine the oropharynx for evidence of palatal petechiae, contusions and swelling, frenulum tears, or broken teeth. Other important sites of examination include the scalp, the neck and shoulders, the breasts, the buttocks, the thighs, and the wrists and ankles. Diagrams and photographs are particularly helpful in ensuring clear documentation as well as for future use should it be necessary to testify. Hospital experts should develop guidelines for the collection of the evidence. Involve the clinical laboratory and the local police. It is helpful to standardize evidence collection with the use of a checklist and a rape kit containing the necessary equipment and to document the evaluation on a standardized form (see Box 151-3). Carefully label all specimens following the specifications of the laboratory (e.g., name, date of birth,

---

*References 4, 11, 20, 33, 37-41, and 43.

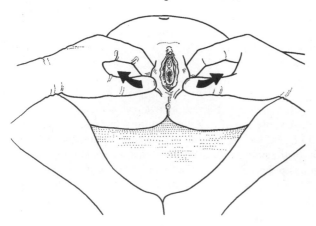

FIG. 151-1 The child in frog-leg position for examination and evidence collection.

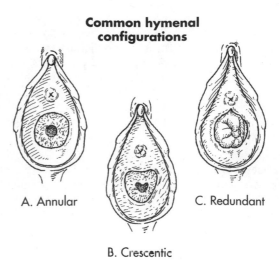

Common hymenal configurations

A. Annular   C. Redundant

B. Crescentic

FIG. 151-3 Configurations of the hymen in prepubertal girl.

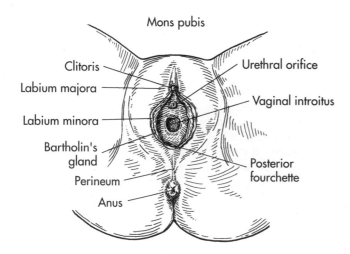

Mons pubis

Clitoris — Urethral orifice

Labium majora — Vaginal introitus

Labium minora —

Bartholin's gland —

Perineum — Posterior fourchette

Anus —

FIG. 151-2 Anatomy of genitalia in prepubertal girl.

date/time of examination, specimen location, medical record number). Finally, seal the specimens and carefully record any change of hands. Remember that this evidence may eventually find its way into a court of law.[4-6,20,43]

GIRLS: PREPUBERTAL AND POSTPUBERTAL. When dealing with an adolescent, take a few minutes to explain the examination to the older child. Ask the mother or other supportive individual to be present for the examination unless the patient chooses otherwise. Examine the prepubertal child in the frog-leg position, the knee-chest position, or both. Some examiners prefer the lateral decubitus position to the knee-chest position, particularly if the patient has been a victim of sodomy. In the frog-leg position, the child can easily see the examiner and participate in the examination and the collection of the evidence (Fig. 151-1). The child can also rest comfortably in the lap of the supportive individual while in this position. In addition, a knowledge of normal anatomy, normal sexual development, and injury patterns of different types of abuse are necessary. Record clinical findings on the physical examination sheet; for girls in the supine position, convention places the posterior fourchette at the 6 o'clock position and the clitoris at the 12 o'clock position.

Visualize the perihymenal tissue and hymenal opening by

exerting outward and downward traction of the labia (see Chapter 75). In the prepubertal girl, carefully inspect each of the following structures: the mons pubis, the labia majora and minora, the urethra, the hymen, the vaginal vestibule, the posterior fourchette, and the perianal region (Figs. 151-2 and 151-3). The hymen has many normal configurations in the prepubertal child, including annular, crescentic, microperforate, septate, cribriform, and imperforate (see Fig. 151-3). The knee-chest or lateral decubitus position allows a careful examination of the perianal area. In addition, in the knee-chest position the anterior vaginal wall is more easily viewed. In experienced hands the culposcope can provide more information and allow documentation through photography. Controversy exists regarding the transverse diameter of the hymen because it is affected by position, examination technique, degree of patient relaxation, and age and size of the child. Currently, it alone is not a single criterion for determining sexual abuse.*

Note the patient's Tanner stage (Fig. 151-4) and degree of estrogenization. Note the presence of any vaginal or perianal discharge. Acute physical findings may include bruises, bite marks, petechiae, discharge, and hymenal, vaginal wall, or rectal tears. Chronic findings may include hypopigmentation or hyperpigmentation, thickened irregular hymenal borders, and an interrupted vascular pattern of the posterior forchette. Asymmetric perianal rugae, nonmidline perianal tags, a diminished anal wink, and anal dilation with an empty ampullae are all consistent with anal penetration† (Box 151-4).

It is best to examine the postpubertal adolescent female with her in the lithotomy position. Just as with the prepubertal girl, begin the examination with careful inspection of the external genitalia. Again, note the degree of estrogenization and the Tanner stage. Palpate the inguinal nodes. Note the clitoral size and examine the perihymenal and hymenal tissues and lower one third of the vagina. It is easy to examine most nulliparous adolescents with the Huffman

---

*References 20, 27, 28, 34, 35, and 39.
†References 3, 7, 11, 15, 16, 20, 32, 36, and 39.

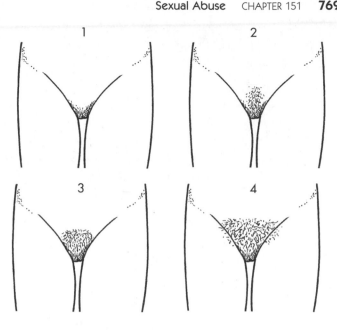

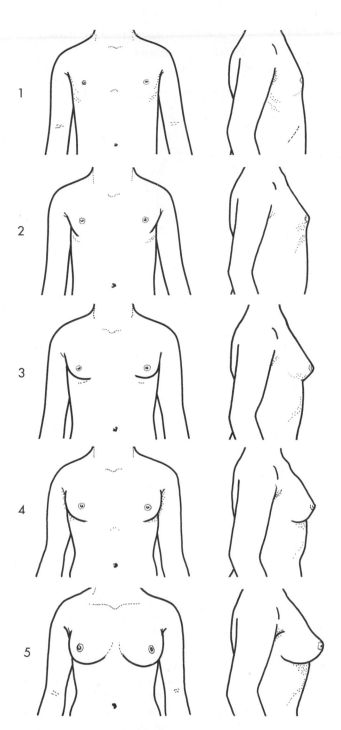

FIG. 151-4   Tanner stages.

(Redrawn from Tanner JM: Growth at adolescence, ed 2, Oxford, 1962, Blackwell Scientific Publications.)

vaginoscope (4½ × ½). Multiparous and larger adolescents may require the Pederson speculum (4½ × ⅞) for better visualization of internal structures. Warm the speculum with water. Avoid using a lubricant because doing so interferes with culture and forensic specimens. To avoid urethral trauma, insert the speculum slowly with downward pressure. Inspect the cervix, ectropion, Nabothian cysts, and vaginal wall; take the necessary specimens. When complete, perform a bimanual examination, and note the presence of tenderness and uterine and adnexal size. Refer the patient to a gynecolo-

---

BOX 151-4   PHYSICAL FINDINGS AND SEXUAL ABUSE

Findings diagnostic of sexual abuse

Acute anal or genital injuries with an inadequate mechanism
Presence of semen, sperm, or acid phosphatase
Pregnancy
N. gonorrhoeae or syphilis beyond the neonatal period
HIV infection without risk factors for transmission
An enlarged hymenal opening associated with disruption, absence, or scars

Findings consistent with sexual abuse

Chlamydia spp., Trichomonas spp., human papillomavirus, herpes simplex virus infection (without perinatal transmission)
Posterolateral thinning or scarring of the hymen
Anal scars or tags outside of the midline
Anal dilation > 15-20 mm without stool in the ampulla

Findings sometimes seen with sexual abuse

Bacterial vaginosis
Extensive labial adhesions
Posterior fourchette friability
Repeated anal dilation <15 mm
Perianal fissures or edema

Findings unlikely to be a result of abuse

Periurethral bands
Small labial adhesions
Erythema of the vestibule
Avascular midline of the posterior fourchette
Perianal erythema/hyperpigmentation
Midline skin tags or folds
Candida albicans dermatitis
Anterior concavities of the hymen
Hymenal mounds on an otherwise normal hymen

Modified from Bays J, Chadwick D: Medical diagnosis of the sexually abused child, *Child Abuse Negl* 17:91-110, 1993.

BOX 151-5 **FINDINGS THAT MAY MIMIC SEXUAL ABUSE**

Lichen sclerosus
Congenital hemangiomas
Urethral prolapse
Periurethral bands
Diastasis ani
Chronic constipation

Straddle injury
Nonspecific vaginitis
Perianal streptococcal infection
Shigella/streptococcal vaginitis
Vaginal foreign body
Chron's disease

BOX 151-6 **CENTERS FOR DISEASE CONTROL AND PREVENTION: GUIDELINES FOR THE EVALUATION OF SEXUALLY TRANSMITTED DISEASES IN PREPUBERTAL CHILDREN**

Cultures for *N. gonorrhoeae* from any site potentially infected*
Cultures for *C. trachomatis* from any site potentially infected*
Examination of vaginal fluid for evidence of *T. vaginalis* or bacterial vaginosis
Gram stain or any genital or anal lesions
Culture of lesions suspicious of herpes simplex virus
Serum for syphilis serology
Serum for HIV†
Store serum for future testing if needed

Modified from Centers for Disease Control and Prevention: 1993 Sexually transmitted diseases: treatment guidelines, *MMWR* 42:97-101, 1993.
*The use of nonculture tests is not recommended. For *N. gonorrhoeae,* culture oropharynx, vagina/meatus, and anus. For *C. trachomatis,* culture vagina/meatus and anus.
†Testing based on local disease prevalence and exposure risk.

gist if significant vaginal/cervical lacerations are present.[5,6,14] Box 151-5 lists conditions that may mimic sexual abuse.

BOYS: PREPUBERTAL AND POSTPUBERTAL. Examination of the male genitalia is straightforward. Note the Tanner stage and whether or not the patient has been circumcised. Observe the inguinal region, urethral meatus, glans, frenulum, shaft, scrotum, testes, and epididymis. Document the presence of discharge, abrasions, bruises, petechiae, or bite marks. Carefully inspect the perianal region and evaluate the rugal pattern, the degree of relaxation of the sphincter muscle, the presence of nonmidline anal tags, subcutaneous fat loss, hyperpigmentation, bruising, abrasions, and lacerations. If there are signs of anal trauma or if there is history of forceful anal penetration, perform a careful rectal and abdominal examination. Anoscopy or sigmoidoscopy is indicated in the case of rectal bleeding, laceration, or hemoccult-positive stool.[6,20]

Sexually Transmitted Diseases/Pregnancy. Obtain cultures if the abusive episode occurred within the preceding 72 hours or if the patient has genital symptoms. Currently, the American Academy of Pediatrics also recommends collecting cultures on any patient with a history of genital contact.[2] A recent report by Siegel et al.[44] found that the presence of abnormal genital findings identified all girls less than 13 years of age who had a sexually transmitted disease. Other investigators' experiences also support a low incidence of sexually transmitted diseases in chronically abused children.[4,20,32] Obtain oropharyngeal, vaginal/cervical, or urethral and rectal cultures for of *Neisseria gonorrhoeae.* Take similar specimens for *Chlamydia trachomatis,* excluding the oropharyngeal site. Collect any discharge for a wet mount, whiff test, Gram stain, and culture. To perform the "whiff test," put some vaginal fluid onto a glass slide and add a drop of 10% potassium hydroxide solution. The amines released account for the characteristic "fishy" odor and aids in the diagnosis of bacterial vaginitis (see Chapter 76). In the prepubertal male, swab the meatus, oropharynx, and rectum for *N. gonorrhoeae;* swab the rectum for *C. trachomatis* if indicated (Box 151-6).

Obtaining culture specimens does not need to be painful. Allow the child to play with the cotton-tipped swabs, and explain the procedures. With downward and outward traction of the labia majora in a cooperative patient, it is easy to view the genitalia, and the hymen relaxes and is open. Slide the cotton-tipped swab through the hymen and into the vagina and rotate it a few times. If performed carefully, the cotton-

tipped swab will not touch the labia or hymenal borders. Also consider carefully applying 1% viscous lidocaine gel to the labia minora and hymenal surface before obtaining cultures or performing vaginal irrigation. Take caution when applying the gel to avoid contaminating the specimen. In prepubertal males, swab the meatus and avoid painful urethral penetration. Directly inoculate swabs obtained for *N. gonorrhoeae* onto chocolate and Thayer-Martin agar plates at room temperature. When a discharge is present, collect a specimen for a Gram stain and look for intracellular gram-negative diplococci. Place swabs for *C. trachomatis* in the appropriate transport media. When obtaining chlamydial specimens, do not use wooden cotton-tipped swabs because doing so inactivates the transport media. For female patients, place swabs for *Trichomonas vaginalis* in 1 to 2 ml of nonbacteriostatic saline; make a slide and view it immediately (see Chapter 76). Even under ideal conditions, wet mounts identify the organism only 60% of the time; a culture is superior. Inspect the wet mount for "clue cells" (epithelial cells studded with bacteria), and perform a "whiff test" by adding potassium hydroxide to the slide and detecting the characteristic amine odor associated with the presence of *Gardnerella vaginalis.* Cultures for the herpes simplex virus are best taken by unroofing new lesions, scraping the base, and placing the swab in the appropriate viral media. A single serology for syphilis at follow-up minimizes venipuncture and diagnoses the disease.*

Culture all postpubertal victims for *N. gonorrhoeae* and *C. trachomatis* from potentially infected sites. Obtain a rapid plasma reagent (RPR) test at the initial visit, and discuss tests for hepatitis B and HIV. Obtain a pregnancy test for young women regardless of the timing of their last menstrual period. Evaluate vaginal pool specimens for the presence of

*References 4, 8, 14, 20, 31, and 33.

BOX 151-7   **CENTERS FOR DISEASE CONTROL AND PREVENTION: GUIDELINES FOR THE EVALUATION OF SEXUALLY TRANSMITTED DISEASES IN POSTPUBERTAL CHILDREN**

Cultures for *N. gonorrhoeae* and *C. trachomatis* from any site of attempted penetration

Pregnancy screening for female patients

Specimens for *T. vaginalis* and bacterial vaginosis in female patients

Consider testing for HIV

Consider testing for hepatitis B

Frozen serum specimen for future testing

Follow-up at 2-3 weeks for repeat cultures

Consider a visit at 2-3 months for repeat RPR, hepatitis B, and HIV testing

Modified from Centers for Disease Control and Prevention: 1993 Sexually transmitted diseases: treatment guidelines, *MMWR* 42:97-101, 1993.

T. vaginalis and *G. vaginalis* (Box 151-7). Save serum from the initial visit for future testing for the human immunodeficiency virus (HIV) or other specific antibodies should the patient develop new symptoms.[5,6,8,29,30]

There is currently no universally accepted policy regarding HIV testing. The prevalence of transmission of the HIV virus through sexual abuse is unknown.[44] A survey by Gellert of child protection services in the United States identified 28 children who acquired HIV through sexual abuse.[19] The Centers for Disease Control and Prevention (CDC) currently recommends testing on the basis of local prevalence of the infection and on the exposure risk and risk factors of the alleged perpetrator, if they are known.[8] Gutman et al make some preliminary recommendations, including testing in children who have another sexually transmitted disease, those with evidence of anal or vaginal injury, those who have had documented invasive abuse, those exposed to an infected perpetrator, and those with confirmation of suspected abuse.[25] For adolescent victims or victims of penetration, save the serum from the first visit for later testing if follow-up tests are positive.

Forensic Evidence. When there is a history of ejaculation or recent penetration, use the rape kit to obtain specimens for determining the presence of sperm or seminal fluid and other foreign debris (see Box 151-3). Always wear gloves throughout the entire examination to prevent contamination of specimens. Eighty percent of all individuals secrete blood-group antigens in bodily fluids, including perspiration. Therefore an examiner's hands may obscure the blood-group typing that may identify the perpetrator. Place the victim's clothes in paper bags, not plastic, to avoid bacterial or fungal overgrowth that may destroy evidence. If the victim was wearing a diaper, tampon, or sanitary napkin during the time of the assault or if such items were used shortly after the assault, send them as evidence. In general, it is better to send too much evidence than too little. Obtain two to three slightly moistened cotton-tipped swabs from each area involved in

the assault; allow them to air dry for 60 minutes before placing them in appropriately labeled specimen containers. Drying prevents the contamination of evidence with bacterial overgrowth. Obtain vaginal specimens with dry or slightly moistened cotton swabs or through vaginal washings. Attach a small catheter to a syringe and instill a few milliliters of saline into the vagina; aspirate the fluid after 1 minute. In small children this same method can be used with an eyedropper. Obtain specimens from the rectum by inserting the cotton-tipped swabs approximately 1 inch into the rectum. Swab the patient's buccal mucosa along the upper and lower molars. Remove areas of dried secretions anywhere on the patient's body with a moistened swab, or scrape the secretions away with a scalpel and capture them in a clean envelope.

A Wood's lamp may aid in the identification of seminal fluid because it fluoresces. Some laboratories prefer that the emergency physician make slides directly with the swabs he or she obtains, while other laboratories prefer to make their own. These slides or swabs are necessary for the detection of sperm, acid phosphatase, P-30, mouse antihuman semen 5, and blood-group antigens. Prepare a wet mount from each area and evaluate immediately for the presence of motile sperm. Sperm remains motile for 6 to 10 hours in the vagina but up to 5 days on the cervix. Nonmotile sperm may be present as long as 72 hours. The time period for the detection of acid phosphatase is approximately 10 hours. Prepare these wet mount slides with Papanicolaou (PAP) fixative and include them with the evidence. Comb the patient's pubic hair and save the debris in a spare envelope; save any pubic hair found on the patient. If necessary, pluck a sample of the patient's pubic hair and scalp hair, including the root. Obtain scrapings underneath the fingernails in the setting of an acute event, particularly if the victim struggled to get away. Obtain a blood sample to determine the patient's blood group. Finally, ask the patient to chew on a few cotton gauze pads to collect a sample of saliva, and place them in a sterile tube. Label each specimen with the patient's name, medical record number, date and time of collection, body part from which it was taken, and the collector's name; place each specimen in a sealed container. Document the transfer of the specimens to the police officer to preserve the chain of evidence.*

Treatment. Although it is rare following rape, discuss the possibility of pregnancy with every postpubertal sexual assault victim and obtain a mandatory pregnancy test at the time of the evaluation. Pregnancy prophylaxis within 72 hours following the event is effective in 99% of all cases. If the patient's pregnancy test is negative, give two tablets of Ovral (norgestrel 0.5 mg, ethinyl estradiol 0.05 mg) twice and 12 hours apart. This drug is recommended for postcoital prevention of pregnancy and is the only drug with this combination of hormones. Concomitant administration of an antiemetic medication is helpful. Repeat pregnancy testing 2 to 3 weeks later at the follow-up visit.[8,12]

Do not begin empiric treatment for sexually transmitted diseases in sexually abused children.[2,3,33,39] In general, these patients are victims of longstanding abuse and need treat-

---

*References 5, 11, 17, 20, 24, and 28.

BOX 151-8 RECOMMENDED TREATMENT OF SEXUALLY TRANSMITTED DISEASES

Uncomplicated *N. gonorrhoeae*, all patients

Ceftriaxone 125 mg IM (children <45 kg)
Ceftriaxone 250 mg IM (all >45 kg)
Ciprofloxacin 500 mg PO (> 15 years)
Ofloxacin 400 mg PO (> 17 years)
Cefixime 400 mg PO
Spectinomycin 2 g IM

Upper genital tract *N. gonorrhaeae*

Ceftriaxone 250 mg IM
Cefoxitin 2 g IV q6h
Clindamycin 900 mg q8h IV and gentamicin 1.5 mg/kg q8h IV

C. trachomatis

Erythromycin 50 mg/kg for 7 days for patients <9 years
Doxycycline 100 mg BID for 7 days
Azithromycin 1 g PO (>15 years)
Ofloxacin 300 mg BID for 7 days
Erythromycin base 500 mg QID for 7 days

T. pallidum

Primary, secondary, and early latent: Benzathine penicillin G, 2.4 million units IM
Latent syphilis: Benzathine penicillin G, 2.4 million units IM 3 consecutive weeks
Neurosyphilis: Aqueous crystalline penicillin G, 12-24 million units q4h IV for 2 weeks

Hepatitis B vaccination

Tetanus prophylaxis (open wounds present)

Modified from Centers for Disease Control and Prevention: 1993 Sexually transmitted disease treatment guidelines, *MMWR*, 42:97-101, 1993.

BOX 151-9 AVAILABLE RESOURCES FOR SEXUAL ABUSE VICTIMS

Child Help's National Child Abuse Hotline
P.O. Box 630
Hollywood, CA 90028
(1-800-4-A-CHILD)

National Coalition Against Sexual Assault
527 E. Capitol Ave., Suite 100
Springfield, IL 62701
(217-753-4117)

National Center for Missing and Exploited Children
1835 K St., NW, Suite 600
Washington, D.C. 20009
(202-634-9821)

---

ment only if the physical examination is suspicious or if genital cultures are positive. Prophylactic treatment prevents few infections. Furthermore, the risk of complications from infection is lower in prepubertal children.

The rate for sexually transmitted diseases following the sexual assault of young women is common and therefore warrants a diagnostic work-up and a thoughtful approach toward treatment (Box 151-8). This age group has a higher incidence of sexually transmitted disease and a lower incidence of compliance with follow-up examination. Experience has revealed that *N. gonorrhoeae* cultures are positive between 2.4% and 12% of the time at the initial visit; at follow-up, 5.6% of the women with a previously negative culture are positive. Ten percent of women have positive *C. trachomatis* cultures at the initial visit; at follow-up an additional 1.5% are positive. *T. vaginalis* and *G. vaginalis* infections are common and are present 5% to 25% of the time at follow-up. The risk of herpes simplex virus and syphilis is very low. The risk of human papilloma virus (HPV) is currently unknown. HIV is not presently a common occurrence in this population.[21,29,30] The efficacy of zidovudine prophylaxis is unknown; do not prescribe it routinely. Recommended treatment regimens appear in Box 151-8. Instruct patients to return for acute vaginal or abdominal symptoms, and advise them to abstain from sexual intercourse or to use condoms. Reinforce the need for follow-up examination with the patient.

Documentation. The medical chart serves two purposes. It is a reflection of the evaluation and treatment in the ED and is a written record to remind the physician of the patient should it become necessary to testify. Legibility is of the utmost importance. Whenever possible, use the patient's own words; document in the first person with the use of quotations. When documenting the physical examination, avoid words such as *normal*. Be descriptive (e.g., no bruising or erythema noted, scant white discharge). The final diagnosis should reflect a complete evaluation that includes the history, physical examination, and laboratory data. Avoid a discharge diagnosis of Rule-out Sexual Abuse. Consider conclusions such as Sexual Abuse Complaint, History of Sexual Abuse and Normal Physical Examination, or Physical Examination Consistent with Sexual Abuse.[11,20,33]

Disposition. In rare instances, a patient may require hospitalization for medical treatment. Otherwise, discharge him or her with an adult who will take responsibility for protecting the child/adolescent from further harm. If such an adult is not available, emergency foster care or hospitalization is necessary. Social work assessment is crucial in each case. Reading material and crisis hotline numbers may be helpful for the adolescent patient and for the parents of the child/adolescent. Refer all pediatric and adolescent patients for counseling (Box 151-9).

Reporting. Every state requires physicians to report *suspected* sexual abuse to the appropriate agencies, including Child Protective Services and the police. Furthermore, the diagnosis of sexual abuse carries with it civil and criminal ramifications. Even if the family or teenager wishes that the physician not report the incident, it is a legal mandate to make the report. The obligation to protect the abused child and other possibly abused children supersedes the patient's right to privacy. Most states require that injuries inflicted in violation of any state penal law be reported. It is the physician's responsibility to be familiar with state law and to comply with it. Failure to report is a misdemeanor that is punishable by fine or imprisonment.[11,20,33]

Follow-up. Medical follow-up by the primary physician or sexual abuse team for reexamination and cultures should occur at 2 weeks and again at 3 months. Refer all patients for a mental health evaluation. At the 2-week follow-up visit, repeat the wet mount and pregnancy test. If antibiotics were not given at the first visit, repeat cultures for *N. gonorrhoeae* and *C. trichomatis* are obtained. Repeat an RPR at 3 months and an HIV test at 3 to 6 months. It is important to emphasize to the patient the need for follow-up for the detection of infections.[8]

REFERENCES

1. American Academy of Pediatrics, Committee on Adolescence: Rape and the adolescent, *Pediatrics* 81(4):595-597, 1988.
2. American Academy of Pediatrics, Committee on Child Abuse and Neglect: Guidelines for the evaluation of sexual abuse of children, *Pediatrics* 87(2):254-260, 1991.
3. Bays J, Chadwick D: Medical diagnosis of the sexually abused child, *Child Abuse Negl* 17:91-110, 1993.
4. Berkowitz CD: Sexual abuse of children and adolescents, *Adv Pediatr* 34:275-312, 1987.
5. Braen GR: Examination of the female rape victim. In Roberts JR, Hedges JR, editors: *Clinical procedures in emergency medicine,* Philadelphia, 1985, WB Saunders.
6. Braen GR: Sexual assault: In Rosen P, Barkin R, editors: *Emergency medicine: concepts and clinical practice,* ed 3, St Louis, 1992, Mosby.
7. Cartwright PS and The Sexual Assault Study Group: Factors that correlate with injury sustained by survivors of sexual assault, *Obstet Gynecol* 70:44-46, 1987.
8. Centers for Disease Control and Prevention: 1993 Sexually transmitted diseases: treatment guidelines, *MMWR* 42:97-101, 1993.
9. Cupoli JM, Sewell PM: One thousand fifty-one children with a chief complaint of sexual abuse, *Child Abuse Negl* 12:151-162, 1988.
10. DeJong AR, Rose M: Frequency and significance of physical evidence in legally proven cases of child sexual abuse, *Pediatrics* 84:1022-1026, 1989.
11. DeJong AR, Finkel MA: Sexual abuse of children, *Current Prob Pediatr* September 1990 pp. 490-567.
12. Dixon GW, et al: Ethinyl estradiol and conjugated estrogens as postcoital contraceptives, *JAMA* 244:1336-1339, 1980.
13. Elam AL, Ray VG: Sexually related trauma: a review, *Ann Emerg Med* 15:576-584, 1986.
14. Emans SJ: Sexual abuse. In Emans SJ, Goldstein DP, editors: *Pediatric and adolescent gynecology,* ed 3, Boston, 1990, Little, Brown.
15. Emans SJ: Vulvovaginitis in the child and adolescent, *Pediatr Rev* 8:12-19, 1986.
16. Emans SJ, et al: Genital findings in sexually abused symptomatic and asymptomatic girls, *Pediatrics* 79:778-785, 1987.
17. Enos WF, Conrath TB, Byer JC: Forensic evaluation of the sexually abused child, *Pediatrics* 78:385-398, 1986.
18. Geist RF: Sexually related trauma, *Emerg Med Clin North Am* 6:439-466, 1988.
19. Gellert GA, et al: Situational and sociodemographic characteristics of children infected with HIV from pediatric sexual abuse, *Pediatrics* 91:31-44, 1993.
20. Giardino AP, Finkel MA, Giardino ER, et al: A practical guide to the evaluation of sexual abuse in the prepubertal child, Philadelphia, 1991, The Children's Hospital of Philadelphia.
21. Glaser JB, Hammerschlag MR, McCormack WM: Sexually transmitted diseases in victims of sexual assault, *N Engl J Med* 315:625-627, 1986.
22. Graves CB, et al: Postcoital detection of a male-specific semen protein, application to the investigation of rape, *N Engl J Med* 312:338-343, 1985.
23. Green AH: Child maltreatment and its victims: a comparison of physical and sexual abuse *Psychiatr Clin North Am* 11:591-610, 1988.
24. Gutman LT, Herman-Giddens ME, McKinney RE: Pediatric acquired immunodeficiency syndrome: barriers to recognizing the role of sexual abuse, *Am J Dis Child* 147:775-780, 1993.
25. Gutman LT, et al: Sexual abuse of HIV-positive children: outcomes of perpetrator and evaluation of other household children, *Am J Dis Child* 146:1185, 1992.
26. Hausler WJ, Herrman KL, Isenberg HD, et al, editors: *Manual of Clinical Microbiology,* ed 5, Washington, DC, 1991, American Society for Microbiology.
27. Herman-Giddens ME, Frothingham TE: Prepubertal female genitalia: examination for evidence of sexual abuse, *Pediatrics* 80:203-208, 1987.
28. Horowitz D: Physical examination of sexually abused children and adolescents, *Pediatr Rev* 9:25-29, 1987.
29. Jenny C: Sexual assault and STD. In Holmes KK, Mardh PA, Sparling PF, et al, editors: *Sexually transmitted diseases,* ed 2, New York, 1990, McGraw-Hill.
30. Jenny C, et al: Sexually transmitted diseases in victims of rape, *N Engl J Med* 332:713-716, 1990.
31. Kreiger JN, et al: Diagnosis of trichomonas: comparison of conventional wet-mount examination with cytologic studies, cultures, and monoclonal antibody staining of direct specimens, *JAMA* 259:1223-1227, 1988.
32. Ladson S, Johnson CF, Doty RE: Do physicians recognize sexual abuse? *Am J Dis Child* 141:411-415, 1987.
33. Ludwig S: Child abuse. In Fleischer GR, Ludwig S, et al, editors: *Textbook of pediatric emergency medicine,* ed 3, Baltimore, 1993, Williams & Wilkins.
34. McCann J: Use of the colposcope in childhood sexual abuse examinations, *Pediatr Clin North Am* 37:873-880, 1990.
35. McCann J, et al: Comparison of genital examination techniques in prepubertal girls, *Pediatrics* 85:182-187, 1990.
36. Muram D: Child sexual abuse-genital tract findings in prepubertal girls. I. The unaided medical examination, *Am J Obstet Gynecol* 160:328-333, 1989.
37. Myers JEB: Role of physician in preserving verbal evidence of child abuse, *J Pediatr* 109:409-411, 1986.
38. Orr DP, Prietto SV: Emergency management of sexually abused children, *Am J Dis Child* 133:628-631, 1979.
39. Paradise JE: The medical evaluation of the sexually abused child, *Pediatr Clin North Am* 37(4)839-862, 1990.
40. Paradise JE, Rostain AL, Nathanson M: Substantiation of sexual abuse charges when parents dispute custody or visitation, *Pediatrics* 81:835-839, 1988.
41. Ricci LR: Child sexual abuse: the emergency department response, *Ann Emerg Med* 15(6)711-716, 1986.
42. Runyan DK, et al: Impact of legal intervention on sexually abused children, *J Pediatr* 113:647-653, 1988.
43. Sgroi SM: *Handbook of clinical intervention in child sexual abuse,* Lexington, Mass, 1983, Lexington Books.
44. Siegel RM, Schubert CG, Myers PA, et al: The prevalence of sexually transmitted diseases in children and adolescents evaluated for sexual abuse in Cincinnati: rationale for limited STD testing in prepubertal girls, *Pediatrics* 96:1090-1094, 1995.
45. Soules MR, et al: The forensic laboratory evaluation of evidence in alleged rape, *Am J Obstet Gynecol* 130:142-147, 1978.
46. Tintinalli JE, Hoelzer M: Clinical findings and legal resolution in sexual assault, *Ann Emerg Med* 14:447-453, 1985.

152 Court Orders

Stephen Ludwig

The rights of a child and his or her parents usually remain harmonious. Parents generally want what is best for their child; sometimes these sets of rights are in conflict. In such cases the laws allow for the representation of children in seeking what is best for them. Children have certain civic rights independent of their parents. There are three situations in which this issue arises most often in the pediatric Emergency Department (ED) or pediatric intensive care unit (PICU): (1) child abuse or neglect,[4] (2) parental refusal of treatment or diagnostic tests, (3) and unavailability of a parent or guardian to sign consent for treatment.[2,3,5]

Indications

In the case of child abuse or neglect, a child's rights are protected from further acts of omission (neglect) or acts of commission on the part of the parents. The child may or may not articulate this right; although it may not be articulated, it is always presumed. Each state in the United States has a child abuse–reporting law, which designates the physician as a mandated reporter. Thus there is a legal requirement that physicians report suspected abuse or neglect. Each state law defines the age of the children to which the law applies, legal protection for reporting in good faith, and legal sanctions for failure to report. Some states go further and give physicians the authority to take children into legal custody. This authority is a broad power and is usually reserved only for police. However, for some physicians working in the ED or PICU, state law allows a child to be hospitalized contrary to the wishes of the parent. Sometimes the particular state law requires that the physician obtain a restraining order to hold the child. In granting a restraining order, the state is not denying the child the right to protection but is keeping the decision-making power in the hands of a judge. In some states, not only do police have the power to take children into custody, but also physicians make child abuse reports from which the police may decide (with the physician's advice) whether or not to hospitalize a child for treatment and protection.

The second major indication for a court order arises when the parent refuses to consent for a diagnostic test or treatment that the physician believes is in the best of interest of the child's health and safety. Such a situation may occur when the physician requests permission to perform a lumbar puncture and the parent refuses or when the physician feels that a blood transfusion is indicated, which goes against the parent's beliefs.[3]

The third indication occurs when the parent is not available to give consent. The ED may need parental consent in situations in which the child arrives at the ED from the scene with an injury or when the parent has left the child in the care of a babysitter or relative. If there is an acute emergency and if the child is already in the ED, it is physician's responsibility to do what is best for the child.[5] However, it is also the hospital's responsibility to go to all lengths possible to obtain parental consent.[2,3,5]

Contraindications/Complications

There are no contraindications per se to obtaining a court order, but there are complications. In general the physician should do everything possible to avoid taking this step but should also be prepared to use a well-formulated and approved protocol when it becomes necessary to do so.

Usually good physician/parent communication can prevent court orders from becoming necessary. In the case of child abuse, good communication is facilitated if the physician avoids taking an accusatory stance with the parent and does not heighten the parent's guilt or fear. Maintain the focus on the health and needs of the child; emphasize common agreeable ground for both the physician and the parent. In obtaining permission for diagnostic tests or procedures, it may be only a matter of explaining the need for the test or treatment and putting it into an understandable context for the parent. Calling in a third party such as a primary care provider with whom the parent has a trusting relationship can often enhance communication. Sometimes a grandparent or a church elder may provide the stable wisdom and maturity that is lacking in a parent who is in crisis because of the child's health.

It is best to avoid court orders because they bring the entire criminal-justice machinery into the health arena. Parents generally resent losing their parental rights and authority. There may be repercussions to losing a long-term therapeutic relationship with a family. In some cases, the violation of religious principles may leave a child alienated from his or her own family and community.

Nevertheless, when there are no other options available, it is important to know how to obtain a court order promptly and efficiently. Each ED should have in its policy and procedure manual a method for getting a court order. The hospital attorney must review and approve the court-order procedure to be sure it conforms to state and regional laws. There should also be a list of on-call hospital attorneys if the physician needs one to intercede in the process. If the emergency physician is equipped with the proper technique and information, the procedure should proceed smoothly.

Techniques

Boxes 152-1 to 152-3 are from the Children's Hospital of Philadelphia Policy & Procedure Manual.[1] Box 152-1 addresses the procedure for gaining telephone consent from a parent who is not present in the ED. Telephone consent provides one way to avoid a full court-order procedure.

Box 152-2 details when to obtain an emergency court order either because of parental absenteeism or refusal to consent. Note that an "emergency" implies the standard for Pennsylvania: "When a physician believes that a medical

BOX 152-1   EMERGENCY ADMISSIONS AND CONSENTS

Consent by telephone or fax

1. Telephone consent permitted in emergency situation only.
2. Attending physician is responsible for obtaining and documenting informed consent.
3. Phone conversation (physician-legal guardian) should be witnessed by MD, RN, clerk.
4. Physician must explain reasons for admission and the risks, benefits, and alternatives such that a reasonable person could make an informed decision.
5. Documentation must include the following:
   a. Date and time
   b. Name of parent/legal guardian spoken with
   c. Relationship to patient
   d. Description of information given to parent/guardian
   e. Whether or not consent was given
   f. Signature of persons making and witnessing call
6. Parents/guardians should sign hospital admission or consent form when they arrive.
7. A faxed copy of consent for admission or treatment may be used after phone conversation between parent/guardian and physician.

From Children's Hospital of Philadelphia: *Administrative policy & procedure manual,* Philadelphia, 1994, Children's Hospital, Philadelphia.

BOX 152-2   EMERGENCY COURT ORDERS—PARENTAL CONSENT REFUSED OR UNAVAILABLE

Summary of procedures

1. Advise parents/guardian of intention to seek court order (if possible)
2. Responsible physician contacts lawyer on call
   a. Hospital administrator, social worker on call may contact attorney for the physician.
   b. Do not leave messages on answering machines.
   c. If attorney is unavailable, proceed to call next attorney on list.
3. Provide attorney with pertinent information about need for treatment and parental/guardian refusal to consent.
4. Provide attorney with phone numbers to reach parent/legal guardian and physician if necessary.
5. Attorney contacts judge and advises the hospital as soon as authorization is received.
6. When oral court order authorizing treatment is obtained, record pertinent information (time of order, scope of authorization) into patient's medical record.
7. When written order is obtained, place a copy into the patient's chart.
8. If no attorney is available, the responsible physician contacts the judge on call directly at City Hall. Document conversation with the judge in the patient's chart, including the following:
   a. Date and time
   b. Parties to the conversation (name of judge, physician)
   c. Substance of conversation
   d. Whether authorization for treatment obtained
   e. Scope of such authorization
9. Inform hospital attorney as soon as possible of oral court order so documents can be filed with the court within 48 hours.

From Children's Hospital of Philadelphia: *Administrative policy & procedure manual,* Philadelphia, 1994, Children's Hospital of Philadelphia.

BOX 152-3   EMERGENCY PETITION FACT SHEET

Contact person at hospital: _____

Telephone number: _____

Patient (full name): _____

Parents: Father: _____

Mother: _____

Address: _____

Telephone number: _____

Who has custody and control of the child? _____

Patient birth date: _____

Date of admission to hospital: _____

Diagnosis: _____

Date of diagnosis: _____

Treatment required: _____

_____

_____

Attending physician: _____

When care of child assumed: _____

Board certification: _____

(If none, fill out below)

Senior attending staff physician: _____

Where licensed: _____

Board certification: _____

Have parents been notified of the procedure? _____

How? When? _____

Who notified them? _____

Why have they not consented? _____

Has court been contacted? _____

Time and date: _____

From Children's Hospital of Philadelphia: *Administrative policy & procedure manual,* Philadelphia, 1994, Children's Hospital of Philadelphia.

emergency requires treatment *to preserve a child's life or prevent immediate, serious, and permanent harm to the child's health. . . .* "Ultimately, the physician must make this statement to the judge to justify the order. In other states physicians must use different terminology and procedures. An oral court order permitting treatment must be followed by the filing of necessary papers within 48 hours to obtain a written court order. Normally the written order is effective only for a set number of days. A new order must be obtained if the need for the medical treatment continues or recurs beyond the specified time period. Boxes 152-1 and 152-2 provide examples of what the hospital should anticipate and plan for long before the need for a court order occurs. Box 152-3 is a simple fact sheet that helps the physician have before him or her pertinent facts for discussion with the judge.

Remarks

The need for a court order is relatively rare. Good communication with parents is essential to avoid this conflict in rights. The focus must remain on the needs of the child. No parent will be angry if the physician shows legitimate concern for the child. Anger is the inevitable product when finger pointing, accusations, guilt, and fear come into the ED or PICU. Anger is not only out of place in the ED or PICU but also is a serious drain on the central mission: the care of children.

Educate parents about the need to provide for consent when they are not present. Schools, daycare centers, and sports programs need to have a way to bring a child to the hospital for emergency health care and to have proper consent to do so. Parents who go away on vacation also need to leave their consent with the person(s) acting in their place. Anticipatory guidance of parents in these issues is helpful to children and to the health-care institution that must treat them.

REFERENCES

1. Children's Hospital of Philadelphia: *Administrative policy & procedure manual,* Philadelphia, 1994, Children's Hospital of Philadelphia.
2. Fleisher G, Ludwig S: *Textbook of pediatric emergency medicine,* ed 3, Baltimore, 1993, Williams & Wilkins.
3. George JE: *Law and emergency care,* St Louis, 1980, Mosby.
4. Ludwig S, Kornberg A: *Child abuse: a medical reference,* ed 2, New York, 1993, Churchill Livingstone.
5. Selbst SM: Treating minors without their parents, *Pediatr Emerg Care* 1:168-173, 1985.

Index